Darling Sarah,

I am sure you will have as much fun doing medicine as I have. You might even find this useful!

All my love

Dad

May 2006.

Oxford Medical Publications

Arthritis in Children and Adolescents

Arthritis in Children and Adolescents

Juvenile Idiopathic Arthritis

Edited by

Ilona S. Szer

*Chief, Pediatric Rheumatology, Children's Hospital San Diego
and Professor of Clinical Pediatrics, University of California,
School of Medicine, San Diego, California, USA*

Yukiko Kimura

*Chief, Pediatric Rheumatology, Joseph M. Sanzari Children's Hospital,
Hackensack University Medical Center and Associate Professor of Pediatrics,
University of Medicine and Dentistry, New Jersey Medical School,
New Jersey, USA*

Peter N. Malleson

*Professor of Paediatrics, Division of Rheumatology, British Columbia
Children's Hospital, University of British Columbia, Vancouver, British
Columbia, Canada*

Taunton R. Southwood

*Professor of Paediatric Rheumatology, University of Birmingham and Head,
Academic Department of Paediatrics Birmingham Children's Hospital,
Birmingham, UK*

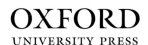

OXFORD
UNIVERSITY PRESS

OXFORD

UNIVERSITY PRESS

Great Clarendon Street, Oxford OX2 6DP

Oxford University Press is a department of the University of Oxford.
It furthers the University's objective of excellence in research, scholarship,
and education by publishing worldwide in

Oxford New York

Auckland Cape Town Dar es Salaam Hong Kong Karachi
Kuala Lumpur Madrid Melbourne Mexico City Nairobi
New Delhi Shanghai Taipei Toronto

With offices in

Argentina Austria Brazil Chile Czech Republic France Greece
Guatemala Hungary Italy Japan Poland Portugal Singapore
South Korea Switzerland Thailand Turkey Ukraine Vietnam

Oxford is a registered trade mark of Oxford University Press
in the UK and in certain other countries

Published in the United States
by Oxford University Press Inc., New York

British Library Cataloguing in Publication Data

Data available

Library of Congress Cataloging in Publication Data

Data available

Typeset by Newgen Imaging Systems (P) Ltd., Chennai, India
Printed in Italy
on acid-free paper by
Lito Terrazzi, Firenze

ISBN 0–19–263292–2   978–0–19–263292–0

10 9 8 7 6 5 4 3 2 1

Remembering Dr Jerry C. Jacobs: A tribute to a mentor

On 6 September 1997, the paediatric rheumatology community lost one of its most energetic advocates and some of us, lost a mentor; a man we called our medical father. We were lucky to have one, and for me it was both a pleasure and a privilege to have been the first of Jerry's fellows in paediatric rheumatology.

Dr Jacobs was born and raised in New York City and received the bachelor of arts and medical degrees from Columbia University. Other than his internship at Bellevue Hospital, Jerry's training in Paediatrics and in Adult Rheumatology was also completed at Columbia Medical Center. Following his training with the adult department of rheumatology, Dr Jacobs established the first Paediatric Rheumatology service which marked the beginning of pediatric rheumatology in New York City. In 1981, the fellowship program was created with Robert Winchester and Leonard Chess providing the research opportunities and experience. Following me, Yukiko Kimura, Suzanne Li, Lisa Imundo, and Karin Peterson, also completed the 3-year fellowship program.

Jerry taught by example; see one, do one, teach one was definitely the modus operandi. When one of our new lupus patients came in for the second time with a pulmonary haemorrhage, I was introduced as the expert having watched Jerry save her life the first time. He was clearly the consummate clinician, the one who sensed the correct diagnosis sooner than most. We all wanted to have that gift. And when we were faced, as we often are in this field, with a diagnostic dilemma, Jerry liked to say "there is an answer for everything, you just have to wait long enough and ask the right questions". He was usually correct.

Jerry's priorities were always clear. Although he moved the fastest around sick children, his family and home life came first. Jerry met his wife Isabel during her first day at Barnard College, the women's college of Columbia University. Isabel and their three children were the center of Jerry's life and we, *the medical daughters* as he referred to us, were welcome and included in the family. Jerry was passionate about travel, great food, and good wine. He managed to partake of all that can be baked, steamed, or served raw, combined with the best there was to drink, and told multiple unsuspecting listeners about it. He was a great story teller.

Dr Jacobs' entire career, which spanned over 30 years, was spent at Columbia University where he was respected as one of its most treasured teachers and clinicians. His early work and writing about Kawasaki disease earned him an international reputation and a friendship with Dr Kawasaki that he treasured. He travelled the globe as a Visiting Professor and his easy going and dynamic lecturing style provided generations of students of medicine with practical and life long lessons in the recognition and care of children with rheumatic diseases.

Through his *Textbook of Pediatric Rheumatology for the Practitioner*, Dr Jacobs' impact has been enormous. Shortly before his death, Jerry requested that his medical daughters write and edit the next edition of the textbook. Thus, writing Part 1 of this textbook, and utilizing most of Jerry's original words and illustrations, has been a labour of love for us. We have preserved, as best as possible, the best of Jerry's writing, namely his logical approach to the sick child and the ability to recognize a particular pattern of symptoms that allows the reader to eliminate the enormous number of possibilities and to arrive at the single correct diagnosis. It has been a pleasure to update Jerry's original writing with information published during the past decade since he wrote the last edition of *Pediatric Rheumatology for the Practitioner*.

Sadly, Dr Jacobs came to know of his enormous influence and respect only in the last few months of his life when many of those whose lives he touched, wrote to him. To me however, his greatest strength and the lesson that I will always be grateful for, is his philosophy of the importance and magic of childhood and the responsibility we all share in that regard. He expressed it in this quote: "the overall management of arthritis in children can be summarized as: life as normal as possible. It's bad enough to have arthritis without having the arthritis ruin the rest of your life. You know, childhood is a preparation for life. You cannot skip childhood. You've got to play, go to school; that's how a child learns to be an adult. If you skip any of that then the child is not going to be a well-functioning adult. So our big job is to make sure that our children are not maimed in terms of function by this disease. We've got to put up with whatever scarring the disease causes in the joints but we don't have to have scars in the child as a person. That's our big job."

Dr Jacobs died very much the way he lived. He was in a hurry to go, not wanting to be remembered ill. He need not have worried; we will always remember him as a dynamic, full of life and vigor, exuberant, and incredibly productive leader of our field.

Ilona S. Szer

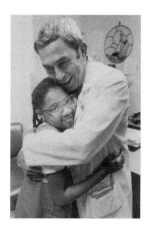

Remembering Vinny: A tribute to Dr Aldo Vincent "Vinny" Londino

Aldo Vincent "Vinny" Londino, Jr. M.D. was born outside of Pittsburgh on May 29, 1952 and left us, much too prematurely, on 17 December 2000. In his short life, Vinny accomplished more than most men aspire to in a lifetime of dreams. He was the consummate physician as he flawlessly blended academic brilliance and clinical acumen with an uncanny sense of the personal needs of his adoring patients. Whether caring for adults or the children with rheumatic diseases who so loved his presence, he left his patients with a sense of comfort and confidence that regularly transformed fear into hope. If the corticosteroids were ineffective the boisterous laugh and gentle touch of Dr Londino were enough to soothe the pain of the young patient with JIA who longed to make the trek to Children's Hospital in Pittsburgh just to see and hug her beloved "Dr Dino." Vinny laboured day and night caring for patients whose diseases often paled in comparison to his own physical ailments. Many who knew him had no idea that Dr Londino himself was chronically ill. He struggled his entire life with cystic fibrosis, and the lung transplant that we hoped and prayed would save his life ended up being too great an obstacle for our courageous friend. His undying devotion to his patients, family, and friends will be the legacy left to those he so tenderly touched in his short life.

Vinny's impact on the students that he taught and the doctors with whom he interacted was powerful. He received numerous clinical excellence and teaching honours and was named "Teacher of the Year" by the paediatric residents at Children's Hospital of Pittsburgh, a distinct and exclusive honour for a physician trained as an internist. He was named the region's top paediatric rheumatologist and would regularly be referred the most challenging and difficult cases to diagnose and manage. Dr Londino's peers would both covet his medical opinions and long to hear his fanciful stories, as did the medical students whom he faithfully mentored for over 17 years.

Yet a litany of medical achievements fails to capture the essence of Vinny Londino. His quick wit and resilient spirit beautifully complemented his marvellous medical skills. His passion for baseball and his love of coaching was a natural extension of his God-given talent to poignantly touch the lives of those who crossed his path. Many young boys on the baseball diamonds of Vinny's neighborhood learned the value of fair play, good sportsmanship, and compassion from the man they revered as "Coach Londino." Vinny realized that his impact and the lasting effect that he would have on the lives of these young boys went far beyond the final score of a baseball game. However, as much as his dedication to his patients and players embodied his public life, it was his undying devotion to his family that epitomized the true nature of Dr Londino. He treasured the time that he would spend with his wife and soulmate, Joanne, and he adored his two young boys, Vinny and Greg, as he skillfully and lovingly taught them that their character must be built slowly and carefully with a firm foundation and from the inside out. We all learned first-hand how Vinny handled the events of his short but fruitful life with a tender heart and open arms and his ability to handle even the most tiresome circumstances are an inspiration to all of us. His deep unconditional love warmed every heart and is the real story behind the doctor, coach, husband, father, and friend whom we affectionately called, "Vinny." When I think of my good friend, I am reminded of the words of a missionary, Jim Elliot, who years ago gave his life preaching to a native tribe in the jungle of Ecuador:

He is no fool who gives what he cannot keep to gain what he cannot lose.

Vinny Londino gave and gave until there was no longer anything else to give, but his labour of love left a legacy that will never die. Those of us who had the privilege and honour to know him will be forever impacted and eternally grateful.

Chester V. Oddis

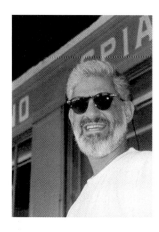

Remembering Barbara: A tribute to Barbara Ansell

When Barbara Ansell died in September 2001, a defining chapter in the history of Paediatric Rheumatology ended. Barbara was born in Warwick in 1923 and received her medical education at the University of Birmingham, graduating with Distinction in 1946. Her initial plan was to become a cardiologist, and after house jobs in Birmingham and at the Hammersmith Hospital, she joined Professor Eric Bywaters, at the Medical Research Council's Unit for the study of Rheumatic Disease in Childhood at Taplow in Berkshire, to study Rheumatic Heart Disease.

Once at Taplow however, she became enchanted by the children with "Still disease" whom she met there. Changing course, she eventually became the Doyenne of Paediatric Rheumatology. The Unit thrived and soon became a world centre of excellence for the treatment of children with what is now known as Juvenile Idiopathic Arthritis. Visitors from all parts of the globe (except Mongolia, she was fond of reminding us) came to visit and learn, and she travelled the world as a Visiting Professor.

In 1976, she moved with her Unit to Northwick Park Hospital in Harrow, which became the National Centre for the Treatment of Rheumatic Diseases in Childhood. At the same time she was appointed Honorary Consultant to Great Ormond Street Children's Hospital and began to establish with local paediatricians a network of Regional Centres throughout the United Kingdom. In the late 1970s she was the driving force responsible for the establishment of the British Paediatric Rheumatology Group (now The British Society for Paediatric and Adolescent Rheumatology) and of the Paediatric Rheumatology European Society.

She worked closely with many organizations focused on arthritis, including the Arthritis Research Campaign, Arthritis Care, and the Children's Chronic Arthritis Association. She was the first Chairperson of the EULAR Standing Committee on Paediatric Rheumatology. She had the very rare distinction of being a Fellow of three Royal Colleges, the College of Physicians, College of Paediatrics, and College of Surgeons. She was an honorary fellow or member of over 16 national and international societies. In 1982, she was awarded the CBE (Commander of the British Empire). She was author of over 360 papers in adult and paediatric rheumatology and her MD Thesis on the Classification of Juvenile Arthritis, based on patterns of disease presentation, still forms the basis of current classifications. When Barbara retired from the National Health Service in 1988, she continued to serve on committees, support colleagues in peripatetic clinics, and was active in private practice until her final illness.

These are the bald facts but they in no way reflect the Barbara we all knew and loved. Succinctly described by one of her former patients, now an adult, as "loud, large, loving and so lovable," she really was larger than life in every respect and lived hers to the full. Barbara lived for her "special children," and was determined that their disease was not going to dominate and spoil their lives. She was as concerned to maximize their social,

emotional, and cognitive development as she was to control their disease and limit their pain and deformity. She inspired, enthused, enabled, and above all, instilled confidence in her patients and in her colleagues and trainees. Nothing was too much trouble for her, and her work load was phenomenal. After a 10 hour day without a break for coffee, lunch, or tea, she would dismiss her team with the words, "off you go; I want to get down to some real work now." She would then often work into the small hours writing papers, responding to numerous requests from colleagues for help with a difficult diagnosis or treatment problem, or perhaps phoning a teenager who needed that extra bit of support and encouragement.

She was an astute and honest clinician, and her judgements were sound and precise. Her memory for clinical detail was legendary, and she was almost invariably right. Demanding the highest standards in her own work, she expected a lot from her team. While she could reduce both patients and staff to tears on occasion, it was clear that her intention was only to get the very best out of them and for them. She had a wonderfully infectious smile and laugh, and was one of the least self regarding people I have ever known. Never allowing herself the luxury of wallowing in a set back, one of her favourite expressions was, "There is nothing you can't overcome by hard work."

Barbara was happily married to Angus Weston, a General Practitioner, whom she met in later life. They did not have children of their own, but she was a devoted and loving stepmother and grandmother. She loved travel, the theatre, opera, and teddy bears, but most of all she loved filling their home with friends. She never missed an opportunity to throw a party, and once told me that her father had suggested that she become a Cook General. Her cooking was of such a high standard that I always rather assumed she had managed to train somewhere along the line.

Shortly before her death, she said that thought she had "helped Paediatric Rheumatology to develop, and that it was now our turn to continue to take it forward." We, your trainees and colleagues, owe you that at the very least, Barbara, and will always remember you as a wonderful mentor and friend.

Ann Hall

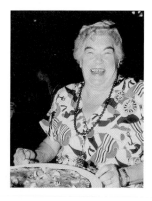

Preface

Ilona S. Szer, Yukiko Kimura, Peter N. Malleson, and Taunton R. Southwood

Musculoskeletal symptoms are an important health burden of children and adolescents. They are the second most common health concern of adolescents, after acne. Musculoskeletal complaints are experienced by up to 30% of all children [1] and rheumatic diseases are one of the most common causes of chronic disability in childhood and adolescence. Despite these clinical imperatives, most medical schools do not teach paediatric rheumatology. As a result, most paediatricians in practice today have had little or no training in the diagnosis and management of rheumatic disorders, or in the proper physical examination of the musculoskeletal system. The differential diagnosis of musculoskeletal pain in children is among the most complex in medicine, with more than one hundred entities to be considered. The treatment of paediatric rheumatic disease is also complex and involves a potentially large interdisciplinary team.

Drs Barbara Ansell and Jerry Jacobs were among the first to recognize these needs and to write about paediatric rheumatology as a specialty subject. They were both wonderful clinicians and were responsible for educating many of the paediatric rheumatologists practising in the world today. This book is our tribute to them as teachers and mentors. In particular, the first section is drawn from Jerry Jacobs' textbook, *Pediatric Rheumatology for the Practitioner*. This book is also a tribute to one of our dear colleagues, Dr. Aldo "Vinny" Londino. As a teacher, clinical paediatric rheumatologist, and friend, he was without peer.

Over the past decade, the number of health professionals interested in paediatric rheumatology has expanded dramatically. This has been reflected in the development of professional qualifications for paediatric rheumatology (e.g. certification in paediatric rheumatology by the American Board of Pediatrics), recognition of rheumatology as a specialty of paediatrics (e.g. Royal College of Paediatrics and Child Health in the UK and Royal College of Physicians and Surgeons of Canada), and the formation of new international paediatric rheumatology societies (e.g. Paediatric Rheumatology European Society: PReS) and discussion groups (e.g. the Paediatric Rheumatology list serve and the Paediatric Rheumatology Discussion Group: PRDG).

In parallel with the broadening appeal of paediatric rheumatology, there has been an expansion of the evidence-base underpinning the specialty, and an increasing number of special interest groups within the specialty, both disease-related (e.g. periodic fever syndromes) and age-specific (e.g. adolescence and transitional care). This textbook aims to reflect both of these trends by employing the principles of evidence-based practice, and by concentrating on only one of the major disease groups in paediatric rheumatology, Juvenile Idiopathic Arthritis (JIA).

Herein lies a dilemma. We have chosen to use the nomenclature of JIA throughout the textbook as a direct substitute for Juvenile Rheumatoid Arthritis (JRA), or Juvenile Chronic Arthritis (JCA), although these terms are not synonymous. We have taken this approach for two reasons: (1) JIA represents the agreed umbrella term of the ILAR classification, the first international consensus about the classification of arthritis in childhood convened under the auspices of the WHO and ILAR; and (2) In order to maximize the internal consistency of the book and minimize potential reader confusion. We recognize, however, that the ILAR classification has yet to be validated for clinical use, and was developed primarily to facilitate international research efforts at understanding the aetiology, pathogenesis, and treatment of JIA. An additional concern is that it has only recently begun to be used in the published literature. In consequence, we (and the chapter authors) have had to bear the risk of inaccurately interpreting some of the evidence-base, especially if it was published under the umbrella terms of either JRA or JCA. In order to minimize confusion with regard to terminology, we have chosen to capitalize only the ILAR classification terminology throughout this book, and to use the JRA and JCA terminology only if those terms are essential to clarify the meaning of the published literature.

The textbook attempts to take a practical, "hands on" approach, with the following twin goals: (1) To assist the clinician in formulating the framework for the differential diagnoses of children and adolescents presenting with symptoms suggestive of arthritis; and (2) To enable the clinician to implement an evidence-based treatment plan. The book primarily targets the paediatric rheumatology fellow/trainee, but we believe that it will also be relevant to all clinicians involved with the care of children. We have endeavored to ensure that each chapter is relatively self-sufficient, to the extent that it might form the basis for a lecture or tutorial.

Part 1 is a compilation of the range of the disorders that need to be considered before arriving at the diagnosis of JIA, using extensive symptom-based algorithms and tables. The algorithms lead the reader from the chief complaint through a suggested scheme of evaluations to the most likely diagnosis. Each diagnosis is then discussed in detail in the following chapters. As the primary focus of the textbook is arthritis, other chronic inflammatory conditions, such as SLE and its variants, inflammatory myopathies and systemic vasculitis syndromes, are considered in broad outline as differential diagnoses rather than in the fine detail one might expect in a textbook covering the whole spectrum of rheumatic disease in children.

Part 2 is devoted to detailed discussion of each of the diseases under the umbrella term of Juvenile Idiopathic Arthritis (JIA). Each subtype of JIA is given its own chapter, in which is discussed the epidemiology, clinical characteristics, complications and monitoring necessary in caring for children with one of these diseases. We have used the nomenclature recommended in most recently revision of the ILAR classification criteria [2].

1. Systemic Arthritis (previously known as Still's disease or systemic onset JRA/JCA)

2. Oligoarthritis (previously known as Pauciarticular onset JRA/JCA) which is itself also sub divisible into Persistent or Extended Oligoarthritis

3. Rheumatoid Factor Negative Polyarthritis (previously known as polyarticular onset JRA/JCA)

4. Rheumatoid Factor Positive Polyarthritis (previously known as polyarticular onset JRA or sometimes simply JRA)

5. Psoriatic Arthritis

6. Enthesitis Related Arthritis (previously known as seronegative enthesitis and arthritis (SEA) syndrome, juvenile spondyloarthropathy or juvenile ankylosing spondylitis)

7. Undifferentiated Arthritis (no previous equivalent term)

In addition, there are 3 chapters in Part 2 devoted to the histopathology, immunology, genetics, cytokine abnormalities, and environmental factors involved in the pathogenesis of childhood arthritis.

Part 3 discusses the evidence-based management of children with JIA. Each chapter is organized to reflect the natural progression of childhood arthritis over time as experienced in clinical practice. Whenever possible, the authors organized each chapter using the same treatment approach employed by the practicing paediatric rheumatologist, which is to start with the management of early arthritis, followed by therapeutic options for established arthritis and then finally discussing approaches to refractory arthritis.

One aspect of clinical progress of the last 15 years is the realization that the true prognosis of childhood arthritis is much worse than previously believed. This has resulted in turning upside down the additive and cautious treatment algorithms of the past, and consideration of remittive therapies much earlier in the disease course for children threatened with future disability. At the same time, our field has experienced a revolution in the availability of new treatment options for childhood arthritis. Fifteen years ago, aspirin was still being used, and slow-acting antirheumatic drugs of poorly documented and questionable efficacy, including intramuscular gold, penicillamine, and hydroxychloroquine, were administered sequentially over periods of years. In contrast, the treatment of children with JIA today is more aggressive and is beginning to be targeted with greater specificity towards fundamental abnormalities in the immune system, including the excessive production or presence of pro-inflammatory cytokines such as TNFα. The therapeutic armamentarium is expanding rapidly, as randomised controlled clinical trials in children with JIA are being completed. The rate of expansion will likely increase further as new and innovative clinical trials are designed and implemented using new international clinical trials infrastructures such as PRINTO (Paediatric Rheumatology International Trials Organization) and CARRA (Childhood Arthritis and Rheumatology Research Alliance) to enable large multicenter studies. The results of these changes are clearly felt, as the use of corticosteroids in JIA has decreased and the amount of disability has dramatically diminished already.

Challenges remain, however. The general public still has little awareness of the existence of arthritis in children, even though it is one of the most common chronic diseases in children. Our current treatment approaches, while achieving much better results, are still unable to "cure" our patients, and we do not completely understand the aetiologies of JIA, or the mechanisms of action of many of the drugs. Drs Ansell, Jacobs, and Londino all faced these challenges and their legacy is evident. We hope this book is a fitting tribute to their memories and a useful contribution to the future of our field.

References

1. Goodman, J. E. and McGrath, P. J. The epidemiology of pain in children and adolescents: a review. *Pain* 1991;46:247–64.

2. Petty, R. E., Southwood, T. R., Manners, P., Baum, J., Glass, D. N., *et al.* International League of Associations for Rheumatology classification of juvenile idiopathic arthritis: second revision Edmonton 2001;31:390–2.

Acknowledgements

All multicontributor books require a huge collaborative effort. This book is no exception. Without the dedicated commitment and patience of our authors, we would never have succeeded in finishing this textbook.

In particular, we would like to thank Helen Liepman and Oxford University Press, our colleagues at work, and most of all, our families:

Paul, Annie, and Kate
Jeff, Nick, and Emi
Roey, Tom, and Sarah
Debbie, Jessica, James, and Romaney

Without the educational grant from Wyeth Pharmaceuticals, the book would lack the integrated colour photographs, which we feel add considerably to its impact. We also thank the PRDG for their enthusiastic and libacious encouragement.

We would like to dedicate this book to our students, past, present, and future, and most of all, to our patients and their families.

Contents

Remembering Dr Jerry C. Jacobs: A tribute to a mentor *v*
Ilona S. Szer

Remembering Vinny: A tribute to Dr Aldo Vincent "Vinny" Londino *vi*
Chester V. Oddis

Remembering Barbara: A tribute to Barbara Ansell *vii*
Ann Hall

Preface *ix*

Acknowledgements *xi*

Contributors *xv*

Part 1 The approach to the child with musculoskeletal complaints

1.1 Clinical skills in the evaluation of arthritis *3*
Ilona S. Szer

1.2 The use of investigations and imaging in the evaluation of arthritis *19*
Ilona S. Szer

1.3 Common presenting problems *24*
Yukiko Kimura

1.4 Acute inflammatory rheumatic syndromes *49*
Ilona S. Szer

1.5 Acute and chronic infections of bones and joints *63*
Yukiko Kimura

1.6 Major rheumatic diseases *86*
Suzanne C. Li and Lisa F. Imundo

1.7 Autoinflammatory diseases and distinct but rare rheumatic conditions *116*
Suzanne C. Li

1.8 Non-inflammatory musculoskeletal disorders *130*
Suzanne C. Li

1.9 Idiopathic pain syndromes *147*
Lisa F. Imundo

1.10 Musculoskeletal and autoimmune manifestations of non-rheumatic disorders *155*
Karin S. Peterson

1.11 Disorders of bone and connective tissue *179*
Karin S. Peterson

Part 2 Juvenile Idiopathic Arthritis in children and adolescents

2.1 Classification of childhood arthritis *205*
Taunton R. Southwood

2.2 Systemic Arthritis *210*
Anne-Marie Prieur, Peter N. Malleson, and Yukiko Kimura

2.3 Oligoarthritis *223*
John J. Miller and Peter N. Malleson

2.4 Rheumatoid Factor Positive Polyarthritis *233*
Janet Gardner-Medwin

2.5 Rheumatoid Factor Negative Polyarthritis *244*
Alberto Martini

2.6 Psoriatic Arthritis *252*
David A. Cabral

2.7 Enthesitis Related Arthritis *259*
Ross E. Petty

2.8 Undifferentiated Arthritis *265*
Taunton R. Southwood and Yukiko Kimura

2.9 Immunopathology of the joint in Juvenile Idiopathic Arthritis *272*
Lucy R. Wedderburn, Kiran Nistala, and Taunton R. Southwood

2.10 Genetic and cytokine associations in Juvenile
     Idiopathic Arthritis *280*
     *Wendy Thomson, Patricia Woo, and
     Rachelle Donn*

2.11 Environmental factors in the pathogenesis of
     Juvenile Idiopathic Arthritis *290*
     *Berent J. Prakken, Salvatore Albani, and
     Wietse Kuis*

**Part 3 The approach to treating
Juvenile Idiopathic Arthritis**

3.1 Introduction *301*
    Peter N. Malleson

3.2 Patient-centred care and the team approach *303*
    Ciarán Duffy

3.3 Adolescent rheumatology services *315*
    Janet E. McDonagh and Patience White

3.4 Disease evaluation *330*
    Lori B. Tucker

3.5 Educational issues *337*
    Laurie Ebner-Lyon and Joy Brown

3.6 Psychosocial aspects *343*
    Karen Shaw

3.7 Pain assessment and management *357*
    *David D. Sherry, James W. Varni, and
    Michael A. Rapoff*

3.8 Pharmacological treatment of early or
    established arthritis *367*
    Peter N. Malleson

3.9 Physiotherapy and occupational therapy *381*
    Gay Kuchta and Iris Davidson

3.10 Nutrition *392*
     Deborah Rothman

3.11 Adjunctive therapies *397*
     Marisa Klein-Gitelman

3.12 Surgical interventions *403*
     Ann Hall

3.13 Clinical trials *414*
     Brian Feldman

3.14 Pharmacological treatment: Approach to the
     management of refractory arthritis *431*
     Nico M. Wulffraat and Berent J. Prakken

     Appendix: Intra-articular
     corticosteroid injections *442*
     *Clive A.J. Ryder, Taunton R. Southwood, and
     Peter N. Malleson*

     Index *447*

Contributors

Salvatore Albani Translational Research Unit, Clinical Investigations Institute, University of California, San Diego, California, USA. (salbani@ucsd.edu)

Joy Brown Parent Liaison, Division of Rheumatology, Children's Hospital and Health Center, San Diego, California, USA. (joy@san.rr.com)

David A. Cabral Clinical Associate Professor and Head, Division of Rheumatology, British Columbia Children's Hospital, University of British Columbia, Vancouver, British Columbia, Canada. (dcabral@cw.bc.ca)

Iris Davidson Physiotherapist, Mary Pack Arthritis Centre, and British Columbia Children's Hospital, Vancouver, British Columbia, Canada. (idavidson@cw.bc.ca)

Rachelle Donn Arthritis Research Campaign, Epidemiology Unit, Division of Epidemiology and Health Science, University of Manchester, Manchester, UK. (rachelle.donn@man.ac.uk)

Ciarán Duffy Head, Division of Rheumatology, Montreal Children's Hospital, University of McGill, Montreal, Quebec, Canada. (ciaran.duffy@muhc.mcgill.ca)

Laurie Ebner-Lyon Division of Rheumatology, Joseph M. Sanzari Children's Hospital, Hackensack University Medical Center, Hackensack, New Jersey, USA. (lebner-lyon@humed.com)

Brian Feldman Associate Professor of Paediatrics, Health Policy Management & Evolution and Public Health Sciences, University of Toronto, Senior Scientist and Staff Rheumatologist, Hospital for Sick Children, Toronto, Ontario, Canada. (brian.feldman@sickkids.on.ca)

Janet Gardner-Medwin Senior Lecturer in Paediatric Rheumatology, University of Glasgow, Department of Child Health, Royal Hospital for Sick Children, Yorkhill, Glasgow, UK. (jgm4w@clinmed.gla.ac.uk)

Ann Hall Consultant Paediatric Rheumatologist, Oxford Paediatric and Adolescent Rheumatology Centre, Nuffield Orthopaedic Centre, Oxford UK. (ann.hall@ukf.net)

Lisa F. Imundo Director, Division of Rheumatology, Morgan Stanley Children's Hospital of New York, Columbia University College of Physicians and Surgeons, New York, NY, USA. (lfi1@columbia.edu)

Yukiko Kimura Chief, Division of Rheumatology, Joseph M. Sanzari Children's Hospital, Hackensack University Medical Center, Hackensack, New Jersey, and Associate Professor of Pediatrics, University of Medicine and Dentistry, New Jersey Medical School, USA. (ykimura@humed.com)

Marisa Klein-Gitelman Assistant Professor of Pediatrics, Division of Immunology/Rheumatology, Children's Memorial Hospital, Northwestern University, Chicago, Illinois, USA. (klein-gitelman@northwestern.edu)

Gay Kuchta Occupational Therapist, Mary Pack Arthritis Centre, and British Columbia Children's Hospital, Hospital, Vancouver, British Columbia, Canada. (gkuchta@cw.bc.ca)

Wietze Kuis Professor of Paediatrics and Head of Department, Wilhemina Children's Hospital, Utrecht, The Netherlands. (w.kuis@wkz.azu.nl)

Suzanne C. Li Division of Rheumatology, Joseph M. Sanzari Children's Hospital, Hackensack University Medical Center, Hackensack, New Jersey, and Assistant Professor of Pediatrics, University of Medicine and Dentistry of New Jersey, New Jersey Medical School, USA. (sli@humed.com)

Peter N. Malleson Professor of Paediatrics, Division of Rheumatology, British Columbia Children's Hospital, University of British Columbia, Vancouver, British Columbia, Canada. (malleson@interchange.ubc.ca)

Alberto Martini Professor and Head, Department of Pediatrics, University of Genova, Pediatria II, IRCCS G. Gaslini, Genova, Italy. (albertomartini@ospedale-gaslini.ge.it)

Janet E. McDonagh Arthritis Research Campaign Senior Lecturer in Paediatric and Adolescent Rheumatology, University of Birmingham, Institute of Child Health, Birmingham, UK. (j.e.mcdonagh@bham.ac.uk)

John J. Miller Emeritus Professor of Pediatrics, Stanford University, Stanford, California, USA. (DrJJMIII@aol.com)

Kiran Nistala Research Fellow in Paediatric Rheumatology, Institute of Child Health, University College London, London, UK. (Kiran.Nistala@bch.nhs.uk)

Chester V. Oddis Professor of Medicine, University of Pittsburgh School of Medicine, Division of Rheumatology and Clinical Immunology, Pittsburgh, PA, USA. (oddis@msx.dept-med.pitt.edu)

Karin S. Peterson Assistant Professor of Pediatrics, Division of Allergy and Immunology, Morgan Stanley Children's Hospital of New York, Columbia University College of Physicians and Surgeons, New York, NY, USA. (ksp4@columbia.edu)

Ross E. Petty Professor Emeritus of Paediatrics, Division of Rheumatology, British Columbia Children's Hospital, and University of British Columbia, Vancouver, British Columbia, Canada. (rpetty@cw.bc.ca)

Berent J. Prakken Wilhemina Children's Hospital, Utrecht, The Netherlands. (b.prakken@wkz.azu.nl)

Anne-Marie Prieur Pediatrician, Medecin des hopitaux, Hôpital Necker Enfants Malades, Unité d'Immunologie, Hématologie et Rhumatologie pediatriques, Paris, France. (anne-marie.prieur@nck.ap-hop-paris.fr)

Michael A. Rapoff Section Chief, Behavioral Pediatrics, Department of Pediatrics, University of Kansas Medical Center, Kansas City, Kansas, USA. (mrapoff@kumc.edu)

Clive A.J. Ryder Head, Department of Rheumatology, Birmingham Children's Hospital – NHS Trust, Birmingham, UK. (clive.ryder@bch.nhs.uk)

Deborah Rothman Director Pediatrics and Rheumatology, Shriners Hospital for Children, Springfield, Massachusetts and Assistant Professor of Pediatrics, University of Massachusetts Medical School, Worcester, Massachusetts, USA. (drothman@shrinenet.org)

Karen Shaw Research Psychologist, School of Health Sciences, University of Birmingham, Birmingham, UK. (k.l.shaw@bham.ac.uk)

David D. Sherry Professor of Pediatrics, Division of Rheumatology, The Children's Hospital of Philadelphia, University of Pennsylvania, Philadelphia, Pennsylvania, USA. (sherry@email.chop.edu)

Taunton R. Southwood Professor of Paediatric Rheumatology, University of Birmingham and Head, Academic Department of Paediatrics Birmingham Children's Hospital, Birmingham, UK. (t.r.southwood@bham.ac.uk)

Ilona S. Szer Head, Division of Rheumatology, Children's Hospital San Diego, and Professor of Clinical Pediatrics, Department of Pediatrics, University of California, San Diego, California, USA. (iszer@chsd.org)

Wendy Thomson Arthritis Research Campaign, Epidemiology Unit, Division of Epidemiology and Health Science, University of Manchester, Manchester, UK. (wendy.thomson@man.ac.uk)

Lori B. Tucker Clinical Associate Professor of Paediatrics, Division of Rheumatology, British Columbia Children's Hospital, Vancouver, British Columbia, Canada. (ltucker@cw.bc.ca)

James W. Varni Professor and Vice-Chair for Research, Department of Pediatrics, and Professor, Department of Landscape, College of Medicine and Urban Planning, College of Architecture, Texas A&M University, College Station, Texas, USA. (jvarni@archmail.tamu.edu)

Lucy R. Wedderburn Reader in Paediatric Rheumatology, Institute of Child Health, University College London, London, UK. (l.Wedderburn@ich.ucl.ac.uk)

Patience White Chief Public Health Officer, Arthritis Foundation, Atlanta, Georgia, and Professor of Medicine and Pediatrics, George Washington School of Medicine and Health Sciences, Washington, D.C., USA. (pwhite@arthritis.org)

Patricia Woo Professor of Paediatric Rheumatology, The Windeyer Institute of Medical Sciences, University College London, London, UK. (patricia.woo@ucl.ac.uk)

Nico M. Wulffraat Department of Pediatric Immunology, University Medical Center, Utrecht, The Netherlands. (n.wulffraat@wkz.azu.nl)

1

The approach to the child with musculoskeletal complaints

1.1 Clinical skills in the evaluation of arthritis
Ilona S. Szer

1.2 The use of investigations and imaging in the evaluation of arthritis
Ilona S. Szer

1.3 Common presenting problems
Yukiko Kimura

1.4 Acute inflammatory rheumatic syndromes
Ilona S. Szer

1.5 Acute and chronic infections of bones and joints
Yukiko Kimura

1.6 Major rheumatic diseases
Suzanne C. Li and Lisa F. Imundo

1.7 Autoinflammatory diseases and distinct but rare rheumatic conditions
Suzanne C. Li

1.8 Non-inflammatory musculoskeletal disorders
Suzanne C. Li

1.9 Idiopathic pain syndromes
Lisa F. Imundo

1.10 Musculoskeletal and autoimmune manifestations of non-rheumatic disorders
Karin S. Peterson

1.11 Disorders of bone and connective tissue
Karin S. Peterson

1.1 Clinical skills in the evaluation of arthritis

Ilona S. Szer

Aims

The aim of this chapter is to fully describe the physical findings in children with Juvenile Idiopathic Arthritis (JIA) and related conditions. Most children with rheumatic conditions have objective physical findings, especially in muscles and joints. Through careful examination and pattern recognition the physician can arrive at the correct diagnosis.

Structure

- Taking the history
- Physical examination
  - Examination of the joints
    - Upper and lower extremity
    - Lumbar spine
  - Tender point exam
- The functional status

Taking the history

The initial consultation visit sets the stage for the future care of the child. The physician should be unhurried and undisturbed. Therapy begins when the physician greets the patient at the doorstep and continues as the history is taken. The interview could be a constructive experience for the patient and family, clearly indicating the physician's compassionate interest in the child and in the details of the problem that has brought the family to the doctor. The parents and the older child are the physician's allies in working out the problem. It is a joint undertaking, a team effort. Skillful interviewing with a thorough approach to organization and analysis, as well as attention to detail, in an effort to ascertain just what is wrong and what steps are needed to further define or treat the problem, convince the family that they are in good hands and encourage cooperation [1,2].

The history of the present illness begins with the invitation, "tell me why you came to see me" and continues with, "can you remember exactly how it all began." It is sometimes important to know whether the pain first appeared on arising or during a mathematics examination. The family is encouraged to provide every bit of information; nothing is considered irrelevant. The physician listens attentively not without diagnostic hypothesis to be explored, but without firmly preconceived diagnostic notions.

The importance of creative analytical listening by a physician, who is intrigued and challenged by the problem and uses reason and imagination in the effort to solve it, cannot be overestimated. An effort is made not to interrupt, but many opportunities arise where the physician can spontaneously interject questions to obtain needed information and help in the organization of the information. If the patient rambles too much, it is helpful to summarize what has been detailed so far, to indicate how the physician is organizing the material provided. A checklist may help in summarizing and recording the information (Table 1.1.1).

Special attention is paid to the signs and symptoms of rheumatic disease, including pain, swelling, limitation of motion, stiffness, gelling after inactivity, and weakness; weakness needs to be separated from fatigue and decreased energy. Skin rashes, eye manifestations, and genital, urinary, and bowel symptoms are specifically inquired about (Tables 1.1.1 and 1.1.2). Special inquiry is made about any injury or illness during the months prior to the onset of the present problem.

Table 1.1.1 Rheumatological disease checklist: history of the present illness and physical signs

Disease	History
Joints	Pain on motion and tenderness, swelling, limitation of motion, gelling or morning stiffness
Muscles	Proximal muscle weakness, atrophy, muscle tenderness, (especially calves)
Skin	Rash or fingernail abnormalities, nodules, alopecia, sclerodactyly, Raynaud phenomenon, oedema, hyper-pigmentation, finger tip or toe ulcers, telangiactasias, calcinosis
Gastrointestinal	Dysphasia, reflux, bloating, abdominal pain, diarrhoea, constipation, dry mouth, mouth sores, salivary gland enlargement, hepatosplenomegaly
Ocular	Dry eyes, blurred vision, red eyes, conjunctivitis, photophobia, blepharitis
Urinary	Dysuria, genital ulcers
Cardiopulmonary	Pericardial or pleuritic chest pain, dyspnea, orthopnea, shortness of breath
Family history	Inflammatory low back pain, heel pain, knee problems, arthritis or other rheumatic disease, inflammatory bowel disease (colitis, ileitis), prostatitis, urethritis, cervicitis, psoriasis

Table 1.1.2 Rheumatological disease checklist: skin and mucus membrane signs of connective tissue disease

Disease	History
Rash	Butterfly, vasculitic, purpuric, evanescent, salmon-pink (typical of Systemic Arthritis), rash; dermatographia, psoriasis, dermal edema, livedo reticularis, heliotrope of the eyelids, Gottron nodules over extensor surfaces of joints (especially knuckles, knees, and elbows), cuticle hyperemia, subcutaneous (rheumatoid) nodules, nodular panniculitis, fingertip ulcers or pitting scars, telangiactasias, discoid lesions of skin or ear pinnae, and rarely keratoderma blenorrhagicum
Hair	Alopecia, frontal hair fracturing
Mucous membranes	Mouth and genital ulcers, tongue lesions, dryness of eyes and mouth, balanitis
Nails	Pitting, onycholysis, clubbing
Raynaud phenomenon	Skin thickening, tightening, contractures, and calcinosis

Especially diarrhoeal illness or change in bowel frequency as well as any flu-like illness, other viral syndrome or vaccination, should be elicited.

Care is taken to establish the family constellation and any history of prior marriages of the parents. The usual family history of disease is embellished with specific questions about rheumatic disease, including, in addition to arthritis and other rheumatic diseases, low back pain, worse on arising, psoriasis, colitis, ileitis, urethritis, iritis, prostatitis, heel pain, and any symptoms similar to those of the child. In childhood rheumatic disease the family history often provides significant relevant information. The social history includes the occupation of the parents and what effect the illnesses is having on their family life. Occupants of the home are determined and sleeping arrangements are established. The child's school grades, performance, and attendance are noted and inquiries are made about any recent change in school. The child's attitude toward the symptoms and any alterations in lifestyle caused by or attributed to them is evaluated. While the routine history of pregnancy, birth, the neonatal period, development, immunizations, allergies, infectious diseases, operations, injuries, and prior illnesses are listed, special attention is paid to any unusual illnesses and to all prior hospitalizations.

After eliciting all of the details of the patient's current illness and the effect that it is having on each member of the family, the response to whatever therapy has been provided, the family history, and the history of prior illnesses the physician generally has an excellent grasp of the problem. An optimal history-taking interview generally provides the diagnostic hypotheses, which can then be confirmed or rejected by physical examination and laboratory studies.

The importance of the history and submitted primary source data in diagnosis depends on the clinical situation. If a physical feature is visible from a distance and provides an obvious diagnosis, the history is taken as an aid to the care of the patient rather than for its diagnostic potency. However, a large number of patients who are brought to the paediatric rheumatologist have mysterious symptoms that have not led to a diagnosis in visits to other physicians. These patients have usually been subjected to repeated physical examinations and laboratory studies; it is unlikely that an additional physical examination or laboratory study will provide the diagnosis. In these cases the history may provide the diagnosis through a process called pattern recognition. This is a somewhat intuitive recognition of the pattern of illness; patterns recognition is an important diagnostic skill in rheumatology and in diagnostic paediatrics (see Part 1, Chapter 1.3, Table 1.3.2) [1].

The history-taking interview provides the physician with more than just an answer to the question, "what is wrong with the patient?." It sets the stage for special emphasis on the physical examination and for laboratory and radiographic studies that may be required. In addition, during this interview one can get an idea of what goals are appropriate for the patient; which joint is affected is not as important as how the child and the family are functioning with the problem. In rheumatological disease, maintenance of function is an important and primary goal, and the interview provides clues as to the strategy that may be adopted by the physician to best achieve that goal [1,2].

Physical examination

Rheumatological diagnosis requires a thorough general physical examination with additional emphasis on the skin and the musculoskeletal system (Tables 1.1.1 and 1.1.2). Special attention is paid to the general appearance of the patient, emotional responses, nutrition and growth chart of height and weight. In addition, in evaluating any evident rashes, the skin is examined for dermatographia, livedo reticularis, nodules, oedema, changes in dermal thickness, tightening, contractures, pigmentation, ungual or dermal telangiactasias, nail changes, alopecia, or new hair growth (see also Part 1, Chapter 1.3, Table 1.3.3). Fingertip circulation, capillary refill, ulceration, and the presence of pitted scars, are noted. Ulcerations are also sought in the mucus membranes; the mouth or genital regions and the eyes and mouth are also examined for unusual dryness. Muscle strength is ascertained by having the child climb up on the table, rise from a supine position, and by instructing the child to rise from a sitting position on the floor observing for the presence of the Gower sign (Figure 1.1.1 (a)–(d)) after first testing the strength and resistance of individual muscles graded in accordance with the commonly used system (Table 1.1.3). Testing of muscle strength takes only a minute and must be part of a physical examination by the rheumatologist. For the busy primary care provider, two excellent manoeuvres that will greatly aid in the identification of the weak child are recommended: (1) Watching a child perform an unassisted sit up and (2) an attempt to overpower the neck flexors while the patient is supine and instructed to hold his head up against the examiner's force.

The most important aspect of the manual muscle exam is placing the patient in a position that allows the examiner to test individual muscle group against gravity (Table 1.1.3). A frequently observed error in the strength exam is testing neck resistance with the patient sitting up; in this position, gravity "helps" the patient exhibit more strength. Neck flexor strength is an important part of the evaluation of a child thought to have weakness from dermatomyositis; neck flexors are usually weak early in the course and often the last muscles to improve after treatment has begun. That combined with an unassisted sit up are excellent clues to an underlying myopathy.

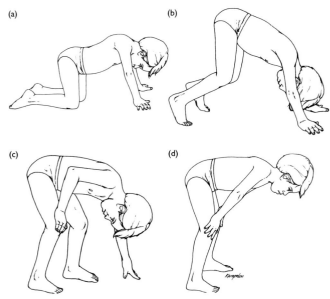

Fig. 1.1.1 Test of muscle strength to elicit a Gower sign. Child is placed supine or sitting cross-legged on the floor and directed to rise. The weak child is unable to rise without first rolling over to the prone position and then gradually pushing himself up, first onto his knees (a), then walking along the floor with his hands (b), then gradually using first one knee (c), and ultimately both knees (d) as aids to hold on to while he pushes himself up to stand. While initially described as the classic sign of children with muscular dystrophy, this sign is very useful in evaluating truncal weakness in general and is of special value in rheumatology in children with dermatomyositis or with steroid-induced myopathy. Sometimes, very weak children will simply refuse to sit on the floor for this test, signifying their inability to rise and the fear of not being able to perform the task, or that they will fall attempting to sit down.

Table 1.1.3 Muscle strength grading chart

Muscle gradations	Description
5 or normal	Complete range of motion against gravity with full resistance
4 or good	Complete range of motion against gravity but not full resistance
3 or fair	Full range of motion against gravity but no resistance
2 or poor	No joint motion against gravity but complete motion when gravity eliminated
1 or trace	Evidence of some muscle contractility but no motion at all
0 or zero	No evidence of contractility

Note: The patient must be positioned against gravity

Physical examination of the joints

Examination of the joints is of particular importance in the diagnosis and management of patients with rheumatic disease. There is no substitute for experience in examining the joints. The purpose of including a discussion of the physical examination of the joints in this book is not to try to make experts of every reader. It is hoped that after reading this oversimplified discussion the primary care provider will be more comfortable examining joints.

The best way to start is with one self, studying the normal appearance and range of motion of each joint when one is at leisure. Then, while examining healthy children when the office schedule is not too hectic, just for fun, one can begin to examine the joints testing the range of motion. In this fashion, the reader can expect to develop sufficient expertise in joint examinations to distinguish normal from abnormal and, to a certain extent, to quantify any functional loss [3–5].

Inspection, palpation, range of motion, and strength

Examination of the joints consists of inspection, palpation, and determining the range of motion possible in the joints (Tables 1.1.4 and 1.1.5). The examination begins with inspection, observing symmetry, loss of normal contour and landmarks, distention and fullness, erythema, atrophy, angulations, and deformities.

The joint and periarticular areas are then palpated, noting pain, tenderness, warmth, and swelling. When examining small joints, it is helpful to encircle the joint with the examiner's fingers to feel the joint margins for the presence of fluid. Effusions in the knees are generally easily felt and may be balloted. Most effusions form in the suprapatellar bursa and need to be "milked" into the joint capsule, followed by lightly tapping on the patella to elicit up and down motion indicative of an effusion. Elbow effusions obliterate the posterior "dimples," seen in full extension in normal elbows on either side of the olecranon. Synovial hypertrophy often extends outside and around the joint and has a doughy (boggy) feel accounting for periarticular thickening and loss of normal landmarks. Bursal and synovial out-pouching are commonly swollen with fluid in children with arthritis and generally have well defined margins. Fluid in the joints may be balloted, whereas synovial thickening and induration are palpable but do not feel like fluid. In the chronically inflamed joint, one often feels both boggy thickening of the synovium and fluid [6].

Bony palpation may be performed with the joint in several positions. If bony tenderness is present, it is often possible to distinguish the point tenderness of metaphyseal osteomyelitis from the more generalized but exquisite tenderness of periostitis. Inconsistent findings are characteristic of complex regional pain syndromes in children who complain of severe pain to the lightest palpation often accompanied by a sharp intake of breath (personal observation by T.R. Southwood).

Table 1.1.4 Examination of the joints

Inspection
Gait
Loss of normal contour and landmarks
Distention and fullness
Angulation and deformity
Palpation
Pain, tenderness, warmth
Effusion and distention
Induration, boggy swelling
Nodules
Movement
Range of motion
Stability
Strength
Manual muscle testing including sit up, neck flexor strength, and Gower sign

Table 1.1.5 Range of motion of various joints in degrees (Modified from J.C. Jacobs)

	Flexion	Extension	Internal rotation	External rotation	Abduction	Adduction
Neck (tilt)	45	50	80 (right)	80 (left)	40 (tilt)	40 (tilt)
TMJ	4 cm (space between the incisors when mouth opened fully)					
MCPs	90	30–45		0		
1st MCP	70 (palmar)	0				
Wrist	80	70			20 (radial)	30 (ulnar)
Elbow	135	0–5	90 (supination)	90 (pronation)		
Shoulder	90	45	>55	>40–45	180	45
Hip	135	30	35	45	45–50	20–30
Knee	135	2–10			0	0
Ankle	50	20	>5 (inversion)	>5 (eversion)	10 (forefoot)	20
1st MTP	45	70–90				

The range of motion is then determined (Table 1.1.5) remembering that flexion contractures are a hallmark of JIA. Motion is tested in all the planes of movement possible for a given joint. Stability and strength can be evaluated at the same time. A joint chart or mannequin is helpful for notation of degrees of lost motion if many joints are affected. (Figure 1.1.2). If active range of motion is limited, passive range of motion can be determined and expressed as the number of degrees of motion lost from normal. The difference in the range of motion between the patient's active range and the examiner's evaluation of passive range may be due to the strength of muscles about the tested joint or the degree of cooperation.

It is extremely important to perform an examination of all joints and not limit the examination to the area of complaint. It is common in examining children with arthritis to discover significantly reduced range of motion, especially in the wrists, elbows, and hips, even though the child has no complaints referable to those areas [7].

Examination of the cervical spine

Paediatricians are accustomed to examining the neck for meningeal signs and are aware that the neck should be able to flex so that the chin touches the chest (Figure 1.1.3 (a)) and that it could extend so that the head can touch the back (Figure 1.1.3 (b)). In the examination for arthritis of the cervical spine, it is noted that normally the neck rotates to either side so that the chin is in line with the shoulder (Figure 1.1.3 (c)) and that the neck can tilt laterally 45° toward each shoulder (Figure 1.1.3 (d)).

Examination of the temporomandibular joints

The temporomandibular joint (TMJ) opens and closes between 1500 and 2000 times daily and is frequently affected in Polyarthritis as well as in some children with Oligoarthritis. The joint may be palpated just anterior to the tragus with the mouth closed and during opening and closing, pain and crepitus may be apparent. The mouth span, asymmetricity, and any hypoplasia of the chin are noted at the same time. Normal TMJ opening is considered to be 4 cm between the incisors (Figure 1.1.4).

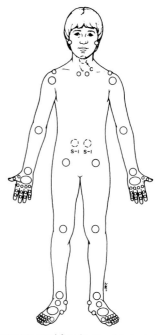

Fig. 1.1.2 Joint mannequin used for charting. Marked circle indicates affected joint or enthesis.

Examination of the upper extremity

Examination of the wrist and hand

The wrist is the most frequently affected upper extremity joint in childhood arthritis and may have considerable hidden abnormalities. This is because the wrist is normally positioned in only mild extension; for children with chronic arthritis, considerable loss of extension is possible without attracting the attention of adults. Children do not realize that they are losing strength in the wrist as a result of the inability to extend. Even synovial swelling of the wrist (Figure 1.1.5) is commonly ignored or it is referred to as "ganglion." True ganglions are probably uncommon in children, and if swelling is associated with loss of motion, the diagnosis is almost certainly arthritis. In addition to 70° of extension the wrist normally flexes 80° (Figure 1.1.6) and deviates

(a) (b) (c) (d)

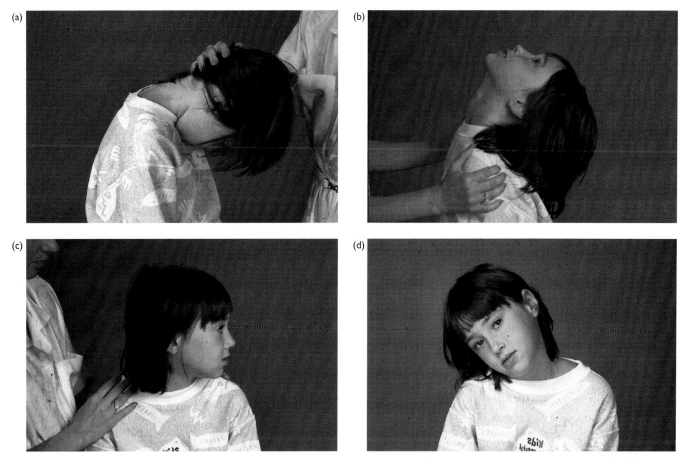

Fig. 1.1.3 Neck flexion (a), extension (b), rotation (c), and lateral tilt (d) are evaluated with the child sitting up on the exam table. Limitation of extension, lateral bending, and subsequently rotation, are common in polyarthritis because of fusion of C2 and C3, as well as in severe juvenile ankylosing spondylitis.

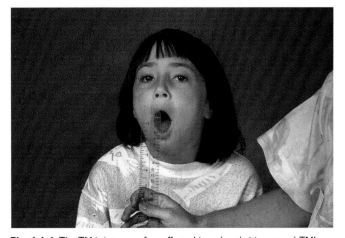

Fig. 1.1.4 The TM joints are often affected in polyarthritis; normal TMJ opening is considered to be 4 cm between the incisors.

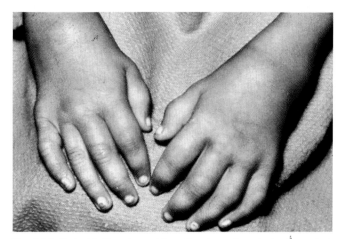

Fig. 1.1.5 Typical finding of synovial swelling above the wrist is often called "synovial pouch" and is a classic finding in children with wrist inflammation. It is often painless.

20° to the radial side and 30° to the ulnar side. Range of motion of the metacarpophalangeal (MCP) joints includes 30° of extension and 90° of flexion (Figure 1.1.7 (a) and (b)). Proximal interphalangeal (PIP) joints normally can flex 100° and extend to zero (Figure 1.1.8 (a) and (b)) while the distal interphalangeal (DIP) joints extend 10° and flex 90° (Figure 1.1.9). The thumb can flex to touch the tips of each finger and

the pad of the base of the fifth finger (Figure 1.1.10 (a)) and can abduct away from the index finger by 50° (Figure 1.1.10 (b)). Arthritis of the fingers is most common in the older child with Polyarthritis. Careful attention to the loss of usual anatomic landmarks such as the lack of skin wrinkling of the PIP joints while the hand is fully extended provides an early clue to the presence of arthritis. Palpation of these

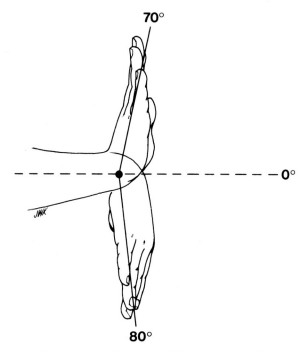

Fig. 1.1.6 The wrist normally flexes to 80° and extends (dorsiflexes) to 70°.

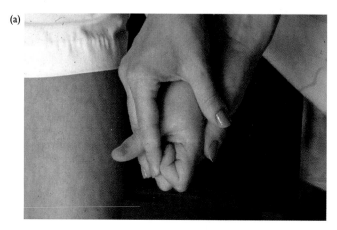

Fig. 1.1.8 PIP joints flex to 100° (a) and extend to 0 (b).

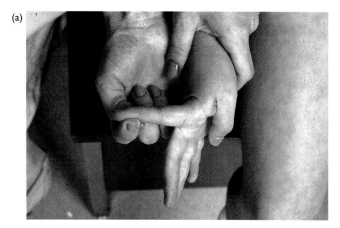

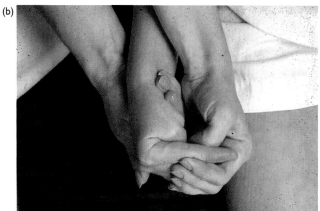

Fig. 1.1.7 MCP joints extend to at least 30° (a) and flex to 90° (b).

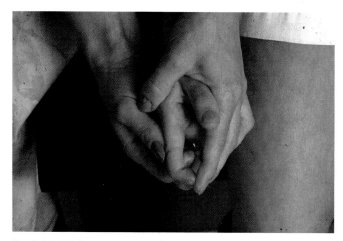

Fig. 1.1.9 DIP flexion is usually 90° while extension is 10°.

joints often provides a feeling of bogginess and not of articulating bones [8].

Examination of the elbow

Swelling may be apparent on inspection especially if unilateral. Warmth and tenderness are evaluated and rheumatoid nodules are felt for at the extensor surface where, if present at all, they are most commonly found (Figure 1.1.11).

The elbow extends to a straight position and flexes 135° (Figure 1.1.12). The test for supination and pronation is done with the

(a)

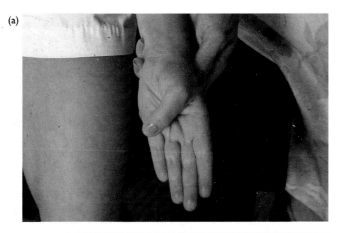

(b)

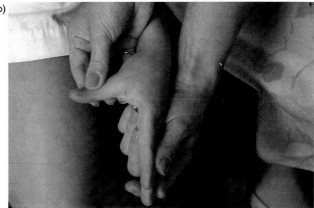

Fig. 1.1.10 The thumb can flex to touch the tips of each finger and the pad of the base of the fifth finger (a) while it abducts away from the index finger by 50° (b).

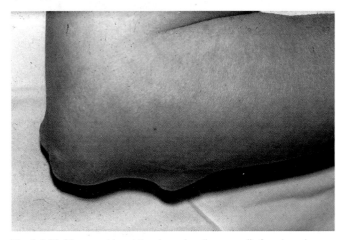

Fig. 1.1.11 Rheumatoid nodules about the elbow, usually found on the extensor surface.

elbow held flexed 90° and against the chest to avoid confusing shoulder motion with elbow motion (Figure 1.1.13 (a) and (b)). Flexion contractures at the elbow and loss of full supination are commonly found in children with arthritis even if there are no complaints referable to the elbow.

Examination of the shoulder

The shoulder is usually involved only in rather severe polyarticular disease especially in children who have Systemic Arthritis.

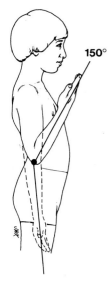

Fig. 1.1.12 As elbow disease progresses in children with arthritis, both extension (0° or 180°) and flexion (150°) may be lost.

Sternoclavicular and acromioclavicular joints may be affected in addition to the glenohumeral (shoulder) joint. Synovial out-pocketing and cystic swellings are sometimes seen in severely affected children and can be documented by ultrasonography. Range of active motion may be conveniently tested by having the child perform three maneuvers: place one hand on the opposite shoulder (Figure 1.1.14 (a)); place one hand behind the head on the opposite shoulder (Figure 1.1.14 (b)); and place the hand behind the back so that the fingers touch the opposite scapula (Figure 1.1.14 (c)). These manoeuvres require 180° of abduction and 45° of adduction, 90° of flexion and 45° of extension, 55° of internal rotation and 40° of external rotation, and test the motion at both the glenohumeral and scapulothoracic articulations. Movement at the sternoclavicular and acromioclavicular joints also takes place during shoulder motion.

Physical examination of the lower extremity and the lumbar spine

Observation of the gait

Lower extremity joints are the most frequently affected in childhood arthritis. Examination of the lower extremity begins with observation of the gait. Pain anywhere in the lower extremity may result in an antalgic gait; that is, the child, when walking, puts weight on the affected extremity for a shorter than normal time to avoid pain. Other common disorders of gait seen in JIA include lateral or posterior lurches as a result of hip disease (Trendelenberg sign) and avoidance of normal heel strike because of pain under the heel or at the Achilles tendon. Metatarsalgia will cause children to avoid push off during the normal gait cycle. Leg length discrepancies secondary to asymmetric growth will also result in an asymmetric gait and may contribute to flexion deformity. With increasing disease in many joints, a combination of abnormalities may occur.

Examination of the hip

The lumbar spine normally curves anteriorly (lumbar lordosis) and flexion deformities of the hip lead to increased lumbar lordosis as a substitute for hip extension; increased lumbar lordosis with exaggerated

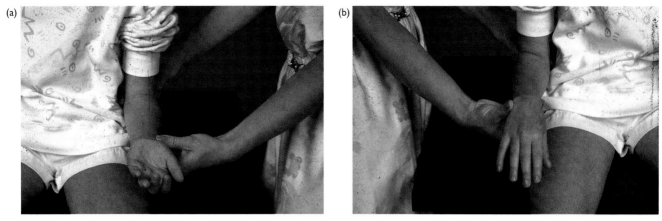

Fig. 1.1.13 The elbow is frequently affected in all forms of JIA and is the most common upper-extremity joint affected in ERA. In cases of what appears to be mono-articular arthritis, evidence of JIA rather than infection, trauma, a foreign body, or orthopaedic pathology can often be obtained by examining the "asymptomatic" elbow. The most common limitation in childhood arthritis is the loss of full supination (a). Tests of pronation (b) and supination are performed with the elbow flexed at 90° and held against the body; a pencil may be held in the hand to evaluate the position.

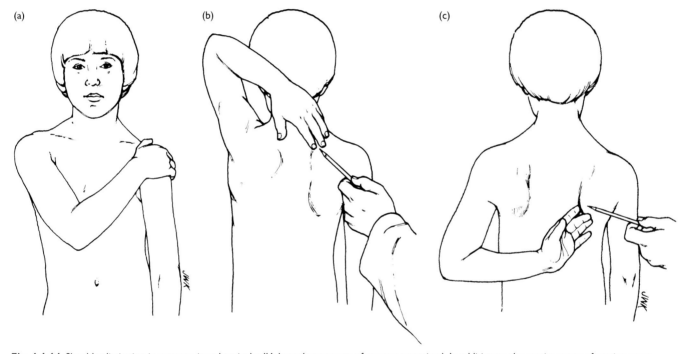

Fig. 1.1.14 Shoulder limitation is common in polyarticular JIA but when present often goes unnoticed. In addition to the passive range of motion exam (see text for details), testing active internal rotation by placing the hand on opposite shoulder (a), external rotation by placing the hand behind the back so the fingers touch the opposite scapula (b), and abduction by placing the hand behind the head and touching the opposite scapula (c).

protrusion of the buttocks may therefore be the first sign of unrecognized arthritis in the hips (Figure 1.1.15).

Bony palpation about the hip includes discriminating the iliac crest, anterior superior iliac spine, pubic tubercles, greater trochanter, ischial tuberosity, posterior iliac spine, vertebral spinous processes, and the sacroiliac joints. Soft tissue palpation includes flexor, extensor, adductor, and abductor muscle groups. The most important part of the examination of the hip for the physician is evaluation of the range of motion (Figure 1.1.16). Paediatricians are generally experienced in this area from examination of the newborn for hip dysplasia. The child should be able to bring the hip across the midline (adduct) 20° with the knee bent (Figure 1.1.16 (a)) and abduct the hip at least 45°

(Figure 1.1.16 (b)). Most children can flex their hips to their chest at least 135° (Figure 1.1.16 (c)) and extend the hip at least 30° (Figure 1.1.16 (d)). The examination of hip extension requires the examiner to put pressure on the buttocks while lifting the entire leg into extension to avoid compensation at the lumbar spine (Figure 1.1.17). To test hip rotation, the child is placed supine on the table with the hip in 90° of flexion. Normally, the leg can rotate externally by 45° (Figure 1.1.18 (a)) and internally by 35° (Figure 1.1.18 (b)). The "screening" for the hip must include internal and external rotation because internal rotation is one of the most sensitive manoeuvre to detect hip abnormalities in children. Muscle strength of the hip flexors, extensors, abductors, and adductors is tested at the same time (Table 1.1.3).

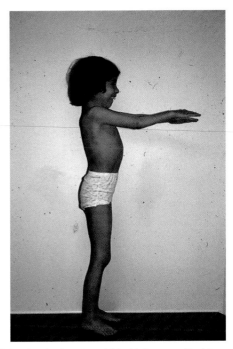

Fig. 1.1.15 Lumbar lordosis in a child with long-standing hip contractures and polyarthritis.

Examination of the knee

The knee is the most frequently affected joint in childhood arthritis and is often the only affected joint at onset. The knee is also the most commonly injured joint, being especially susceptible because of its reliance on the capsule, tendons, and ligaments to ensure joint stability and the great stress to which it is subjected. The knee bends and straightens over 100 times per minute during walking and is subjected to greater stress in running, jumping, and twisting.

Children with chronic knee complaints, especially those who limp and have unilateral involvement, usually develop atrophy of the quadriceps muscle above the affected knee. This can be documented by measuring the circumference of the thigh several centimeters above the upper pole of the patella (Figure 1.1.19 (a)) and comparing it to the other, unaffected side (Figure 1.1.19 (b)). This measurement may provide a helpful clue in children who cannot identify the knee as the source of pain or in children who present to the primary physician with a painful leg. Patients with an affected knee often stand with a slightly bent knee (Figure 1.1.20). Weakness of the quadriceps muscle and inability of the knee to fully extend result in an unstable knee at the time the heel strikes the ground.

In addition, the involved leg may be longer than the uninvolved or less involved one (see also Part 2, Chapter 2.3). This may result in an increased flexion contracture or valgus deformity of the more involved knee to compensate for the extra length when walking or standing. Excessive valgus angulation of the knee may also result from disease at the hip that, by causing limitation of external rotation, requires valgus positioning of the knee for balance.

The measurement of leg length (the span from anterior iliac crest to the middle of the malleolus, Figure 1.1.21) is a routine part of the physical exam for children with chronic arthritis. It is important to note, that patients with significant leg length discrepancy have a pelvic tilt while standing. Any tilt can be "corrected" by placing the shorter extremity on a "block" using standard size blocks. If a leg length discrepancy is

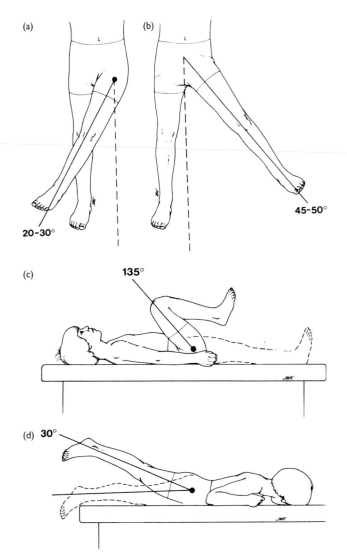

Fig. 1.1.16 Each leg should be able to be adducted across the opposite leg at least 20° (a) and abducted laterally from the midline about 45° (b). Children usually can flex their hips so as to draw their knees right up to the chest, or at least 135° (c), and extend the hip at least 30° (d).

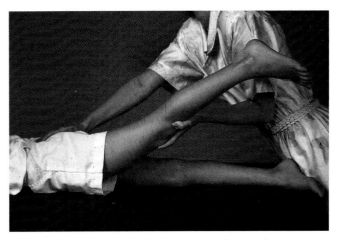

Fig. 1.1.17 The hand should be placed on the child's buttocks when full hip extension is examined to avoid lifting the entire pelvis and missing potential hip flexion contracture.

(a)

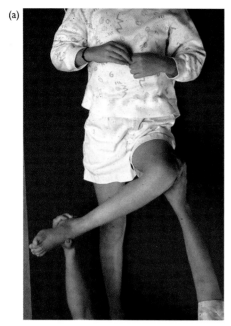

(b)

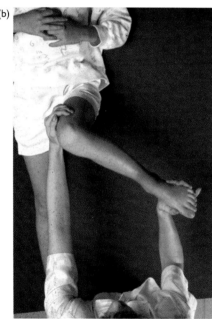

Fig. 1.1.18 With the knee bent and the child in the supine position, the hip should externally rotate at least 45° (a) while internal rotation should be 35° (b).

(a)

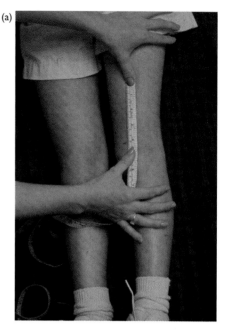

(b)

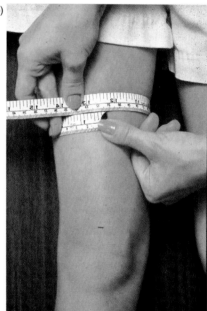

Fig. 1.1.19 Looking for muscle atrophy above the affected knee requires that the examiner place a landmark several centimetres above the upper surface of the patella (a) and then compares the circumference of the thighs (b).

documented, a heel lift is placed on the sole of the shoe worn on the uninvolved leg (Figure 1.1.22) with care taken to match the lift to the sole.

Swelling of the knee may be either localized, a result of fluid accumulation in one of the bursea about the knee (prepatellar, suprapatellar, infrapatellar, pes anserine, or gastrocnemius-semimembranous (Baker cyst), or may be generalized due to fluid in the joint itself or a combination of fluid in the joint and inflammation in the bursae and soft tissues around the joint.

The suprapatellar bursa usually communicates with the articular synovial space and is generally thought of as a pouch of the knee rather than a bursa. This is by far the most common area of fluid accumulation in chronic childhood arthritis (Figure 1.1.23). In childhood arthritis, a ball valve mechanism sometimes seems to result in more

fluid in the pouch than in the knee itself, allowing the examiner to ballotte the knee, after milking the fluid from the suprapatellar bursa into the joint capsule. An analogous swelling occurs in some cases of Baker cyst where the cyst communicates directly with the joint, really representing an out-pouching of synovial membrane that creates a synovial pouch behind the knee.

Examination of the knee generally begins with palpation of the bursae and out-pocketings and then proceeds to palpation of the synovial membrane. The suprapatellar pouch is compressed first, and the joint may then be lightly palpated with the thumb and forefinger of the right hand for fluid and for synovial thickening. It is difficult to distinguish fluid from synovial thickening, and both are often present simultaneously. When there is sufficient fluid, the patella is ballottable

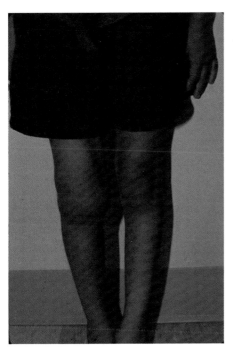

Fig. 1.1.20 Typical stance of a child with Oligoarthritis and a knee flexion contracture.

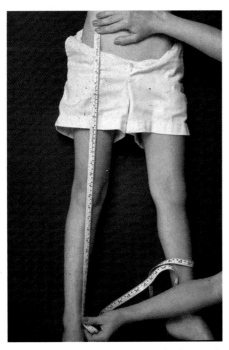

Fig. 1.1.21 Leg length measurement comparing the distance between the superior anterior iliac crest to the middle of the medial malleolus.

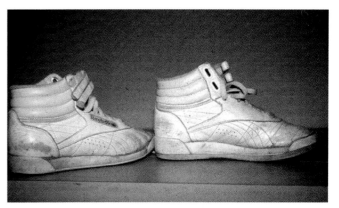

Fig. 1.1.22 Invisible lift matching the colour of the sole of the shoe custom made for a child with leg length discrepancy resulting from asymmetric arthritis of the lower extremities.

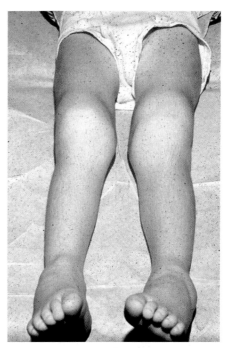

Fig. 1.1.23 Typical accumulation of fluid in the suprapatellar bursa in a child with knee arthritis.

(it rebounds after being pushed down as a result of fluid being first pushed to the side and then flowing back under the patella).

The patella must be separately evaluated when examining the knee. It plays an important role in knee function. If infected, it may be the primary cause of knee effusion. Prepatellar septic bursitis and patellar osteomyelitis can usually be distinguished from pathology in this joint by careful palpation (see Part 1, Chapter 1.5).

Anterior knee pain syndrome (patellofemoral syndrome) is a common cause of knee pain in teenagers especially if there is associated diffuse hypermobility. Helpful physical signs include grating of the undersurface of the patella when the knee is flexed and extended or when the patella is pushed against the femur; this may be quite painful. In addition, pain may be reproduced by palpation of the medial undersurface of the patella, and inhibition of patellar motion by pushing against the patella while the patient contracts the quadriceps muscle (Figure 1.1.24). Pushing the patella laterally may create the so-called "patella apprehension" sign consistent with the patient's fear of dislocation.

Range of motion of the knee is then tested. This is best accomplished while the child is supine on the table. The knee may normally be flexed so the heel touches the buttock (Figure 1.1.25 (a)) and may be extended a little beyond neutral (Figure 1.1.25 (b)). Hypermobile children have more than 10° of hyperextension and may stand with their knees locked behind them and hyper extended. There is also about 10° of internal or external rotation possible with the femur held

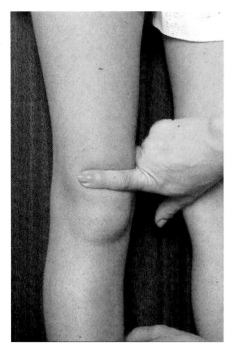

Fig. 1.1.24 While the examiner places the hand over the patella to prevent it from riding upward, the patient is asked to fully extend the knee. This "patellar inhibition" may elicit symptoms of anterior knee pain aka patello-femoral syndrome.

(a)

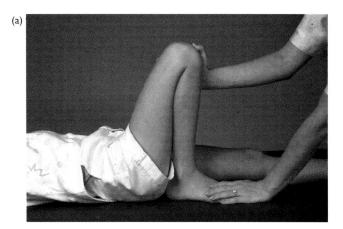

(b)

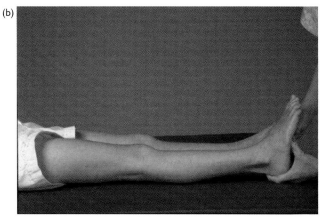

Fig. 1.1.25 The knee flexes to 135° (a) and often hyper-extends by about 10° (b).

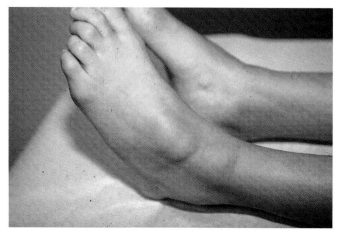

Fig. 1.1.26 Tenosynovitis of the ankle joint seen frequently in Polyarthritis, akin to the wrist pouches (see Figure 1.1.5).

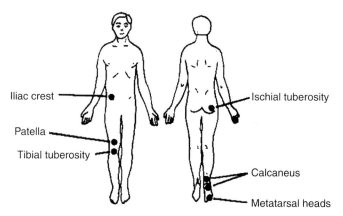

Fig. 1.1.27 Sites of tendon insertions into the bone (enthesis) palpated in children with ERA who often have enthesitis.

in a fixed position. If there are symptoms to suggest knee instability, further investigations may be justified.

Examination of the foot and ankle

The ankle and the foot are commonly involved in childhood arthritis especially in children with Enthesitis Related Arthritis (see Part 2, Chapter 2.7). Swelling of the ankle joint with tenosynovitis may be visible to inspection (Figure 1.1.26). Palpation may reveal bony tenderness in the calcaneus, especially near the sites of insertion of the Achilles tendon or the plantar fascia prone to enthesitis. Pain and crepitus on motion of the first metatarsal should especially be evaluated, since extension at this joint is critical for normal gait. The Achilles tendon may also be tender and thickened, and the retrocalcaneal bursa, palpated behind the Achilles tendon, may become inflamed as well. Spurs may form at the inflamed attachments (entheses) of the Achilles tendon and plantar fascia to the calcaneus. Inflammation at the enthesis is the hallmark of ERA. Periosteal pain, bone pain from erosions, and pain in the tendons and fascia can all be demonstrated at the insertions of the Achilles tendon and plantar fascia into the calcaneus (Figure 1.1.27).

The range of motion of the ankle involves dorsiflexion (20°, Figure 1.1.28 (a)) and plantar flexion (50°, Figure 1.1.28 (b)) at the ankle mortise (articulation of the tibia and fibula with talus), and eversion (5°, Figure 1.1.29 (a)) and inversion (5°, Figure 1.1.29 (b)) at

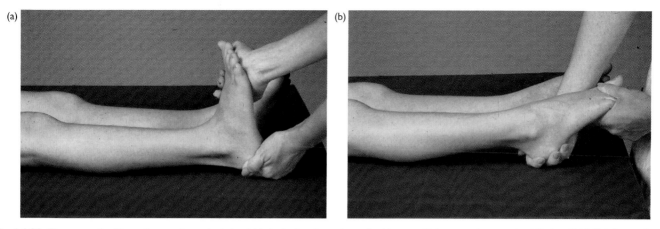

Fig. 1.1.28 The range of ankle motion can be evaluated quickly by having the patient raise his toes off the ground to test dorsi-flexion ((a) 20°, influenced not only by ankle motion but also by the length of Achilles tendon) and push up on his toes to test plantar flexion ((b) at least 50°).

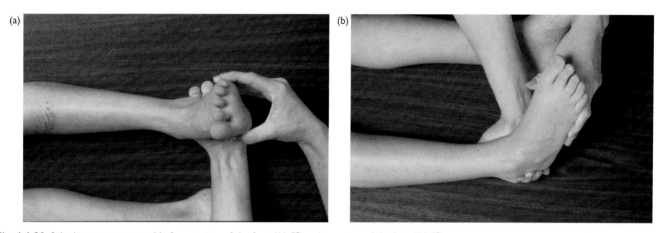

Fig. 1.1.29 Subtalar joint is responsible for eversion of the foot ((a) 5°) and inversion of the foot ((b) 5°).

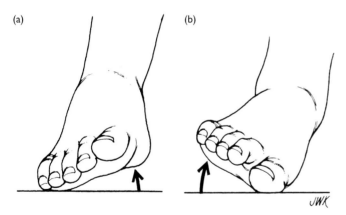

Fig. 1.1.30 The forefoot should also be able to be abducted 10° (a) and adducted 20° (b) by the examiner.

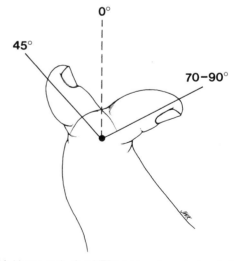

the subtalar joint. Forefoot abduction (10°, Figure 1.1.30 (a)) and adduction (20°, Figure 1.1.30 (b)) requires motion at the mid-tarsal (talonavicular and calcaneocuboid) joints.

The first metatarsal joint normally flexes 45° (Figure 1.1.31(a)) and extends 70–90° (Figure 1.1.31(b)); normal toe-off for proper gait cycle requires a minimum of 35° of extension of the large toe. Unlike the other toes, there is normally no extension at the proximal PIP joint of the great toe.

Fig. 1.1.31 Motion at the first MTP joint is an important part of the examination since this joint is frequently affected in ERA and sometimes is the sole affected joint at the time of the first visit. The joint should be able to flex 45° (a) and extend at least 70° (b).

Metatarsalgia is a hallmark of Polyarthritis. It can be elicited by squeezing the metatarsal heads together or by watching the child walk without shoes. Custom-made shoe inserts are recommended and relieve pain by taking the weight off the metatarsophalangeal (MTP) heads and providing shock absorption.

Examination of the lumbar spine

Paravertebral muscle spasm results in awkward or unnatural movements during undressing and bending. Paravertebral muscles in spasm and pelvic tilt may be grossly visible. The vertebral bodies should be palpated. Pain from discitis or tumors invading the spinal cord may be referred to the hip, thigh, or even the knee. Simple manoeuvres such as deep knee bends and touching the toes provide an opportunity for the examiner to observe evidence of abnormality in the spine, hips, and knees. Normally, the child can extend the back 30° at the lumbar area (Figure 1.1.32 (a)), bend forward and touch the toes (Figure 1.1.32 (b)), move it laterally 50° to each side (Figure 1.1.32 (c)), and rotate the lumbar area 30° to each side. When the paravertebral muscle spasm is present, or there is limitation of lumbar spine flexion as seen in early ERA, the patient may bend solely at the hips, maintaining a straight back (lumbar lordosis) instead of developing the smooth curve that is normally seen on bending forward. To evaluate for the presence of decreased lumbar spine flexion, the modified Schober test is used (Figure 1.1.33). While the patient stands with the back to the examiner, the posterior superior iliac spines (underneath the dimples of Venus) are identified and a mark is placed at this level over the lumbar spine (Figure 1.1.33 (a)). Next, the examiner measures 10 cm above and 5 cm below the initial mark, creating a 15 cm span (Figure 1.1.33 (a)). The patient is then instructed to bend forward with knees straight and the span is remeasured (Figure 1.1.33 (b)). Normal expansion is at least 6 cm (from 15 to 21 cm); anything less implies decreased lumbar flexion and provides a clue to an underlying inflammation. Most healthy children have "generous" motion at the lumbar spine. Equally important is assessing the lateral profile of the lower spine when the patient is bending forward. Normally, there is a smooth, continuous curve from the sacrum to the cervical spine. In restricted spinal movement, the curve is replaced by visible areas of flattening (see Part 2, Figure 2.7.1).

The sacroiliac joint is the articulation of the bony pelvis with the sacrum and transmits the weight from the entire upper body to the pelvis and lower extremities. Some motion exists in these joints in children and in young adults. Palpation of the sacroiliac joint is important since it is sometimes tender in ERA. Septic sacroiliitis also occurs in children; the exquisite tenderness of the infected sacroiliac joint is easily differentiated from the more subtle pain of inflammatory sacroiliitis of ERA. Pain in the sacroiliac joint can be elicited by compressing or distracting the pelvis. The most sensitive test is probably direct pressure over the sacrum while the child is lying prone. Raising the straight leg with the patient supine may produce pain in the back and all along the course of the sciatic nerve if there is disc or sciatic nerve disease. If the leg is lowered to where the pain disappears and the foot is then dorsi-flexed, reproducing the sciatic pain, this increases the likelihood of disease process affecting the sciatic nerve. Pain in the opposite leg with the straight leg-raising test suggests a space-occupying lesion such as a herniated disk in the lumbar spine.

Hamstring tightness (less than 70° during the straight leg raise, Figure 1.1.34) is quite common; interestingly, it may be an isolated finding or discovered in association with diffuse hypermobility. It is also common in both long-standing dermatomyositis and arthritis.

Examination of tender points

The examiner needs experience with the technique of identifying and locating tender points, often present in children and adolescents with fibromyalgia (Figure 1.1.8). Although various sets of "best" tender points have been proposed, the presence of 11 out

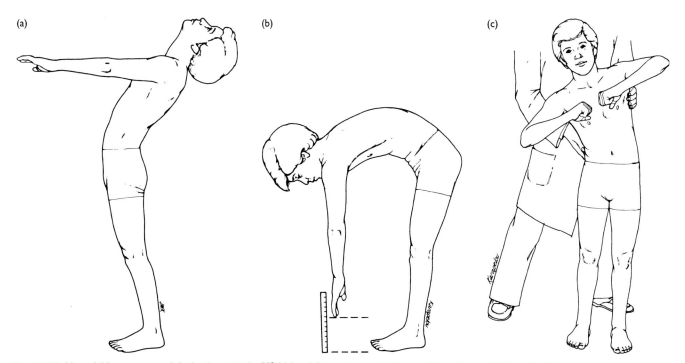

Fig. 1.1.32 Most children can extend the lumbar spine by 30° (a) bend forward to touch the toes (b), and move 50° laterally (c).

(a)

(b)

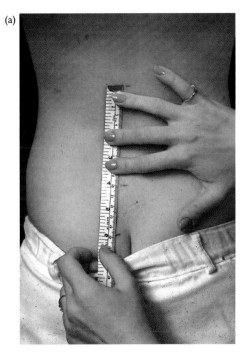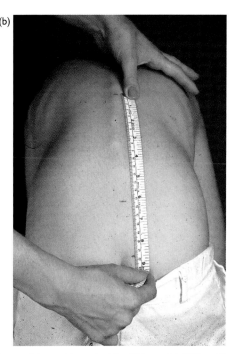

Fig. 1.1.33 The measurement of flexion of the lumbar spine (the modified Schober test) is most important in children with ERA and has been undervalued as part of the paediatric physical examination. With the patient standing with his/her back to the examiner (a), the dimples of Venus, L4 level, are identified and a mark is placed on the spine at that level. Subsequent mark is placed 10 cm above and 5 cm below. The child is then instructed to bend forward (b) without bending the knees and the examiner remeasures the 15 cm span. A subsequent measurement of at least 21 cm is considered normal lumbar spine flexion in adolescents and the test works well for young children as well. This measurement is useful in evaluating progression or remission of disease and may be used as a measure of drug efficacy [9].

of 18 possible tender points is most commonly used (see Part 1, Chapter 1.9). The patient should be seated comfortably on the examination table and queried as to the presence of pain following the palpation of each bilateral anatomic site. Palpation should be done with the thumb or forefinger, applying pressure approximately equal to the force of 4 kg, as excessive force may elicit pain in anyone. A systematic palpation of each site, beginning at the suboccipital muscle insertion at the posterior skull, progressing to the medial fat pad of the knee, should be followed. Control anatomic sites, such as over the thumbnail, or forehead should also be palpated. These sites are not as painful on pressure as the selected anatomic sites, although most patients with fibromyalgia are more tender to palpation at many muscle and soft tissue sites than are normal controls [10].

Evaluation of posture

The child should be observed in a lateral position for any forward tilting of the head with flattening of the anterior chest wall; thoracic kyphosis and loss of lumbar lordosis are characteristic of the posture in ERA. Children with ERA and other patients with hip disease often stand leaning forward a bit with flexed knees because of flexion contractures of the hips. Similarly, children with knee flexion contractures tend to stand with hips flexed, while children with metatarsalgia stand with their toes off the ground and walk using small shuffling steps to avoid bearing weight on the inflamed metatarsal heads.

Chest expansion can be evaluated and measured with a tape measure in teenagers and compared in repeated visits. The measurement

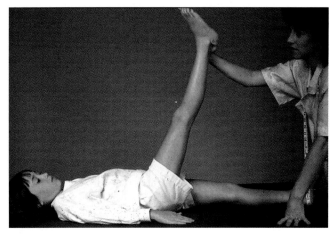

Fig. 1.1.34 Most children can bend to touch their toes without bending their knees unless their hamstrings are tight (straight leg raise should be at least 70°).

is performed at the nipple line after instructing the patient to breathe out fully and then take a maximal breath.

Evaluation of the functional state of the patient

Once the history is taken and the physical examination has been performed the physician can make a determination about the functional state of the patient. Is the child functioning normally

Table 1.1.6 Evaluation of functional state in musculoskeletal disease

	JIA	Mechanical injury	Psychogenic pain
Pain	+/−	+	++++ (8–10/10)
Swelling	++	+	−
LOM	++	−	−
Limp	++	+	++++ (bizarre)
Muscle atrophy	++	−	−
Disability	−	−	++++
School absence	−	−	++++
Sleep disturbance	−	−	+++

despite the disease? If not, is the loss of function proportional to visible disability? How does this child function in comparison to other children with the same evidence of the physical disease (Table 1.1.6). A variety of functional tools have been developed to assess functioning in children with arthritis (see Part 3, Chapter 3.4).

When organic disease is obvious, such an evaluation leads to setting up reasonable goals of therapy and helps the physician judge the need for specific medications and treatment and whether the child or family is so distressed that psychiatric help is needed to restore them to optimal function despite the illness. The physician must guard against the natural concern only with "organic" disease and the tendency to "reject" the patient who is disabled but does not have a "disease." The nonfunctioning child is ill; if one cannot find a disease to explain this illness, it does not mean that there is nothing wrong or that the child does not require treatment. Physicians have the responsibility to be nonjudgmental and to try to heal the patient whether there is a physical disease or not. Some children who are disabled with musculoskeletal complaints have no evidence of organic disease on physical examination or on laboratory studies. Their limited function may be worse than that seen in children with severe rheumatic disease. A physician accustomed to caring for chronically ill children who are attending school each day and enjoying reasonable lifestyles may be confronted with a homebound child who has no discernable findings. The problem of children out of school for months or in bed with withdrawal and depression is accentuated by the physician who has to be certain there is no physical illness present at all before deciding to deal with the disability or to send the patient somewhere where the disability can be dealt with. This error is avoided by taking simultaneous steps both to continue to explore the possibility of physical illness and to get the patient back in the main stream, whether or not there is any physical illness. While this problem exists in rheumatology with patients of any age, the problem of recognizing disability out of proportion to the visible evidence of disease is exaggerated in children and

adolescents because others are not dependant on that "sick individual" for support. Physicians forget that a child not attending school daily is the equivalent of an adult not going to work.

Families often state that nonfunction is the result of physician instruction not to function; this usually means that some physician has "read the child's mind" or the parent's and prescribed what was sought as the prescription. Nonfunction is accepted at face value and dealt with directly; if the child can return to school the next day and live a normal life, then no other resources may be necessary. If there is obviously no chance of the child returning to a lifestyle appropriate for visible and comprehensible disability, then the synthesis of that problem should be achieved at the time of the first visit and appropriate action taken to find the help needed to get the child functioning again [1,11].

References

1. Jacobs, J.C. Clinical techniques in pediatric rheumatology. In J.C. Jacobs, ed. *Pediatric Rheumatology for the Practitioner*. New York: Springer-Verlag, 1992; pp.1–22.

2. Smith, R.C. and Hopp, R.B. The patient's story: integrating patient and physician centered approaches to interviewing. *Ann Int Med* 1991; 15: 470–7.

3. Liang, M.H. and Sturrock, R.D. Evaluation of the musculoskeletal system. In J.H., Klippel and P.A., Dieppe eds., *Rheumatology*. New York: Mosby, 1998; pp.2.1.1–18.

4. Polley, H.F. and Hunder, G.G. Rheumatologic interviewing and physical examination of the joints, 2nd edn. Philadelphia, PA: Saunders, 1978.

5. Bickley, L.S. The musculoskeletal system. In *Bates' Pocket Guide to Physical Examination and History Taking*, 3rd edn. Philadelphia, PA: Lippincott, 2000.

6. Southwood, T.R. and Malleson, P.N. The clinical history and physical examination. In T.R., Southwood and P.N., Malleson eds. *Arthritis in Children and Adolescents. Bailliere's Clinical Pediatrics*. London: Bailliere Tindall, 1993;1:3:637–64.

7. McGhee, J.L. Burks, F.N. Sheckels, J.L. and Jarvis, J.N. Identifying children with chronic arthritis based on chief complaints: absence of predictive value for musculoskeletal pain as an indicator of rheumatic disease in children. *Pediatrics* 2002;110:354–9.

8. Siegel, L.B. and Gall, E.P. A systematic approach to the physical examination in rheumatoid arthritis. Part 1: the head, neck, torso, and upper extremities. *J Musculoskeletal Med* 1999;16:329–35.

9. Merritt, J.L. *et al.* Measurement of trunk flexibility in normal subjects: reproducibility of three clinical methods. *Mayo Clin Proc* 1986;61:192–7.

10. Wolfe, F. Smythe, H.A. Yunus, M.B. *et al.* The American College of Rheumatology 1990 Criteria for the classification of fibromyalgia: report of the Multicenter Criteria Committee. *Arthritis Rheum* 1990;33:160–71.

11. Szer, I.S. Musculoskeletal pain syndromes affecting adolescents. In E.R. Stiehm ed. *Archives of Pediatric and Adolescent Medicine*, 1996; 150: 740–7.

The use of investigations and imaging in the evaluation of arthritis

Ilona S. Szer

Aim

The aim of this chapter is to describe the laboratory and imaging evaluation for the child who is suspected of having Juvenile Idiopathic Arthritis.

Structure

- Synovial fluid analysis
- Acute phase reactants
- White blood cell count
- Haemoglobin
- ANA
- RF
- Imaging techniques

Laboratory evaluation

Introduction

Laboratory tests are not usually helpful in positively establishing the diagnosis of Juvenile Idiopathic Arthritis (JIA) but they are helpful in excluding other disorders and providing evidence for the presence and extent of other chronic rheumatic conditions. Laboratory studies may help in determining the type of JIA such as Rheumatoid Factor (RF) Positive Polyarthritis, or HLA B27 associated arthritis. Specific rheumatic tests are reserved for children in whom there is strong clinical suspicion suggested by a constellation of signs and symptoms, or in establishing prognosis in limited circumstances but they are of little value in "screening" for a rheumatic illness. Generally speaking, there are few serologic tests in rheumatic conditions that are diagnostic.

Laboratory tests are also helpful in screening for organ involvement and in "staging" in systemic rheumatic illnesses such as systemic lupus erythematosus (SLE) and dermatomyositis that may affect organ systems not clinically apparent or symptomatic.

Synovial fluid analysis

Examination of the joint fluid is essential when monoarticular arthritis suggests the possibility of an infection. Arthrocentesis should generally be performed by the person who has the most experience in that procedure; often, in community settings, the orthopaedic surgeon. The fluid is examined for volume, viscosity, color, clarity, cell count, protein,

and sugar; a smear is made for staining and fluid is sent for culture in all appropriate media. The mucin clot test has not been found useful in paediatrics and because gout is not usually seen in children, tests for uric acid crystals are not necessary. Tests on the synovial fluid for complement, immune complexes, antinuclear antibodies, and rheumatoid factors (RF) are hard to interpret and are not considered useful in clinical medicine [1].

The primary purpose of arthrocentesis is to exclude infection (see Part 1, Chapter 1.3, Algorithm 1.3.1). Fluid with a white blood cell (WBC) count over 100,000/ml (mostly polymorphonuclear) is usually septic and should be considered so until proven otherwise. Lower synovial fluid cell counts do not exclude the possibility of infection. Septic fluid tends to have a very high protein and a glucose more than 25% below simultaneously obtained blood glucose. The specimen drawn for cell count should be obtained in a syringe containing an anticoagulant to prevent clotting. No procaine containing preservatives that may sterilize the culture artificially should be injected into the joint or area to be aspirated until after the specimen for culture is obtained. Sterile joint fluid does not assure the physician that the patient does not have osteomyelitis in a bone where the infected metaphysis is outside of the joint, such as of the knee. Septic arthritis may be proven by examination of joint fluid but a negative Gram stain or culture do not rule out this diagnosis (see Part 1, Chapter 1.5).

Other laboratory investigations

Four basic characteristics of diagnostic tests help judge their usefulness in the evaluation of patients: sensitivity, specificity, plus positive, and negative predictive value [2]. *Sensitivity* is the likelihood of a positive test resulting in a person with the disease (the true positive rate of a diagnostic test) and is reported as the percentage of positive results in patients known to have the disease. A test with a sensitivity of 90% has a true positive rate of 90% and a false negative rate of 10%. *Specificity* is the likelihood of a negative test occurring in a patient without the disease (the true negative rate of a test). Specificity is reported as the percentage of true negative results in patients known to be free of the disease. A test with a specificity of 90% has a false positive rate of 10%.

While tests are usually described in terms of their sensitivity and specificity, the clinician is more interested in the predictive value of a test or the probability that the patient has a disease given a positive test result. Similarly, if the test is negative what is the probability that the patient does not have the disease? The positive predictive value of a test is the probability of a disease if the test is positive while the negative predictive value of a test is the probability of a disease being absent if the test is negative. Using Bayes' theorem one can determine the predictive value (positive or negative) of a test if one knows its sensitivity and specificity, and the prevalence of the disease in the population.*

Reasonable laboratory studies to be performed in patients being evaluated for rheumatic diseases are listed (Table 1.2.1) and the approach to the work up of common presenting complaints is outlined in appropriate algorithms (see Part 1, Chapter 1.3). The significance of specific laboratory studies is discussed in the chapters on the individual diseases. All laboratory studies ordered must be individualized for a given patient; no scheme may be applied to every patient. Only several of the most frequently ordered laboratory tests are discussed here.

Acute phase reactants

Acute phase reactants (APR) are plasma proteins made in the liver that usually increase during inflammation or tissue necrosis and may parallel chronic inflammation. They form a heterogeneous group comprised of coagulation and transport proteins, complement components, protease inhibitors, and others such as albumin, fibronectin, and serum amyloid-A related protein. Of these, the most frequently used are the erythrocyte sedimentation rate (ESR) which reflects the presence of several proteins whose concentrations increase during inflammation and the C-reactive protein (CRP), a single 105 kDa protein with five linked subunits. The CRP is more rapidly responsive to inflammation than the ESR. The ESR is frequently used by practitioners to document inflammation even though data suggest that the ESR is not useful in distinguishing inflammatory arthritis from other causes of joint symptoms; it may be normal in inflammatory arthritis and elevated in the absence of clinical disease [3]. In addition, it may be falsely low in conditions associated with abnormal red cells or in patients in congestive heart failure, and falsely elevated in pregnancy or while oral contraceptives are used. CRP concentration may increase 100–1000 fold, while the ESR measures proteins whose concentrations rise only 2–4 fold. The ESR is often less sensitive and "lags behind" the patient's clinical status. For example, early in the course of reactive arthritis, both ESR and CRP are elevated but as the inflammation subsides, the ESR remains elevated while the CRP returns to normal. Neither the ESR nor the CRP provides clues to where the inflammation is.

The ESR is usually elevated in children with Systemic Arthritis and SLE but much less frequently in children with Oligoarthritis, Henoch–Schönlein Purpura (HSP), or dermatomyositis. The CRP also varies in different clinical situations. As a screening test for the presence of inflammation it may be a highly informative study. Because of its sensitivity to change, reflecting ongoing changes more accurately, it correlates more closely with the course of the chronic inflammation in Systemic Arthritis or Polyarthritis; in SLE however, an elevated CRP in the presence of normal or mildly elevated ESR suggests an intercurrent infection and not a flare of underlying disease; the latter being more closely associated with an elevated ESR.

WBC count

WBC count rises during the inflammatory response and tends to be elevated in children with acute inflammatory conditions. For this reason, a low or normal WBC count should raise clinical suspicion

*Positive predictive value of a test = sensitivity (prevalence of the disease)/ sensitivity (prevalence) + (1 − specificity)(1 − prevalence).

Table 1.2.1 Laboratory and radiographic studies in paediatric rheumatology (these lists are suggestions and may not all be applicable in every clinical situation)

Initial evaluation (see Part 1, Ch 1.3)
  CBC with differential count done manually and reticulocyte count
  ESR or CRP
  Urinalysis
  Metabolic and chemistry panel including renal and liver function tests
  Anti-streptococcal antibodies
  Lyme antibodies (in endemic area only)
  PPD skin test

Testing for possible SLE (see Part 1, Chapter 1.6)
  ANA
  Coomb test
  Platelet count and Reticulocyte count
  C3 and C4 or the total haemolytic complement
  PTT, lupus anticoagulant, anti-cardiolipin antibody, VDRL, RVVT, anti-beta 2 glycoprotein
  Anti-ds DNA, anti-ENA (SSA, SSB, Sm, and RNP)
  24-h urine for protein and creatinine (if UA abnormal).
  Chest X-ray

For possible dermatomyositis (see Part 1, Chapter 1.6)
  AST, ALT, CPK, Aldolase, LDH
  ANA, anti-ENA
  Nail fold capillaroscopy
  EMG (if typical rash absent)
  Muscle biopsy (if typical rash absent or muscle enzymes normal)
  TSH and free T4
  Toxoplasmosis
  Chest X-ray

For possible Systemic Arthritis (see Part 2, Chaper 2.2)
  Fibrin degradation products or d-dimers, ferritin
  Chest X-ray
  ECG
  2D-echocardiogram
  Urinary catecholamine
  Abdominal ultrasound
  Technetium bone scan
  Bone marrow examination
  Small intestinal series
  CT and MRI studies

For other forms of JIA (see Part 2)
  ANA
  RF
  HLA B27
  TSH, Free T4
  Slit lamp exam

For Kawasaki disease (see Part 1, Chapter 1.4)
  ECG
  Chest X-ray
  2D-echocardiogram
  Slit lamp exam

For possible Systemic Sclerosis (see Part 1, Chapter 1.6)
  Esophogram
  Chest X-ray
  Anti-ENA, Anti-SCL-70, Anti-centromere
  Nail fold capillaroscopy

Table 1.2.1 (*Continued*)

For possible systemic vasculitis syndromes
   ANCA
   Immune complex assays
   All tests done for SLE
   Hepatitis antigens and antibodies
   Cryoglobulins
   Consider EMG and Nerve Conduction Studies, MRA, MRV, aortogram, angiogram, skin, muscle, kidney and/or sural nerve biopsy
Chest X-ray

for acute lymphocytic leukemia in a young child with fever and musculoskeletal pain (see Part 1, Chapter 1.3, Algorithm 1.3.1) and SLE in an adolescent. In viral syndromes, the WBC may also be low but the leucopaenia is associated with a relative lymphocytosis while in SLE, there is more likely to be absolute lymphopaenia. Indeed, lymphopaenia (absolute lymphocyte count of <1200) is one of the 11 classification criteria for SLE and if present on the initial CBC, provides support for further evaluation for SLE.

Similarly, low or normal platelet count may provide a clue to an underlying malignancy or to autoimmune cytopenia seen in SLE; platelet count typically rises in inflammation as seen during the second week of Kawasaki disease (KD) (see Part 1, Chapter 1.4) or at any time in active Systemic Arthritis. A low or low normal platelet count in face of a raised ESR or CRP is suggestive of either SLE or childhood leukaemia.

Haemoglobin

Most children with inflammatory conditions develop anaemia of inflammation; serum iron level, iron binding capacity, and the reticulocyte counts are low. In contrast, children with nutritional, iron deficiency also have low iron and reticulocyte count but have an elevated iron binding capacity. In autoimmune conditions, particularly SLE, haemoglobin drops secondary to peripheral destruction (Coomb positive haemolytic anaemia) and reticulocytosis is present. In vasculitis syndromes or thrombotic thrombocyclopenic purpura (TTP), haemoglobin may fall secondary to micro-angiopathic haemolysis. Children with inflammatory bowel disease (IBD) have low haemoglobin and low iron stores secondary to chronic bleeding from the GI tract (see Part 1, Chapter 1.4).

The antinuclear antibody test (ANA) and the rheumatoid factor (RF)

One of the favourite tests of the primary care physician is the antinuclear antibody test (ANA), often used as a screening study for all rheumatic diseases in children. While it is true that many patients who have a chronic rheumatic illness test positive for the ANA, the ANA is neither a specific nor a useful diagnostic tool unless the physician is strongly considering SLE because the patient already exhibits one or more classification criteria for SLE (see Part 1, Chapter 1.6). The finding of a positive ANA simply creates anxiety and the "need" to immediately refer the child to the sub-specialist. Depending on the assay and the substrate used, positive ANA have been identified in healthy individuals of any age; using the Hep-2 assay, up to 30% of healthy individuals test positive at a titre of 1:40; 10–15% at a titre of 1:80, and 5% at 1:160 while specific autoantibodies (Sm/RNP,

anti-dsDNA, SSA, SSB and others) cannot be found [4]. In a healthy child with positive ANA, there is no need for additional studies; the ANA may be repeated 3–4 months later to ascertain whether or not it is transient. If still positive, it simply becomes part of the patient's medical profile, to be interpreted appropriately at any time of future clinical concern, but not repeated again unless there is a clinical change and suspicion for SLE has once again arisen. Longitudinal studies have shown that children with positive ANA do not frequently develop rheumatic illnesses later in life [5,6].

Similarly, the RF has no utility in the initial evaluation of a child with musculoskeletal complaints; only those children who have symmetric arthritis of multiple joints need to be tested, primarily for prognostic reasons. The RF, an autoantibody directed against the Fc portion of IgG, is sometimes positive in children who have disorders other than JIA and is usually negative in children with JIA except in the older female adolescent (see RF Positive Polyarthritis, in Part 2, Chapter 2.4). The child with a positive RF may have either an acute or chronic infection, (SBE, EBV, hepatitis, tuberculosis, syphilis, Lyme disease, multiple parasitic infections), SLE, sarcoidosis, localized scleroderma, or Sjögren syndrome. In one retrospective analysis, in no case was RF testing helpful in either establishing a diagnosis of chronic arthritis or in ruling it out [7].

Imaging techniques in childhood rheumatic disease

Radiographs are not useful in making an early diagnosis of any of the childhood rheumatic diseases but may be helpful in providing clues favoring another diagnosis. Therefore, X-rays of the symptomatic joint should nearly always be obtained. Plain radiographs show bone best and the soft tissues less well. The earliest finding that may be useful in the diagnosis of JIA is ostoepenia. Radiographs are not useful in osteomyelitis or septic arthritis because in the initial stages they are usually normal (see Part 1, Chapter 1.5).

In more advanced disease, radiographs provide an objective measure of severity; they should be taken infrequently to avoid unnecessary radiation but generally speaking radiographs contribute substantially to the management of JIA especially at times of making decisions to escalate or discontinue treatment (see Part 3, Chapter 3.8 and Part 2, Chapters 2.2–2.7).

A chest X-ray is obtained in Systemic Arthritis, SLE, dermatomyositis, scleroderma, when sarcoidosis is a consideration, when the tuberculin test is positive or when otherwise clinically required.

Small bowel and colon barium studies are obtained when IBD is a possibility; endoscopy with intestinal biopsy is sometimes diagnostic of IBD when other studies are negative. An abdominal ultrasound is obtained if neuroblastoma is a consideration. Ultrasound is also useful in demonstrating hidden pelvic and abdominal abscess, pyomyositis, and coronary aneurysms in Kawasaki disease. Small amounts of pericardial fluid may be demonstrated in Systemic Arthritis and cardiac myxoma while cardiac valves are evaluated in acute rheumatic fever.

The role of ultrasonography, CT, and MRI in early JIA

The ultrasound is an excellent technique for imaging the soft tissues but interpretation of this test is difficult and requires special expertise [8]. In studies, ultrasound was used effectively to identify synovial "pouches" about the wrist, extremely common in Polyarthritis and at

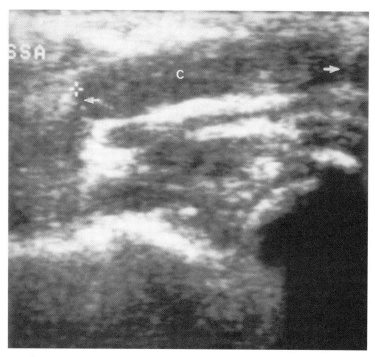

Fig. 1.2.1 Ultrasound longitudinal view of posterior knee in a boy with ERA: an oval hypolucent cyst (c) is seen posterior to the joint space.

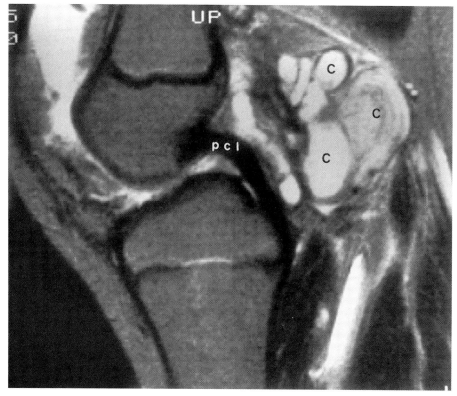

Fig. 1.2.2 MRI of same joint: transverse view of posterior knee showing an oval mass adjacent to a relatively dark medial condyle.

the knees (Figure 1.2.1). The CT scan is particularly useful for visualizing the spine and for assessing the integrity of the intervertebral discs, and contrast enhancement may show spinal compression. However, images of the peripheral joints are difficult to interpret and expose the patient to large doses of radiation.

MRI provides the earliest evidence of cartilage and bone loss in children with chronic arthritis and is now used extensively to image joints and soft tissues that may be affected by rheumatic disease, especially initially when trauma and ligamentous tears are also considered. The introduction of more powerful magnets has allowed high definition of soft tissues and the detection of early bony erosions and Baker cysts (Figure 1.2.2). Enhancement of the MRI images by gadolinium-DPTA allows the detection of early synovitis and enables disease progression to be monitored. The MRI also has a role in establishing the diagnosis of dermatomyositis in children who are clinically strong. T2 images show enhancement of inflamed muscles and can be used to guide the muscle biopsy. (see Part 1, Chapter 1.6) Long-term studies are still required to determine the value of this technique in following disease progression and the effects of treatment

Radionuclide scanning may be helpful in identifying hidden abscess, malignancy, and bone infection or osteoid osteoma. Computerized axial tomography and magnetic resonance imaging are aides to the exclusion or localization of hidden infection or tumour that might otherwise be mistaken for JIA.

Magnetic resonance angiography (MRA, MRV) is valuable in assessing for vasculitis. Proton Emission Tomography (PET) has been studied in patients with CNS lupus [9]. Clinical usefulness remains limited; the studies are expensive and the spectrum of normal is still evolving.

References

1. Swan, A., Amer, H., and Dieppe, P.A. The Value of Synovial Fluid Assays in the Diagnosis of Joint Disease: a literature review, www.annrheumdis.com. *Ann Rheum Dis* 2002;61:493–8.

2. ARA Glossary Committee. *Dictionary of the Rheumatic Diseases: Volume II: Diagnostic testing.* New York: Contact Associates, 1985.

3. Sox H.C. Jr. and Liang M.H. The ESR: guidelines for rational use. *Ann Intern Med* 1986;104:515–23.

4. Solomon, D.H., Kavanaugh, A.J., Schur, P.H., and ACR ad hoc committee on immunologic testing guideline. Evidence-based guidelines for the use of immunologic tests: ANA Testing. *Arthritis Rheum* 2002;47:434–44.

5. Cabral, D.A., Petty, R.E., Fung, M., and Malleson, P.N. Persistent antinuclear antibodies in Children without Identifiable Inflammatory rheumatic or Autoimmune Disease. *Pediatrics* 1992;89:441–4.

6. Deane, P.M.G., Liard, G., Sigel, D.M., and Baum, J. The outcome of children referred to a pediatric rheumatology clinic with positive ANA test but without an autoimmune disease. *Pediatrics* 1995;95:892–5.

7. Eichenfield, A.H., Athreya, B.H., Doughty, R.A., and Randall, C.C. Utility of rheumatoid factor in the diagnosis of juvenile rheumatoid arthritis. *Pediatrics* 1986;78:480–4.

8. Szer, I.S., Klein-Gitelman, J., DeNardo, B.S., and McCauley, R. Ultrasonography in the study of prevalence, and clinical evolution of popliteal cysts in children with arthritis. *J Rheumatol* 1992;19:458–62.

9. Reiff, A., Miller, J., Shaham, B., Bernstein, B., and Szer, I.S. Childhood CNS Lupus: longitudinal assessment using single photon emission tomography. *J Rheumatol* 1997;24:2461–5.

1.3 Common presenting problems

Yukiko Kimura

Aim

The aim of this chapter is to guide the reader in formulating a logical work-up of the extensive differential diagnosis of childhood arthritis, using symptom-based algorithms and tables, with emphasis on pattern recognition.

Structure

- Algorithms
  - The child with fever, musculoskeletal pain, and dysfunction
  - The child with musculoskeletal pain and dysfunction without fever
  - The child with back pain
  - The child with musculoskeletal pain and dysfunction following trauma
- Tables
  - Arthritis syndromes associated with infections
  - Joint pain and symptom patterns
  - Skin manifestations associated with rheumatic diseases
  - The child with hip pain

Introduction

This chapter is the key to the rest of this textbook. Ideally, it will guide the reader through some common clinical situations towards a working differential diagnosis of a child presenting with musculoskeletal complaints. Once candidate diagnoses have been determined, the reader will then be referred to the disease-specific chapters in the book, which will describe each disorder in more detail, allowing the reader to decide whether a given diagnosis fits the clinical picture at hand. The basic idea behind this chapter is to guide the practitioner through a large differential diagnosis, and then to narrow down the diagnosis based on key historical or physical clues using algorithms and tables of clinical pearls until the correct diagnosis can be reached. Our hope is that these algorithms and clinical pearls will allow the reader to 'think like a paediatric rheumatologist' when faced with a given set of presenting complaints, since an experienced paediatric rheumatologist can be difficult to access for many practitioners outside of major tertiary care centres.

Two main algorithms provide the backbone for this chapter. These are Algorithm 1.3.1, 'The Child with Fever and Musculoskeletal Pain/Dysfunction' and Algorithm 1.3.2, 'The Afebrile Child with Musculoskeletal Pain/Dysfunction'. From these algorithms, the reader will be referred when appropriate to the other two algorithms as well as Tables 1.3.1–1.3.4. The other two algorithms are: Algorithm 1.3.3, 'The Child with Back Pain', and Algorithm 1.3.4, 'The Child with Musculoskeletal Pain Following Trauma'. In addition to the algorithms, the Tables present sets of clinical circumstances that should lead the reader to consider certain diagnoses. There are four

Tables: Table 1.3.1, 'Arthritis Syndromes associated with Infections', Table 1.3.2, 'Joint Pain and Symptom Patterns', Table 1.3.3, 'Skin Manifestations Associated with Rheumatic Diseases', and Table 1.3.4, 'The Child with Hip Pain'. Although both Tables 1.3.2 and 1.3.3 are quite lengthy, they are to be read thoroughly, as they provide very specific clues that may be central to a specific diagnosis.

When reading the algorithms and tables in this chapter, the reader should be aware that these are only general guidelines. The danger of algorithms is that they tend to oversimplify and reduce to black and white situations that may be more ambiguous and complex. There are many 'real life' situations to which these algorithms may not necessarily apply, and so adhering to the algorithms too rigidly would be a mistake. Nothing (not even algorithms) should take the place of good clinical judgement. In addition, it should be noted that in the interest of simplification and space, there are some extremely rare conditions that have been omitted from the tables and algorithms. These rare conditions are listed and discussed in specific disease-related chapters later in this book.

Please note that this chapter is organized in the following order:

(1) Descriptions and explanations of each of the algorithms and tables

(2) Algorithms

(3) Tables

(4) Colour figures representing some of the characteristic skin findings described in Table 1.1.1, "Skin manifestations associated with rheumatic diseases."

The child with fever and musculoskeletal pain/dysfunction (Algorithm 1.3.1)

A common problem faced by paediatricians and other primary care physicians is the child who presents with musculoskeletal pain or limping accompanied by fever. Although this is a common presentation of Systemic Arthritis, the first and foremost diagnoses to consider in this situation are infection (especially serious infections such as osteomyelitis and septic arthritis), and malignancy. Once these have been excluded, either because of the clinical circumstances, or through blood and imaging tests, many other diagnostic considerations will emerge to be considered and then excluded before one can finally make the diagnosis of Systemic Arthritis.

The child with musculoskeletal pain/dysfunction without fever (Algorithm 1.3.2)

Musculoskeletal pain or dysfunction in a child without a history of fever presents a different set of differential diagnoses to consider, although there is considerable overlap. Infectious causes of pain and limping, as well as malignancies, may present without fever, but it would be unusual. Certainly most bacterial infections would cause fever. Most forms of Juvenile Idiopathic Arthritis (JIA) are not associated

ALGORITHM 1.3.1
The Child with Fever And Musculoskeletal Pain/Dysfunction

*Important notes:

Children with significant continued fever and musculoskeletal pain should have the following during the work-up:

- Complete blood count with differential
- Acute phase reactants (ESR, C-reactive protein)
- Routine serum chemistries (including creatinine, muscle, and liver enzymes)
- Urinalysis
- ASO titre
- Cultures as appropriate (blood, urine, throat); if considering endocarditis, obtain at least two blood cultures from separate sites (remember that endocarditis can present with polyarthritis and fever and sometimes a positive rheumatoid factor)
- PPD with controls
- Imaging studies of involved area (plain X-rays, other tests as indicated in algorithm)
- Immunoglobulins and other immunodeficiency studies as appropriate

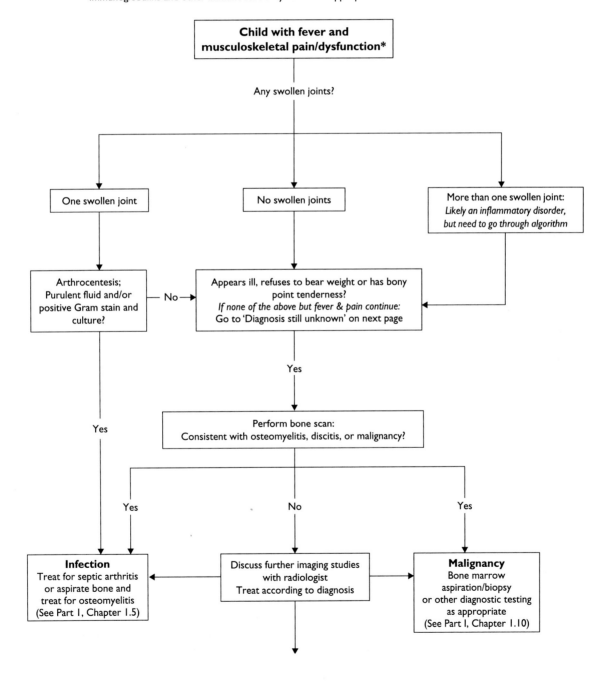

Algorithm 1.3.1 *continued*

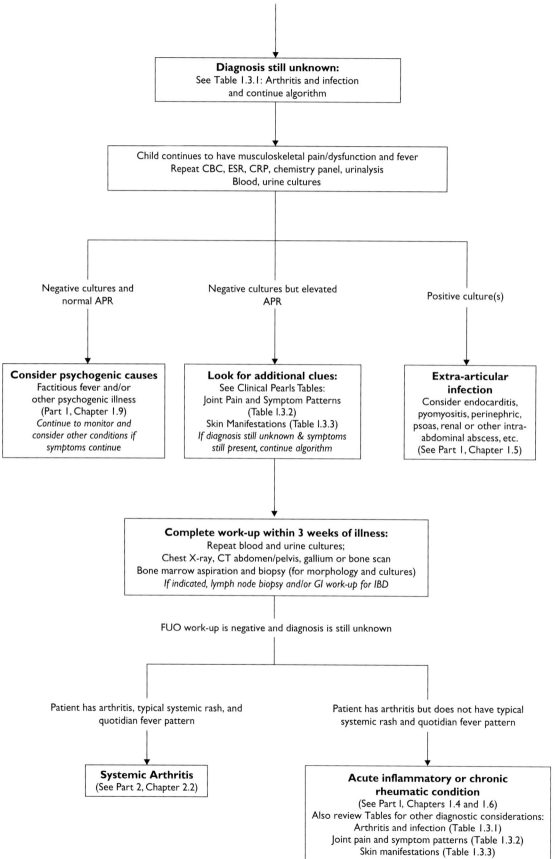

ALGORITHM 1.3.2
The Afebrile Child with Musculoskeletal Pain/Dysfunction

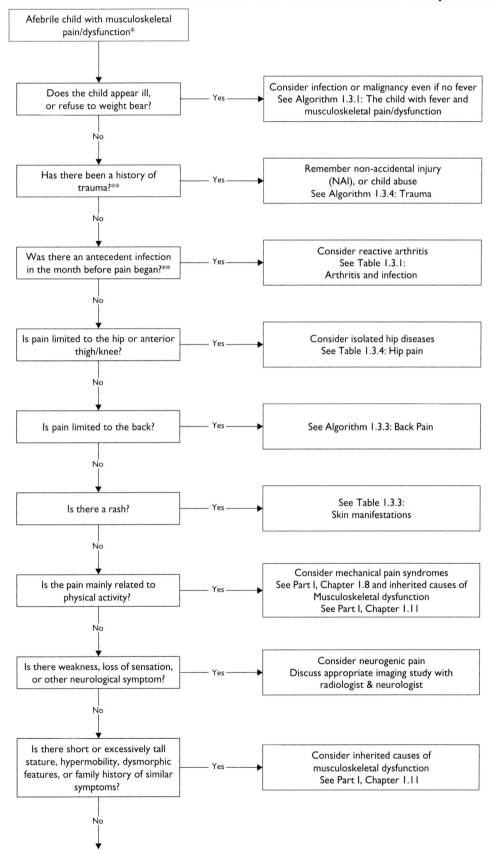

Afebrile child with musculoskeletal pain/dysfunction*

Does the child appear ill, or refuse to weight bear? — Yes → Consider infection or malignancy even if no fever
See Algorithm 1.3.1: The child with fever and musculoskeletal pain/dysfunction

No

Has there been a history of trauma?** — Yes → Remember non-accidental injury (NAI), or child abuse
See Algorithm 1.3.4: Trauma

No

Was there an antecedent infection in the month before pain began?** — Yes → Consider reactive arthritis
See Table 1.3.1: Arthritis and infection

No

Is pain limited to the hip or anterior thigh/knee? — Yes → Consider isolated hip diseases
See Table 1.3.4: Hip pain

No

Is pain limited to the back? — Yes → See Algorithm 1.3.3: Back Pain

No

Is there a rash? — Yes → See Table 1.3.3: Skin manifestations

No

Is the pain mainly related to physical activity? — Yes → Consider mechanical pain syndromes
See Part I, Chapter 1.8 and inherited causes of Musculoskeletal dysfunction
See Part I, Chapter 1.11

No

Is there weakness, loss of sensation, or other neurological symptom? — Yes → Consider neurogenic pain
Discuss appropriate imaging study with radiologist & neurologist

No

Is there short or excessively tall stature, hypermobility, dysmorphic features, or family history of similar symptoms? — Yes → Consider inherited causes of musculoskeletal dysfunction
See Part I, Chapter 1.11

No

*Important notes:
Children with persistent musculoskeletal pain should have the following work-up considered:
- Complete/full blood count with differential
- Acute phase reactants (ESR, C-reactive protein)
- Routine serum chemistries (including creatinine, liver and muscle enzymes)
- Urinalysis
- Imaging studies (plain X-rays of involved area, other studies as indicated in the algorithm(s))
- PPD with controls

**Caveats:
- Minor trauma and infections are common in children and may not necessarily be related to the diagnosis
- Remember infection, malignancy, and non-accidental injury (child abuse) at each stage

Algorithm 1.3.2 *continued*

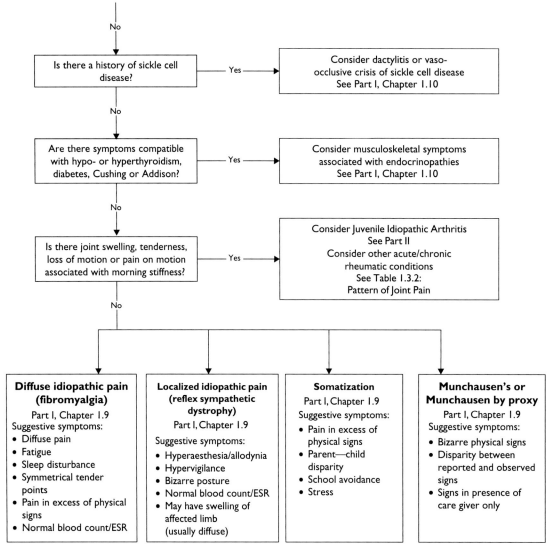

with fever, but depending on the clinical circumstances, there are many traumatic, mechanical, rheumatic, and other causes of pain that need to be excluded before the diagnosis of JIA can be made.

The child with back pain (Algorithm 1.3.3)

Back pain is not an unusual complaint in older children and adolescents, many of whom have non-specific back pain. However, back pain can also be a presenting manifestation of a tumour, malignancy, infection, and Enthesitis Related Arthritis, among other disorders. There are warning signs that often accompany these more serious causes, which indicate the need for a more thorough and aggressive investigation.

The child with musculoskeletal pain/dysfunction following trauma (Algorithm 1.3.4)

Physicians who care for children and adolescents often make the mistake of attributing all their patients' musculoskeletal complaints to trauma or other orthopaedic causes. This is likely because children

by nature are quite active and prone to minor injuries. Although traumatic causes of musculoskeletal pain must be considered when there has been a significant traumatic event, or when there are physical signs of trauma or abuse, incidental minor trauma is unlikely to lead to chronic musculoskeletal complaints. Conversely, significant trauma may cause transient joint swelling which may be mistaken for inflammatory arthritis.

Arthritis syndromes associated with infections (Table 1.3.1)

Table 1.3.1 summarizes the clinical patterns, causative agents, and diagnostic evaluations for acute arthritis associated with infections. Acute bacterial infectious causes of arthritis and musculoskeletal pain are emergencies that must be considered first in the differential diagnosis of a child with fever and limping, and are not addressed in this table. However, there are many infectious agents that are known to cause joint symptoms and arthritis, either through direct infection (as in Lyme arthritis or syphilis) or as a post-infectious phenomenon (acute rheumatic fever or Parvovirus arthritis).

Algorithm 1.3.3
The Child with Back Pain

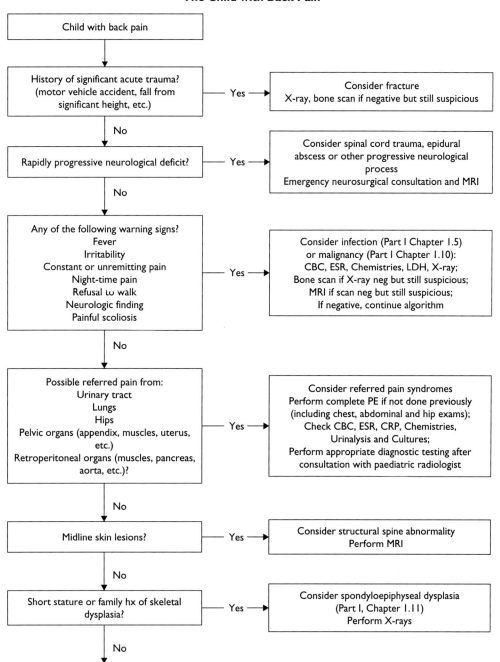

Algorithm 1.3.3 *continued*

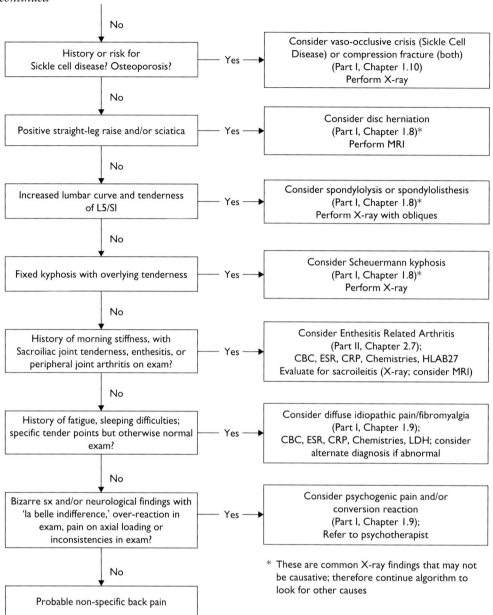

* These are common X-ray findings that may not be causative; therefore continue algorithm to look for other causes

ALGORITHM 1.3.4
The Child with Musculoskeletal Pain or Dysfunction following Trauma

*Important notes:
- Minor trauma is common in children/adolescents and may not necessarily be related to the diagnosis
- Always remember to consider non-accidental trauma (child abuse). The following are clues:
  - Any trauma that is poorly explained
  - X-rays show bone chips, multiple fractures at various stages of healing
  - Multiple 'hot spots' on bone scan
  - Multiple bruises and/or scars
- If intra-articular haemorrhage, consider haemophilia or other bleeding disorder

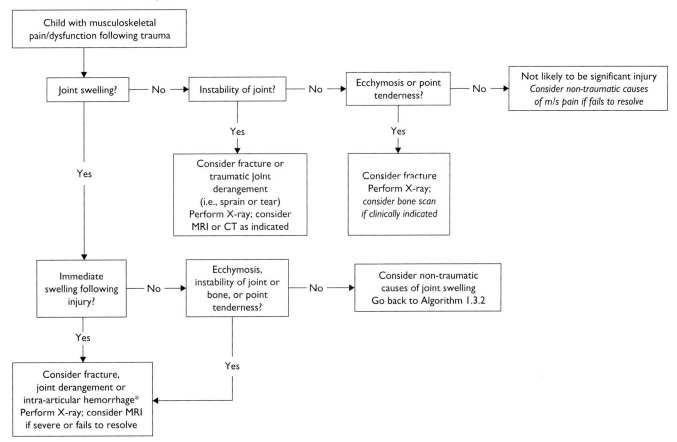

Joint pain and symptom patterns (Table 1.3.2)

Table 1.3.2 is an extensive but important table that combines historical clues with physical findings that are tip-offs to various disorders. These patterns are a critical part of the knowledge base that allow experienced paediatric rheumatologists to focus on a specific diagnosis. It is organized so that more acute causes of joint pain are presented first, followed by sub-acute or chronic causes. In addition, these disorders are in the order found in the rest of the textbook. If a pattern is found that fits a specific diagnosis, the reader should refer to those chapter(s) later in the book that will have detailed descriptions of each disorder.

Skin manifestations associated with rheumatic diseases (Table 1.3.3)

During an initial evaluation, paediatric rheumatologists will always ask about and look carefully for rashes and other cutaneous lesions.

This is because skin manifestations can be invaluable clues in the diagnosis of many rheumatic diseases. Table 1.3.3 groups skin manifestations associated with arthritis and other rheumatic complaints into categories by appearance, the various diseases with which these rashes are associated, and common clinical patterns that point to a specific diagnosis (see also Figures 1.3.1 to 1.3.34).

The child with hip pain (Table 1.3.4)

The hip is the largest joint in the body and is often affected by various mechanical and inflammatory conditions. In addition, because of its somewhat deep, 'hidden' location, infection and inflammation outside but near the hip can be mistakenly thought to originate in the hip joint. Conversely, hip pathology may 'refer' to other locations, most notably the anterior thigh and knee in younger children. Table 1.3.4 highlights the typical age and gender characteristics of various hip conditions along with their usual signs and symptoms, thereby allowing the reader to initiate the appropriate diagnostic work-up.

Table 1.3.1 Arthritis syndromes associated with infections

Clinical symptoms	Causative agent	Investigations
Post-streptococcal syndromes (Part 1, Chapter 1.4) Acute rheumatic fever: Acute migratory polyarthritis and fever 1–3 weeks after Strep infection; may have carditis, nodules, and typical rash; arthritis 'melts away' with treatment Post-streptococcal reactive arthritis: Acute arthritis (usually of large weight-bearing joints) following Strep infection; arthritis lasts for months even when treated	*Group A Streptococcus*	Anti-Streptolysin O titre Anti-DNase B titre Throat culture High ESR and other APR 2D-echocardiogram EKG
Parvovirus associated arthritis (Part 1, Chapter 1.5) Fever and rash followed or accompanied by arthritis, often affecting multiple small joints Occasionally (especially in children) pauciarticular, large joint arthritis Can be confused with systemic lupus erythematosus	*Parvovirus B19*	Parvovirus B19 IgM and IgG titres
Disseminated gonococcal infection (Part 1, Chapter 1.5) Fever, pustular rash, additive polyarthritis, often with wrist tenosynovitis in a sexually active patient	*Neisseria gonorrhoea*	Urethral, rectal, throat, and cervical cultures
Tuberculosis (Part 1, Chapter 1.5) Septic arthritis: Chronic monarthritis, often without fever Poncet disease: Reactive arthritis involving many joints in patients with active TB	*Mycobacterium tuberculosis*	PPD (with controls) Chest X-ray Biopsies of synovium or bone may be necessary
Reactive arthritis (Part 1, Chapter 1.5) Lower extremity oligoarthritis following enteric or sexually transmitted infection (although in children many other infections have been known to cause reactive arthritis); may have uveitis or conjunctivitis	*Enteric pathogens (salmonella, shigella, yersinia, campylobacter); Chlamydia trachomatis*	Stool cultures Urethral, rectal, throat, and cervical cultures HLA B27
Rubella arthropathy (Part 1, Chapter 1.5) Typical rash and lymphadenopathy associated with arthritis (of multiple joints in young women; may be oligoarticular, in the knees in younger children)	*Rubella*	Rubella IgM and IgG titres
Varicella reactive arthritis (Part 1, Chapter 1.5) Oligoarticular lower extremity arthritis following varicella infection Note: Varicella is a risk factor for bacterial septic arthritis (because of breaks in skin)	*Varicella zoster*	Physician documented varicella Varicella IgM titre
Lyme disease (Part 1, Chapter 1.5) Acute: May have joint and muscle pain, not arthritis, with erythema migrans and fever Chronic: Large effusions, usually of knees, weeks to months after infection Usually spontaneously resolves, but recurs if not treated. Not associated with fever	*Borrelia burgdorferi*	Lyme ELISA (measures IgG antibodies to B. burgdorferi) Perform Western blot if positive
Hepatitis prodrome (Part 1, Chapter 1.5) Acute polyarthritis, rash (maculopapular or urticarial) and fever preceding jaundice	*Hepatitis A and B viruses*	Liver function tests Hepatitis A and B IgM and IgG titres
Hepatitis C associated vasculitis (Part 1, Chapter 1.6) With chronic infection, multiple rheumatic syndromes described, such as arthralgias and arthritis, mixed cryoglobulinemia and Sjögren syndrome	*Hepatitis C*	Liver function tests; Hepatitis C IgM and IgG; ANA; anti-smooth muscle, anti-liver-kidney-microsomal; ANCA
Autoimmune hepatitis (Part 1, Chapter 1.6) Hepatitis associated with joint pain and mild systemic symptoms	*Hepatitis B or C*	Liver function tests; Hepatitis B and C IgM and IgG; ANA; anti-smooth muscle; anti-liver-kidney-microsomal; ANCA; Liver biopsy
Syphilis (Part 1, Chapter 1.5) Congenital: Pseudoparalysis, sometimes with joint swelling. X-rays show perostitis Clutton joints in older children with inadequately treated syphilis Secondary: Polyarthralgias and polyarthritis (symmetrical and non-migratory) accompanied by generalized lymphadenopathy, maculopapular rash and oral mucous plaques	*Treponema pallidum*	VDRL and FTA
Whipple disease (Part 1, Chapter 1.5) Diarrhoea, weight loss, fever, transient attacks of arthritis and neurological symptoms	*Tropheryma whippelii*	Intestinal biopsy Tissue PCR

Table 1.3.2 Joint pain and symptom patterns

Historical clues	Physical findings	Diagnosis	Investigations
Acute syndromes			
Prior history of antibiotic therapy Sudden onset of hives, joint pain, and often fever	Urticarial skin rash (including erythema multiforme) swelling of hands and feet	**Serum sickness** (Part 1, Chapter 1.4)	May have elevated acute phase reactants (APR), eosinophilia or elevated IgE
Joint pain and swelling with purpuric rash below waist following URI or strep pharyngitis May have crampy abdominal pain	Joint swelling, purpuric rash below the waist May have oedema of feet and other areas	**Henoch–Schönlein Purpura** (Part 1, Chapter 1.4) (Figures 1.4.5–6, 1.4.8–9)	APR normal or mildly elevated May have haematuria May have elevated IgA Skin biopsy: leukocytoclastic vasculitis with IgA deposits on IF
Prolonged high fever, rash, red eyes and oral mucosal inflammation Often has joint pain and irritability	Bilateral non-exudative conjunctivitis Variable rash starting in groin Strawberry tongue and red, cracked lips May have unilateral cervical lymphadenopathy, red palms and soles, arthritis	**Kawasaki Disease** (Part 1, Chapter 1.4) (Figures 1.4.13–23)	Elevated ESR, CRP Elevated WBC Platelets often very elevated after the first week of illness May have elevated ALT, AST, and sterile pyuria 2D-echocardiogram may show coronary artery abnormalities
Joint pain beginning days to weeks after an infectious illness (Table 1.3.1)	Asymmetrical large joint arthritis; may have associated conjunctivitis, urethritis, rash	**Reactive arthritis** (Part 1, Chapter 1.4) (Figure 1.4.4)	APR may be elevated
Acute migratory polyarthritis and fever, exquisitely responsive to anti-inflammatory agents	Joints are extremely tender to touch and movement Joint(s) affected one day may be completely normal the next day May have a new murmur, nodules, or erythema marginatum	**Acute rheumatic fever** (Part 1, Chapter 1.4) (Figure 1.4.2)	APR very elevated ASO titre usually very high May have first degree heart block or valvulitis May have positive throat culture for Group A Strep
One swollen joint accompanied by refusal to bear weight or move the extremity and fever	Irritable and ill-appearing; with red, hot, swollen and extremely tender joint with barely any mobility	**Septic arthritis** (Part 1, Chapter 1.5) (Figures 1.5.17, 1.5.20)	Joint aspiration for cell count and culture, blood culture, CBC and ESR, X-ray MRI if osteomyelitis a possibility
Pain with diaper changing or parent holding leg Fine when picked up under arms, but uncomfortable when cuddled	Irritable baby/child Refusal to bear weight	**Discitis** (Part 1, Chapter 1.5)	Spine X-rays may show decreased disc space (Figure 1.5.9) Bone scan, MRI more sensitive early
Recurrent bone pain and tenderness (sterile osteomyelitis) in various locations	Bony tenderness and swelling over affected bones Clavicle often involved	**Chronic Recurrent Multifocal Osteomyelitis** (Part 1, Chapter 1.5) (Figures 1.5.13–14)	Bone scan may show multiple areas of increased uptake X-ray may show Brodie abscess (Figure 1.5.11)
Episodic large joint effusions (especially knee) in a patient who has been in a Lyme endemic area (+/− history of deer tick bite)	4+effusions of large joints, usually knees, often without much pain	**Lyme arthritis** (Figure 1.5.22) (Part 1, Chapter 1.5) (Intermittent joint symptoms, but usually without large effusions, can also be seen in Enthesitis-Related Arthritis, Part 2, Chapter 2.7)	APR may be elevated Lyme IgG titre and Western blot positive
Complete or intermittent refusal to bear weight	Irritable and ill-appearing child, may have fever, may or may not have joint swelling(s)	**Malignancy or tumour** (Part 1, Chapter 1.10) **Osteomyelitis or retroperitoneal abscess** (Part 1, Chapter 1.5) (Figure 1.5.7) **Discitis** (Part 1, Chapter 1.5) (Figure 1.5.9) **Occult fracture**	X-rays may be abnormal More sensitive: bone scan, MRI (Figures 1.5.2, 1.5.4) CT (discuss with radiologist) Other (i.e. bone marrow) as indicated
Sudden onset of bilateral calf pain and tenderness, often with refusal to walk during or shortly after flu-like illness	Severe tenderness of calves Pain in calf with dorsiflexion of ankles	**Benign viral myositis** (Part 1, Chapter 1.5)	Elevated CK, Aldolase

Table 1.3.2 (*Continued*)

Historical clues	Physical findings	Diagnosis	Investigations
Episodic joint pain +/− swelling accompanied by recurrent high fevers and abdominal pain	Joint swelling and pain disappear completely during afebrile periods May have other symptoms: rash, serositis, lymphadenopathy, pharyngitis, or stomatitis (depending on the syndrome)	**Familial Mediterranean Fever** **TRAPS** Hyper-IgD syndrome (HIDS) PFAPA syndrome (Part 1, Chapter 1.7)	APR, WBC elevated during attacks, returning to normal when well Elevated IgD level (HIDS) Identification of gene mutation associated with FMF, TRAPS, HIDS
Pain and swelling of hands and feet in an infant/toddler, especially with family history of sickle cell disease	Diffuse swelling and pain of all fingers and toes (dactylitis)	**Sickle cell disease** (Part 1, Chapter 1.10)	Coombs negative haemolytic anaemia Positive sickle preparation and haemoglobin electrophoresis
Haemarthrosis without significant trauma	May have discolouration of skin overlying affected joint May have joint hypermobility and skin laxity (Ehlers–Danlos)	**Haemophilia** (Part 1, Chapter 1.10) **Synovial haemangioma** (Part 1, Chapter 1.10) **Ehlers–Danlos syndrome** (Part 1, Chapter 1.11) **PVNS** (Part 1, Chapter 1.10)	Bloody joint fluid Bleeding dyscrasia (PT, PTT) MRI may reveal joint derangement (trauma) or haemosiderin in Pigmented Villonodular Synovitis (PVNS)
Recurrent episodes of burning pain, redness, and heat in extremities exposed to warmth and relieved by ice	Red, warm, swollen hands, and feet	**Erythromelalgia**	May be associated with thrombocythemia and rarely SLE
Sub-acute and chronic syndromes			
Multi-systemic illness (including arthritis, rash, fevers, malaise, and weight loss) especially in an adolescent female	Malar rash most typical but other rashes occur May have alopecia, oral and/or nasal ulcerations, serositis, arthritis, lymphadenopathy, hepatosplenomegaly	**Systemic lupus erythematosus** (Part 1, Chapter 1.6) (Figures 1.6.2–3)	Pancytopenia Elevated APR (ESR, not CRP) Proteinuria and haematuria,+ ANA, anti-DNA, and low complement levels
Clinical features of several connective tissue diseases Often Raynaud, arthritis, interstitial lung disease, muscle weakness and constitutional symptoms	May have tight, shiny skin, and abnormal nailfold capillaries Nodular polyarthritis SLE and/or dermatomyositis rash	**Mixed Connective Tissue Disease** (Part 1, Chapter 1.6)	Positive ANA, anti-RNP May have positive anti-DNA and other markers of various connective tissue diseases
Rash and proximal muscle weakness (difficulty with stairs, opening heavy doors, sitting up from supine position) May have arthritis	Gottron papules on extensor aspect of finger joints Periorbital oedema and heliotrope rash of eyelids Nailfold telangiectasias Proximal muscle weakness	**Dermatomyositis** (Part 1, Chapter 1.6) (Figure 1.6.14)	Elevated muscle enzymes (ALT, AST, LDH, CK, Aldolase) APR may be elevated ANA may be positive
Severe chronic upper respiratory tract disease: sinusitis or otitis media refractory to antibiotics, recurrent epistaxis, arthritis, often with weight loss and fever	May have nasal septal perforations May have arthritis	**Wegener granulomatosis** (Part 1, Chapter 1.6) (Figure 1.6.21)	Elevated APR Haematuria and proteinuria + C-ANCA (anti-proteinase 3) Bony destruction of sinuses and pulmonary granulomas Biopsy: necrotizing granulomatous vasculitis Renal biopsy: crescentic pauci-immune glomerulonephritis
Recurrent painful oral ulcerations May have genital ulcerations Other symptoms: joint pain, eye inflammation, rashes, recurrent aseptic meningitis	Large painful oral or genital ulcers May have uveitis May have erythema nodosum, pustular lesions or pyoderma gangrenosum	**Behçet disease** (Part 1, Chapter 1.6)	Elevated APR Neutrophilic infiltration in skin lesions Occlusive vasculitis in arterioles and veins
Fevers, weight loss, myalgias (especially calf), and arthralgias, rash, testicular pain in boys	Nodular skin lesions	**Polyarteritis nodosa** (Part 1, Chapter 1.6)	Elevated APR Anaemia; May have + P-ANCA (anti-myeloperoxidase) Necrotizing vasculitis on skin or nerve/muscle biopsy

Table 1.3.2 (*Continued*)

Historical clues	Physical findings	Diagnosis	Investigations
Unexplained fever and weight loss Claudication	Hypertension, bruits, decreased/asymmetric pulses	**Takayasu arteritis** (Part 1, Chapter 1.6)	Elevated APR Anaemia Aortogram or MR Angiogram will show stenotic lesions of the great vessels and other major arteries
Multi-organ system dysfunction in a child with chronic asthma	Rashes, arthritis, mononeuropathy	**Churg Strauss Syndrome** (Part 1, Chapter 1.6)	Hypereosinophilia Fleeting pulmonary infiltrates Renal dysfunction
Ear redness, swelling, and pain with residual deformity May have other cartilage inflammation (i.e. nose, trachea, joints)	Deformed ear or nasal cartilage	**Relapsing Polychondritis** (Part 1, Chapter 1.6)	Elevated APR Inflammatory perichondritis on biopsy
Raynaud phenomenon May have heartburn and dyspnoea on exertion	Tight, shiny skin distally Abnormal nailfold capillaries	**Systemic sclerosis** (Part 1, Chapter 1.6)	May have positive ANA, anti-SCL70 antibody Interstitial lung disease on CT scan Restrictive lung disease with low DLCO May have pulmonary hypertension
Raynaud phenomenon May have heartburn, dysphagia, and dyspnoea on exertion	Sclerodactyly Telangiectasias Abnormal nailfold capillaries Subcutaneous calcifications	**CREST syndrome** (Part 1, Chapter 1.6)	May have positive ANA, anti-centromere antibody Interstitial lung disease on CT scan Restrictive lung disease with low DLCO
Arthritis, uveitis, erythema nodosum	Boggy synovitis Nodular skin lesions Red eyes	**Sarcoidosis** (Part 1, Chapter 1.7)	Elevated Calcium, ACE level, and lysozyme May have hilar adenopathy Biopsy: non-caseating granuloma
Fever, severe uveitis, rash, and arthritis in a young child (usually less than 5)	Boggy synovitis Variable rash Red eyes	**Early onset sarcoidosis** (Part 1, Chapter 1.7)	Elevated ACE Elevated APR Biopsy shows non-caseating granuloma
Weight loss or growth failure (may be only symptom) Other symptoms: fever, abdominal pain, +/− diarrhea, arthritis	May have arthritis, oral ulcers, and uveitis May have erythema nodosum, pustular lesions or pyoderma gangrenosum May have abdominal tenderness	**Inflammatory bowel disease** (Part 1, Chapter 1.7)	Elevated APR Anaemia May have + P-ANCA (anti-myeloperoxidase), ASCA Occult blood + stool Abnormal small bowel series
Recurrent transient synovitis of hip(s) (irritable hip) Often with family history of enthesitis related arthritis and inflammatory back pain	Enthesitis and inflammatory spine/SI pain in addition to hip limitation	**Enthesitis Related Arthritis** (Part 2, Chapter 2.7)	HLA B27 often positive X-ray may show sacroileitis
Short-lived recurrent leg pain, bilateral and not well-localized, occurring only at night (no daytime symptoms)	Completely normal physical examination without any joint or bone tenderness or abnormality	**Growing pains**	Normal blood counts, APR, X-rays
Pain usually occurs after physical activity	Joint hypermobility Look at skin elasticity, abnormal scarring, arachnodactyly, pectus excavatum)	**Benign joint hypermobility** (Part 1, Chapter 1.8) Consider other syndromes associated with hypermobility (i.e. Marfans, Ehlers–Danlos) (Part 1, Chapter 1.11)	Normal blood tests and X-rays Genetics work-up Consider cardiac and ophthalmology work-up
Pain usually occurs after physical activity	Variable	**Mechanical pain syndromes** (Part 1, Chapter 1.8)	Variable
Limping without pain	Limitation of motion of hip or leg length discrepancy	**Legg-Calve-Perthes** (Part 1, Chapter 1.8)	X-rays show avascular necrosis Early on, MRI more sensitive
Severe pain of one extremity with complete disuse and bizarre posturing	Severe hyperesthesia with diffuse oedema, temperature and colour changes	**Localized idiopathic pain** (Part 1, Chapter 1.9)	Bone scan may show diffusely increased uptake X-ray may show regional osteoporosis

Table 1.3.2 (*Continued*)

Historical clues	Physical findings	Diagnosis	Investigations
Diffuse stiffness and pain with fatigue, depression, and difficulty sleeping	Normal examination except for the presence of specific tender points	**Diffuse idiopathic pain** (Part 1, Chapter 1.9)	Normal labs
Pain in excess of physical signs Bizarre unexplained symptoms Family conflict School avoidance	Excessive reaction to examination 'La bell indifference' Bizarre or incongruous physical findings	**Psychogenic rheumatism** (Part 1, Chapter 1.9)	Normal labs (sometimes may be abnormal with Munchausen or Munchausen's by proxy)
Night-time, localized pain Often relieved with aspirin or NSAIDs	May have localized tenderness over bone	**Osteoid osteoma** (Part 1, Chapter 1.10)	Normal blood counts, APR X-rays may show lesion Bone scan/CT if X-rays are normal
Joint swelling and stiffness without much pain; associated with weight gain, constipation, cold intolerance	Synovial thickening without tenderness Enlarged thyroid	**Hypothyroidism** (Part 1, Chapter 1.10)	Thyroid function tests Anti-thyroid antibodies
Chronic arthritis in a patient with recurrent infections	Variable arthritis Some immunodeficiencies may be associated with specific physical findings	**Arthritis associated with immune deficiencies** (Part 1, Chapter 1.10)	Variable defects in immunity depending on the disease (immunoglobulins, T cells, neutrophils, etc.)
Poor growth Malabsorption syndrome or Chronic abdominal pain Chronic joint pain and swelling	Arthritis in a few joints	**Coeliac disease** (Part 1, Chapter 1.10)	Anti-gliadin antibodies Anti-tissue transglutaminase IgA Abnormal small intestinal biopsy
Severe limb pain, usually symmetrical and distal May be associated with cystic fibrosis, inflammatory bowel disease, biliary atresia, cyanotic heart disease, malignancies with lung metastases	Clubbing Severe tenderness of long bones Occasionally arthritis	**Hypertrophic osteoarthropathy** (may be primary or secondary) (Part 1, Chapter 1.10)	X-rays show periosteal new bone formation
Painless firm lump on or near joint	Firm, soft-tissue mass (often not contiguous with joint)	**Malignant synovial tumours** (Part 1, Chapter 1.10)	X-ray, MRI, biopsy
Episodic attacks of excruciating pain after mild trauma	Mild swelling of affected joint with discoloration of skin	**Synovial haemangioma** (Part 1, Chapter 1.10)	Bloody joint fluid X-ray may show calcification MRI
Diffuse joint pain and stiffness May have family history of skeletal dysplasia	Short stature May have dysmorphic facies or other features	**Skeletal dysplasia** (Part 1, Chapter 1.11)	Typical X-ray abnormalities
Excruciating hip, knee, and/or thigh pain, sometimes with fever	Bone tenderness Splenomegaly	**Gaucher Disease** (Part 1, Chapter 1.10)	X-rays show widened distal femur (Erlenmeyer-flask sign) Bone marrow
Recurrent episodes of localized fascial and fibrous tissue inflammation and swelling often presenting with torticollis	Localized swelling, pain, and severe stiffness Small great toes bilaterally	**Fibromyositis Ossificans Progressiva** (Part 1, Chapter 1.11)	X-rays show heterotopic bone formation in soft tissues Synostosis of the phalanges of the great toes
Joint swelling without pain	Swollen, non-tender joints, and distal necrosis of toes and fingers	**Congenital indifference to pain** (Part 1, Chapter 1.11)	Bizarre destructive and sclerotic X-ray changes of extremities
Morning stiffness or stiffness after periods of inactivity (gelling)	Swollen joint(s) and two of the following: tenderness, limitation of motion, pain on motion or heat	**Chronic inflammatory arthritis of any kind** (Part 2)	APR may or may not be elevated X-rays normal (unless long-standing)
High spiking daily fevers (1–2 spikes a day with normal temperatures in between), rash and arthritis	Evanescent salmon-coloured macular rash May have Koebner phenomenon Arthritis of one or more joints May have generalized lymphadenopathy and hepatosplenomegaly	**Systemic Arthritis** (Part 2, Chapter 2.1)	Leukocytosis, anaemia and thrombocytosis Extremely elevated APRs, ferritin levels Positive D-dimer May have a pericardial or pleural effusion on chest X-ray

Table 1.3.3 Skin manifestations associated with rheumatic diseases

Rash appearance or type	Possible diagnoses	Details
Urticarial	**Serum sickness** (Figure 1.3.1) (Part 1, Chapter 1.4)	Acute onset of pruritic hives that may progress to erythema multiforme, often with fever, hand, and foot swelling (self-limited)
	Prodromal hepatitis (Part 1, Chapter 1.5)	Pruritic, hive-like rash associated with joint pain prior to the onset of clinical hepatitis and jaundice
	Urticarial vasculitis (Figure 1.3.2) (Part 1, Chapter 1.6)	Recurrent episodes of burning urticarial skin lesions associated with joint pain, chest pain, and sometimes pulmonary disease (may rarely be a manifestation of lupus)
	Muckle–wells syndrome (Part 1, Chapter 1.7)	Familial periodic fevers associated with urticaria and limb pain accompanied by progressive nerve deafness and CIASI gene mutations
Annular	**Rheumatic fever** (erythema marginatum) (Part 1, Chapter 1.4) (Figure 1.4.2)	Circular rash with distinct serpiginous borders associated with fever, migratory polyarthritis, carditis
	SLE (subacute cutaneous lupus, SCLE or discoid lupus DLE) (Part 1, Chapter 1.6) (Figure 1.3.3)	SCLE: Diffuse annular, often violaceous lesions with raised borders. DLE: Chronic, scarring annular lesions with scaling and central atrophy
	Acute Lyme disease (erythema migrans) (Part 1, Chapter 1.5) (Figures 1.5.24(a) and (b)	Large annular lesion originating at the tick bite, with central clearing and expanding borders; may be multiple
	Granuloma annulare (pseudo rheumatoid nodules) (Part 1, Chapter 1.7) (Figure 1.3.4)	Annular erythematous lesions with nodular borders, often around a pseudo rheumatoid nodule
Morbilliform	**Kawasaki disease** (Part 1, Chapter 1.4) (Figure 1.4.14)	Erythematous, diffuse rash often beginning in or more intense in the groin (many different rashes may be seen with Kawasaki Disease (KD))
	Drug reaction (Part 1, Chapter 1.4)	Diffuse erythematous rash, often with fever, temporally associated with drug intake
Vesicular	**Viral** (especially herpesviruses, enteroviruses) (Part 1, Chapter 1.5) (Figure 1.3.5)	Vesicles (clear or pustular) with erythematous base in a typical distribution, associated with other viral symptoms and rarely arthritis
	Mucha–Habermann (Part 1, Chapter 1.4) (Figure 1.4.27)	Varicella-like rash, which becomes atrophic, associated with arthritis and fever
Scarletiniform	**Streptococcal infection** (scarlet fever)	Diffuse, sandpapery erythematous rash, with Pastia lines (accentuation in creases) and circumoral pallor
	Kawasaki disease (Part 1, Chapter 1.4)	Same as above; this is a common rash seen in KD
Nodular (painful) See also Part 1, Chapter 1.7, Table 1.7.2 for complete discussion of nodules and association to rheumatic disease	**Erythema nodosum** (Part 1, Chapter 1.4) (Figures 1.3.6 and 1.4.25)	Acute, large, erythematous nodules occurring on anterior shins
	Inflammatory bowel disease (Part 1, Chapter 1.7)	Erythema nodosum associated with fevers, GI symptoms, uveitis, weight loss, and arthritis
	Sarcoidosis (Part 1, Chapter 1.7)	Erythema nodosum associated with prolific synovitis, uveitis, and hilar adenopathy (or fevers in a young child)
	Polyarteritis nodosa (Part 1, Chapter 1.6)	Painful subcutaneous non-erythematous nodules often in calves and feet associated with fevers, weight loss, arthralgias, myalgias
	Pernio (Chilblains) (Part 1, Chapter 1.6) (Figure 1.3.7)	Painful reddish purple papules on fingers or toes after cold exposure; may occur in association with lupus
	Weber–Christian disease (Part 1, Chapter 1.7)	Fluctuant subdermal nodular panniculitis associated with arthralgia, myalgia, fever and fatigue (often with visceral inflammatory involvement)
	Reactive arthritis (Part 1, Chapter 1.4)	Erythema nodosum in association with reactive arthritis
	Behçet Disease (Part 1, Chapter 1.6) (Figure 1.3.8)	Erythema nodosum-like tender nodules in association with recurrent oral/genital ulcerations, uveitis, and other symptoms (joints, CNS)
	Endocarditis (Part 1, Chapter 1.5)	Osler nodes and Janeway lesions occurring in a child with fever, new murmur, and sometimes arthralgias/arthritis
	SLE (Part 1, Chapter 1.6) (Figure 1.3.9)	Nodular endocarditis-like lesions in the distal extremities may occur in active SLE
Nodular (not painful) See also Part 1,	**Rheumatic fever** (Part 1, Chapter 1.4) (Figure 1.3.10)	Small, hard, non-erythematous nodules in association with fever, migratory polyarthritis and carditis which disappear with treatment

Table 1.3.3 (*Continued*)

Rash appearance or type	Possible diagnoses	Details
Chapter 1.7 Table 1.7.2 for complete discussion of nodules and association to rheumatic diseases	**RF-positive Polyarthritis** (Part 2, Chapter 1.5)	Small, non-erythematous nodules in protruding areas: elbows, feet
	Pseudorheumatoid nodules (Part 1, Chapter 1.7) (Figure 1.3.11)	Single or multiple non-tender nodules often on shins, feet, and hands Sometimes associated with granuloma annulare rash (See Figure 1.3.4)
	Multicentric reticulohistiocytosis (Part 1, Chapter 1.10)	Pruritis followed by brownish wart-like nodules on face, ears and hands and mutilating DIP arthritis
	Farber (in infants) (Part 1, Chapter 1.10)	Subcutaneous nodules, joint swelling and contractures, poor growth and development, hoarse voice
Erysipeloid	**Rheumatic fever** (Erythema marginatum) (Part 1, Chapter 1.4)	Circular rash with distinct serpiginous borders associated with fever, migratory polyarthritis, carditis
	Familial Mediterranean Fever (Part 1, Chapter 1.7) (Figures 1.7.1–2)	Erysipelas-like rash associated with periodic fevers, abdominal pain, and elevated APR
Purpuric, petechial, or ecchymotic	**Henoch-Schonlein Purpura** (Part 1, Chapter 1.4) (Figure 1.3.12)	Bruise-like purpuric lesions mostly from the waist down associated with arthritis, and peripheral swelling, often with abdominal pain and haematuria
	SLE (Part 1, Chapter 1.6)	Petechiae may be due to thrombocytopenia or vasculitis Purpuric lesions occur in active lupus vasculitis
	Other vasculitis (Part 1, Chapter 1.6) (Figure 1.3.13)	Purpuric lesions are common in active vasculitis
	Endocarditis (Part 1, Chapter 1.4)	Conjunctival petechiae, splinter haemorrhages, tender purpuric lesions on hands and feet
	Malignancy (Part 1, Chapter 1.10)	Petechiae and ecchymoses due to thrombocytopenia
	Fabry Disease (Part 1, Chapter 1.10)	Hundreds of tiny red or blue-black flat spots or papules (angiokeratoma) between the waist and knees associated with excruciating burning pain in fingers an toes with multiple joint contractures
Pustular	**Gonococcal arthritis** (Part 1, Chapter 1.5)	Pustulo-vesicular lesions associated with fever and arthritis in a sexually-active patient
	Inflammatory bowel disease (Part 1, Chapter 1.7)	Various pustular skin lesions, including pyoderma gangrenosum, may occur
	Behçet disease (Part 1, Chapter 1.6)	Various pustular skin lesions, including pyoderma gangrenosum, may occur
	SAPHO syndrome and CRMO (Part 1, Chapter 1.5)	Palmoplantar pustulosis or severe acne in association with chronic recurrent multifocal osteomyelitis and hyperostosis
	PAPA (Pyogenic sterile arthritis, pyoderma gangrenosum and acne) (Part 1, Chapter 1.10)	Pyarthrosis and recurrent pyoderma gangrenosum following minor trauma
Reticular or lacy	**Parvovirus infection** (Part 1, Chapter 1.5)	Lacy reticular rash on trunk, extremities often associated with a 'slapped cheek' appearance of the face
	Vasculitis (livedo reticularis) (Part 1, Chapter 1.6) (Figure 1.3.14)	Lacy reticular rash with 'broken circles', is a common skin manifestation of vasculitis
	Anti-phospholipid antibody syndrome (Part 1, Chapter 1.6)	Lacy reticular rash with 'broken circles', is seen in patients with anti-phospholipid antibody syndrome
Bullous	**SLE or other vasculitis** (Part 1, Chapter 1.6) (Figure 1.3.15)	Severe skin vasculitis may develop into bullae
	Staphylococcal infection	Bullae are characteristic of a staphylococcal skin infection
Scaly erythematous papules on extensor aspects of joints, especially hands	**Dermatomyositis** (Part 1, Chapter 1.6) (Figure 1.3.16)	Gottron papules are diagnostic of dermatomyositis
	Mixed connective tissue disease (MCTD) (Part 1, Chapter 1.6)	Lupus syndromes which overlap with dermatomyositis may have similar rashes
Heliotrope rash of eyelids	**Dermatomyositis** (Part 1, Chapter 1.6)	Violaceous upper eyelids (often with enlarged capillaries) can be seen in dermatomyositis

Table 1.3.3 (*Continued*)

Rash appearance or type	Possible diagnoses	Details
	Mixed connective tissue disease (MCTD) (Part 1, Chapter 1.6)	Lupus syndromes which overlap with dermatomyositis may have similar rashes
Malar rash	**Parvovirus** (Fifth disease) (Part 1, Chapter 1.5) (Figure 1.5.25)	'Slapped cheek' appearance of face is typical of Fifth disease; Parvovirus often causes arthritis
	SLE (Part 1, Chapter 1.6) (Figure 1.3.17)	Erythematous butterfly rash extending from cheeks to bridge of nose, sparing the nasolabial folds
	Dermatomyositis (Part 1, Chapter 1.6) (Figure 1.3.18)	Dermatomyositis may cause a photosensitive rash very similar to that of lupus
Non-specific maculopapular	**Viral arthritis** (Part 1, Chapter 1.5)	Viral exanthems may be associated with virally induced arthritis
	Kawasaki disease (Figures 1.4.13–23) (Part 1, Chapter 1.4)	Many rashes can be seen with KD, including non-specific MP rashes. Usually begins in groin area
	NOMID/CINCA (Part 1, Chapter 1.7)	Rash and fevers begin in infancy in these children who develop severe arthropathy, dysmorphic features, epiphyseal changes, and mental retardation
Hyperaemic cuticles with enlarged capillaries	**Dermatomyositis** (Part 1, Chapter 1.6) (Figure 1.3.19)	Enlarged nailfold capillaries visible to the naked eye are common in dermatomyositis
	MCTD and SLE (Part 1, Chapter 1.6)	Nailfold capillary changes with dilatation and drop-out visible with magnification are common in lupus and MCTD, scleroderma and CREST
	Systemic sclerosis (Part 1, Chapter 1.6)	Same as above
	CREST syndrome (Part 1, Chapter 1.6)	Same as above
Evanescent, pink macular rash	**Systemic Arthritis** (Part 2, Chapter 1.1) (Figures 1.3.20 and 1.4.1)	Round to oval macules which are slightly raised and sometimes pruritic which are accentuated during fever spikes and by stroking skin (Koebner phenomenon)
Plaque-like lesions	**Psoriatic Arthritis** (Part 2, Chapter 1.6) (Figure 1.3.21)	Scaly erythematosus plaques often on extensor surfaces of joints, scalp, buttock crease, or umbilicus, associated with arthritis
	Morphea (Part 1, Chapter 1.6) (Figure 1.3.22)	Erythematous, oedematous plaques that evolve into firm, waxy, ivory, and shiny lesions with a violaceous border
	Sweet syndrome (Part 1, Chapter 1.7) (Fig 1.4.29)	Raised painful plaques associated with fever, arthralgias, and arthritis
Fingertip or toe ulcerations	**SLE** (Part 1, Chapter 1.6) (Figure 1.3.23)	A manifestation of small vessel vasculitis that can cause distal necrotic lesions
	Vasculitis (Part 1, Chapter 1.6) (Figure 1.3.24)	Same as above
	MCTD (Part 1, Chapter 1.6)	Same as above
	Scleroderma (with severe Raynaud's) (Part 1, Chapter 1.6) (Figure 1.3.25)	Severe arterial insufficiency due to Raynaud in scleroderma can cause digital pitting (from necrosis) or even necrosis of entire digit(s)
Panniculitis	**Erythema nodosum** (Part 1, Chapter 1.4) (Figures 1.3.6, 1.4.25–26)	Tender erythematosus coin-sized nodules on anterior shins
	Weber–Christian (Part 1, Chapter 1.7)	Fluctuant subdermal nodular panniculitis associated with arthralgias, myalgias, fever and fatigue (often with visceral inflammatory involvement)
	Rothman–Makai (Part 1, Chapter 1.7)	Circumscribed panniculitis of the legs with multiple painless lumps, leaving atrophic depressions
Tight, shiny skin	**Scleroderma** (Part 1, Chapter 1.6)	Tightening of the skin beginning distally and moving proximally is characteristic of scleroderma
	MCTD (Part 1, Chapter 1.6)	Overlap syndromes can look very much like scleroderma

Table 1.3.3 (*Continued*)

Rash appearance or type	Possible diagnoses	Details
	Eosinophilic fasciitis (Part 1, Chapter 1.6)	Rapid onset of diffuse skin tightening can be confused with scleroderma; there is often associated morphea
Excessive skin elasticity	**Ehlers–Danlos syndrome** (Part 1, Chapter 1.11) (Figure 1.3.26)	Excessive joint hypermobility with velvety soft skin which is hyper-elastic and cigarette-paper scars is typical of EDS
	Cutis Laxa (Part 1, Chapter 1.11)	Lax, not hyperelastic skin with drooping and sagging facial skin not associated with hypermobility
Plaques of tight, shiny skin with erythematous borders	**Localized scleroderma** (Part 1, Chapter 1.6) (Figure 1.3.27)	Both morphea and linear scleroderma cause localized areas of skin tightening
	Lichen atrophicus (Chronic Lyme) (Part 1, Chapter 1.5)	A rare manifestation of Lyme disease looks very much like morphea
Skin ulcerations	**Inflammatory Bowel Disease** (Part 1, Chapter 1.4)	Pyoderma gangrenosum is a ulcerating pustular lesion associated with IBD
	Behcet (Part 1, Chapter 1.6)	Pyoderma gangrenosum
	Polyarteritis nodosa (PAN) and other vasculitis (Part 1, Chapter 1.6) (Figure 1.3.28)	Vasculitis may cause necrotic skin lesions
	SLE (Part 1, Chapter 1.6) (Figure 1.3.29)	Necrotic skin lesions due to vasculitis
	Dermatomyositis (Part 1, Chapter 1.6)	Small necrotic skin lesions occur commonly, but severe skin and visceral ulcerations may also be seen
Lipodystrophy	**Dermatomyositis** (Part 1, Chapter 1.6) (Figure 1.3.30)	Diffuse or localized loss of subcutaneous fat in patients due to lipodystrophy
	Rothman–Makai (Part 1, Chapter 1.7)	Circumscribed panniculitis of the legs with multiple painless lumps, leaving atrophic depressions
Subcutaneous calcifications	**Dermatomyositis** (Part 1, Chapter 1.6) (Figure 1.3.31)	A variety of calcification patterns can be seen in long-standing dermatomyositis (tumourous, along fascial planes, etc.)
	CREST syndrome (scleroderma) (Part 1, Chapter 1.6)	Subcutaneous calcifications are typical of CREST
	Fibromyositis ossificans progressiva (Part 1, Chapter 1.11)	Painful swelling often begins behind the neck with eventual heterotopic bone formation, which can occur in other locations
	Weber–Christian disease (Part 1, Chapter 1.7)	Fluctuant subdermal nodular panniculitis associated with arthralgia, myalgia, fever, and fatigue (often with visceral inflammatory involvement), followed by formation of subcutaneous calcification
Raynaud phenomenon	**Scleroderma** (Part 1, Chapter 1.6) (Figure 1.3.32)	Tri- or biphasic colour changes of fingers or toes in response to cold temperatures are common in scleroderma
	SLE (Part 1, Chapter 1.6)	Similar changes are also common in lupus patients
Nail pitting	**Psoriatic Arthritis** (Part 2, Chapter 2.6) (Figure 1.3.33)	Multiple tiny 'pits' in the nail are associated with psoriasis even if there are no typical skin lesions

Table 1.3.4 The child with hip pain*

Clinical symptoms	Physical findings	Typical age/sex	Diagnosis	Investigations
May be asymptomatic	'Clunking' sensation with hip abduction	Infancy (but can be missed so may present later)	**Congenital hip dysplasia** (Part 1, Chapter 1.9)	X-rays
Antecedent upper respiratory infection Limping and pain, worse with activity Often has low-grade fever Self-limited	Limited range of motion of hip	3–10 years Boys > Girls	**Transient synovitis (Irritable hip)** (Part 1, Chapter 1.4)	Normal labs (ESR and/or WBC can be mildly elevated) X-ray normal or shows widened joint space Ultrasound shows fluid in hip
Joint pain and stiffness (usually of multiple joints) Short stature and limbs Usually familial (autosomal dominant)	Limitation of motion	Toddler-school age	**Epiphyseal dysplasia** (Part 1, Chapter 1.11)	X-rays show flattened, sclerotic epiphyses
Hip, knee, or groin pain with activity, intermittent limping Can be bilateral Little pain	Limited internal rotation and abduction Affected leg may be shorter	Preschool-school age Boys > Girls	**Legg–Calve–Perthes** (Part 1, Chapter 1.8) Also consider inherited causes of osteonecrosis (Part 1, Chapter 1.11)	Normal labs X-ray abnormal late Early detection by MRI
Hip, thigh, or knee pain with activity; can be insidious in onset Can be bilateral Limping	Obese Limited range of motion of hip Affected leg may be shorter	Preteen-teenage Boys > Girls	**Slipped Capital Femoral Epiphysis** (Part 1, Chapter 1.8)	Normal labs X-rays show subluxation of femoral head epiphysis Early detection by USG, bone scan, MRI
Sudden onset of hip pain following activity (such as doing a 'split')	Limited range of motion of hip	Preteen-teenage	**Acute chondrolysis of hip** (Part 1, Chapter 1.8)	X-rays show severe narrowing of hip joint
Insidious onset of anterior or medial thigh pain, limp Can be bilateral	Limited range of motion of hip Muscle spasm Affected leg may be shorter	Preteen-teenage Girls > boys	**Idiopathic chondrolysis of hip** (Part 1, Chapter 1.8)	Normal labs X-rays show demineralization of femoral head, joint space narrowing
Morning and inactivity stiffness May complain of heel pain or lower back pain and stiffness Positive family history of ERA and related conditions such as inflammatory bowel disease	Limitation of motion of hip May have enthesitis May have spine or SI tenderness and limitation Affected leg may be longer Other joints may be involved	Preteen-teenage commonly, but younger children can of affected Boys > girls	**Enthesitis Related Arthritis** (ERA) (Part 2, Chapter 2.7)	X-rays may show widened joint space initially and fluid on ultrasonogram Other changes typical of arthritis after many years Sacroileitis may be present HLA B27 often be positive
History of trauma Severe hip pain and limping	Limited range of motion of hip with debilitating pain	Teenage	**Transient demineralization of hip** (Part 1, Chapter 1.8)	Normal labs X-rays: dramatic regional osteoporosis
Acute onset of hip pain following an infectious illness May have fever	Pain and limitation of motion of hip Other joints may be involved May have associated conjunctivitis and/or urethritis	Any age	**Reactive arthritis** (Part 1, Chapter 1.4)	APR often elevated X-rays may show widened joint space initially and fluid on ultrasonogram
Hip/anterior knee pain with activity and limping Risk factors: corticosteroid use, sickle cell disease, systemic lupus erythematosus, Cushing syndrome	Limited range of motion of hip Affected leg may be shorter	Any age	**Osteonecrosis of hip** (Part 1, Chapter 1.8) Also consider inherited causes of osteonecrosis (Part 1, Chapter 1.11)	X-ray abnormal late Early detection by MRI

Notes:
• Trauma (fracture), malignancy, and infection (septic arthritis of the hip, osteomyelitis of the femur as well as the pelvic bones, and soft-tissue infections in and near the hip, such as retroperitoneal or pelvic muscle abscess and sacroiliac septic arthritis) are important causes of hip pain at any age that need to be considered first in the differential diagnosis of hip pain.
• Hip pain in children is often perceived as pain in the anterior knee or anterior thigh.
• Consider hip as the source of pain in an infant who does not move a leg but no abnormality is obvious.
• Groin pain and pain on internal rotation of the hip are clues to hip joint involvement.

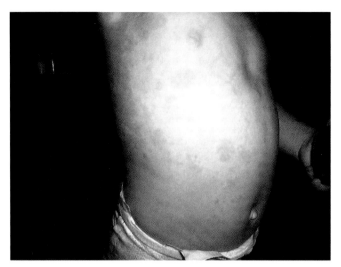

Fig. 1.3.1 Erythema multiforme in a child with serum sickness.

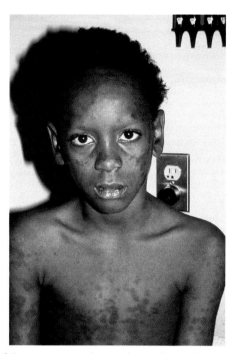

Fig. 1.3.3 Subacute cutaneous lupus rash in an 8 year-old with SLE. This rash can be mistaken for erythema multiforme because of its annular appearance.

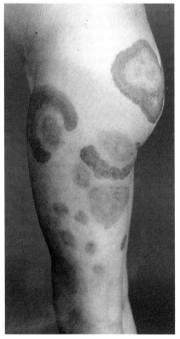

Fig. 1.3.2 Urticarial vasculitis (courtesy of T.R. Southwood).

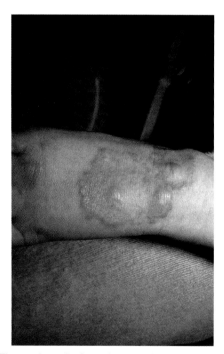

Fig. 1.3.4 The annular rash of granuloma annulare overlying pseudo rheumatoid nodules on the foot.

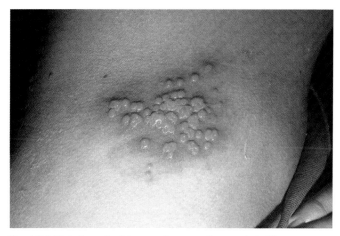

Fig. 1.3.5 Vesicular rash with an erythematous base, typical of herpes zoster.

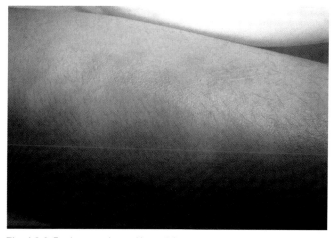

Fig. 1.3.8 Erythema nodosum-like nodules in a patient with Behçet disease.

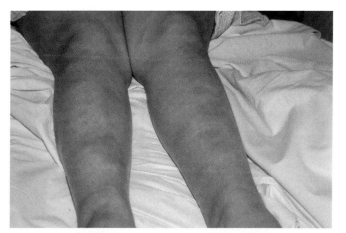

Fig. 1.3.6 Erythema nodosum causes tender coin-sized erythematous nodules on the shins.

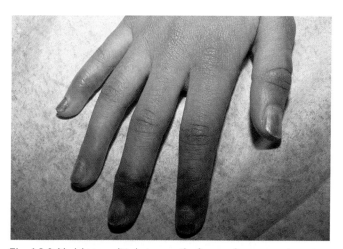

Fig. 1.3.9 Nodular vasculitic lesions on the fingers of a young patient who was eventually diagnosed with SLE.

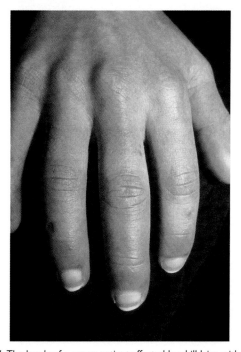

Fig. 1.3.7 The hands of a young patient affected by chilblains with characteristic swelling and erythema.

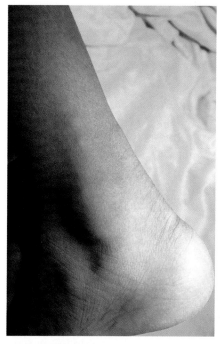

Fig. 1.3.10 Small non-tender nodules on the tendons of the ankle of a patient with acute rheumatic fever.

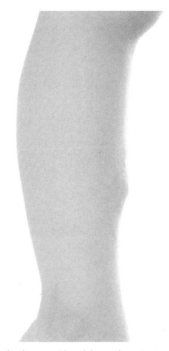

Fig. 1.3.11 Pseudo rheumatoid nodule on the anterior tibia (courtesy of T.R. Southwood).

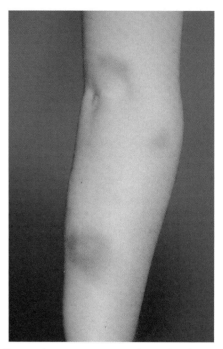

Fig. 1.3.13 Purpuric lesions in a patient with vasculitis (courtesy of T.R. Southwood).

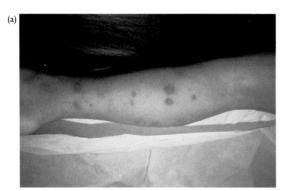

(a)

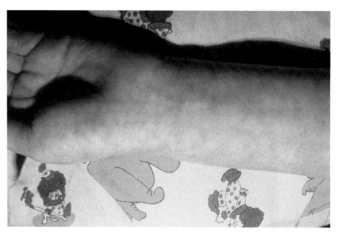

Fig. 1.3.14 Livedo reticularis in an 8 year old girl with vasculitis.

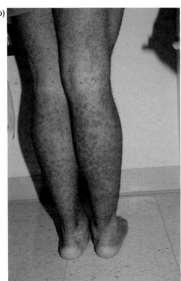

(b)

Fig. 1.3.12 (a) Purpuric lesions in varying stages on the legs of a patient with Henoch–Schönlein Purpura. (b) More superficial purpuric lesions and swelling of the right leg in another patient with Henoch–Schönlein Purpura.

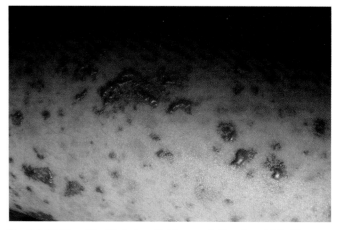

Fig. 1.3.15 Vasculitic skin lesions that became bullous in a child with Henoch–Schönlein Purpura.

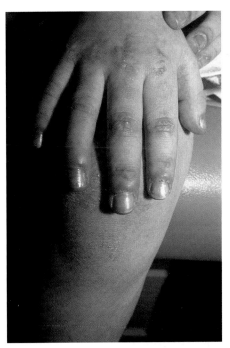

Fig. 1.3.16 Scaly erythematous papules on the extensor surfaces of the fingers (Gottron papules) and the knee in this young patient with dermatomyositis.

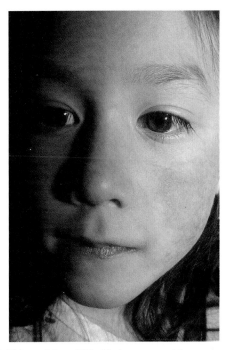

Fig. 1.3.18 Malar rash in a child with dermatomyositis.

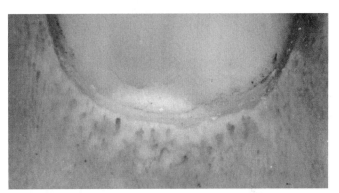

Fig. 1.3.19 Dilatation and drop-out of nailfold capillary loops in dermatomyositis (courtesy of T.R. Southwood).

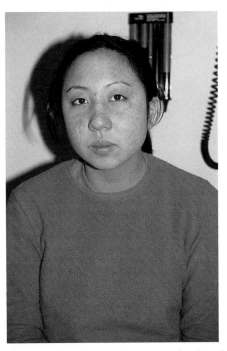

Fig. 1.3.17 Characteristic 'butterfly' rash in a young female with SLE, crossing the bridge of the nose and sparing the nasolabial folds.

Fig. 1.3.20 The rash of Systemic Arthritis consisting of slightly-raised irregularly sized pink macules that come and go and often display the Koebner phenomenon with stroking the skin.

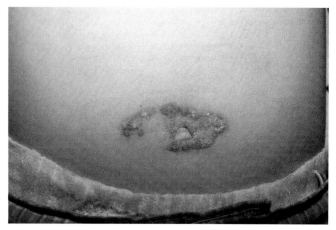

Fig. 1.3.21 Psoriatic plaque around the umbilicus in a girl with dactylitis of the toes (see Figure 2.6.1).

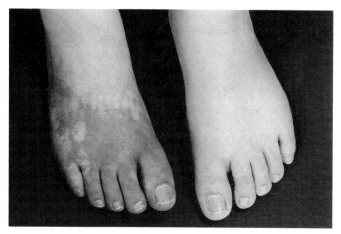

Fig. 1.3.24 Necrosis of the entire right forefoot in a patient with polyarteritis nodosa (courtesy of T.R. Southwood).

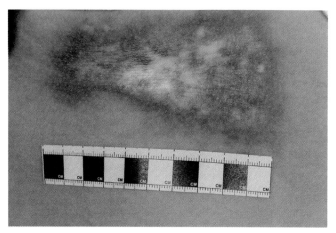

Fig. 1.3.22 Morphea, a form of localized scleroderma (courtesy of T.R. Southwood).

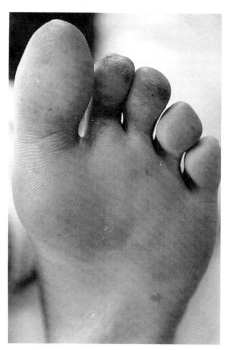

Fig. 1.3.25 Ischemic necrosis secondary to severe Raynaud phenomenon in a patient with systemic sclerosis (courtesy of T.R. Southwood).

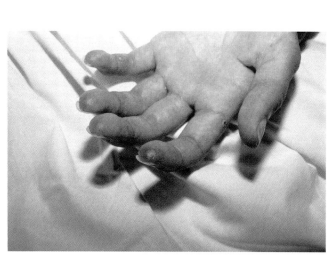

Fig. 1.3.23 Small area of necrosis on the finger tip of this patient with SLE.

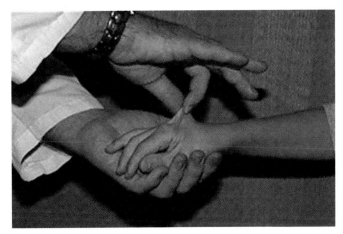

Fig. 1.3.26 Excessive skin elasticity in a patient with Ehlers–Danlos Syndrome.

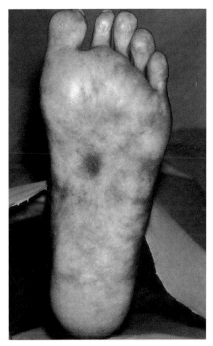

Fig. 1.3.28 There is a necrotic ulcer due to vasculitis in the sole of this patient's foot (courtesy of T.R. Southwood).

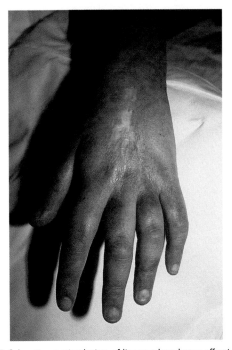

Fig. 1.3.27 Sclerotic scarring lesion of linear scleroderma affecting the hand (the lesion extended to the shoulder in this patient).

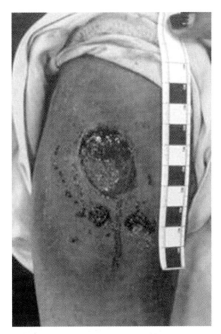

Fig. 1.3.29 A large necrotic ulcer on the arm of a patient with SLE (courtesy of T.R. Southwood).

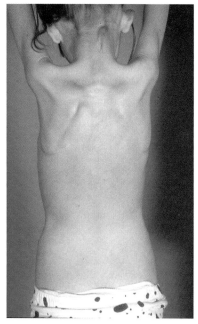

Fig. 1.3.30 Lipodystrophy of the soft-tissues of the trunk in this young girl with dermatomyositis (courtesy of T.R. Southwood).

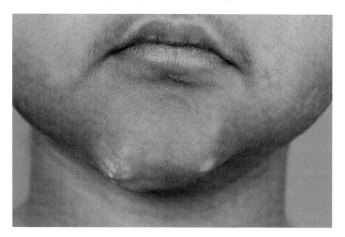

Fig. 1.3.31 Calcinonsis on the chin of a patient with dermatomyositis (courtesy of T.R. Southwood).

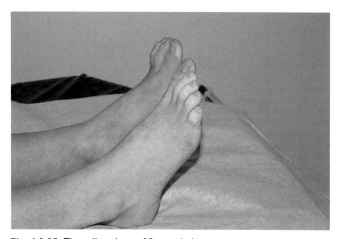

Fig. 1.3.32 The pallor phase of Raynaud phenomenon is seen on the toes of the right foot.

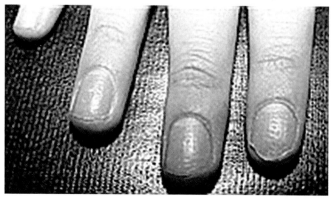

Fig. 1.3.33 Nail pitting is characteristic of psoriasis and may precede the development of skin lesions (courtesy of T.R. Southwood).

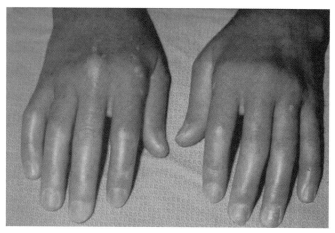

Fig. 1.3.34 Tight, shiny skin of the extremities is quite characteristic of systemic sclerosis (from J.C. Jacobs).

1.4   Acute inflammatory rheumatic syndromes

Ilona S. Szer

Aim

The aim of this chapter is to describe the acute and usually self limited inflammatory conditions of children which are manifested by arthritis and must be ruled out before chronic rheumatic conditions, such as Juvenile Idiopathic Arthritis, may be considered.

Structure

- Acute rheumatic fever
- Post-streptococcal reactive arthritis
- Other reactive arthritis
- Arthritis associated with Inflammatory Bowel Disease
- Transient Synovitis of the Hip
- Henoch–Schönlein Purpura
- Hemorrhagic oedema of infancy
- Hypersensitivity vasculitis
- Serum sickness type reactions
- Kawasaki disease
- Erythema nodosum
- Mucha–Habermann
- Acute parapsoriasis
- Sweet syndrome

Introduction

The differential diagnosis of childhood arthritis is extensive, as can be appreciated from algorithms found in Chapter 1.3. To date, over 110 distinct disorders that include arthritis have been identified. Some of these conditions have not yet been recognized in children and some have only been seen in children and not in adults. The paediatrician faced with a child who has developed joint swelling has a formidable job. One must remember that all chronic illnesses, including JIA, have a beginning. However, the many acute conditions presenting with transient arthritis are much more common than chronic conditions, and a careful evaluation for those which occur and resolve in the first few weeks of illness, is of paramount importance to prevent over-treatment, reduce hospitalizations, and initiate appropriate therapy.

This chapter will focus on the acute and self-limited inflammatory conditions of children (Table 1.4.1) while the chronic inflammatory rheumatic conditions will be discussed in subsequent chapters.

Most of these acute conditions are not rare, and with the exception of Mucha–Haberman disease and Sweet syndrome, every paediatrician can expect to see patients with these disorders from time to time in a busy practice.

Acute rheumatic fever

Improved socioeconomic conditions, prompt diagnosis, the prevention of recurrent attacks by prophylactic penicillin, and adequate treatment of streptococcal pharyngitis resulted in greatly lowered incidence of acute rheumatic fever (ARF) from 1970 to 1984 [1]. Since 1985 there has been a resurgence of epidemic rheumatic fever in the continental United States. The physician should have no trouble diagnosing a child with obvious valvular carditis following a streptococcal pharyngitis. This is not the usual situation however. Erythema marginatum, chorea, and rheumatic nodules are definitive diagnostic findings, but they are seen so infrequently now that they may not be recognized even when present. The more frequent diagnostic problem initially confronting the paediatrician is a child with polyarthralgia and an elevated ESR who does not yet fulfill the modified Jones classification criteria developed by the American Heart Association [2] as a useful guide to the diagnosis of ARF (Table 1.4.2).

In some joints, such as the hip or the neck, swelling cannot be demonstrated on physical examination. The differentiation of arthralgia from arthritis in these joints is often solely dependent on demonstrating a range of motion limited by pain. Many children said to have polyarthralgia can be demonstrated to have arthritis provided all of the joints are carefully subjected to range of motion examination (see Part 1, Chapter 1.1). Any joint may be affected in ARF, although the most frequently involved sites are the knees, ankles, elbows, and wrists.

The acute and migratory quality of the arthritis in ARF helps to differentiate it from JIA (Table 1.4.3) in which the arthritis is present persistently for over 6 weeks. In contrast, in ARF, the joint that was so painful yesterday is often painless today, even though some swelling may persist. Yesterday's painful joint is likely to be better today even without therapy even though another joint has now become tender and has limited motion. This migratory quality sets this syndrome apart from others. It has been observed that in ARF, adequate doses of aspirin is usually rapidly effective. In older children, additive rather than migratory arthritis may cause confusion. Children with Lyme arthritis (see Part 1, Chapter 1.5) also have transient synovitis of large joints, but the nature of this arthritis is recurrent and not migratory, and the presence of pain is not the most impressive feature, while children with ARF may be so sensitive to pain as not to be able to tolerate the sheet over the involved joint.

Table 1.4.1 Clinical features of acute rheumatic conditions, in addition to fever

Acute rheumatic fever	Migratory polyarthritis
	Acute carditis
	Chorea
	Erythema marginatum
	Rising anti-streptococcal antibody titers
	Elevated APRs (ESR, CRP)
Post-streptococcal arthritis	Rash
	Joint swelling and pain
	Elevated ASO
	No carditis or other major criteria for ARF
Other reactive arthritis	Preceding illness and/or antibiotic treatment
	Rash (+/−)
	Arthritis
	Elevated APRs
Arthritis associated with inflammatory bowel disease	Poor growth and/or weight loss
	Anemia
	Elevated APR
	Abdominal pain +/− diarrhoea
	Erythema nodosum
Transient synovitis of the hip	Preceding history of viral illness
	Sudden onset of inability to move hip or to ambulate
Henoch–Schönlein purpura	Purpuric rash on lower extremities
	Abdominal colic
	Large joint arthritis
	Haematuria
Haemorrhagic edema of infancy	Purpuric rash, generalized
	large joint arthritis
Hypersensitivity vasculitis (HV)	Older patients
	Purpuric rash
	Leukocytoclastic vasculitis
	Renal disease
Serum sickness type reactions	Migratory polyarthritis
	Drug reactions
	HV
	Erythema multiforme
	Angioneurotic oedema
Kawasaki Disease	Polymorphous rash
	Cervical lymphadenopathy
	Conjunctival hyperemia
	Cracked lips, mucositis (strawberry tongue)
	Erythematous palms and soles
	Oedema of dorsum of palms and soles
	Irritability
Erythema Nodosum	Nodular panniculitis on extensor surfaces of the legs
	Arthritis
	May be associated with: tuberculosis, streptococcal infection, IBD, sarcoid, fungi, drug reactions (BCP, PTU, other)
Mucha–Habermann acute parapsoriasis	Episodic chickenpox type rash
	Elevated ESR
Sweets syndrome	Rash (painful plaques)
	Arthralgia/arthritis,
	Elevated ESR

Table 1.4.2 Revised Jones Criteria for guidance in the diagnosis of ARF

Major criteria	Minor criteria
Carditis	Fever
New or changing murmurs	Arthralgia
Cardiomegaly, congestive heart failure	History of prior attack of rheumatic fever
Pericarditis	
Migratory polyarthritis	Elevated ESR, CRP
Chorea	Prolonged PR interval on ECG
Erythema marginatum	
Subcutaneous nodules	

Diagnosis is likely with two major criteria or one major and two minor criteria and documentation of preceding Group A Streptococcal Infection. Diagnosis is doubtful when evidence of recent streptococcal illness cannot be documented by history of scarlet fever or isolation of Group A streptococcus from throat culture, or rising titre of anti-streptococcal antibodies (Circulation 69:204A–208A, 1984)(2).

In some children with fever and polyarthritis, Systemic Arthritis is a more reasonable early diagnostic consideration than ARF. In children under the age of 4, for example, ARF is very rare; most young children with persistent polyarthritis in this age group do turn out to have JIA. This is even more likely if they also have pericarditis without mitral valvulitis. Pericardial effusions are almost never seen as an isolated cardiac manifestation of ARF but are a common feature of early Systemic Arthritis. The typical rash of Systemic Arthritis (Figure 1.4.1 and Part 2, Chapter 2.2), provided it can be differentiated from erythema marginatum (Figure 1.4.2), will also help differentiate these conditions (Table 1.4.3). Nodules (Figure 1.4.3) that appear soon after the onset of arthritis always indicate ARF. In JIA, nodules associated with late onset RF positive Polyarthritis (see Figure 1.11, Part 1, Chapter 1.1 and Part 2, Chapter 2.5), are a late manifestation, seen in patients in whom the diagnosis of chronic, rather than acute disease, is obvious. In addition, subcutaneous nodules in Polyarthritis are not usually accompanied by fever.

After adequate blood cultures have been obtained, children thought to have ARF are started on salycylates and full doses of penicillin to treat the previously undiagnosed Streptococcal infection. Prophylactic doses are initiated only after completion of a full 10-day course of penicillin aimed at eradicating streptococci from the nasopharynx. Corticosteroids are reserved for patients whose rheumatic carditis is accompanied by congestive heart failure or pericarditis. The commitment to rheumatic prophylaxis can always be changed if it becomes apparent that a presumptive diagnosis of ARF was erroneous. In the past, fear of labeling a patient or treating a patient with a presumptive diagnosis of ARF, led to unnecessary hospitalizations and sometimes resulted in a recurrent attack of rheumatic carditis [3].

The arthritis of ARF rarely continues for more than 3 weeks when untreated; the elevated ESR rarely persists for more than 6 weeks. With consistent salycylates treatment (100 mg/kg/day), the arthritis of ARF promptly disappears. Once the ESR has returned to normal, salycylate dose can be reduced gradually over a period of a few weeks in an effort to avoid a rebound of arthritis and carditis. Abrupt withdrawal of aspirin in children with subclinical rheumatic carditis may precipitate pancarditis [4]. Other nonsteroidal anti-inflammatory drugs that have replaced salycylates in other settings, have not been studied in children with ARF; there is no evidence that these agents are any less efficacious than salycylates but clinicians who care for these children tend to treat with salycylates.

Rheumatic fever may occur with acute glomerulonephritis in the same patient at the same time but this is extraordinarily rare. Second attacks of rheumatic fever, now being seen most often in inner-city

Table 1.4.3 Acute fever and rash in young children

	KD	Stevens–Johnson	ARF	Systemic Arthritis	Measles	TSS
Fever	++	+	++	++	+	+
Rash	++	+	+	+	+	+++
Adenopathy	++	+/−	+/−	++	+/−	−
Conjunctivitis	++	++	−	−	++	+
Extremities						
Swelling	++	−	+	+/−	−	+
Peeling	++	−	+	−	−	+
Mouth						
Lip fissures	++	++	−	−	−	−
Strawberry tongue	++	++	+	−	−	−
Arthritis	Transient	−	Migratory	Persistent	−	−

Abbreviation: KD: Kawasaki Disease, Mucocutanous Lymph Node Syndrome; TSS: Toxic Shock Syndrome; ARF: Acute Rheumatic Fever.

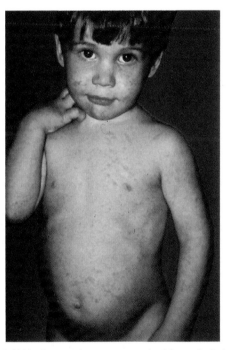

Figure 1.4.1 Mild salmon pink evanescent rash of Systemic Arthritis (from J. Jacobs).

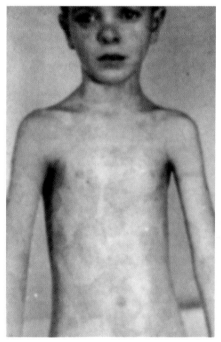

Figure 1.4.2 ARF Erythema Marginatum—typical erythema marginatum rash in a 9-year-old boy with acute rheumatic fever (from J. Jacobs).

immigrant populations in which the initial attack was unrecognized, often have a more fulminant presentation, sometimes with rheumatic pneumonia and/or galloping carditis.

Post-streptococcal reactive arthritis

Patients who develop polyarthritis days after Group A beta-haemolytic streptococcal infection and who do not fulfill the modified Jones criteria for a diagnosis of acute rheumatic fever, have been classified as having post-streptococcal reactive arthritis (PSRA) [5]. Of 25 children described in one series, the arthritis lasted from 5 days to 6 months and followed sore throat by an average of 7 days; all patients had an elevated ASO titre, and most had an elevated ESR. One of these children developed mitral regurgitation [6]. However, other published series of such patients report a relatively high risk (6–7%) of subsequent attack of rheumatic fever with

carditis, in this population [7,8]. Just as patients with what was once thought to be rheumatic chorea or "scarletina"-associated arthritis bear a significant risk of subsequent rheumatic heart disease, so do those children who have what has been called PSRA. It is probably best to provide penicillin prophylaxis for such patients to prevent streptococcal sore throats and recurrent attacks of rheumatic fever. The length of prophylaxis in these children is still being debated. Although some experts advocate 1–2 years of prophylaxis and discontinuation if there is no evidence of heart involvement [8], evidence over time may suggest otherwise and indefinite prophylaxis may prove to be best in the long term.

Other reactive arthritis

The paediatrician is frequently worried by a child who has fever, joint pain with swelling, and a recent history of a viral-like or other intercurrent

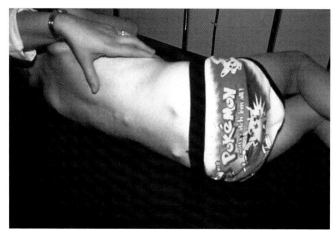

Figure 1.4.3 Rheumatic nodules found on many extensor surfaces and on the spine of a child with ARF (courtesy of Y. Kimura).

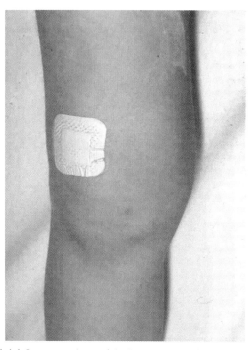

Figure 1.4.4 Reactive arthritis of the knee in a young boy that resolved 2 weeks after onset (courtesy of T. R. Southwood).

illness, including dysentery. Most of these children continue to ambulate and do not appear ill. They may have a swollen knee (Figure 1.4.4) or ankle, and may limp but continue to attend school and to play. There is usually only mild tenderness and the range of motion is usually well preserved. The classical triad of post-dysenteric reactive arthritis, with arthritis, conjunctivitis and urethritis is seldom seen in children, but can occasionally occur. Laboratory studies confirm elevated acute phase reactants (APR) comparable with Systemic Arthritis but unlike in Systemic Arthritis, the inflammatory reaction responds dramatically to anti-inflammatory drugs and the entire illness usually resolves quickly with all symptoms gone within 2–4 weeks of onset. Although stool and throat cultures may be positive for a pathogen (bacterial or viral), the diagnosis of a viral associated reactive arthritis is often presumptive; the diagnosis is made retrospectively because the child had a short-lived illness [9].

Arthritis associated with Inflammatory Bowel Disease

Clinical features of acute and chronic arthritis are well recognized but relatively uncommon manifestations of inflammatory bowel disease (IBD) in children and adolescents [10]. There appears to be an important aetio-pathogenic overlap between reactive arthritis, the arthritis of IBD, and Juvenile Idiopathic Arthritis (JIA). In some children, an acute arthritis, which appears to be associated with clinical features of a preceding gastrointestinal infection, may eventually turn out to have the more chronic manifestations of IBD. Additionally, several investigators have demonstrated sub-clinical features of intestinal inflammation in patients with an established diagnosis of JIA. Increased gut permeability, as manifest by a significant increase in urinary lactulose/ mannitol ratio, has been found in patients with Oligoarthritis and Enthesitis Related Arthritis, comparable to that found in IBD patients [11]. The increased permeability was shown to be independent of the use of NSAIDs.

Occasionally, a child presenting with acute arthritis may be exhibiting the first features of IBD, particularly if they also have prominent constitutional features of poor growth, mild fever and pallor. Enquiries for abdominal pain and changes in bowel habit should always be made, especially in older children and adolescents who may be reluctant to volunteer such information. Other clinical manifestations may be very helpful in pointing the clinician towards the correct diagnosis of an underlying IBD, including the presence of oral ulcerations, static weight gain or weight loss, dactylitis, a tender abdominal mass, or erythema nodosum.

Investigations should include a full blood count, which is likely to reveal anaemia of greater severity than may have been expected, and measures of acute phase reactants, which again are often much higher than expected in IBD. Plain radiographs of the abdomen are unlikely to be useful, but barium studies will usually reveal upper or lower gastrointestinal pathology in the child with IBD. Some authors have suggested that leucocyte scintigraphy may not only highlight the extent of bowel inflammation, but also may reveal joint involvement [12]. The investigation of choice, although not usually considered in the front line of the acute arthritis work up, is gastrointestinal endoscopy and mucosal biopsy. Typically, these reveal macroscopic inflammatory changes of the bowel wall, and microscopic evidence of dense lymphocytic infiltrate with granuloma formation.

Arthralgia and arthritis are reported as important complications of established IBD. These typically appear to follow one of two patterns; peripheral arthritis or axial arthritis. In younger children with IBD, symptoms of peripheral, large joint, lower limb arthralgia are the most common musculoskeletal manifestations. The physical examination may reveal an overt arthritis, most often of the knee or ankle, but this is usually transient, self-limiting, and non-destructive. Commonly, such manifestations appear to parallel the extent of inflammation in the gastrointestinal tract, and wax and wane in direct correlation with the IBD symptoms. In a prospective study of musculoskeletal manifestations in 521 patients with IBD in older children, adolescents and adults, peripheral arthralgia is found in 12% of IBD patients, whereas objective evidence of arthritis is much less frequent (only 4 patients, giving a point prevalence of 0.8%) [13]. The treatment of this form of arthritis usually involves intermittent use of NSAIDs (while being aware that these may contribute to clinical features of abdominal pain) and intra-articular depot corticosteroids. If disease modifying drug treatment is required for the IBD, sulfasalazine is probably of greater benefit for the arthritis than non-sulfa containing salicylic acid preparations (see also Part 3, Chapter 3.8).

Axial arthritis, while less common, is a much more worrying musculoskeletal feature of IBD. Typically, this begins as a peripheral arthritis in the older child or adolescent, with persistent objective swelling of one or more lower limb joints. The hip, sacroiliac joint or lumbosacral spine may be involved relatively early in the disease course, and, in distinction to the isolated peripheral arthritis mentioned above, there is little evidence of clinical fluctuation in concert with the activity of the IBD. This form of arthritis has been associated with the presence of HLA-B27 and appears to progress inexorably to ankylosing spondylitis (AS) in a small number of IBD patients (3.7%) [14]. AS has been found in both ulcerative colitis (2.6%) and Crohn disease (6%), and no correlation between the location or extent of IBD has been shown. The prevalence of undifferentiated spondyloarthropathy in IBD is much higher, up to 22% of patients, but it is important to be aware that clinical features of inflammatory back pain may indicate a chronic idiopathic pain syndrome such as fibromyalgia (see also Part 1, Chapter 1.9). The treatment of this form of arthritis usually involves intermittent intra-articular depot corticosteroids and sulfasalazine (see also Part 3, Chapter 3.8). There may also be a role in this situation for biologic agents such as anti-TNF monoclonal antibodies, which are effective in both Crohn disease and AS.

Transient synovitis of the hip (irritable hip, toxic synovitis of hip)

Paediatricians often see a child, typically a young boy, who awakens with sudden onset of hip pain and limp or inability to bear weight which persists for a few days. Although dramatic in its presentation, this entity is not often associated with fever, leukocytosis, or elevation of ESR [15]. A few days of anti-inflammatory therapy enables almost complete recovery without using the old remedies of bed rest, and traction. Bacterial joint infection is usually easily distinguished by the presence of high fever, and more impressive physical and laboratory abnormalities. Some children who cannot bear weight should be appropriately assessed for intra-articular infection (see Part 1, Chapter 1.3, Table 1.3.4). Recurrent episodes of hip pain may represent the onset of Enthesitis Related Arthritis (ERA, Part 2, Chapter 2.7), and occasionally of Legg-Perthes disease (Part 1, Chapter 1.7), Lyme arthritis (Part 1, Chapter 1.5), Gaucher disease (Part 1, Chapter 1.10), or osteoid osteoma (Part 1, Chapter 1.9).

Henoch–Schönlein Purpura

Arthritis, colicky abdominal pain, and a characteristic lower-extremity (Figure 1.4.5) and buttock (Figure 1.4.6) papular, often palpable, purpuric rash, constitute the diagnostic triad of Henoch–Schönlein Purpura (HSP). Abdominal colic often precedes the rash and arthritis (Table 1.4.4). Young children, especially boys, are most frequently affected.

HSP is a small vessel vasculitis, associated with alternate complement pathway mediated IgA immune complex vasculitis that can be set off by a variety of infectious and noninfectious stimuli. When the dermal vasculitis is severe, there may be considerable oedema, especially of the dorsum of the hands (Figure 1.4.7) and feet or in the scrotum, forehead, and periorbital areas.

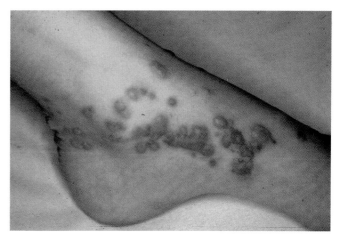

Figure 1.4.5 Palpable purpura near the ankle joint typical of HSP, in a child with abdominal colic and arthritis.

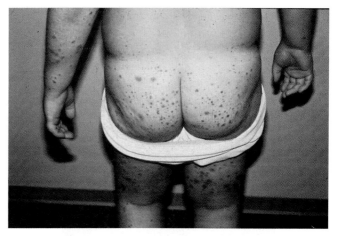

Figure 1.4.6 Typical purpuric rash of HSP localized to buttocks (the dependent area of the body).

Table 1.4.4 Clinical manifestations of Henoch–Schönlein Purpura

	% at onset	% during course
Purpura (normal platelet count)	50	100
Subcutaneous nodules	10–20	20–50
Arthritis of large joints	25	60–85
Abdominal pain, bloody stools	30	85
Renal, haematuria	?	10–50
GU, (R/O testicular torsion)	?	2–35
Pulmonary (decreased DLCO)	?	95
CNS, headache, organic brain syndrome	?	rare

R/O = rule out

Hematuria and mild gastrointestinal bleeding are common. Rarely, life threatening pulmonary haemorrhage or CNS vasculitis may occur.

The diagnosis of HSP is not difficult when the rash is apparent. However, in those cases in which arthritis precedes the rash, it is impossible to recognize that the arthritis is a feature of this syndrome. Unlike JIA, arthritis of HSP is transient. It is characterized by pain, stiffness,

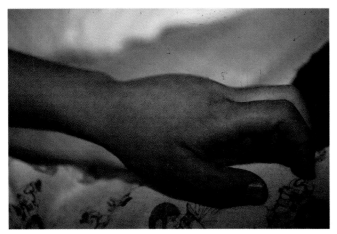

Figure 1.4.7 Painful subcutaneous oedema over the wrist in a 14-year-old boy with HSP whose pain resolved completely with a short course of corticosteroids.

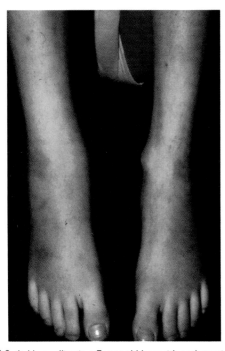

Figure 1.4.8 Ankle swelling in a 7-year-old boy with ecchymotic purpura, colicky abdominal pain and arthritis.

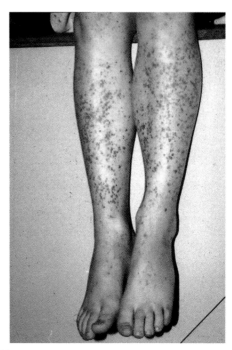

Figure 1.4.9 Extensive palpable purpura extending from feet to buttocks in a 10-year-old girl with 24 months of recurrent crops of lesions after minor upper respiratory infections. She eventually recovered without sequelae.

and effusions in the large joints of the lower extremities and sometimes in the wrists and elbows, often with periarticular swelling. It may be quite subtle (Figure 1.4.8). Without treatment, it may come and go over a period of weeks, and recurrences of the whole syndrome are not rare within a period of 6 months after onset; occasional patients have recurrences as late as 2 years after the initial episode (Figure 1.4.9).

When arthritis is present alone, it is usually easily controlled with anti-inflammatory drugs. There is no evidence that corticosteroids improve the rash of HSP, or any other manifestations except perhaps subcutaneous oedema [16], and possibly abdominal pain. Evidence suggests that children with abdominal pain treated with corticosteroids have a statistically faster recovery than children who are not treated. However, at 72 hours after the onset of abdominal pain, both groups of patients are indistinguishable [17]. Short courses of corticosteroid, at 1 mg/kg/day, is often used successfully and is not associated with

detrimental side-effects. There is some evidence that children treated with steroids do not develop intussusception, reported in approximately 2% of children with HSP [16]. If arthritis is present with colic, it resolves quickly with steroids.

The only children with HSP who carry a guarded prognosis are those patients who present with severe renal disease, including nephrotic range proteinuria, renal insufficiency, or renal failure. Their renal biopsy, often documenting crescenteric glomerulonephritis, is indistinguishable from adult IgA nephropathy, and carries a poor prognosis for renal recovery.

There is a paucity of reports documenting long-term renal outcome in children with HSP. A recent retrospective cohort study suggests that the presence of renal disease 1 month after onset of HSP is predictive of who is at risk for ongoing problems. If there is evidence of renal disease after 1 month, the children need long-term follow-up with attention to blood pressure and urine findings [18].

Acute haemorrhagic oedema of infancy (AHE)

An entity known as acute haemorrhagic oedema (AHE), described almost exclusively in the European literature in children under 24 months of age, may or may not represent HSP in infants [19]. The manifestations of AHE are oedema, target like purpura on the limbs (Figure 1.4.10) and buttocks (Figure 1.4.11) that becomes ecchymotic in dependent areas of the body (Figure 1.4.12). Most patients have a history of either a recent illness, drug exposure or immunization. Systemic symptoms such as bloody stools or renal involvement occur less frequently in AHE than in HSP, although these symptoms are also uncommon in infants and toddlers thought to have HSP [16]. Spontaneous and complete resolution occurs within 1–3 weeks but one to three recurrences are frequent. Leukocytoclastic vasculitis is seen when a skin biopsy is obtained but it is not clear whether or not AHE is an IgA-related vasculitis.

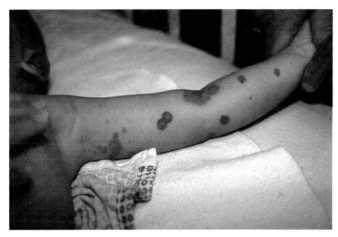

Figure 1.4.10 Toddler with AHE, target-like purpura over the arms.

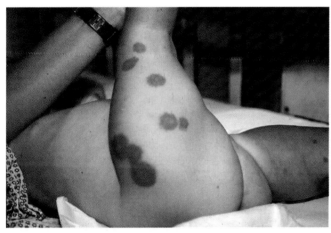

Figure 1.4.11 Same child with purpura over the buttocks and thighs.

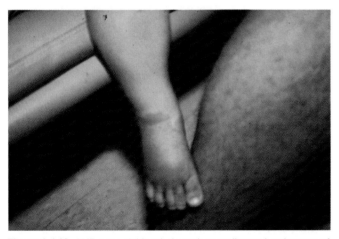

Figure 1.4.12 AHE, same child with dependent swelling and ecchymosis of the foot.

Hypersensitivity vasculitis

Recently, a subcommittee of the American College of Rheumatology (ACR) defined criteria for the classification of several forms of vasculitis in adults, including HSP and hypersensitivity vasculitis (HV, Table 1.4.5) [20]. Because the two entities share many clinicopathological

Table 1.4.5 Criteria for the classification of Hypersensitivity Vasculitis

Older than 16 years of age at onset

Medication at onset that may have triggered the episode

Palpable purpura, non-blanching, with normal platelet count

Maculopapular rash, flat lesions present over one or more areas of body

Biopsy of skin documenting the presence of granulocytes in perivascular or extravascular location.

A patient can be classified as having HV if at least three of the five criteria are present. Any three or more criteria yield a sensitivity of 71% and specificity of 83.9% (20)

Table 1.4.6 Criteria for differentiating Henoch–Schönlein Purpura from HV

Criterion	Definition
Palpable purpura	Slightly elevated purpuric rash over one or more areas of the skin not related to thrombocytopenia
Bowel angina	Diffuse abdominal pain worse after meals or bowel ischemia usually including bloody diarrhoea
GI bleeding	GI bleeding, including melena, hematochezia or positive test for occult blood in the stool
Haematuria	Gross hematuria or micro-haematuria (>1/hpf)
Age at onset <20	Development of first symptoms at age 20 or less
No medications	Absence of any medication at onset of disease which may have been a precipitating factor

The presence of any three or more of the six criteria yields a correct classification of HSP in 87.1%. The presence of two or fewer criteria yields a correct classification of HV in 74.2%.

Source From: Calabrese *et al.* The ACR 1990 criteria for the classification of hypersensitivity vasculitis. *Arthritis Rheum* 1990;33:1108–13 (20).

features and HSP is often considered a type of HV in the adult population, an effort has been made to define HV and HSP as separate and definable clinical syndromes (Table 1.4.6). Both disorders share the common feature of leukocytoclastic vasculitis of small vessels with prominent skin involvement however, major differences exist with respect to frequency and type of other organ involvement as well prognosis, suggesting that indeed these are distinct entities. Although haematuria and proteinuria are more often seen in HSP, elevated urea and creatinine, as features reflecting functional renal impairment (and likely to reflect a worse prognosis), are significantly more frequent in HV. Generally, important organ involvement occurs more often in HV (pleuritis, pericarditis, congestive heart failure, with more extensive involvement of skin, mucosa, and muscle). Similarly, tests, which classically reveal active inflammatory processes, that is, ESR and C4 levels, are more frequently abnormal in patients with HV than those with HSP. Frank arthritis is significantly more common in HSP whereas arthralgia is reported more frequently in HV. HSP in adults tends to affect organs more extensively and the prognosis appears to be worse with regard to renal disease when compared with children and adolescents with HSP [21].

Drug reactions, serum sickness, erythema multiforme, angioneurotic oedema

Most mild cases of erythema multiforme (Figure 1.3.1) are precipitated by herpes simplex virus infections. Serum sickness, the classic form of antigen-antibody mediated immune complex disease, which results from the infusion of heterologous serum, is rarely seen today. However, similar allergic reactions for which serum sickness is the model, are common. With the increase in the use of sulfa and other drugs, many more cases of serum sickness-like reactions are seen. Most are mild, manifested mostly with urticaria, (Figure 1.3.2) and few other symptoms, and disappear promptly following withdrawal of the drug or other allergen. Some reactions more closely resemble true serum sickness with sudden onset of urticarial or erythema multiforme skin lesions, angioneurotic oedema, lymphadenopathy, arthritis, and polyserositis. In addition to the swelling of the fingers, which is associated with angioneurotic oedema, the large joints are frequently effused, stiff, and painful, usually without heat or redness. The ESR is generally normal, but the total haemolytic complement or C4 level is sometimes low due to binding in immune complexes; these laboratory determinations may be helpful in the differential diagnosis.

Most of these reactions are mild and are easily controlled with antihistamines and an anti-inflammatory drug after the offending agent has been withdrawn. Corticosteroids are reserved for use in only the most severe cases. A few children, however, develop the more serious drug or infection-induced vasculitis such as Stevens–Johnson syndrome, which is characterized by severe mucocutanous lesions (Table 1.4.3).

Occasionally children seem to go through a stage in which erythema multiforme with arthralgia or arthritis follows each presumed viral illness. Sometimes the offending agent is something special given to the child only during an intercurrent illness. In one such patient, ingestion of certain brands of cherry soda or cherry flavoured medications produced the reaction. Extensive detective work established that almond extract, often used in cherry flavours, was the culprit [22].

Kawasaki disease

In the initial report published in Japanese in 1967, Dr Tomisaku Kawasaki was able to gather data on 50 children with mucocutaneous lymph node syndrome, later re-named Kawasaki disease. Nationwide surveys have been regularly conducted in Japan since 1970; over 100,000 cases have been recorded to date [23].

The clinical manifestations are protean and the true clinical spectrum is still emerging as more children who with few clinical symptoms do develop coronary artery aneurysms come to our attention (Table 1.4.7) [24].

The illness begins with unexplained fever, sometimes with striking cervical lymphadenopathy (Figure 1.4.13). Frequently, the adenitis is unilateral and simulates a cervical gland abscess. After a few days, a polymorphous rash appears all over the body (Figure 1.4.14). The conjunctivae become hyperemic (Figure 1.4.15 and 1.4.16). The oral mucosa and lips are red and the tongue is described as "strawberry" in appearance (Figure 1.4.17). The lips fissure and crack (Figure 1.4.18). Striking indurative oedema appears on the dorsa of the hands and feet (Figure 1.4.19). The palms and soles become red, often with a sharp line of color demarcation at the wrists and ankles in a glove like distribution (Figure 1.4.20). Similar redness may be seen about the genitalia; the perineal rash is a useful diagnostic feature. During the recovery period, desquamation occurs in the areas that were previously red. The desquamation often begins under the finger or toe nails producing a distinctive appearance (Figure 1.4.21). Some children develop sheet-like desquamation (Figure 1.4.22). In severe cases, transverse grooves or furrows known as Beau lines, (Figure 1.4.23) are seen on the fingernails 1–2 months after the illness.

Table 1.4.7 Clinical Manifestations of KD

Manifestation (%)	Characteristics
Fever (95)	Spiking to 104 F, unresponsive to NSAID, lasts 5–23 days in untreated children
Rash (92)	Polymorphous: papular, morbiliform, multiforme, raised plaques, scarletiniform; perineal accentuation, site of BCG vaccination may develop Arthus-like reaction pruritic, followed by desquamation
Lymphadenopathy (75)	Mostly cervical; may be unilateral Single nodes may be very large and simulate abscess Frequently subsides early in the course
Conjunctival Hyperaemia (88)	Suffused bulbar conjunctivae without exudates Uveitis
Extremity changes (94)	Induration of the hands and feet (76) Erythema of the palms and soles (88) Typical desquamation of fingers and toes in the convalescent period (94) Beau lines (transverse grooves) in nails later in the recovery period in severe cases
Mouth lesions (90)	Erythema and fissuring of the lips and oropharynx Strawberry tongue
Associated features	Arthralgia or arthritis Aseptic meningitis Abdominal pain, obstructive jaundice, intestinal perforation, hydrops of gall bladder Myocarditis, pericarditis, tamponade, cardiac failure, arrhythmia, acute mitral insufficiency, myocardial infarction
Laboratory features	Leukocytosis with left shift, high ESR, high CRP, elevated liver enzymes, sterile pyuria, and CSF pleocytosis. EKG and 2D Echocardiographic abnormalities Ultrasound documenting hydrops Thrombocytosis in the second week of illness

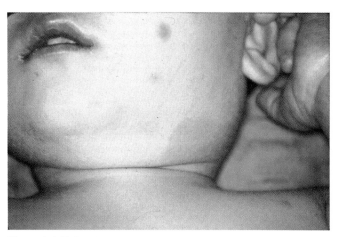

Figure 1.4.13 Toddler with KD and dramatically enlarged cervical node (from J. Jacobs).

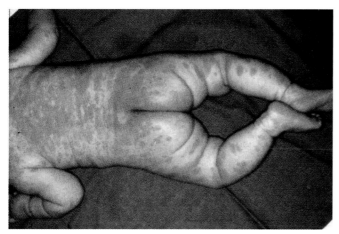

Figure 1.4.14 Morbiliform rash typical of KD (from J. Jacobs).

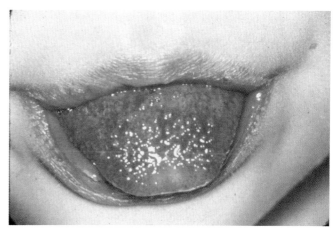

Figure 1.4.17 Strawberry tongue of KD.

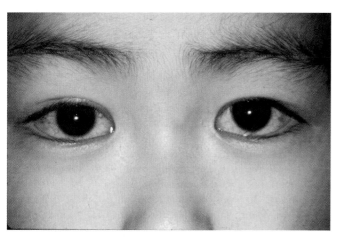

Figure 1.4.15 Red eyes associated with KD (from J. Jacobs).

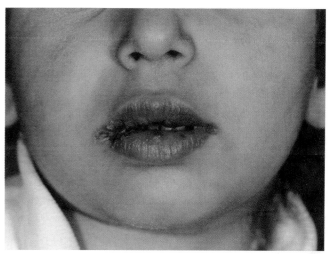

Figure 1.4.18 Mucositis of KD (courtesy of Y. Kimura).

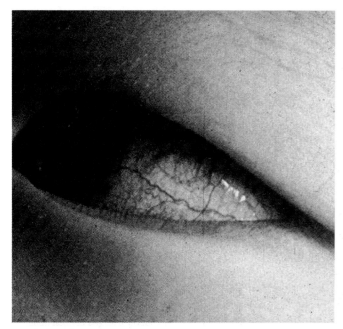

Figure 1.4.16 Kawasaki eye showing vascular dilatation and tortuosity.

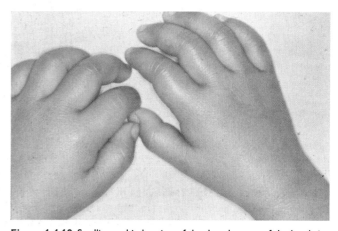

Figure 1.4.19 Swelling and induration of the dorsal aspect of the hands in a child with KD (from J. Jacobs).

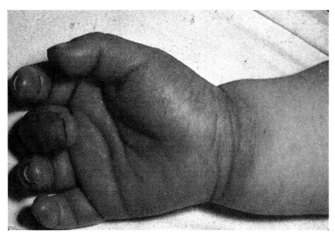

Figure 1.4.20 Redness over the palmar aspect of the hand in KD (from J. Jacobs).

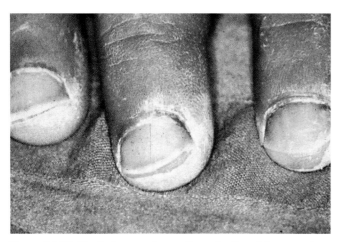

Figure 1.4.21 Classic desquamation starting under the nail in a young boy with KD (from J. Jacobs).

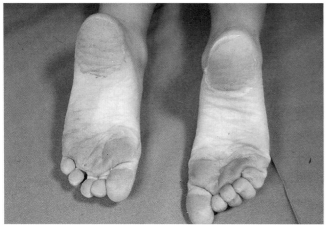

Figure 1.4.22 Sheet-like peeling of the skin where rash had been (courtesy of T. R. Southwood).

Not every patient has every feature, and there is variability in the persistence of each clinical manifestation. Lymphadenopathy may be present only for a day, and the rash on the palms and soles may be disappearing by the time the patient is examined. Paediatricians who have seen a prior case tend to suspect the diagnosis promptly. The illness may be confused with measles, toxic shock syndrome, scarlet

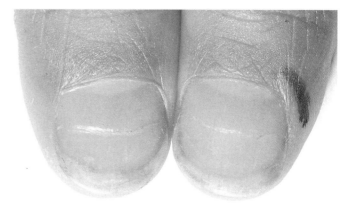

Figure 1.4.23 Beau lines in a child with severe KD (courtesy of T. R. Southwood).

fever, Stevens–Johnson's and other drug eruptions, Systemic Arthrits, reactive anthritis, infectious mononucleosis, Rocky Mountain spotted fever, yersiniosis, and leptospirosis (Table 1.4.8). Despite some overlapping features, distinction from these disorders is actually not difficult where measles has been eradicated. KD is considerably more common than most of the disorders in the differential diagnostic list, especially in infancy. Caution is needed when evaluating children with "atypical Kawasaki disease." The full spectrum of this illness is still evolving; it is hard to call an illness atypical if its spectrum is still not fully appreciated [25]. One of the more useful tests has been the ESR, aided by the CRP, which are both greatly elevated in KD and may help to distinguish this disorder in its early stages from the various viral illnesses affecting children. A febrile infant with no source to explain the fever, should undergo a 2-dimensional echocardiography. Elevated peripheral WBC count with a left shift also suggests that the child does not have a simple viral illness. The distinction from Systemic Arthritis is more difficult in those children whose rash is less prominent and who develop arthritis during the acute presentation. At times, it is the failure of IV IgG to control the illness, that the thought of Systemic Arthritis is entertained. However, the rash associated with Systemic Arthritis is fleeting, appearing during the fever spikes and the temperature pattern of JIA is hectic while in KD both fever and rash are persistent features. The platelet count is usually normal during the first week of illness and rises over time, peaking in the recovery phase.

The diagnosis of KD is based on the presence of five of six criteria (Table 1.4.9) [26]. As in many other rheumatic conditions, some patients do not all have the classical features and yet clearly have the illness as demonstrated by the development of aneurysms, suggesting that one must consider KD, especially in young infants and toddlers, who may only have had fever and rash or red eyes, or enlarged lymph nodes. Failure to recognize KD places these children at high risk for morbidity from unrecognized aneurysms (Figure 1.4.24). Striking enlargement of the liver may occur and is associated in some children with hydrops of the gallbladder. Chemical evidence of hepatitis is frequent during the first week of illness. Diarrhoea is common as well. Intestinal obstruction and ischemic vasculitis with perforation may occur. Pancreatitis occurs occasionally.

Arthritis is a frequent manifestation, either as part of the early course of disease when it is largely overshadowed by other features, or rarely as a late manifestation in the third week of disease especially in untreated patients or children whose salicylate was rapidly weaned after. The early arthritis is mainly in the fingers while the knees and the ankles are the joints most frequently affected in the convalescent

Table 1.4.8 Differentiation of KD from other exanthemas, and mucocutanous syndromes

	Different characteristic(s)	Absent findings	Laboratory aides
Erythema Multiforme, Serum sickness, Stevens–Johnson	Rare in infants; conjunctival discharge; Aphthous-like mouth ulcers; bullous and target skin lesions.	Lymphadenopathy; redness of hands and feet.	Occasional low C4.
Scarlet fever	Scarletiniform rash with Pastia lines and circumoral pallor; streptococcal pharyngitis; rare in infants.	Conjunctival hyperemia; lip fissures; swelling and redness of hands and feet;	Positive throat culture Rising antibody titre.
Toxic shock syndrome (TSS)	Rapid onset; erythroderma; confusion; shock; rare in infants	Lymphadenopathy	Renal insufficiency; thrombocytopenia; Presence of TSS toxin (TSST)
Leptospirosis	Rare in infants	Lip fissures; swelling and redness of hands and feet; Lymphadenopathy	Acute and convalescent serologies.
Reactive arthritis	Conjunctival discharge; Severe polyarthritis; Evanescent rash or keratoderma blenorrhagicum.	Lip fissures; strawberry tongue; diffuse mouth erythema; nodes	HLA-B27
Rocky mountain spotted fever	Tick exposure; older children; stupor; Spotted rash on palms and soles	Lip fissures; strawberry tongue; mouth erythema; nodes	Acute and convalescent serologies.
Measles	Profuse conjunctival and nasal discharge; cough; Koplik spots	Lip fissures; swelling and redness of hands and feet;	Leucopenia; Measles IqM
Systemic Arthritis	Quotidian fever; typical rash with Koebner phenomenon;	Conjunctivitis; mucositis; swelling and redness of hands and feet	Extremely elevated ferritin

Table 1.4.9 Criteria for diagnosis of KD

Bilateral conjunctival injection (80–90%)

Changes in the or pharyngeal mucous membranes (including one or more of: injected and/or fissured lips, strawberry tongue, injected pharynx) (80–90%)

Changes in the peripheral extremities, including erythema and/or edema of the hands and feet (acute phase) or periungual desquamation (convalescent phase) (80%)

Polymorphous rash, primarily truncal; nonvesicular (>90%)

Cervical lymphadenopathy with at least one node >1.5 cm (50–75%)

Fever ≥5 days plus at least four of the following clinical signs (4 days if treatment with IVIG eradicates fever), not explained by another disease process (numbers in parentheses indicate the approximate percentage of children with KD who display the criterion):

Source: Modified from Centers for Disease Control: Revised diagnostic criteria for KD (26).

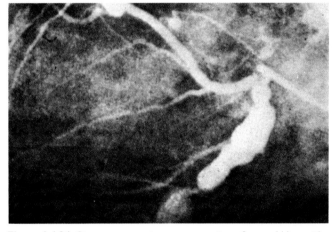

Figure 1.4.24 Giant coronary artery aneurysms in an 8-year-old-boy with "atypical" KD. The diagnosis was delayed by several weeks; the aneurysms resolved after several months (from J. Jacobs).

period. Irritability and aseptic meningitis are very frequent. Older children may report urethral discomfort. Sterile pyuria is demonstrated in over half of patients and mild transient proteinuria is common. Mild anterior uveitis is very common during the acute illness when the eyes are still red and the slit lamp is a useful test if the diagnosis is not clear. This acute, symptomatic uveitis is unlike the inflammation of the uveal tract described in JIA; chronic anterior uveitis associated with Oligoarthritis is asymptomatic, while Systemic Arthritis is rarely if ever complicated by uveitis. Without treatment, fever and other symptoms may continue for several weeks and arthritis may even appear as the patient seems to be improving. Sometimes a recrudescence of symptoms and fever occurs after the patient has recovered.

In some cases, the diagnosis can only be established during the convalescent period, when typical finger desquamation is observed; this applies especially to patients who do not have other extremity changes during the acute period. It is important, therefore, to advise parents of those children to look for the peeling of the fingers and toes and to advise the physician of its occurrence.

Histological examination of the affected arteries in KD reveals a pan-arteritis; initially the microvasculature is affected but within days, both small to medium sized vessels with particular predilection for the main coronary arteries become inflamed. Although the skin, mucous membranes and heart are most frequently affected, arteries everywhere may have lesions that can result in occlusive or ischemic manifestations, either during the acute phase or at some time later in life. Arteritis of the main coronary arteries may lead to myocardial ischemia [27].

It is generally agreed that children diagnosed with Infantile Polyarteritis Nodosa (see Part 1, Chapter 1.7) had KD. The original descriptions of these infants reveal fever, red eyes and rash indistinguishable from the clinical descriptions of Kawasaki Disease.

Treatment of KD includes IV IgG, given once and repeated if there is not a desired clinical response [28]. Recalcitrant KD may respond to high doses of corticosteroids with or without high dose aspirin. Anecdotal reports of successful treatment of refractory KD with anti-TNF agents supports clinical trials in KD.

Erythema nodosum

Erythema Nodosum is a dramatic clinical syndrome characterized by the sudden appearance of fever and a crop of typical warm, red, tender cutanous nodules on the extensor surfaces of the anterior tibiae (Figure 1.4.25). In severe cases, lesions may extend up both the arms and legs (Figure 1.4.26). The skin lesions are frequently associated with arthralgia and joint effusions. The pathologic finding of perivascular granulomatous septal panniculitis is consistent with a delayed hypersensitivity reaction.

Erythema Nodosum may be a reaction to many specific infectious agents, including streptococcus, tuberculous and lepromatous bacillus, leptospirosis, psittacosis, yersinia, cytomegalovirus, and fungal agents, including those causing coccidiomycosis, blastomycosis, and

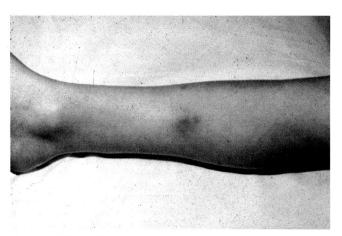

Figure 1.4.25 Painful nodule over the extensor surface of the tibia shortly following streptococcal infection.

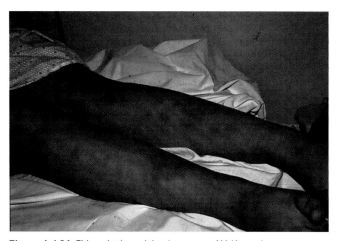

Figure 1.4.26 EN, multiple nodules (courtesy of Y. Kimura).

Table 1.4.10 Differential diagnosis of erythema nodosum in children

Infectious triggers	Other triggers
Streptococcal infection	Inflammatory bowel disease
Tuberculosis	Sarcoid
Leprosy	Drugs, including oral contraceptives
Leptospirosis	
Psittacosis	
Yersiniosis	
Cytomegalovirus infection	
Fungal infections: coccidiomycosis, blastomycosis, histoplasmosis	

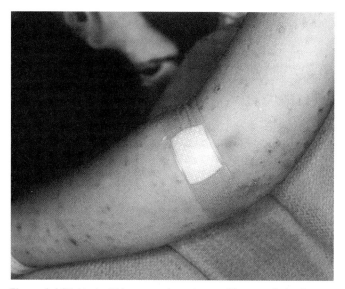

Figure 1.4.27 Mucha–Habermann; the rash resembles varicella but has vasculitic features in addition (from J. Jacobs).

histoplasmosis (Table 1.4.10). In the San Joaquin Valley, 80% of the cases are due to coccidiomycosis. In most cases however, no underlying inciting disease is found. However, when an aetiology can be established, the single most frequent primary diagnosis in children is inflammatory bowel disease (IBD), and this diagnosis must be considered in every patient (see section earlier in this chapter). Sarcoidosis is the most common single aetiology in young adults followed in frequency by IBD and drug allergy, especially allergy to oral contraceptives (also Part 1, Chapter 1.7).

Although new crops of lesions appear and the "attack" usually lasts for a few weeks, the lesions very rarely ulcerate, and the process is self-limited. NSAID therapy is adequate for most children, but corticosteroids may be used in the most severe cases after the tuberculin skin test is shown to be negative.

Mucha–Habermann disease [acute parapsoriasis, Pithyriasis Lichenoides Et Varioliformis Acuta (PLEVA)]

Mucha–Habermann is a little recognized form of cutaneous vasculitis. Also known as Acute Parapsoriasis, this illness is characterized by

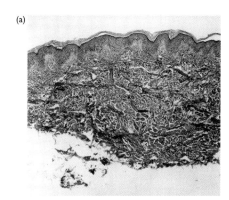

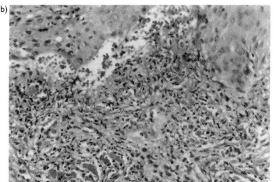

Figure 1.4.28 Histologic section from lesion shown in Figure 1.4.27 documents perivascular lymphocytic infiltrate and extravasated erythrocytes characteristic of Mucha–Habermann disease. (a) Low power ×40 and (b) high power ×250 (from J. Jacobs).

Table 1.4.11 Disorders in which arthritis may be associated with inflammatory dermatoses.

Mucha–Habermann disease (PLEVA)

Sweet syndrome

Inflammatory bowel disease

Intestinal bypass syndrome

Erythema elevatum diutinum

Leukocytoclastic angiitis

Erythema nodosum

Pyoderma gangrenosum

Behçet syndrome

Pancreatitis

Acne fulminans

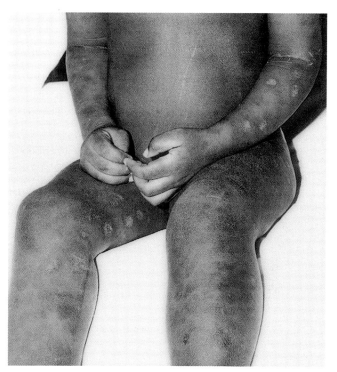

Figure 1.4.29 Five-year-old African-American female with typical raised, painful plaques which began at 10 months of age and stopped following a short course of corticosteroids when the diagnosis of Sweet syndrome was established years later (from J. Jacobs).

the development of recurrent crops of vesicular lesions resembling varicella (Figure 1.4.27), associated with pain and effusions in the large joints with slightly elevated ESR [29]. The diagnosis is established by a punch biopsy of the lesion; histopathologic examination shows a V-shaped perivascular lymphocytic infiltrate about normal blood vessels (Figure 1.4.28(a,b)), the aetiology is unknown. Mucha–Habermann disease is one of a group of inflammatory dermatoses (Table 1.4.11) that may be associated with arthritis. The arthritis seen in Mucha–Habermann disease is mild and transient and responds well to NSAIDs but may recur with each recurrent crop of skin lesions. Although the illness usually subsides within a few months, some children may suffer recurrent episodes for many years.

Sweet syndrome

This acute febrile neutrophilic dermatosis is another disorder characterized by crops of skin lesions associated with fever, myalgia, arthralgia, and occasionally, arthritis. The skin lesion is clinically distinctive and consists of raised painful plaques (Figure 1.4.29) that on histological examination, show a dense neutrophilic small vessel perivascular infiltrate in the mid and upper dermis (Figure 1.4.30(a; b)). Polymorphonuclear cells generally predominate, and some are disrupted, creating nuclear fragments and dust about the vessel (Figure 1.4.30(c)). There are no changes in the blood vessels themselves. The whole syndrome is responsive to a brief course of corticosteroid therapy. In some cases, a single brief course of treatment is curative, but there may be recurrent episodes over a period of years. Untreated episodes often last for two months [30].

Similar or identical syndromes occur after ileojejunal bypass surgery and in association with malignancy, Fanconi and other anemias, chronic recurrent multifocal osteomyelitis (CRMO, see Part 1, Chapter 1.5), and Behçet disease (Part 1, Chapter 1.7).

References

1. Eshel, G., Barr, J., Azizi, E., Aladgem, M., Algom, M., and Mundel, G. Acute Rheumatic Fever in the young: Changing prevalence and pattern. *Eur J Pediatr* 1988;148:208–10.

2. Committee on Prevention of Rheumatic Fever and Bacterial Endocarditis of the American Heart Association. Prevention of Rheumatic Fever. *Circulation* 1984;70:1123A.

3. Stollerman, G.H. Current issues in the prevention of rheumatic fever. *Minerva Med* 2002;93:371–87.

4. Camara, E.J., Braga, J.C., Alves-Silva, L.S., Camara, G.F., and da Silva Lopes, A.A. Comparison of an intravenous pulse of methylprednisolone versus oral corticosteroid in severe acute rheumatic carditis: a randomized clinical trial. *Cardiol Young* 2002;12:119–24.

5. Ayoub, E.M. and Majeed, H.A. Poststreptococcal reactive arthritis. *Curr Opin Rheumatol* 2000;12:306–10.

6. De Cunto, C.L., Giannini, E.H., Fink, C.W., Brewer, E.J., and Person, D.A. Prognosis in children with poststreptococcal reactive arthritis. *Pediatr Infect Dis J* 1988;7:683–6.

7. Tutar, E., Atalay, S., Yilmaz, E., Ucar, T., Kocak, G., and Imamoglu, A. Poststreptococcal reactive arthritis in children: is it really a different entity from rheumatic fever? *Rheumatol Int* 2002;22:80–3.

8. Shulman, S.T. and Ayoub, E.M. Poststreptococcal reactive arthritis. *Curr Opin Rheumatol* 2002;14:562–5.

9. Kunnamo, I., Kallio, P., and Pelkonen, P. Incidence of arthritis in urban Finnish children. A Prospective study. *Arthritis Rheum* 1986;29:1232–8.

10. Cabral, D.A., Malleson, P.N., and Petty, R.E. Spondyloarthropathies of childhood. *Pediatric Clinics of North America* 1995;42:1051–70.

11. Picco, P., Gattorno, M., Marchese, N., Vignola, S., Sormani, M.P. *et al.* Increased gut permeability in juvenile chronic arthritis. A multivariate analysis of the diagnostic parameters. *Clin Exp Rheumatol* 2000;18:773–8.

12. Papos, M., Varkonyi, A., Lang, J., Buga, K., Timar. F. *et al.* HM-PAO-labeled leukocyte scintigraphy in pediatric patients with inflammatory bowel disease. *J Pediatr Gastroenterol Nutr* 1996; 23:547–52.

13. Palm, O., Moum, B., Jahnsen, J., Gran, J.T. The prevalence and incidence of peripheral arthritis in patients with inflammatory bowel disease, a population based study (the IBSEN study). *Rheumatology* (Oxford) 2001;40:1256–61.

14. Palm, O., Moum, B., Ongre, A., Gran, J.T. Prevalence of ankylosing spondylitis and other spondyloarthropathies among patients with inflammatory bowel disease: a population study (the IBSEN study). *J Rheumatol* 2002;29:511–5.

15. Waters, E. Toxic synovitis of the hip in children. *Nurse Pract* 1995;20:44–51.

16. Szer, I.S. HSP: when and how to treat. *J Rheumatol* 1996:23;1661–5.

17. Rosenblum, N.D. and Winter, H.S. Steroid effects on the course of abdominal pain with HSP. *Pediatrics* 1987;79:1018–21.

18. Ronkainen, J., Nuutinen, M., and Koskimies, O. The Adult Kidney 24 years after Childhood HSP: A retrospective cohort study. *Lancet* 2002;360:666–70.

19. Caksen, H., Odabas, D., Kosem, M. *et al.* Report of eight infants with acute infantile hemorrhagic edema and review of the literature. *J Dermatol* 2002;29:290–5.

20. Calabrese, L.H., Michel, B.A., Bloch, D.A. *et al.* The ACR 1990 criteria for the classification of Hypersensitivity Vasculitis. *Arthritis Rheum* 1990:3:1108–13

21. Szer, I.S. Gastrointestinal and renal involvement in vasculitis: management strategies in HSP. *Cleveland Clin J Med* 1999;66:312–7.

22. Jacobs, J.C. Erythema Multiforme, Stevens Johnson's Syndrome and Angioneurotic Edema. In *Pediatric Rheumatology for the Practitioner*, 2nd ed. New York: Verlag, 1992, pp. 34–5.

23. Burns, J.C. Kawasaki disease. *Adv Ped* 2001;48:157–88.

24. Newburger, J. Kawasaki Disease: Who is at risk? *J Pediatr* 2000;13:149–52.

25. Hsieh, Y.C., Wu, M.H., Wang, J.K., Lee, P.I., Lee, C.Y., and Huang, L.M. Clinical features of atypical Kawasaki disease. *J Microbiol Immunol Inf* 2002;35(1):57–60.

26. *MMWR* 1990;39(44–13):27–8.

27. Kato, H. *et al.* Fate of coronary aneurysms in Kawasaki disease: serial coronary angiography and long-term follow-up study. *Am J Cardiol* 1982;49:1758–66.

28. Newburger, J. *et al.* The treatment of Kawasaki syndrome with intravenous immunoglobulin. *New Eng J Med* 1986;315(6):341–7.

29. Korppi, M., Tenhola, S., and Hollmen, A. Mucha–Habermann Disease: a diagnostic possibility for prolonged fever associated with systemic and skin symptoms. *Pediatr Derm* 1991;8:151.

30. Cohen, P.R., Kurzrock, R. Sweet's Syndrome: a review of current treatment options. *Am J Clin Dermatol* 2002;3:117–31.

1.5 Acute and chronic infections of bones and joints

Yukiko Kimura

Aim

The aim of this chapter is to discuss all of the infectious conditions that may present with musculoskeletal manifestations and must be "ruled out" early in the evaluation of the child with arthritis.

Structure

- Pyogenic bone infections
- Pyogenic joint infections
- Lyme and other non-bacterial arthritis
- Soft tissue infections around joints
- Foreign body synovitis
- Fungal, parasitic and other rare infectious causes of arthritis

Introduction

When a child presents with fever and a limp or limb pain, the first and most urgent diagnostic consideration should be that of a serious bacterial infection (see Part 1, Chapter 1.3, Algorithm 1.3.1, "The Child with Musculoskeletal Pain/Dysfunction and Fever"), rather than Juvenile Idiopathic Arthritis (JIA). Bacterial musculoskeletal infections such as osteomyelitis and septic arthritis, which occur commonly in children, can cause serious morbidity if not recognized, diagnosed, and treated promptly and appropriately. In addition to the physical damage to the affected bone and/or joint, these infections have the potential to be associated with distant organ disease as well as causing septic shock and death, because they are almost always the result of bacteraemia in children. In addition to bacterial infections, viral and other infections of bones and joints in children, as well as other common musculoskeletal syndromes related to infection are important to differentiate from JIA and will be discussed in this chapter.

Osteomyelitis

Acute haematogenous osteomyelitis

General considerations

Although osteomyelitis is not rare, it is still commonly either misdiagnosed or delayed in diagnosis (Table 1.5.1). In a series from Jacobs's original textbook [1], only 13 of 79 patients with osteomyelitis were diagnosed correctly at the onset. Jacobs theorized that perhaps

Table 1.5.1 Primary diagnosis made in 79 children with osteomyelitis at Columbia-Presbyterian Medical Center, 1965–74 [1]

Diagnosis	Number of patients
Trauma	24 (30.4%)
Viral syndrome or upper respiratory tract infection	19 (24.1%)
Cellulitis	14 (17.7%)
Osteomyelitis	13 (16.5%)
Other	4 (5.1%)
Acute rheumatic fever	3 (3.8%)
Rheumatoid arthritis	2 (2.5%)
Osteomyelitis considered at first but rejected	18

the frequency with which children limp after minor trauma or have fever as a result of an insignificant viral illness interferes with recognition of the seriousness of this symptom complex. Although rapid diagnosis and institution of intravenous antibiotics are critical to the outcome of osteomyelitis, late diagnosis has been the rule in most published series, with subsequent increased morbidity for the patient [1–3]. With a better understanding of some of the pitfalls of making a diagnosis of osteomyelitis, both early recognition and improved outcome should be possible.

Presentation

The usual presentation of osteomyelitis is the sudden onset of fever and limb pain, often after an inconsequential injury (Table 1.5.2). The degree and character of the pain is an important clue: children with osteomyelitis have tremendous pain. They typically refuse to bear weight on the affected extremity and will not even be able to limp, a symptom which should always be of great concern. In contrast, children with JIA may limp and have difficulty in walking, but will very rarely absolutely refuse to bear weight. There is usually no break in the skin, because osteomyelitis in children is most often the result of a haematogenous infection which often settles in the metaphysis of a long bone (Figure 1.5.1).

Examining the bone

Point tenderness over the affected bone is diagnostic of osteomyelitis but may be hard to demonstrate, especially in a young child. A slow and thorough examination of the suspected bone, starting far away

Table 1.5.2 Presenting complaints in children with osteomyelitis (percentages)

Symptoms	Jacobs [1] (n = 79)	Bonhoeffer [9] (n = 81)	Dahl [7] (n = 80)	Karwowska [10] (n = 146)
Bone pain and limp or disuse	100	95	91	84
Fever	86	80	75	40
Joint pain	65	60	ND	35
History of injury >24 h	33	ND	ND	ND
History of injury <24 h	13	ND	ND	ND

ND = No data.

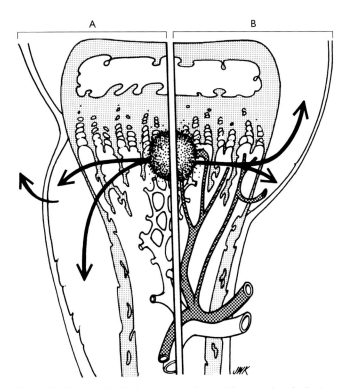

Fig. 1.5.1 Diagram of differing patterns of spread from a nidus of infection located at the metaphysis of a long bone, depending on whether the metaphysis is located within the joint capsule or outside the capsule. The metaphysis is the most common site for acute osteomyelitis, presumably because of capillary looping, as shown. If the metaphysis is outside the joint capsule (A), as at the knee, infection can spread subperiosteally down the bone and can ultimately form soft-tissue abscesses by rupturing through the periosteum. However, although a sympathetic joint effusion may be present, joint fluid is sterile. Aspiration of sterile joint fluid from the knee is often misinterpreted as evidence against bacterial infection, although a sterile knee effusion is a characteristic finding in osteomyelitis of the distal femur or proximal tibia. If the infected metaphysis is within the joint space, (B), as at the hip, infection commonly spreads laterally, through the cortex into the joint. Joint fluid will be purulent. The finding of purulent fluid in the hip always indicates the possibility of osteomyelitis in the proximal femur. Since the treatment regimen for osteomyelitis is different from that of septic arthritis without bone infection, it is important to exclude bone infection in patients with septic arthritis. (From J. Jacobs.)

from the affected area, will go a long way toward calming the child, thereby allowing an accurate examination. Periosteal rebound tenderness can sometimes be demonstrated in the area of maximal point tenderness. While osteomyelitis usually affects the long bones, other smaller bones may also be affected (Table 1.5.3). Bony point tenderness in a febrile child is quite specific for osteomyelitis, whereas in leukemia, bone pain may be seen without fever. In contrast, the pain and tenderness in inflammatory arthritis is much more diffuse, centred around the joint line rather than in a focal area of the bone, and worsens with movement of the joint.

Significance of adjacent joint effusions

Since osteomyelitis most commonly starts in the metaphysis of a bone, the nearby joint may also be involved (Figure 1.5.1). When the metaphysis sits outside the joint capsule, as it does at the knee, the effusion is often "sympathetic" and not septic. Therefore, aspiration of sterile joint fluid does not exclude bacterial infection in the bone. Conversely a septic knee joint is not likely to be associated with adjacent osteomyelitis. Careful palpation of the adjacent bones (including the patella) should be performed to assess for point tenderness of each of the bones surrounding the swollen joint.

The situation is different when the metaphysis is inside the joint capsule, as in the hip and shoulder joints, which may result in both septic arthritis and osteomyelitis (Figure 1.5.2). Therefore, when aspiration of the hip or shoulder demonstrates infection, evaluation should also be undertaken for osteomyelitis in one of the adjacent bones. This is critical, as osteomyelitis will require a longer duration of antibiotic treatment. In addition, not uncommonly, hip, groin, buttock, and abdominal pain may all be manifestations of pelvic osteomyelitis, including sacroiliac osteomyelitis.

Systemic manifestations

High fever is almost always present in acute osteomyelitis. If there is sustained bacteremia, more than one bone and/or joint may be infected, making the diagnosis much more difficult. Such an illness can sometimes be mistaken for rheumatic fever or Systemic Arthritis. However, children with osteomyelitis tend to remain febrile throughout the day, while patients with Systemic Arthritis typically have a quotidian fever pattern of one or two spikes of high fever daily with the temperature returning to normal (or subnormal) in the interim. In addition, when the infection becomes life-threatening as a result of septic embolization to the lung, endocardium, and kidney, the primary focus in bone may be missed.

Laboratory studies

Blood should be obtained for a complete blood count (CBC) and erythrocyte sedimentation rate (ESR), both of which may sometimes be normal, especially early in the illness. The CRP (C-reactive protein) may be a more sensitive and earlier indicator of acute inflammation. In addition, whereas the results of the ESR can be understated if the test is not run promptly after blood drawing (as can be the case when the test is transported to distant commercial laboratories), the CRP is more reliable. A blood culture should also be obtained. If there is a joint effusion, fluid should be aspirated and tested for cell count, Gram stain, and culture, as well as for glucose level (Table 1.5.4). In addition to obtaining joint fluid and blood for culture, it is critical that every attempt is made to isolate the pathogenic organism from the bone and periosteum by aspiration or biopsy.

Table 1.5.3 Distribution of bones affected in childhood osteomyelitis (%)

	Jacobs [1] (n = 79)	Fink [2] (n = 316)	Cole [8] (n = 76)	Bonhoeffer [9] (n = 81)	Karwowska [10] (n = 146)	Dahl [7] (n = 80)
Femur	20	27	29	24	14	35
Tibia	21	25	22	18	32	28
Pelvis (incl. SI)	13	5	11	13	8	9
Fibula	11	5	12	2	5	NR
Humerus	7	12	7	5	6	19
Radius	5	4	4	NR	4	1
Vertebra	4	2	NR	2	NR	NR
Patella	4	<1	0	NR	NR	NR
Calcaneus	4	5	9	(10)[a]	13	NR
Metatarsus, metacarpus, phalanx	4	4		(10)[a] (3)[b]	9	16 (foot or hand)
Rib	5	<1	NR	NR	NR	NR
Tarsal	1	1	4	(10)[a]	NR	NR
Ulna	1	2	1	NR	NR	NR
Sternum	<1	<1	NR	NR	NR	NR
Mandible	<1	<1	NR	NR	NR	1
Scapula	<1	<1	NR	NR	NR	NR
Clavicle	<1	<1	NR	5	2	1
Other	NR	NR	NR	NR	4	NR

NR = not reported.

[a] 10% had "foot" involvement.

[b] 3% had "hand" involvement.

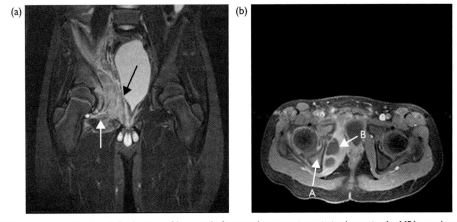

Fig. 1.5.2 This 12-year-old boy presented with a 1-day history of low-grade fever and progressive pain in the groin. An MRI was done which revealed osteomyelitis of the acetabulum, as well as extension of the infection into the adjacent muscle and joint. (a) Coronal fast STIR images reveals oedema in the iliacus and obturator internus muscles, a fluid collection in the right side of the pelvis that is displacing the bladder and oedema in the bone of the right acetabulum as well as fluid in the hip joint. (b) Axial T1 GRE with gadolinium administration reveals enhancement in the bone of the acetabulum (A), as well as rim enhancement medial to the hip joint in the obturator internus muscle which is seen displacing the bladder (B).

Table 1.5.4 Comparison of clinical features of septic arthritis, osteomyelitis, and JIA

	Septic arthritis	Osteomyelitis	Oligoarthritis
Predominant sign/symptom	Hot, swollen, very painful joint with little mobility and refusal to bear weight	Disuse of affected limb with point tenderness of bone; may have associated joint swelling (can be septic or sterile)	Swollen and moderately tender (may be warm) joint with mild–moderate limitation but able to use affected limb; morning and inactivity stiffness prominent
Fever	++	+++	− If Systemic Arthritis: +++
WBC	++	++	− If Systemic Arthritis: ++
Acute phase reactants	++	+++	+/− If Systemic Arthritis: +++
Joint fluid white count	+++	−[a]	++
Joint fluid Gram stain	+	−[a]	−
Decreased joint fluid glucose	+	−[a]	−
Bone scan	Diffusely increased uptake on both sides of joint	Focal increased uptake only in affected bone	Diffusely increased uptake on both sides of joint
MRI	Joint effusion and soft-tissue swelling Synovial enhancement with gadolinium	Abnormal marrow signal in affected bone No synovial enhancement with gadolinium	Joint effusion and soft-tissue swelling Synovial enhancement with gadolinium

[a] Unless the infection has also extended to the joint (especially in the hip).

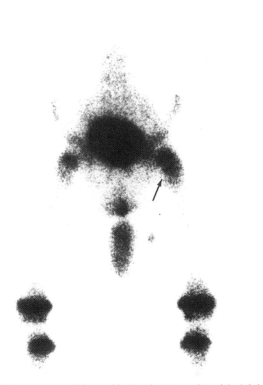

Fig. 1.5.3 Bone scan in a 1½ year old girl with osteomyelitis of the left femur. The scan was positive at the time of presentation, with mild monarticular synovitis of the left hip. (From J. Jacobs.)

Radiographic studies

Plain radiographs are not useful in the diagnosis of acute osteomyelitis, as X-ray changes may not occur until 10–21 days after onset of symptoms. Occasionally, oedema in the soft tissues close to the periosteum, causing a loss of clear bone definition, can suggest osteomyelitis before overt bony radiographic changes have occurred. However, they should be obtained to rule out preexisting disease, associated bone pathology, and fractures. A technetium-99-m bone scan should be performed as soon as possible. Combined blood pool and bone imaging often confirm the clinical diagnosis of osteomyelitis. While bone scans are excellent imaging procedures that provide support for the early diagnosis of osteomyelitis (Figure 1.5.3), they are not a substitute for a skillful history and physical examination. There may also be certain technical problems with bone scans. For example, at some institutions bone scans may not be immediately available, and in addition, bone scans may be negative during the first 24–48 h of illness. Therefore, while a positive bone scan is helpful in establishing the diagnosis of osteomyelitis, a negative bone scan does not necessarily exclude it.

In very early osteomyelitis and in situations when the bone scan is negative but osteomyelitis is still strongly suspected, an MRI (magnetic resonance imaging) should be obtained [4,5]. This imaging test is quite sensitive in detecting osteomyelitis, which will manifest as areas of bone marrow oedema due to accumulation of purulent material (Table 1.5.4 and Figure 1.5.4). At times, it may be difficult to distinguish osteomyelitis from leukemic infiltration by MRI (Figure 1.5.5). In contrast, an MRI of inflammatory arthritis will usually not show extensive marrow changes (Figure 1.5.6). Instead, it will document fluid in the joint space and gadolinium enhancement of the synovium.

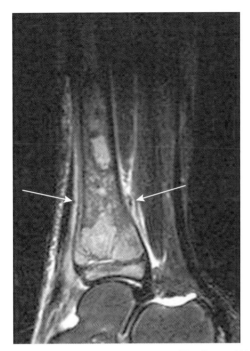

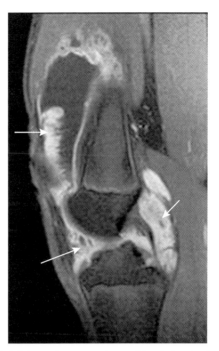

Fig. 1.5.4 MRI of osteomyelitis of the distal tibia. This 8-year-old boy developed fever to 103, vomiting, diarrhoea, and a rash. He was treated with penicillin by his pediatrician. The rash and GI symptoms resolved, but he developed pain and swelling of his left ankle which progressed over a 10-day period so that he was unable to bear weight on his left leg. The WBC was 17.0, platelet count 1,038,000, and the ESR was 105. He had exquisite tenderness of his left distal tibial metaphysis, as well as 3+ swelling, warmth, and erythema of his ankle. An X-ray of his ankle revealed a linear lucency along the metaphysis of the medial tibia. The MRI revealed extensive marrow signal abnormality involving the distal tibial diaphysis, metaphysis, and epiphysis with generalized periosteal elevation, joint fluid, and subperiosteal edema. Aspiration of the distal tibia confirmed the diagnosis of osteomyelitis.

Fig. 1.5.6 Gadolinium enhancement is a useful technique to demonstrate synovial inflammation, such as seen in JIA. This MRI of the knee in a boy with Polyarthritis showed marked enhancement of the proliferated synovium (see arrows) as well as a joint effusion.

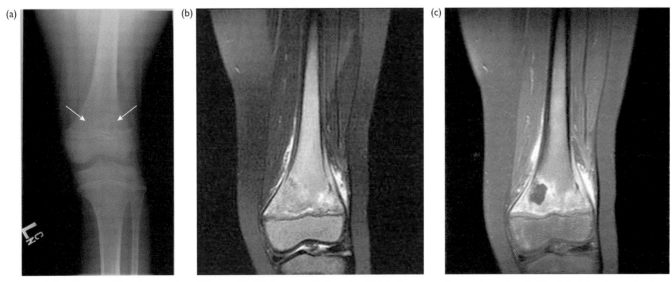

Fig. 1.5.5 This 9-year-old female was referred for possible JIA because of joint pain which had progressed over a 6-week period to include her knees, hands, wrists, ankles, and feet. She had morning stiffness and swelling of the joints, and difficulty in walking. On examination, she had significant pain, and had great difficulty bearing weight. There were multiple swollen joints which were extremely tender and warm. The CBC had a WBC of 7.4 (normal differential), hemoglobin 10.2, platelet count 288,000. The ESR was 115, and the LDH was normal. (a) X-ray of the left knee showed a mottled distal femoral metaphysis with cortical disruption both medially and laterally. (arrows) (b) and (c) An MRI was then obtained, which showed inhomogeneity and increased signal within the marrow space of the distal femoral metaphysis with periosteal reaction and fluid in the knee joint. The bone marrow confirmed the diagnosis of acute lymphoblastic leukaemia.

Table 1.5.5 General treatment guidelines for bacterial osteomyelitis

Time frame	Action	Comments
Immediate	Obtain cultures of bone and blood	
	Begin intravenous antibiotics with anti-Staphylococcal antibiotic	Consider adding *H. influenzae* coverage in immunocompromised or unimmunized children; add *Salmonella* coverage in patients with sickle-cell disease
	Place PPD and control antigens	
Within a week	Once organism identified, tailor antibiotic regimen	
Up to 6 weeks	Continue IV antibiotics	
	Follow temperature curve, ESR as guide to response	If not responding, perform MRI; if abscess has formed, consider surgical drainage

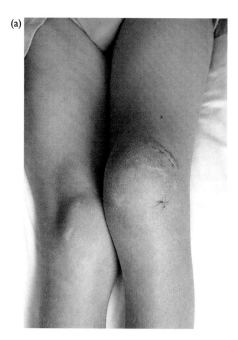

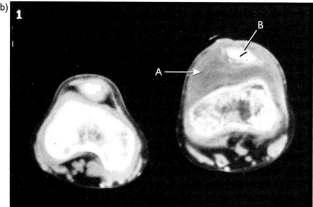

Fig. 1.5.7 (a) Osteomyelitis of the patella presenting as a large solitary knee effusion which was thought to be due to Oligoarthritis until an MRI was performed. (b) This showed a large joint effusion (A) and irregularity and destruction of the patella (B). (Courtesy of T. R. Southwood.)

Treatment

Treatment is generally straightforward (Table 1.5.5). The critical point for the treating physician is to work with the orthopaedic surgeon to obtain a culture (either by aspiration or biopsy) of the bone prior to treatment in order to identify the pathogenic organism. Blood cultures alone are not sufficient, because they are only positive in about 30% of patients with osteomyelitis. In contrast, bone aspiration will yield the organism in at least 80% of patients [2,3,6–10]. If treatment is begun empirically without a specific organism having been isolated, the patient will often require broad-spectrum intravenous antibiotics for the entire treatment course, which can be as long as 6 weeks. In addition, if the patient fails to respond to the initial antibiotic treatment, or develops allergy to the antimicrobial agent, it is difficult to choose an alternate antibiotic regimen without a specific pathogen identified.

Subacute osteomyelitis of the patella

Infections of the patella must be distinguished from infection within the knee joint, which can sometimes be difficult. Most cases of osteomyelitis of the patella occur in children between the ages of 4 and 15 years and are usually due to *Staphylococcus aureus*. Because these tend to be low-grade infections that are accompanied by sterile knee effusions, they are often confused with Oligoarthritis. This infection should be considered if there is tenderness of the patella to direct palpation; a finding that is not present in JIA. The bone scan and MRI are the most useful imaging techniques to confirm the diagnosis (Figure 1.5.7). When radiographs are taken, it is important to obtain lateral films of the contralateral, unaffected patella for comparison, especially in a child whose patella is not yet completely ossified.

Osteomyelitis in the sacroiliac area

Pelvic osteomyelitis in the bones articulating at the sacroiliac joint is not rare (Table 1.5.3). The initial physical findings are quite characteristic: fever, limp, and buttock pain, often with radicular sciatic pain. Most

patients will not be able to walk, and have exquisite point tenderness over the affected bone. In contrast, patients with Enthesitis Related Arthritis (ERA); (see Part 2, Chapter 2.7) may also have sacroiliac pain and tenderness, but the tenderness is not exquisite and there is usually no associated fever. Additionally, other signs of ERA such as peripheral arthritis or enthesitis, will generally be present. In addition, patients with ERA tend to have bilateral sacroiliac involvement, whereas sacroiliac osteomyelitis is usually unilateral. The techniques for diagnosis and management of patients with presumed osteomyelitis are identical to infection in any other location, although the bone scan may be negative in up to 40% of these patients.

Vertebral osteomyelitis

Osteomyelitis of the vertebral body is unusual in children. Patients typically present with an indolent course of low-grade fever and dull back pain that may continue for months [11,12]. There is often localized tenderness of one particular vertebral body and percussion of the specific spinous process involved may elicit exquisite tenderness.

X-rays may initially show a localized radiolucency followed by involvement of adjacent vertebrae. Although radionuclide bone scan and gallium scan may be positive, MRI is a more sensitive imaging study [11,12]. *Staphylococcus aureus* is the most likely organism, but occasionally urinary tract pathogens have been isolated, particularly in adults. In addition, tuberculous vertebral osteomyelitis (Pott disease—Figure 1.5.8) should always be considered in the differential diagnosis. Although lumbar spine tenderness and limitation of flexion are both features of ERA (see Schober test, Part 1, Chapter 1.1, Figure 1.1.7), the tenderness is not localized to one vertebral body, and fever is not usually present.

Other unusual organisms can occasionally be responsible for vertebral osteomyelitis. *Pseudomonas* infection (most often associated with a history of intravenous drug abuse), fungi and *Brucella* have been documented. Rarely, vertebral osteomyelitis and paravertebral soft-tissue collections associated with cat-scratch disease (*Bartonella henselae*) may occur in children with a history of prior exposure to multiple cat scratches followed by regional lymphadenopathy.

Discitis

Infection of the intervertebral disc in young children is not rare and constitutes a condition requiring special consideration. It generally begins with vague leg, hip, or low back pain but may progress over a period of weeks to inability to walk, then sit, and ultimately to immobility. The children typically cry when being cuddled or while their diaper is changed, but then become less irritable when picked up under the arms, presumably because pressure on the spine is relieved. Diagnosis can be difficult, especially because discitis tends to affect younger children who cannot verbally localize their discomfort [13]. Referred abdominal pain, radicular symptoms, and meningeal irritation are less common signs. In the past, the diagnosis was sometimes extraordinarily difficult, and as a result an extensive

literature of untreated children exists [12]. Without treatment, after 2–14 weeks, disc-space narrowing will become apparent on X-ray (Figure 1.5.9). Earlier detection is now possible using bone scan and MRI (Figure 1.5.10). After obtaining a blood culture, treatment should begin with an anti-*Staphylococcal* antibiotic.

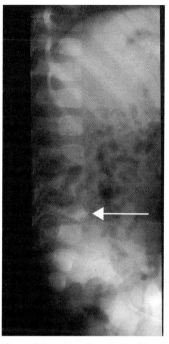

Fig. 1.5.8 Lateral X-ray of the spine of a patient with tuberculous vertebral osteomyelitis. There is destruction and loss of height of the L5 vertebral body with narrowing of the adjacent L5/S1 interspace with irregularity of the inferior end plate of L5. (Courtesy of T.R. Southwood.)

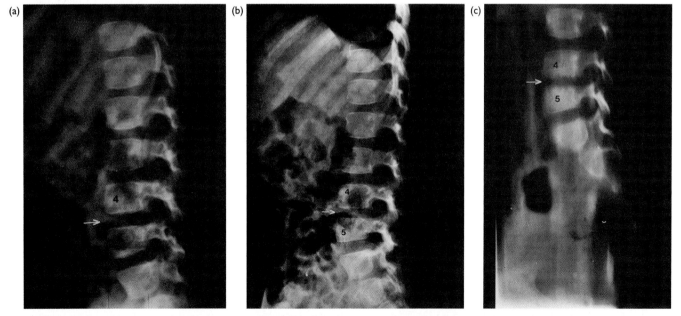

Fig. 1.5.9 Radiographic progression of discitis in a 4-year-old girl. The illness began with a limp in late February and progressed to refusal to walk and then to sit up in bed. Films pictured are from March 5 and 23 and April 20. The initial X-ray (a) is normal. The intermediate film (b) shows the beginning of narrowing of the L4–5 disc that was too subtle to be recognized. Film 4 weeks later (c) shows obvious narrowing of the disk space with erosions of both adjacent vertebral endplates, a typical radiographic progression of discitis. (From J. Jacobs.)

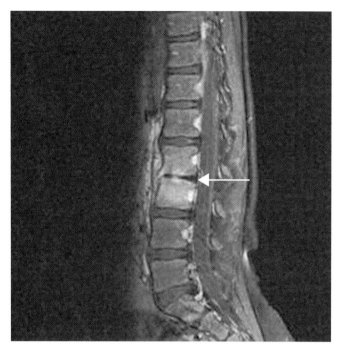

Fig. 1.5.10 This 5-year-old girl developed hip pain without fever which progressed over ensuing weeks so that she appeared to have a "pregnant walk," according to the mother. X-rays of her hips and spine were normal, but she had an ESR of 87. Hip MRI was normal. Finally, a bone scan was done which revealed increased uptake involving L2 and L3, following which an MRI confirmed the diagnosis of discitis, which showed loss of intervertebral disc space height at L2–3 (see arrow) with abnormal T2 hyperintensity involving the vertebral bodies of L2 and L3, as well as enhancing soft-tissue material encompassing the L2–3 intervertebral disc space anteriorly. Interestingly, her younger brother was diagnosed at the time of her initial symptoms with a Brodie abscess of the distal tibia (see Figure 1.5.12), and initially her symptoms were thought to be attention-seeking behaviour.

Although extension of the infection to the adjacent vertebral bodies and subsequent vertebral osteomyelitis are well documented, in many series of untreated children, the course is surprisingly benign [12], leading some to question the infectious aetiology of discitis. Despite this, most experts currently advocate antibiotic treatment for this disorder.

Subacute osteomyelitis

Some children with acute osteomyelitis may improve, even without treatment, and then go on to develop subacute osteomyelitis. More commonly, however, children are given antibiotics for another concomitant infection such as otitis media, thereby partially treating the osteomyelitis, which recurs again when the antibiotics are discontinued. The signs of subacute osteomyelitis are usually limited to minimal tenderness and local heat, but when these bone infections are in or near the knee or ankle joints, they are frequently associated with a knee or ankle effusion and may easily be mistaken for Oligoarthritis. X-rays may be helpful in this situation, but may take months to demonstrate a typical Brodie abscess (Figure 1.5.11). An MRI should be done if this is suspected (Figure 1.5.12). Therefore, in selected patients with monoarticular arthritis who have a history of being treated with antibiotics just prior to the onset of the arthritis,

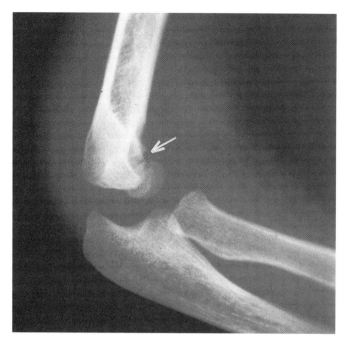

Fig. 1.5.11 Cystic osteomyelitis (Brodie abscess) of the distal femoral epiphysis, which presented with a monarticular knee effusion. These lesions are sometimes mistaken for tumours. (From J. Jacobs.)

an MRI may be indicated to rule out subacute osteomyelitis of adjacent bone.

Osteomyelitis following puncture wounds of the foot

A unique form of osteomyelitis is seen following puncture wounds, primarily of the feet. The usual history is recurrence of pain after a puncture wound has improved, usually days to weeks later. The puncture may be as trivial as an insect bite, or may be completely unnoticed. Most, but not all of these puncture wound infections, are caused by *Pseudomonas*, especially if the penetration occurred through the sole of a sneaker or shoe. *Pseudomonas* appears to cause an osteochondritis rather than a true osteomyelitis, primarily because of this organism's predilection to infect cartilage. Simple surgical debridement and a short course of an anti-*Pseudomonas* antibiotic may be sufficient to cure this infection. Less commonly, other organisms including atypical mycobacteria have been reported. As in other causes of osteomyelitis, debridement and culture must be performed prior to the institution of antibiotic therapy in order to identify the responsible organism.

Chronic osteomyelitis

Fortunately, this complication of inadequately treated acute or subacute osteomyelitis is now rare. Patients usually present with a non-functioning, painful extremity and a sinus tract in the involved limb, which chronically drains purulent material. Cultures usually grow *Staph. aureus*. X-rays often reveal the presence of a necrotic bone (the sequestrum) which requires surgical debridement. These patients need prolonged treatment with antibiotics, which unfortunately often fails to cure the infection permanently. Prevention of chronic osteomyelitis is one of the most important reasons for making certain that patients with acute osteomyelitis are treated appropriately from the onset.

(a)

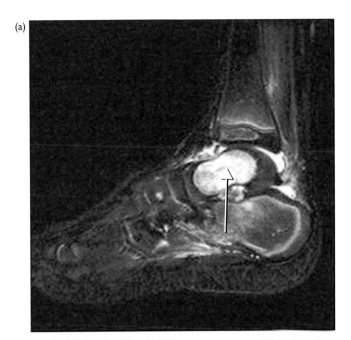

(b)

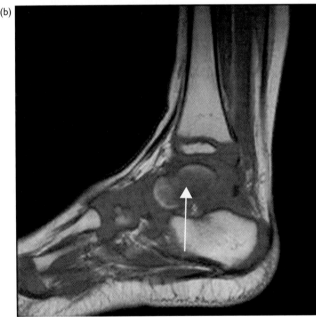

Fig. 1.5.12 This 20-month-old boy suddenly developed non-weight bearing of the right foot that continued for 3 weeks, not associated with fever. He began crawling instead of walking. He then developed fever to 103 and swelling of the ankle, which was aspirated and was clear. X-rays and WBC were normal, but the ESR was 50. On examination, he was playful, but could bear weight only momentarily if holding on, and the right ankle was very swollen and warm. There was no discernable point tenderness. (a) An MRI with STIR images was done and revealed fluid in the ankle joint and abnormal signal intensity within the ossified portion of the talus, consistent with a Brodie abscess. (b) The regular T1 weighted images show decreased signal within the ossified talus because of replacement of normal fatty marrow. The bone aspirate grew *Staph. aureus*. Interestingly, his 5-year-old sister developed discitis during the same period of time (see Figure 1.5.10).

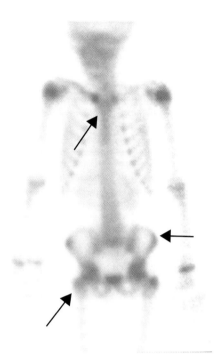

Fig. 1.5.13 This 7-year-old girl had been previously diagnosed with osteomyelitis of her toe, which was found to be sterile. Several months later, she developed back pain. A bone scan was performed, which revealed increased uptake (arrows) in the right iliac bone, left greater trochanter, and the right clavicle, consistent with a diagnosis of chronic recurrent multifocal ostemyelitis. (Courtesy of K. A. Haines.)

Chronic recurrent multifocal osteomyelitis

Chronic Recurrent Multifocal Osteomyelitis (CRMO) is not an infection, but a chronic inflammatory disorder of bone that is characterized by recurrent attacks of bone pain lasting from 1 to 12 weeks and is associated with radiographic evidence of multifocal osteolytic lesions, which are sterile (Figure 1.5.13) [14]. These lesions are most frequent in the clavicles (Figure 1.5.14) and in the distal metaphyses of long bones, but may also occur in the spine. There may be local and systemic signs of inflammation, but there is no response to antibiotics. The clinical course may be prolonged, often lasting years, and is characterized by relapses and remissions. Most patients have been reported to respond to nonsteroidal anti-inflammatory drugs (NSAIDs), but some may need treatment with corticosteroids. Other treatments reported to be of benefit include alpha-interferon, calcitonin, and bisphosphonates.

In some children, CRMO has been associated with sterile pustular lesions of the palms and soles—palmoplantar pustulosis. Some of these patients may evolve into the so-called SAPHO Syndrome (synovitis, acne, pustulosis, hyperostosis, and osteitis) (Figure 1.5.15) [15]. It has also been suggested that CRMO may evolve into ERA [16].

Septic arthritis

Acute septic arthritis

Like osteomyelitis, septic arthritis is an important differential to consider in any patient who presents with a single swollen joint, especially when fever is present. About one-third of all cases of septic arthritis occur in children. Seventy-five percent of cases affect large weight-bearing joints such as the knee, hip, and ankle (Table 1.5.6).

Large joints of the upper extremity (elbow, wrist, and shoulder) make up almost all of the other affected joints, with the elbow involved two to three times as frequently as the shoulder or the wrist [17–21]. Less commonly, other joints, such as the sacroiliac joint or symphysis pubis, can be affected (Figure 1.5.16).

The typical presentation is an acutely painful, tender, and warm joint with associated muscle spasm and severe limitation of motion in a patient with fever (Table 1.5.4). Although patients with Oligoarthritis may also present with a single swollen joint, there is usually no accompanying fever and the arthritis does not present as acutely. Systemic Arthritis, on the other hand, typically does present with high fever, and occasionally with monoarticular arthritis, making the distinction between septic arthritis and Systemic Arthritis difficult. However, the joint in Systemic Arthritis is not quite as "hot" and acutely painful as in septic arthritis, and the quotidian pattern of fever and the rash typical of Systemic Arthritis would not be expected to be features of septic arthritis. Lastly, patients with reactive arthritis and patients with acute rheumatic fever may also present both with fever and acute joint swelling, making it difficult at times to distinguish these conditions from septic arthritis.

Radiographic tests may help, but the results are usually nonspecific. X-rays of septic joints are initially normal, or may show widening of the joint space (Figure 1.5.17), and are occasionally helpful in disclosing some other cause for these symptoms such as a fracture or a radiopaque foreign body in the joint. Bone scans (Figure 1.5.18) show increased uptake on both sides of the joint, rather than in a single focus in the bone, which would be more suggestive of osteomyelitis. MRI is useful in ruling out the presence of osteomyelitis, but other than disclosing the presence of fluid in the joint, does not have specific findings for acute septic arthritis. However, ultrasonograms can be helpful in children with hip involvement, because it can identify the presence of fluid, which cannot be detected on physical examination of the hip (Figure 1.5.19). Although the presence of fluid is not diagnostic of infection, and may simply be an indicator of inflammation, it does help to narrow down the causes of hip pain and dysfunction (see Part 1, Chapter 1.3, Table 1.3.4, "The Child with Hip Pain").

(a)

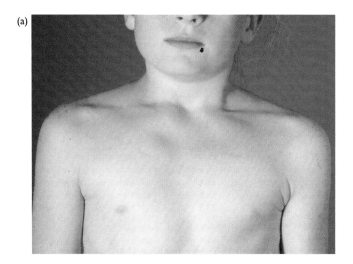

(b)

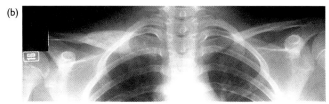

Fig. 1.5.14 (a) This young boy developed hyperostosis of the right clavicle, a typical location of bony involvement in CRMO. AP view of the clavicles (b) radiograph shows expansion, inhomogeneity, and sclerosis of the medial half of the right clavicle, consistent with the diagnosis of CRMO. (Courtesy of T.R. Southwood.)

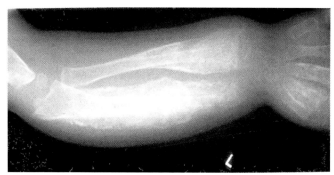

Fig. 1.5.15 X-ray of a patient with SAPHO syndrome reveals marked periosteal reaction involving the radial and ulnar shafts as well as the third and fourth metacarpals. Expansion of contour, and in places, complete obscuration of the underlying normal contour has occurred. (Courtesy of T.R. Southwood.)

Table 1.5.6 Distribution of joints affected in septic arthritis (%)

	Fink [2] (n = 646)	Christiansen [3] (n = 48)	Speiser [18] (n = 86)	Nelson [17] (n = 136)	Welkon [19] (n = 95)
Knee	40	48	30	44	49
Hip	23	17	29	14	27
Ankle	13	2	17	17	17
Elbow	14	10	11	12	9 (shoulder or elbow)
Shoulder	4	NR	2	6	
Wrist	4	NR	1	6	NR
Hand/foot	1	NR	10	1	NR
Other	1	8	NR	NR	5

NR = not reported.

(a)

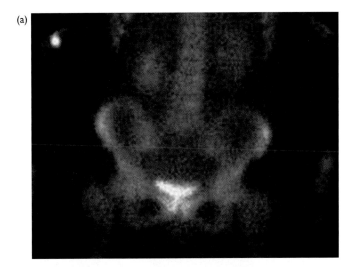

(b)

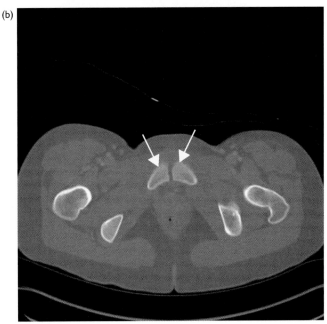

Fig. 1.5.16 This 16-year-old female developed bilateral groin pain, which worsened over the next few days so that at times she was unable to sit up or stand. She then developed chills and fevers to 103. An ultrasound examination of the pelvis was normal at another hospital, as was an MRI of the pelvis. However, the ESR was 127, and the WBC was 8.0 with 25% bands. On examination, she had severe pain and was unable to even sit up. There was lower abdominal tenderness with mild rebound and pronounced tenderness of the suprapubic area. The hip examination was normal. (a) A bone scan revealed increased uptake on either side of the symphysis pubis. (b) A CT scan showed irregularity of the anterior aspect of both sides of the symphysis pubis, and a fluid collection in the same area with edema in the soft tissue anterior to the pubic symphysis. Both a blood culture and joint fluid culture were positive for *Staph. aureus*.

In any child in whom septic arthritis is suspected, aspiration of the affected joint must be performed. The fluid should be examined for cell count, Gram's stain, culture, glucose, and protein. Typically, the fluid is grossly purulent, with WBCs of >50,000/mm³. However, since very high synovial WBCs can also be seen in inflammatory arthritis, this test may not distinguish between septic arthritis and JIA. In septic arthritis, the glucose level is usually quite low and protein level is high

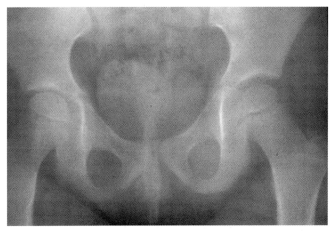

Fig. 1.5.17 This is an AP view of the pelvis in a boy with septic arthritis of the left hip, which shows widening of the joint space as well as displacement of the femoral head relative to the acetabulum. (Courtesy of T.R. Southwood.)

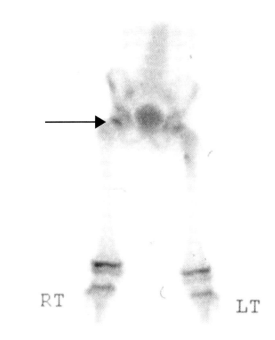

Fig. 1.5.18 Bone scan of septic arthritis of the right hip, which shows increased uptake of both the right femoral head as well as acetabulum. (Courtesy of T.R. Southwood.)

(Table 1.5.4). The Gram stain and culture are usually positive, but the incidence of culture negative joint fluid in septic arthritis ranges from as high as 70% [21] to the more commonly reported values of 30–40% [2,17–20,22].

When the hip joint is involved, surgical decompression should be performed regardless of whether the infection is primarily in the joint (i.e. septic arthritis), or secondary to osteomyelitis of the femur. All other joints may need to be aspirated repeatedly in order to keep the pressure in the joint low, although this approach remains controversial [22,23]. Surgical drainage usually needs to be performed in cases where there has been an unsatisfactory clinical response to antibiotics alone.

(a)

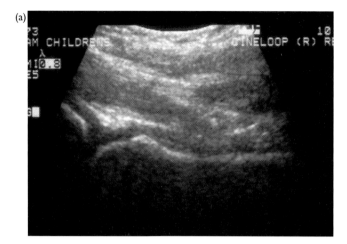

(b)

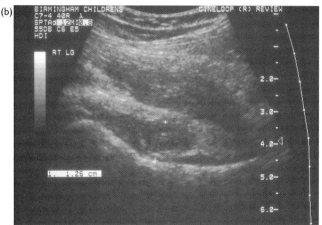

Fig. 1.5.19 (a) Normal hip ultrasound. (b) In contrast, in this ultrasound of the hip, there is elevation of the joint capsule by relatively hypoechoic material, which is consistent with a joint effusion. (Courtesy of T.R. Southwood.)

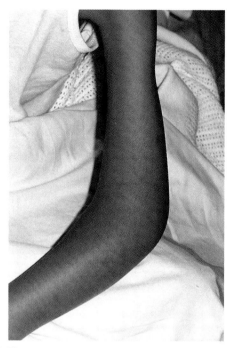

Fig. 1.5.20 This youngster with known sickle-cell disease developed sudden onset of elbow pain, swelling, and fever. Aspiration of the joint revealed a high WBC and a positive Gram stain for Gram-negative rods. The culture subsequently grew *Salmonella*. (Courtesy of T.R. Southwood.)

In areas of the world where infants are routinely immunized against *Hemophilus influenzae*, *Staph. aureus* is almost always the causative agent. However, among nonimmunized individuals, especially young infants, *H. influenzae* should be considered. As in osteomyelitis, septic arthritis in children is usually a consequence of bacteremia rather than an extension of a local injury, except in the occasional patient with *Pseudomonas* arthritis in the metatarsophalangeal (MTP) joint following puncture wounds of the foot (see "Puncture wounds of the feet" above). In children with sickle-cell disease, antibiotic coverage for *Salmonella* is important (Figure 1.5.20).

As soon as the diagnosis is made clinically and both a blood culture and joint aspirate have been obtained for culture, treatment should be started with intravenous anti-*Staphylococcal* antibiotics. However, if either the hip or shoulder joint is involved, infection of an adjacent bone is likely high, because of the placement of the metaphysis within the joint capsule in these locations. In this situation, there should be an assessment for bone involvement with an MRI, and if suspected, bone aspiration should be performed prior to starting antibiotics. Antibiotics should be continued for 3 weeks (unless osteomyelitis is present, when the treatment should be continued for at least 6 weeks), or until the ESR has returned to normal and all clinical findings have resolved.

Prolonged immobilization is probably unnecessary [23] but may be used for a day or two to lessen pain with movement. Physical therapy should be encouraged as soon as possible to prevent contractures, and NSAID therapy may be added during the recovery period when postinfectious inflammatory synovitis and/or reactive arthritis contribute to the symptoms.

Septic arthritis and immunodeficiencies

Patients with congenital and acquired immunodeficiencies, such as those secondary to human immunodeficiency virus (HIV), chronic granulomatous disease, hypo- or agammaglobulinaemia, may be at increased risk for musculoskeletal infections, particularly septic arthritis. The infections are often due to the same bacteria seen in immunocompetent patients, but can also be caused by less common organisms such as Candida, mycoplasma, or ureaplasma. The possibility that unique aetiological agents may be responsible makes precise microbiologic diagnosis particularly critical in this population. Conversely, all patients with musculoskeletal infections involving unusual organisms, or with a history of recurrent infections or suspicious symptoms or signs (diffuse lymphadenopathy, candidiasis, weight loss, lymphopenia, hyper- or hypogammaglobulinaemia) should undergo a prompt work-up for possible immunodeficiency (see Part 1, Chapter 1.10).

The gonococcal arthritis–dermatitis–tenosynovitis syndrome

Disseminated gonococcal infection is a common cause of infectious arthritis or tenosynovitis in sexually active women. The usual clinical presentation consists of a migratory or additive polyarthritis with fever and chills, often starting 1 week after menses. The arthritis tends to localize to one or two large joints. Painful crops of skin lesions appear, primarily on the extremities. These lesions characteristically begin as a macule or a small purpuric spot and progress through a papular–vesicular stage to a pustule. Many patients develop painful tenosynovitis, often involving the wrists and appearing as tender erythema overlying the tendon sheaths.

Diagnosis is usually made on the basis of the characteristic clinical syndrome [24]. Cultures of the blood, genitourinary tract, throat, and/or rectum are positive in less than 50% of cases. Although all patients are presumed to have septicaemia, the arthritis is usually sterile and is therefore most likely secondary to immune-complex disease. The response to appropriate antibiotic treatment is usually prompt.

The clinical picture of chronic meningococcaemia is similar, with sterile effusions commonly seen [25]. Joint damage is usually insignificant in these cases even when the joint is truly infected.

Tuberculosis

Tuberculosis of the bones and joints should always be considered in the differential diagnosis of arthritis in children. In addition to typical mycobacteria, atypical organisms have been reported in children with immunodeficiencies, and are occasionally reported secondary to dissemination from BCG (*Bacillus Camille-Guérin*) vaccination. Because tuberculous arthritis is not an acute, febrile illness, it can be confused with Oligoarthritis (Figure 1.5.21). Indeed, a recent report of several children with tuberculous arthritis from one center demonstrates how easily a mistaken diagnosis of Oligoarthritis can be made [26]. The tuberculin test is a simple screen which should ideally be performed in all children presenting with arthritis with or without

fever. Tuberculous osteomyelitis can occur as well, and the spine can be affected (Pott disease) (Figure 1.5.8). In addition to primary infection of the bones and joints, tuberculous rheumatism, or Poncet disease, is a reactive polyarthritis secondary to tuberculosis which is occasionally seen.

Lyme arthritis

Lyme arthritis is a late manifestation of Lyme disease (Table 1.5.7), the most common tick-borne infection in the United States, and is caused by the spirochete *Borrelia burgdorferi*. Interestingly, the initial cases were in children: an "epidemic" of Juvenile Rheumatoid Arthritis (JRA) was reported to health authorities by the mother of one child in Old Lyme, Connecticut, and led to recognition of the disorder as an entity. Although all of the children were initially thought to have JRA, none of them had persistent arthritis for at least 6 weeks; a requirement for the diagnosis of JRA/JIA, demonstrating the importance of this criterion. In fact, as opposed to children with Oligoarthritis (the type most commonly confused with Lyme arthritis) who have chronic persistent synovitis, children with Lyme arthritis generally have recurrent brief episodes of joint swelling, most often of the knees, lasting from a few days to a few weeks. In addition, the arthritis is usually not accompanied by much pain, despite the large effusions that are typical of Lyme arthritis (Figure 1.5.22).

Infections are most common in the north-eastern United States, from Cape Cod to southern New Jersey, and have also been reported in areas of northern California, Oregon, Minnesota, Wisconsin, Georgia, and Nevada, as well as in Europe, Asia, and Australia. The tick, usually an *Ixodes* spp. (Figure 1.5.23), must be attached to the host for a minimum of 36–48 h in order to successfully transmit *B. burgdorferi* infection [27].

(a)
(b)

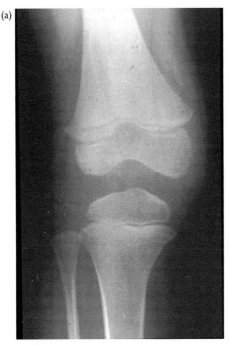
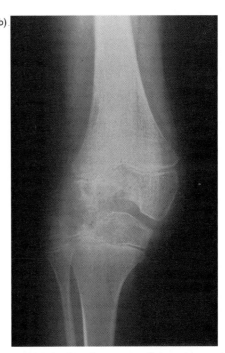

Fig. 1.5.21 Although the initial X-ray (a) in this patient who was eventually diagnosed with tuberculous septic arthritis was normal, 3 years later (b), there is joint space loss of the lateral compartment and apposition of the distal femur and proximal tibial epiphyses, which are irregular in contour and have erosive changes. (Courtesy of T.R. Southwood.)

Table 1.5.7 Clues to the diagnosis of Lyme disease

Acute Phase (first few weeks after tick bite; usually late spring, summer, early autumn)	History of a tick bite in an endemic area EM (a distinctive red expanding circular skin lesion up to 20 inches in diameter, up to 1 month after the bite) Flu-like illness (fever, arthralgias, and myalgias)
Late Phase (weeks to months after tick bite)	Episodic large effusion(s) of large joints, especially knees Neurological manifestations (Bell palsy, peripheral neuropathy, aseptic meningitis, pseudotumor cerebri) Cardiac arrhythmias (especially atrioventricular (AV) conduction defects)

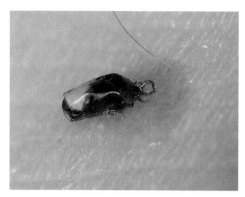

Fig. 1.5.23 Appearance of the deer tick (*Ixodes scapularis*). (Courtesy of T.R. Southwood.)

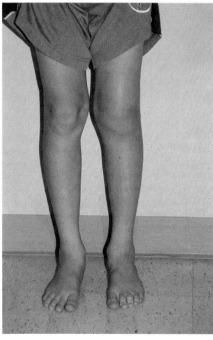

Fig. 1.5.22 This 10-year-old girl had recurrent left knee swelling. She had one previous episode of knee swelling 3 months before which lasted for a week and then disappeared without treatment. On examination, she had an enormous effusion of her left knee, without much tenderness or pain on motion. She had been to a camp in southern New York State 6 months before, but did not recall a tick bite or rash. Her Lyme titre was positive, however, and her Western blot revealed the presence of 10 bands, consistent with the presence of true Lyme antibody. She was treated with a 4-week course of oral antibiotics with complete resolution of her symptoms.

Early localized disease

A characteristic skin lesion, erythema migrans (EM), occurs at the site(s) of the tick bite in an estimated 40–50% of patients who are infected. EM consists of a circular erythematous lesion, often with a pale centre, that may grow in diameter over a period of days or weeks to a distinctive bright red expanding circle 3–20 inches in diameter (Figure 1.5.24(a) and (b)). In some cases, multiple lesions may appear in various locations, presumably as a result of spirochetemia. EM occurs days to weeks following the tick bite, and is often associated with fever, myalgias, and arthralgias, constituting a short-lived and

(a)

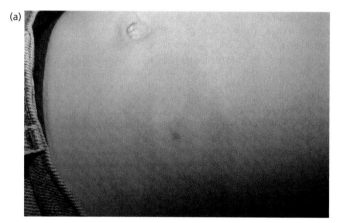

(b)

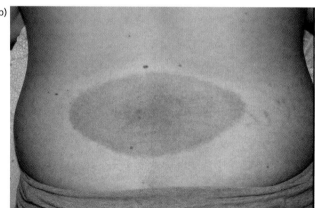

Fig. 1.5.24 Erythema migrans, the characteristic dermal manifestation of acute Lyme disease that may later be followed weeks or months later by arthritis, neurological, and sometimes cardiac manifestations. This rash usually begins at the site of the tick bite, where there may be a papule, (a) and spreads concentrically to a large diameter (3–20 in.) during the next few days to a week with central clearing, causing the typical "bulls eye" appearance (b). During this time, the patient may have a flu-like illness with fever, fatigue, myalgias, and arthralgias.

self-limited "flu-like" illness in the late spring, summer, and early fall months.

Early disseminated disease

Some patients develop neurological or cardiac abnormalities several weeks following the acute infection. Early neurological Lyme disease includes meningoencephalitis, cranial neuropathy (most commonly unilateral or bilateral facial nerve palsy), and/or radiculoneuropathy. The most common cardiac manifestations are atrioventricular conduction defects, but rarely, myocarditis has also been reported.

Late persistent disease

Weeks to months (occasionally years) after the initial infection, a small percentage of untreated patients develop late sequelae of Lyme disease, most commonly recurrent arthritis. Lyme arthritis is classically manifested by brief, intermittent, acute synovitis. Typically, there is a sudden onset of a large, obvious effusion lasting several days to weeks which then resolves spontaneously, only to recur again days, weeks, or months later, unless the patient receives appropriate treatment. Large weight-bearing joints, most often the knee, are most commonly affected. Occasionally, more than one joint is involved, but this is rare. In fact, it is often confused with Oligoarthritis because of the mono- or oligoarticular pattern of joint involvement. However, unlike patients with Lyme arthritis, children with JIA have chronic and persistent, not intermittent, swelling of their joints with early flexion contractures and synovial thickening. Interestingly, despite the degree of swelling usually present, patients with Lyme arthritis usually report little pain or stiffness. Systemic symptoms, such as fever, are not present at the time the arthritis develops, and involvement of small joints (such as the finger joints) does not occur. Acute phase reactants such as the ESR may be elevated.

Chronic neurological and skin manifestations also occur, but are much less common than arthritis. The incidence of chronic Lyme encephalopathy, characterized by neuropsychiatric manifestations such as headaches, fatigue, memory lapses, and depression is debated; a few controlled studies of patients treated with longer than standard antibiotic courses have not shown clinical efficacy [28]. Rarely, patients develop a late skin lesion called acrodermatitis chronica atrophicans which resembles morphea, a form of localized scleroderma.

Diagnosis

The diagnosis of Lyme disease should be reserved only for patients who have an appropriate clinical presentation, and live in, or have travelled to, endemic areas (Table 1.5.7) and have positive laboratory evidence. Serologic diagnosis involves a two-step process, an enzyme immunoassay (EIA), followed by a confirmatory immunoblot, or Western blot, if the EIA is positive [29]. A Lyme EIA which is indeterminate or positive with a negative Western blot is considered a false positive test.

Early in the disease course (within a month after the acute infection), the Lyme IgG EIA may not yet be positive, unless the patient has been exposed previously. At this point in the illness, the Lyme IgM may be positive, but this is not a reliable test and can be often falsely positive. However, by the time a patient develops arthritis (a later finding), high levels of IgG antibodies can almost always be detected, and the Western blot is highly positive, with the presence of multiple specific bands. The Center for Disease Control in the United States requires the presence of five or more typical IgG bands in the Western blot to confirm the presence of true Lyme antibody.

A caveat is that as many as 20% or more of healthy, asymptomatic individuals who live in a Lyme endemic area may test positive for the antibody. Therefore, seropositivity alone does not mean that the patient's symptoms are necessarily due to Lyme disease. If the patient does not have a clinical syndrome typical of Lyme disease, even if the patient is seropositive, further work-up for other causes of the patient's symptoms should be undertaken. Testing during the acute phase (the first 4 weeks after the tick bite) is not useful except for demonstrating prior serologic status. Other testing methods, such as polymerase chain reaction (PCR), have not been standardized and do not always correlate with active infection. A urine antigen test for Lyme has been popularized by some practitioners, but has not been approved for use and has been found to be associated with frequent false positive results [30].

Treatment

Oral antibiotics are sufficient to treat most cases of Lyme disease, whether in the early or late stages. Treatment consists of oral doxycycline for patients over 9 years of age, amoxicillin or a macrolide antibiotic (for penicillin-allergic patients) for those 8 years and younger, for a duration of 2–4 weeks [31]. Patients with definite neuroborreliosis (i.e. meningitis, meningoencephalitis, or facial nerve palsy associated with meningitis) should be treated with intravenous ceftriaxone for a total of 4 weeks. Occasionally, there are patients with Lyme arthritis who do not respond or who relapse following treatment with a month of oral antibiotic therapy, and need to be treated with intravenous antibiotics. Many patients with adequately treated Lyme arthritis may have persistent mild but asymptomatic swelling. Retreatment should only be considered after at least 3 months have elapsed. Although some physicians prescribe prolonged treatment with IV or oral antibiotics, there is no evidence that more than a 4-week course is of added benefit.

Prevention and prognosis

The infection may be prevented by careful daily checks for ticks, as it has been shown that 36–48 h of attachment must occur for successful transmission of the infection to the human host [27]. Lyme vaccine may reduce the risk of infection by 70%, but has been recently withdrawn because of poor demand fueled by controversy regarding possible side effects of immunization.

The prognosis for children with Lyme arthritis is excellent, and full recovery without residua should be expected [32]. However, there are patients with Lyme arthritis who have gone on to develop antibiotic-resistant chronic erosive arthritis which is pathologically indistinguishable from rheumatoid arthritis, after 4–24 months of recurrent transient attacks of arthritis. Susceptibility to chronic arthritis appears to be enhanced by the presence of the *HLA DR4* allele. These patients appear to have excessive T cell response to the infection [33].

Viral arthritis

Arthritis may be associated with, or follow, a variety of viral illnesses. The literature is replete with reports of transient arthritis associated with documented mumps, varicella, rubella, parvovirus B19, coxsackie, ECHO, alpha viruses, adenovirus, herpesvirus, Epstein–Barr virus,

Table 1.5.8 Causes of viral arthritis and principal extra-articular manifestations

Clinical symptoms	Causative agent	Diagnostic test
"Slapped cheek" rash on face and reticular rash on extremities +/− fever preceding the arthritis	Parvovirus B19	Parvovirus B19 IgM Parvovirus PCR
Typical maculopapular rash beginning at the hairline and lymphadenopathy	Rubella	Rubella IgM
Urticarial or maculopapular rash and arthritis preceding clinical jaundice	Hepatitis viruses	Hepatitis virus A or B IgM
Typical crops of vesicular skin lesions fever preceding arthritis	Varicella	Varicella IgM and IFA from lesion
Typical vesicular rash on palms, soles, and pharynx	Coxsackievirus	Coxsackie IgM Viral culture
Exudative pharyngitis, fever, lymphadenopathy, and splenomegaly	Epstein–Barr virus	Atypical lymphocytes on blood smear Heterophile antibody EBV VCA IgM
Exudative pharyngitis and lymphadenopathy	Cytomegalovirus	CMV IgM Urine viral culture
Exudative conjunctivitis, fever	Adenovirus	Viral culture of nasopharynx or conjunctivae
Typical painful oral or genital vesicles	Herpesvirus	Herpes IgM Viral culture of unroofed vesicle
Arthritis and variable rash that lasts for 1–2 weeks (mostly in Australia and South Pacific)	Alphaviruses	Alphavirus IgM

hepatitis A, B, and C, cytomegalovirus, vaccinia, and smallpox (Table 1.5.8).

Several different pathogenic mechanisms may be operative in viral arthritis. Rarely, as in vaccinia, the arthritis is a result of direct viral invasion of synovial tissue, causing local inflammation and cell necrosis. Arthritis caused by other viruses, such as rubella, probably results from local host immune response to the virus or viral products in the joint space. In most cases, however, the pathogenic mechanism is probably a systemic serum sickness-like reaction, as in hepatitis, with formation of immune complexes that are demonstrable in both serum and synovial fluid. Non-necrotizing vasculitis may be seen in synovial membrane biopsy specimens obtained from these patients.

Viral arthritis may vary in severity and course, and may affect any number of joints. It may therefore resemble septic arthritis, migratory arthritis as in acute rheumatic fever, or be mistaken for drug allergy or rheumatoid arthritis. Cases may be sporadic or epidemic. The process is generally brief, although occasional patients may have intermittent symptoms for a year, usually with a decrescendo quality.

When arthritis has the benign quality typical of most viral arthritis, or if the etiology of the underlying illness is apparent because of a viral exanthem or other distinctive clinical feature, the list of possible causes is often short. However, 24% of children with osteomyelitis in one series had been misdiagnosed initially as having a viral illness (Table 1.5.1) [1]. Even the most experienced physician may have difficulty in distinguishing septic from viral arthritis when only a single joint is affected, so if there is consideration of septic arthritis or osteomyelitis, the joint should be aspirated and a bone scan or MRI ordered to evaluate the possibility of osteomyelitis. The synovial fluid is generally "benign" in viral infections and often contains a preponderance of mononuclear cells.

Three distinctive viral arthritis syndromes deserve special emphasis: Parvovirus B19, hepatitis, and rubella.

Parvovirus B19

Parvovirus B19 causes a variety of clinical syndromes: epidemic erythema infectiosum or Fifth ("slapped cheek") disease (Figure 1.5.25), aplastic crises in children with hemolytic anemia, hydrops fetalis, and arthritis. In adult women, arthropathy occurs in 60% of cases, while in adult men it is less common (30%). Arthropathy is even less common in children (less than 10% of those infected) [34]. Attacks of pain and swelling in the small joints of the hands and feet occur soon after the onset of the typical rash. The arthritis is usually brief and self-limited, lasting less than 10 days. Although polyarthritis affecting the small joints is most common, especially in adults, any joint can be affected. Young children tend to have arthritis in only a few joints. Some patients have recurrent episodes of arthritis, each less severe and of shorter duration than the prior attack (similar to rubella). The brief duration of the arthritis and the rash that precedes it differentiates parvovirus arthritis from JIA. In adolescent females, systemic lupus erythematosus (SLE) is an important diagnostic consideration, as the clinical features (facial rash and arthritis) can be similar, and transiently positive antinuclear antibody (ANA) and even anti-DNA antibody have been reported [35]. It should be noted that various rashes have been associated with parvovirus infection, including petechial, purpuric, or nonspecific maculopapular eruptions. Therefore, any rash preceding the onset of arthritis should raise the possibility for parvovirus infection.

Since up to 30% of the general population have antibodies to parvovirus as adults, acute arthritis due to parvovirus is probably quite common. Live virus has not been recovered from joint fluid, but parvovirus B19 DNA has been detected in the joint fluid of affected individuals through the use of PCR. Joint symptoms occur less frequently in children infected with Parvovirus, but the exact incidence is not known. Although acute transient arthritis is the rule, about 10% of adult women go on to develop a chronic arthritis indistinguishable from rheumatoid arthritis. As in adults, parvovirus B19 has been suggested as a possible cause of some cases of chronic arthritis in children [36].

The spectrum of disease caused by parvovirus B19 is still expanding. In addition to its implication in the possible etiology of rheumatoid arthritis, Parvovirus B19 has been associated with, or reported in, children with Kawasaki disease, Henoch–Schönlein purpura, polyarteritis nodosa, systemic lupus erythematosus, and Wegener granulomatosis.

Hepatitis viruses

Acute polyarthritis and rash may be a prodrome of hepatitis A, B, or C infection. Serum complement levels are low, and the phenomenon seems similar to serum sickness (Part 1, Chapter 1.4). It subsides as jaundice appears and hepatitis becomes clinically apparent. The arthritis may be quite severe and may precede other manifestations by weeks. The rash may be urticarial but is often maculopapular and sometimes petechial. Immune-complex nephritis occasionally occurs, causing a hepatorenal syndrome.

Both circulating and tissue-fixed complement-binding viral antigen–antibody complexes have been demonstrated in association with this syndrome. When it is secondary to hepatitis B, up to 30% of patients may have these immune complexes [37]. Although acute polyarthritis was initially associated specifically with hepatitis B infection, there is increasing evidence of similar syndromes occurring with hepatitis A and C infection, as well as an association with the development of autoimmune hepatitis, vasculitis, and cryoglobulinemia [38]. In addition, there have been occasional reports of arthritis, mostly of the benign reactive type, following hepatitis B vaccination.

Rubella: the "catcher's crouch" syndrome

Brief episodes of polyarthritis are commonly seen in epidemic rubella; adult women are much more prone to developing rubella-associated arthritis than children. Occasionally, the arthritis precedes other clinical manifestations, but usually it accompanies the rash or follows it by only a few days. Most patients improve within 2 weeks. Rubella-associated arthritis is rare in countries where there is universal vaccination in children.

Rubella vaccine has been reported to cause arthritis, but this is uncommon, as current strains have been developed to have minimal potential to cause arthritis. When children do develop rubella vaccine arthritis, they often have a rather distinctive syndrome. They awake in the morning with pain in the knees out of proportion to visible swelling, and they stand with the knees flexed. This position has been termed the "catcher's crouch" [39]. Tenosynovitis may also be seen over the dorsum of the hands. There may be an associated neuritis, primarily manifested as painful paraesthesias of the hands or feet. The history of recent immunization, characteristic morning stance, and unusual neuritis generally make the correct diagnosis apparent.

Other infections that mimic septic arthritis or osteomyelitis

Suppurative prepatellar bursitis

Infection of the patella must be differentiated from suppurative prepatellar bursitis, a complication of "housemaid's" or "football-player's" knee. In suppurative prepatellar bursitis, the bursa generally appears tensely swollen and obviously infected (Figure 1.5.26); this clinical impression can be confirmed by aspiration of purulent material from the bursa. A similar lesion, "student's elbow," is occasionally seen at

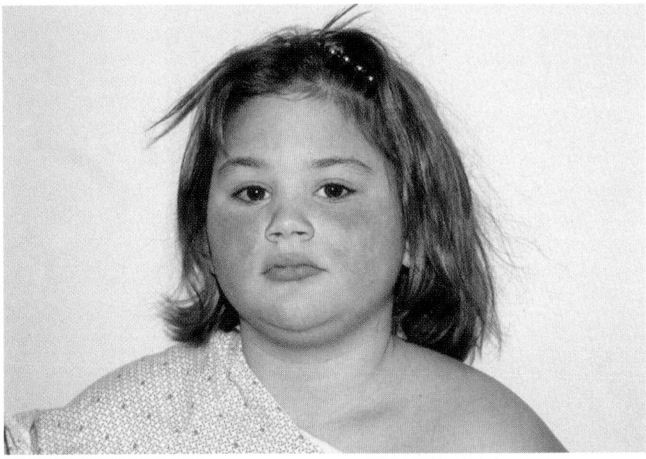

Fig. 1.5.25 This 12-year-old girl was referred with a diagnosis of lupus because of the sudden onset of facial rash, fatigue, polyarticular arthritis, and a positive ANA. However, she was found to have a positive Parvovirus B19 IgM, and eventually her symptoms resolved without treatment.

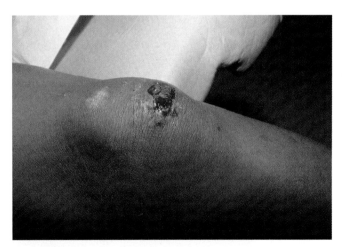

Fig. 1.5.26 This young patient developed knee pain, swelling, and fever. However, the pain and swelling were all anterior to the patella, and did not involve the knee joint. The patient was able to ambulate, and the range of motion of the knee was not greatly affected. Aspiration of the prepatellar bursa revealed pus, confirming the diagnosis of prepatellar bursitis.

the olecranon bursa. Septic bursitis generally responds well to oral antibiotics after aspiration. Bursitis is exceedingly rare in young children.

Suppurative iliac lymphadenitis and retroperitoneal (psoas) abscess

These infections may simulate osteomyelitis of the pelvic bones or septic arthritis of the hip. In general, however, the clinical picture is less acute, so that the child often limps, complaining of vague hip, back, and abdominal pain, and low-grade fever for a week or two prior to admission to the hospital. In contrast to the patient with a septic hip, in whom hip range of motion is extremely limited by pain in all directions, these children have little pain with hip abduction and adduction, but great pain when the hip is extended. Computed tomography (CT) scan of the abdomen and pelvis is the most reliable imaging test for confirming the correct diagnoses.

Pyomyositis

The clinical picture of pyomyositis is that of a toxic-appearing child with severe pain and an enlarging area of erythema, tenderness, and swelling in one or both thighs. Although the affected muscle is extremely tender, there is no localized bone pain, which differentiates this infection from osteomyelitis. In some cases, there is a history of trauma 1–3 days prior to the onset of the excruciating pain and toxic appearance. Although the thigh muscles are most commonly affected (Figure 1.5.27), other muscles, such as the smaller pelvic muscles, can sometimes be involved.

The diagnosis can usually be confirmed by MRI of the muscle (Figure 1.5.28), and by aspirating the abscess. Blood cultures are rarely positive. Pyomyositis requires prompt surgical drainage in addition to intravenous antibiotics. This infection is almost always caused by *Staph. aureus*, but cases due to Gonococcus and other bacteria have been reported. In addition, there is an increasing incidence of pyomyositis associated with HIV infection in the paediatric population [40].

Benign viral myositis

Benign viral myositis is a common entity during influenza season [41]. Typically, immediately following an acute flu-like illness with high fever, myalgias, and arthralgias, the child complains of pain in both calves. The pain and tenderness become quite pronounced, so that the child is often unable to straighten the legs or walk. There is severe tenderness of both calves, not associated with oedema or erythema, and dorsiflexion of the ankles causes considerable pain. Blood tests document elevated muscle enzymes: creatine phosphokinase (CPK), aldolase, lactate dehydrogenase (LDH), and transaminases. Fortunately, the symptoms resolve over a period of days while the child is treated symptomatically with a nonsteroidal anti-inflammatory drug. The acute onset of pain and lack of skin findings and proximal muscle weakness differentiates this entity from dermatomyositis (see Part 1, Chapter 1.6).

Less common infections of bones and joints

A summary of the symptoms and diagnostic tests of unusual infections causing musculoskeletal complaints can be found in Table 1.5.9. A few of these unusual musculoskeletal infections are discussed in more detail below.

Brucellosis

Children who drink raw milk or eat cheese made from unpasteurized milk may develop arthritis and osteomyelitis as manifestations of *Brucella melitensis* sepsis. Diagnosis is usually a result of serologic testing but the organism can be grown from joint fluid, bone, or blood. The arthritis is most often monoarticular (hip or knee), but two or more joints have been reported in some cases.

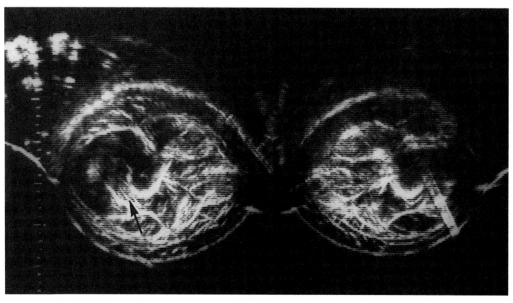

Fig. 1.5.27 A patient presented with high fever and an erythematous, tender, swollen left thigh. An ultrasound examination easily demonstrated a fluid collection within the thigh muscle, which was surgically drained. (From J. Jacobs.)

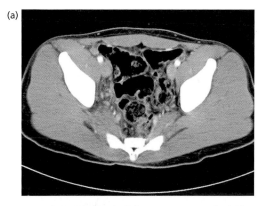

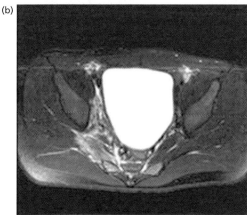

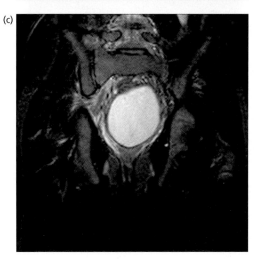

Fig. 1.5.28 This 16-year-old male developed severe right-sided low back and right hip pain, along with fever and weight loss, over 1 week's time. An MRI of the hip suggested right lower quadrant inflammation consistent with appendicitis or ileitis, and a CT of the abdomen was suggestive of appendicitis. An appendectomy was performed but the appendix was normal, and he continued to have severe pain and fever. His examination revealed severe tenderness on palpation of the right flank over the iliac crest and sacrum with pain on flexion of the right hip. Hip joint aspiration was negative, but a blood culture grew *Staph. aureus*. An indium-tagged WBC study revealed increased uptake of the right side of the pelvis overlying the area of the iliac bone. (a) A CT scan of the pelvis with contrast showed thickening of the right pyriformis muscle with adjacent streaky inflammation. The MRI (b) revealed abnormal signal intensity within the right pyriformis muscle as well as soft-tissue swelling medial to the acetabulum with a mass effect on the bladder. (c) This shows similar findings on a coronal plane. Aspiration of the muscle confirmed the diagnosis of pyomyositis of the pyriformis muscle.

Salmonellosis

Bone and joint infection with *Salmonella* is rare in children, even among those with sickle-cell disease, who have an increased susceptibility to *Salmonella* infections. Nevertheless, if osteomyelitis or septic arthritis is documented in a child with sickle-cell disease, the chances of the infection being caused by *Salmonella* is greater than from any other organism (Figure 1.5.20).

Cat-scratch disease

This common illness is usually characterized by regional lymphadenitis occurring 1 or 2 weeks after a cat scratch. Occasional patients may present with bone/joint pain secondary to osteolytic bone lesions. X-rays are initially negative, but after several weeks, a lytic lesion can be demonstrated. Diagnosis in patients with a lytic bone lesion is achieved by integrating the history of a cat scratch, purulent but "sterile" lymphadenitis, plus a compatible histologic picture of granulomas with central necrosis surrounded by epithelioid cells and lymphocytes. These lesions generally heal spontaneously, but children with abscesses of the liver and spleen, overwhelming pneumonia, or encephalitis may be very ill and can resemble patients with systemic vasculitis [42]. Vertebral osteomyelitis secondary to cat-scratch disease has also been reported (see "Vertebral osteomyelitis" above). The diagnosis can be made serologically.

Foreign-body synovitis

Wood splinters and plant thorns (such as from palm or blackthorn) may penetrate the skin and lead to chronic synovitis or tendonitis. Plant-thorn synovitis is not rare in children [43]. When the inflammation is severe, periosteal new bone may be noted, and when a thorn is sticking into the bone, a lytic lesion stimulating osteomyelitis or tumour may be seen radiographically (Figure 1.5.29).

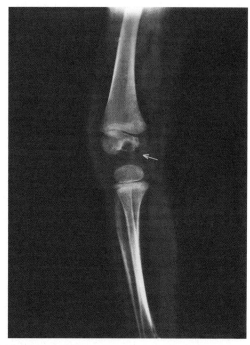

Fig. 1.5.29 An X-ray demonstrating erosion of the distal humerus caused by inflammation around a plant thorn. This cause of monoarticular arthritis may mimic septic arthritis or JIA. (From J. Jacobs.)

Table 1.5.9 Unusual infections with musculoskeletal manifestations

Clinical symptoms	Syndrome	Causative agent	Diagnostic test
Arthralgias and fevers after travel to endemic areas	**Babesiosis**	*Babesia microti*	Blood smear Babesia titre
Fever, monoarticular arthritis and/or osteomyelitis in children who consume unpasteurized milk or cheese	**Brucellosis**	*Brucella melitensis*	Brucella titres Cultures of bone, joint or blood
Osteomyelitis in long bone or vertebra associated with lymphadenitis following cat scratch	**Cat-scratch disease**	*Bartonella henselae*	*Bartonella henselae* IgM Characteristic histology of lymph node
Reactive arthritis following psittacosis or Chlamydia pneumonia	**Chlamydia pneumonia Psittacosis**	*Chlamydia psittaci* and *pneumoniae*	Specific Chlamydia titres
Arthritis and erythema nodosum. Isolated limb pain and swelling (osteomyelitis) with abnormal chest X-ray in patient who lives in an endemic area	**Coccidioidomycosis**	*Coccidioides immitis*	Coccidioidomycosis *titre*
Sudden fever, headache, rash, musculoskeletal pain, haemorrhage, shock Arthritis occurs rarely	**Dengue fever**	*Dengue viruses*	Dengue serology
Chylous arthritis of knee secondary to lymphatic obstruction	**Filariasis**	*Wuchereria bancrofti*	Identification of microfilariae in blood samples
Rare arthritis in a patient with abdominal pain and diarrhoea who has been in endemic area	**Giardiasis**	*Giardia lamblia*	Giardia immunofluorescent antibody (IFA) of stool
Fever, malaise, and other organ system involvement Arthritis and pericarditis can occur rarely	**Histoplasmosis**	*Histoplasma capsulatum*	Histoplasma titre Culture of affected site Histology
Seronegative arthritis, reactive arthritis syndrome, vasculitis, Psoriatic Arthritis, or Sjögren like-syndrome in an individual at risk for HIV	**HIV and AIDS**	*HIV*	HIV serology HIV viral load (RNA PCR)
Fever, uveitis, rashes, lymphadenopathy, GI, CNS symptoms, and sometimes arthritis	**Leptospirosis**	*Leptospira* spp.	Leptospira titres
Inguinal adenopathy associated with proctitis, arthritis, erythema, nodosum, in sexually active or abused patients	**Lymphogranuloma venereum**	*Chlamydia trachomatis*	Biopsy
Arthralgias associated with high fevers, anemia, hepatosplenomegaly in patients who live in or travel to endemic areas	**Malaria**	*Plasmodium* spp.	Blood smear for malaria
Arthritis preceded by respiratory illness, especially pneumonia	**Mycoplasma**	*Mycoplasma* spp.	Cold agglutinin antibody Mycoplasma titres
Fever, malaise, cough, maculopapular rash, and occasionally arthritis, which can be septic, following rat bite	**Rat-bite fever**	*Spirillum minor* *Streptococcus moniliformis*	Typical syndrome, blood and synovial fluid cultures
Fever, arthralgia, myalgia, headache, swelling of hands and feet; rash beginning on the extremities Arthritis occurs rarely	**Rocky Mountain Spotted Fever**	*Rickettsia rickettsii*	Rickettsia serologies IFA staining of skin biopsy PCR of blood or tissue
Pseudoparalysis of arm or leg Osteochondritis, periostitis, dactylitis, metaphysitis on X-ray Clutton joints (gummatous arthritis of knees and elbows)	**Congenital syphilis**	*Treponema pallidum*	VDRL Fluorescent treponemal antibody (FTA)
Symmetrical, nonmigratory arthritis of the knees associated with generalized lymphadenopathy, maculopapular rash	**Secondary syphilis**	*Treponema pallidum*	VDRL FTA
Transient attacks of arthritis with diarrhea, fever, weight loss, and sometimes central nervous system (CNS) symptoms	**Whipple disease**	*Tropheryma whippelii*	Typical histology of intestinal biopsy

Most often, the history of injury has been forgotten, and months may elapse between entry of the fragment and its dissection into the joint. Standard imaging studies may fail to show any abnormality other than inflammation of the affected joint which is indistinguishable from Oligoarthritis. Careful history-taking in a patient with monoarticular arthritis is therefore essential (Figure 1.5.30).

The diagnosis is easier when the foreign body is radio-opaque, such as glass or metal, and is apparent on X-ray. In other cases, CT, MRI, and ultrasonogram may aid in localization [44]. Surgical removal of the foreign body is the only effective therapy; careful surgical exploration may be necessary to prove the diagnosis.

Fungal arthritis

Fungi may cause arthritis by several different mechanisms [45–47]:

1. Direct invasion into a joint either from infected adjacent bone or from the skin as in Madura foot.

2. Association with erythema nodosum (see Part 1, Chapter 1.4).

3. Haematogenous spread with formation of granulomas in the joints.

4. Very rarely as a complication of intra-articular injection of corticosteroids.

Coccidioidomycosis is a common infection in the south-western region of the United States. It may become clinically apparent many years (and in another location) after the initial infection. Of the 14 recently reported childhood cases, 3 presented with musculoskeletal complaints, including knee, thigh, and hand pain and swelling, all documented as manifestations of chronic fungal osteomyelitis [47]. Chest radiographs show nodular infiltrates and the diagnosis is confirmed

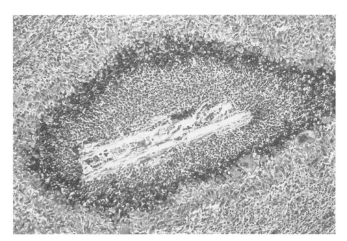

Fig. 1.5.30 A photomicrograph of the synovium of a patient with plant thorn synovitis (note the thorn in the middle of the picture). This was taken from a 6-year-old boy who developed swelling of the right knee. He was referred to an orthopaedist who aspirated the joint. There were less than 20,000 WBC in the fluid, and the culture was negative. X-ray and bone scan were normal. The child was placed on ibuprofen and eventually referred to paediatric rheumatology. A history was then obtained that 6 months previously he had fallen into a large cactus plant, and had to be taken to an Emergency Room to have multiple thorns removed. He had developed the knee swelling 1 month later. There was no history of joint stiffness, and he had little pain. He had a large boggy joint without limitation of motion. He was sent back to the orthopaedist with a diagnosis of plant thorn synovitis, and an arthroscopic debridement was performed. (Courtesy of I. S. Szer.)

with serologic testing and the demonstration of the organism in pathologic specimens. Skin tests are often negative in disseminated coccidiomycosis.

Parasitic arthritis

Immune-complex formation occurs in many parasitic infections [48]. As a consequence of immune-complex deposition, arthralgia is frequent in malaria and babesiosis; arthritis has occasionally been reported in association with giardiasis, blastocystis hominus, and in overwhelming *Strongyloides* and *Taenia* infections. Lymphatic obstruction caused by systemic filariasis may be associated with chylous arthritis of the knee.

Syphilis and other infections caused by flexibacteria

Both congenital and acquired syphilis may present with a variety of musculoskeletal manifestations. The diagnosis of childhood syphilis was easier years ago when physicians were more familiar with the broad clinical spectrum of syphilis. Recently trained physicians may fail to recognize the infection despite its resurgence in the past few years.

Congenital syphilis classically presents with pseudo paralysis of an arm or leg, sometimes associated with joint swelling. Syphilitic invasion of bone results in osteochondritis, periostitis, dactylitis, and metaphysitis, which cause the musculoskeletal symptoms and are demonstrable radiographically. These manifestations may occur later in childhood if congenital syphilis is not adequately treated in infancy.

In addition, another form of syphilitic arthritis occurs in older children, usually those between ages 8 and 16, who have inadequately treated congenital syphilis. These gummatous infections, called Clutton joints, most commonly present with isolated knee effusions; occasionally, the elbows are also involved. Although Clutton joints were originally said to be painless, they can be associated with some pain and other minimal inflammatory signs. Diagnosis is based on serologic tests for syphilis. Both the infantile forms of congenital syphilis and Clutton joints respond to treatment with penicillin.

Paediatricians may also see secondary syphilis in children who are sexually active, or who have been sexually abused. Polyarthralgias are a common manifestation of secondary syphilis, and the clinical picture may resemble subacute bacterial endocarditis, acute rheumatic fever, or Systemic Arthritis. When arthritis occurs, it tends to be symmetrical and nonmigratory, settling most frequently in the knees and resembling Clutton joints. Sometimes the arthritis is accompanied by tenosynovitis; in general, the tenosynovitis associated with secondary syphilis is "cold" in contrast to the heat and erythema that is characteristic of the gonorrhoeal tenosynovitis–arthritis syndrome. Secondary syphilis is usually accompanied by generalized lymphadenopathy; the posterior auricular nodes tend to be especially large, tender, and boggy. This characteristic posterior auricular lymphadenopathy is sometimes accompanied by a maculopapular rash and infectious oral mucous plaques which are all clues to the diagnosis of secondary syphilis. Similar manifestations may also occur in yaws.

Migratory arthralgias or arthritis has been seen in other flexibacterial diseases including rat-bite fever, Haverhill fever, and leptospirosis.

Whipple's disease

Whipple's disease is a rare manifestation of a systemic bacterial infection with *Tropheryma whippelii* [49]. The clinical syndrome includes diarrhoea, weight loss, fever, arthralgias/arthritis, and sometimes CNS symptoms. It may be fatal if untreated, and tends to be more common in white, middle-aged males. However, it occasionally occurs in children, and should be ruled out in any child who presents with failure to thrive, chronic diarrhoea, malnutrition, and arthralgias or arthritis. Unlike the more persistent arthritis of JIA or arthritis associated with inflammatory bowel disease, this arthritis tends to occur in transient attacks, lasting only a few hours or days. Joint symptoms may precede gastrointestinal manifestations by years. *T. whippelii* is extremely difficult to culture, but can be identified in involved tissue using PCR. The diagnosis is generally made by histologic examination of intestinal biopsy specimens. Various antibiotic regimens are rapidly effective and curative.

Acknowledgments

The author wishes to thank Melissa Liebling, MD, for her invaluable assistance in selecting appropriate imaging studies for this chapter, and Jeffrey R. Boscamp, MD, for his careful review and editorial comments.

References

1. Jacobs, J.C. The differential diagnosis of arthritis in childhood. In J.C. Jacobs ed. *Pediatric Rheumatology for the Practitioner*, 2nd edn. New York: Springer-Verlag, 1993; pp. 25–230.

2. Fink, C.W. and Nelson, J.D. Septic arthritis and osteomyelitis in children. *Clin Rheum Dis* l986;12:423–35.

3. Christiansen, P. Frederiksen, B., Glazowski, J. et al. Epidemiologic, bacteriologic and long-term follow-up data of children with acute hematogenous osteomyelitis and septic arthritis: A ten-year review. *J Pediatr Orthop B* 1999;8:302–5.

4. Mazur, J.M., Ross, G., Cummings, J., Hahn, G.A., and McCluskey, W.P. Usefulness of magnetic resonance imaging for the diagnosis of acute musculoskeletal infections in children. *J Pediatr Orthop* 1995;15:144–7.

5. Jaramillo, D., Treves, S.T., Kasser, J.R., et al. Osteomyelitis and septic arthritis in children: Appropriate use of imaging to guide treatment. *Am J Roentgenol* 1995;165:399–403.

6. Dich, V.D., Nelson, J.D., and Haltalin, K.C. Osteomyelitis in infants and children. *Am J Dis Child* 1975;129:1273–8.

7. Dahl, L.B., Hyland, A.L., Dramsdahl, H., and Kaaresen, P.I. Acute osteomyelitis in children: A population-based retrospective study 1965–1994. *Scan J Infect Dis* 1998;30:573–7.

8. Cole, W.B., Dalziel, R.E., and Leitl S. Treatment of acute osteomyelitis in childhood. *J Bone Joint Surg* 1982;64B:218.

9. Bonhoeffer, J., Haeberle, B., Schaad, U.B., and Heininger, U. Diagnosis of acute haematogenous osteomyelitis and septic arthritis: 20 years experience at the University Children's Hospital Basel. *Swiss Med Wkly* 2001;131:575–81.

10. Karwowska, A., Davies, H.D., and Jadavji T. Epidemiology and outcome of osteomyelitis in the era of sequential intravenous-oral therapy. *Pediatr Infect Dis J* 1998;17:1021–6.

11. Fernandez, M., Carrol, C.L., and Baker, C.J. Discitis and vertebral osteomyelitis in children: An 18-year review. *Pediatrics* 2000;105:1299–304.

12. Boscamp, J.R., and Steigbigel, N.H. Disk space infection. In D. Schlossberg ed., *Orthopedic Infection*. New York: Springer-Verlag, 1988; pp. 49–68.

13. Brown, R., Hussain, M., McHigh, K., Novelli, V., and Jones, D. Discitis in young children. *J Bone Joint Surg Br* 2001;83:106–11.

14. Sonozaki, H., Mitsui, H., Miyanaga, Y., et al. Clinical features of 53 cases with pustulotic arthro-osteitis. *Ann Rheuma Dis* 1981;40:547.

15. Beretta-Piccoli, B.C., Sauvain, M.J., Gal, I., et al. Synovitis, acne, pustulosis, hyperostosis, osteitis (SAPHO) syndrome in childhood: A report of ten cases and review of the literature. *Eur J Pediatr* 2000;159:594–601.

16. Bittecoq, O., Said, L.A., Michot, C., et al. Evaluation of chronic recurrent multifocal osteitis toward spondylarthropathy over the long term. *Arthritis Rheum* 2000;43:109–19.

17. Nelson, J.D. and Koontz, W.C. Septic arthritis in infants and children: A review of 117 cases. *Pediatrics* 1966;36:370–3.

18. Speiser, J.C., Moore, T.L., Osborn, T.G., et al. Changing trends in pediatric septic arthritis. *Semin Arthritis Rheum* 1985;15:132–8.

19. Welkon, C.J., Long, S.S., Fisher, M.C., et al. Pyogenic arthritis in infants and children: A review of 95 cases. *Pediatr Infect Dis* 1986;5:669–76.

20. Shetty, A.K., and Gedalia, A. Septic arthritis in children. *Rheum Dis Clin North Am* 1998;24:287–304.

21. Lyon, R.M. and Evanich, J.D. Culture-negative septic arthritis in children. *J Pediatr Orthop* 1999;19:655–9.

22. Wilson, N.I. and DiPaola, M. Acute septic arthritis in infancy and childhood. 19 years' experience. *J Bone Joint Surg Br* 1986;38:584–7.

23. Donatto, K.C. Orthopedic management of septic arthritis. *Rheum Dis Clin North Am* 1998;24:275–86.

24. Hook, E.W., III and Holmes, K.K. Gonococcal infections. *Ann Intern Med* 1985;102:229–43.

25. Schaad, U.B. Arthritis in disease due to *Neisseria meningitides*. *Rev Infect Dis* 1980;2:880–7.

26. Al-Matar, M.J., Cabral, D.A., and Petty RE. Isolated tuberculous monoarthritis mimicking oligoarticular juvenile rheumatoid arthritis. *J Rheumatol* 2001;28(1):204–6.

27. Schwan, T.G., Piesman, J., Golde, W.T., Dolan, M.C., and Rosa, P.A. Induction of an outer surface protein on *Borrelia burgdorferi* during tick feeding. *Proc Natl Acad Sci* 1995;92:2909–13.

28. Klempner, M.S., Hu, L.T., Evan, J., et al. Two controlled trials of antibiotic treatment in patients with persistent symptoms and a history of Lyme disease. *N Engl J Med* 2001;345:85–92.

29. Tugwell, P., Dennis, D.T., Weinstein A, et al. Guidelines for laboratory evaluation in the diagnosis of Lyme disease. *Ann Intern Med* 1997;127:1106–8.

30. Klempner, M.S., Schmid, C.H., Hu L., et al. Intralaboratory reliability of serologic and urine testing for Lyme disease. *Am J Med* 2001;110:217–9.

31. Wormser, G.P., Nadelman, R.B., Dattwyler, R.J., et al. Practice guidelines for the treatment of Lyme disease: The Infectious Diseases Society of America. *Clin Infect Dis* 2000;31 (Suppl.):1–14.

32. Szer, I.S., Taylor, E., and Steere, A.C. The long-term course of Lyme arthritis in children. *N Engl J Med* 1991;325:159–63.

33. Kalish, R.A., Leong, J.L., and Steere, A.C. Association of treatment-resistant chronic Lyme arthritis with HLA-DR4 and antibody reactivity to Osp A and Osp B of *Borrelia burgdorferi*. *Infect Immun* 1993;61:2774–9.

34. Torok, T.J. Parvovirus B19 and human disease. *Adv Inter Med* 1992;37:3952–6.

35. Nesher, G., Osborn, T.G., and Moore, T.L. Parvovirus infection mimicking systemic lupus erythematosus. *Semin Arthritis Rheum* 1995;24:297–303.

36. Nocton, J.J., Miller, L.C., Tucker, L.B., and Schaller, J.G. Human parvovirus B19-associated arthritis in children. *J Pediatr* 1993;122:186–90.

37. Wands, J.R., Mann, E., Alpert, E., et al. The pathogenesis of arthritis associated with acute hepatitis B surface antigen-positive hepatitis. *J Clin Invest* 1975;55:930–6.

38. Buskila, D. Hepatitis C-associated arthritis. *Curr Opin Rheumatol* 2000;12:295–9.

39. Spruance, S.L., Metcalf, R., Smith, C.B., et al. Chronic arthropathy associated with rubella vaccination. *Arthritis Rheum* 1977;20:741–7.

40. Gardiner, J.S., Zauk, A.M., Minnefor, A.B., *et al.* Pyomyositis in an HIV-positive premature infant: case report and review of the literature. *J Pediatr Orthop* 1990;10:791–3.

41. Middleton, P.J., Alexander, R.M., and Szymanski, M.T. Severe myositis during recovery from influenza. *Lancet* 1970;2:533–5.

42. Margileth, A.M., Wear, D.J., and English, C.K. Systemic cat scratch disease: Report of 23 patients with prolonged or recurrent severe bacterial infection. *J Infect Dis* 1987;155:390–402.

43. Sugarman, M., Stobie, D.G., Quismorio, F.P., Terry, R., and Hanson V. Plant thorn synovitis. *Arthritis Rheum* 1977;20:1125–8.

44. Stevens, K.J., Theologis, T., and McNally, E.G. Imaging of plant-thorn synovitis. *Skeletal Radiol* 2000;29:605–8.

45. Katzenstein, D. Isolated Candida arthritis: Report of a case and definition of a distinct clinical syndrome. *Arthritis Rheum* 1985; 28: 1421–4.

46. Rosenthal, J., Brandt, K.D., Wheat, L.J., and Slama, T.G. Rheumatologic manifestations of histoplasmosis in the recent Indianapolis epidemic. *Arthritis Rheum* 1983;26:1065–70.

47. Kafka, J.A. and Catanzaro, A. Disseminated coccidioidomycosis in children. *J Pediatr* 1981;98:355–61.

48. Bocanegra, T., Espinoza, L.R., Bridgeford, P., *et al.* Reactive arthritis induced by parasitic infection. *Ann Int Med* 1981;94:207–9.

49. Relman, D.A., Schmidt, T.M., MacDermott, R.P., and Falkow, S. Identification of the uncultured bacillus of Whipple's disease. *N Engl J Med* 1992;327:293–301.

1.6   Major rheumatic diseases

Suzanne C. Li and Lisa F. Imundo

Aims

The aims of this chapter are to discuss the major rheumatic diseases that may present with features similar to those seen in Juvenile Idiopathic Arthritis (JIA). These major systemic rheumatic diseases include systemic lupus erythematosus, neonatal lupus erythematosus, mixed connective tissue disease, dermatomyositis, scleroderma, and vasculitis. Some of the less common rheumatic diseases will also be discussed. Clinical characteristics and laboratory studies that can be used to distinguish between JIA and these other childhood rheumatic diseases will be discussed.

Structure

- Systemic lupus erythematosus
- Neonatal lupus erythematosus
- Mixed connective tissue disease
- Chronic cutaneous lupus erythematosus
- Subacute cutaneous lupus erythematosus
- Drug-induced lupus
- Antiphospholipid antibody syndrome
- Dermatomyositis
- Polymyositis
- Amyopathic dermatomyositis
- Scleroderma
- CREST syndrome
- Eosinophilic fasciitis
- Vasculitis
- Polyarteritis Nodosa
- Microscopic Polyarteritis
- Wegener granulomatosis
- Limited Wegener granulomatosis
- Takayasu arteritis
- Behçet syndrome
- Churg–Strauss syndrome
- Cogan syndrome
- Relapsing polychondritis
- MAGIC syndrome: mouth and genital ulcers with inflamed cartilage syndrome

Systemic lupus erythematosus

Introduction

Systemic Lupus erythematosus (SLE) should be considered in the differential diagnosis of an adolescent girl presenting with musculoskeletal complaints and constitutional symptoms. Although both SLE and JIA are associated with immunological disturbances such as altered cytokine profiles, SLE is the prototypical autoimmune disease characterized by a high level and range of autoantibody production. Pathological findings include inflammation, vascular abnormalities (vasculopathy, vasculitis), and immune complex deposition. As these lesions can occur anywhere in the body, the symptoms of lupus are extremely varied, but frequently include constitutional symptoms such as fatigue, weight loss, malaise, and anorexia as well as rash and arthralgia/arthritis (Table 1.6.1 (HLA, family history, ethnicity, and risk factors based on References 1–7)). Many genes have been identified that increase susceptibility to SLE, while only a few have been identified for JIA, and patients with SLE are much more likely to have a family history of autoimmune disease. SLE is also more likely to develop in blacks, Hispanics, and Asians, while JIA most commonly develops in Caucasians (Table 1.6.1). About 10–15% of all cases of SLE have their onset in childhood [8]. Similar to adult patients, girls are more likely to develop SLE than boys. However, this difference is only four to five fold compared with the six to ten fold differences in adults; very young patients with SLE have an even lower ratio. Unlike Systemic Arthritis, which occurs throughout childhood, SLE is extremely rare before 5 years of age and infrequent before 10 years of age. Therefore, for a very young child presenting with musculoskeletal complaints and constitutional symptoms, SLE would be an unlikely diagnosis. In contrast, an adolescent girl with musculoskeletal and constitutional symptoms needs to be carefully evaluated for Systemic Arthritis and RF+ Polyarthritis as well as for SLE. In some patients, the pattern of symptoms may change and overlap these different diseases during the course of illness. Careful monitoring, as well as laboratory studies are critical in determining the appropriate diagnosis.

Diagnosis

The American College of Rheumatology (ACR) established a set of "classification" criteria that have 90% sensitivity and 96–99% specificity for SLE [9]. These criteria, developed for classification of patients into studies, have been validated in children [10]. The criteria were updated in 1997 (Table 1.6.2 [11]), but these modifications have not yet been validated in children or in adults. A major criticism of the ACR criteria has been that they do not identify patients early enough and that up to one-third of patients with SLE do not fulfill

Table 1.6.1 Childhood systemic lupus erythematosus versus juvenile idiopathic arthritis

	Systemic lupus erythematosus	**Systemic Arthritis**	**RF positive Polyarthritis**
Age distribution	Increased in adolescence Uncommon < 5 year	No peak, throughout childhood; usually younger	Generally >=8 year
Sex	F > M 4.5:1	F = M	F >>> M
Arthritis pattern	nondeforming, small joints, Jaccoud's	oligo or poly oligo: large joints poly: symmetrical, small	Symmetrical involvement of five or more small joints, erosions
Extra-articular manifestations	Constitutional symptoms: anorexia, fatigue, fever, weight loss oral ulcers Raynaud phenomenon	Fever (quotidian) with improved activity in-between fever spikes HSM, LA, pericarditis, pleuritis	May have low-grade fever, anorexia, fatigue LA, HSM subcutaneous nodules
Rash	Malar, photosensitive Vasculitic lesions, Raynaud phenomenon, telangiectasia	Fluctuates with fever Salmon-pink, evanescent	Can get vasculitic lesions
Labs			
Hb	↓	↓	↓, milder
WBC	↓	↑	±
Plt.	↓ often	↑	±
ESR	↑	↑	↑
CRP	often normal	↑	↑
U/A	+cells, protein	−	−
LFTs	↑ often	↑	↑ sometimes
ANA	+	uncommon	+, majority
RF	+ often	−	+
dsDNA ab	+	−	−
anti-Sm ab	+	−	−
HLA	DR2, DR3 Caucasians DR2, DR7 AfricanAm	DRB1*0405, DQB1* 0401 may be associated with Japanese Systemic Arthritis. No consistent findings in other Systemic Arthritis	DR4
Family Hx (FHx)	20–27% have FHx of autoimmune disease	rare	rare
Ethnicity	African American, African Caribbean, Asian, Hispanic >Caucasians	Predominantly Caucasian	Predominantly Caucasian
Immunodeficiencies associated with increased risk of developing disease (see also Part 1, Chapter 1.10)	All complement components; highest for C1q, C4, C1r/s, C2 IgA IgG and IgG subclasses CVID, CGD	IgA	IgA
Other associated factors	TNFa2 allele FcγRII, FcγRIII low affinity alleles Specific Il-10, IL-1ra, IL-4, Il-6, TNF R polymorphisms may affect severity UV light Some chemicals/drugs	Specific IL6 polymorphisms are found in Systemic Arthritis patient that present before 5 years of age Specific TNFα polymorphisms are associated with Japanese Systemic Arthritis	Specific TNFα, IL-1β, IL-4 polymorphisms are associated with disease severity

ANA = antinuclear antibody; anti-Sm ab = anti-smith antibody; CGD = chronic granulomatous disease: CGD is more commonly associated with discoid lupus than SLE; mothers of patients with CGD also have a higher incidence of discoid lupus; CVID = common variable immunodeficiency; ds DNA ab = anti-double stranded DNA antibody; ESR = sedimentation rate; Hb = haemoglobin; HSM = hepatosplenomegaly; LA = lymphadenopathy; LFTs = liver function tests; plt = platelet count; pop = population; RF = rheumatoid factor; U/A = urinanalysis; UV = ultraviolet light.

Table 1.6.2 The 1982 revised criteria for the diagnosis of systemic lupus erythematosus

Mucocutaneous Lesions
1. Butterfly rash
2. Discoid Lupus
3. Photosensitivity
4. Oral or nasopharyngeal ulcers (usually painless)

Musculoskeletal manifestations
5. Arthritis (non-erosive)

Serositis
6. Pleuritis (pleuritic pain/rub or pleural effusion) or pericarditis

Renal disease
7. Proteinuria (>0.5 g/day) or cellular casts (red cell, haemoglobin, granular, tubular, or mixed)

Haematologic abnormalities
8. Haemolytic anaemia (with reticulocytosis) or leukopenia (<4 K/mm^3 on two or more occasions) or lymphopenia (<1.5 K/mm^3 on two or more occasions) or thrombocytopenia (<100 K/mm^3)

Immunologic abnormalities
9. Positive fluorescence test for ANA
10. LE cells or anti-ds DNA antibodies or anti-Sm antibodies or chronic false-positive test for syphilis

Neurologic manifestations
11. Psychosis or convulsions: both in absence of known metabolic derangements or precipitating drugs

    Cerebral arteritis, transverse myelitis, peripheral neuropathy are also suggestive of SLE but are not part of the official 1982 ACR criteria [10].

Note: four of 11 items listed above are ultimately present in 96% of SLE patients; specificity is 96–99%.
The criteria were modified in 1997, but only the 1982 criteria have been validated in children with SLE [11].
The principal changes in the 1997 criteria involve the immunologic abnormalities. The presence of LE cells
was eliminated and testing for antiphospholipid antibodies was expanded to:

(1) Abnormal serum level of IgG or IgM anticardiolipin antibodies,

(2) Positive test result for lupus anticoagulant using a standard method, or

(3) False-positive serological test for syphilis known to be positive for at least 6 months and confirmed by *Treponema pallidum* immobilization or fluorescent treponemal antibody.

these criteria at the time of the first visit to the physician. These criteria were intended for the classification of groups of patients rather than for individual diagnosis. Patients meeting some but not four or more of these criteria need to be monitored for disease progression and have their symptoms treated as required. The hallmark of childhood SLE is the presence of multi-system involvement, which requires prompt diagnosis based on recognition of distinct pattern of symptoms (Table 1.6.1).

Clinical manifestations

Musculoskeletal

Arthritis/arthralgia

The most common musculoskeletal symptoms in SLE are pain, morning stiffness, and joint swelling, all of which may be suggestive of mild JIA. However, unlike Oligoarthritis or positive Polyarthritis, the pain is often disproportionate to the degree of arthritis. Joint swelling is generally transient with little demonstrable arthritis at the time of examination. Permanent deformity, erosions, and scarring are rarely found in children with SLE, unlike the pattern found in children with positive Polyarthritis. Rheumatoid factor (RF) can be demonstrated in the serum of about 20% of children with SLE, but its presence does not correlate with the destructive arthritis seen in patients with RF positive Polyarthritis [12–17]. A distinctive deformity of the hands has been

reported in SLE (the "lupus hand") that is characterized by ulnar deviation, swan neck deformity of the fingers, and subluxations. These features have been described under the eponym Jaccoud arthropathy or arthritis [18]. Jaccoud arthropathy resembles that found in RF positive Polyarthritis, but unlike RF positive Polyarthritis, erosions and synovitis are usually absent. In addition, the joint deformities found in the SLE are usually correctable, at least initially, while those of JIA are fixed. Patients with Jaccoud arthropathy are more likely to have anti-U1 RNP antibodies [1] and less likely to have renal disease, similar to the pattern found in mixed connective tissue disease (MCTD, see next section). Others have found an increased frequency of antiphospholipid antibodies and antiphospholipid antibody syndrome (APLS, see following section) in patients with Jaccoud arthropathy [18]. Another deformity associated with RF positive Polyarthritis that can occur in SLE is the boutonniere deformity (Figure 1.6.1)).

Occasionally, patients have flexion contractures and an arthritic picture indistinguishable from severe RF positive Polyarthritis at onset and for varying periods of time, even years, before other manifestations of SLE became apparent. Others have reported similar cases [19]; hypertension and renal disease are less frequent in these patients with SLE with severe arthritis. In other patients, SLE has only become manifest years after presentation with other symptoms such as haemolytic anaemia and immune thrombocytopenia (Evan syndrome). Close monitoring of all patients for changes in symptoms and labs is

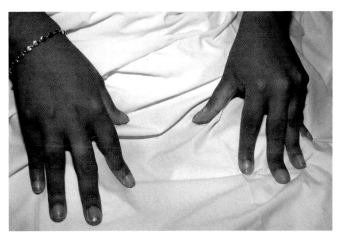

Figure 1.6.1 SLE arthritis: This 17-year-old Hispanic girl was initially given the diagnosis of Systemic Arthritis at age 7 years, when she presented with fever, weight loss, polyarthralgias, and pericarditis. Her hands show flexion of the MCPs and hyperextension of the DIPs; these deformities can be correctable.

important; if these markers change significantly, repetitive serological studies are used to determine if the patients have "evolved" into SLE or another rheumatic disease.

Myalgia

Myalgias are common in childhood SLE, but are rare in Systemic Arthritis. Occasionally, children with SLE have weakness due to muscle inflammation and necrosis with elevation of muscle enzyme levels in blood [1,12]. Some patients with JIA may also have myositis, but this is not associated with elevated muscle enzyme levels. Children with SLE or JIA who are steroid-dependent may also develop steroid myopathy, and in this case, the weakness will be associated with normal muscle enzymes. Severe myositis is also found in patients with dermatomyositis, polymyositis, and MCTD (see following sections); serological tests and other symptoms are helpful in distinguishing among these different rheumatic conditions. A more common muscle problem in patients with JIA is muscle atrophy and weakness secondary to active arthritis in the adjacent joint; this is not usually seen in patients with SLE.

Osteonecrosis of bone

Osteonecrosis of bone is a troublesome complication of both steroid administration and SLE [20]. Studies have found that up to 40% of children with SLE develop osteonecrosis, but only 4.5% have symptoms [12]. Some studies have found an association between the development of osteonecrosis and SLE features such as Raynaud phenomenon, Cushingoid habitus, antiphospholipid antibodies, and active vasculitis; however, other studies have not found any correlation [21]. Steroid treatment increases the risk of osteonecrosis, but it is not clear if the risk is related to the individual or cumulative dose of steroids, or if the route of administration affects the risk [20,21]. The risk from steroids is greatly increased in patients who have a systemic illness [21], so steroid-dependent patients with Systemic Arthritis also have an increased risk for osteonecrosis. The course of osteonecrosis is variable. Most patients are asymptomatic, and the lesion is found only because of a radiological survey. In contrast to the pain caused by inflammation in JIA, patients with symptomatic osteonecrosis can present with sudden, severe, deep pain localized to

bone. This pain is out of proportion to any evidence of arthritis physical, and is aggravated by activity [21]. Hips, knees and shoulders are most frequently affected, and a mild reactive effusion may occur in adjacent joints.

Symptoms may antedate radiographic manifestation by many months. X-rays most commonly show a crescentic area of rarefaction in subchondral bone, but there may be patchy sclerosis of the femoral head or irregularity and flattening of the epiphysis. Earlier diagnosis is possible with MRI [21]. Some patients progress rapidly to total joint destruction requiring joint replacement. The risk of epiphyseal collapse appears lower in growing children presumably because of increased blood supply to the growing epiphysis. The pain is treated with nonsteroidal antiinflammatory drugs with full weight bearing and normal activities as tolerated, as the natural history of the disease does not appear to be altered by reduction of weight bearing. Core decompression may decrease pain [20,21], but is relatively contraindicated in growing children.

Constitutional

Fever

Fever is one of the most common presenting symptoms, occurring in 55–76% of all children with SLE [12,14–17,22,23]. In contrast, to the hectic quotidian or bi-quotidian, high-grade fever found in Systemic Arthritis, the fever in SLE is usually low grade, and may be intermittent or continuous. A child with Systemic Arthritis typically feels very ill during the fever, and fairly well in between spikes, and the fever spikes are usually accompanied by the characteristic Still's rash (Figure 1.3.20, Part 1 and see Part 2, Chapter 2.2). In contrast, the malaise and constitutional symptoms of SLE are sustained. Some patients will have daily spikes to 104° or higher, similar to the pattern found in Systemic Arthritis [19].

Weight loss and anorexia

Both SLE and JIA may present with weight loss and anorexia. Weight loss is related to fever, anorexia, and, in SLE, mouth sores, but seems more prominent in SLE than in JIA. Weight loss does not usually exceed 10% of total body weight in SLE, although great emaciation (25–30%) occasionally occurs. Children presenting with musculoskeletal complaints and weight loss should also be evaluated for inflammatory bowel disease (IBD). Patients with IBD are more likely to have changes in their bowel pattern, cramping abdominal pain, bloody stools, and vomiting than patients with SLE or JIA. Growth retardation and weight loss are usually greater in IBD than in SLE (see also Part 1, Chapter 1.4) [24].

Skin

There are several differences between the rash found in SLE and that found in Systemic Arthritis. There are a variety of rashes found in SLE; the characteristic butterfly rash found in 50–70% of children with SLE [10,12,13,16,17,23,25] is a well-demarcated, erythematous rash found on the malar area, which usually spares the nasolabial folds (Figure 1.6.2(a)). In most cases, the rash is maculopapular with fine scales (Figure 1.6.2(b)); occasionally there are discoid lesions or only an erythematous blush [26,27]. In contrast, the typical Systemic Arthritis rash is found most commonly on the trunk and proximal extremities, and consists of multiple, discrete small salmon-pink macules, which are evanescent [28]. An erythematous facial rash is also characteristic of dermatomyositis. Both the SLE and dermatomyositis rash may be photosensitive (Figure 1.6.3, 1.6.14); both diseases

(a)

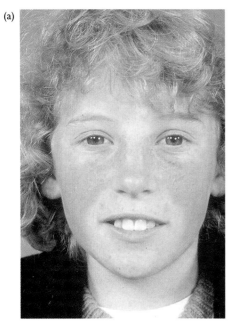

(a)

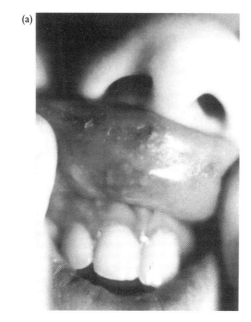

(b)

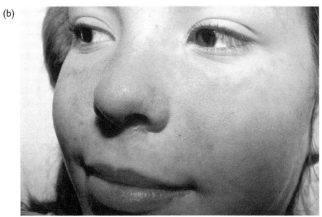

(b)

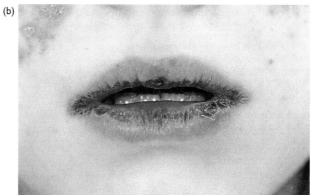

Figure 1.6.2 Malar rash. (a) Typical rash of childhood systemic lupus; note the sparring of the nasolabial fold area (Courtesy of T. R. Southwood). (b) This 17-year-old patient presented with fever, arthritis, weight loss, and malaise in addition to this malar rash.

(c)

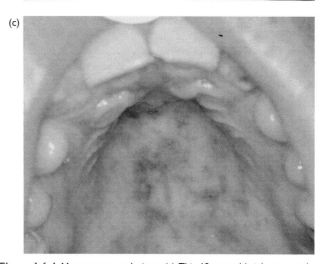

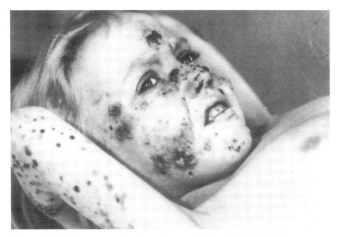

Figure 1.6.3 Photosensitive ulcerating rash. This child with SLE had an exacerbation of her rash and SLE after sun exposure (Courtesy of J. Jacobs).

Figure 1.6.4 Mucocutaneous lesions. (a) This 13-year-old girl presented with fever, malar rash, anorexia, weight loss, and arthritis. She had a +ANA, anti-ds DNA, low complement proteins, and antiphospholipid antibodies. She subsequently developed ulcers of the lip and buccal mucosa (From J. Jacobs). (b) This child shows some of the lip changes that can be seen in SLE (Courtesy of T. R. Southwood). (c) This patient with SLE developed numerous ulcers on her palate (Courtesy of D. Sherry).

can therefore show a similar distribution of rash in other sun exposed areas such as the anterior chest, extensor surfaces of the arm, and ear pinnae [1]. Hispanic children with SLE appear to have a higher incidence of photosensitivity than other ethnic groups [13,16,17,22]. In contrast to the SLE rash, the facial rash associated with dermatomyositis tends to extend down the nasolabial folds and is less well demarcated (see Figure 1.6.14(c)). In addition, facial lesions in dermatomyositis include heliotrope discolouration of the upper eyelids, which are usually swollen (Figure 1.6.14(a)); this rash is not associated with SLE.

Unlike children with JIA, children with SLE often develop mucocutaneous lesions of the buccal mucosa, lips, gums, palate, and occasionally, vulva [26]. These lesions may be painless, and can appear with exacerbations of disease (Figure 1.6.4). IBD and Behçet (see following section) also present with mucocutaneous lesions. In IBD, these tend to consist of apthous stomatitis, rather than the larger ulceration often seen in SLE. Children with Behçet develop painful clusters of oral lesions compared to the usually more limited, but larger, oral lesions seen in children with SLE.

Other skin lesions found in SLE include hyperpigmentation at sites of prior skin lesions, ulcerated infarcted lesions (Figure 1.6.5(a,c)), palmar erythema (Figure 1.6.5(b)), subungual hemorrhages, and nailfold telengiectasias[26,27]. Ulcerated or severe vasculitic lesions may also be seen in severe RF positive Polyarthritis, as well in dermatomyositis, but these types of lesions are generally not seen in Systemic Arthritis. Less commonly seen lesions include petechial and purpuric rashes not associated with thrombocytopenia or trauma. Similar lesions can be found in Henoch–Schönlein Purpura (see Part 1, Chapter 1.4), but in the latter condition, these painless lesions are generally localized to dependent or pressure-bearing areas. Subcutaneous nodules caused by panniculitis, rheumatoid nodules, and bullous lesions (pemphigoid-like) can occasionally also occur in SLE [26] (see Part 1, Chapter 1.3, Table 1.3.3).

Other findings seen in SLE but not in JIA include alopecia and Raynaud phenomenon [26,27]. A history of some hair loss may be elicited from about a third of children with SLE (range 20–58% [13–16,23,25]). There may be generalized thinning or patches of hair loss but total alopecia does not occur (Figure 1.6.6). Only 15–20% of children with SLE develop Raynaud phenomenon (see following section (Figure 1.6.7), which may precede the appearance of other signs of SLE by many years. Raynaud phenomenon is more commonly found in MCTD and scleroderma) (see following sections); serology and other symptoms should help distinguish amongst these conditions.

Cardiac

Patients with either Systemic Arthritis or SLE can develop cardiovascular complications, the most common of which is pericarditis. The pericarditis can range from a small, asymptomatic effusion to life-threatening cardiac tamponade. Pericarditis is more common, and more likely to be associated with cardiomegaly and a friction rub, in Systemic Arthritis than in SLE. Myocarditis occurs in a minority of patients with either Systemic Arthritis or SLE; it is often subclinical but can be associated with congestive heart failure or other potentially life-threatening problem [28]. Anti-Ro and anti-La antibodies are associated with an increased incidence of cardiac disease in paediatric patients with SLE; in adult patients, anti-Ro antibodies are associated

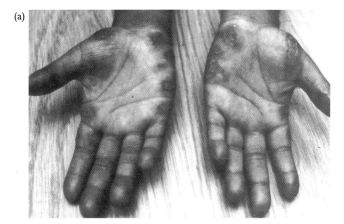

(a)

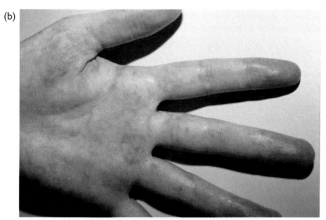

(b)

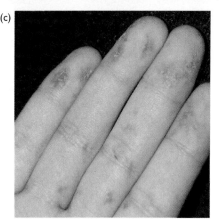

(c)

Figure 1.6.5 Digital and palmar vasculitis. (a) This 10-year-old African American girl presented with swelling and pain in her hands, anorexia, arthritis, and a facial rash (Courtesy of J. Jacobs). (b) This adolescent Asian American girl presented with recurrent facial and palmar rashes, malaise, and weight loss (Courtesy of Y. Kimura). (c) This patient had deeper vasculitic lesions on her fingers (Courtesy of D. Sherry).

with a higher likelihood of developing myocarditis and cardiac conduction defects [12,29]. Children with SLE as young as 1 year old can develop the vegetative valvular lesions of Libman–Sachs endocarditis; valvular lesions are also more likely to occur in patients with antiphospholipid antibodies (see following section) [30].

Treatment with corticosteroids in either Systemic Arthritis or SLE is associated with an increased risk of atherosclerosis. However,

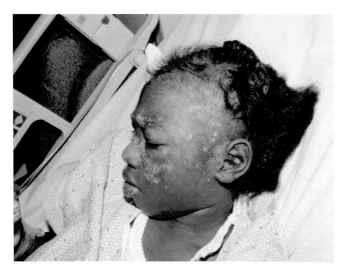

Figure 1.6.6 Alopecia and frontal hair fracturing. This 11-year-old girl presented with malar and discoid rashes, alopecia, fever, fatigue, weight loss, Raynaud phenomenon, and arthritis (Courtesy of Y. Kimura).

(a)

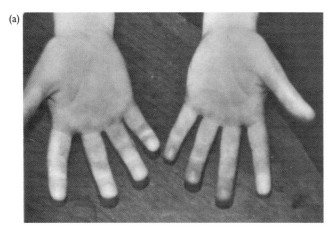

(b)

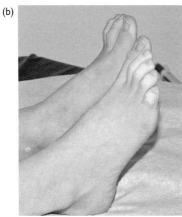

Figure 1.6.7 Raynaud phenomenon. (a) This 9-year-old boy with MCTD shows simultaneous pallor and reactive hyperemia in his hands (Courtesy of J. Jacobs). (b) This child had Raynaud phenomenon in both her hands and feet (Courtesy of Y. Kimura).

patients with SLE are more likely to suffer a myocardial infarction because of additional risk factors such as hypertension, dyslipoprotienaemia from active disease, and coronary artery narrowing from vasculitis or thromboembolism (antiphospholipid antibodies) [31]. It is not known whether alternate-day corticosteroid regimens reduce the coronary risk factors inherent to corticosteroid use. However, diabetes mellitus and hypertension, two known risk factors for atherosclerotic heart disease, both occur less frequently in patients receiving alternate-day corticosteroid therapy [32].

Reticuloendothelial

Lymphadenopathy/splenomegaly

Patients with either SLE or Systemic Arthritis may present with significant lymphadenopathy, although this is more commonly seen in Systemic Arthritis (70%) than SLE (25–30%) [12,13,28]. Lymph nodes may become as large as several centimeters in diameter and suggest the possibility of lymphoma. Biopsies show oedema and sinus hyperplasia similar to that seen in JIA, but sometimes necrosis with hematoxylin bodies are seen. Lymphoma or leukaemia may be associated with positive LE cells raising diagnostic confusion. Lymph-node biopsies and bone marrow aspirations may be necessary in patients with lymphadenopathy with either JIA or SLE. A few cases have been reported in which Hodgkin lymphoma or acute leukaemia was present with, or mimicked, childhood SLE [12].

Splenomegaly is also found in children with either SLE or Systemic Arthritis; again the frequency is higher in Systemic Arthritis (50%) than SLE (19–33%) [16,28,33]. Children with SLE may develop functional asplenia and are at increased risk for developing overwhelming pneumococcal sepsis [12,34]. Functional asplenia has not been seen in JIA [1].

Hepatic

Both Systemic Arthritis and SLE may present with significant hepatomegaly as well as with mild abnormalities in liver function tests [12,25,28]. In Systemic Arthritis, severe liver dysfunction may occur with complications such as macrophage activation syndrome (MAS) or disseminated intravascular coagulopathy (DIC), or secondary to drug toxicity (NSAID or methotrexate)[28] (See Part 3, Chapter 3.8). Jaundice is rare in both diseases. In the absence of severe haemolytic anaemia, the presence of jaundice suggests that the patient does not have SLE but rather may have autoimmune chronic active hepatitis, an illness that resembles SLE and may also be associated with antinuclear and anti-DNA antibodies [35]. In patients in whom jaundice and liver disease are the most prominent manifestations, but who have serologic evidence of SLE, the distinction between chronic active hepatitis and SLE has generally been made on the basis of the liver biopsy. Piecemeal liver necrosis with plasma cell and lymphocyte infiltration are pathognomonic of chronic active hepatitis [35]. Patients with autoimmune chronic active hepatitis rarely have significant renal disease or other major organ involvement typical of SLE. Occasionally, a patient with typical SLE also has chronic active hepatitis as one feature of their disease.

Haematological

Haematological abnormalities are commonly found in both Systemic Arthritis and SLE. Anaemia (haemoglobin <10 g) occurs in 40–50% of children with SLE [12,14,23,25] and, when severe or accompanied by jaundice, is primarily due to autoimmune Coombs test positive, haemolytic anaemia. Autoimmune haemolytic anaemia may be the initial presenting sign of childhood SLE, and years may elapse before other symptoms of lupus occur. However, other factors (e.g. chronic disease, iron deficiency, decreased life span of red blood cells, decreased bone-marrow activity, and renal failure) may also contribute to anemia. Children with Systemic Arthritis also frequently have anaemia with Hb in the 7–10 g range, generally from "anaemia of chronic disease", although it may be complicated by iron deficiency [28]. The markedly elevated ferritin level found in Systemic Arthritis is related to disease activity rather than to the iron store status. Occasionally, red cell or marrow hypoplasia or pancytopenia due to hemophagocytosis is seen in children with SLE. The rare MAS complication of Systemic Arthritis is also associated with haemophagocytosis and pancytopenia [28]. In both SLE and Systemic Arthritis, bone marrow dysplasia may develop from medications such as cyclophosphamide.

In contrast to the marked leukocytosis found in Systemic Arthritis, leukopenia is typically found in SLE (30–55% incidence [10,13,16,23,25]). The white blood cell count is generally between 2500 to 3500/mm^3. There is usually a greater degree of lymphopenia than granulocytopenia. The leukopenia may be due to antileucocyte antibodies, lymphocytotoxic antibodies, as well as antibodies against growth factors [12,36]. Only a few patients with JIA have been reported to develop Felty syndrome, which is associated with leukopenia; this syndrome is seen in about 1% of adult patients with rheumatoid arthritis [37].

While Systemic Arthritis usually presents with marked thrombocytosis, thrombocytopenia is more commonly found in SLE. If the thrombocytopenia is sufficiently severe, the patient may present with petechiae, purpura, haemorrhagic vesicles and bullae on the skin, and bleeding from the gums and GI tract. Thrombocytopenia is found in 10–35% of children with SLE and occasionally is the major presenting manifestation [10,12–15,23]. Some patients with Idiopathic Thrombocytopenic Purpura (ITP) develop SLE after several years [38]. Patients with ITP that have +ANA should be screened for other evidence of autoimmune and systemic symptoms, including more specific autoantibodies (such as anti-double stranded DNA antibody, antiphospholipid antibodies, and Coombs), complement protein levels, complete blood count with differential and platelet count, ESR, C-reactive protein, urinanalysis, serum creatinine, and liver function tests. If other abnormalities are found, the patient should be carefully monitored for the development of autoimmune symptoms.

Evans syndrome, or the combination of autoimmune haemolytic anaemia and thrombocytopenia, may be the sole presenting manifestation of some patients with SLE. Not all patients with Evans syndrome evolve into SLE and overall, patients with lupus presenting only with haematological abnormalities have a milder course except for a strong association with APLS (see following section) [30]. Occasionally, a child with a haemoglobinopathy also develops SLE, a possibility that must be considered when a child with known sickle-cell disease develops arthritis.

Thrombotic thrombocytopenic purpura is a rare, potentially fatal disease that may occur by itself, or as a life-threatening manifestation of SLE. In some patients, its appearance may precede the development of SLE. Patients present with a pentad of symptoms: thrombocytopenic purpura, microangiopathic haemolytic anaemia, fever, renal disease, and varying neurological signs or symptoms [39]. Laboratory studies show leukocytosis, thrombocytopenia, in addition to the usually Coombs negative hemolytic anaemia. Rigorous treatment, including fresh-frozen plasma, plasma exchange, glucocorticoids, anticoagulants, and/or splenectomy, has improved the outcome in some patients.

Pulmonary

In both SLE and Systemic Arthritis, patients may present with pleuritic chest pain secondary to serositis, constrictive pericarditis, costochondritis, or muscle inflammation. Although pleuropulmonary disease occurs in most children with SLE, it rarely occurs in children with JIA, and patients with JIA are much more likely to have pleural rather than parenchymal disease [28]. Up to 77% of children with SLE have abnormal pulmonary function tests (PFT), typically showing restrictive disease and/or diffusion defects [40]. Although many patients with JIA also have abnormal PFTs, these abnormalities are milder, typically consisting of a mild decrease in FVC secondary to respiratory muscle weakness [41].

Children with SLE are therefore much more likely to develop symptoms of "breathlessness", tachypnea, cyanosis, and respiratory distress. In SLE, these symptoms can represent a range of problems such as acute lupus pneumonia, interstitial pneumonitis (Figure 1.6.8), diaphragmatic muscle dysfunction, pulmonary emboli, pulmonary haemorrhage, or pulmonary hypertension. A few of these conditions (interstitial pneumonitis, diaphragmatic muscle dysfunction, and pulmonary haemorrhage), as well as other parenchymal diseases such as rheumatoid nodules, lymphoid hyperplasia, lymphoid bronchiolitis, and obliterative bronchiolitis, have been reported in JIA [1]. In both diseases, life-threatening respiratory distress can also be caused by cricoarytenoid arthritis; patients will present with stridor, dyspnea, and cyanosis [42].

Because immunosuppressive drugs such as corticosteroids and cyclophosphamide are used to treat both SLE and Systemic Arthritis, patients with either disease can develop pneumonia, a lung abscess, or an empyema. However, the risk of infection is higher in SLE than JIA due to the multiple immune defects associated with SLE. These include functional asplenia, low levels of complement, leukopenia, lymphopenia, and abnormally functioning immune cells; all of these defects are increased in patients with active disease. Furthermore, some patients with SLE have congenital deficiencies of complement or immunoglobulins, both salmonella risk factors for infections. Children with SLE are especially susceptible to pneumococcal, salmonella, meningococcal, and gonococcal infections [12,34]. Tuberculosis should also be considered in the differential diagnosis of parenchymal lung disease in SLE.

Gastrointestinal

Abdominal complaints are more common in SLE than in Systemic Arthritis. In both diseases, complaints may be related to the use of medicines such as steroids and NSAIDs. SLE, however, also directly leads to various GI manifestations such as serositis, vasculitis, pancreatitis, splenic infarcts, lymphadenitis, peritonitis, and protein-losing enteropathy [12]. Episodes of abdominal pain ("gastrointestinal crises") in childhood lupus may be confused with appendicitis or other acute abdominal problems. Vasculitis of the mesentery and bowel wall may lead to bowel haemorrhage, infarction, and perforation.

(a)

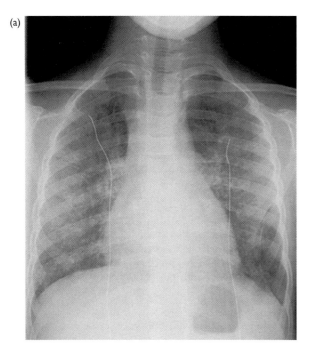

(b)

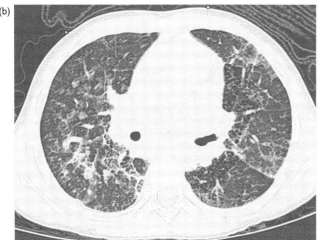

Figure 1.6.8 Interstitial pneumonitis. This 8-year-old boy developed fever, abdominal discomfort, peripheral and facial edema, and exertional dyspnea. He had rales, decreased breath sounds, +ANA, +anti-ds DNA ab, low complement proteins, and Class IV lupus nephritis. His CXR (a) showed diffuse hazy pulmonary infiltrates and his high-resolution chest CT (b) showed bilateral thick interstitium with multiple foci of hazy ground glass appearance.

Severe abdominal conditions, such as peritonitis, have only been rarely reported in JIA. Patients with Systemic Arthritis may also develop abdominal pain in association with the rare complication of amyloidosis [1,28].

Diarrhoea is not a common manifestation of childhood lupus, but occasionally a child presents in a fashion similar to ulcerative colitis or Crohn Disease (see also Part 1, Chapter 1.4). There have been a few cases reported of coexistence of both IBD and SLE [1]. Pancreatitis occasionally occurs as a manifestation of SLE or may be a complication of steroid therapy [12]. Patients with pancreatitis present with severe epigastric pain, nausea, vomiting, and elevated amylase and

lipase levels. Some develop a concurrent acute respiratory distress syndrome resembling hyaline membrane disease [12]. Acute or chronic pancreatitis may be associated with fever, subcutaneous nodules, and an arthritis-like picture related to fat necrosis. Laboratory studies and other symptoms allow this condition to be distinguished from SLE. Severe abdominal pain and diarrhoea may also be a side-effect of medication. Both diarrhoea and pancreatitis are very uncommon in Systemic Arthritis.

In addition to the acute abdominal crises of untreated or poorly controlled SLE and those associated with pancreatitis, a third form of abdominal crisis is that associated with overwhelming sepsis, to which these patients are prone. In both JIA and SLE, patients are at increased risk for infections secondary to immunosuppressive therapies. Sepsis associated with peritonitis in SLE may be due to pneumococci, staphylococci, streptococci, as well as gram-negative bacteria [12,34]. While acute appendicitis or other coincidental abdominal problems may occur in a child with lupus, abdominal problems are usually directly related to the SLE. Surgery should only be performed when it is essential, as children ill with acute lupus and/or sepsis represent a significant surgical risk.

Renal

Renal abnormalities are commonly found in children with SLE (50–60%) [10,12–14,16,23,25], but are not associated with any form of JIA. All patients with SLE should regularly have routine urinalyses to evaluate for the presence of abnormal sediment (white blood cells, red blood cells and cellular casts) and protein. Urinary findings in mildly affected individuals vary, from one urinalysis to the next, and repeat samples are needed to more accurately reflect the activity of the disease. Infection must be excluded in all patients with abnormal urinalyses, and obviously the possibility of menstrual red cells must also be excluded. Patients with significant urine sediment or protein abnormalities warrant a renal biopsy to characterize the renal disease. Renal involvement is classified on the basis of the World Health Organization (WHO)-proposed classification criteria. These histological classes provide information on disease severity, chronicity, and activity, and are important for treatment purposes [1,43].

Proteinuria is almost always present in patients with severe renal disease. While urinary protein determinations with "dipsticks" are easily performed, they are not reliable in the low range. Orthostatic proteinuria is common in adolescents; a timed collection may provide a more accurate measurement. The ratio of protein to creatinine in spot urine samples is another accurate way to monitor a patient's proteinuria. Although the advent of proteinuria or increases in the amount of mild proteinuria are cause for concern, and reduction in the amount of protein in the urine is a good sign, persistence of proteinuria is not necessarily of consequence. Renal-vein thrombosis must be ruled out in patients with sudden massive increases in proteinuria [12]. Patients with nephrotic syndrome, with or without antiphospholipid antibodies, are prone to renal-vein thrombosis and pulmonary emboli. Proteinuria due to renal-vein thrombosis does not respond to prednisone or immunosuppressive therapy, but instead requires anticoagulation [12].

Hypertension (HTN) is very uncommon in JIA except during treatment with daily corticosteroids or cyclosporin. In contrast, it develops in 40–60% of children with SLE during the course of the illness. HTN may be a prominent and life-threatening symptom of SLE and its persistence is usually a poor prognostic sign [12,14,16,25].

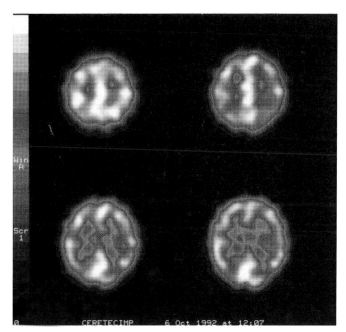

Figure 1.6.9 SPECT scan. Asymmetric cerebral perfusion defects in a 14-year-old girl with ophthalmitis and encephalopathy whose contrast enhanced CT and MR studies were normal (Courtesy of I. Szer).

Neuropsychiatric

Neuropsychiatric manifestations are common in SLE and absent in JIA, except as part of the rare complication of MAS. Between 25% and 95% of children with SLE have neuropsychiatric symptoms [44]. These symptoms include headache, mood disorders, cognitive disorders, seizures, acute confusional state, anxiety disorder, peripheral nervous system disorder (including Guillain–Barré syndrome), cerebral vascular disease, psychosis, chorea, demyelinating syndrome and myelopathy [44,45]. Abnormal MRI and SPECT (Figure 1.6.9) brain imaging studies have been found in many patients with SLE that lack overt neuropsychiatric symptoms; however, the significance of these findings is not clear [34,40]. Unfortunately, central nervous system (CNS) disease in SLE is often difficult to diagnose because of the lack of specific tests, and the lack of correlation between other manifestations of SLE and CNS disease [34,40]. In addition, CNS symptoms may be secondary to a variety of other problems, such as infections, side effects from drug therapy, or emotional stress. In children, antiphospholipid antibodies have been associated with cerebrovascular disease, chorea, myelopathy, and migraine headaches [46], while headache, cerebrovascular disease, seizure, and cranial neuropathy have been associated with these antibodies in adult patients with SLE [47].

Headache is a prominent symptom in children with active SLE and frequently is one of the presenting complaints [34,45]. The headaches usually subside as other manifestations of disease activity disappear. In some cases, the pattern of headache is identical to that of migraine with a visual aura. Headache may also be a manifestation of elevated blood pressure, intracranial haemorrhage, and meningitis (septic and aseptic), or may be a sign of increased intracranial pressure from pseudotumor cerebri due to SLE, steroid withdrawal, or hypersensitivity to nonsteroidal anti-inflammatory drugs. Seizures have been reported to occur at presentation in 23% of Dutch children with SLE, but other studies report a lower incidence [12,15,45]. There

are many potential causes of seizures in SLE including vasculitis, injury caused by previously active vasculitis, azotemia, fluid and electrolyte abnormalities, hypertension, hemorrhage, and infection. Chorea is not a common manifestation of SLE but, when present, tends to occur early in the disease, often before the diagnosis of SLE has been established. Patients with chorea should also be evaluated for acute rheumatic fever (ARF); unfortunately, since chorea is a late manifestation of ARF, diagnosis may be difficult (see also Part 1, Chapter 1.4). However, the presence of cardiac valve anomalies suggests ARF as the most likely diagnosis. As with chorea, when transverse myelopathy is a feature of SLE, it is often part of the presenting syndrome.

In SLE, eye inflammation may involve all parts of the eye in contrast to the anterior chamber inflammation seen in Oligoarthritis. Although iritis and uveitis may occur in SLE, more common findings include keratoconjunctivitis sicca, lupus retinopathy, and retinal vasculitis [48,49]. Other eye symptoms include choroidopathy, episcleritis, scleritis, interstitial keratitis, conjunctivitis, optic neuritis, and internuclear opthalmoplegia. Eye inflammation may precede the development of other signs of SLE by several years, and the appearance of scleritis or retinal disease may serve as an indication of impending systemic or CNS exacerbation [48,49].

Endocrine

Although children with Systemic Arthritis or RF positive Polyarthritis may have impaired growth and delayed sexual development, these conditions are due to active disease, corticosteroid side-effects, and insufficient nutrition rather than to endocrine abnormalities. Children with SLE may have similar defects in growth and development; a small percentage may also have hypo- or hyperthyroidism [8,34]. Many more patients with SLE have antithyroglobulin and antimicrosomal antibodies while they remain euthyroid. Patients with SLE and thyroid disease have also been found to have a higher frequency of concommitant Sjogren syndrome [43].

Laboratory findings

When a child presents with musculoskeletal and constitutional symptoms, and is found to have abnormalities in complete blood count, urinanalysis, serum creatinine level, ESR, C-reactive protein, or liver function tests (LFTs), further screening for SLE should be considered. Similar to patients with Systemic Arthritis, children with SLE often have an elevated ESR and may have an elevated ferritin level. Unlike Systemic Arthritis, SLE may present with a normal CRP even when the ESR is elevated except when there is a concomitant infection [43]. More specific tests to evaluate patients for SLE include complement, and autoantibody measurements. Low levels of total hemolytic complement activity or CH50, and/or individual complement components C1q, C4, C2, or C3 have been shown to reflect disease activity. Close monitoring of complement levels is important for assessing disease activity as a fall in their levels may precede disease flares [12]. Immunodeficiencies in complement and immunoglobulin production predispose individuals to SLE Table 1.6.1 [1,2].

Among the different autoantibody tests, the anti-nuclear antibody (ANA) is commonly used for screening as it detects nearly all patients with SLE (>95% [8,10,13,14,16]). A positive test is one of the ACR classification criteria for SLE (Table 1.6.2), but it is not required for the diagnosis nor is it considered any more important than any of the other criteria. This test is commonly reported as a titre, which is an indication of the level of antibody found; the minimal value is usually 1:40 or 1:80. The pattern of ANA staining is reported, with homogeneous and speckled accounting for the majority of patterns seen in SLE. However, although the ANA is a very sensitive screening test, it is not at all specific for SLE. The ANA is found in other rheumatic diseases such as Oligoarthritis and positive Polyarthritis, MCTD, dermatomyositis, as well as in chronic active hepatitis, and transiently after certain viral infections [50]. In addition, about 5–10% of healthy children have +ANA, and may even have a very elevated ANA titre [51,52]. In the absence of other findings or laboratory abnormalities, these children are not at risk for developing subsequent disease [50,53]. Unless SLE is suspected based on clinical and physical findings, the ANA test should not be done routinely.

The different patterns of ANA staining correlate with the presence of autoantibodies to specific components of the nucleus. Among these, anti-double stranded DNA (anti-ds DNA) and anti-Sm (Smith) antibody have high specificity for SLE, although they are not found in all patients (75–90% for anti-ds DNA antibodies, 15–50% for anti-Sm [8,10,13,15,17,22]). Patients who have these autoantibodies are likely to have SLE rather than another rheumatic disease. The titre of the anti-ds DNA antibody is correlated with disease activity in most children with SLE. A rise in anti-ds DNA antibody is associated with a fall in complement levels (C3, C4, or total CH50), and both tests are useful for monitoring changes in disease activity [12]. Other antinuclear autoantibodies include anti-RNP, anti-histone, anti-Ro (anti-SSA), anti-La (anti-SSB), and anti-scl70. All of these antibodies may also be found in SLE patients, but some, such as anti-RNP, are more likely to be associated with MCTD (see following section) [54–56], while the presence of anti-histone antibodies in the absence of anti-ds DNA and anti-Sm antibodies is more suggestive of drug-induced lupus (DIL; see following section) [7,57]. The anti-Ro antibody is found in nearly all of the ANA negative SLE, as well as in most patients with subcutaneous lupus erythematosus (SCLE; see following sections). The presence of Ro and La antibodies has also been associated with an increased incidence of cardiac disease [8,12,13,17,22,29].

Systemic lupus erythematosus is often associated with autoantibodies reactive with specific cells, such as erythrocytes (Coombs) or leukocytes, or specific molecules, such as phospholipids (APLA; see following section) and immunoglobulins. One of these, rheumatoid factor is more likely to be associated with SLE (12–50%) than with JIA (10% for RF positive Polyarthritis, much lower for other JIA subtypes) in the paediatric population [12–16]. Interestingly, this marker may be less common in Asian children with SLE [22,33]. The patient's clinical pattern (i.e. anaemia with evidence for haemolysis, symptoms suggestive of thrombosis) will determine which additional autoantibodies should be screened for. Two tests that were previously used in screening for SLE, the LE prep and lupus band test, are no longer performed because of the availability of specific autoantibody tests. Whenever possible, all newly diagnosed patients with SLE should have a PPD planted prior to beginning immunosuppressive therapy.

Treatment and prognosis

With more aggressive and improved treatment, the prognosis of childhood SLE has improved greatly, with 5 year survival reported

Table 1.6.3 Medications commonly used to treat systemic lupus erythematosus

Medication	Indications
Corticosteroids	Most manifestations of SLE; pulse doses for severe flares
NSAIDs	Musculoskeletal, mild serositis, fever
Hydroxychloroquine	Rash, arthritis, constitutional symptoms
Methotrexate	Corticosteroid sparing, arthritis
Azathioprine	Corticosteroid sparing, mild nephritis
Cyclophosphamide	Progressive or severe disease, especially of the kidney, central nervous system, or lung
Cyclosporin A	Renal disease, thrombocytopenia, corticosteroid sparing
Mycophenolate mofetil	Renal disease and other active manifestations
Intravenous gammaglobulin	Immune thrombocytopenia, immune leukopenia
Anti-CD20 Mab	Haemolytic anaemia, thrombocytopenia

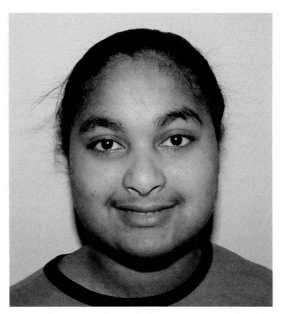

Figure 1.6.10 Cushingnoid facies. This Hispanic teenage girl with SLE developed cataracts and Cushingnoid facies, and striae while on corticosteroid treatment.

between 85% and 93% [8,34,58]. Because the manifestations of SLE can vary tremendously, treatment needs to be individualized and based upon the specific symptoms of the patient. General goals of therapy are to control disease manifestations, to allow the child to lead a normal life without major exacerbations, to prevent scarring in any organ and to prevent intolerable side-effects of the therapeutic regimen. Table 1.6.3 lists drugs that are commonly used to treat childhood SLE [1,40,58]. Unfortunately, because of the seriousness of the disease, immunosuppressant agents are usually required which increases the risk of developing secondary infections and malignancy. Corticosteroids have been very helpful in the treatment of SLE, but their use

Table 1.6.4 Steroid side-effects that can mimic SLE symptoms

Steroid side-effect	SLE symptom
Myopathy	Myositis
Psychosis and emotional liability	Same
Osteonecrosis	Arthritis, osteonecrosis from SLE
Infection: pneumonia, sepsis	Lupus pneumonitis, severe flare
Hypertension	Same
Atherosclerosis/coronary artery disease	Same
Pancreatitis	Same
Peptic ulcer disease/gastrointestinal bleeding	Gastrointestinal vasculitis
Pseudotumor cerebri (from steroid withdrawal)	Pseudotumor cerebri

is associated with many unpleasant and/or serious side effects in children (see also Part 3, Chapter 3.8) (Figure 1.6.10). Another difficulty with steroid use is that some of its side effects mimic specific SLE symptoms (Table 1.6.4).

Neonatal lupus erythematosus

Neonatal lupus erythematosus is associated with transplacental transfer of maternal anti-Ro/SSA and anti-La/SSB antibodies. At the time of delivery, only a minority of the mothers have SLE, most have another rheumatic disease (Sjögren syndrome, undifferentiated autoimmune syndrome) [59]. In addition, most of the asymptomatic mothers will develop a rheumatic disease within 5 years of delivery [59]. The risk for recurrence of NLE in future pregnancies is increased in all of these women [59,60]. The NLE rash consists of long-lasting, discrete erythematous, annular, mostly macular lesions that may have a central clearing (Figure 1.6.11). The rash usually involves the face (Figure 1.6.11b), and is commonly found in the periorbital area and on the scalp, but may involve the whole body [59]. The NLE rash is often triggered by UV exposure. Fever is uncommon in NLE.

Complete congenital heart block (CCHB) is the most common lesion in NLE. Evidence suggests that the cardiac disease may be due to direct binding of the autoantibodies to fetal heart tissue [60]. Other less common NLE manifestations include Coombs positive haemolytic anaemia, thrombocytopenia, leukopenia, transient hypocalcaemia with seizures, myelopathy, and neonatal hepatitis with cholestasis [60]. NLE typically presents around 6 weeks of life (range 0–20 weeks). Noncardiac symptoms resolve in about 6 months time, but 25% of infants with cutaneous NLE have residual sequela (telangiectasia, dyspigmentation, pitting/scarring/atrophy) [59]. Very few babies with neonatal lupus require treatment for noncardiac lupus symptoms. A few children with NLE later developed SLE, and in one study, 2/57 children with NLE subsequently developed Systemic Arthritis [59].

Mixed connective tissue disease

Mixed connective tissue disease is a disease that has combined features of SLE, progressive systemic sclerosis (PSS; see following section), and

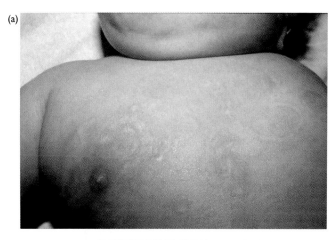
(a)

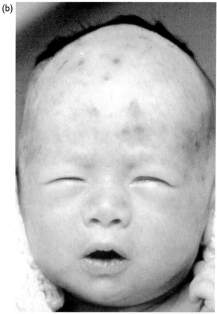
(b)

Figure 1.6.11 Neonatal LE. (a) At 2 weeks of life, this infant developed an erythematous, annular rash, and was found to have anti-Ro and anti-La antibodies. The child's mother had no known rheumatic disease at the time of delivery (Courtesy of Y. Kimura) (b) The neonatal lupus rash is frequently an erythematous, photosensitive maculopapular rash that presents on the face (Courtesy of T. R. Southwood).

polymositis/dermatomyositis (see following section) (Table 1.6.5; referenced in Kotajima *et al.* [54]). Patients with MCTD, similar to many patients with Systemic Arthritis or RF positive Polyarthritis, frequently present with polyarthritis, rash, and fever. However, the pattern of these symptoms is more similar to SLE than to JIA. Although most patients with MCTD have a +RF, systemic symptoms of rash, muscle weakness, and pain are much more prominent than their arthritis. The arthritis associated with MCTD is rarely erosive, and is more similar to the Jaccoud arthritis of SLE than to that associated with RF positive Polyarthritis [54,55]. The rashes seen in patients with MCTD differ from the transient Still rash, and instead resemble either SLE or dermatomyositis. Other skin changes commonly seen in MCTD include Raynaud phenomenon (Figure 1.6.7), and swelling of the hands with tightening, thickening, and loss of elasticity [61]; changes similar to those seen in PSS. Two other common MCTD symptoms, myositis

Table 1.6.5 Preliminary diagnostic criteria for mixed connective tissue disease

I. Common symptoms
   1. Raynaud phenomenon
   2. Swollen fingers or hands

II. Anti-nRNP antibody

III. Mixed findings
   A. Systemic lupus erythematosus-like findings
     1. Polyarthritis
     2. Lymphadenopathy
     3. Facial erythema
     4. Pericarditis or pleuritis
     5. Leukopenia ($<$4,000/mm^3) or thrombocytopenia ($<$100,000/mm^3)
   B. Systemic sclerosis-like findings
     1. Sclerodactyly
     2. Pulmonary fibrosis, restrictive change of the lung (%VC $<$ 80%), or reduced diffusion capacity (DLCO $<$ 70%)
     3. Hypomotility or dilation of the oesophagus
   C. Polymyositis-like findings
     1. Muscle weakness
     2. Increased serum levels of myogenic enzymes (CPK)
     3. Myogenic pattern in electromyography

Requirements for MCTD
   1. Positive in either one or two common symptoms
   2. Positive anti-RNP antibodies
   3. Positive in one or more findings in two or three disease categories of A, B, and C.

associated with muscle weakness and elevated muscle enzymes, and abnormal esophageal motility [54,61], are also unlikely in JIA. Similar to SLE, nearly all patients with MCTD have +ANA. Other autoantibodies that can be found in both diseases include RF, anti-RNP, but rarely anti-dsDNA or anti-Sm antibodies. The frequency and titre of anti-RNP antibodies is much higher in MCTD than SLE [54,55,61,62]. None of these autoantibodies are found in the patient with Systemic Arthritis. Patients with either SLE or MCTD may develop restrictive lung disease and decreased diffusing capacity as well as renal disease [54–56]. Lung disease is more commonly associated with pulmonary hypertension in MCTD than SLE, while renal disease is more common in SLE than MCTD. Patients with MCTD rarely have thrombocytopenia or CNS disease [61]. Treatment is aimed at specific symptoms using many of the same drugs used for SLE. Long-term outcome is variable; many patients do well, but the development of pulmonary hypertension is associated with a poor prognosis [54,55,61,62].

Chronic cutanenous lupus erythematosus

In chronic cutaneous lupus erythematosus (CCLE), the major manifestations are limited to the skin and mucous membranes. A variety of skin lesions are found, none of which resemble the rash of Systemic Arthritis. Discoid lupus erythematosus (DLE) is the most common form of CCLE, and is characterized by persistent local erythema, adherent scales, follicular plugging, telangiectasia, and atrophy [26]. The face, ears, chest, arms, scalp, and mucous membranes are most frequently affected (Figure 1.6.12). Some patches resolve, but most

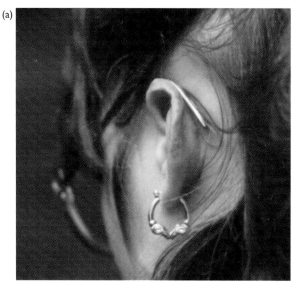

(a)

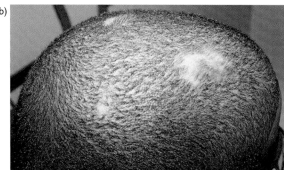

(b)

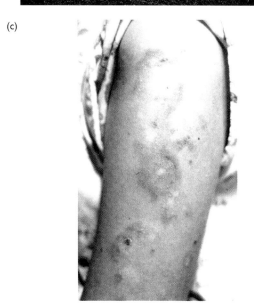

(c)

Figure 1.6.12 Discoid lupus. (a) This adolescent girl developed progressive discoid lesions on her scalp and ear (Courtesy of J. Jacobs). (b) An African American boy with discoid lupus presented with complaints of alopecia. (c) An African American girl had papules and hyperpigmented lesions typical of discoid lupus on the extensor surface of her arms as well as on her face (Courtesy of J. Jacobs).

leave flat, white scars, while others result in diffuse hyperpigmentation [26]. During the acute phase, the lesions are elevated and form ugly red oedematous plaques that may enlarge peripherally and coalesce into bizarre patterns.

DLE is uncommon in childhood. Unlike adult disease, childhood DLE does not show a female predominance, has a low incidence of photosensitivity (30% versus 60%), and frequently progresses to SLE at an early age (50% in 1 study) [63]. The SLE course may be severe, with all major organs involved (renal, CNS, cardiac, pulmonary). Both DLE and Systemic Arthritis may present with an elevated ESR, and high gamma globulin. However, similar to SLE and unlike Systemic Arthritis, DLE is also associated with a +ANA, antiphospholipid antibodies, and mild leukopenia. Other forms of CCLE include hypertrophic (verrucous) LE, chilblain LE or pernio, and lupus panniculitis [26].

Subacute cutaneous lupus erythematosus

Subacute cutaneous lupus erythematosus (SCLE) is another rheumatic disease whose manifestations are primarily limited to the skin and minor organs such as joints. This disease is much more commonly seen in adults than children. The typical lesion is a chronic erythematous papulosquamous patch that resembles that seen in psoriasis, different than the rash seen in Systemic Arthritis. The rash mainly occurs on sun-exposed areas (trunk, limbs, face, palms) [26] (Figure 1.6.13). Other skin manifestations include non-scarring alopecia, Raynaud phenomenon, periungal telengiectasias, painful violaceous, and atrophic finger pads secondary to vasculopathy, oral ulcers, and livedo reticularis [64]. The majority of patients have +ANA and anti-Ro/SSA antibodies and many have musculoskeletal complaints; only 5% have anti-dsDNA antibodies.

Drug-induced lupus

Many drugs have been associated with the development of a lupus-like syndrome (Table 1.6.6 [7,57,65]), which is generally milder than SLE. The most common symptoms are musculoskeletal (arthralgia, myalagia, arthritis), fever and weight loss, pleuritis and pleural effusions. The arthritis affects multiple joints (hands, wrists, elbows and, less commonly larger joints) similar to the pattern seen in RF positive Polyarthritis. However, similar to SLE and in contrast to JIA, the arthritis is non-deforming [7]. Life-threatening pericarditis may occur with either DIL or Systemic Arthritis; in DIL, it is most commonly associated with procainamide or hydralazine [7]. Unlike JIA, DIL is associated with lupus-like skin rashes (discoid, malar, and maculopapular rashes), photosensitivity, Raynaud phenomenon, mucosal ulcers, renal involvement, and neuropsychiatric symptoms [7], but these occur less frequently in DIL than in SLE. Nearly all patients with DIL develop a +ANA (exceptions are those induced by minocycline or quinidine) of a homogenous pattern, and most have anti-histone antibodies [7,57]. Generally, patients with DIL do not have anti-ds DNA or anti-Sm antibodies; antibodies that are most specific for SLE. Patients with DIL may have an elevated ESR, mild anaemia (normochromic, normocytic), and a +RF, but unlike Systemic Arthritis, DIL is usually associated with mild leukopenia rather than leukocytosis [7]. Some patients have been found to have lupus anticoagulants (LA) and other antiphospholipid antibodies, although only rarely has their presence been associated with thrombosis [7].

The criteria for the diagnosis of DIL have not yet been established, and patients with DIL usually have less than 4 of the 11 ACR criteria

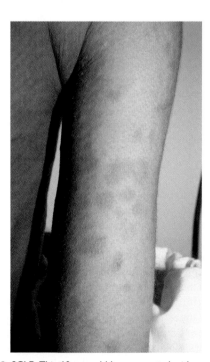

Figure 1.6.13 SCLE. This 10-year-old boy presented with a rash on his face that subsequently involved his arms and chest. He had a +ANA, oral sores, and alopecia (Courtesy of Y. Kimura).

Table 1.6.6 Medications associated with drug-induced lupus

Anticonvulsants
  carbamazepine
  ethosuximide
  phenytoin

Antimicrobials
  isoniazid
  minocycline

Antidepressants/antipsychotics
  chlorpromazine

Antihypertensive and cardiotonic
  hydralazine
  procainamide
  quinidine
  methyldopa
  acebutolol
  captopril

Anti-inflammatory/antirheumatic
  d-penicillamine
  sulfasalazine
  antitumour necrosis factor-α (infliximab, etanercept)

bold = drugs associated with the highest risk for development of drug-induced lupus.
For a more comprehensive list, see References 7, 57, and 65.

for the classification of SLE (Table 1.6.2). Diagnosis requires a temporal association of symptoms with drug treatment (weeks to months), and gradual resolution of symptoms after discontinuation of the drug [7,57]. DIL is more frequent in individuals who are genetically slow acetylators. Both sexes are affected relatively equally, and Caucasians are more likely to be affected than blacks [7]. Symptoms of DIL usually resolve within a few weeks after the causative agent is removed, although laboratory abnormalities may persist longer. In some cases, the symptoms may continue for over a year [7]. Some drugs, such as phenobarbitol and isoniazid are associated with a high incidence of inducing a +ANA, but not with actually triggering the development of DIL [7]. Therefore, +ANA in the absence of other symptoms is not an indication to change the current medication. Instead, patients should be monitored for other symptoms, and a treatment change considered if DIL symptoms develop. Mild symptoms of DIL can be treated with NSAIDs.

Antiphospholipid antibody syndrome

Antiphospholipid antibodies (aPL), have been associated with an increased risk for the development of recurrent vascular thrombosis and/or pregnancy loss [66], and include Lupus anticoagulant LA, anticardiolipin (aCL), and VDRL. Screening tests for aPL antibodies should also include APTT and PT, both of which can be prolonged. Antiphospholipid antibody syndrome (APLS) can be primary, or secondary to other autoimmune diseases, infections (HIV, parvovirus, Lyme, TB, streptococcus, and others), drugs (phenothiazines, procainamide, anticonvulsants, oral contraceptives), or, in adults, malignancies. Not all patients that have aPL will have a thrombotic event; and only those patients that are clinically symptomatic are considered to have APLS. Table 1.6.7 [66] shows a recent classification criteria for APLS; other criteria have also included the presence of clinical symptoms such as thrombocytopenia, haemolytic anaemia, and livedo reticularis in the classification criteria, but these features may not be as specific [66]. Between 19% and 87% of paediatric patients with SLE have aPL, and up to 44% of these patients had a thrombotic event [46]. Low dose aspirin and hydroxychloroquine may be helpful in preventing thrombosis in asymptomatic patients with SLE and aPL [67]. Many patients with JIA (13–50%) also have aPL; however, thrombotic

complications are extremely rare in JIA compared with SLE [46,68]. Other diseases associated with aPL include Sjögren syndrome, dermatomyositis, Takayasu arteritis (TA), Henoch–Schönlein purpura, insulin dependent diabetes mellitus, spondyloarthropathies, and IBD [46].

Patients with aPL are at risk for deep vein thrombosis, pulmonary emboli, strokes, transient ischaemic attacks, renal artery or vein thrombosis, pulmonary hypertension, cerebral venous sinus thrombosis, myocardial infarct, and gangrene/ischaemia of the limbs [46]. APLS is associated with autoimmune thrombocytopenia (platelets $50–150 \times 10^3$), and bleeding can also occur in these patients if they have hypoprothrombinaemia (increased PT). Some patients may develop cardiac valve vegetations or regurgitation, chorea, transverse myelopathy, or migraine headaches [46,69]. Catastrophic APLS is rare but often fatal; patients present in acute medical collapse with severe thrombocytopenia, acute respiratory distress syndrome, multi-organ failure, often with hypertension, or evidence of multiple vessel occlusions [46]. Children with Systemic Arthritis and disseminated intravascular coagulopathy may present with a similar picture, as can patients with SLE or thrombotic thrombocytopenic purpura.

Dermatomyositis
Introduction

Juvenile Dermatomyositis (JDM) is an autoimmune inflammatory disease of skin and muscle (myositis), characterized by proximal muscle weakness. Children with JDM may initially appear to have JIA because of the poorly defined extremity pain and functional disabilities such as difficulty in climbing stairs or trouble with walking and running. In addition, arthritis may also be present as a disease manifestation. Subtle signs and symptoms of proximal muscle weakness must often be teased out of the history and physical examination. (Table 1.6.8) [1,70–79]. However, experienced physicians can make the diagnosis promptly because of the typical distribution of the rash (Figure 1.6.14).

Although the etiology is not known, there is likely a role of infection and environmental triggers. Dermatomyositis symptoms may also occur in the context of SLE and MCTD. The illness is most common in children 10–14 years of age but also occurs in younger children. The incidence in children under 16 years of age is 1.9–3.0 per million.

Diagnosis

The diagnosis of dermatomyositis is based on the presence of the characteristic rash and myositis in the absence of laboratory evidence of SLE or MCTD (Table 1.6.9, [80]). Some children present with an *acute onset* with high fever, prostration, rash, and profound muscle weakness but this is quite rare. Most patients have a more *insidious onset* in which the rash precedes obvious muscle weakness by months. Unusual distribution of the rash should still alert the clinician to the possibility of JDM, particularly if associated with periorbital oedema. In those with insidious onset, diagnosis is frequently delayed and the rash is ascribed to eye or skin allergies, prolonged viral infection such as EBV, Systemic Arthritis if there is sufficient accompanying arthritis, or blamed on behavioral problems as children become more and more irritable and frustrated. Inability to take the big step onto the school bus, or to open the refrigerator door, and stumbling with a tendency

Table 1.6.7 Preliminary criteria for the classification of the antiphospholipid syndrome (Sapporo criteria)

Clinical criteria:
  A. Vascular thrombosis: one or more clinical episodes of arterial, venous, or small vessel thrombosis, in any tissue or organ. Thrombosis must be confirmed by imaging or Doppler studies or histopathology, with the exception of superficial venous thrombosis.
  B. Pregnancy morbidity

Laboratory criteria:
  A. Anticardiolipin antibody of IgG and/or IgM isotype in medium or high titer, on two or more occasions, at least 6 weeks apart
  B. Lupus anticoagulant present in plasma, on two or more occasions at least 6 weeks apart; other coagulopathies should be excluded

Definite antiphospholipid antibody syndrome is considered to be present if at least one of the clinical criteria and one of the laboratory criteria are met.
For details on pregnancy morbidity, and lupus anticoagulant testing, see Reference 66.

Table 1.6.8 Comparison of JIA with juvenile dermatomyositis, Wegener granulomatosis, and polyarteritis nodosa

	Systemic Arthritis	Positive polyarthritis	Juvenile dermatomyositis	Wegener granulomatosis	Polyarteritis nodosa
Age	No peak, throughout childhood; usually younger	Generally >8 years	Males: peak onset 6 years, and 11 years Females: peak onset 6 years, and 11–12 years	Mean: 12.7 years	Median 5–10 years
Sex	F = M	F >>> M	F:M varies from 1:1–5:1	F > M varies from 1.1–2.1:1	F = M
Arthritis pattern	Oligo or poly: oligo: large joints Poly: symmetrical, small	Polyarticular, symmetrical, small joints Erosions	Nondeforming, nondestructive Large and small joints	Arthralgia > arthritis (ankles, knees, hips, wrists) Nonerosive	Arthritis: large joints of leg May be localized, diffuse, or migratory
Extraarticular manifestations	Fever(quotidian) with improved physical activity in between fever spikes HSM, LA, pericarditis, pleuritis	May have low-grade fever, LA, HSM, anorexia, fatigue Subcutaneous nodules	May have fever, fatigue, myalgia, LA proximal muscle weakness, mouth ulcers, GI symptoms, calcinosis, lipodystrophy	Fever, fatigue, weight loss Sinusitis, OM, rhinitis, epistaxis, saddle nose Cough, subglottic stenosis, dyspnea, stridor, abnl CXR Conjunctivitis, scleritis, uveitis, proptosis Mouth ulcers Myalgia, abdominal pain	Fever, weight loss, LA, hepatomegaly, Myalgia, weakness, leg tenderness Abdominal pain, Hypertension HA, neuropathy, psychosis, seizures
Rash	Fluctuates with fever Salmon-pink, evanescent	Can get vasculitic lesions	Gottron papules Heliotrope rash Nailfold capillary changes Photosensitive, erythematous rash	Purpura Vescicles Papules Nodules	Painful subcutaneous nodules, purpura, splinter haemorrhage, livedo reticularis
Labs					
Hb	↓	↓, milder	May be nl or mildly ↓	↓	↓
WBC	↑	+/−	nl	nl or ↑	↑
Plt	↑	+/−	nl	↑	↑
ESR	↑	↑	nl or ↑	↑↑	↑↑
U/A	nl	nl	nl	haematuria, RBC casts, proteinuria	haematuria, proteinuria
Transaminases	↑	↑	↑, from muscle	nl	nl
CK, aldolase	nl	nl	↑	nl	nl
GGTP	↑	↑	nl	nl	nl
ANA	−	+ majority	+ 6–70%	−	uncommon
RF	−	+	−	−	−
Other			↑ vwf	+ANCA (c > p)	+/− ANCA, ↑ vwf
Family Hx	Rare	Rare	Increased incidence of autoimmune disease	Rare	Rare
Ethnicity	Predominantly Caucasian	Predominantly Caucasian	Caucasians >> Hispanic > African American	None	None

Abnl = abnormal; ANA = antinuclear antibody; ANCA = antineutrophil cytoplasmic antibodies; CK = creatinine kinase; CNS = central nervous system; CXR = chest X-ray; ENT = ears, nose, throat; GGTP = gamma glutamyl transpeptidase; GI = gastrointestinal; Hb = haemoglobin; HSM = hepatosplenomegaly; Hx = history; LA = lymphadenopathy; nl = normal; OM = otitis media; plt = platelet count; RBC = red blood cells; RF = rheumatoid factor; sx = symptoms; U/A = urinanalysis; vwf = von Willebrand factor

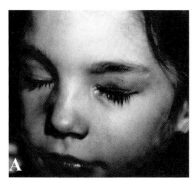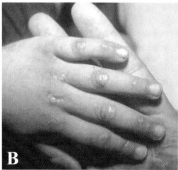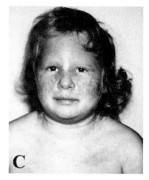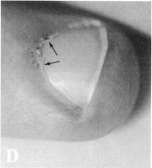

Figure 1.6.14 Dermatomyositis. (a) Heliotrope rash: A 7-year-old girl with dermatomyositis demonstrates a violaceous hue with prominent telangiectasias on her eyelids and a vasculitic pit in the inner acanthal fold. (b) Gottron papules. These lesions are flat, scaly, and may resemble psoriasis. They are found on the extensor surfaces of the PIPs, MCPs, DIPs, elbows, and knees. Although this case of Gottron papules is obvious, many children with dermatomyositis have only a few isolated papules. (Courtesy of Y. Kimura) (c) Dermatomyositis rash. This child has a generalized erythematous scaly rash. In most cases, the rash is confined to sun-exposed areas such as around the face and neck. However, some children have a widespread rash that can resemble severe eczema. (d) Telangiectasias. These can be seen, upon magnified examination, in the periungal skin in most children with dermatomyositis. Severe cases are associated with vessel drop out and thrombosis. The children's cuticles may become thickened and ragged, looking as if the child has been biting and peeling their fingertips.

Table 1.6.9 Diagnostic criteria for juvenile dermatomyositis

A diagnosis of juvenile dermatomyositis requires the presence of the rash plus two other criteria [81].

- A. Symmetrical weakness of the proximal musculature
- B. Characteristic cutaneous changes consisting of heliotrope discoloration of the eyelids with periorbital oedema, and an erythematous, scaly rash over the dorsal aspects of the metacarpophalangeal and proximal interphalangeal joints (Gottron papules)
- C. Elevation of the serum level of one or more of the skeletal muscle enzymes: creatine kinase, aspartate aminotransferase, lactic dehydrogenase, and aldolase.
- D. Electromyographic demonstration of the characteristics of myopathy and denervation
- E. Muscle biopsy documenting histologic evidence of necrosis and inflammation

Note: Criteria D and E are not usually required to make a diagnosis of JDM

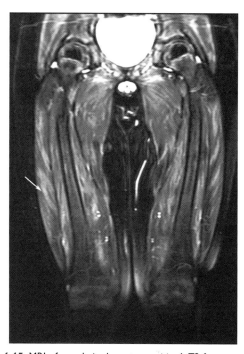

Figure 1.6.15 MRI of muscle in dermatomyositis. A T2 fat suppressed MRI of an affected proximal quadriceps muscle shows white signal indicating inflammation in contrast to the dark signal seen in normal muscle.

to fall have been some of the complaints that have first brought these children to the attention of physicians. Occasionally the presenting complaint of muscle pain or arthritis might suggest the diagnosis of JIA, but careful examination will usually reveal proximal muscle weakness (see Part 1, Chapter 1.1). A characteristic rash and disability out of proportion to concomitant arthritis are important clues to distinguish dermatomyositis from Systemic Arthritis. Conversely, all children with arthritis should have careful testing of proximal and distal muscle groups to elicit subtle weakness.

The classic diagnostic criteria includes presence of rash, typical weakness, and elevation of serum muscle enzymes (AST, ALT, LDH, CPK, and aldolase) due to inflammation (Table 1.6.9) [81]. A negative EMG and/or biopsy does not exclude the diagnosis; biopsy selection artifact results in at least 20% false negatives in well-documented cases [82]. Inflammation in the muscles may be documented with MRI—a T2 fat suppressed image will have a characteristic diffuse symmetric enhancement of muscle, and also may show skin enhancement and oedema [83] (Figure 1.6.15). Indeed, revised clinical criteria have now become the standard of care at many centres [72]; for children with

typical rash, weakness, muscle enzyme elevation, a positive diagnostic MRI can supplant the EMG and muscle biopsy and spare the patient the discomfort of invasive testing. However, if the patient lacks the typical rash an EMG or muscle biopsy may still be necessary.

Clinical manifestations

Rash (Figure 1.6.14)

Swelling of the eyelids and supraorbital areas is the most common early dermal manifestation and can usually be seen even if there are no other dermal manifestations. There is often a characteristic heliotrope hue to the upper eyelids, a dusky lilac discolouration with telangiectasias. In addition, a mild butterfly eruption on the face is common and can resemble the malar rash seen in SLE. However, the facial rash of dermatomyositis often travels down the nasolabial folds while these areas tend to be spared in SLE. Some patients have a more severe vasculitic rash with eschar formation (Figure 1.6.14). An erythematous/violaceous maculopapular eruption also appears in the periphery, especially over the extensor surfaces of the interphalangeal (PIP) joints, the elbows, and knees—called Gottron papules (Figure 1.6.14(b)). In some cases, there is an extensive rash in the V area of the chest. Red and swollen cuticles are almost always found and represent periungual vasculitis, sometimes visible in the form of vertical telangiectasia in the cuticles (Figure 6.14(d)); magnified nailfold capillaroscopy may be needed to demonstrate this sign.

Muscle weakness

Early in the disease there may be considerable pain in the proximal muscles. The myopathy is symmetric and proximal and usually spares distal muscles. The proximal muscle disease may be demonstrated by difficulty with prolonged elevation of the head while supine, or maintaining outstretched arms while sitting. Truncal weakness produces the Gower sign, an inability to rise from the floor without "climbing up" with hands over legs. Inability to do an unassisted sit up from the lying position is another excellent test of truncal strength. These simple manoeuvres should be performed in any child with swelling or periorbital or extensor surface rash (see also Part 1, Chapter 1.1).

Arthritis

Arthritis, manifested by joint effusion, pain and limitation can precede muscle weakness. Over 60% of JDM patients have arthritis, 2/3 oligoarticular and 1/3 polyarticular [83]. A few patients may have intermittent arthritis, with flares of myositis, and then continue to have arthritis after the myositis has resolved. The arthritis often includes small joints of the hand. Most children with arthritis improve quickly after corticosteroids are initiated. When arthritis is present, particularly if associated with Raynaud phenomenon, MCTD and SLE must be excluded through serologic testing. However, most children with JDM are younger than the typical adolescent with SLE or MCTD.

Gastrointestinal problems

Dysphagia, as a result of myopathy of palatal muscles, is common, especially in profoundly weak children, and these children are at risk for aspiration. Many children develop a nasal speech pattern with a decrease of voice volume—a sign of pharyngeal involvement that should not be ignored. Pneumatosis, air in the bowel wall demonstrated on X-ray, can be missed if the patient has no abdominal symptoms. Gastrointestinal (GI) bleeding and pain is not uncommon and complications of steroid therapy need to be distinguished from GI vasculitis. GI perforation from bowel-wall infarction and ulceration is now extremely rare but remains an important cause of death [85].

Lung disease

Weakness of the primary and accessory respiratory muscles may interfere with respiration and cough, which fosters aspiration, formerly a common cause of death in severely affected children. Interstitial pneumonia/fibrosis (fibrosing alveolitis) is probably more common

than had been previously recognized, but raises the possibility of MCTD. A small series found that half of JDM patients had asymptomatic lung disease on PFT testing [86].

Laboratory findings

Assay for creatinine phosphokinase (CPK) is commonly used in the diagnosis of skeletal or cardiac muscle diseases, but may be elevated in a variety of additional conditions such as exercise, insertion of needle into muscle (EMG), head injury or cerebral insult, infections, hypokalaemia, hypothyroidism, pulmonary disease, asthma treatment, and drug abuse (cocaine, alcohol). In this case an elevated CPK without manifestations of proximal muscle weakness or rash cannot be diagnosed as dermatomyositis and further evaluation is needed. Elevated LDH, ALT (SGOT), and AST (SGPT) can be muscular in origin. GGT, a more specific liver enzyme is not elevated in myositis and can help differentiate liver from muscle as the source of elevated enzyme. It should be noted that mild myositis, demonstrated by biopsy and by MRI, may also exist without muscle enzyme elevation [87]. Von Willebrand antigen, a marker of endothelial cell activation may be useful for following vasculitic complications of dermatomyositis, particularly when muscle enzymes are not revealing. ESR is not a good marker of muscle inflammation and is often normal even in very active disease.

Late complications

Calcinosis (Figure 1.6.16)

Children with dermatomyositis are prone to calcify skin, fascia, subcutaneous tissue, and fat, particularly during the healing phase of JDM. The extremities and trunk, pelvis, and neck may be affected. Most of the calcium deposits are small, punctate or clumpy, popcorn-like superficial lumps. The most superficial ones may become painful and then open, discharging calcium with relief of pain. Sheets of calcium are occasionally laid down, forming an exoskeleton that prevents adequate mobility of the joints. Recently, the presence of calcinosis has been linked to active myositis requiring treatment of underlying myopathy. With time many lesions improve with almost total disappearance of the sheets of calcium and improvement in function as a result. Tumorous calcinosis occurs occasionally and in rare cases requires surgical removal to improve local function.

Lipodystrophy

Some patients with a chronic or more severe course of disease may develop either generalized lipodystrophy or partial lipodystrophy [88]. Children with lipodystrophy have a characteristic loss of subcutaneous fat. Partial lipodystrophy is easily recognized in the extremities as deep, painless indentations without associated rash. Diffuse lipodystrophy is harder to recognize because these patients take on a leaner, atrophied appearance, but unusually defined muscles and vasculature can be seen (Figure 1.6.17). These patients often have associated insulin resistance, hyperinsulinaemia, diabetes, hypertriglyceridaemia, hypertension, and liver disease in addition to short stature.

Course, treatment, and prognosis

Most of the children are ill for a number of years. The disease may be uniphasic, polyphasic, or continuous [89]. There may be relative exacerbations and remissions while it is active or a polyphasic course may

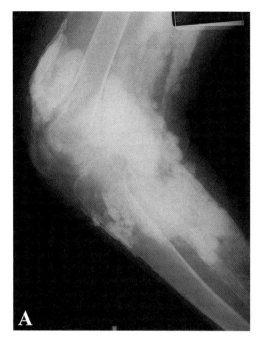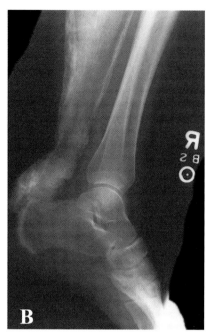

Figure 1.6.16 (a, b) Calcinosis. This girl was initially thought to have osteomyelitis after she presented with a limp and positive bone scan. Her dermatomyositis rashes had been unrecognized for years, and although she was not weak, her muscle enzymes were significantly elevated. Over the next 6 months, she developed widespread calcium deposits, which left her immobilized.

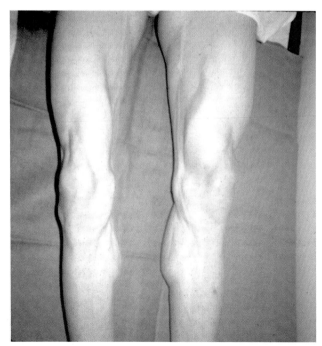

Figure 1.6.17 Lipodystrophy. This teenager presented simultaneously with dermatomyositis and diffuse lipodystrophy. Lipodystrophy can be localized or diffuse, and can occur at any point during the disease course. The elevation of liver enzymes associated with lipodystrophy can be confused with a flare of dermatomyositis (Courtesy of J. Jacobs) (see also Part I, Chapter 1.3, Fig 1.3.30).

be created by premature withdrawal of medications. Most children recover within 5 years with minimal or no residua. Some patients have contractures from arthritis, and up to one quarter develop persistant calcifications [90]. The goal of treatment should be the normalization of strength and muscle enzymes. Therapy should be escalated if palatal dysfunction or vasculitis is present. Corticosteroids are the mainstay of treatment, and methotrexate or intravenous gammaglobulin used as additional medications [91]. Very few children with dermatomyositis now die of the disease.

Polymyositis

Polymoysitis is rare in children, accounting for less than 10% of inflammatory myopathies [92], and often representing dermatomyositis with difficult to appreciate rash due to dark skin, or delayed onset of rash. Differentiating polymyositis from Polyarthritis requires a thorough joint exam, detailed testing of muscle strength, and laboratory studies. Polymyositis in children is identical in clinical presentation and radiographic findings to dermatomyositis excluding the dermatologic findings. Muscle biopsy is necessary to confirm this diagnosis. Polymyositis may be less responsive to steroid treatment than dermatomyositis.

Amyopathic dermatomyositis (JDM sine myositis)

Amyopathic dermatomyositis describes a subset of patients who present with the classic dermatologic manifestations of dermatomyositis without any evidence of myositis on physical or laboratory exam. A recently published series discovered that many of these patients were found to have subtle signs of myositis when investigated fully, mild weakness, abnormal MRI or muscle biopsy [93]. In fact, because approximately half the patients with JDM develop a rash even as long as 2 years prior to muscle weakness, distinction of amyopathic from JDM may be impossible. Those patients with subtle myositis should be treated. The patients without myositis may not require treatment. Patients with amyopathic dermatomyositis do not present with arthritis, and the rash is usually easily distinguished from rashes seen in Systemic Arthritis.

Scleroderma

Introduction

The hallmark of the heterogeneous but related group of disorders called scleroderma is the presence of hard, tight, inelastic (hidebound) skin and subcutaneous tissue, and refers to two distinctly different syndromes: (1) localized scleroderma and (2) Systemic Sclerosis (SSC). These disorders are easy to distinguish. The localized form does not affect internal organs and favourable prognosis is the norm, whereas SSC is a rare, devastating disorder with a very poor prognosis. In both disorders, at least two-thirds of affected children are girls but familial cases are rare. Joint involvement in scleroderma is usually a contracture secondary to affected skin overlying joints, rather than widespread inflammatory synovitis. Differentiation from JIA and Oligoarthritis is not difficult and the pattern of autoantibodies allows these conditions to be distinguished from SLE and MCTD. There are other disorders that can mimic cutaneous and systemic scleroderma [94,95].

Systemic sclerosis (SSC, also known as Progressive systemic sclerosis—PSS)

Systemic sclerosis is extremely rare in childhood. The initial symptom is almost always Raynaud phenomenon (see section "Raynaud Phenomenon") followed by an oedematous inflammatory phase. Skin involvement is generally easily recognized, and a skin biopsy is frequently unnecessary. The diagnosis of systemic sclerosis is generally made on the basis of generalized bilateral symmetrical sclerodermatous skin changes proximal to the MCP or MTP joints. Patients with SSC may have severe and frequent episodes of Raynaud phenomenon that lead to tissue compromise and ulcerations, and occasionally even the reabsorption of the distal phalanges (Figure 1.6.18(c,d)).

Clinical manifestations

Raynaud phenomenon

Raynaud phenomenon includes three phases: pallor (complete spasm of the vessel), cyanosis (partial spasm), and hyperaemia (reactive dilatation). Not only skin vessels are affected; 38% of otherwise normal individuals may have decreased lung vital capacity, especially when exposed to cold [96].

The use of Raynaud phenomenon as a marker of PSS is complex, because the phenomenon, albeit rare in young children, is common in

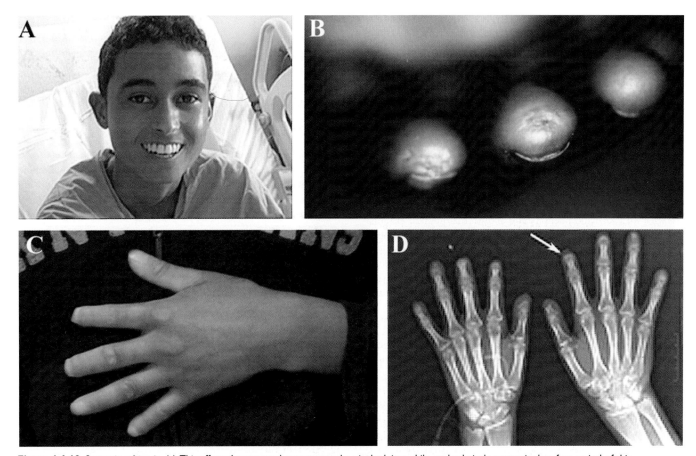

Figure 1.6.18 Systemic sclerosis. (a) This affected teenager demonstrates the pinched, immobile, and relatively expressionless face typical of this disease; his mouth cannot be fully opened. (b) Digital pits: This boy also had frequent episodes of Raynaud phenomenon, and had digital pits and loss of subcutaneous tissue from his fingertips. (c) Shortening of the digits resulted in loss of function. (d) An X-ray shows the bony changes associated with reabsorption of the distal phalanges.

Table 1.6.10 Differential diagnosis of Raynaud phenomenon

Condition resembling Raynaud Phenomenon	Mechanism	Associated finding
Acrocyanosis	Vasoreactive; may be induced by sympathomimetic drugs	Symmetric blueness of nailbeds slower in onset than Raynaud phenomenon and related to duration of cold exposure
Pheochromocytoma/Carcinoid	Vasospastic	Cool, painful, cyanotic extremities associated with hypertension/flushing/syncopy and high urine VMA
Migraine related	Vasospastic	Headaches
Cryoglobulinemia, Polycythaemias Cold agglutinin disease	Abnormal blood viscosity	Cold agglutinins, high hematocrit, cryoglobulins
Thoracic outlet, Crutch syndrome Vibration induced	Mechanical	Often associated with specific activities
Cold injury/frostbite	Vasculopathy of small vessels	Prolonged redness and pain after cold exposure (see also Part I, Chapter 1.8)
Primary hyperoxaluria	Vascular insufficiency	Renal failure and gangrene secondary to oxalate deposition
Reflex sympathetic dystrophy	Neurovascular reflex	Pain, allodynia, coolness, and swelling Vascular insufficiency, gangrene (see also Part I, Chapter 1.9)
Erythromelalgia	Neurovascular reflex	Episodic burning, erythematous swelling often associated with diabetes
Solitary mastocytoma	Vasospastic secondary to histamine release	Pink-brown skin lesions develop vesiculations or wheal and flare with rubbing Generalized flushing may be accompanied by diarrhoea, vomiting, pain, headache, high fever, convulsions

teenage girls (1.9–4.6% of the population) (Figure 1.6.7). Onset is usually at puberty and female to male ratio is 20:1. Most patients develop the episodes while in cold ambient temperature or under stress. The presence of ANA, (especially anticentromere antibodies or antitopoisomerase) or of nailfold capillary abnormalities, has consistently identified a sub-population at increased risk for developing systemic scleroderma or other connective-tissue diseases [97]. However, nailfold telangiectasia does not invariably progress to PSS. Digital tip pitting (ulcerations) or scars (Figure 1.6.18(b)), decreased oesophageal motility, and decreased pulmonary diffusing capacity identify a subset of patients with Raynaud at higher than usual risk for development of systemic disease [98]. An analysis of many studies suggests that for a teenager with Raynaud phenomenon and normal physical examination, the risk of later developing a connective tissue disease is about 3% while in the presence of physical findings or laboratory markers of increased risk, 25% of teenagers later develop clear autoimmune disease [99–101]. The differential diagnosis of illnesses that resemble Raynaud syndrome is presented in Table 1.6.10.

Skin findings

Children with swelling of the hands are often referred to the rheumatologist to rule out scleroderma or arthritis (Table 1.6.11). In PSS, there may be striking oedematous swelling of the fingers that lasts for several weeks before it is replaced by thick, tight, non-pliable skin that becomes increasingly taut, shiny, and atrophied. After a period of months or years, the skin of fingers and hands then becomes diffusely thickened. Often, there are pigmentary changes, either hypo or hyperpigmentation. When scleroderma affects the face, the patient can develop a pinched, immobile and expressionless facade and lose the ability to fully open the mouth (Figure 1.6.18(a)). Nailfold telangiactasias and Raynaud phenomenon usually precede these changes in the skin.

Joint problems

Joints may be limited and symptomatic as a result of overlying scleroderma. Occasional patients may have arthritis resembling that seen in RF positive Polyarthritis. Brief episodes of monoarticular inflammation occur in some children.

Gastrointestinal

Abnormal oesophageal motility occurs in almost all patients with systemic sclerosis, sometimes with oesophageal erosions. Hypomobility of the small intestine may also result in dilatation of the duodenum and result in malabsorption and wasting. Patients often have bloating, abdominal cramps, diarrhoea, or severe constipation.

Cardiac and pulmonary

Most children with SSC have impairment of gas exchange and decreased vital capacity as a result of pulmonary fibrosis. Dyspnoea may be a prominent symptom, although the child may be unaware of changes in lung physiology because they have already restricted their activities [102]. Pulmonary fibrosis or pulmonary vascular hypertension may also occur. Pulmonary hypertension may present with syncopal episodes. Myocarditis and pericarditis may be early manifestations. Cardiac decompensation (pericardial tamponade) has been the most common cause of death in children with PSS.

Localized scleroderma—morphea, linear scleroderma

In 10% of children, localized scleroderma begins with arthritis, in a clinical presentation indistinguishable from Oligoarthritis, and the diagnostic skin lesions appear months or years later [103]. Alternatively

Table 1.6.11 Differential diagnosis of hand swelling

Aetiology	Distribution	Clinical characteristics
Scleroderma	Symmetric: digits, hands, face	May be initial presentation, acute onset of dramatic warm tender swelling. May last weeks to months
Frostbite—cold injury	Area of cold exposure	Persistent colour changes, coolness of extremity pain; severe cases can have gangrenous changes
Hypertrophic osteoarthropathy	Clubbing fingers/toes Symmetric	Can be associated with chronic lung disease, inflammatory bowel disease, cyanotic congenital heart disease or malignancy
Dactylitis—sickle cell disease spondyloarthritis	Isolated to one or several digits	Painful sausage-like digits, usually red
Diabetes mellitus	Cheiroarthropathy	Painless stiffness and swelling of digits with restricted ROM
Child abuse	Localized to areas of trauma; in hands, can be dorsal hand and knuckles	Painful, discoloration over abused area. X-rays can show fractures, bone chips, periosteal new bone formation
Allergic reaction/ hereditary angioedema/ Cold-induced urticaria	Can be localized or diffuse	May respond to antihistamines; pruritis is present. Often associated with urticaria
Reflex sympathetic dystrophy	Generally part of one extremity	Pain, allodynia, change in color and temperature of the affected region
Erythromelagia	Distal extremities, both hands and feet	Erythematous, warm, and swollen extremities associated with painful burning sensation
Thiemann disease	PIP joints hands > feet	Relatively painless, firm, symmetrical swelling of PIP joints, with typical X-ray changes of irregular epiphyses (see also Part 1, Chapter 1.8)

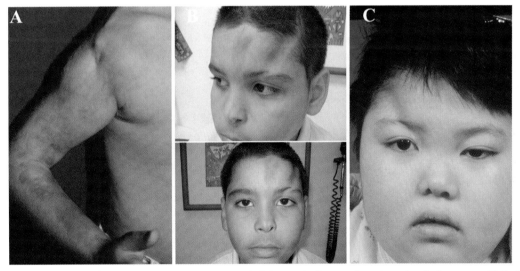

Figure 1.6.19 Linear scleroderma. (a) This child has severe involvement, which has resulted in atrophy and arm length discrepancy. (b) En Coup de Sabre. This child had a linear lesion that crossed his forehead and nose. The nasal ostia and teeth were affected. (c) Parry Romberg Syndrome. Facial hemiatrophy with coup de sabre-like indentation of the right side of face without sclerodermatous features (Courtesy of J. Jacobs).

joint contractures may be present when the abnormal skin overlies a joint. Localized scleroderma rarely may precede systemic sclerosis in the setting of an overlap syndrome [104].

Clinical manifestations

Flesh-colored or erythematous oedematous plaques that evolve into firm, waxy ivory, or yellow-white shiny lesions, sometimes with a violaceous border, are called morphea. Lesions may be single or multiple and they may coalesce. Linear scleroderma lesions sometimes

resemble morphea at onset but have a linear configuration that appears as a broad band, often running along an entire extremity (Figure 1.6.19(a)). The initial inflammatory phase may be accompanied by more generalized oedema. Unlike morphea, linear scleroderma is not limited to the skin, but the involvement of the underlying fat, muscle, fascia, and sometimes bone may result in severe growth deformities or mutilation. A particular localized form of this lesion termed "coup de sabre" (Figure 1.6.19(b)) appears in the forehead and scalp and may extend down into the face and be accompanied by morphea. This lesion may distort the orbit, sinuses, and nares. There might be ipsilateral brain lesions which possibly result in seizures [105]. Facial hematrophy the Parry-Romberg syndrome (Figure 1.6.19(c)) may be a consequence of linear scleroderma (coup de sabre). Children with localized scleroderma may have arthritis, oesophageal dysfunction, and coup-de-sabre-induced CNS manifestations, but they do not have the other systemic manifestations characteristic of PSS [106]. Nailfold changes and telangiectasias are not seen in morphea.

CREST syndrome

CREST, a variant of systemic scleroderma, is very rare in children. This condition is characterized by prominent Calcinosis (C), Raynaud phenomenon (R), oesophageal dysmotility (E), sclerodactyly (S), and telangiectasia (T). The classical autoantibody associated with CREST is the antibody to centromere. Patients with CREST syndrome tend to have a slower, more indolent course than those with PSS, but the disease may suddenly become aggressive and indistinguishable from PSS. Thickened skin may also be seen as a feature of other indurative diseases (see also Part 1, Chapter 1.3, Table 1.3.3).

Eosinophilic fasciitis

Eosinophilic fasciitis is characterized by painful, generalized, indurated, scleroderma-like swelling of the hands and feet following exercise. The progressive swelling of the extremities is so dramatic that pitting oedema is often demonstrable. These patients can rapidly develop extensive flexion contractures. In some cases, the face and trunk are also involved. There is impressive eosinophilia in the peripheral blood representing 8–29% of white blood cells. The ESR is elevated and hypergammaglobulinaemia is usually present. Biopsy must be deep and include fascia otherwise the pathologic lesion may be missed [107]. Some children have localized scleroderma lesions (morphea and/or linear scleroderma) preceding diffuse fasciitis [108]. Most patients respond quickly to a course of high-dose corticosteroids.

Vasculitis

Introduction

Most systemic vasculitis syndromes are uncommon in children except for Kawasaki Disease and Henoch–Schönlein Purpura (Part 1, Chapter 1.4) [76]. The diagnosis of systemic vasculitis is suspected (in the absence of SLE, MCTD, and JDM) when (1) several organ systems are simultaneously or consecutively affected and (2) the clinical manifestations include myalgia, arthralgia/arthritis, rash, and other symptoms (Table 1.6.12). The physician evaluating a child with possible systemic vasculitis should also consider Systemic Arthritis. Both diseases can share common symptoms such as arthritis, fever, weight loss, and malaise. In addition, elevated acute phase reactants are commonly seen in both illnesses. However, the rash of Systemic Arthritis is quite characteristic (Part 2, Chapter 2.1) and does not occur in vasculitis. In addition, the arthritis associated with systemic vasculitis tends to be painful but not erosive, and arthralgias are more common than arthritis.

Table 1.6.12 Clinical features suggesting systemic vasculitis in children

Multiple organ systems[a]	Clinical features
Rheumatic	Fever, myalgia, arthritis, abdominal pain, high ESR out of proportion to physical findings
Skin	Rash, ulceration, erythema nodosum
Renal	Nephritis, hypertension
Respiratory	Nasal congestion, pulmonary infiltrates, eosinophilia
Neurological	Multiple neurological manifestations of CNS and peripheral
Cardiovascular	Pulse deficits, pericarditis, heart failure, coronary artery disease

[a] Simultaneous or consecutive involvement.

Diagnosis

Diagnosis depends upon a high level of clinical awareness and pattern recognition by an astute clinician. Classical examples of systemic vasculitis include: a teenage girl with failure to thrive, unexplained fevers and vague musculoskeletal complaints, may have Takayasu arteritis even before the characteristic loss of peripheral pulses. The combination of glomerulonephritis and nasal serosanguinous discharge in an adolescent raises the possibility of Wegener granulomatosus, whereas a younger child with renal and CNS features may have polyarteritis nodosa. Very rarely, the child with asthma and nodular skin rash may have Churg–Strauss syndrome.

Polyarteritis Nodosa (PAN)

Introduction

PAN occurs only rarely under the age of 18 years and is characterized by hypertension, renal arteritis, and frequent neurologic involvement [109]. Vasculitis of skin, muscle, testes, and joints is common, and aneurysms may occur in medium-sized renal, visceral (especially hepatic), and cerebral arteries. Males are slightly more frequently affected than females. In children, this illness usually begins with unexplained fevers associated with arthralgia, abdominal pain, and severe myalgia [110–112]. In males, testicular pain may be a helpful diagnostic clue. When present, it is usually an early manifestation, preceding fever, but it is often mistaken for torsion of the testis. Some children have obvious vasculitic or purpuric skin lesions. In some patients, vasculitis in the extremities is severe enough to cause periosteal new-bone formation and exquisite bone tenderness.

Similar to patients with Systemic Arthritis, patients with PAN often have anaemia, leukocytosis, and an elevated ESR (Table 1.6.8, [1, 70–79]). Nonspecific symptoms such as myalgia and fatigue often precede more specific symptoms by a year or more [113]. Arthritis occurs in 30% of patients and involves large joints. However, unlike Systemic Arthritis, PAN frequently is associated with other major organ involvement including nerve and muscle. All layers of arteries are affected with resulting fibrinoid necrosis, thrombosis, and infarction. Aneurysms form in weakened arterial walls. The vascular lesions

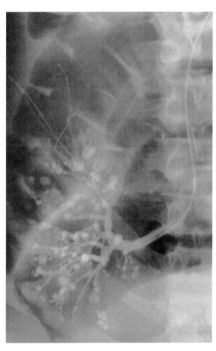

Figure 1.6.20 Polyarteritis nodosa. This teenager presented with fevers, renal disease, and elevated liver function tests. An angiogram revealed grape-like aneurysms in his liver and kidneys. The patient had a spontaneous subscapsular bleed in one kidney, which was electively embolized to present uncontrollable haemorrhage.

are usually segmental, tend to be most apparent at the bifurcations and branchings of small- and medium-sized arteries, and are simultaneously seen in all stages of development (Figure 1.6.20). Appropriate radiological investigations may include MRA or an angiogram.

Course and prognosis

Without prompt treatment, PAN may be fatal. The high mortality rate in children is often due to under recognized and under-treated disease. Cyclophosphamide and high-dose corticosteroids are the treatment of choice for life-threatening necrotizing vasculitis. Recent experience suggests that long-term clinical remission or cure is possible. Severe aneurysms seen in abdominal vessels can regress. Thus, the historically grave prognosis for PAN does not seem appropriate, provided patients are diagnosed early and treated aggressively.

Microscopic polyangiitis

Children with microscopic polyangiitis (MPA) may present with features similar to those seen with PAN, however, MPA typically involves small vessels and causes pulmonary and interstitial kidney involvement [100]. Patients often present with alteration in renal function, and proteinuria. Rapidly progressive glomerulonephritis and renal failure are characteristic of MPA [114]. Antineutrophilic cytoplasmic antibodies (ANCA) with myeloperoxidase specificity (pANCA) are found in 40–80% of patients. ANCA are not typical of PAN and can be used as a differentiating test. The treatment of both syndromes is similar. Diagnosis is most often confirmed by finding necrotizing vasculitis of small vessels on renal biopsy.

Wegener granulomatosis

Introduction

Wegener granulomatosis (WG) is a clinical triad consisting of disseminated, ANCA positive, small-vessel vasculitic granulomas of both the upper and lower respiratory tracts, associated with renal disease [115]. Most patients have fever, purpuric skin lesions, myositis sinusitis, otitis, nasopharyngeal symptoms, haemoptysis and/or pulmonary infiltrates. WG is extremely rare in children, and is more commonly seen in the adolescent. Boys and girls are equally affected, unlike adults where there is a significant male predominance.

Most present with unexplained fever, anorexia, weight loss, cough, chest pain, pulmonary haemorrhage, myalgia, and arthritis or arthralgia. In our experience, nasal symptoms, although frequently ignored by the physician, are the most important clue to this diagnosis in a child with mysterious multisystem disease [76]. On occasion the arthritis is the first presenting symptom and half of patients complain of lower extremity pain [73]. The features that are distinct from RF positive Polyarthritis and Systemic Arthritis are presented in Table 1.6.8 [1,70–79].

Diagnosis

Childhood onset WG is similar to adult onset disease, however, children are more likely to have subglottic stenosis and nasal deformities [74]. Nasal mucosal ulceration, nasal obstruction or mucosal lesions, and serous otitis media may accompany sinusitis. Destruction of the bony walls of the sinuses and of the nasal septum may result in the characteristic saddle nose deformity (Figure 1.6.21). Childhood onset WG can have severe pulmonary manifestations with haemoptysis, pulmonary haemorrhage, and severe impairment of pulmonary function. Pulmonary lesions may sometimes be demonstrated radiographically or on pulmonary function testing even in the absence of pulmonary symptoms. Renal disease often occurs later than other symptoms of WG.

Eye lesions are common and include lesions of the conjunctiva, cornea, and sclerae as well as uveitis and pseudotumour of the orbit; some children present with only sinus and orbital lesions. About 25% of WG patients have haemoptysis, 25% have cardiac manifestations, and at least 25% have neurological manifestations. The most common neurological symptom is mononeuritis multiplex, but occasionally there are CNS granulomatous lesions. Anaemia, leukocytosis, hypergammaglobulinaemia, and an elevated ESR are commonly demonstrated. Renal lesions are segmental and focal pauci-immune crescentic glomerulonephritis.

Laboratory findings

Antineutrophilic cytoplasmic antibodies initially were reported to be diagnostic of WG, with a sensitivity of 97%; these antibodies may disappear with treatment and reappear as predictors of exacerbation. Most patients with active WG have a positive ANCA, predominantly to proteinase 3 (c-ANCA) [116]. The ANCA pattern helps to differentiate the renal disease of WG from MPA. In the absence of characteristic renal and pulmonary findings diagnosis depends on the demonstration of characteristic giant-cell vasculitic granulomas in the upper respiratory tract or lungs.

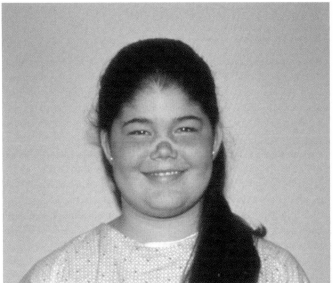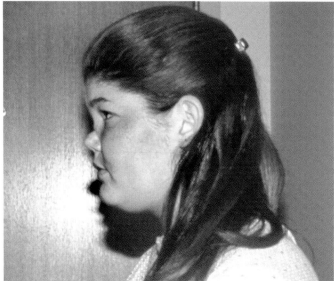

Figure 1.6.21 Saddle nose deformity. This 12-year-old girl with limited Wegener granulomatosis had aggressive sinus disease, which progressed to a saddle nose deformity and hearing loss (Courtesy of Y. Kimura).

Limited Wegener granulomatosis

The "limited" form of WG is defined by lesions only in the orbit and respiratory tract (lung, sinuses, and other mucosal surfaces) without involvement of the kidneys or the vascular system. In contrast to the generally rapid progression of generalized WG, the limited forms of disease usually evolve slowly, but destruction of the sinuses and hearing loss do occur and these patients require aggressive therapy.

The diagnosis of limited WG may be difficult because ANCA testing is usually negative. It is important to remember that the diagnosis of limited WG is not dependent upon the finding of vasculitis but rather on the demonstration in biopsy of typical foci of necrosis, palisading granulomas, and giant cells. The prognosis of limited WG is better than systemic WG but relapses are common [75].

Takayasu arteritis

Takayasu arteritis, originally called "pulseless disease" is characterized by inflammation of the aorta and its major branches including the pulmonary arteries [117]. The majority of patients with TA are young women (post-pubertal). Asians, particularly Japanese, are especially susceptible. The disease usually has a chronic onset with anorexia, malaise, fatigue, slowing of linear growth, and failure to gain weight. However, these symptoms may be so mild that they are initially missed. Arthralgia, unexplained fever, and brief episodes of arthritis occur in some patients. The only clues to the extent of the process are the finding of a greatly elevated ESR and greatly increased levels of gamma globulin. The chronic pre-pulseless phase may persist for years before an acute exacerbation demands diagnosis. The usual setting for diagnosis is the finding of diminished peripheral pulses, and a dilated aorta on chest radiograph. Alternatively, hypertension is a presenting symptom [118] and maybe associated with mid-aortic lesions, that can be found during renal evaluation. Children with lesions of the mid-aorta alone do not have diminished peripheral pulses.

Unfortunately, the diagnosis is often established following acute hypertensive encephalopathy with seizures or during profound congestive heart failure due to hypertension from renal and systemic arterial occlusion. There may also be aortic valvulitis with aortic insufficiency and pulmonary artery obstruction. Syncopal spells and sudden episodes of paroxysmal hypertension characterized by tachycardia with palpitations, headache, dyspnea, precordial pain, choking sensations, sweating, and flushing of the face may be caused by aortic arch lesions that alter carotid sinus baroreceptor sensitivity. These spells may be set off by sudden changes in posture or by micturition.

Diagnosis may be suspected on blood vessel ultrasound studies and must be promptly confirmed by MRI/MRA. Studies show irregularity, occlusion, stenosis, post-stenotic dilation, and aneurysms of the proximal portions of branches of the aorta (Figure 1.6.22). Segmental mural inflammation can be demonstrated on special sequence MRI, which is particularly useful in following disease activity [119,120].

Behçet syndrome

Behçet syndrome is characterized by recurrent genital and oral ulceration with relapsing iritis, and/or conjunctivitis [121]. Recurrent mouth ulcers can be the only manifestation of disease in many children [122]. Ocular disease may occur less frequently in children than in adults but when it occurs it can be severe and refractory to treatment [123,124]. In addition to the mucocutaneous-ocular symptom complex, patients with Behçet syndrome also develop articular, intestinal, neurologic, and vasculitic manifestations [125]. If arthritis and uveitis occur together, these children are generally thought to have Oligoarthritis. It is only later, when genital ulcers appear that the syndrome is recognized.

Joint pain in Behçet syndrome is prevalent, occurring in 79% of children with Behçet in one series [126]. Arthritis occurs in about one-third of patients and tends to be oligoarticular primarily in the knees

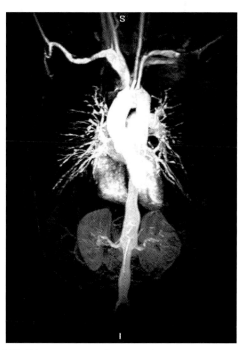

Figure 1.6.22 Takayasu arteritis. The MRI of this patient with Takayasu arteritis shows ectasia and narrowing of the aorta, as well as aneurysms at the branch points of the subclavian, brachial, and pulmonary arteries. This patient also had coronary artery aneurysms.

and ankles, and hip. Mild and recurrent episodes resemble those seen in patients with Enthesitis Related Arthritis. Radiographic changes are rare, and when sacroiliac changes are demonstrable, they are generally very mild. The most commonly affected upper-extremity joints are the wrists and elbows. Papulopustular skin lesions and arthritis are concurrent in many Behçet patients [127].

Gastrointestinal complaints are common in Behçet syndrome and resemble those seen in patients with IBD (see also Part 1, Chapter 1.4). At colonoscopy, the findings in these patients are sometimes indistinguishable from Crohn Disease or ulcerative colitis. However, severe oesophageal ulcers are more common in Behçet syndrome, and discrete vesicles and localized ulceration may be demonstrated at various sites within an otherwise completely normal GI tract. These lesions resemble the aphthous ulcers seen in the mouth and genitals and suggest this diagnosis.

Rashes occur in the majority of patients over the course or their illness, but there are no characteristic biopsy findings. During acute exacerbations of Behçet syndrome the skin may show a peculiar hyperreactivity to needle puncture, which is called pathergy. Within 24 h, a pustule surrounded by a red halo appears at the site of the puncture. Erythema nodosum, pyoderma, and dermal vasculitis are other dermatological manifestations. Erythema nodosum may accompany the bowel symptoms or herald their appearance.

Neurologic manifestations occur in about 25% of patients with Behçet syndrome at some time during the disease and may wax and wane along with the other manifestations. Aseptic meningitis is the most frequent CNS manifestation, but transient ocular palsies, cerebellar ataxia, cerebral venous sinus thrombosis, cerebral vasculitis, and corticospinal-tract involvement resulting in hemi- or quadriparesis may occur. Aortitis, vena caval obstruction from thrombophlebitis,

multiple pulmonary artery aneurysms, and other arterial aneurysms may occur. Coronary arteritis is rare.

Churg–Strauss syndrome

The usual presentation is the sudden onset of fever, pulmonary infiltrates, vasculitic skin lesions (especially subcutaneous nodules), pericarditis and congestive heart failure in a child who has had asthma [128,129]. Peripheral neuropathy (mononeuritis multiplex) and signs of gastrointestinal vasculitis are common. Although there is sometimes clinical overlap with PAN, a distinct combination of features including asthma, allergic features and peripheral eosinophilia (generally higher than $1500/\text{mm}^3$) is characteristic of Churg–Strauss syndrome (CSS) and not PAN [130]. CSS has been associated with positive p-ANCA directed against myeloperoxidase in about 70% of patients. Arthralgias and arthritis are noted in approximately 20% of patients, which are sometimes migratory and transient.

Cogan syndrome

Bilateral nerve deafness and interstitial keratitis (without syphilis) constitute Cogan syndrome. Occasionally, the keratitis is accompanied by iritis. Patients tend to have recurrent attacks resulting in progressive deafness and threatening vision. Vertigo, tinnitus, and ear pain also occur. One-fourth of patients has been reported to have musculoskeletal manifestations, usually arthralgia or mild arthritis. In a paediatric review 20% of reported cases were associated with life-threatening aortic insufficiency, which sometimes occurred suddenly and unexpectedly [131]. Associated symptoms included fever, weight loss, hepatosplenomegaly, and lymphadenopathy.

Iritis and sensorineural deafness are seen in relapsing polychondritis (RP); Enthesitis Related Arthritis; Heerfordt syndrome (with seventh nerve palsy); Vogt–Koyanagi syndrome (with alopecia, poliosis, and vitiligo); and Harada syndrome (with cells and protein in spinal fluid). Other causes of autoimmune hearing loss are listed in Table 1.6.13.

Relapsing polychondritis

Relapsing polychondritis (RP) is a relatively rare, episodic, but generally progressive disorder characterized by destructive inflammation of cartilage. Ear cartilage is most commonly affected, and the children

Table 1.6.13 Causes of secondary immune mediated hearing loss

Antiphospholipid antibody syndrome
Cogan Syndrome
Inflammatory bowel disease
Muckle–Wells Syndrome
Polychrondritis
Sjögren syndrome
Enthesitis Related Arthritis
Vogt–Koyanagi–Harada syndrome
Wegener granulomatosis

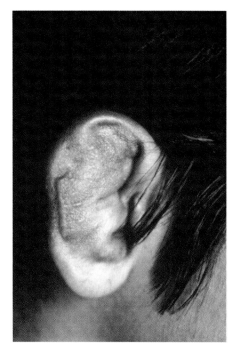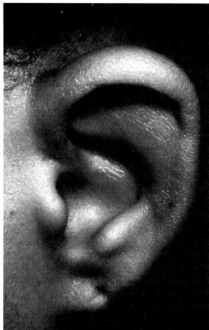

Figure 1.6.23 Relapsing polychondritis, The effect of destructive inflammation of the cartilage is obvious in these patient's deformed pinnae (Courtesy of J. Jacobs).

generally present with recurrent inflammation of the cartilaginous portion of the ear pinnae that ultimately leads to almost total loss of ear cartilage (Figure 1.6.23). In most cases, the diagnosis is obvious and need not be confirmed by biopsy. Other common manifestations of RP include nasal chondritis that may cause a saddle-nose deformity, respiratory obstruction from laryngotracheobronchial chondritis (that can be life-threatening and require intubation), ocular inflammation (conjunctivitis, scleritis, iritis, keratitis) [132], and auditory and vestibular impairment that may result from meatal narrowing and inflammation.

Arthritis in RP tends to be intermittent and migratory with attacks that last from several days to weeks and then resolve spontaneously only to recur again months later. Large and small joints of all extremities may be involved, usually in an asymmetrical fashion. The parasternal joints (costochondral cartilages) are involved in 30–60% of the attacks [133]. In young children, metaphyseal inflammation during growth may result in deformity with a unique radiographic appearance characterized by severe cartilaginous destruction with little or no involvement of adjacent bone or joint. The joint fluid is non-inflammatory. Laboratory studies are not helpful in RP; the only consistent abnormality is an elevated ESR. However, laboratory studies are obtained to help exclude other disorders.

MAGIC syndrome: mouth and genital ulcers with inflamed cartilage syndrome

MAGIC syndrome is a term applied to patients with overlap syndromes between polychondritis and Behçet disease. A review of patients with Behçet and polychondritis has indicated overlap of symptoms and a common immunologic target (Elastin) has been proposed. In the reported series of patients with MAGIC, only one child (10 years old, female) was described. Steroids have been used successfully to control inflammation [134].

References

1. Cassidy, J. and Petty, R. *Textbook of Pediatric Rheumatology.* Philadelphia, PA.: W. B. Saunders Co., 2001.

2. Sullivan, K. Complement deficiency and autoimmunity. *Curr Opin Pediatr* 1998;10:600–6.

3. Date, Y., Seki, N., Kamizono, S. *et al.* Identification of a genetic risk factor for systemic juvenile rheumatoid arthritis in the 5′-Flanking region of the TNFalpha gene and HLA genes. *Arthritis Rheum* 1999;42:2577–82.

4. Arnett, F. Genetic studies of human lupus in families. *Int Rev Immunol* 2000;19:297–317.

5. Cantagrel, A., Navaux, F., Loubet-Lescoulie, P. *et al.* Interleukin-1beta, interleukin-1 receptor antagonist, interleukin-4, and interleukin-10 gene polymorphisms: relationship to occurence and severity of rheumatoid arthritis. *Arthritis Rheum* 1999;42:1093–100.

6. Cvetkovic, J., Wallberg-Jonsson, S., Stegmayr, B., Rantapaa-Dahlqvist, S., and Lefvert, A. Susceptibility for and clinical manifestations of rheumatoid arthritis are associated with polymporphisms of the TNF-alpha, IL-1beta, and IL-1Ra genes. *J Rheumatol* 2002;29:212–19.

7. Yung, R. and Richardson, B. Drug-induced lupus. *Rheum Dis Clin North Am* 1994;20:61–86.

8. Tucker, L., Menon, S., Schaller, J., and Isenberg, D. Adult- and childhood-onset systemic lupus erythematosus: a comparision of onset, clinical features, serology, and outcome. *Br J Rheumatol* 1995;34:866–72.

9. Tan, E., Cohen, A., and Fries, J. The 1982 revised criteria for the classification of systemic lupus erythematosus. *Arthritis Rheum* 1982;25:1271–77.

10. Bosi Ferraz, M., Goldenberg, J., Hilario, M. *et al.* Evaluation of the 1982 ARA lupus criteria data set in pediatric patients. *Clin Exp Rheumatol* 1994;12:83–87.

11. Hochberg, M. Updating the American College of Rheumatoloy revised criteria for the classification of systemic lupus erythematosus. *Arthritis Rheum* 1997;40:1725.

12. DeMarco, P. and Szer, I. Systemic lupus erythematosus in childhood. In R., Lahita, ed., *Systemic Lupus Erythematosus*. New York: Academic Press, 2004, pp. 485–514.

13. Gedalia, A., Molina, J., Molina, J., Uribe, O., Malagon, C., and Espinoza, L. Childhood-onset systemic lupus erythematosus: a comparative study of African Americans and Latin Americans. *J Natl Med Assoc* 1999;91:497–501.

14. Marini, R. and Lavras Costallat, L. Young age at onset, renal involvement and arterial hypertension are of adverse prognostic significance in juvenile systemic lupus erythematosus. *Rev Rhum* (Engl Ed) 1999;66:303–9.

15. Rood, M., ten Cate, R., van Suijlekom-Smit L, *et al.* Childhood-onset systemic lupus erythematosus. *Scand J Rheumatol* 1999;28:222–6.

16. Caeiro, F., Michielson, F., Bernstein, R., Hughes, G., and Ansell, B. Systemic lupus erythematosus in childhood. *Ann Rheum Dis* 1981;40:325–31.

17. Font, J., Cervera, R., Espinosa, G., *et al.* Systemic lupus erythematosus (SLE) in childhood: analysis of clinical and immunological findings in 34 patients and comparison with SLE characteristics in adults. *Ann Rheum Dis* 1998;57:456–9.

18. van Vugt, R., Derksen, R., Kater, L., and Bijlsma, J. Deforming arthropathy or lupus and rhupus hands in systemic lupus erythematosus. *Ann Rheum Dis* 1998;57:540–4.

19. Ragsdale, C., Petty, R., Cassidy, J., and Sullivan, K. The clinical progression of apparent juvenile rheumatoid arthritis to systemic lupus erythematosus. *J Rheumatol* 1980;7:50–55.

20. Mont, M. and Jones, L. Management of osteonecrosis in systemic lupus erythematosus. *Rheum Dis Clin North Am* 2000;26:279–309.

21. Assouline-Dayan, Y., Chang, C., Greenspan, A., Shoenfeld, Y., and Gershwin, M. Pathogenesis and natural history of osteonecrosis. *Semin Arthritis Rheum* 2002;32:94–124.

22. Chandrasekaran, A., Rajendran, C., Ramakrishnan, S., Madhavan, R., and Parthiban, M. Childhood systemic lupus erythematosus in South India. *Indian J Pediatr* 1994;61:223–9.

23. Chen, J-H., Lin, C-Y., Chen, W-P., Tang, R-B., and Hwang, B. Systemic lupus erythematosus in children. *Chinese J Microbiol Immunol* 1987;20:23–8.

24. Motil, K., Grand, R., Davis-Kraft, L., Ferlic, L., and Smith, E. Growth failure in children with inflammatory bowel disease: a prospective study. *Gastroenterology* 1993;105:681–91.

25. Cassidy, J., Sullivan, D., Petty, R., and Ragsdale, C. Lupus nepritis and encephalopathy: prognosis in 58 children. *Arthritis Rheum* 1977;20:315–22.

26. Laman, S. and Provost, T. Cutaneous manifestations of lupus erythematosus. *Rheum Dis Clin North Am* 1994;20:195–211.

27. Wananukul, S., Watana, D., and Pongprasit, P. cutaneous manifestations of childhood systemic lupus erythematosus. *Pediatr Dermatol* 1998;15:342–6.

28. Schneider, R. and Laxer, R. Systemic onset juvenile rheumatoid arthritis. *Bailliere's Clin Rheumatol* 1998;12:245–71.

29. Oshiro, A., Derbes, S., Stopa, A., and Gedalia, A. Anti-Ro/SS-A and Anti-La/SS-B antibodies associated with cardiac involvement in childhood systemic lupus erythematosus. *Ann Rheum Dis* 1997;56:272–4.

30. Amigo, M-C. and Khamashta, M. Antiphospholipid (Hughes) syndrome in systemic lupus erythematosus. *Rheum Dis Clin North Am* 2000;26:331–48.

31. Ilowite, N. Premature atherosclerosis in systemic lupus erythematosus. *J Rheumatol* 2000;27 (Suppl 58):15–19.

32. Davisson, N., Westervelt, F., and Bolton, W. Comparison of alternate day steroids and daily steroids in renal transplant recipients. *Proc Clin Dial Transplant Forum* 1980;10:150–154.

33. Lee, B., Yap, H., Yip, W., *et al.* A 10 year review of systemic lupus erythematosus in Singapore children. *Aust Paediatr* J 1987;23:163–165.

34. Klein-Gitelman, M., Reiff, A., and Silverman, E. Systemic lupus erythematosus in childhood. *Rheum Dis Clin North Am* 2002;28:561–577.

35. Mackay, I. Auto-immune (lupoid) hepatitis: an entity in the spectrum of chronic active liver disease. *J Gastroenterol Hepatol* 1990;5:360–361.

36. Hellmich, B., Csernok, E., Schatz, H., Gross, W., and Schnabel, A. Autoantibodies against granulocyte colony-stimulating factor in Felty's syndrome and neutropenic systemic lupus erythematosus. *Arthrities Rheum* 2002;46:2384–91.

37. Bloom, B., Smith, P., and Alario, A. Felty syndrome complicating juvenile rheumatoid arthritis. *J Pediatr Hematol Oncol* 1998;20:511–13.

38. Zimmerman, S. and Ware, R. Clinical significance of the antinuclear antibody test in selected children with idiopathic thrombocytopenic purpura. *J Pediatr Hematol Oncol* 1997;19:297–303.

39. Brunner, H., Freedman, M., and Silverman E. Close relationship between systemic lupus erythematosus and thrombotic thrombocytopenic purpura in childhood. *Arthrities Rheum* 1999;42:2346–55.

40. Arkachaisri, T., and Lehman, T. Systemic lupus erythematosus and related disorders of childhood. *Curr Opin Rheumatol* 1999;11:384–392.

41. Knook, L.M., de Kleer, I.M. van der Ent, C.K. van der Net, J.J., Prakhen, B.J. and Kuis. W. Lung function abnormalities and respiratory muscle weakness in children with juvenile chronic arthritis. *Eur Respir J* 1999;14:529–33.

42. Malleson, P., Riding, K., and Petty, R. Stridor due to cricoarytenoid arthritis in pauciarticular onset juvenile rheumatoid arthritis. *J Rheumatol* 1986;13:952–3.

43. Wallace, D. and Hahn, B. *Dubois' Lupus Erythematosus*. Philadelphia, PA: Lippincott Williams and Wilkins, 2002:1348.

44. Sibbitt, Jr., W., Brandt, J., Johnson, C., *et al.* The incidence and prevalence of neuropsychiatric syndromes in pediatric onset systemic lupus erythematosus. *J Rheumatol* 2002;29:1536–42.

45. Quintero-Del-Rio, A. and Miller, V. Neurologic symptoms in children with systemic lupus erythematosus. *J Child Neurol* 2000;15:803–7.

46. Ravelli, A. and Martini, A. Antiphospholipid antibody syndrome in pediatric patients. *Rheum Dis Clin North Am* 1997;23:657–76.

47. Sanna, G., Bertolaccini, M., Cuadrado, M., *et al.* Neuropsychiatric manifestations in systemic lupus erythematosus: prevalence and association with antiphospholipid antibodies. *J Rheumatol* 2003;30:985–92.

48. Foster, C. Systemic lupus erythematosus, discoid lupus erythematosus, and progressive systemic sclerosis. *Int Ophthalmol Clin* 1997;37:93–110.

49. Hamideh, F. and Prete, P. Ophthalmologic manifestations of rheumatic diseases. *Semin Arthritis Rheum* 2001;30:217–41.

50. Deane, P., Liard, G., Siegel, D., and Baum, J. The outcome of children referred to a pediatric rheumatology clinic with a positive antinuclear antibody test but without an autoimmune disease. *Pediatrics* 1995;95:892–5.

51. Perilloux, B., Shetty, A., Leiva, L., and Gedalia, A. Antinuclear antibody (ANA) and ANA profile tests in children with autoimmune disorders: a retrospective study. *Clin Rheumatol* 2000;19:200–3.

52. Solomon, D., Kavanaugh, A., and Schur, P., Guidelines AAHCoIT. Evidence-based guidelines for the use of immunologic tests: antinuclear antibody testing. *Arthritis Rheum* 2002;47:434–4.

53. Cabral, D., Petty, R., Fung, M., and Malleson, P. Persistent antinuclear antibodies in children without identifiable inflammatory rheumatic or autoimmune dsease. *Pediatrics* 1992;89:441–4.

54. Kotajima, L., Aotsuka, S., Sumiya, M., Yokohari, R., Tojo, T., and Kasukawa, R. Clinical features of patients with juvenile onset mixed connective tissue disease: analysis of data collected in a nationwide collaborative study in Japan. *J Rheumatol* 1996;23:1088–94.

55. Tiddens, H., van der Net, J., de Graeff-Meeder E, *et al.* Juvenile-onset mixed connective tissue disease: Longitudinal follow-up. *J Pediatr* 1993;122:191–7.

56. Yokota, S., Imagawa, T., Katakura, S., *et al.* Mixed connective tissue disease in childhood: a nationwide retrospective study in japan. *Acta Paediatr Jpn* 1997;39:273–76.

57. Rubin, R. Etiology and mechanisms of drug-induced lupus. *Curr Opin Rheumatol* 1999;11:357–63.

58. Shaham, B. and Bernstein, B. The rheumatic diseases of childhood. In Weisman M., Weinblatt M., Louie, J., eds. *Treatment of the Rheumatic Diseases*. New York: W.B. Saunders company, 2001, pp. 423–45.

59. Neiman, A., Lee, L., Weston, W., and Buyon, J. Cutaneous manifestations of neonatal lupus without heart block: characteristics of mothers and children enrolled in a national registry. *J Pediatr* 2000;137:674–80.

60. Tseng, C.-E. and Buyon, J. Neonatal lupus syndromes. *Rheum Dis Clin North Am* 1997;23:31–54.

61. Yokota, S. Mixed connective tissue disease in childhood. *Acta Paediatr Jpn* 1993;35:472–79.

62. Mier, R., Ansell, B., Hall, M., *et al.* Long term follow-up of children with mixed connective tissue disease. *Lupus* 1996;5:221–6.

63. George, P. and Tunnessen, W. Childhood discoid lupus erythematosus. *Arch Dermatol* 1993;129:613–17.

64. Parodi, A., Caproni, M., Cardinali, C., *et al.* Clinical, histological and immunopathological features of 58 patients with subacute cutaneous lupus erythematosus. *Dermatology* 2000;200:6–10.

65. Favalli, E., Sinigaglia, L., Varenna, M., and Arnoldi, C. Drug-induced lupus following treatment with infliximab in rheumatoid arthritis. *Lupus* 2002;11:753–5.

66. Wilson, W., Gharavi, A., Koike, T., *et al.* International consensus statement on preliminary classification criteria for definite antiphospholipid syndrome. *Arthritis Rheum* 1999;42:1309–11.

67. Alarcón-Segovia, D., Boffa, M., Branch, W., *et al.* Prophylaxis of the antiphospholipid syndrome: a consensus report. *Lupus* 2003;12:499–503.

68. von Scheven, E., Athreya, B., Rose, C., Goldsmith, D., and Morton, L. Clinical characteristics of antiphospholipid antibody syndrome in children. *J Pediatr* 1996;129:1–10.

69. Chapman, J., Rand, J., Brey, R., *et al.* Non-stroke neurological syndromes associated with antiphospholipid antibodies: evaluation of clinical and experimental studies. *Lupus* 2003;12:514–17.

70. Pachman, L. Juvenile dermatomyositis: immunogenetics, pathophysiology, and disease expression. *Rheum Dis Clin North Am* 2002;28:579–602.

71. Ramanan, A. and Feldman, B. Clinical features and outcomes of juvenile dermatomyositis and other childhood onset myositis syndromes. *Rheum Dis Clin North Am* 2002;28:833–57.

72. Ramanan, A. and Feldman, B. Clinical outcomes in juvenile dermatomyositis. *Curr Opin Rheumatol* 2002;14:658–62.

73. Belostotsky, V., Shah, V., and Dillon, M. Clinical features in 17 paediatric patients with Wegener granulomatosis. *Pediatr Nephrol* 2002;17:754–61.

74. Rottem, M., Fauci, A., Hallahan, C., *et al.* Wegener's granulomatosis in children and adolescents: clinical presentation and outcome. *J Pediatr* 1993;122:26–31.

75. Stegmayr, B., Gothefors, L., Malmer, B., Müller Wiefel, D., Nilsson, K., and Sundelin, B. Wegener granulomatosis in children and young adults. *Pediatr Nephrol* 2000;14:208–13.

76. Sundel, R. and Szer, I. Vasculitis in childhood. *Rheum Dis Clin North Am* 2002;28:625–54.

77. Al Mazyad, A. Polyarteritis nodosa in Arab children in Saudi Arabia. *Clin Rheumatol* 1999;18:196–200.

78. Bakkaloglu, A., Ozen, S., Baskin, E. *et al.* The significance of antineutrophil cytoplasmic antibody in microscopic polyangitis and classic polyarteritis nodosa. *Arch Dis Child* 2001;85.

79. Athreya, B. Vasculitis in children. *Pediatr Clin N Am* 1995;42:1239–61.

80. Bohan, A. and Peter, J. Polymyositis and dermatomyositis. *N Engl J Med* 1975; 292:344.

81. Bohan, A. and Peter, J.B. Polymyositis and dermatomyositis (second of two parts). *N Engl J Med*, 1975; 292(8):403–7.

82.. Pachman, L.M. *et al.* Juvenile dermatomyositis at diagnosis: clinical characterisics of 79 children. *J Rheumatol*, 1998;25(6):1198–204.

83. Kimball, A.B., *et al.* Magnetic resonance imaging detection of occult skin and subcutaneous abnormalities in juvenile dermatomyositis. Implications for diagnosis and therapy. *Arthritis Rheum* 2000;43(8):1866–73.

84. Tse, S. *et al.*, The arthritis of inflammatory childhood myositis syndromes. *J Rheumatol* 2001;28(1):192–7.

85. Schullinger, J.N., Jacobs, J.C., and Berdon, W.E. Diagnosis and management of gastrointestinal perforations in childhood dermatomyositis with particular reference to perforations of the duodenum. *J Pediatr Surg* 1985; 20(5):521–4.

86. Trapani, S., *et al.* Pulmonary involvement in juvenile dermatomyositis: a two-year longitudinal study. *Rheumatology* (Oxford), 2001;40(2):216–20.

87. Rider, L.G., Outcome assessment in the adult and juvenile idiopathic inflammatory myopathies. *Rheum Dis Clin North Am*, 2002;28(4): 935–77.

88. Huemer, C. *et al.* Lipodystrophy in patients with juvenile dermatomyositis—evaluation of clinical and metabolic abnormalities. *J Rheumatol* 2001;28(3):610–15.

89. Spencer, C.H. *et al.* Course of treated juvenile dermatomyositis. *J Pediatr* 1984;105(3):399–408.

90. Huber, A.M. *et al.* Medium- and long-term functional outcomes in a multicenter cohort of children with juvenile dermatomyositis. *Arthritis Rheum* 2000;43(3):541–9.

91. Oddis, C.V. Idiopathic inflammatory myopathy: management and prognosis. *Rheum Dis Clin North Am* 2002;28(4):979–1001.

92. Rider, L.G. and Miller, F.W. Classification and treatment of the juvenile idiopathic inflammatory myopathies. *Rheum Dis Clin North Am* 1997; 23(3):619–55.

93. Plamondon, S. and Dent, P.B. Juvenile amyopathic dermatomyositis: results of a case finding descriptive survey. *J Rheumatol* 2000;27(8): 2031–4.

94. Jablonska, S. and Blaszczyk, M. Scleroderma-like disorders. *Semin Cutan Med Surg* 1998;17(1):65–76.

95. Harper, J.I. Cutaneous graft versus host disease. *Br Med J (Clin Res Ed)* 1987;295(6595):401–2.

96. Groen, H. *et al.* Pulmonary diffusing capacity disturbances are related to nailfold capillary changes in patients with Raynaud's phenomenon with and without an underlying connective tissue disease. *Am J Med* 1990;89(1):34–41.

97. Weiner, E.S. *et al.* Prognostic significance of anticentromere antibodies and anti-topoisomerase I antibodies in Raynaud's disease. A prospective study. *Arthritis Rheum* 1991;34(1):68–77.

98. Fitzgerald, O. *et al.* Prospective study of the evolution of Raynaud's phenomenon. *Am J Med* 1988;84(4):718–26.

99. Jung, L.K. and Dent, P.B. Prognostic significance of Raynaud's phenomenon in children. *Clin Pediatr* (Phila), 1983;22(1):22–5.

100. Duffy, C.M. *et al.* Raynaud syndrome in childhood. *J Pediatr* 1989;114(1): 73–8.

101. DeCross, A.J. and Sahasrabudhe, D.M. Paraneoplastic Raynaud's phenomenon. *Am J Med* 1992; 92(5):p. 571–2.

102. Garty, B.Z. *et al.* Pulmonary functions in children with progressive systemic sclerosis. *Pediatrics* 1991; 88(6): 1161–7.

103. Cassidy, J.T. *et al.* Scleroderma in children. *Arthritis Rheum* 1977;20(2 Suppl):351–4.

104. Birdi, N. *et al.* Localized scleroderma progressing to systemic disease. Case report and review of the literature. *Arthritis Rheum* 1993; 36(3): 410–5.

105. Chung, M.H. *et al.* Intracerebral involvement in scleroderma en coup de sabre: report of a case with neuropathologic findings. *Ann Neurol* 1995; 37(5): 679–81.

106. Dehen, L. *et al.* Internal involvement in localized scleroderma. *Medicine* (Baltimore), 1994;73(5):241–5.

107. Farrington, M.L. *et al.* Eosinophilic fasciitis in children frequently progresses to scleroderma-like cutaneous fibrosis. *J Rheumatol* 1993;20(1):128–32.

108. Miller, J.J., 3rd. The fasciitis-morphea complex in children. *Am J Dis Child* 1992;146(6):733–6.

109. Lightfoot, R.W., Jr., *et al.* The American College of Rheumatology 1990 criteria for the classification of polyarteritis nodosa. *Arthritis Rheum* 1990; 33(8):1088–93.

110. Ozen, S., *et al.* Diagnostic criteria for polyarteritis nodosa in childhood. *J Pediatr* 1992;120(2 Pt 1):206–9.

111. Magilavy, D.B. *et al.* A syndrome of childhood polyarteritis. *J Pediatr* 1977; 91(1):25–30.

112. Ettlinger, R.E. *et al.* Polyarteritis nodosa in childhood a clinical pathologic study. *Arthritis Rheum* 1979;22(8):820–5.

113. Agard, C. *et al.* Microscopic polyangiitis and polyarteritis nodosa: how and when do they start? *Arthritis Rheum* 2003;49(5):709–15.

114. Jennette, J.C. *et al.* Nomenclature of systemic vasculitides. Proposal of an international consensus conference. *Arthritis Rheum* 1994;37(2):187–92.

115. Leavitt, R.Y. *et al.* The American College of Rheumatology 1990 criteria for the classification of Wegener's granulomatosis. *Arthritis Rheum* 1990; 33(8):1101–7.

116. Bartunkova, J., Tesar, V., and Sediva, A. Diagnostic and pathogenetic role of antineutrophil cytoplasmic autoantibodies. *Clin Immunol* 2003;106(2): 73–82.

117. Arend, W.P. *et al.* The American College of Rheumatology 1990 criteria for the classification of Takayasu arteritis. *Arthritis Rheum* 1990;33(8): 1129–34.

118. Jain, S. *et al.* Takayasu arteritis in children and young indians. *Int J Cardiol* 2000;75 (Suppl 1):S153–S157.

119. Itazawa, T. *et al.* Magnetic resonance imaging for early detection of Takayasu arteritis. *Pediatr Cardiol* 2001,22(2):163 4.

120. Aluquin, V.P. *et al.* Magnetic resonance imaging in the diagnosis and follow up of Takayasu's arteritis in children. *Ann Rheum Dis* 2002; 61(6):526–9.

112. Criteria for diagnosis of Behcet's disease. International Study Group for Behcet's Disease. *Lancet* 1990;335(8697):1078–80.

122. Kim, D.K., *et al.* Clinical analysis of 40 cases of childhood-onset Behcet's disease. *Pediatr Dermatol* 1994;11(2):95–101.

123. Kone-Paut, I., *et al.* Familial aggregation in Behcet's disease: high frequency in siblings and parents of pediatric probands. *J Pediatr* 1999;135(1):89–93.

124. Tugal-Tutkun, I. and Urgancioglu, M. Childhood-onset uveitis in Behcet disease: a descriptive study of 36 cases. *Am J Ophthalmol* 2003;136(6): 1114–19.

125. Lang, B.A., *et al.* Pediatric onset of Behcet's syndrome with myositis: case report and literature review illustrating unusual features. *Arthritis Rheum* 1990;33(3):418–25.

126. Krause, I., *et al.* Childhood Behcet's disease: clinical features and comparison with adult-onset disease. *Rheumatology* (Oxford), 1999;38(5):457–62.

127. Yurdakul, S., Hamuryudan, V., and Yazici, H. Behcet syndrome. *Curr Opin Rheumatol* 2004;16(1):38–42.

128. Oermann, C.M., *et al.* Pulmonary infiltrates with eosinophilia syndromes in children. *J Pediatr* 2000;136(3):351–8.

129. Masi, A.T. *et al.* The American College of Rheumatology 1990 criteria for the classification of Churg–Strauss syndrome (allergic granulomatosis and angiitis). *Arthritis Rheum* 1990;33(8):1094–100.

130. Abril, A., Calamia, K.T., and Cohen, M.D. The Churg–Strauss syndrome (allergic granulomatous angiitis): review and update. *Semin Arthritis Rheum* 2003;33(2):106–14.

131. Olfat, M. and Al-Mayouf, S.M. Cogan's syndrome in childhood. *Rheumatol Int* 2001; 20(6):246–9.

132. Isaak, B.L., Liesegang, T.J., and Michet, C.J., Jr., Ocular and systemic findings in relapsing polychondritis. *Ophthalmology* 1986;93(5):681–9.

133. Balsa, A., *et al.* Joint symptoms in relapsing polychondritis. *Clin Exp Rheumatol* 1995;13(4):425–30.

134. Firestein, G.S., *et al.* Mouth and genital ulcers with inflamed cartilage: MAGIC syndrome. Five patients with features of relapsing polychondritis and Behcet's disease. *Am J Med* 1985;79(1):65–72.

1.7 Autoinflammatory diseases and distinct but rare rheumatic conditions

Suzanne C. Li

Aim

The aim of this chapter is to describe a number of diseases occurring in children that may mimic JIA particularly Systemic Arthritis. These diseases are frequently hereditary and their genetic basis is becoming increasingly understood.

Structure

- Definition of autoinflammatory diseases
- Periodic fever syndromes
  - PFAPA
  - Cyclic neutropenia
  - FMF
  - HIDS
  - TRAPS
- Other hereditary febrile syndromes
  - Familial urticarial syndromes
  - Muckle–Wells
  - ADPF
  - CINCA/NOMID
  - PAPA
- Granulomatous diseases
  - Sarcoidosis
  - Blau syndrome
- Hyperostosis syndromes
  - Goldbloom syndrome
  - Caffey–Silverman syndrome

Definition of autoinflammatory diseases

In addition to rheumatic conditions, such as systemic lupus erythematosus, dermatomyositis, and vasculitis syndromes discussed in Chapter 1.6, there are a number of other systemic inflammatory conditions that can present with features suggestive of Systemic Arthritis. These include the periodic fever syndromes, sarcoidosis, CINCA/NOMID, Blau syndrome, Caffey disease, and Goldbloom syndrome, all of which will be discussed in this chapter. Recent studies have identified the genes responsible for a number of the hereditary periodic fever

syndromes. Many of the identified genes are suspected to be involved in regulating inflammation or apoptosis. Nearly all of the hereditary periodic fever syndromes, and many chronic systemic inflammatory conditions, such as Crohn disease, Behçet syndrome, CINCA/NOMID, and Blau syndrome are proposed to comprise a new disease category called autoinflammatory diseases. Autoinflammatory diseases are systemic conditions characterized by inflammation not due to autoreactive B or T lymphocytes [1–4]. Other diseases that are likely candidates for this category include PFAPA and sarcoidosis. Interestingly, with the identification of genes involved in many of these syndromes, it has become clear that a number of patients with phenotypic features of autoinflammatory diseases do not have mutations in any of the identified candidate genes. Thus, it is likely that additional genes will be identified that give rise to similar disease phenotypes, and that future classification of these illnesses will involve both genetic and phenotypic markers.

Periodic Fever Syndromes

Introduction

Periodic fever syndromes (PFS) are distinct from other chronic inflammatory conditions and fever of unknown origin in that the patient is relatively healthy in between episodes. Children with periodic fever syndromes usually have normal laboratory studies and exams when they are not sick. Besides systemic arthritis, other diseases that should be considered in the child who presents with recurrent fever include infections (viruses, bacterial, or parasitic), neoplasm, inflammatory bowel disease, and Behçet syndrome. Periodic fever syndromes include PFAPA (Periodic Fever, Apthous stomatitis, Pharyngitis and Adenitis), FMF (Familial Mediterranean Fever), HIDS (Hyper IgD Syndrome), TRAPS (tumour necrosis factor receptor1 associated periodic syndrome), cyclic neutropenia, MWS (Muckle–Wells Syndrome), and FCAS (Familial Cold Autoinflammatory Syndrome) (Table 1.7.3).

Periodic fever, aphthous stomatitis, pharyngitis, adenitis (PFAPA)

When a young child (2–5 years average, range 6 months to 7 years) presents with recurrent, brief episodes of fever primarily associated with aphthous stomatitis, pharyngitis, or cervical adenopathy, the diagnosis is more likely to be Periodic Fever, Aphthous Stomatitis, Pharyngitis, Adenitis (PFAPA) [5] than Systemic Arthritis (Table 1.7.1). Although some children with PFAPA can have arthralgias, arthritis has not been described, and the oral mucosal features

Table 1.7.1 PFAPA criteria

Diagnostic criteria for PFAPA
Regularly recurring fevers with an early age of onset (<5 years)

Constitutional symptoms in the absence of upper respiratory infection with at least one of the following clinical signs
    Apthous stomatitis
    Cervical lymphadenitis
    Pharyngitis

Exclusion of cyclic neutropenia
Completely asymptomatic interval between episodes
Normal growth and development
Other criteria include exclusion of other episodic syndromes, such as FMF, HIDS, Behçet.

Table 1.7.2 Criteria for the diagnosis of familial mediterranean fever (FMF)

Major

Typical attacks of
    Peritonitis (generalized)
    Pleuritis (unilateral) or pericardial
    Monoarthritis (hip, knee, ankle)
    Fever alone
    Incomplete abdominal attacks

Minor

Incomplete attacks in the
    Chest
    Joint
    Leg (exertional pain)
    Favourable response to colchicine

Requirement for the diagnosis of FMF are the presence of one major criterion or two minor criteria. Typical attacks are defined as recurrent (three at the same site), febrile (> = 38 °C rectal temperature), and short (lasting 12 h to days). Incomplete attacks are defined as painful and recurrent attacks differing from typical attacks in one or two features as follows: (1) temperature is normal or lower than 38 °C, (2) attacks are longer or shorter than specified (but not shorter than 6 h or longer than a week), (3) no signs of peritonitis are recorded during the abdominal attacks, (4) the abdominal attacks are localized, and (5) the arthritis involves joints other than those specified. Attacks not fulfilling this definition of typical incomplete attacks are not counted. [5,14,67].

classically associated with PFAPA are not seen in Systemic Arthritis. The clinical pattern associated with both diseases includes high fevers, malaise, and irritability. However, in PFAPA, these episodes are brief (average 4–5 days) and recur at regular 3–6-week intervals in contrast to the prolonged and sustained fevers in flares of Systemic Arthritis that occur at unpredictable intervals. Patients with PFAPA are usually well in between episodes, while children with Systemic Arthritis often develop generalized adenopathy, hepatosplenomegaly, and a characteristic rash which can persist for weeks to months. Children with PFAPA only develop cervical adenopathy, rarely have a rash, and are more likely to have nausea, abdominal pain, and headache (Table 1.7.3) [6,7]. Other symptoms associated with PFAPA and uncommon for Systemic Arthritis include diarrhoea, cough, and coryza [7].

In both diseases, an elevated ESR, leukocytosis, and neutrophilia are seen, although these markers are often only mildly elevated in PFAPA [6,7]. The thrombocytosis and anaemia seen in Systemic Arthritis are usually not found in PFAPA, and patients with PFAPA have normal laboratory studies in between episodes. Similar to Systemic Arthritis, no ethnic predisposition or familial pattern is found, although unlike Systemic Arthritis, there is a slight male predominance in PFAPA. Patients with PFAPA have an excellent prognosis, with about 50% of children going into remission within 5 years. Those that continue to have episodes do not have problems with general health, growth, or development [7]. Treatment with one or two doses of corticosteroids can induce dramatic resolution of fever and shorten the length of the episode. However, corticosteroid treatment also appears to shorten the interval between episodes. Some patients have gone into remission following treatment with cimetidine for 6–8 months or following tonsillectomy [6,7].

Cyclic neutropenia

When an infant presents with recurrent episodes of fever, fatigue, and lymphadenopathy associated with oral mucosal problems, such as ulcerations, gingivitis, pharyngitis, or tonsillitis, cyclic neutropenia as well as immunodeficiencies should be considered in the differential diagnosis. Patients with cyclic neutropenia usually present during the first few months of life in contrast to the later onset typical of Systemic Arthritis. These patients will have leukopenia and neutropenia in contrast to the leukocytosis and neutrophilia seen in Systemic Arthritis (Table 1.7.3). Cyclic neutropenia, also known as cyclic haematopoiesis, is characterized by precisely regular oscillations (average 21 days, range 18–24 days) in the production of all blood cells in the bone marrow [8]. However, it is the periodic neutropenia that is the most

serious feature of this illness because the nadir is in the range of 0–200/mm^3. The actual neutropenia generally lasts 3–6 days at which time the patient is at increased risk for opportunistic infections that frequently affect the oral mucosa or skin, and less commonly the joints, blood, or peritoneum. Patients can therefore present with myalgia, bone pain, headache, and abdominal pain. At the time of infection, the patient's neutrophil count is usually rising requiring serial complete blood counts with differential counts to document the neutropenia [8]. About one-third of cases are familial (autosomal dominant) and have been found to have a mutation in the *ELA2* gene (neutrophil elastase) gene [9].[1] In some of the adult-onset sporadic cases, patients have been found to have malignancies, but this has not been reported in children. Once diagnosed, patients can be treated with granulocyte colony stimulating factor (G-CSF) to decrease the severity and length of neutropenia.

Familial Mediterranean Fever (FMF)

When a young child (often 5 years or less) presents with fever, arthritis, and severe abdominal pain, familial mediterranean fever (FMF) should be considered in the differential diagnosis especially if the family is of Sephardic Jewish, Armenian, Arabic, or Turkish ethnicity (Table 1.7.2). Patients with this autosomal recessive illness can have marked elevation in the acute phase reactants, leukocytosis, and neutrophilia, similar to Systemic Arthritis patients. However, these blood tests will tend to revert to normal in between episodes, and both thrombocytosis and anaemia are absent. In contrast to the lengthy episodes of Systemic Arthritis, those of FMF usually only last 2–3 days, although the arthritis may last longer (Table 1.7.3) [5,14,67].

The majority of patients with FMF have arthritis, with typical symptoms of tenderness, warmth, and limitation of movement, but these symptoms usually improve after the first 24 h. The most common pattern is monoarticular arthritis of the knee, ankle, or hip, which leaves no permanent damage and resolves within a week [5,10]. Unfortunately, some patients have prolonged (months) monoarticular arthritis of the hip that may result in articular damage, or a prolonged (6–12 week) migratory arthritis that resembles acute rheumatic fever, or a polyarticular pattern similar to Enthesitis Related Arthritis (ERA). The arthritis pattern includes sacroiliitis, enthesitis, and back/neck pain, but patients are HLA-B27 negative. FMF patients with these patterns of arthritis can be distinguished from JIA by the episodic nature of the fever and the presence of serositis. The serositis can manifest as sterile peritonitis or pleuritis [11]. Nearly all patients have abdominal pain which can be very severe, and associated with diarrhoea, nausea, vomiting, and constipation; symptoms uncommon in Systemic Arthritis. The abdominal symptoms with ERA-type arthritis may suggest inflammatory bowel disease, however, patients with FMF generally do not have weight loss or abnormal growth, and are asymptomatic between episodes. Similar to Systemic Arthritis, many children with FMF (up to one-third) develop chest pain; this is usually due to unilateral pleuritis versus the pericarditis more commonly seen in Systemic Arthritis (see Part 2, Chapter 2.2).

Rashes can be seen in both FMF and Systemic Arthritis, but the typical FMF rash is an erysipelas-like eruption over the lower extremities (Figures 1.7.1 and 1.7.2) in contrast to the predominantly truncal macular or maculopapular rash associated with Systemic Arthritis (Fig 1.4.1 and 1.3.20) [12]. Unlike Systemic Arthritis, patients with FMF do not have lymphadenopathy although splenomegaly occurs in up to 50%. Acute scrotal swelling and tenderness are reported in only a small percentage of boys with FMF [13], but are unlikely in Systemic Arthritis; these symptoms should suggest FMF or TRAPS. Myalgia occurs in up to 25% of children with FMF; in some, it is precipitated by exercise, while others may develop severe myalgia with fever that lasts up to 6 weeks [15].

Patients with FMF are at a much higher risk for developing the potentially fatal complication of amyloidosis than patients with Systemic Arthritis. Corticosteroids do not help reduce attacks or symptoms, but treatment with colchicine can prevent the development of amyloidosis and reduces the frequency of attacks in nearly all patients. Gene mapping studies have identified mutations in the *MEFV* gene as the cause of FMF [13,15,16].[2] A significant percentage of children of Mediterranean ethnicity who have functional abdominal pain, but no other symptoms of FMF, have been found to have mutations in one or both alleles of their *MEFV* gene [17]. These children presumably have a milder form of FMF, and colchicine treatment may be warranted.

Hyperimmunoglobulinaemia D syndrome (HIDS)

Hyperimmunoglobulinaemia D syndrome and Systemic Arthritis are both associated with recurrent episodes of fever, arthritis, rash, and hepatosplenomegaly. In HIDS, the arthritis, which usually involves the large joints, is limited to the duration of the febrile episode and is non-destructive, unlike the prolonged, frequently destructive, arthritis found in JIA. Various rashes are seen in HIDS including erythematous macules, papules, urticaria, erythematous nodules, palpable purpura, and annular erythema (Figure 1.7.3) [18], and unlike Systemic

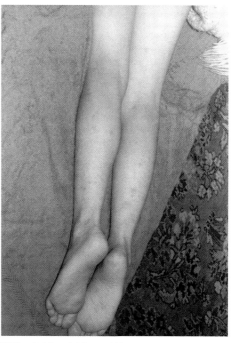

Fig. 1.7.2 FMF rash. This child with FMF develops a diffuse erythematous erysipeloid rash of the lower extremities associated with painful vasculitic lesions with each febrile episode. (Courtesy of J. Jacobs.)

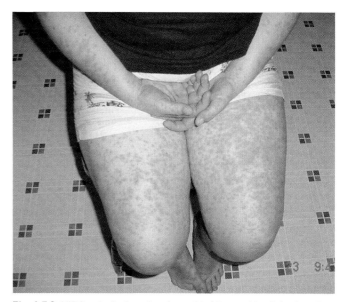

Fig. 1.7.3 HIDS rash: At 6 weeks of age, this 14-year-old girl developed fever, diarrhoea, and an erythematous maculopapular rash on her extremities. These symptoms occur every 4 to 6 weeks, along with arthralgia, myalgia, oral ulcers, and tender cervical lymph nodes. (Courtesy of D. Kastner.)

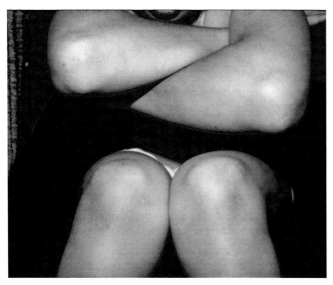

Fig. 1.7.1 FMF erysipelas rash. This boy with FMF gets erysipelas on his elbows during his attacks. (Courtesy of Y. Kimura.)

Arthritis, the lesions occur predominantly on the extremities and not the trunk. Although lymphadenopathy and hepatosplenomegaly are seen in both diseases, the lymphadenopathy is tender in HIDS [19]. Other features that distinguish HIDS from Systemic Arthritis include the prodromal and abdominal symptoms, and the precipitation of many HIDS episodes by childhood vaccination or stress, such as surgery. The prodrome consists of headache, fatigue, congestion, dry throat, and vertigo, and attacks are usually accompanied by abdominal pain, diarrhoea, and vomiting [20].

Patients with HIDS usually present in the first year of life, an uncommon age of presentation for Systemic Arthritis, and the episodes are much briefer (3–7 days) than those associated with JIA (Table 1.7.3). In both diseases, laboratory studies show an elevated ESR, leukocytosis, and neutrophilia. However, the characteristic finding in patients with HIDS is an elevated IgD level (>100 IU/ml) [19] that is not reported in Systemic Arthritis. Other laboratory findings in HIDS include elevated serum IgA levels and urine mevalonic acid levels during episodes of fever. The long-term prognosis is good, with the frequency and severity of attacks tending to decrease with age. NSAIDs and corticosteroids have been used to treat the arthritis; colchicine has generally not been helpful. Genetic analyses have identified mutations in the MVK gene (mevalonate kinase) as the cause of this disease [15].[3]

TNF-receptor-associated periodic syndrome (TRAPS)

TNF-receptor-associated periodic syndrome is an autosomal dominant periodic fever previously known as familial Hibernian fever, autosomal dominant periodic fever with amyloidosis, and benign autosomal dominant familial periodic fever [1,21]. With the identification of mutations in the TNFRSF1A gene (which encodes the p55 receptor for TNFα) as the cause, the name has been changed accordingly.[4] Similar to Systemic Arthritis, patients can present with prolonged episodes (weeks) of fever, arthritis, lymphadenopathy, and rash (Table 1.7.3). However, patients with TRAPS more typically have severe myalgia (Figure 1.7.4) and large joint arthralgia rather than arthritis, and the arthritis does not result in joint damage (Figure 1.7.5) [15,21]. The lymphadenopathy affects the cervical, axillary, and inguinal areas and, unlike Systemic Arthritis, is not associated with hepatosplenomegaly.

The TRAPS associated rash is also different from that seen in Systemic Arthritis; it is generally an erysipelas-like, warm, tender, oedematous rash that usually begins on the proximal limbs, and migrates peripherally (Figure 1.7.6(a), (b)) [22]. The rash and myalgia are co-localized, and migrate together; the severe pain is usually associated with stiffness or spasticity, and decreased limb movement. In addition, unlike Systemic Arthritis, TRAPS, similar to FMF, is usually associated with severe abdominal pain, with vomiting, nausea, diarrhoea, or constipation. Chest pain can occur in both diseases; in TRAPS, it is often associated with breathlessness and is felt to be due to chest wall muscle inflammation, rather than to lung or cardiac problems. Other common TRAPS associated symptoms include painful or stinging conjunctivitis, unilateral or bilateral periorbital oedema (Figure 1.7.7), and testicular pain in 50% of males [15,21]; these symptoms are all atypical of Systemic Arthritis.

Many of the patients with TRAPS present at an earlier age than commonly seen for Systemic Arthritis. In one study, >80% of patients developed rash and fever by 2 years of age [22], and in another study, about 20% of the patients developed episodes during the first year of life [21]. In both diseases, laboratory studies show elevated acute phase reactants and leukocytosis; patients with TRAPS are also likely to have increased immunoglobulin levels, especially IgA. About 14–25% of patients with TRAPS develop amyloidosis; the rest generally have a good prognosis although the prolonged episodes can be debilitating [15,23]. Genotype analyses indicate that patients with cysteine mutations in the p55 TNF receptor have an increased risk of amyloidosis [23]. Colchicine has not proven effective, but corticosteroids have been helpful in reducing the symptoms of the attacks. Recent studies suggest that anti-TNFα treatment can reduce clinical symptoms and shorten episodes; in one patient, AA amyloidosis was reversed [2,15,24].

Other hereditary febrile syndromes

These autosomal dominant syndromes are characterized by episodes of fever, joint symptoms, and rash that are generally less periodic than those associated with the periodic fever syndromes. These syndromes include the familial urticarial syndromes Familial Cold Autoinflammatory Syndrome (FCAS), Muckle–Wells Syndrome (MWS), and autosomal dominant periodic fever with amyloidosis (ADPF) and CINCA/NOMID. The genes involved in all four syndromes have been mapped to chromosome 1q44, and recently, mutations of the same gene (NALP3/CIAS1/PYPAF1) have been found in all four syndromes [25–28].[5]

Familial cold autoinflammatory syndrome (FCAS)

Familial cold autoinflammatory syndrome, also known as familial cold urticaria, is characterized by recurrent episodes of fever, rash, myalgia, and arthralgia/arthritis (Table 1.7.3) [29]. However, unlike Systemic Arthritis, these symptoms are triggered exclusively by cold exposure, ranging from 5 min to 3 h, and the febrile symptoms persist for 12–24 h in contrast to the weeks of fever commonly seen in children with Systemic Arthritis. The rash associated with FCAS is usually associated with a burning sensation, and consists of erythematous papules or plaques that begin on the extremities before spreading to other areas (Figure 1.7.8). The arthritis seen in both diseases can be associated with joint stiffness, swelling, tenderness, and synovial thickening, and affects similar joints (hands, wrists, elbows, knees, and ankles). Although the arthralgia can be debilitating, unlike Systemic Arthritis, the arthritis is short-lived (hours to days) [30]. Patients with FCAS generally present at an earlier age (most by 6 months) with symptoms uncommon for Systemic Arthritis. These include painful, watery eyes, with conjunctivitis and blurred vision, profuse sweating, extreme thirst, extremity swelling, and nausea. In both diseases, laboratory studies show leukocytosis, neutrophilia, and elevated acute phase reactants, but patients with FCAS do not have the thrombocytosis or anemia seen in Systemic Arthritis [29,30]. Patients with FCAS rarely develop amyloidosis, and most have a normal lifespan. NSAIDs may relieve arthralgia but do not improve other symptoms. High dose corticosteroids may help a subset of patients, while colchicine does not have any benefit [29,31]. Treatment with an anti-IL1 agent prevents the onset of symptoms [68].

Muckle–Wells syndrome (MWS)

Muckle–Wells Syndrome is an autosomal dominant disease characterized by recurrent episodes of fever, rash, and arthralgia; (Table 1.7.3) [32] symptoms similar to those seen in Systemic Arthritis. The erythematous macular or maculopapular rash seen in MWS can resemble that found in Systemic Arthritis. In both diseases, the rash occurs with the fever episodes, may persist between episodes, and tends to change its

Table 1.7.3 Characteristic features of the Periodic Fever Syndromes and hereditary febrile syndromes

	FMF	HIDS	TRAPS	PFAPA	Cyclic neutropenia	Muckle–Wells syndrome	FCAS	CINCA/NOMID
Major symptoms	Fever, abd.pain, chest pain, arthritis	Fever, abd. pain, arthritis, LA, HSM	Fever, abd. pain, localized myalgia, chest pain, arthralgia, periorbital oedema, conjunctivitis	Fever, pharyngitis, aphthous stomatitis, cervical LA	Fever, stomatits, pharyngitis, skin infections, diarrhoea	Fever, arthralgia, conjunctivitis, hearing loss	Fever, arthralgia, conjunctivitis	Fever, chronic meningitis, LA, HSM, arthralgia/arthropathy, eye lesions, hearing loss
Arthritis patterns	Acute or protracted; monoarthritis in large joint	Acute; oligo, symmetrical in large joints	Uncommon	None	Can have septic arthritis	Oligo or mono, large joints, can be symmetrical	Occasionally	Arthralgia. joint effusion, joint contracture, and/or arthropathy
Rash	Erysipelas-like erythema, purpuric rash on lower leg	Eryth. macules and papules on extremities	Generalized migratory eryth. plaques or patches	Rash in minority	Can get skin infections	Eryth. macules, macularpapular, or urticaria	Eryth. papules or plaques on extremities	Non-pruritic, migratory eryth. papules, or urticaria
Length of attacks (days)	1–3	3–7	7–21	4–5	3–6	1–3	Most < 1	Persistent rash and joint sx; variable febrile episodes
Interval between attacks	Weeks to months	4–8 weeks	Weeks to months	2–8 weeks	18–24 days	1 to a few weeks	Depends upon exposure to cold	Fever can be episodic or chronic
Laboratory findings	↑Acute phase reactants; ↑wbc; ↑ IgD in 13%	↑Acute phase reactants; ↑wbc (neutrophils); ↑ IgD (> 100 IU) in 95%;↑ IgA in many	↑Acute phase reactants; ↑wbc (neutrophils); ↑ IgD in 10%	± ESR, mild ↑wbc (neutrophils); ↑IgD in some	Low to no neutrophils	↑Acute phase reactants; ↑wbc (neutrophils)	↑Acute phase reactants; ↑wbc (neutrophils)	↑Acute phase reactants; ↑wbc (neutrophils and eosinophils), ↑plt, hypochromic anaemia
Presenting age (years)	50% by 5	< 1	Most < 10	≤ 5	< 1	Infancy to mid-childhood	< 0.5	Majority have rash at birth; others within first year
Family history	+	+	+	–	+	+	+	+/–
Ethnicity	Sephardic Jews, Arabs; Turkish, Armenian	Dutch, French, other European	Any but especially Irish, Scottish	None	Predominately Caucasian	Northern European	Predominantly N. American, European	Predominantly Caucasian
Genetics, associated gene	AR, 16p13.3 MEFV	AR, 12q24 MVK	AD, 12p13.3 TNFRSF1A	Unknown	AD, 19p13.3 ELA2	AD, 1q44 NALP3/CIAS1/PYPAF1	AD, 1q44 NALP3/CIAS1/PYPAF1	AD, 1q44 NALP3/CIAS1/PYPAF1
Treatment	Colchicine	NSAIDs, corticosteroids[1]	Corticosteroids, anti-TNFα	Cimetidine, corticosteroids	G-CSF	Unknown anti-IL-1*	Corticosteroids anti-IL-1*	Corticosteroids anti-IL-1*
Sequelae	Amyloidosis	None usually	Amyloidosis in 25%	None except from corticosteroids	Sepsis, intestinal perforation, chronic gingivitis	Amyloidosis, deafness	Amyloidosis uncommon	Amyloidosis, growth retardation, joint deformities, mental retardation, blindness, deafness

Abbreviations: abd. pain = abdominal pain, AD = Autosomal Dominant, AR = Autosomal Recessive, CINCA/NOMID = Chronic Neurological Cutaneous and Articular syndrome/Neonatal Onset Multisystem Inflammatory disease, *ELA2* = neutrophil elastase, [1] eryth. = erythematous, FCAS = Familial Cold Autoinflammatory syndrome, FMF = Familial Mediterranean Fever, G-CSF = granulocyte colony stimulating factor, HIDS = Hyper IgD syndrome, HSM = hepatosplenomegaly, LA = lymphadenopathy, count, *MEFV* = Mediterranean fever gene (pyrin/marenostin),[2] mono = monoarticular, *MVK* = mevalonate kinase,[3] *NALP3/CIAS1/PYPAF1* = cryopyrin,[5] oligo = oligoarticular, plt = platelets, sx = symptoms, TNFα = tumor necrosis factor alpha, *TNFRSF1A* = tumour necrosis factor receptor 1 (p55, CD120a);[4] TRAPS = TNF-receptor-associated periodic syndrome, wbc = white blood count
* anti-IL-1 treatment has been reported to be effective in a small number of patients with these diseases.

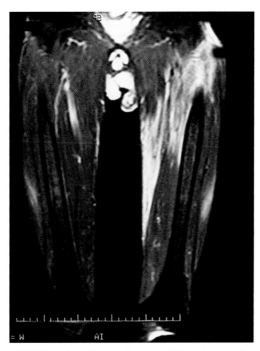

Fig. 1.7.4 TRAPS myalgia: This man has had a lifelong history of periodic episodes of fever, severe abdominal pain, rash, and myalgia. The myalgia was due to fascitis of his muscles as seen on the MRI. His rash was located over the fascitis. (Courtesy of D. Kastner.)

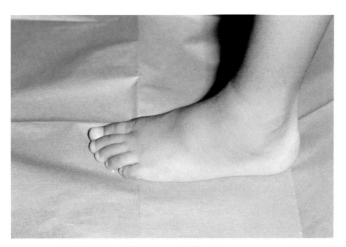

Fig. 1.7.5 TRAPS arthritis. This 6-year-old boy has intermittent episodes of fever and rash associated with arthritis of his foot. (Courtesy of D. Kastner.)

(a)

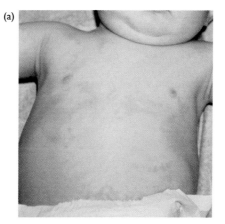

(b)

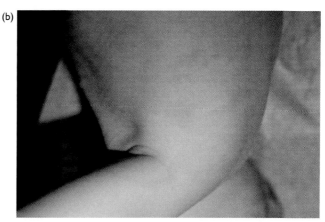

Fig. 1.7.6 TRAPS rash. a, b. This 6-month-old infant developed recurrent episodes of fever and rash beginning at 1 month of life. (Courtesy of B. Athreya.)

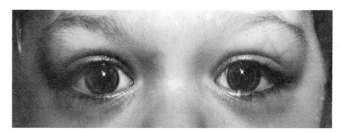

Fig. 1.7.7 TRAPS periorbital oedema. This toddler has recurrent episodes of fever, rash, conjunctivitis, arthralgia, and abdominal pain. Her father and three siblings are similarly affected. (Courtesy of D. Kastner and the Archives of Dermatology.)

appearance over time. An urticarial rash is more commonly seen in patients with MWS than patients with Systemic Arthritis. In contrast to Systemic Arthritis, the rash associated with MWS is often painful or pruritic, aggravated by heat or cold exposure, and tends to be less evanescent than the rash of Systemic Arthritis (Figure 1.7.9). Differences between the two diseases can also be seen in the fever pattern and its duration. In contrast to the high, spiking quotidian fever pattern seen in Systemic Arthritis, MWS is associated with low-grade fever. The febrile episodes are also shorter in duration than those commonly seen in Systemic Arthritis (1–3 days versus weeks). Episodes of MWS recur every one to several weeks, and are characterized by malaise, abdominal

pain, arthralgias, and occasionally myalgias [32–34]. The abdominal pain can be severe, and is often accompanied by vomiting and diarrhoea, symptoms uncommon for Systemic Arthritis.

Patients with either disease can have large joint arthritis associated with pain, tenderness, swelling, and erythema, and the arthritis can persist between attacks in MWS (Figure 1.7.10). However, patients with MWS more typically have aching distal limb pain and swelling as well as large joint arthralgia instead of arthritis [34]. Other differences from Systemic Arthritis include the age of onset (first year of life for MWS versus mid-childhood for Systemic Arthritis), symptoms of red, painful eyes (due to episcleritis and conjunctivitis), and sensorineural

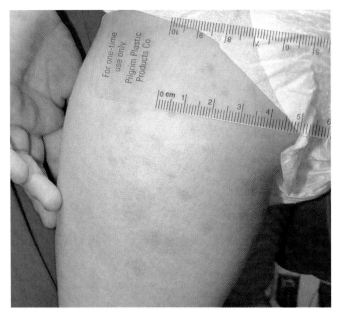

Fig. 1.7.8 FCAS rash. This child shows the typical rash seen in familial cold autoinflammatory syndrome. (Courtesy of H. Hoffman.)

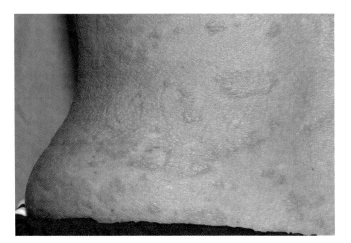

Fig. 1.7.9 Muckle–Wells rash: This child presented with urticarial lesions within hours of birth. She has had almost daily recurrence of this rash, often accompanied by fever. At age 9 she began to develop hearing loss, and at age 11, she developed arthritis and headaches secondary to papilloedema. (Courtesy of D. Kastner.)

deafness. In both diseases, laboratory studies commonly show elevated acute phase reactants, hypergammaglobulinaemia, polymorphonuclear leukocytosis, thrombocytosis, and sometimes anaemia. The elevated ESR and hypergammaglobulinaemia can persist between attacks of MWS [34]. The long-term outcome for the patients with MWS is guarded due to the high incidence of amyloidosis [33]. Treatment with an anti-IL1 agent completely reduced disease symptoms in three family members with MWS [69].

Autosomal dominant periodic fever with amylodosis

A recently described autosomal dominant periodic fever syndrome (ADPF) has so far been identified in one Indian family [35]; this

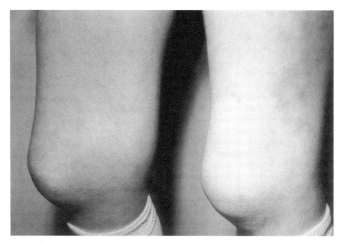

Fig. 1.7.10 Muckle–Wells arthritis. This young girl presented with recurrent episodes of knee arthritis, vasculitic rash, keratitis, and nerve deafness since early infancy (Courtesy of J. Jacobs).

syndrome is different than the ADPF related to TRAPS. The Indian ADPF is characterized by prolonged episodes of fever (1–4 weeks), urticarial skin rash, periorbital oedema, conjunctivitis, and arthralgia/ arthritis. The length of the episodes can be similar to that seen in Systemic Arthritis, but the symptoms of periorbital oedema and conjunctivitis are not associated with Systemic Arthritis. The arthralgia/ arthritis affects the knees and elbows initially, and later includes the wrist and hand joints. Unlike Systemic Arthritis, destructive arthritis is not seen and the arthralgia is often moderate to severe. Other differences include a later disease onset for ADPF (average of 10 years), increased severity of symptoms in males versus females, and increased risk of amyloidosis. In both illnesses, laboratory studies show markedly elevated acute phase reactants. The prognosis is primarily dependent on the development of amyloidosis [35].

Chronic Infantile Neurological Cutaneous and Articular syndrome (CINCA), Neonatal Onset Multisystem Inflammatory Disease (NOMID)

Chronic Infantile Neurological Cutaneous and Articular syndrome, also called Infantile-Onset Multisystem Inflammatory Disease or Neonatal Onset Multisystem Inflammatory Disease [36–38] is a rare inflammatory condition, which can resemble Systemic Arthritis. Patients with CINCA can present with high spiking fevers with a quotidian pattern, lymphadenopathy, and hepatosplenomegaly (Figure 1.7.11(a), (b)). However, the episodes of fever tend to be shorter than those of Systemic Arthritis. Unlike Systemic Arthritis, CINCA is complicated by neurologic symptoms such as seizures, transient hemiplegia, leg spasticity, and headaches secondary to sterile, neutrophil-associated meningitis (Table 1.7.3) [36–38]. Sensorineural hearing loss and eye involvement are also common in CINCA [39]. The majority of patients have optic disc involvement, and about half have anterior uveitis. Similar to the anterior uveitis associated with Oligoarthritis, the disease in CINCA can progress to band keratopathy, synechiae, and cataracts [40].

The onset of symptoms is typically earlier in CINCA than in Systemic Arthritis, with the rash present at birth in two-thirds of

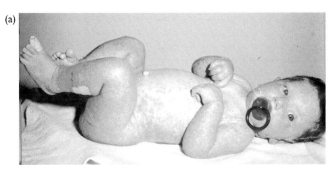
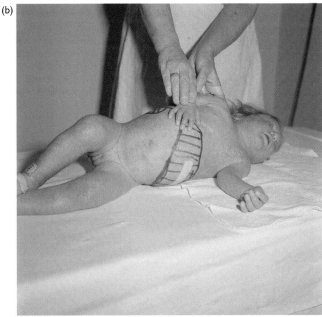

Fig. 1.7.11 (a), (b) CINCA rash and hepatosplenomegaly. This infant presented with rash in the newborn nursery, and then developed episodes of high fever within a few months. She also had lymphadenopathy, hepatosplenomegaly, and periosteal new-bone formation in her long bones and phalanges (Courtesy of J. Jacobs).

patients, and occurring within one year in the remainder. The rash is a nonpruritic, migratory erythema or urticaria, which can resemble the Systemic Arthritis rash; however, the CINCA rash is present every day (Figure 1.7.11(a,b)) [39,41]. Joint symptoms vary from arthralgia, transient swelling, to severe symmetrical polyarthropathy affecting the knees, ankles, feet, elbows, wrists, and hands(Figure 1.7.12(a)). Unlike Systemic Arthritis, there is rarely involvement of the spine, hips, or shoulders, and patients do not have morning stiffness [39,41]. Radiographic changes are also quite distinctive in CINCA; characteristic findings include enlarged epiphyses with irregular ossification, flared, irregular, and cupped metaphyses, and extreme patellar over growth with premature ossification (Figure 1.7.12b) [38]. Patients often develop joint contractures. Despite these abnormalities, these children tend not to complain of morning stiffness. Skull anomalies are often seen and include frontal bossing and late closure of the anterior fontanelle. Some patients may develop a saddle nose.

Children with CINCA show a more severe failure to thrive and greater growth retardation than is usually seen in Systemic Arthritis. In both diseases, laboratory studies document elevated acute phase reactants, leukocytosis, neutrophilia, hypergammaglobulinaemia, and

thrombocytosis. However, patients with CINCA also have eosinophilia, and eosinophils are seen in tissue biopsies. Patients with CINCA have a poor prognosis, with life-long inflammation, risk of secondary amyloidosis, severe growth retardation, and persistent neurological symptoms sometimes associated with mental retardation, deafness, or blindness [37,39]. NSAIDs are only effective against pain, corticosteroids may reduce fever and pain but do not control the more serious symptoms [39]. Recent experience suggests that treatment with an anti-IL-1 agent is effective in dramatically reducing symptoms [70]. Although mutations in the *CIAS1* have been identified in many patients with CINCA [26,27], in one study, half of the patients did not have a mutation in this gene implying that mutations in other genes may give rise to a similar phenotype [26].

Pyogenic sterile arthritis, pyoderma gangrenosum, and acne syndrome (PAPA)

Another inflammatory condition that often presents during infancy is pyogenic sterile arthritis, pyoderma gangrenosum, and acne. This autosomal dominant condition is associated with severe, intermittent arthritis that typically is a monarthritis of the elbow, knee, or ankle [42–45]. Episodes can be associated with low-grade fevers, an elevated ESR, leukocytosis, elevated aldolase, and mild anaemia. The ESR and leukocytosis can resolve in between episodes of arthritis. In contrast to Oligoarthritis, the arthritis of PAPA is intermittent, migrates, and is associated with erythema. Affected joints usually contain a sterile seropurulent or purulent material, and patients may require surgical drainage and intra-articular corticosteroids in order to improve. Later in childhood (ages 8–13 years), the patients develop the skin manifestations of pyoderma gangrenosum and severe acne (Figure 1.7.13) [42,43]. This syndrome was originally described as streaking leukocyte factor by Jerry Jacobs (see Part 1, Chapter 1.10, Figure 1.10.16). Treatment with corticosteroids may reduce the acute symptoms of the arthritis, but progressive joint destruction is common. An anti-IL-1 agent was found to effectively treat one patient with steroid resistant PAPA associated arthritis [71]. Recently, mutations in the *CD2BP1* gene have been found in these patients [44].[6]

Granulomatous diseases

Sarcoidosis

Sarcoidosis is a systemic disease of unknown aetiology characterized by the presence of noncaseating granulomas in multiple organs. Children under the age of 4 develop an early onset form which differs clinically from the late onset type seen in the older child and adult [45,46]. Both types share features seen in Systemic Arthritis, such as fever, rash, arthritis, and adenopathy. However, in both early and late forms, the arthritis is characterized by much larger swelling than is usually seen in JIA. Sarcoid arthritis tends to present with large, boggy synovial thickening and effusions affecting both joint synovia and tendon sheaths [46,47]. Surprisingly, patients generally have minimal pain or joint limitation. Some patients develop morning stiffness and pain, but X-rays usually remain normal for years. In early-onset sarcoidosis (EOS), the arthritis is initially in only a few joints, but over time develops into symmetric polyarthritis affecting large and small joints especially

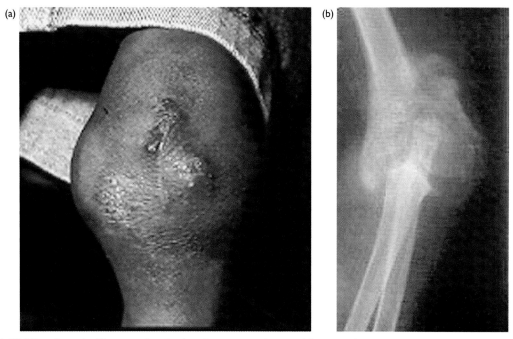

Fig. 1.7.12 (a), (b) CINCA arthropathy. This young boy developed persistent arthritis and fevers in infancy; his X-ray is shown in 7.12b. (Courtesy of D. Goldsmith.)

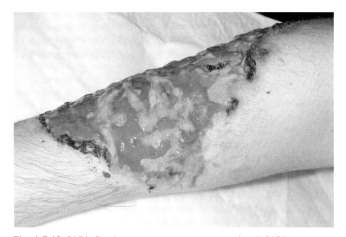

Fig. 1.7.13 PAPA. Pyoderma gangrenosum associated with PAPA siyndrome. (Courtesy of D. Kastner.)

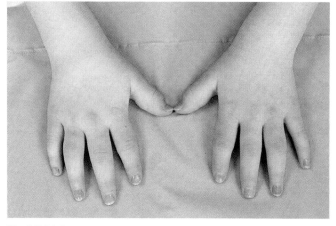

Fig. 1.7.14 Sarcoid arthritis. This child has symmetrical polyarthritis of her hands. Her hands show synovial thickening and effusions of the joints and tendons, features characteristic of sarcoidosis. (Courtesy of T. R. Southwood.)

wrists, ankles, knees, and elbows (Figure 1.7.14). This pattern of poly-arthritis is also typical for late onset sarcoidosis. After many years, patients may develop pain and marked joint destruction and impairment. Sarcoid arthritis, unlike JIA, does not respond well to NSAIDs.

In addition to arthritis, EOS is characterized by rash and uveitis. Unlike the rash seen in Systemic Arthritis, the EOS rash is usually an erythematous follicular, scaling erythema that lasts months to years, and leaves a residual of hyperkeratotic dry skin [48,49]. The rash often presents in the first year of life, earlier than the usual onset of Systemic Arthritis. Eye findings can be similar to those seen in Oligoarthritis, including keratic precipitates, synechiae, band keratopathy, and cataracts, but the uveitis of sarcoidosis may also affect the posterior segment which does not occur in JIA, and may produce symptoms in contrast to the painless uveitis seen in Oligoarthritis. In addition,

sarcoidosis of the eye is characterized by conjunctival granuloma, and a different pattern of synechiae and keratic precipitates than seen in JIA, and is more likely to involve the retina and optic nerve [46,50]. Fever, lymphadenopathy, and hepatosplenomegaly are less frequent than in Systemic Arthritis. Patients with either disease can present with pericarditis. Pulmonary involvement is uncommon in EOS in contrast to late onset sarcoidosis. Parotid swelling may occur in early and late sarcoidosis but would be very atypical of Systemic Arthritis. In both Systemic Arthritis and EOS, patients may have elevated acute phase reactants; other laboratory abnormalities, such as thrombocytosis or leukocytosis are usually not seen in EOS. The vast majority of patients with EOS have significant sequelae from inflammation affecting the eyes, joints, and other organs, and overall prognosis is poor [48,49].

Similar to Systemic Arthritis, patients with late onset childhood sarcoidosis (LOS) usually have peripheral lymphadenopathy, hepatosplenomegaly, fever, and fatigue, and about 50% develop arthritis. Unlike Systemic Arthritis, however, LOS is more commonly associated with weight loss, fatigue, cough, parotid swelling, and uveitis. In addition, the pattern of arthritis and uveitis, as described above, is different [45,46]. Chest radiographs show bilateral hilar lymphadenopathy and/or interstitial disease, and about one-half of the children have restrictive lung disease on pulmonary function tests. Up to 40% of these patients also have a rash, usually red to brownish/violaceous, flat-topped papules or nodules, or erythema nodosum [46]; lesions very different from those usually seen in Systemic Arthritis. Neurologic symptoms, such as seizures, encephalopathy, and cranial neuropathy, are more likely to be found in LOS than in Systemic Arthritis, while pericarditis is less likely to be seen in sarcoid. In both diseases, there is an elevation of acute phase reactants and hypergammaglobulinemia, but patients with late onset sarcoidosis more commonly have leukopenia and eosinophilia rather than the leukocytosis and neutrophila found in Systemic Arthritis. Most LOS patients, unlike those with EOS or Systemic Arthritis, also have an elevated angiotensin converting enzyme (ACE) levels, and may have hypercalcemia and/or hypercalciuria and decreased creatinine clearance [46]. Most patients with LOS improve, although some have complications from the eye or lung inflammation.

Blau syndrome (Familial granulomatous arthritis)

Young children with this autosomal dominant illness can present with arthritis, rash, and uveitis (Fig 1.7.15). Patients with Blau syndrome often do not have fever. Similar to sarcoidosis and different from JIA, the uveitis associated with Blau syndrome affects both the anterior and posterior segments [51,52]. In both Systemic Arthritis and Blau syndrome, the arthritis is commonly polyarticular, affecting wrists, ankles, knees, elbows, as well as small joints of the hands and feet. However, patients with Blau syndrome can progress from painless cysts and mild "boutonniere-deformities" of fingers, to camptodactyly and giant cyst formation [52]. Other patients with Blau syndrome develop extremity pain followed sequentially by erythema, oedema, giant cyst formation, and contractures. The maculopapular or papuloerythematous rash associated with Blau syndrome is different than the transient, salmon-coloured rash of Systemic Arthritis although both are painless and can be easily missed. The rash associated with Blau syndrome may appear in the first year of life, but more commonly appears later in childhood, followed by the development of arthritis and uveitis (Figure 1.7.15). A skin biopsy shows noncaseating granulomas, with multinucleated giant cells, findings similar to those seen in sarcoid. Patients with Blau syndrome generally have normal laboratory studies; about one-half have elevated gammaglobulinaemia (IgG and/or A), and only a minority have a mildly elevated ESR, raised ACE level, or are ANA positive [52]. Mutations in the CARD15 gene have been identified in patients with Blau syndrome and in some patients with familial Crohn disease [53].[7] Because of the overlap in symptoms between early onset sarcoidosis and Blau syndrome, there has been conjecture about the relationship between these two illnesses. Recently, mutations in the CARDIS gene have also been found in 9 out of 10 patients with EOS [72].

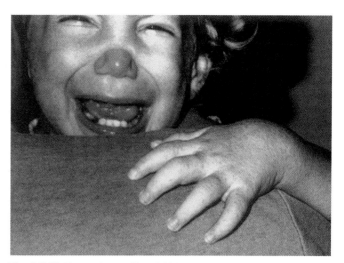

Fig. 1.7.15 Blau syndrome: This child, her two siblings, mother, and grandmother had a similar sarcoid-like rash and arthritis. (Courtesy of C. Balakrishnan.)

Hyperostosis syndromes

Idiopathic Periosteal Hyperostosis with dysproteinemia (Goldbloom Syndrome)

When confronted with a child between the age of 3–12 years with severe extremity pain and fever, the differential diagnosis should include Goldbloom syndrome in addition to malignancy, osteomyelitis, and Systemic Arthritis. Similar to children with Systemic Arthritis, children with Goldbloom syndrome have prolonged fever and fatigue as well as elevated acute phase reactants, leukocytosis, and normochromic, normocytic anaemia. Patients with Goldbloom syndrome, however, do not have thrombocytosis, and show a dysproteinaemia including hypergammaglobulinaemia, hypoalbuminaemia, and variations in alpha 1, alpha 2, and beta globulins [54,55]. Although the patient with Goldbloom syndrome may refuse to walk, this is not due to arthritis, but rather to periostitis which leads to a tender, warm, indurated, and painful extremity[54,55]. X-rays show periostitis in the long bones, fingers, or feet, while a bone scan shows increased uptake in these areas (Figure 1.7.16(a), (b)). A bone biopsy documents periosteal new bone, increased plasma cells in the marrow, and no inflammatory infiltrate. Patients recover spontaneously, and symptoms often respond to NSAIDs.

Infantile cortical hyperostosis (Caffey disease, Caffey–Silverman syndrome)

When children present with severe extremity pain, irritability, anorexia, and fever during the first year of life, the evaluation should include infantile cortical hyperostosis, or Caffey disease, in addition to malignancy and Systemic Arthritis. Unlike Systemic Arthritis, the fever associated with Caffey disease is low grade, and the patients develop symptoms at an earlier age (often within the first 6 months) than is typical for JIA [56]. Unlike JIA, patients do not have arthritis, but rather have hyperostosis due to obliteration of small arteries in the bone, leading to hypoxia, and hyperostosis [57]. These children present with soft tissue swelling and tenderness, and a biopsy shows an

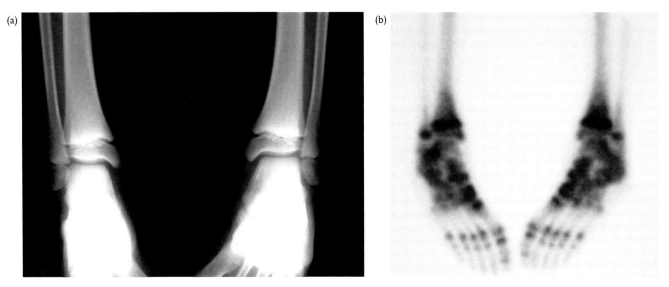

Fig. 1.7.16 Goldbloom syndrome: This 9 1/2-year-old boy developed fatigue, malaise, daily fevers, and knee and ankle discomfort without swelling. (a) His X-rays showed hyperostosis of the distal metaphyses of the tibiae, talus, and navicular bones, and a triple phase bone scan (b) documented increased uptake at these areas. Symptoms abated after 6 months without sequelae. (Courtesy of D. Goldsmith.)

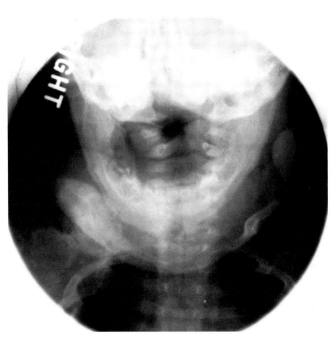

Fig. 1.7.17 Multifocal Caffey disease. This infant developed pain at 5 weeks of age and initially had normal X-rays. At 4 months of age, radiographs show involvement of the right mandible and clavicle. (Courtesy of Children's Hospital of NY-Presbyterian.)

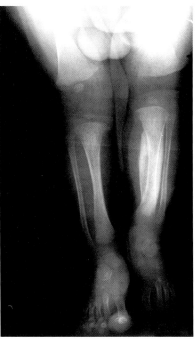

Fig. 1.7.18 Unifocal Caffey disease. This infant developed unifocal leg swelling at 14 day of his life; an X-ray at that time showed a mild periosteal reaction and the ESR was 3. Two weeks later, a repeat X-ray shows extensive periosteal reaction and leg length discrepancy. (Courtesy of Children's Hospital of NY-Presbyterian.)

inflammatory infiltrate unlike the biopsy seen in Goldbloom syndrome. Radiographs show subperiosteal new-bone growth, and cortical thickening (Figures 1.7.17 and 1.7.18). Both familial (autosomal dominant) and sporadic types occur, with the familial affecting the tibia and lower extremity more frequently than the mandible (Figure 1.7.18), while the sporadic form affects the mandible more than the tibia (Figure 1.7.17) [56]. Clavicles, scapulas, ulna, and the ribs may be affected in both types. The familial form also occurs at an earlier age, with an average age of onset of 6–7 weeks, with some cases diagnosed in utero. In both Systemic Arthritis and Caffey disease, patients have elevated acute phase reactants, thrombocytosis, anaemia, and leukocytosis. However, infants with Caffey's may have thrombocytopenia, often a normal ESR, and a very elevated alkaline phosphatase. Patients tend to have recurrent episodes until the age of three followed by spontaneous resolution, but may develop complications, such as leg length inequity, synostosis between tibia and fibula and/or radius and ulna, facial asymmetry, and bowing of the long bones [56]. In addition, prenatal cases may be associated with polyhydramnios and fetal anasarca. NSAIDs may help relieve symptoms [58].

Notes

1. *ELA2* encodes a neutrophil elastase (aka leukocyte elastase, elastase 2, and medullasin). Neutrophil elastase is a serine protease found in neutrophil and monocyte granules, and is present in promyelocytes at an early stage of neutrophil development [59]. It is postulated that this protein affects the survival of the early myeloid precursor cell as this precursor cell has been shown to have a shortened survival time in patients that have cyclic neutropenia. If neutrophil synthesis is regulated by a feedback mechanism, then a decrease in survival of the neutrophil precursor would lead to a cycling pattern in neutrophil numbers [59].

2. The *MEFV* (Mediterranean fever gene, pyrin or marenostrin) gene encodes a novel inflammatory regulator expressed in peripheral neutrophils, eosinophils, and monocytes. The pyrin protein has several different protein motifs, one of which has been labeled the PYRIN (also known as PyD, PAAD, DAPIN) domain. This domain resembles the death domain found in proteins involved in apoptosis, and is important for protein–protein interactions. Recent studies have shown that PYRIN can interact with the ASC apoptosis protein via its PYRIN domain [2,4]. The expression of pyrin is upregulated by proinflammatory cytokines, such as TNFα and IFNγ, and it is postulated that pyrin functions as a downregulator of inflammation [3]. Over 25 different mutations have been identified in the pyrin gene. The risk of amyloidosis appears to be increased in patients that are homozygous for the M694V, M694I, and M680I mutations, or have a combination of mutations at codon 694 and 680 [60]. These patients may also have an earlier disease onset and are more likely to have arthritis. In contrast, patients with the E148Q mutation are more likely to have a milder course; in one series, 55% of patients homozygous for E148Q were asymptomatic [60]. However, other factors, such as ethnicity and genetic modifiers, appear to affect the phenotypes associated with the different mutations [60,61]. Some patients with typical FMF symptoms have only one mutated allele of *MEFV* [13,62].

3. The mevalonate kinase (*MVK*) gene encodes the protein that catalyzes the conversion of mevalonic acid to 5-phospho-mevalonic acid. This pathway is important in the biosynthesis of cholesterol and nonsterol isoprene compounds. How this genetic defect leads to the inflammatory symptoms of HIDS is not known [63]. An increased level of one inflammatory cytokine, IL-1beta, was found to be produced by mevalonate kinase deficient cells [64]. The elevated levels of IgD found in these patients may also contribute to inflammation. Mutations in other genes may also give rise to the HIDS phenotype, as some patients with typical features of HIDS do not have mutations in their *MVK* gene [63].

4. The *TNFRSF1A* gene encodes the tumor necrosis factor receptor 1 which is known to bind TNFα. TNFα is a proinflammatory cytokine, and its biologic effects include leukocyte activation, pyrexia, anaemia, cachexia, and host resistance to intracellular pathogens. Some of the identified *TNFRSF1A* mutations are thought to result in decreased receptor shedding from the cell surface [2]. This may lead to a prolonged period of TNFα signaling through the p55 receptor on the cell surface, and thereby increase the inflammatory response [1,2]. Other *TNFRSF1A* mutations may affect ligand binding, or have other effects on receptor assembly [2].

5. The *CIAS1* gene, also known as *NALP3* and *PYPAF1*, encodes cryopyrin. Cryopyrin is expressed in peripheral blood leukocytes and contains a pyrin-like domain, a motif also seen in the gene associated with FMF. Cryopyrin has a nucleoside triphosphatase (NTPase) domain that belongs to the NACHT (NAIP, CIIA, HET-E, and TP-1) family of NTP'ases [65]. Both the PYRIN and NACHT domains have been found in other proteins associated with apoptosis and inflammation [3,65]. The gene associated with MWS, FCAS, ADPF, and CINCA/NOMID has been identified to be the same *NALP3/CIAS1/PYPAF1*gene [26–29]. These findings suggest that different mutations in this gene can lead to different phenotypes. In addition, some mutations have been identified in more than one disease; mutation D303 is associated with both CINCA/NOMID and MWS [26], mutation R260W is associated with both MWS and FCAS [66], and mutation R262W is associated with both MWS and the Indian family with ADPF [25]. This suggests that other genes are also important for determining disease phenotype.

6. The CD2-binding protein 1 gene (CD2BP1) encodes an adaptor protein found in T lymphocytes; this protein interacts with PEST-type protein tyrosine phosphatases (PTP) [44]. The mutations identified in this gene in patients with PAPA results in a decreased interaction between the CD2BP1 protein and PTP. The CD2BP1 protein has also been found to bind pyrin, the protein encoded by the *MEFV* gene [2]. It is postulated that mutations in CD2BP1 may lead to defective regulation of proliferation of inflammatory cells, resulting in the observed increase in neutrophil accumulation in the skin lesions and affected joints in patients with PAPA [2,44].

7. The *CARD15* gene, also known as *NOD2*, is a member of CED4/APAF1 family of apoptosis regulators and is expressed in monocytes [53]. The protein has two caspase recruitment domains (CARDs), a nucleotide-binding site (NBS), and a leucine rich region (LRR) [2]. Other CARD proteins are involved in apoptosis or NFkB activation [4]. Mutations have been found in the NBS in Blau syndrome [53]. This gene is also mutated in some familial cases of Crohn disease, but in the LRR portion of the protein [2].

References

1. Galon, J., Aksentijevich, I., McDermott, M., O'Shea, J., and Kastner, D. *TNFRSF1A* mutations and autoinflammatory syndromes. *Curr Opin Immunol* 2000; 12:479–86.
2. Hull, K., Shoham, N., Chae, J., Aksentijevich, I., and Kastner, D. The expanding spectrum of systemic autoinflammatory disorders and their rheumatic manifestations. *Curr Opin Rheumatol* 2003; 15:61–9.
3. Kastner, D. and O'Shea, J. A fever gene comes in from the cold. *Nature Genet* 2001; 29:241–2.
4. McDermott, M. and Aksentijevich, I. The autoinflammatory syndromes. *Curr Opin Allergy Clin Immunol* 2002; 2:511–16.
5. Brik, R., Shinawi, M., Kasinetz, L., and Gerhoni-Baruch. The musculoskeletal manifestations of familial mediterranean fever in children genetically diagnosed with the disease. *Arthritis Rheum* 2001; 44:1416–19.
6. Padeh, S., Brezniak, N., Zemer, D., *et al.* Periodic fever, aphthous stomatitis, pharyngitis, and adenopathy syndrome: clinical characteristics and outcome. *J Pediatr* 1999; 135:98–101.
7. Thomas, K., Feder, H., Jr, Lawton, A., and Edwards, K. Periodic fever syndrome in children. *J Pediatr* 1999; 135:15–21.
8. Palmer, S., Stephens, K., and Dale, D. Genetics, phenotype, and natural history of autosomal dominant cyclic hematopoiesis. *Am J Med Genet* 1996; 66:413–22.
9. Horwitz, M., Benson, K., Person, R., Aprikyan, A., and Dale, D. Mutations in *ELA2*, encoding neutrophil elastase, define a 21-day biological clock in cyclic haematopoiesis. *Nature Genet* 1999; 23:433–6.
10. Majeed, H. and Rawashdeh, M. The clinical patterns of arthritis in children with familial mediterranean fever. *Q J Med* 1997; 90:37–43.
11. Ben-Chetrit, E. and Levy, M. Familial mediterranean fever. *Lancet* 1998; 351:659–64.
12. Majeed, H., Quabazard, Z., Hijazi, Z., Farwana, S., and Harshani, F. The cutaneous manifestations in children with familial mediterranean fever (recurrent hereditary polyserosis): a six-year study. *Q J Med New Series* 1990; 75:607–16.

13. Samuels, J., Aksentijevich, I., Torosyzan, Y., *et al.* Familial mediterranean fever at the millennium. *Medicine* 1998; 77:268–97.

14. Majeed, H., Al-Qudah, A., Qubain, H., and Shahin, H. The clinical patterns of myalgia in children with familial mediterranean fever. *Semin Arthritis Rheum* 2000; 30:138–143.

15. Drenth, J. and van der Meer, J. Hereditary periodic fever. *N Engl J Med* 2001; 345:1748–57.

16. Centola, M., Wood, G., Frucht, D., *et al.* The gene for familial mediterranean fever, *MEFV*, is expressed in early leukocyte development and is regulated in response to inflammatory mediators. *Blood* 2000; 95:3223–31.

17. Brik, R., Litmanovitz, D., Berkowitz, D., *et al.* Incidence of familial Mediterranean fever (FMF) mutations among children of Mediterranean extraction with functional abdominal pain. *J Pediatr* 2001; 138:759–62.

18. Drenth, J., Boom, B., Toonstra, J., van der Meer, J., and Group IHIS. Cutaneous manifestations and histological findings in the hyperimmunoglobulinemia D syndrome. *Arch Dermatol* 1994; 130:59–65.

19. Drenth, J., Haagsma, C., van der Meer, J., and Group IHIS. Hyperimmunoglobulinemia D and periodic fever syndrome. *Medicine* 1994; 73:133–44.

20. Frenkel, J., Houten, S., Waterham, H., *et al.* Clinical and molecular variablity in childhood periodic fever with hyperimmunoglobulinaemia D. *Rheumatol* 2001; 40:579–84.

21. McDermott, E., Smillie, D., and Powell, R. Clinical spectrum of familial hibernian fever: a 14-year follow-up study of the index case and extended family. *Mayo Clin Proc* 1997; 72:806–17.

22. Toro, J., Aksentijevich, I., Hull, K., Dean, J., and Kastner, D. Tumor necrosis factor receptor-associated periodic syndrome: a novel syndrome with cutaneous manifestations. *Arch Dermatol* 2000; 136:1487–94.

23. Aksentijevich, I., Galon, J., Soares, M., *et al.* The tumor-necrosis-factor receptor-associated periodic syndrome: new mutations in *TNFRSF1A*, ancestral origins, genotype-phenotype studies, and evidence for further genetic heterogeneity of periodic fevers. *Am J Hum Genet* 2001; 69:301–14.

24. Hull, K. and Kastner, D. Hereditary periodic fever. *N Engl J Med* 2002; 346:1415.

25. Aganna, E., Martinon, F., Hawkins, P., *et al.* Association of mutations in the *NALP3/CIAS1/PYPAF1* Gene with a broad phenotype including recurrent fever, cold sensitivity, sensorineural deafness and AA amyloidosis. *Arthritis Rheum* 2002; 46:2445–52.

26. Aksentijevich, I., Nowak, M., Mallah, M., *et al.* De novo *CIAS1* mutations, cytokine activation, and evidence for genetic heterogeneity in patients with neonatal-onset multisystem inflammatory disease (NOMID). *Arthritis Rheum* 2002; 46:3340–8.

27. Feldman, J., Prieur, A., Quartier, P., *et al.* Chronic infantile neurological cutaneous and articular syndrome is caused by mutations in *CIAS1*, a gene highly expressed in polymorphonuclear cells and chondrocytes. *Am J Hum Genet* 2002; 71:198–203.

28. Hoffman, H., Mueller, J., Broide, D., Wanderer, A., and Kolodner, R. Mutation of a new gene encoding a putative pyrin-like protein causes familial cold autoinflammatory syndrome and Muckle-Wells syndrome. *Nature Genet* 2001; 29:301–305.

29. Hoffman, H., Wanderer, A., and Broide, D. Familial cold autoinflammatory syndrome: phenotype and genotype of an autosomal dominant periodic fever. *J Allergy Clin Immunol* 2001;108:615–20.

30. Commerford, P. and Meyers, O. Arthropathy associated with familial cold urticaria. *S Afr Med J* 1977;51:105–8.

31. Zip, C., Ross, J., Greaves, M., Scriver, C., Mitchell, J., and Zoar, S. Familial cold urticaria. *Clin Exp Dermatol* 1993;18:338–41.

32. Muckle, T. The 'Muckle-Wells' syndrome. *Br J Dermatol* 1979;100:87–92.

33. Cuisset, L., Drenth, J., Berthelot, J.M., *et al.* Genetic linkage of the Muckle-Wells syndrome to chromosome 1q44. *Am J Hum Genet* 1999;65:1054–9.

34. Watts, R., Nicholls, A., and Scott, D. The arthropathy of the Muckle-Wells syndrome. *Br J Rheumatol* 1994;33:1184–7.

35. McDermott, M., Aganna, E., Hitman, G., Ogunkolade, B., Booth, D., and Hawkins, P. An autosomal dominant periodic fever associated with AA amyloidosis in a north Indian family maps to distal chromosome 1q. *Arthritis Rheum* 2000;43:2034–40.

36. De Cunto, C., Liberatore, D., San Román, J., Goldberg, J., and Morandi, A., G.F. Infantile-onset multisystem inflammatory disease: a differential diagnosis of systemic juvenile rheumatoid arthritis. *J Pediatr* 1997;130:551–6.

37. Prieur, A., Griscelli, C., Lampert, F., *et al.* A chronic, infantile, neurological, cutaneous and articular (CINCA) syndrome. A specific entity analysed in 30 patients. *Scand J Rheumatol* 1987;(Suppl) 66:57–68.

38. Torbiak, R., Dent, P., and Cockshott, W. NOMID—a neonatal syndrome of multisystem inflammation. *Skeletal Radiol* 1989;18:359–64.

39. Prieur, A. A recently recognised chronic inflammatory disease of early onset characterized by the triad of rash, central nervous system involvement and arthropathy. *Clin Exp Rheumatol* 2001;19:103–6.

40. Dollfus, H., Häfner, R., Hofmann, H., *et al.* Chronic infantile neurological cutaneous and articular/neonatal onset multisystem inflammatory disease syndrome. *Arch Ophthalmol* 2000;118:1386–92.

41. Huttenlocher, A., Frieden, I., and Emery, H. Neonatal onset multisystem inflammatory disease. *J Rheumatol* 1995;22:1171–3.

42. Lindor, N., Arsenault, T., Solomon, H., Seidman, C., and McEvoy, M. A new autosomal dominant disorder of pyogenic sterile arthritis, pyoderma gangrenosum, and acne: PAPA syndrome. *Mayo Clin Proc* 1997;72:611–15.

43. Wise, C., Bennett, L., Pascual, V., Gillum, J., and Bowcock, A. Localization of a gene for familial recurrent arthritis. *Arthritis Rheum* 2000;43:2041–5.

44. Wise, C., Gillum, J., Seidman, C., *et al.* Mutations in CD2BP1 disrupt binding to PTP PEST and are responsible for PAPA syndrome, an autoinflammatory disorder. *Hum Mol Genet* 2002;11:961–9.

45. Pattishall, E. and Kendig, E., Jr. Sarcoidosis in children. *Ped Pulmonol* 1996;22:195–203.

46. Shetty, A. and Gedalia, A. Sarcoidosis in children. *Curr Probl Pediatr* 2000;30:153–76.

47. North, A., Jr, Fink, C., Gibson, W., *et al.* Sarcoid arthritis in children. *Am J Med* 1970;48:449–55.

48. Fink, C. and Cimaz, R. Early onset sarcoidosis: not a benign disease. *J Rheumatol* 1997;24:174–7.

49. Vogel, R. Sarcoidosis of early onset. A challenge for the pediatric rheumatologist. *Clin Exp Rheumatol* 1993;11:685–91.

50. Lindsley, C., and Godfrey, W. Childhood sarcoidosis manifesting as juvenile rheumatoid arthritis. *Pediatrics* 1985;76:765–8.

51. Manouvrier-Hanu, S., Puech, B., Piette, F., *et al.* Blau syndrome of granulomatous arthritis, iritis, and skin rash: a new family and review of the literature. *Am J Med Genet* 1998;76:217–21.

52. Raphael, S., Blau, E., Zhang, W., and Hsu, S. Analysis of a large kindred with Blau syndrome for HLA, autoimmunity, and sarcoidosis. *Am J Dis Child* 1993;147:842–8.

53. Miceli-Richard, C., Lesage, S., Rybojad, M., *et al.* CARD15 mutations in Blau syndrome. *Nature Genet* 2001;29:19–20.

54. Cameron, B., Laxer, R., Wilmot, D., Greenberg, M., and Stein, L. Idiopathic periosteal hyperostosis with dysproteinemia (Goldbloom's syndrome): case report and review of the literature. *Arthritis Rheum* 1987;30:1307–12.

55. Gerscovich, E., Greenspan, A., and Lehman, W. Idiopathic periosteal hyperostosis with dysproteinemia-Goldbloom's syndrome. *Pediatr Radiol* 1990;20:208–11.

56. Borochowitz, Z., Gozal, D., Misselvitch, I., Aunallah, J., and Boss, J. Familial Caffey's disease and late recurrence in a child. *Clin Genetics* 1991;40:329–35.

57. Saul, R., Lee, W., and Stevenson, R. Caffey's disease revisited. *Am J Dis Child* 1982;136:56–60.

58. Thometz, J. and DiRaimondo, C. A case of recurrent Caffey's disease treated with naproxen. *Clin Orthop Rel Res* 1996; 323:304–9.

59. Dale, D., Person, R., Bolvard, A., *et al.* Mutations in the gene encoding neutrophil elastase in congenital and cyclic neutropenia. *Blood* 2001; 96:2317–22.

60. Touitou, I. The spectrum of familial mediterranean fever (FMF) mutations. *Eur J Hum Genet* 2001;9:473–83.

61. Gershoni-Baruch, R., Shinawi, M., Shamaly, H., Katsinetz, L., and Brik, R. Familial mediterranean fever: the segregation of four different mutations in 13 individuals from one inbred family: genotype-phenotype correlation and intrafamilial variability. *Am J Med Genet* 2002;109:198–201.

62. Livneh, A., Aksentijevich, I., Langevitz, P., *et al.* A single mutated *MEFV* allele in Israeli patients suffering from familial mediterranean fever and Behçet's disease (FMF-BD). *Eur J Hum Genet* 2001;9:191–6.

63. Simon, A., Cuisset, L., Vincent, M.-F., *et al.* Molecular analysis of the mevalonate kinase gene in a cohort of patients with the hyper-IgD and periodic fever syndrome: its application as a diagnostic tool. *Ann Intern Med* 2001;135:338–43.

64. Frenkel, J., Rijkers, G., Mandey, S., *et al.* Lack of isoprenoid products raises ex vivo interleukin-1beta secretion in hyperimmunoglobulinemia D and periodic fever syndrome. *Arthritis Rheum* 2002;46:2794–803.

65. Koonin, E. and Aravind, L. The NACHT family-a new group of predicted NTPases implicated in apoptosis and MHC transcription activation. *TIBS* 2000;25:223–4.

66. Dodé, C., Le Dû, N., Cuisset, L., *et al.* New mutations of *CIAS1* that are responsible for Muckle-Wells syndrome and familial cold urticaria: a novel mutations underlies both syndromes. *Am J Hum Genet* 2002;70: 1498–1506.

67. Lineh, A., Langevitz, P., Zemer, D., *et al.* Criteria for the Diagnosis of familial Mediterranean Fever. *Arthritis Rheum* 1997;40:1879–85.

68. Hoffmann., H., Rosengren, S., Boyle, D., *et al.* Prevention of cold-associated acute inflammation in familial cold autoinflammatory syndrome by interleukin-1 receptor antagonist. *Lancet* 2004:364:1779–85.

69. Hawkins, P., Lachmann, H., Aganna, E., *et al.* Spectrum of clinical features in Muckle-Wells syndrome and response to anakinra. *Arthritis Rheum* 2004;50:607–12.

70. Lovell D., Bowyer, S., Solinger, A. Interleukin-1 blockade by anakinra improves clinical symptoms in patients with neonatal-onset multisystem inflammatory disease. *Arthritis Rheum* 2005;52:1283–6.

71. Dierselhuis, M.P., Frenkel, J., Wulffraat, N. M., *et al.* Anakinra for flares of pyogenic arthritis in PAPA syndrome. *Rheumatology* 2005;44:406–8.

72. Kanazawa, N., Okafuji, I., Kambe, N., *et al.* Early-onset sarcoidosis and CARD15 mutations with constitutive nuclear factor-kappaB activation: common genetic etiology with Blau syndrome. *Blood* 2005;105:1195–7.

1.8 Non-inflammatory musculoskeletal disorders

Suzanne C. Li

Aim

The aim of this chapter is to describe those diseases of bones and soft tissues that are not usually associated with an inflammatory arthropathy, but that are causes of persistent or recurrent musculoskeletal pain, and that may, in some cases, be associated with the development of deformities.

Structure

- Benign limb pains
  - Growing pains
  - Benign hypermobility syndromes
- Musculoskeletal syndromes localized to the hip
  - Osteonecrosis
    - Legg–Calvé–Perthes and Meyer Dysplasia
    - Osteonecrosis associated with corticosteroids
  - Slipped capital femoral epiphysis
  - Chondrolysis of hip/transient demineralization of the hip
  - Apophysitis
  - Stress fractures
  - Snapping hip
  - Osteoarthritis
- Musculoskeletal syndromes localized to the knee
  - Knee problems secondary to bone problems
    - Osgood–Schlatter disease
    - Sinding–Larsen–Johansson
    - Bipartite patella
    - Medial tibial stress syndrome (shin splints)
    - Stress fractures
    - Osteochondritis dissecans
    - Osteoarthritis
  - Knee pain secondary to patella tracking/alignment problems
    - Patellofemoral pain syndrome
    - Recurrent patellar dislocation/subluxation
  - Knee pain secondary to soft tissue injuries
    - Meniscal problems
    - Ligament injury
    - Synovial plica syndrome
    - Iliotibial band friction syndrome
  - Other causes of swelling around the knee
    - Popliteal cyst
    - Eosinophilic synovitis
- Musculoskeletal syndromes localized to the foot
  - Osteochondroses
    - Freiberg disease
    - Kohler disease
  - Apophysitis
  - Stress fracture
  - Tarsal coalition
  - Accessory bones
  - Osteochondritis dissecans
- Musculoskeletal syndromes localized to the back
  - Spondylolysis/spondylolisthesis
  - Scheuermann disease
  - Disk herniation
  - Apophyseal ring fracture
  - Osteoporosis
- Musculoskeletal syndromes localized to the shoulder or elbow
  - Physiolysis of the proximal humerus
  - Overuse injuries to the elbow
  - Stress fractures
- Musculoskeletal syndromes localized to the hand or wrist
  - Physeal injuries
- Thiemann disease
- Congenital indifference to pain (Charcot disease)
- Frostbite arthropathy and phalangeal microgeodic syndrome
- Child abuse
- Cracking joints

Introduction

Musculoskeletal pain is a common complaint in the paediatric population, of which only a small percentage will be found to be due to a chronic rheumatic condition. Many of the musculoskeletal complaints are secondary to mechanical or noninflammatory causes. Some complaints will be related to overuse or trauma, while others are related to the increased joint laxity found in many children. Compared to adults, children are more susceptible to bone injuries than ligamentous injuries owing to the relative strength of the tendons and ligaments as compared with the epiphyseal plate [1]. With children participating in more competitive sports and training, overuse injuries are becoming more common. These affect the lower extremities more frequently than the upper extremities, with the knee being the most commonly injured joint in the lower extremity [1]. A careful history taking and examination can help distinguish most of these conditions from Juvenile Idiopathic Arthritis (JIA).

Benign limb pains

Growing pains

Between 4.2–33.6% of children develop the benign condition known as growing pains (Table 1.8.1) [2,3]. The name is a misnomer, as children usually do not develop growing pains during peak periods of growth. Instead, symptoms usually develop between 3 and 5 years, or 8 and 12 years of age. These children complain of intermittent, dull, aching, or boring pain, localized to their calves, front of the thighs, behind the knees, or, rarely, in the arms [2]. Both right and left limbs are affected, although often not during the same episode. The pains generally occur at the end of the day, and classically awaken the child

Table 1.8.1 Criteria for the diagnosis of growing pains (Naish and Apley [3]):

At least a 3-month history of pain
Intermittent pain with symptom-free intervals of days, weeks, or months
Pain late in day or awakening child at night
Pain not specifically related to joints
Pain of significant severity to interrupt such normal activity as sleep
Normal physical exam, laboratory data, and roentgenograms

from sleep. In contrast, the pain of JIA is typically worse in the mornings, and rarely awakens the child from sleep. In older children, the pain can resemble cramps, creeping sensations, or restless legs. Girls are affected more often than boys. Children with growing pains have a normal physical exam with no evidence of swelling, tenderness, limitation of movement, limping, or erythema. All laboratory and X-rays are within normal limits. Children with growing pains also have a higher frequency of headaches and stomach aches [3].

The aetiology is not known, and no long-term ill effects are noted in the child's growth or development. Symptoms generally decrease in frequency over a 12–24-month period without treatment. No specific treatment is available or needed, but if the child complains of severe pain, acetaminophen, gentle massage, or warm soaks, may help. One study found a decline in the frequency of painful episodes in patients who carried out a twice-daily muscle-stretching program with their parents [4].

Other conditions that can present with nocturnal pain include nocturnal leg cramps, osteoid osteoma, and malignancies, both primary bone tumours, such as Ewing sarcoma or osteogenic sarcoma, and secondary malignancies, such as lymphoblastic leukaemia or neuroblastoma. Children with nocturnal leg cramps present with night-time cramping pain with a contracted calf muscle. These cramps generally occur after vigorous daytime activity. Adolescents with osteoid osteoma present with pain localized to one anatomic area, sometimes with a sympathetic joint effusion in the adjacent joint. A dramatic, prompt response to an NSAID is a good clue. Malignancies and osteoid osteomas are discussed in Part I, Chapter 1.10.

Benign hypermobility syndromes

Joint hyperextensibility can be found in a number of diseases, such as Marfan, Ehlers–Danlos, Down syndrome, Larsen syndrome, cutis laxa, and osteogenesis imperfecta. Children with these conditions may have damage to their joints as a result of recurrent subclinical dislocations. However, mild, generalized, and often familial ligamentous laxity is relatively common in the general population and can be demonstrated in 10–34% of children [5] (Figure 1.8.1(a), (b)). Girls are more

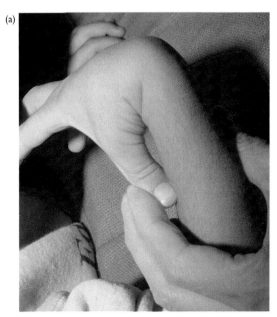 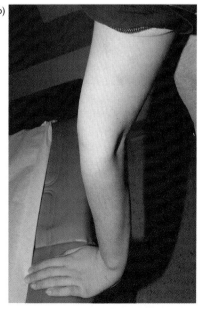

Fig. 1.8.1 Benign hypermobility: (a) This 4-year-old boy is able to appose his thumb to his forearm, one of the measures of the Beighton score. (b) This 9-year-old boy is able to hyperextend his elbows, knees, and other joints. He can easily put his palms on the floor.

Table 1.8.2 Revised (Brighton 1998) criteria for the diagnosis of benign joint hypermobility syndrome

Major criteria

Beighton score of 4/9 or greater;

Arthralgia for >3 months in four or more joints.

Minor criteria

A Beighton score of 1–3/9;

Arthralgia ≥3 months in 1–3 joints or back pain ≥3 months, or spondylosis, or spondylolisthesis;

Dislocation or subluxation in more than one joint, or in one joint on more than one occasion;

Three or more soft tissue rheumatism lesions (e.g. tenosynovitis, bursitis, epicondylitis);

Marfanoid habitus (span/height >1.03, upper:lower segment ratio <0.89, arachnodactyly);

Abnormal skin: striae, hyperextensibility, thin skin, papyraceous scarring;

Eye signs: drooping lids or myopia or anti-mongoloid slant;

Varicose veins or hernia or uterine/rectal prolapse.

Beighton score: Maximum of 9 points: 1 point for each of the following: passively dorsiflex either 5th MCP to ≥90°, appose either thumb to volar aspect of ipsilateral forearm, hyperextend either elbow to ≥10°, hyperextend either knee to ≥10°, place hands on floor without bending knees.

Benign joint hypermobility syndrome is diagnosed in the presence of two major criteria, or one major and two minor criteria, or four minor criteria. Two minor criteria suffice where there is an unequivocally affected first-degree relative. BJHS is excluded by the presence of Marfan or Ehlers–Danlos syndrome. Criteria Major 1 and Minor 1 are mutually exclusive, as are Major 2 and Minor 2 [6].

commonly affected than boys, and the frequency of hypermobility generally decreases with age. The diagnosis of benign joint hypermobility syndrome (BJHS) can be made using the Brighton criteria (Table 1.8.2) [6], and these criteria were recently validated in over 700 Dutch children [7]. Pes planus (flat feet) is a common finding in patients with hypermobility. If the patient's foot is flexible and an arch forms when the patient is lying down or standing on her toes, then the pes planus is not pathological. Individuals with hypermobility and pes planus may, however, develop an overuse injury in their feet. Problems also arise if the patient has pes planus with a tight heel cord or hamstring (see Part 1, Chapter 1.1, Figure 1.1.34).

Children with BJHS, as well as children who have significant joint hypermobility in a limited number of joints, can develop recurrent bland effusions and arthralgias. Unlike patients with JIA, hypermobile children tend to develop pain localized to the joint later in the day or in the evening, especially after vigorous exercise earlier in the day. The effusions and pain usually resolve by the following morning. The overall prognosis for patients with BJHS or joint hypermobility is favourable. Increased susceptibility to injury is not usually significant and rarely, if ever, requires restriction from sports. There have been reports of an association between hypermobility and juvenile episodic arthritis/arthralgias, chronic fatigue syndrome, and increased susceptibility to fibromyalgia, but these associations require further study [5,8,9].

Musculoskeletal syndromes localized to the hip

Introduction

Few children with JIA present with isolated hip pain, while several different noninflammatory conditions can present this way (see Part 1,

Chapter 1.3, Table 1.3.4). Both Legg–Calvé–Perthes (LCP) and slipped capital femoral epiphysis (SCFE) are diseases in which early diagnosis can significantly improve the long-term outcome. Both conditions present with pain during walking or climbing, and can be associated with limping. In contrast, pain associated with JIA often increases with rest or inactivity. The pattern of pain in transitory demineralization of the hip and acute chondrolysis also differs from that found in JIA. In these conditions, patients present with a sudden onset of pain and limited mobility following intense physical activity. Osteoarthritis can present as intermittent episodes of pain and limp, and can develop in patients with long-standing JIA, as well as in patients with other prior hip problems. Severe nocturnal pain may be due to benign tumours, such as aneurysmal bone cysts or osteoid osteoma, or malignant bone tumours, such as Ewing sarcoma or osteogenic sarcoma. Severe pain with constitutional symptoms may be due to malignant tumours or infection. In addition, discomfort in the hip may represent referred pain from the knee or the back. Cases of delayed diagnosis of LCP or SCFE still occur because the pain was localized to the knee, misleading the physician evaluating the patient.

Osteonecrosis

Children with osteonecrosis have a different pattern of pain than that found in children with JIA. The pain associated with osteonecrosis initially occurs during standing or walking, and is absent at rest and at night. Osteonecrosis occurs in a number of clinical settings in children (Table 1.8.3). Osteonecrosis secondary to heritable defects or rheumatic disease is discussed elsewhere (see Part 1, Chapter 1.10). The aetiology of osteonecrosis is not known; it was initially thought to be secondary to circulatory compromise and inadequate nutrition of cancellous bone (avascular necrosis), but it is not clear if the circulatory compromise is primary or secondary [10]. Diagnosis depends on imaging studies. Radiographs, however, may remain normal for several weeks. MRI allows early diagnosis, and is more sensitive than bone scan or CT.

Table 1.8.3 Factors and conditions associated with osteonecrosis in children

Antiphospholipid antibodies

Congenital disorders
  Blood disorders: haemoglobinopathies (SS, SC, SD, SA), polycythemia, haemophilia
  Gaucher's, Fabry's, skeletal dysplasias, familial dysautonomia

Coagulopathies

Drugs (corticosteroids, low-molecular weight heparin)

Hyperlipidaemia

Infections (HIV, meningococcus)

Inflammatory bowel disease

Leukaemia/lymphoma

Orthopaedic problems
  Congenital dysplasia of the hip
  Legg–Calvé–Perthes
  Slipped capital femoral epiphysis

Rheumatic disease or vasculitis (SLE, JIA, Sjögren, Raynaud)

Trauma

Based on [10,12,57,58].

Legg–Calvé–Perthes and Meyer dysplasia

Legg–Calvé–Perthes (LCP) is an osteochondrosis of the hip, that is, the most common type of hip osteonecrosis in children. Osteochondroses are idiopathic conditions in which there is a disturbance in endochondral ossification that leads to bone necrosis. Some arise from trauma, while others may be related to vascular insufficiency. LCP predominantly occurs in young boys (majority between 4–9 years of age) and is bilateral in 10% of patients [11]. Importantly, boys with bilateral disease should be evaluated for hypothyroidism and skeletal dysplasia (Part 1, Chapter 1.10). Painless limp alone is the clinical presentation in 25% of these patients, but hip or knee pain with activity and limping form the more frequent pattern of presentation. A few patients (2–3%) will present following transient synovitis. Limp may arise from pain, leg length discrepancy, or from limited ROM (see Part 1, Chapter 1.1, Fig. 1.1.16 and 1.1.18). AP and frog leg view hip X-rays, when abnormal, initially show a smaller femoral head and widening of the cartilage space, followed by a radiolucent cleft in the femoral head, fragmentation, and lastly, deformity of the femoral head [11] (Figure 1.8.2). Bone scan and MRI allow an earlier diagnosis at a time when radiographs are normal or only questionably abnormal. Laboratory tests will be normal. Possible aetiologies include an increased thrombophilic tendency predisposing to venous occlusion of the femoral vessels and synovitis of the hip leading to increased pressure with a resultant reduced blood flow [12]. Patients with a mild degree of femoral head involvement may be managed non-surgically, and outcome is better in patients who present at a younger age and have minimal distortion of the femoral head. Most patients who had a normal or flattened head were pain-free and without signs of osteoarthritis 30–50 years later, whereas those that had an irregular or very deformed head, had a high incidence of osteoarthritis and hip replacement [13].

Young children (≤5 years) who present with limping or an abnormal gait and are found to have hip abnormalities on radiographs may have Meyer's dysplasia (dysplasia epiphysealis capitis femoris) rather than LCP (Figure 1.8.3). Boys are more likely to be affected than girls and the dysplasia can be bilateral. In contrast to LCP, patients with Meyer's dysplasia are found to have normal bone marrow signals on bone scan or MRI. This condition typically resolves spontaneously by the age of 6 [14].

Osteonecrosis associated with corticosteroids

Children with asthma and other disorders treated with corticosteroids, such as SLE and juvenile dermatomyositis, may develop osteonecrosis, especially of the hips [15] (Figure 1.8.4). Patients with a vasculitis may have an inherently increased risk of developing osteonecrosis, and this risk is probably increased further by treatment with corticosteroids [10]. Neither, the mechanism nor the exact incidence of osteonecrosis among patients treated with corticosteroids is known. It remains unclear whether the dose, duration of corticosteroid treatment, or a

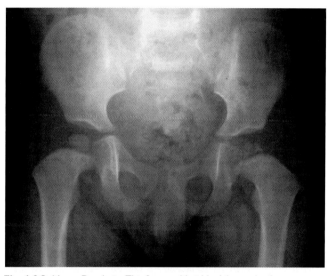

Fig. 1.8.3 Meyer Dysplasia. This 2-year-old girl had 1 month of an intermittent, painless limp following a minor fall. She had pain with full ROM of her L hip. Her X-ray shows a smaller and fragmented L femoral head epiphysis, but her T2 weighted MRI showed normal marrow signal and preservation of the cartilage in the hip.

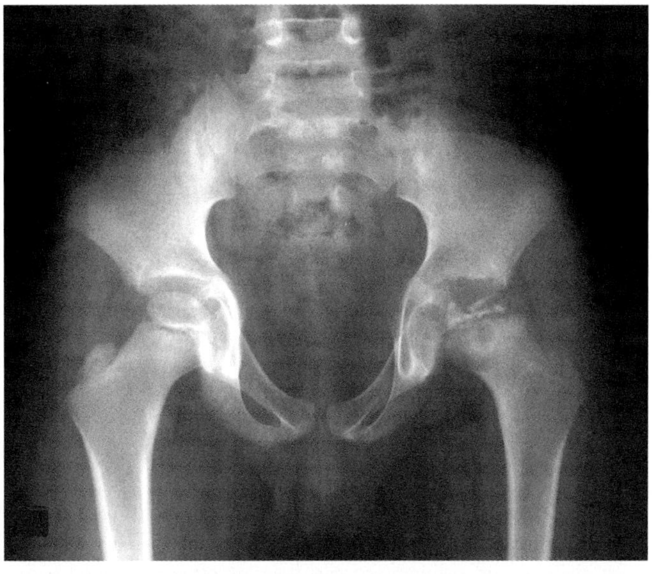

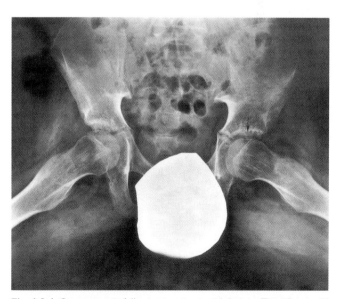

Fig. 1.8.2 Legg–Calvé–Perthes. This 9-year-old boy developed nocturnal pain in his thigh and knee, knee pain with activity, and a limp. Initial X-rays done only of his femur and knee were normal. His symptoms persisted, and a hip X-ray 6 months later showed sclerosis and a reduced femoral head.

Fig. 1.8.4 Osteonecrosis following corticosteroid therapy. This 15-year-old boy developed hip pain and limitation following corticosteroid therapy for a brain tumour. His X-ray shows flattening of the femoral head with a subchondral curved lucency (arrow). (Courtesy of J. Jacobs.)

combination of both leads to an increased risk of osteonecrosis [10,12]. Different non-surgical and surgical treatments have and continue to be studied, but none have shown clear benefit. Remineralization without sequelae is possible in milder cases. Most orthopedic surgeons recommend non-weight bearing for a variable time period. Rheumatologists tend to believe that NSAIDs are helpful, both in relieving pain and reducing the associated synovitis which may contribute to a poor outcome.

Slipped capital femoral epiphysis

Similar to LCP, patients with slipped capital femoral epiphysis (SCFE) present with groin, medial thigh, or knee pain that is worsened by walking or climbing, and improved by rest. The onset of SCFE can be insidious with either little or no hip pain initially, or a dull, aching hip, groin, thigh, or knee pain associated with activity. Later, patients present with external rotation of hip, decreased internal rotation and flexion, and a shorter affected leg. Weeks to months may pass before a diagnosis is reached. This condition typically affects overweight adolescent and preadolescent children (7–15 yr); these children are also usually >90th percentile for height for their age [11]. Boys are more likely to be affected than girls. SCFE can occur bilaterally in up to 60% of the cases. AP and frog leg view X-rays show a widened and irregular physis, and displacement of the proximal femoral metaphysis anterolaterally and superiorly [11] (Figure 1.8.5). The greater the displacement of the slip, the worse is the long-term prognosis. Radiographs may miss the diagnosis in 20% of patients with early SCFE; ultrasonography or MRI may be more sensitive [16].

Prompt surgical treatment is required if the slip is more than very minor to try to avoid the three major complications of a slip: acute chondrolysis, osteonecrosis of the femoral head, and late osteoarthritis [12,16]. Risk factors for chondrolysis include African-American race, female sex, and more severe slips. Conditions associated with SCFE include cryptorchidism, growth hormone therapy, hypothyroidism, hypopituitarism, hypogonadism, acromegaly, Klinefelter syndrome, trisomy 21, and coxa vara [17]. SCFE may also arise from delayed treatment of septic arthritis of the hip [12].

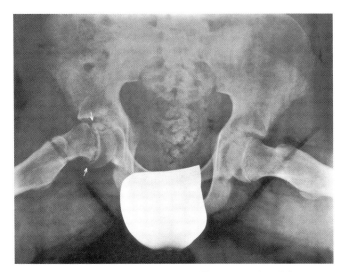

Fig. 1.8.5 Slipped capital femoral epiphysis; This overweight, adolescent boy presented with thigh pain that was aggravated by activity. Arrows point to the slip of the femoral head. (Courtesy of From J. Jacobs.)

Chondrolysis of the hip/transient demineralization of the hip

Two conditions which usually have a clear history of precipitating trauma are acute chondrolysis of the hip (juvenile lamellar coxitis) and transient demineralization of the hip. Following sudden extreme motions, such as jumping into a swimming pool or doing a "split", patients immediately complain of pain and have limited hip movement. In acute chondrolysis, X-rays show evidence of cartilage dissolution (joint space narrowing and irregularity). In transient demineralization, X-rays show demineralization of the femoral head. With weight bearing and anti-inflammatory drug therapy, both symptoms and X-rays return to normal in several months.

In addition to acute chondrolysis from trauma, chondrolysis or destruction of articular cartilage can occur in patients who have had SCFE, LCP, infection, prolonged immobilization, or severe lower extremity burns [18]. There is also a form of chondrolysis (idiopathic) for which there is no known cause or precipitating factor; this tends to occur in adolescent girls, and is often bilateral [19]. African Americans may be at increased risk. Idiopathic chondrolysis, unlike acute chondrolysis, presents with an insidious onset of anterior or medial pain in the thigh or hip. Patients have limited ROM, joint stiffness, and limping; these symptoms can be similar to those found in patients with JIA. Within months, patients may develop a flexion contracture. Laboratory studies are usually normal, but hip X-rays show joint space narrowing, as well as osteopenia and other findings (Figure 1.8.6(a)) [19]. Long-term prognosis is variable; some patients recover, while others develop hip ankylosis or osteonecrosis (Figure 1.8.6(b)). Various treatments have been tried with generally only limited success [19].

Apophysitis

Apophyses are bone outgrowths that have their own center of ossification and often serve as sites of tendon attachments. Apophysitis is pain at the site of the apophysis. The aetiology is unknown but may be due to microfracture and/or avulsion secondary to repeated trauma. In the pelvis, runners are most likely to develop apophysitis of the iliac crest, while dancers are more likely to develop ischial apophysitis. Adolescent boys are the group most likely to develop hip apophysitis [20]. These patients complain of a low level of pain that is worsened by activity, in contrast to patients with JIA who have pain at rest. Because children with more serious conditions, such as SCFE and LCP may present similarly, X-rays and careful evaluation are always needed. X-rays are usually normal with apophysitis unless there is avulsion of the apophysis. Patients who have an apophyseal avulsion will usually have a sudden sharp pain, feel a pop, and be unable to continue an activity [20]. They complain of direct point tenderness and swelling at the site. Avulsions and apophysitis of the hip and pelvis tend to resolve spontaneously with activity modification and symptomatic treatment.

Stress fractures

Stress fractures occur in the femoral bones of children (5–16 years) involved in repetitive activities, such as running, jumping, dancing, roller skating, and riding a scooter; they are often associated with a recent increase in activity [21,22]. The children complain of hip or groin pain and may develop limping; however, most of them are able (a)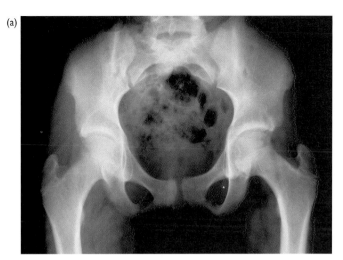

(b)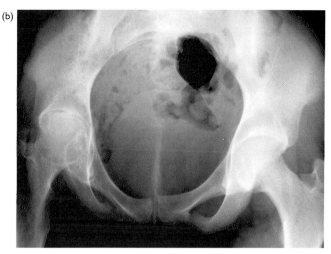

Fig. 1.8.6 Idiopathic chondrolysis of the hip. (a) This 14-year-old girl presented with insidious onset of aching hip pain. Her initial X-ray shows dome loss of the femoral head medially and mild sclerosis of the right hip. (b) Her follow-up X-ray 15 months later shows progressive destruction of her right hip, with loss of joint space and deformity of the femoral head. (Courtesy of C. Rose.)

to continue most of their normal activities for weeks to months before the diagnosis is made. Similar to other overuse injuries, the pain is worsened by activity and relieved by rest. If the child continues to be active, a complete fracture may occur. Fractures most frequently occur in the femoral neck, but can also be seen in the femoral diaphysis and mid-femur [21]. Stress fractures have also been reported in the sacrum [23]. X-rays or bone scans confirm the diagnosis. Patients generally recover with reduced weight bearing.

Snapping hip

Some children, especially adolescent girls, can produce a snapping sound in their hip which may be associated with pain. Snapping can occur bilaterally, and is often produced when the hip is extended from a flexed abducted and externally rotated position. The sound is due to abnormal movement of the iliotibial band over the greater trochanter or of the iliopsoas tendon over the pelvis [24]. A minority of patients may have an associated bursitis. Most will improve with conservative treatment and reassurance.

Osteoarthritis (OA)

Primary OA is a disorder of aging not seen in children except as a rare feature of progeria or its adolescent equivalent, Werner syndrome. However, once the joint cartilage is damaged as a result of any primary process, secondary degenerative changes may take place, especially in weight-bearing joints. Secondary osteoarthritis is seen in children following septic hips, LCP, SCFE, JIA, and other disorders (Table 1.8.4). These children present with episodes of "traumatic synovitis" associated with sudden increase in pain and limitation of motion. If the inflammation is sufficiently severe, there may also be systemic signs, such as fever and an elevated ESR. The possibility of reactivation of a previous infection or the development of a new infection must always be considered. The history of prior joint damage and lack of evidence for arthritis elsewhere make JIA an unlikely aetiology. In patients who already have JIA, the acute onset of severe pain should prompt evaluation for osteonecrosis, OA, infection, or other problems. In OA, X-rays show joint space narrowing and bony hypertrophy

Table 1.8.4 Types of OA seen in children

Primary
  Progeria
  Werner syndrome

Secondary
  Septic hip
  Legg–Calvé–Perthes
  Congenital dislocation of the hip
  SCFE
  JIA
  Metabolic
  Sports/trauma

(Figure 1.8.7). Attacks are usually brief, and NSAIDs can be used to relieve the pain of the acute episodes. Chronic administration of NSAIDs is rarely necessary.

Musculoskeletal syndromes localized to the knee

Introduction

Knee pain in children is often related to mechanical disorders, such as overuse and trauma. Overuse-related conditions include stress fractures, shin splints, Osgood–Schlatter, Sinding–Larsen–Johansson, as well as injuries of the meniscus and ligaments. Overuse related pain usually increases during activity, and improves, at least initially, with rest. Bony tenderness or pain localized to one side of a joint should help in the differentiation of these conditions from JIA. As discussed earlier, children with hypermobility often have knee pain, especially if associated problems, such as recurrent patellar dislocation or subluxation, occur as well. Because knee pain may represent referred pain from the hip or foot, these adjacent joints must also be carefully evaluated.

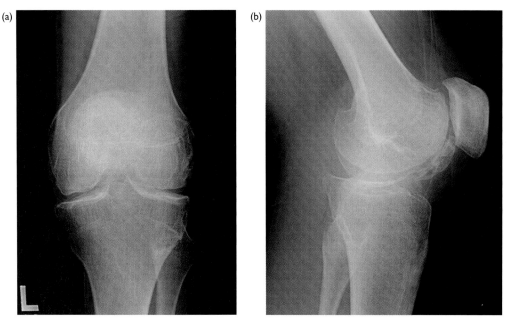

Fig. 1.8.7 Secondary osteoarthritis. This teenage boy with long-standing, poorly controlled, polyarticular JIA shows bony hypertrophy of his tibia and femur, in addition to joint space narrowing and erosions of the distal femur.

Knee pain secondary to bone problems

Osgood–Schlatter disease

Osgood–Schlatter disease (OSD) is a traction apophysitis of the tibial tubercle that typically affects 10–15 year-old children (10–11-year-old girls, 13–14-year-old boys); boys are more likely to be affected than girls. Patients complain of pain, tenderness, and swelling at the tibial tuberosity [21] (Figure 1.8.8). This condition is commonly found in children who play sports that involve running and jumping. Both knees are involved in up to 30% of boys with OSD [25]. Some patients have a history of familial occurrence. X-rays (AP and lateral) may show a partial avulsion of the tibial tuberosity or ossicle formation at the site, but are often normal. Patients with OSD are treated with activity modification, quadriceps strengthening and stretching exercises, and NSAIDs. Patients improve with time, but it may take months to years for full recovery.

Sinding–Larsen–Johansson

Sinding–Larsen–Johansson is a traction apophysitis of the distal pole of the patella. Patients have similar symptoms to those seen in Osgood-Schlatter, except that the pain and tenderness is localized to the inferior pole of the patella. A lateral X-ray may show irregularity at the inferior pole of the patella, or separation of part of the patella. Adolescent males who are involved in jumping sports are commonly affected [25,26]. This condition usually resolves completely within 3 to 12 months, and patients can be treated similarly to those with OSD with modification of activities, quadriceps strengthening exercises, and NSAIDs.

Bipartite patella

During early adolescence, secondary ossification centers develop in the patella. If these secondary centres fail to fuse to the primary ossification centers, the patient will have a bipartite patella [25]. This is usually asymptomatic. However, some patients may have pain because of

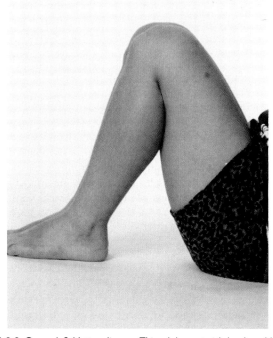

Fig. 1.8.8 Osgood–Schlatter disease. This adolescent girl developed knee pain with hyperextension, and a swollen, painful tibial tuberosity. (Courtesy of T.R. Southwood.)

motion between the two centres or because of poor alignment of the secondary center with the rest of the knee joint. The bipartite patella may also fracture following minor trauma [25]. The pain is usually located at the superiolateral pole of the patella, and there may be swelling over the patella, and tenderness of the adjacent synovium and joint capsule. Unlike children with JIA involving the knee, patients with a bipartite patella do not have a joint effusion. X-rays show the bipartite patella. Patients are treated symptomatically, and rarely require surgery.

Medial tibial stress syndrome (shin splints)

Adolescents who participate in sports such as running and jumping may develop a periostitis along the posterior medial tibia [27]. Patients with shin splints tend to complain of sharp pain that is aggravated by activity, and have tenderness along the posterior medial tibial border in the distal third of the tibia, or along the anterior medial border rather than in the joint. The pain is worsened by active ankle dorsiflexion and is often bilateral. X-rays may be normal, or show periosteal new bone, or calcification, in the area of tenderness; bone scan often documents a linear increased area of uptake along the tibia [27].

Stress fractures

Stress fractures occur in normal bone subjected to repeated episodes of minor stress associated with the normal daily activities of an athletic child or adolescent. Younger children typically develop stress fractures in the tibia. Adolescent runners and basketball players develop stress fractures in their proximal tibiae, as well as in the patellae and distal femoral physes, while ice skaters develop stress fractures in their fibulae [26]. Boys and girls are equally affected. Children complain of well-localized pain, swelling, and tenderness at the site of the fracture. The onset of pain is usually insidious and associated with activity; later, the pain may be constant and the patient may develop a limp. Unlike the patient with JIA, the pain and tenderness are adjacent to, rather than within, the joint; these symptoms may be mistaken for subacute osteomyelitis (see Part 1, Chapter 1.5). X-rays may be normal for many weeks, and then show radiolucency along the edge of the site followed by periosteal new-bone formation. MRI, CT, or bone scan allow

earlier diagnosis [1]. Patients are treated symptomatically; healing occurs in 2 weeks to 3 months.

Osteochondritis dissecans

Osteochondritis dissecans (OD) is an idiopathic condition involving sequential necrosis of subchondral bone and articular cartilage; different etiologies have been postulated including trauma, ischaemia, and genetic predisposition [28]. Up to 20–30% of children have bilateral disease, and up to 50% have multiple areas of OD lesions although some of these may be asymptomatic [25,26]. Some families appear to have an autosomal dominant form of OD [25]. OD is uncommon in children less than 10 years of age, and is most common in athletic adolescent boys, during the growth spurt [28,29]. The knee is the most commonly affected area, with OD occurring at the lateral aspect of the medial femoral condyle, lateral condyle, or patella. The patient with OD, similar to patients with JIA, may present with anterior knee pain, joint effusion, limited ROM, and quadriceps atrophy [26,29], but the patient with OD has knee pain with activity rather than at rest, especially with movements involving rotation, and may also have a sensation of popping, locking, or giving way [25]. X-ray findings are variable; during early disease, there may be soft tissue swelling and no bony changes. Later, X-rays may show irregularity of the articular surface, sclerosis, and separation of fragments of bone (Figure 1.8.9). MRI allows earlier detection of OD [25]. Patients are treated with modification of activities until the lesion heals; if the patient remains symptomatic, surgery may be needed to prevent future problems [25].

Osteoarthritis

Secondary OA, as discussed in the hip pain section, may occur in any joint with pre-existing damage.

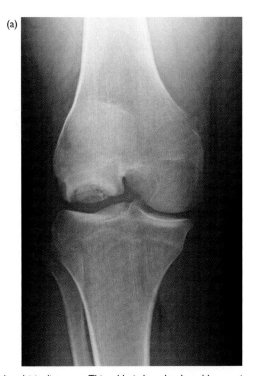
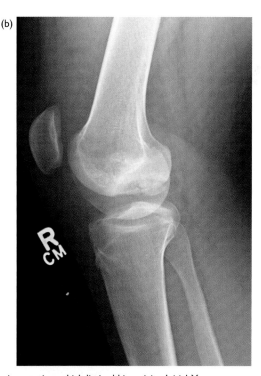

Fig. 1.8.9 Osteochondritis dissecans. This athletic boy developed knee pain during running, which limited his activity. Initial X-rays were normal; a repeat X-ray ((a) = AP, (b) = lateral) after several months showed sclerosis and bone fragments. (Courtesy of Children's Hospital of NY-Presbyterian.)

Knee pain secondary to patella tracking/alignment problems

Patellofemoral pain syndrome, patellofemoral syndrome, or idiopathic anterior knee pain syndrome

Patellofemoral pain is commonly reported by athletic adolescents, and is one of the most common causes of anterior knee pain. Girls are more frequently affected than boys. The cause is not known, but malalignment/poor tracking of the patella and vastus medialis muscle dysfunction are thought to contribute to the syndrome [26,30]. The pain is often poorly localized and related to activities, such as stair climbing/descending or squatting, as well as prolonged sitting [26]. There may be tenderness over the inferomedial side of the patella [26], or with pressure applied to the patella during medial or lateral displacement [see Part 1, Chapter 1.1 (Figure 1.1.24) 30]. The onset of pain may be acute or gradual, and often follows an increase in physical activity. Patients may feel that their knee "catches" or "gives way", or that it locks [30]. In contrast to patients with JIA, there is usually no joint effusion. This condition is benign, and patients are treated with activity modification, NSAIDs, quadriceps strengthening, and hamstring stretching excercises; bracing or taping to improve patellar tracking may help. Full recovery may take years. Only a minority of patients has chondromalacia in which there is damage to the articular cartilage, and some of these patients may require surgery [30].

Recurrent patellar dislocation and subluxation

Patients with joint laxity are particularly prone to dislocation of the patella, which occurs laterally and is often precipitated by a twisting motion. The patient has a sensation that the knee is "going out of place" and then "popping back in", and the knee appears abnormal at the time of the dislocation [29]. Patients who have patellar subluxation have similar complaints, but here the knee spontaneously reduces, and the appearance of the knee is not distorted. Subluxations most commonly occur in adolescent girls, who report that running, jumping, and climbing aggravate their parapatellar pain. Following the subluxation or dislocation, patients may develop small to large joint effusions and medial patellar tenderness [29]. However, unlike the patient with JIA, these patients have pain and guarding related to patellar maneuvers during joint movement, and can trace their pain to specific activities. Patients are usually treated initially with immobilization or splinting. Strengthening the vastus medialis muscle may help reduce the likelihood of recurrence; more severe cases may require surgical intervention.

Knee pain secondary to soft tissue injuries

Meniscal problems

Younger children rarely develop meniscal injuries unless they have a congenital anomaly, such as a discoid meniscus [25]. It is typically the lateral meniscus that is affected. The discoid meniscus is thicker and less stable than the normal meniscus, and is thus more easily injured. The risk of injury is also increased if the meniscus lacks posterior tibial attachments [31]. Adolescents may tear their meniscus following a twisting motion of the flexed knee [25]. Patients with a torn meniscus complain of pain, clicking, clunking, or snapping as the knee is moved. Both JIA and meniscal injury can present with a joint effusion, but the patient with a meniscal tear also complains of severe tenderness along the joint line, lateral bulging, and clunking during ROM, as well as locking and limited knee extension [31]. The bulge along the lateral joint line will often disappear during full extension. MRI is the preferred imaging technique (Figure 1.8.10). Surgical treatment may be needed for more serious injuries.

Ligament injury

Ligament injuries are more common in athletic than nonathletic children. Breaststroke swimmers using the whip-kick technique can develop sprains of the medial collateral ligament (MCL) and have pain and tenderness over the medial knee along the MCL. Injury of the MCL is usually caused by a valgus or rotational force. Minor tears may be treated conservatively, while more serious ones require bracing or surgery [26]. Anterior cruciate ligament (ACL) injuries can occur following jumping, pivoting, or twisting motions [32]. Girls are

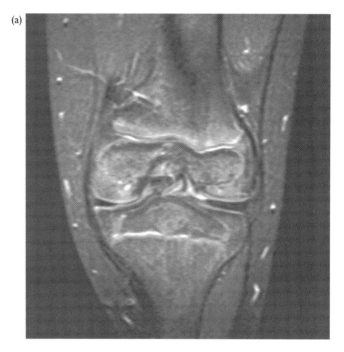

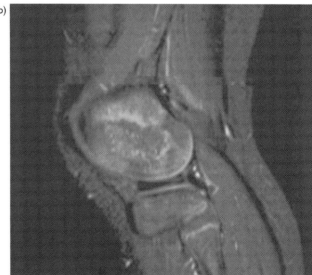

Fig. 1.8.10 Discoid meniscus. This 5-year-old boy had a 6-month history of bilateral knee pain that worsened with activity. His MRI ((a) = AP, (b) = lateral) shows a thicker lateral meniscus with a tear. (Courtesy of M. Liebling.)

more likely to be affected than boys; in boys, the injury is usually contact-related [32]. The patient may feel a "pop" and develop acute joint swelling, diffuse tenderness around the knee, and limited motion [25,26]. Knee laxity can be assessed on physical exam (Lachman, pivot-shift, anterior drawer tests), and MRI shows the extent of the ligament defect. ACL injuries are more serious than MCL injuries, and patients need vigorous rehabilitation, and possibly surgery. There may be an increased risk for the later development of articular cartilage damage [26].

Synovial plica syndrome

Most children who have a synovial plica are asymptomatic. However, with trauma or overuse, children may develop inflammation and pain related to the synovial plica. This condition usually develops during adolescence in youngsters involved in running and jumping sports [29]. Patients develop a dull, aching pain in the medial knee, and medial parapatellar tenderness of the often-palpable thickened plica. They may complain of a snapping or "catching" sensation due to the thickened plica moving over the medial condyle during knee extension and flexion [25,29]. Symptoms usually improve with conservative treatment although some patients may need surgical excision of the plica.

Iliotibial band friction syndrome

Iliotibial band friction syndrome is seen in adolescent runners. Patients have pain over the lateral knee, especially when running downhill. Physical exam reveals tenderness over the lateral condyle [27]. Most patients improve with conservative treatment.

Other causes of swelling around the knee

Popliteal cyst

Popliteal or Baker cysts usually present as painless, firm, mobile swellings located medially in the popliteal space behind the knee. Patients generally do not have any limitation in motion unless the cyst extends into the calf or is very large. If the cyst is very large, or ruptures, patients may develop compartment syndrome or pseudothrombophlebitis syndrome [33]. Cysts are commonly found in children with knee arthritis, especially those with a large effusion, but may occur as an isolated finding unrelated to arthritis at the knee [34]. X-rays should be obtained to evaluate for other lesions or malignancy. Ultrasonography (Figure 1.8.11) and MRI can be used to exclude other processes if there are atypical symptoms. No treatment is usually needed as most cysts resolve spontaneously, and many recur following surgery [25]. Healing may be hastened by wrapping the calf with an ace bandage starting at the ankle and "milking" the fluid back into the joint capsule. Rarely, it may take years for the cyst to resolve completely.

Eosinophilic synovitis

Patients with eosinophilic synovitis present with recurrent episodes of acute, large monoarticular swelling that lacks warmth or redness; some patients feel severe pain while others feel no pain [35,36]. The knee is frequently involved. Aspiration of joint fluid usually reveals a predominance of eosinophils(up to 95%), with leukocyte count varying from 1.2 K/mm^3 to more than 10 K/mm^3 [35,37]. Mild peripheral eosinophilia (mean 6%) may be seen in some patients [37]. The maximal swelling occurs within 12–24 h; in some cases it will disappear within 24 h, while in others, the swelling remains for 1–2 weeks. Girls are more frequently affected than boys.

Synovial fluid eosinophilia may also be found in patients with septic arthritis, parasitic infections, Lyme disease, tuberculosis, atopic

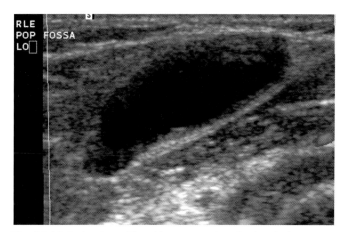

Fig. 1.8.11 Popliteal cyst. This athletic teenage boy developed a large cyst, which extended into his calf. (Courtesy of Children's Hospital of NY-Presbyterian.)

allergy, malignancy, hypereosinophilic syndrome, or rheumatoid arthritis [35,37]. In many of these other diseases, however, other types of leukocytes will predominate in the joint. Rarely, patients develop eosinophilic synovitis following trauma. NSAIDs relieve most symptoms, and diethylcarbamazine may also help [37].

Musculoskeletal syndromes localized to the foot

Introduction

Pain localized to the foot can represent the enthesitis associated with Enthesitis Related Arthritis (ERA see Part 2, Chapter 2.7), or may represent overuse or trauma-related problems. Overuse and trauma-related conditions include osteochondrosis, stress fractures, tenosynovitis, congenital indifference to pain and frostbite. Congenital indifference to pain and frostbite are discussed in the Hand section below. Foot pain may also arise from congenital anomalies, such as tarsal coalition and accessory bones. As with other joints, pain in the foot may be referred from the adjacent joint, which in this case is the knee. Evaluation of the foot should also include evaluations for infections more specific to the foot including nail puncture or splinter wounds (see Part 1, Chapter 1.5).

Osteochondroses

Osteochondroses of the foot include Freiberg and Kohler disease. Freiberg disease, or infraction, most commonly involves the second or third metatarsal head, but can also affect the other metatarsal heads. This condition most commonly affects adolescent girls, who will complain of pain, swelling, and tenderness on the plantar side of the metatarsal head and may limp. X-rays show flattening of the metatarsal head and widening of the joint space. Treatment is symptomatic [38].

Patients with Kohler disease complain of foot pain and tenderness on the dorsal surface of the navicular bone. Although patients may limp from the pain, this condition, which affects children between the ages of 2 and 9 years, is usually self-limited [38]. X-rays show fragmentation and patchy sclerotic changes in the navicular bone.

Apophysitis

Sever apophysitis results from repetitive stress injury to the calcaneal tuberosity at the site of the Achilles tendon insertion into the calcaneus [39]. The physeal plate at this site can fragment, most commonly in children who participate in sports, such as soccer, basketball, and gymnastics; the peak incidence occurs between ages 9 and 11 years [30,39]. Boys are more likely to be affected than girls, and complain of heel pain with tenderness over the posterior and inferior heel. Patients with ERA may have pain in a similar area secondary to enthesopathy, but the pattern of pain will be different. Similar to other overuse conditions, patients with Sever disease have increased pain with exercise and decreased pain with rest, without joint effusions or Achilles tendon tenderness. Patients with Sever disease may develop dorsiflexion weakness and Achilles tendon contracture [39]. These children should avoid strenuous activity, but often benefit from stretching/strengthening exercises; they may also benefit from heel inserts. The condition is benign and self-limited.

Stress fracture

Stress fractures occur in the metatarsals, and similar to those seen in the tibia, are more common in adolescent runners. Patients complain of localized tenderness, initially related to activity. Later, the pain can become constant and may be associated with swelling.

Tarsal coalition

Tarsal coalition refers to a soft tissue or bony connection between two or more tarsal bones, usually arising from a congenital defect, but occasionally secondary to arthritis, trauma, infection, or degenerative joint disease [40]. Most patients are between 9–14 years of age [39]. Similar to children with JIA affecting the subtalar joint, children with tarsal coalition have limitation in subtalar or midfoot movement. Most children with tarsal coalition, however, are asymptomatic; some complain of an insidious, aching pain in the hindfoot, midfoot, or ankle, that worsens with activity and is lessened by rest, unlike the pain associated with JIA. The pain can be episodic and patients may give a history of recurrent ankle sprains [38]. This condition can be inherited in an autosomal dominant fashion, and is present bilaterally in half of the patients [40].

Two main types of tarsal coalition have been described: calcaneonavicular and talocalcaneal [39]. Calcaneonavicular coalition leads to loss of motion, and talocalcaneal coalition results in a rigid flat foot. Oblique X-ray often documents the calcaneonavicular coalition, while coronal sections by CT are best for talocalcaneal coalition (Figure 1.8.12) [39]. Patients improve with adjustment in activities, NSAIDs, shoe inserts, and/or cast. Surgery may be needed for those with recurrent or severe pain that interferes with activity.

Accessory bones

Most children with an accessory navicular bone remain asymptomatic. However, some patients develop pain from: (1) an inflammatory traction apophysitis at the tendon insertion into the accessory navicular and navicular bones; (2) mechanical irritation over the junction of the accessory navicular and navicular; and/or (3) an associated flat foot [20]. Children may present with pain with activity, tenderness over the posterior tibial tendon insertion into the navicular, and swelling over this area of the navicular base. Children often respond to immobilization of the area and rehabilitation; more severe cases may require surgery.

Another accessory bone that can give rise to foot pain is the os trigonum, which is adjacent to the posterior talus [39]. Ballet dancers,

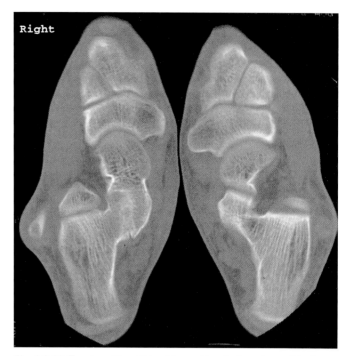

Fig. 1.8.12 Tarsal coalition. This adolescent boy had persistent right foot pain and was found to have a talocalcaneal coalition on CT. (Courtesy of Children's Hospital of NY-Presbyterian.)

gymnasts, and other athletes who place their feet in maximal flexion may develop posterior ankle pain. Patients generally improve with conservative treatment.

Osteochondritis dissecans

Athletic adolescents develop ankle pain secondary to osteochondritis dissecans (OD) in either the medial or lateral articular surface of the talus [39]. The lesions in the posteromedial area tend to be asymptomatic while those in the anterolateral site usually cause pain. Similar to the pain seen in patients with JIA, children with osteochondritis dissecans (OD) may have joint effusions and tenderness. However, children with OD have more localized tenderness, and movement aggravates their pain; in addition, there may be crepitus during ankle flexion. These patients report a catching sensation with movement, and usually have a preceding history of trauma [28]. Depending upon the stage of the disease, X-ray findings vary from compression of the subchondral bone to complete detachment of an osteochondral fragment with a corresponding defect of the talus. Mild lesions may be treated symptomatically, or with restriction from sports for several months, while more severe lesions may require surgery [39].

Musculoskeletal syndromes localized to the back

Introduction

Back pain is a common complaint during childhood, occurring in 11–36% of school-age children [41], and may be due to such conditions as discitis, tumour, sacroiliac enthesitis associated with ERA, and fibromyalgia. The child with back pain should be evaluated according to Algorithm 1.3.3 in Part 1, Chapter 1.3 Although earlier studies suggested that the underlying cause of the back pain could be identified in most children, a more recent review found a specific diagnosis for only 22% of the patients [42]. Nocturnal or constant pain and a short duration of symptoms (< 3 months), are suspicious and warrant more complete studies to rule out tumour as a cause of the back pain [42]. In the older child and adolescent, back pain can arise from injury and overuse syndromes, such as spondylolysis/spondylolisthesis, disk herniation, muscle or ligament sprains, stress fracture of the sacrum, apopyseal ring fracture, or from Scheuermann kyphosis. Back pain may also represent referred pain from the thorax, abdomen, retroperitoneum, or pelvis. Some studies have found an association between psychosocial factors, such as conduct problems or hyperactivity and low back pain [59]. Although back stiffness and pain can occur in the older child with ERA, back pain is uncommon in most other forms of JIA.

Spondylolysis/spondylolisthesis

Spondylolysis is a common cause of back pain in athletic children and adolescents. Spondylolysis is a defect in the pars interarticularis of the L4 or L5 vertebra, that can result from overuse/trauma. It rarely occurs before the age of 5 years [41], and is most commonly found during the adolescent growth spurt [26]. Children who participate in sports that involve repeated lumbar hyperextension, such as gymnasts, soccer players, dancers, figure skaters, and football linemen, are at the highest risk for spondylolysis [26]. If the vertebral body slips forward, the condition is referred to as spondylolisthesis. With either condition, patients may complain of aching back, especially with hyperextension, have paraspinal tenderness at the L5-S1 level, and hamstring tightness [26]. The pain may radiate to the buttock or leg, and is exacerbated by activity. The patient may also have secondary postural changes, such

as increased lumbar lordosis. Lateral X-rays of the lumbar spine document the defect and indicate the degree of slip (Figure 1.8.13). Bone scan and MRI detect the defect earlier. If the slippage is mild, activity modification followed by rehabilitation may relieve symptoms.

Scheuermann Disease (juvenile kyphosis)

Early adolescents may develop this kyphotic deformity of the thoracic or thoracolumbar spine, which becomes more pronounced during the adolescent growth spurt. The deformity is often thought to be due to poor posture, but unlike postural kyphosis, Scheuermann deformity is fixed and accentuated by forward bending (Figure 1.8.14). Patients often develop a compensatory cervical and lumbar hyperlordosis and hamstring tightness secondary to pelvic tilt. About one-third of patients also have mild to moderate scoliosis. These adolescents may present with aching pain at the site of the deformity or in the lower back; the pain is worsened by prolonged sitting, standing, and performing strenuous activities. Some patients also complain of fatigue later in the day [41]. Although patients with ERA (see also Part 2, Chapter 2.7) may complain of back pain, the marked, fixed deformity seen in Scheuermann disease distinguishes it from ERA. Patients with Scheuermann disease may also have spondylolysis and spondylolisthesis [44].

AP and lateral X-rays show narrowing of the intervertebral disk space, decreased vertebral height with anterior wedging of 3 adjacent vertebrae by 5° or more, irregular vertebral end plates, and sometimes Schmorl nodes [43]. Different aetiologies have been proposed including avascular necrosis, mechanical trauma, and abnormal local growth, but none has been conclusively proven. Patients with a mild degree of kyphosis may be monitored, while patients with more severe kyphosis require bracing. Children with similar clinical and radiographic findings in only one or two vertebrae, do not fulfil classical criteria for Scheuermann disease but presumably have the same condition.

(a)

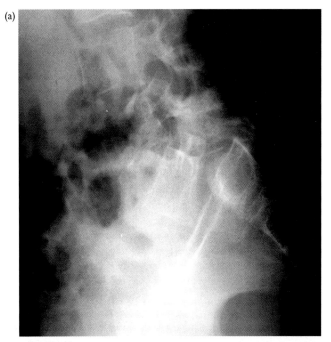

(b)

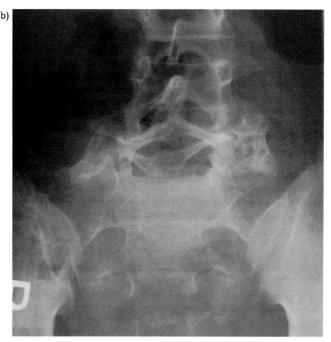

Fig. 1.8.13 Spondylolisthesis. (a) The lateral X-ray of this adolescent patient shows a marked slippage at L5-S1. (b) The AP view shows the "upside-down Napoleon's hat" sign due to the displacement of the vertebral body. (Courtesy of M. Liebling.)

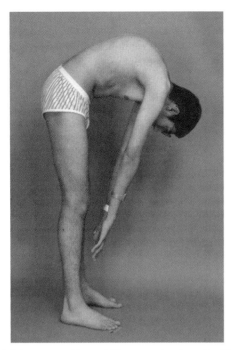

Fig. 1.8.14 Scheuermann disease. This teenage boy has a fixed kyphotic deformity in his thoracic spine. (Courtesy of T.R. Southwood.)

Disk herniation

Disk herniation is uncommon in children, but it may occur secondary to trauma [44]. Most herniations affect the lumbar region, particularly in adolescents. The back pain may be acute or insidious, is worsened by exercise, sneezing, coughing, and improved by rest. Some children have buttock, hamstring, or radicular pain, and there is usually tenderness over the lumbar spine and pain along the sciatic nerve. There may also be neurological signs and secondary spinal deformity (scoliosis, flattening of the lumbar spine). L4–5 or L5-S1 are the most commonly affected disks. X-rays are often normal, and diagnosis may require MRI studies. Most patients improve with rest, limited activities, NSAIDs, and rehabilitation [45]. Whereas disk herniation in adults is due to mechanical fatigue of the disc, disk herniation in children is more commonly due to apophyseal ring fracture.

Apophyseal ring fracture

This injury related problem occurs in adolescent boys who participate in activities, such as weight lifting. The pattern of pain is more similar to the pattern seen with disc herniation than to that seen with JIA; pain is aggravated by activity, and may be associated with sciatica. Onset of pain is usually acute, and the pain is often described as constant and burning. The posterior portion of the lumbar apophysis fractures, followed by partial disk herniation into the spinal canal most commonly at L4. These changes can be seen on a lateral X-ray or by CT scan [44].

Osteoporosis

Idiopathic juvenile osteoporosis is a rare cause of back pain in otherwise healthy children [44]. Preadolescents to adolescent youngsters (8–14 years) present with back, knee, and ankle pain and then develop growth arrest. Some children may also present with an abnormal gait, or progressive kyphosis [46]. X-rays show osteopenia, and there may be multiple compression fractures as well as fractures of the long bones, especially

around the joints. The aetiology is unknown, but since patients recover during adolescence, after puberty, there is presumably a temporary hormonal imbalance that leads to the accelerated rate of bone resorption or decreased bone formation. Other disorders that cause osteoporosis such as leukaemia, Cushing disease, thyroid disease, diabetes mellitus, growth hormone deficiency, homocystinuria, osteogenesis imperfecta, and dietary deficiencies (calcium, vitamin D, vitamin C) need to be excluded (see Part 1, Chapter 1.10 and 1.11). In addition, adolescent girls with behavioral eating disorders are at increased risk for osteopenia from reduced levels of oestrogen, testosterone, and insulin-like growth factor 1 (IGF-1) [46]. For the patient with JIA receiving chronic corticosteroid treatment, care must be taken to monitor for and correct osteoporosis to try to prevent secondary problems, such as vertebral collapse.

Musculoskeletal syndromes localized to the shoulder or elbow

Introduction

Children may develop pain in the shoulder or elbow from repetitive stress to these areas during sports. Shoulder pain may also result from inflammation in the rotator cuff tendons, or from stress injury to the proximal humerus physis. Patients with shoulder hypermobility may have pain from recurrent episodes of shoulder subluxation or dislocation. They may complain of a popping sensation during abduction and external rotation [47]. Traction apophysitis can develop at the elbow. Other children may have pain related to stress fractures in the upper extremity.

Physiolysis of the proximal humerus (Little leaguer's shoulder)

This condition is seen in athletic adolescents (usually 11–16 years) who are involved in overhead throwing activities [30]. These include baseball pitching, racquet sports, gymnastics, volleyball, and swimming. As with other repetitive stress injuries, and unlike JIA, pain is associated with activity and relieved by rest; patients also have tenderness in the shoulder or lateral proximal humerus but maintains full range of motion. With continued activity, the pain may become constant. The patient should refrain from pitching until the X-ray shows resolution of the growth plate changes (widening and irregularity), and should then undergo rehabilitation [26].

Overuse injuries to the elbow (Little leaguer's elbow)

Children (8–12 years) who participate in sports that involve pitching and throwing, apply stress to the medial aspect of the elbow. With overuse, this can lead to apophysitis of the medial epicondyle [47]. There is pain and tenderness at the medial epicondyle, sometimes with associated swelling [20]. X-rays show widening of the growth plate, and fragmentation and sclerosis at later stages [47]. There may also be complete avulsion of the medial epicondyle. Patients are treated with rest, and modification of their throwing style [26].

Other forms of little leaguer's elbow include Panner disease and osteochondritis dissecans of the capitellum. Panner disease is an osteochondrosis of the capitellum that usually develops in 4–12 year old children. Repetitive throwing can cause compression of the capitellum and lead to avascular necrosis. Similar to the patient with JIA, the patient with Panner disease develops diffuse swelling, joint effusion, and limitation of extension [47]. The pain is usually dull and aching. Physical examination, unlike in JIA, reveals tenderness localized to the lateral elbow; X-rays show flattening, and sclerosis of the capitellum. Patients generally improve with modification of activity.

Osteochondritis dissecans is a more serious condition of the elbow that develops in children aged 12 years and older who are involved in repetitively throwing activity [28]. The lateral or central capitellum becomes fragmented, and the resulting loose bodies cause pain and locking. Patients have decreased flexion and extension as well as swelling and tenderness [47]. X-rays show radiolucency of the capitellum initially, and loose bodies at advanced stages [28]. The capitellum can spontaneously reossify, but there may be long-term problems or limitations of movement and function [47].

Stress fractures

Stress fractures have been reported in the radius in gymnasts, tennis players, and cyclists. Tennis players are also at risk for stress fractures in the ulna and humerus. Olecreanon stress fractures have been reported in gymnasts and athletes performing throwing motions [48]. As with other stress fractures, the pain is usually a dull ache that worsens with exercise, and improves with rest. There may be tenderness and swelling at the affected site, similar to JIA, but these findings are in the bone rather than the joint, and the tenderness is well localized. The fracture is typically precipitated by a recent increase in the training regimen. Most patients improve with conservative treatment.

Musculoskeletal symptoms localized to the hand or wrist

Introduction

Pain in the hand/wrist may also be related to overuse syndromes. In the radius, and the phalanges, repetitive stress may lead to the more serious consequence of premature closure of the growth plate. Other conditions that may result in hand abnormalities include congenital indifference to pain, frostbite arthropathy, phalangeal microgeodic syndrome, and child abuse. Some parents will also request an evaluation because of the voluntary or involuntary knuckle "cracking" practiced by many children.

Physeal injuries

Gymnasts develop wrist pain from many conditions including physiolysis of the distal radius. This is most likely to occur in adolescent girls (12–14 years) who participate in gymnastics for more than 35 h/week [32]. Patients complain of tenderness over the distal dorsal radius, and have limited mobility of their wrist; 30% have bilateral involvement [30]. A frequent physical exam finding is a prominent radius. X-rays show growth plate widening and irregularity. Although mild cases may improve with rest, this condition has been reported to lead to premature closure of the radial growth plate, overgrowth of the ulna, and later development of arthritis [26].

Premature closure of the distal phalanx growth plate of the thumb has been reported in an adolescent pianist, who had been playing piano for 10 years, up to 6 h/day [49]. He developed intermittent pain, warmth, and swelling of one of his thumbs; X-rays revealed closure of its distal growth plate. Presumably, the child's repetitive stress to this joint from piano practising led to the defect.

Thiemann Disease

The typical features of Thiemann disease are relatively painless, symmetrical, firm swelling of proximal inter phalangeal joints associated with X-ray changes of irregular epiphyses with sclerosis, fragmentation and joint space narrowing. The feet are occasionally affected. The underlying pathology is unclear, but avascular necrosis may play a role. Most affected individuals are young men between the ages of 11 and 19 years. There is a familial predisposition, and autosomal dominance has been reported. [50]

Congenital indifference to pain (Charcot disease)

Swollen but painless joints with distal necrosis of the toes and fingers together with bizarre destructive and sclerotic radiographical changes seen in the fingers and toes are characteristic of this rare inborn incapacity to feel pain (Figure 1.8.15). Children often perform "daring feats" or have scars from unrecognized burns or injuries, including auto amputations, to fingers or tongue (Figure 1.8.16(a)). Many will also have anhidrosis and mental retardation [51]. These patients do not have joint stiffness or pain typical of JIA.

Neurogenic arthropathy may also be seen in lesions of the spinal cord, diabetes mellitus, familial dysautonomia, or any other condition in which there is impairment of deep sensation in a joint. Because children with congenital indifference to pain are susceptible to recurrent fractures and skin infections, an abnormal joint may represent a fracture, septic arthritis, osteomyelitis, or neurogenic arthropathy (Charcot joint) (Figure 1.8.16(b)) [50]. The diagnosis of neurogenic arthropathy is suggested by the characteristic X-ray findings of (1) erosion of articular cartilage, (2) subchondral sclerosis, (3) periosteal new-bone formation, and (4) loose bodies (bone shards) and marginal fractures, in the absence of pain complaints. Abused children may present with similar X-ray findings (Figure 1.8.20(b)).

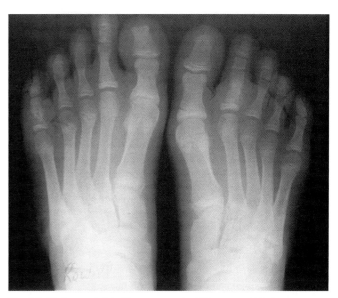

Fig. 1.8.15 Congenital indifference to pain. This young girl had worn away the end of her distal first toe phalanx, and had bizarre fractures and periosteal new-bone. These foot lesions were presumably from overly vigorous bowling; she also had lesions in her hands from unrecognized trauma. The patient was referred for evaluation because the appearance of her fingers and toes raised a question of JIA. (From J. Jacobs.)

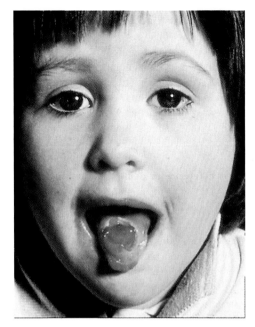

(b)

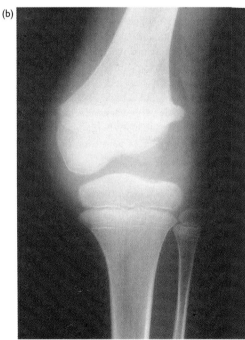

Fig. 1.8.16 Congenital indifference to pain. (a) This young girl has a lesion on her tongue from repeatedly biting it. (b) She has damaged her knee joints from repeated injuries. (Courtesy of T.R. Southwood.)

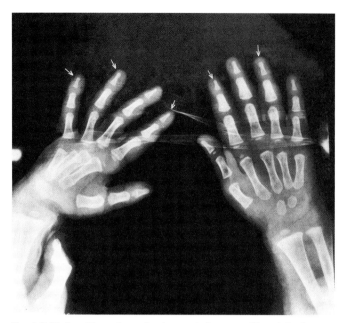

Fig. 1.8.17 Frostbite arthropathy. Arrows indicate penciling of distal phalanges in a toddler following unrecognized frostbite. This boy was referred for Raynaud phenomenon because of vascular instability in the fingers. (Courtesy of J. Jacobs.)

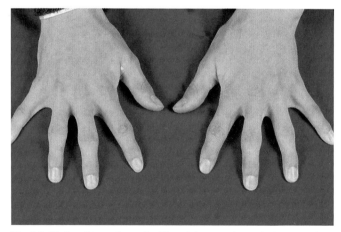

Fig. 1.8.18 Frostbite arthropathy. This adolescent shows thickened PIPS and short fingers secondary to frostbite injury as a young child. (Courtesy of T.R. Southwood.)

Frostbite arthropathy and phalangeal microgeodic syndrome

Occasionally, a small child presents with swollen red fingers and color changes suggestive of Raynaud syndrome months to years after cold exposure. Cold injury to immature digital blood vessels may lead to Raynaud-like hypersensitivity for months or years thereafter. Radiographs may show narrowed "pointing" of the terminal phalanges (Figure 1.8.17). In more severe cases, the child has shortened fingers due to epiphyseal cold injury causing premature closure of epiphyses and growth deformities (Figure 1.8.18). Injury to subchondral bone and articular cartilage may lead to arthritic manifestations, with radiographic changes, such as juxta-articular bone and subchondral cysts similar to those seen in osteoarthritis [52]. Unlike osteoarthritis, however, frostbite arthritis does not have bony sclerosis or osteophytes, and is usually asymmetric.

Some cases of phalangeal microgeodic syndrome may represent a milder form of cold trauma. This syndrome has been reported in children in the wintertime, primarily in Japan [53]. Children present with red, swollen, warm fingers with minimal tenderness. Radiographs show widening of the phalanges and lacunae in the phalanges (Figure 1.8.19). A biopsy shows newly formed bone, proliferation of fibrous connective tissue, and no inflammation or

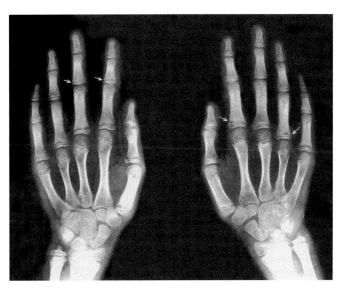

Fig. 1.8.19 Phalangeal microgeodic (holes in stone) syndrome. This 10-year-old girl developed multiple lytic lesions at the ends of the phalanges (arrows), accompanied by periosteal new-bone formation, and an elevated ESR, several weeks after a streptococcal sore throat. The lesions subsided after several months, leaving no sequelae. (Courtesy of J. Jacobs.)

infection agents. Symptoms resolve spontaneously within 2 months. Other cases of phalangeal microgeodic syndrome may be due to bone infarction following an episode of bacterial sepsis. Patients often have a high ESR, but recover spontaneously without treatment.

Child abuse

Abused children may present with thick, brawny induration over and just proximal to the second through fifth proximal interphalangeal joints due to repeated beatings across the hands with a hard object, such as a ruler (Figure 1.8.20(a)). X-rays show thick, dense phalangeal bones suggesting chronic hyperaemia; there may also be bone chips and periosteal new bone formation (Figure 1.8.20(b)). Other clues to the diagnosis include evidence of new and old fractures, specific patterns of fracture (metaphyseal-epiphyseal, ribs, scapular, sternal, and skull) [54], poor explanation for fractures, recurrent mouth lesions, burns, and other recurrent injuries. One case of self-mutilation produced the same findings. When the children are removed from the abusive environment, the fingers may return to normal (Figure 1.8.20(c)).

Cracking joints

Crepitus may signify loss of cartilage and apposition of underlying bone or synovial hypertrophy with alteration of joint mechanics. Some children voluntarily "crack" their knuckles (metacarpophalangeal joints), by applying traction on their joints, causing the formation of a gas bubble in the joint space. Release of the tension collapses the bubble, producing the cracking noise. Transient symptom-less cracking occurs in some children, especially those with hypermobility, and may be caused by tendon movement over a bony prominence [55,56]. Sometimes these movements are associated with pain (see snapping hip, p. 134). Children with ERA may also crack

(a)

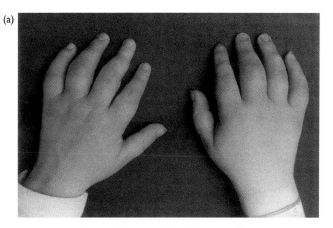

(b)

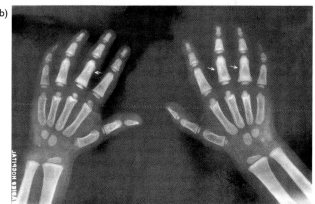

(c)

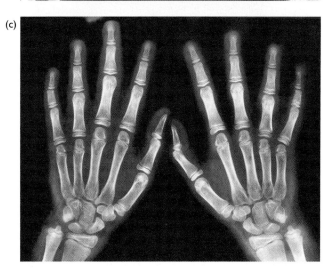

Fig. 1.8.20 Child abuse. (a) This child was beaten across the fingers with a ruler, resulting in brawny induration over and just proximal to the second through fifth proximal interphalangeal joints (b) An X-ray of the hands shows increased density and thickening of the proximal phalanges together with periosteal reaction (arrows). Bone shards are sometimes also found. (c) Follow-up films 9 years later show remodelling to normal. (Courtesy of J. Jacobs.)

joints not affected by objective signs of disease (personal observation). Parents and patients may be concerned about these various cracking sounds; however, in the absence of other evidence of disease, the child and parents may be reassured.

References

1. Bruns, W. and Maffulli, N. Lower limb injuries in children in sports. *Clin Sports Med* 2000;19:637–42.

2. Peterson, H. Growing pains. *Pediatr Clin North Am* 1986;33:1365–72.

3. Naish, J. and Apley, J. "Growing Pains": a clinical study of non-arthritic limb pains in children. *Arch Dis Child* 1951;26:134–40.

4. Baxter, M. and Dulberg, C. "Growing Pains" in childhood—a proposal for treatment. *J Pediatr Orthop* 1988;8:402–6.

5. Gedalia, A. and Brewer, E. Joint hypermobility in pediatric practice—a review. *J Rheumatol* 1993;20:371–4.

6. Grahame, R., Bird, H., Child, A., *et al.* The Revised (Brighton 1998) Criteria for the Diagnosis of Benign Joint Hypermobility Syndrome(BJHS). *J Rheumatol* 2000;27:1777–9.

7. van der Giessen, L., Liekens, D., Rutgers, K., Hartman, A., Mulder, P., and Oranje, A. Validation of Beighton Score and Prevalence of connective tissue signs in 773 Dutch children. *J Rheumatol* 2001;28:2726–30.

8. Barron, D., Cohen, B., Geraghty, M., Violand, R., and Rowe, P. Joint Hypermobility is more common in children with chronic fatigue syndrome than in healthy controls. *J Pediatr* 2002;141:421–5.

9. Klemp, P. Hypermobility. *Ann Rheum Dis* 1997;56:573–5.

10. Mont, M. and Jones, L. Management of osteonecrosis in systemic lupus erythematosus. *Rheum Dis Clin North Am* 2000;26:279–309.

11. Koop, S. and Quanbeck, D. Three common causes of childhood hip pain. *Pediatr Clin North Am* 1996;43:1053–66.

12. Assouline-Dayan, Y., Chang, C., Greenspan, A., Shoenfeld, Y., and Gershwin, M. Pathogenesis and natural history of osteonecrosis. *Semin Arthritis Rheum* 2002;32:94–124.

13. Lecuire, F. The long-term outcome of primary osteochondritis of the hip (Legg-Calvé-Perthes disease). *J Bone Joint Surg Br* 2002;84:636–40.

14. Taybi, H. and Lachman, R. *Radiology of syndromes, metabolic disorders, and skeletal dysplasias*. Chicago: Year Book Medical Publishers, Inc., 1990.

15. Mont, M. and Hungerford, D. Non-traumatic avascular necrosis of the femoral head. *J Bone Joint Surg Am* 1995;77-A:459–74.

16. Reynolds, R. Diagnosis and treatment of slipped capital femoral epiphysis. *Curr Opin Pediatr* 1998;11:80–3.

17. Causey, A., Smith, E., Donaldson, J., Kendig, R., and Fisher, L., III. Missed slipped capital femoral epiphysis: illustrative cases and a review. *J Emerg Med* 1995;13:175–89.

18. Roy, D., and Crawford, A. Idiopathic chondrolysis of the hip: management by subtotal capsulectomy and aggressive rehabilitation. *J Pediatr Orthop* 1988;8:203–7.

19. Rowe, L. and Ho, E. Idiopathic chondrolysis of the hip. *Skeletal Radiol* 1996;25:178–82.

20. Micheli, L. The traction apophysitises. *Clin Sports Med* 1987;6:389–404.

21. Toren, A., Goshen, E., Katz, M., Levi, R., and Rechavi, G. Bilateral femoral stress fractures in a child due to in-line (roller) skating. *Acta Paediatr* 1997;86:332–3.

22. St. Pierre, P., Staheli, L., Smith, J., and Green, N. Femoral neck stress fractures in children and adolescents. *J Pediatr Orthop* 1995;15:470–3.

23. Lam, K. and Moulton, A. Stress fracture of the sacrum in a child. *Ann Rheum Dis* 2001;60:87–8.

24. Pelsser, V., Carnnal, E., Hobden, R., and Ankur, B. Extraarticular snapping hip: sonographic findings. *Am J Roent* 2001;176:67–73.

25. Davids, J. Pediatric knee: clinical assessment and common disorders. *Pediatr Clinics North Am* 1996;43:1067–90.

26. Saperstein, A. and Nicholas, S. Pediatric and adolescent sports medicine. *Pediatr Clin North Am* 1996;43:1013–33.

27. Martin, T. and Martin, J. Special issues and concerns for the high school- and college-aged athletes. *Pediatr Clin North Am* 2002;49:533–52.

28. Schenck, R., Jr and Goodnight, J. Current concept review-osteochondritis dissecans. *J Bone Joint Surg Am* 1996;78-A:439–56.

29. Thabit, G., III and Micheli, L. Patellofemoral pain in the pediatric patient. *Orthop Clin North Am* 1992;23:567–85.

30. Patel, D. and Nelson, T. Sports injuries in adolescents. *Med Clin N Am* 2000;84:983–1007.

31. Kelly, B., and Green D. Discoid lateral meniscus in children. *Curr Opin Pediatr* 2002;14.

32. Loud, K. and Micheli, L. Common athletic injuries in adolescent girls. *Curr Opin Pediatr* 2001;13:317–27.

33. Gomez, J., Kattamis, A., and Schenck, R., Jr. Pseudothrombophlebitis in an adolescent without rheumatic disease: A case report. *Clin Orthop Rel Res* 1994;308:250–3.

34. Szer, I.S., Klein-Gitelman, M., DeNardo, B., and McCauley, R. Ultrasonography in the study of prevalence and clinical evolution of popliteal cysts in children with knee effusions. *J Rheumatol* 1992;19:458–62.

35. Atanes, A., Fernández, V., Núñez, R., *et al.* Idiopathic eosinophilic synovitis. *Scand J Rheumatol* 1996;25:183–5.

36. Brown, J., Rola-Pleszczynski, M., and Ménard, H.-A. Eosinophilic synovitis: clinical observations on a newly recognized subset of patients with dermatographism. *Arthritis Rheum* 1986;29:1147–51.

37. Tauro, B. Eosinophilic synovitis. *J Bone and Joint Surg Br* 1995;77:654–6.

38. Griffen, L. Common sports injuries of the foot and ankle seen in children and adolescents. *Orthop Clin North Am* 1994;25:83–93.

39. Marsh, J. and Daigneault, J. Ankle injuries in the pediatric population. *Curr Opin Pediatr* 2000;12:52–60.

40. Bohne, W. Tarsal coalition. *Curr Opin Pediatr* 2001;13:29–35.

41. King, H. Back pain in children. *Orthop Clin North Am* 1999;30:467–74.

42. Feldman, D., Hedden, D., and Wright, J. The use of bone scan to investigate back pain in children and adolescents. *J Pediatr Orthop* 2000;20:790–5.

43. Ali, R., Green, D., and Patel, T. Scheuermann's kyphosis. *Curr Opin Pediatr* 1999;11:70–5.

44. Ginsburg, G. and Bassett, G. Back pain in children and adolescents: evaluation and differential diagnosis. *J Am Acad Orthop Surg* 1997;5:67–78.

45. Kraft, D. Low back pain in the adolescent athlete. *Pediatr Clin North Am* 2002;49:643–53.

46. Kauffman, R., Overton, T., Shiflett, M., and Jennings, J. Osteoporosis in children and adolescent girls: case report of Idiopathic Juvenile Osteoporosis and review of the literature. *Obstetr Gynecol Surv* 2001;56:492–504.

47. Gómez, J. Upper extremity injuries in youth sports. *Pediatr Clin North Am* 2002;49:593–626.

48. Brooks, A. Overuse injuries in the upper extremity. *Clin Sports Med* 2001;20.

49. Attkiss, K. and Buncke, H. Physeal growth arrest of the distal phalanx of the thumb in an adolescent pianist: a case report. *J Hand Surg-Am* 1998;23:532–5.

50. Kotevoglu-Senerdem, N., Toygar, B. Thiemann Disease. *J Clin Rheumatol* 9:359–61.

51. Bar-On, E., Weigl, D., Parvari, R., Katz, K., Weitz, R., and Steinberg, T. Congenital insensitivity to pain. *J Bone Joint Surg Br* 2002;84:252–7.

52. Carrera, G., Kozin, F., and McCarty, D. Arthritis after frostbite injury in children. *Arth Rheum* 1979;22:1082–7.

53. Kaibara, N., Masuda, S., Katsuki, I., *et al.* Phalangeal microgeodic syndrome in childhood: report of seven cases and review of the literature. *Eur J Pediatr* 1981;136:41–6.

54. Cramer, K. Orthopedic aspects of child abuse. *Pediatr Clin North Am* 1996;43:1035–51.

55. Watson, P. and Mollan, R. Cineradiography of a cracking joint. *Br J Radiol* 1990;63:145–7.

56. Unsworth, A., Dowson, D., and Wright, V. 'Cracking joints'. *Ann Rheum Dis* 1971;30:348–58.

57. Petri, M. Pathogenesis and treatment of the antiphospholipid antibody syndrome. *Med Clin North Am* 1997;81:151–77.

58. Schroer, W. Current concepts on the pathogenesis of osteonecrosis of the femoral head. *Orthop Rev* 1994;23:487–97.

59. Jones, G., Macfarlane, G. Epidemiology of low back pain in children and adolescents. *Arch Dis Child* 2005;90:312–6.

Idiopathic pain syndromes

Lisa F. Imundo

Aim

The aim of this chapter is to familiarize the reader with the spectrum of childhood conditions characterized by severe disability out of proportion to physical findings. It provides a balanced discussion of several frequently encountered painful conditions and offers an approach to management based in large part on JIA experience gleaned from children with painful and disabling conditions who happily attend school regularly and participate fully in after school programs.

Structure

- Fibromyalgia (diffuse idiopathic pain)
- Reflex sympathetic dystrophy (RSD) (localized idiopathic pain)
- Chronic fatigue syndrome (CFS)
- Chronic Lyme disease and post-Lyme syndrome
- Conversion disorders
- Munchausen syndrome

Introduction

Up to 30% of children report chronic or recurrent musculoskeletal pain [1]. The differential diagnosis is quite broad (see Part 1, Chapter 1.3) and includes acute and chronic inflammatory, infectious and metabolic conditions as well as, growing pains, overuse injuries, hypermobility, and mechanical orthopaedic syndromes. These latter conditions are discussed in detail in Part 1, Chapter 1.8. A subset of chronic or recurrent pain conditions, referred to collectively as the "idiopathic pain syndromes" is discussed in this chapter.

Idiopathic pain syndromes are characterized by lack of abnormal physical or laboratory findings in the context of severe complaints and a striking degree of disability [2]. Indeed, the degree of pain and disability in the idiopathic group is surprisingly high when compared to that reported by children with Juvenile Idiopathic Arthritis (JIA) or other chronic rheumatic conditions. Chronic pain, disability out of proportion to physical findings, the sensation of pain to non-painful stimuli, psychological distress, inappropriate affect, significant family history of disability or chronic pain, the presence of multiple other somatic complaints, and enmeshment with the mother are all typical associations found in idiopathic pain syndromes [3,4]. Prolonged or repeated hospitalizations that provide secondary gain or relief of some unbearable stress on the family or on the child may be seen in the most severe cases.

An important, clearly defined etiological component of the idiopathic pain syndromes is depression [5]. While it is often clear to the physician that unexplained or bizarre physical symptoms in an adolescent suffering mood changes, loss of interest in normal activities, and withdrawal to home or bed are not typical symptoms of a physical illness, parents of these patients may ascribe these behavioral changes to a mysterious physical disease [2] rather than to classical forms of depression with somatization. Indeed, a significant problem in the diagnosis of idiopathic pain syndrome is the presumed, but often unproven association of the painful symptom with some physical cause of the illness. To date, these associations have not been fully established, while the overlap of idiopathic pain and depression has, in contrast, been very well documented.

Given the lack of definitive etiology and a large number of associated illnesses, idiopathic pain syndromes have been called by many names despite the possibility that they all represent variations of a similar process. In addition, each condition has a long list of synonyms. For example, fibromyalgia (FMS) is also called diffuse idiopathic pain, fibrositis, myofascial pain syndrome, pain amplification syndrome, and diffuse wide spread myofascial pain. Similarly, reflex sympathetic dystrophy (RSD) may be referred to as localized idiopathic pain, chronic regional pain syndrome type 1, reflex neurovascular dystrophy (RND), causalgia, and Sudeck atrophy. To add to the confusion, chronic fatigue syndrome (CFS), chronic Lyme disease, conversion disorders, Munchausen syndrome and Munchausen syndrome by proxy all fall under the differential diagnoses of idiopathic pain syndromes (Table 1.9.1) and while it is clear that both conversion disorders and Munchausen syndrome by proxy have a large psychological and emotional component, their true aetiology is not known. Conversion disorders present with a myriad of physical manifestations including dramatic onset of pain and frequent inability to walk [6]. Repetitive, poorly explained injuries or illnesses that are either self-inflicted or induced by a parent, (Munchausen syndrome and Munchausen by proxy, respectively) are difficult to diagnose and require a large index of suspicion.

A further problem in understanding these conditions and establishing reliable criteria for diagnoses is that the current definitions have been derived from adult patients and may not necessarily apply to children. Newer nomenclature of diffuse and localized musculoskeletal pain syndromes (Table 1.9.2) has been developed but not yet validated in children [7]. Some authors suggest that precise classification in young people is unnecessary because of overlap in clinical

Table 1.9.1 Idiopathic pain syndromes versus JIA

	Systemic Arthritis (see Part 2, Chapter 2.2)	RF Positive Polyarthritis (see Part 2, Chapters 2.4 and 2.5)	Enthesitis Related Arthritis (see Part 2, Chapter 2.7)	Hypermobility syndrome (see Part 1, Chapter 1.8)	Growing pains	Localized idiopathic pain (RSD)	Diffuse idiopathic pain (FMS)
Age	Throughout childhood; usually young children	Generally >= 8 years	Generally > 8 years	2–8 years	3–5, 9–12 years	Late childhood adolescence	Late childhood adolescence
Sex	F = M	F>>>M ratio	F < M	F = M	F = M	F > M	F>>>M
Family history	Rare	Rare	Common	Common	Common	None	Common
Presence of Arthritis	Yes	Yes	Yes	No, but can have small effusions	No	No, but can have diffuse oedema of affected limb	No
Laboratory tests	Elevated ESR, platelets and WBC Anaemia	Elevated ESR and platelets Anaemia	HLA-B27 often positive	Normal	Normal	Normal	Normal
X-rays	Normal, or changes consistent with arthritis	Normal, or changes consistent with arthritis	Normal, or changes consistent with arthritis, and sacroilitis	Normal	Normal	Normal, or diffuse osteopenia of affected limb	Normal
Pain pattern	Stiffness/pain worse after inactivity which improves with activity	Stiffness/pain worse after inactivity which improves with activity	Stiffness/pain worse after inactivity which improves with activity, and inflammatory back pain common	Pain after physical activities, more often in lower extremity	Poorly localized pain of lower extremity, always at night	Pain out of proportion to triggering event Allodynia (extreme pain to touch) Refusal to move, or weight bear on on affected limb	Complains of severe pain but does not appear in distress Can have morning stiffness Pain in muscles as well as joints Headaches and abdominal pain common

Table 1.9.2 The definition of the idiopathic pain syndromes in children

Diffuse idiopathic musculoskeletal pain
These children have both:
   Generalized musculoskeletal aching at three or more sites for at least 3 months
   Exclusion of other diseases that could reasonably explain the symptoms

Localized idiopathic musculoskeletal pain
These children have all three:
   Pain localized to one limb persisting
      1 week with medically directed treatment or
      1 month without medically directed treatment
   Absence of prior trauma that could reasonably explain the symptoms
   Exclusion of other diseases that could reasonably explain the symptoms

presentation and the fact that approach to treatment is similar for all of the painful conditions [8].

Despite the confusion in description, classification, and aetiology, an experienced clinician should be able to recognize and diagnose idiopathic pain, based on the history and physical examination and a minimal amount of testing.

Fibromyalgia (diffuse idiopathic pain)

Presentation

Fibromyalgia (FMS) is a descriptive term for a syndrome of wide-spread musculoskeletal pain, fatigue, and multiple discrete tender points. While the diagnostic guidelines were developed for adults [9] FMS is also seen in children. FMS is now the third most common condition in some paediatric clinics [10–13]. The mean age of onset is 12.6 years and most patients are Caucasian preadolescent and adolescent girls, who tend to be high achievers. The prevalence of depression is higher in teenage girls with FMS than in adults with FMS but it is not clear whether the onset of depression precedes the onset of FMS or is a consequence of chronic pain [5]. There is often a parental history of chronic pain and FMS [14]. Trauma has been proposed as a risk factor.

FMS is common and should be considered in any child with wide-spread pain that is not responsive to the usual anti-inflammatory medications that usually is effective in relieving pain from rheumatologic conditions such as JIA, or orthopaedic syndromes such as hypermobility [15–17].

Clinical features

Children with FMS report widespread pain involving the entire body [18]. The neck and the upper back are most often affected in terms of tender points. In general, children tend to have fewer tender points than adults [11], but many develop the requisite number (11 out of 18 trigger points) over time. Most patients feel worse after exertion, exercise, or massage and prefer not to be touched or examined. Some children complain that routine physical examinations induce severe pain for days afterward. Other associated complaints frequently include headaches (daily, usually frontal, and often lasting for hours), abdominal pain, and intense menstrual cramps. Some patients complain of numbness, paresthesias, or vertigo [19]. Others feel alterations of cold and hot. None of the complaints, including headaches, abdominal pain, diffuse aches, and menstrual cramps, respond to over-the-counter medications or other common pain interventions.

It is well documented that patients with FMS report disturbed sleep patterns [20]. Complaints of non-restorative sleep are prominent in children; they report both difficulty falling asleep as well as frequent awakening. Loss of sleep contributes to an inability to concentrate and to poor school performance; withdrawal from school and school non-attendance is common. It has been suggested that children with FMS have more stress than their peers and less pain coping mechanisms than age-matched controls. In one study, children with FMS were found to be more disabled and distressed than children with JIA [21]. Indeed, a study of health-related quality of life in children with rheumatic and other conditions documented the worst quality of life in patients with FMS even when compared to children with leukaemia receiving chemotherapy [22]. This suggests that although we have no ability to accurately measure the degree of pain in these patients, there are tools that may accurately reflect how poorly they are feeling.

Evaluation

Patients with FMS should be evaluated to exclude other causes of fatigue and pain, including psychiatric and rheumatologic syndromes [23], especially because FMS not uncommonly occurs in patients with SLE and JIA. A detailed history and physical examination is usually diagnostic; routine screening laboratory tests should include CBC, chemistry panel, ESR, and urinalysis. Some children may require additional testing of thyroid function, muscle enzymes, EBV, and/or Lyme titres depending on the clinical situation. These patients routinely have normal or negative laboratory and radiographic tests and no underlying physiologic pathology can be demonstrated. Most children have specific tender points (Figure 1.9.1) on physical examination, which are usually the only physical findings.

Treatment and prognosis

Management of FMS requires a comprehensive treatment plan that takes into account factors that influence the perception of pain, such as cultural, biochemical, and behavioural/psychiatric components (Table 1.9.3) cognitive behavioural therapies and exercise are thought to be helpful [24]. Sherry *et al.* recommend an extremely vigorous

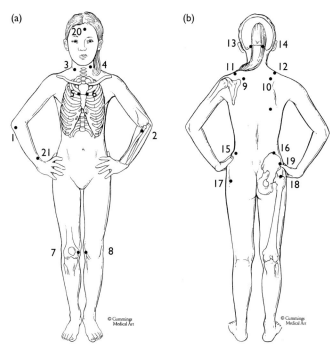

Fig. 1.9.1 Diagram of painful points in fibromyalgia depicted on an adolescent girl. Points 19, 20 and 21 are control points that should not be tender (drawing by Sally Cummings reprinted with permission from The Journal of Musculoskeletal Medicine).

Table 1.9.3 Management approach to fibromyalgia

Reassure the patient and family that
- Symptoms are typical for diffuse idiopathic pain
- These syndromes are difficult to treat but the long-term outcome is better than in adults
- The goal is to optimize function and minimize disability despite continuing symptoms

The treatment protocol includes:
- Educational material with written material for patients
- Mandatory school attendance
- Physical therapy with aerobic exercises to steadily increase endurance

Psychological support with:
- Evaluation for coexisting conditions (depression, anxiety, school phobia or avoidance)
- Cognitive behavioural treatment of sleep disturbances (biofeedback, self hypnosis, relaxation techniques)
- Improving coping and communication skills

Medications may include:
- NSAIDs
- Tramadol hydrochloride
- Tricyclic antidepressants at low doses at night
- Other antidepressants if indicated (with careful monitoring)

exercise program under the supervision of an experienced inpatient team. Although difficult to implement, this structured program for children and adolescents reported an excellent outcome with short-term resolution of symptoms [25]. Alternative therapies have not been proven to improve symptoms. To date, pharmacological interventions remain largely ineffective in controlling pain. However, medications such as tricyclic antidepressants may have a role in normalizing sleep and this intervention alone is helpful in a subset of patients with FMS.

Although there is no universally effective pharmacological treatment, simply providing the patient with a name for their symptoms and reassurance allows many patients to stop their search for other illnesses. Many patients erroneously labelled with chronic fatigue syndrome (CFS), and/or chronic Lyme disease have FMS and this ought to be clearly articulated to the patient and the family [26,27]. Patients should be told that their condition is not mysterious or made up. They must be supported in their successful reentry to school by providing whatever accommodations are needed, such as an extra set of school books, modified physical education program, or beginning classes later in the morning. Limited studies in children have indicated improvement in symptoms and resumption of function in the majority of patients after 2 years [28]. Neither the rate of relapse nor long-term functional outcome is known.

Reflex sympathetic dystrophy (localized idiopathic pain)

Clinical features

Reflex sympathetic dystrophy (RSD) is not rare in childhood but is often misdiagnosed [29–31] (Figure 1.9.2). The important diagnostic clue is that the child suddenly assumes an immobile posture of a hand or foot followed by swelling and continuous burning pain that is greatly intensified by light touch (allodynia). The swelling is often accompanied by color and temperature changes from vascular changes secondary to heightened sympathetic nervous system tone; most often the limb is cool, swollen, and discoloured (Table 1.9.3). RSD usually involves one distal extremity and extends proximally. The child refuses to move the hand or foot, or holds it in an uncomfortable or bizarre posture. Effort is obviously required to maintain the limb position. In contrast, children with JIA have pain localized to the involved joint, and rarely refuse to weight bear or to move the extremity. In addition, children with JIA do not have allodynia.

RSD occurs predominantly in pre-teen and teenage girls. There has been considerable argument over the aetiology and pathogenesis

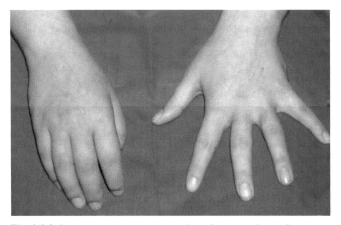

Fig. 1.9.2 Severe pain was associated with coolness, purple mottling, swelling and decreased pulses in the affected hand (courtesy of T. R. Southwood).

of this syndrome. Most affected children have no history of trauma or a precipitating event. In rare instances, RSD may be an unusual response to a minor injury. Onset after trauma is less common in children than in adults but occasionally, immobilization required to control pain from acute flare of arthritis or a fracture may result in RSD once the cast is removed; orthopaedic surgeons tend to recognize this particular presentation in children and adolescents. As it is not clear to what extent the sympathetic nervous system is involved in this condition, the term localized idiopathic pain syndrome may be preferable to RSD.

Not surprisingly, the pathogenesis of RSD in childhood includes a psychological component [32]. The classic profile of the patient with RSD, as in FMS, tend to be high achievers and are frequently involved in a wide variety of extracurricular activities including sports. These children and adolescents tend to be extremely compliant and have difficulty expressing their own needs. There is often an inappropriate closeness and involvement of the child in the parents' affairs and of the parents in the child's decision-making. This family "enmeshment" usually involves the mother and the daughter. Quite frequently RSD appears to "help" the child avoid certain activities. Paradoxically, these are often cited by both patient and her mother as the ones she "loves" and cannot live without.

Investigations

Diagnostic studies should include a radiograph of the involved area to exclude a local lesion that may be precipitating an RSD-like episode. In a classic case, additional radiographic testing is not necessary and should be done only if there is a clinical suspicion of infection, injury, or malignancy. One diagnostic difficulty is that while most imaging studies are normal, abnormalities may occur after a period of time. Radiographs may reveal patchy demineralization while an ultrasound or bone scan may show changes reflecting excessive autonomic activity with increased or decreased blood flow. A technetium bone scan or an MRI can be helpful in distinguishing RSD from bone infection, although clinically this differentiation should be obvious: children with RSD appear well, have no systemic symptoms of fever and their laboratory studies confirm normal acute phase reactants. A technetium bone scans in children with RSD may show increased or decreased and delayed uptake involving the entire leg [33]. Magnetic resonance imaging may be normal or may show dermal enhancement and oedema in affected areas. It is important not to misinterpret these abnormal non-specific radiologic findings as indicative of other disorders. Repeated investigations by physicians inexperienced in this condition who are made anxious by the bizarre symptoms and signs may actually prolong the illness. Prompt, confident diagnosis prevents harmful treatments and procedures that may result in delay of resolution of symptoms. Rarely, long-standing intractable RSD results in significant limb atrophy.

Treatment and prognosis

Familiarity with the disorder and immediate implementation of a well-organized treatment plan is essential (Table 1.9.4). A non-pressured discussion of psychologic stressors as well as to develop a sense of family dynamics should take place. Most children remember the exact moment the pain started, and a discussion of the incident and what happened before and after the disability started often leads to additional insight.

Table 1.9.4 Early signs of RSD

Bizarre posture of a hand or foot with refusal to move the extremity
Diffuse, swelling, and vasomotor changes
Continuous burning pain greatly intensified by light touch and associated with numbness and tingling
Tenderness frequently variable in extent

Table 1.9.5 Guidelines for diagnosis of CFS

Diagnostic steps
History
Physical examination
Mental status examination
Screening laboratory tests (CBC, metabolic panel, urinalysis, thyroid functions)
Fatigue
    New onset of unexplained fatigue
    Not the result of ongoing exertion
    Not substantially alleviated by rest
    Results in a substantial reduction in activities

Symptom criteria (At least four of eight)
Cognitive dysfunction
Sore throat
Tender cervical or axillary lymph nodes
Myalgia
Multi-joint arthralgia without swelling or redness
Headaches of a new pattern
Unrefreshing sleep
Postexertional malaise

Source: Adapted from Fukuda, K., Straus, S.E., Hickie, I., et al. Ann Intern Med 1994;121:953–9, with permission; and adapted from Bell, D.S.: Chronic fatigue syndrome in children and adolescents: a review. Focus Opin Pediatr 1995;1:412–20.

Any form of immobilization is contraindicated. Immediate initiation of desensititization aimed at encouraging motion is of undisputed benefit [34,35]. When the condition is not advanced, gentle massage of the extremity and passive motion are employed in the examining room to show how motion relieves pain and swelling and provides immediate and profound relief. Emphasizing that the problem is relatively common and well recognized is also helpful. Indeed, the complaint nature of the child can be put to good use by physiotherapists who have observed that these girls perform their exercises with fewer complaints than patients with arthritis. Most children and adolescents respond completely to exercise and physiotherapy.

Once the symptom has become "fixed" for a long period of time, however, more intensive pain relief and long-term physical therapy may be required. Refractory cases have been treated with a variety of aggressive interventions including sympathetic blockade, sympathectomy, spinal cord stimulation, and baclofen injections. Small uncontrolled studies in adults have indicated limited therapeutic success. Preventative treatment with an intensive rehabilitation/exercise program is helpful, and concurrent psychological support, and pain management should also be provided. Maintenance therapy and a home program can prevent relapse and should be continued for several weeks after an acute episode.

Chronic fatigue syndrome

Chronic fatigue syndrome (CFS) is defined as debilitating fatigue of greater than 6 months duration. The criteria for CFS overlap with those for FMS and depression (Table 1.9.5 [36–38]). Similar to FMS, demographics indicate a predominance of female, Caucasian, middle class patients. The age of onset of CFS is usually between 20–50 years, but children aged 7–20 years have been reported. As with other idiopathic pain syndromes, it is not clear that the existing definition should be extended to children.

Most patients describe the onset of symptoms after a preceding illness, often pharyngitis and fever. Up to one-third continue to complain of low grade fevers, pharyngitis, adenopathy, and weakness but the fevers are usually not documented on examination. Eighty percent of patients with CFS also report fatigue, difficulty sleeping, abdominal pain, cognitive difficulty, and inability to tolerate activity. Previously, many patients with CFS were found to suffer from depression, anxiety, and somatoform disorders; the current criteria of CFS require the exclusion of diagnosable psychiatric illnesses. Other possible occult causes of fatigue must also be excluded, such as drug or alcohol use, as well as medical conditions, such as mononucleosis, thyroid disease, and rheumatologic or inflammatory conditions.

Many adolescent patients do have a history of preceding problems with school attendance and/or performance [39]. After the onset of

illness, the average length of school missed is 1 year, representing a massive amount of disability compared to their peers with other chronic diseases, such as rheumatic diseases [40]. This is often the most severe consequence of the illness.

In long-term follow up, these children do not appear to develop other diseases. No treatment protocols have been completely successful, but incorporating psychological support and exercise reduces disability. A higher percentage of children than adults will improve over 1–4 years [26,27].

In sum, there is some support for placing CFS into the idiopathic pain syndrome category, since the approach to the diagnosis and treatment is similar.

Chronic Lyme disease and post-Lyme syndrome

Paediatric rheumatologists who practice in Lyme endemic areas often evaluate children for Lyme disease (see Part 1, Chapter 1.5). Most paediatricians recognize and treat uncomplicated Lyme disease without the consultation with a paediatric rheumatologist. However, there is a group of patients with chronic pain and/or fatigue, usually from affluent families, whose symptoms are ascribed to Lyme disease. Some unscrupulous physicians reinforce this notion by prescribing long courses of intravenous and oral antimicrobial therapy each time the patient complains of pain. These patients believe that their mysterious illness is caused by late sequelae of untreated *Borrelia burgdorferi* infection. However, evidence-based recommendations presented by the Infectious Disease Society of America indicated that in the vast majority of cases, 14–28 days of antibiotic treatment is sufficient to eradicate the Lyme spirochete, and prolonged courses of antibiotics are almost never justified [41].

There are well-known chronic sequelae to Lyme disease, such as arthritis, which have straightforward treatment guidelines (Part 1, Chapter 1.5). In the long-term follow-up study of untreated patients, the symptoms of Lyme disease and Lyme arthritis usually resolved over time [42], even without appropriate treatment.

The literature now includes descriptions of late sequelae of Lyme disease currently called the post-Lyme syndrome. This condition seems to be reported with increasing frequency following full treatment of documented Lyme disease, including Lyme arthritis. It is characterized by continued and persistent, sometimes disabling arthralgias and myalgias. Patients also complain of fatigue, headache, sleep disturbances, paresthesias, poor concentration, and poor school performance. Patients do not have arthritis or neurological deficits on physical examination but do report more anxiety and depression [43]. The symptoms are not prevented with early treatment with antibiotics, and in blinded studies, they have been shown to improve with long-term antibiotic treatment [44]. Symptoms usually improve spontaneously with time over months to years [45].

Finally, there are patients who present to the paediatric rheumatologists with symptoms that are similar to post-Lyme syndrome (fatigue, headache, inability to concentrate, arthralgia, and myalgia [56]) and have even been treated with multiple courses of oral or intravenous antibiotics. This syndrome has been called "chronic Lyme". However, remarkably, as many as 60% of patients treated for "chronic Lyme" disease do not have any evidence of ever having had Lyme disease. They are usually being treated on the basis of uncertified testing (urine antigen tests), or solely on the basis of a positive serology [47]. It is important to remember that positive serology is indicative of past exposure to the spirochete and is not necessarily an indicator of active disease; in addition, a positive serology may not become negative with treatment [48]. "Chronic Lyme" disease is in some aspects similar to CFS and FMS and often fulfills the diagnostic criteria for these syndromes [49,50].

In sum, the relationship between Lyme disease and symptoms that are called post-Lyme and "chronic Lyme" syndromes remain uncertain, in the same way that the relationship between viral infections and CFS remains uncertain. What is certain, however, is that these potential, but still unsubstantiated linkages, have been widely misconstrued by the lay public and some physicians, and this has lead to unnecessary treatment and expense of time and effort.

Conversion disorders

Conversion reactions involving the musculoskeletal system occur in children. Manifestations may include paralysis, gait disturbance, visual problems, and pain. Every paediatrician sees youngsters with vague or bizarre complaints of musculoskeletal pain or neuromuscular symptoms without evidence of organic disease on physical examination and with normal X-ray and laboratory studies. Inconsistent or no physiologic findings are common on careful exam. "La belle indifference" and absent gag reflex are often found in these patients [2]. Again, reasonable diagnostic studies are unavoidable, but the child must be directed into a treatment program as soon as possible. A full psychiatric evaluation and ongoing treatment must be obtained immediately if conversion disorder seems likely, but, an underlying psychological explanation cannot always be identified [51]. Physical rehabilitation and pain management in addition to psychotherapy is almost always necessary for resolution of symptoms and return to full function.

Munchausen syndrome

Most psychiatrically determined musculoskeletal illnesses may be classified as malingering (conscious and volitional, sometimes factitious), hysterical (non-volitional and unconscious), or a combination of these mechanisms. Occasionally, illness may be self-inflicted; this rare syndrome was named for Baron von Munchausen, who was famous for telling tall tales. Paediatricians may also be confronted with parentally inflicted illness, a form of child abuse termed Munchausen syndrome by proxy. The child may have a chronic medical illness that requires frequent interaction with medical professionals. In Munchausen by proxy the parent involved most often is the mother, who may have a medical background. These cases are more common than has been recognized, and may be more prevalent in children under 1 year of age. The parent may lie, tamper with laboratory specimens, or directly harm the child by repeated poisonings or suffocation.

The difficulty of diagnosis of Munchausen syndrome can be illustrated by a report of a teenager who repetitively self-injected fecal material into her joints. That patient had 23 hospitalizations and 13 major surgical procedures before the diagnosis was confirmed by finding the syringe with a feculent suspension among her possessions [52]. A high index of suspicion is necessary to make this diagnosis, and physicians have to overcome a natural reluctance to consider self-inflicted illness or child abuse [53,54]. In addition to psychological evaluation, Munchausen by proxy patients must be removed from the perpetrators care.

Conclusion

When disability exceeds visible evidence of organic disease, the child must be directed back to full activities. Repeated studies have demonstrated that long school absence for any reason indicates a poor prognosis for later achievement in life. Occasionally, the child, the family, and their physicians limit the child's activities (or accede to a demand for limitations), and the rheumatologist is then confronted with a totally disabled child without any evidence of organic disease.

When health providers remember that even severely disabled children with JIA and other rheumatic diseases almost always are able to attend school daily, it is easy to recognize children whose musculoskeletal pain results in school, or life, avoidance. It is useful to identify two separate problems in the discussions with these families: (1) the problem of the child's physical symptoms and the possibility that some organic process may exist despite an inability to document such a process at this time; and (2) the emotional problem, the withdrawal from normal activities and the loss of normal socialization. It is crucial to emphasize that despite physical symptoms, it is possible and necessary for the child to return to full-time schooling. Prolonged absences from school result in the secondary problem of anxiety on re-entry (school phobia). Often, a confident assurance that such return is possible and not damaging to the child's well being is all that is necessary; however, not infrequently, intervention from a psychologist or psychiatrist is needed.

These severe disabilities do not occur in a vacuum. Parents obsessed with obtaining medical care for their children have been known to seek out consultation from 10 to 30 specialists at multiple medical centres, and parental anxiety may inadvertently foster school absence.

It is easier to prevent these situations than to treat them. Prevention requires that the physician have an expectation that all children should be able to function fully with little or no restrictions. There is almost no place for limiting activities of children with chronic musculoskeletal complaints. The physician's role is to promote, not restrict function, to enable disabled children to have as full a life as possible change to, and to not contribute to crippling, either physical or emotional.

Overall the prognosis for idiopathic pain syndromes in children is good especially if appropriate treatment is initiated in a timely manner.

References

1. Malleson, P.N., Fung, M.Y., and Rosenberg, A.M. The incidence of pediatric rheumatic diseases: results from the Canadian Pediatric Rheumatology Association Disease Registry. *J Rheumatol* 1996;23(11): 1981–7.

2. Jacobs, J.C. *Pediatric Rheumatology for the Practitioner*, 2nd edn. New York: Springer-Verlag, 1992.

3. Croft, P., Burt, J., Schollum, J., Thomas, E., Macfarlane, G., and Silman, A. More pain, more tender points: is fibromyalgia just one end of a continuous spectrum? *Ann Rheum Dis* 1996;55(7):482–5.

4. Martinez-Lavin, M. Is fibromyalgia a generalized reflex sympathetic dystrophy? *Clin Exp Rheumatol* 2001;19(1):1–3.

5. Benjamin, S., Morris, S., McBeth, J., Macfarlane, G.J., and Silman, A.J. The association between chronic widespread pain and mental disorder: a population-based study. *Arthritis Rheum* 2000;43(3):561–7.

6. Garralda, M.E. Practitioner review: assessment and management of somatisation in childhood and adolescence: a practical perspective. *J Child Psychol Psychiatry* 1999;40(8):1159–67.

7. Malleson, P.N., al-Matar, M., and Petty, R.E. Idiopathic musculoskeletal pain syndromes in children. *Rheumatol* 1992;19(11):1786–9.

8. Isenberg, D. and Miller, J. *Adolescent Rheumatology*. London: Dunitz; Malden, MA, 1999.

9. Wolfe, F., Smythe, H.A., Yunus, M.B., Bennett, R.M., Bombardier, C., Goldenberg, D.L., Tugwell, P., Campbell, S.M., Abeles, M., Clark, P., *et al*. The American College of Rheumatology Criteria for the Classification of Fibromyalgia. Report of the Multicenter Criteria Committee. *Arthritis Rheum* 1990;33(2):160–72.

10. Bowyer, S. and Roettcher, P. Pediatric rheumatology clinic populations in the United States: results of a 3 year survey. Pediatric Rheumatology Database Research Group. *J Rheumatol* 1996;23(11):1968–74.

11. Yunus, M.B. and Masi, A.T. Juvenile primary fibromyalgia syndrome. A clinical study of thirty-three patients and matched normal controls. *Arthritis Rheum* 1985;28(2):138–45.

12. Siegel, D.M., Janeway, D., and Baum, J. Fibromyalgia syndrome in children and adolescents: clinical features at presentation and status at follow-up. *Pediatrics* 1998;101(3 Pt 1):377–82.

13. Buskila, D., Neumann, L., Hershman, E., Gedalia, A., Press, J. and Sukenik, S. Fibromyalgia syndrome in children—an outcome study. *J Rheumatol* 1995;22(3):525–8.

14. Schanberg, L.E., Keefe, F.J., Lefebvre, J.C., Kredich, D.W., and Gil, K.M. Social context of pain in children with Juvenile Primary Fibromyalgia Syndrome: parental pain history and family environment. *Clin J Pain* 1998;14(2):107–15.

15. Schikler, K.N. Is it juvenile rheumatoid arthritis or fibromyalgia? *Med Clin North Am* 2000;84(4):967–82.

16. Gedalia, A., Press, J., Klein, M., and Buskila, D. Joint hypermobility and fibromyalgia in schoolchildren. *Ann Rheum Dis* 1993 Jul;52(7):494–6.

17. Akkasilpa, S., Minor, M., Goldman, D., Magder, L.S., and Petri, M. Association of coping responses with fibromyalgia tender points in patients with systemic lupus erythematosus. *J Rheumatol* 2000;27(3): 671–4.

18. Wolfe, F. The relation between tender points and fibromyalgia symptom variables: evidence that fibromyalgia is not a discrete disorder in the clinic. *Ann Rheum Dis* 1997;56(4):268–71.

19. Rusy, L.M., Harvey, S.A., and Beste, D.J. Pediatric fibromyalgia and dizziness: evaluation of vestibular function. *J Dev Behav Pediatr* 1999;20(4):211–15.

20. Roizenblatt, S., Tufik, S., Goldenberg, J., Pinto, L.R., Hilario, M.O., and Feldman, D. Juvenile fibromyalgia: clinical and polysomnographic aspects. *J Rheumatol* 1997;24(3):579–85.

21. Conte, P.M., Walco, G.A., Kimura, Y. Temperament and stress response in children with juvenile primary fibromyalgia syndrome. *Arthritis Rheum* 2003;48:2923–30.

22. Varni, J.W., Seid, M., Smith, K.T., Burwinkle, T., Brown, J., and Szer, I.S. The PedsQL in pediatric rheumatology: reliability, validity, and responsiveness of the Pediatric Quality of Life Inventory Generic Core scales and Rheumatology Module. *Arthritis Rheum* 2002;46(3):714–25.

23. Mikkelsson, M., Sourander, A., Piha, J., and Salminen, J.J. Psychiatric symptoms in preadolescents with musculoskeletal pain and fibromyalgia. *Pediatrics* 1997;100(2 Pt 1):220–7.

24. Walco, G.A. and Ilowite, N.T. Cognitive-behavioral intervention for juvenile primary fibromyalgia syndrome. *J Rheumatol* 1992; 19(10):1617–9.

25. Sherry, D.D. An overview of amplified musculoskeletal pain syndromes. *J Rheumatol* 2000,27 (Suppl 58):44–8.

26. Bell, D.S., Bell, K.M., and Cheney, P.R. Primary juvenile fibromyalgia syndrome and chronic fatigue syndrome in adolescents. *Clin Infect Dis* 1994;18 (Suppl 1):S21–3.

27. Breau, L.M., McGrath, P.J., and Ju, L.H. Review of juvenile primary fibromyalgia and chronic fatigue syndrome. *J Dev Behav Pediatr* 1999;20(4):278–88.

28. Siegel, D.M., Janeway, D., and Baum, J. Fibromyalgia syndrome in children and adolescents: clinical features at presentation and status at follow-up. *Pediatrics* 1998;101(3 Pt 1):377–82.

29. Ruggeri, S.B., Athreya, B.H., Doughty, R., Gregg, J.R., and Das, M.M. Reflex sympathetic dystrophy in children. *Clin Orthop* 1982(163):225–30.

30. Silber, T.J. and Majd, M. Reflex sympathetic dystrophy syndrome in children and adolescents. Report of 18 cases and review of the literature. *Am J Dis Child* 1988;142(12):1325–30.

31. Ashwal, S., Tomasi, L., Neumann, M., and Schneider, S. Reflex sympathetic dystrophy syndrome in children. *Pediatr Neurol* 1988;4(1):38–42.

32. Sherry, D.D. and Weisman, R. Psychologic aspects of childhood reflex neurovascular dystrophy. *Pediatrics* 1988;81(4):572–8.

33. Bernstein, B.H., Singsen, B.H., Kent, J.T., Kornreich, H., King, K., Hicks, R., and Hanson, V. Reflex neurovascular dystrophy in childhood. *J Pediatr* 1978;93(2):211–5.

34. Lee, B.H., Schar, H.L., Sethna, N.F. *et al.* Physical therapy and cognitive-behavioral treatment for complex regional pain syndromes. *J Pediatr* 2002;141:135–40.

35. Sherry, D.D., Wallace, C.A., Kelley, C., Kidder, M., Sapp, L. Short- and long-term outcomes of children with complex regional pain syndrome type I treated with exercise therapy. *Clin J Pain* 1999;15:218–23.

36. Fukuda, K., Straus, S.E., Hickie, I., Sharpe, M.C., Dobbins, J.G., and Komaroff, A. The chronic fatigue syndrome: a comprehensive approach to its definition and study. International Chronic Fatigue Syndrome Study Group. *Ann Intern Med* 1994 15;121(12):953–9.

37. Bell, D.S., Bell, K.M., and Cheney, P.R. Primary juvenile fibromyalgia syndrome and chronic fatigue syndrome in adolescents. *Clin Infect Dis* 1994;18(Suppl 1):S21–3.

38. Komaroff, A.L., Fagioli, L.R., Geiger, A.M., Doolittle, T.H., Lee, J., Kornish, R.J., Gleit, M.A., and Guerriero, R.T. An examination of the working case definition of chronic fatigue syndrome. *Am J Med* 1996;100(1):56–64.

39. Krilov, L.R., Fisher, M., Friedman, S.B., Reitman, D., and Mandel, F.S. Course and outcome of chronic fatigue in children and adolescents. *Pediatrics* 1998;102(2 Pt 1):360–6.

40. Bell, D.S., Jordan, K., and Robinson, M. Thirteen-year follow-up of children and adolescents with chronic fatigue syndrome. *Pediatrics* 2001;107(5):994–8.

41. Wormser, G.P., Nadelman, R.B., Dattwyler, R.J., Dennis, D.T., Shapiro, E.D., Steere, A.C., Rush, T.J., Rahn, D.W., Coyle, P.K., Persing, D.H., Fish, D., and Luft, B.J. Practice guidelines for the treatment of Lyme disease. The Infectious Diseases Society of America. *Clin Infect Dis* 2000; 31 (Suppl 1):1–14.

42. Szer, I.S., Taylor, E., and Steere, A.C. The long-term course of Lyme arthritis in children. *N Engl J Med* 1991;325(3):159–63.

43. Shadick, N.A., Phillips, C.B., Sangha, O., Logigian, E.L., Kaplan, R.F., Wright, E.A., Fossel, A.H., Fossel, K., Berardi, V., Lew, R.A., and Liang, M.H. Musculoskeletal and neurologic outcomes in patients with previously treated Lyme disease. *Ann Intern Med* 1999 21;131(12):919–26.

44. Klempner, M.S., Hu, L.T., Evans, J., Schmid, C.H., Johnson, G.M., Trevino, R.P., Norton, D., Levy, L., Wall, D., McCall, J., Kosinski, M., and Weinstein, A. Two controlled trials of antibiotic treatment in patients with persistent symptoms and a history of Lyme disease. *N Engl J Med* 2001 12;345(2):85–92.

45. Wang, T.J., Sangha, O., Phillips, C.B., Wright, E.A., Lew, R.A., Fossel, A.H., Fossel, K., Shadick, N.A., Liang, M.H., and Sundel, R.P. Outcomes of children treated for Lyme disease. *J Rheumatol* 1998;25(11):2249–53.

46. Steere, A.C. A 58-year-old man with a diagnosis of chronic Lyme disease. *JAMA* 2002 28;288(8):1002–10.

47. Steere, A.C., Taylor, E., McHugh, G.L., and Logigian, E.L. The overdiagnosis of Lyme disease. *JAMA* 1993 14;269(14):1812–6.

48. Tugwell, P., Dennis, D.T., Weinstein, A., Wells, G., Shea, B., Nichol, G., Hayward, R., Lightfoot, R., Baker, P., and Steere, A.C. Laboratory evaluation in the diagnosis of Lyme disease. *Ann Intern Med* 1997 15;127(12):1109–23.

49. Sigal, L.H. Summary of the first 100 patients seen at a Lyme disease referral center. *Am J Med* 1990;88(6):577–81.

50. Sigal, L.H. and Patella, S.J. Lyme arthritis as the incorrect diagnosis in pediatric and adolescent fibromyalgia. *Pediatrics* 1992;90(4):523–8.

51. Hsu, V.M., Patella, S.J., and Sigal, L.H. "Chronic Lyme disease" as the incorrect diagnosis in patients with fibromyalgia. *Arthritis Rheum* 1993;36(11):1493–500.

52. Calvert, P. and Jureidini, J. Restrained rehabilitation: an approach to children and adolescents with unexplained signs and symptoms. *Arch Dis Child* 2003;88:399–402.

53. Reich, P. and Gottfried, L.A. Factitious disorders in a teaching hospital. *Ann Intern Med* 1983;99(2):240–7.

54. Zitelli, B.J., Seltman, M.F., and Shannon, R.M. Munchausen's syndrome by proxy and its professional participants. *Am J Dis Child* 1987;141(10):1099–102.

55. Fliege, H., Scholler, G., Rose, M., Willenberg, H., and Klapp, B.F. Factitious disorders and pathological self-harm in a hospital population: an interdisciplinary challenge. *Gen Hosp Psychiatry* 2002; 24(3):164–71.

1.10 Musculoskeletal and autoimmune manifestations of non-rheumatic disorders

Karin S. Peterson

Aim

The aim of this chapter is to provide a comprehensive discussion of disorders that may occasionally manifest with secondary musculoskeletal complaints and mimic Juvenile Idiopathic Arthritis.

Structure

- Malignancies
- Hypertrophic osteoarthropathy
- Primary blood disorders
- Kashin–Beck and Mselini joint diseases
- Endocrine disorders
- Metabolic bone diseases
- Excess vitamin intake
- Hyperuricemia
- Alcaptonuria, Lowe syndrome, familiar hypercholesterolemia
- Metabolic storage disorders
- Immunodeficiency disorders
- Dialysis related arthritis
- Primary tumors of bone and joints.

Introduction

Musculoskeletal pain, arthritis or autoimmune phenomena are sometimes encountered in a child already diagnosed with another disorder, such as diabetes, cystic fibrosis, or an immunodeficiency. In most instances this is not the occurrence of a second disease but a symptom related to the underlying disorder or, occasionally, its treatment. Sometimes, a non-rheumatic disease presents with musculoskeletal symptoms, for example, the joint or bone pain that may be misdiagnosed as arthritis in a child with an undiagnosed malignancy. It is important to distinguish these secondary forms of rheumatic disease from the primary ones to ensure that an appropriate therapeutic approach is taken.

Malignancies with secondary effects on the musculoskeletal system

Introduction

Bone pain, arthritis, or periarticular swelling may be the presenting manifestations of a malignancy that originates from a site outside of the musculoskeletal system (Figure 1.10.1(a) and (b)). Of all the disorders discussed in this chapter, the most common to be confused with JIA is cancer, in particular leukaemia, lymphoma, and neuroblastoma. Indeed, the first entity to consider in a child with bone pain, especially with episodic refusal to walk or to use an arm, is malignancy. In particular, when Systemic Arthritis is considered one should always keep in mind the possibility of an underlying malignancy. An extensive workup is usually necessary before the diagnosis of Systemic Arthritis is made (Part 2, Chapter 2.2). A bone marrow biopsy is always recommended prior to initiation of corticosteroids in a child with suspected Systemic Arthritis. If not done, the correct diagnosis of a malignancy may be considerably delayed. A lymph node biopsy should be obtained if the child has lymphadenopathy.

Leukaemia

Leukaemias are the most common childhood cancers, accounting for more than 30% of paediatric malignancies with acute lymphoblastic leukemia (ALL) constituting the majority. Incidence is highest around age 4. Bone pain and arthralgias occur in 20–40% of children diagnosed with ALL along with other symptoms of the disease. However, in some children with ALL (and also in those with other types of cancer) the presenting symptoms may be limited to bone pain, sympathetic effusion, arthralgias, and, sometimes, a low-grade fever prompting referral to a rheumatologist [1,2]. It has been estimated that up to 1% of patients referred for paediatric rheumatology consultation have an underlying malignancy. Bone pain and tenderness to palpation out of proportion to visible signs of arthritis, unexplained fever, or abnormal blood smear always suggest the possibility of cancer (Table 1.10.1). For example, laboratory findings of low/normal white blood cell count and thrombocytopenia would be highly unlikely in a child with Systemic Arthritis, in which both these parameters are usually elevated. Night sweats and/or persistent, low-grade fever, rather than daily spikes of high temperature, should also lead to consideration of disorders other than Systemic Arthritis. The bone pain may awaken the child from sleep; a finding more characteristic of cancer than JIA. Nonspecific radiographic abnormalities that may indicate the presence of a malignancy are listed in Table 1.10.1 (Figure 1.10.2). However, children with cancer and bone pain may not have radiographic evidence of bone involvement and approximately half of those with radiographic evidence of skeletal lesions do not complain of bone pain [3]. Bone scan is the preferred initial imaging technique in children with widespread and diffuse bone pain [2]. The musculoskeletal symptoms result from leukaemic infiltration of the perichondral bone or joint or from expansion of the marrow or periostitis (Table 1.10.2). The bone is osteoporotic and a pathologic

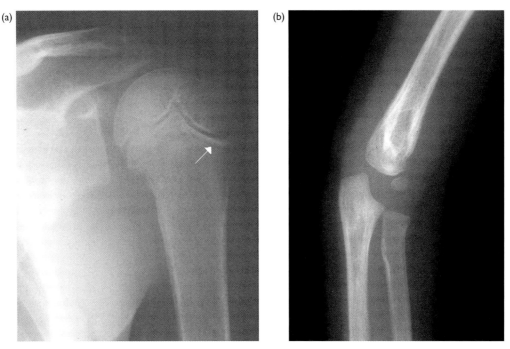

Fig. 1.10.1 (a) ALL presenting with pain and arthralgias of the shoulder. The radiograph shows the lytic lesions and metaphyseal lucent lines (arrow). (Courtesy of Y. Kimura.) (b) Mixed lytic and sclerotic lesions of metastatic neuroblastoma involving the humerus and ulna in a child who presented with monoarticular arthritis of the elbow. (Courtesy of T.R. Southwood.)

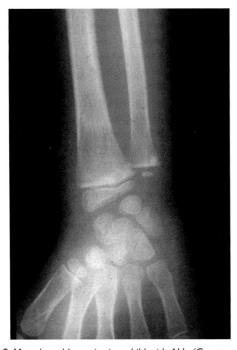

Fig. 1.10.2 Metaphyseal lucencies in a child with ALL. (Courtesy of T.R. Southwood.)

Table 1.10.1 Diagnostic features suggesting malignancy rather than JIA

Weight loss[a]
Low-grade, persistent fever
Night sweats and night pain
Bone pain out of proportion to visible arthritis
Refusal to walk
Isolated back pain

Laboratory studies:
　Severe anaemia[a]
　Low/normal WBC
　Thrombocytopenia[b]
　Elevated serum uric acid
　Elevated serum LDH[b]

Radiographs:[c]
　Generalized osteopenia
　Periosteal bone reaction
　Osteolytic lesions
　Metaphyseal radiolucent bands (metaphyseal rarefaction)

[a] Also common in Systemic Arthritis.

[b] The simultaneous presence of high LDH and elevated ESR or thrombocytopenia and elevated ESR are particularly suggestive of a malignancy and should lead to additional investigations.

[c] These four types of radiographic lesions are commonly seen in children with leukaemia and musculoskeletal symptoms, however, they are not specific.

fracture may occur. Hypertrophic osteoarthropathy is another, rare cause of bone pain in children with a malignancy (see below). Bone marrow examination proves the correct diagnosis in most cases, but it is important to be aware of the child with early leukaemia who may have a normal CBC and peripheral blood smear, and even a normal bone marrow examination.

Lymphoma

Lymphoma is relatively common in childhood and accounts for approximately 10% of paediatric malignancies. Lymphoma also occurs with increased frequency in individuals with immunodeficiency disorders. Non-Hodgkin lymphomas in children are often extra-nodal and

Table 1.10.2 Causes of musculoskeletal pain in childhood malignancy

Bone infarction from marrow or cortical invasion
Hypertrophic osteoarthropathy
Immune complexes in synovium
Invasion of synovium and soft tissues by malignant cells
Periostitis
Referred pain from spinal-cord tumors
Secondary gout in leukaemia

a common primary location is the abdomen; clinical presentation depends on both site and pattern of spread. Hodgkin disease usually originates in a lymph node and the most common presentation is with painless enlargement of one or many nodes; bone pain may result from direct invasion of the cortex or marrow by the tumor or from intrathoracic involvement causing hypertrophic osteoarthropathy (see below). Rheumatic symptoms do not occur as commonly in association with lymphoma as with ALL but the spectrum of musculoskeletal symptoms is similar [2].

Neuroblastoma

Neuroblastoma is the most frequent solid tumor outside of the CNS in children and the most common tumor in infants. Ninety percent of all neuroblastomas are diagnosed before the age of two. The tumour originates in the sympathetic nervous system and clinical manifestations vary depending on the location of the mass and its secretory characteristics. Most often, the primary tumour is located in the abdomen, usually in the adrenal gland. Bone pain results from metastatic spread to the skeleton and the bone marrow, and 75% of affected children have metastatic disease at the time of diagnosis. Urinary excretion of the catecholamine metabolites (vanillylmandelic acid (VMA) and homovanillic acid (HVA)) may indicate the presence of disease. Lytic bone lesions are typically found on radiographs (Figure: 1.10.1(b)), while bone scanning may detect early lesions. Figure 1.10.3 shows a series of imaging studies that were obtained in the diagnostic work-up of a 26-month-old child who presented with fever and back pain.

Hypertrophic osteoarthropathy

Most paediatricians associate hypertrophic osteoarthropathy with clubbed fingers and cardiopulmonary disease. The full syndrome includes periostitis with new bone formation (hyperostosis) and bone pain, arthralgias in large joints, and occasional autonomic dysfunction (flushing, blanching, sweating). The arthralgias often occur without clubbing especially in children with an underlying malignancy. Familial and secondary forms of hypertrophic osteoarthropathy are described in Table 1.10.3. The pathogenesis of both primary and secondary forms of hypertrophic osteoarthropathy remains unclear.

Hereditary hypertrophic osteoarthropathy

There are two rare, hereditary forms of hypertrophic osteoarthropathy that appear to occur with more severity in males. Pachydermoperiostosis (OMIM 167100 [4]) becomes symptomatic in late childhood with periostitis mainly of the distal parts of the extremities and often presents with sympathetic effusions of knees and ankles. Clubbing of the fingers, hyperhidrosis, seborrhoea, pachyderma

and thickening of the skin are other characteristic features. The hands and feet become enlarged as a result of increased soft tissue and bone, and the affected individual may develop an acromegalic appearance. Primary hypertrophic osteoarthropathy without pachyderma (OMIM 119900 [4]) is even less common than that associated with thickening of the skin and is characterized by clubbing in infancy.

Secondary hypertrophic osteoarthropathy

Secondary hypertrophic osteoarthropathy is by no means rare in children and constitutes an important and under-recognized form of musculoskeletal pain (Table 1.10.3). The radiographic demonstration of periostal new bone formation along the shaft of long and tubular bones is diagnostic (Figure 1.10.4) but depends on radiographs being taken at the stage when new-bone formation has taken place. Technetium bone scan, showing uptake in areas of new-bone formation, is more sensitive in detecting early lesions but may occasionally also be negative in the acute stage. Acute periostitis is very painful and patients fear the slightest touch, requiring elevation even of the bed sheets. The pain may have a migratory quality and the severe complaints, in the absence of visible arthritis or radiographic evidence of periostitis may seem puzzling and suggest non-organic pain. Once recognized, the pain is often responsive to treatment with a nonsteroidal anti-inflammatory drug.

Hyperostosis with bone pain may occur in Goldbloom syndrome (Part 1, Chapter 1.7) and some of the osteochondrodysplasias (Part 1, Chapter 1.11) where it may be a presenting symptom.

Cystic fibrosis (CF)

The two most common types of musculoskeletal disease in children with cystic fibrosis are hypertrophic osteoarthropathy, sometimes with clubbing and/or radiographic evidence of periostitis (Figure 1.10.4) and episodic, short-lived attacks of an asymmetric, effusive and nonerosive synovitis involving large and small joints [5]; erythema nodosum has been described as an associated feature in some of these individuals belonging to the latter group. The attacks last from hours to weeks and can usually be controlled with nonsteroidal anti-inflammatory agents. The syndrome may be related to the chronic pulmonary infections that occur in cystic fibrosis and may be caused by an immune-complex induced reaction. Vasculitic rashes have been described in some patients [6] and may have a similar etiology. There has been a report of one child with cystic fibrosis who has developed Rheumatoid Factor Positive Polyarthritis (see Part 2, Chapter 2.4) with nodules [7].

Decreased bone mineral density is common in children with cystic fibrosis and with increased survival, osteoporosis has become an important problem in the adolescent and young adult with CF. Excessive kyphosis, back pain, and an increased fracture rate have been reported to complicate long-standing disease [8]. Risk factors include malnutrition, lack of physical activity, and corticosteroid therapy.

Coeliac disease

Arthritis [9], alopecia areata, autoimmune thyroid disease, and other autoimmune disorders occur with increased frequency in patients with celiac disease. Rheumatic symptoms may accompany any bowel inflammation and the association between inflammatory bowel disease and spondyloarthritis is well recognized (Part 1, Chapter 1.4 and Part 2,

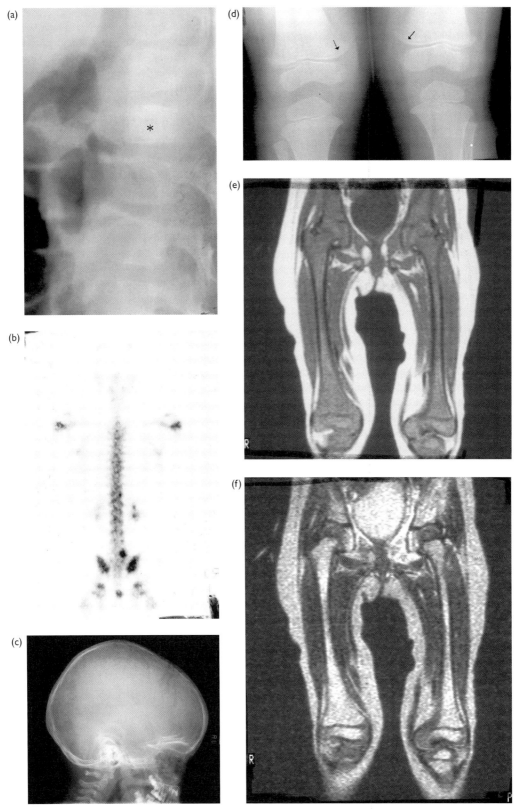

Fig. 1.10.3 (a) Radiograph of the spine in a 26 month-old male who presented with fever and back-pain shows a dense vertebral body (asterix), initially diagnosed as osteomyelitis of the spine not metastatic neuroblastoma. (b) Bone scan shows increased uptake in nearly all of the vertebral bodies. (c) Radiograph of the skull shows the moth-eaten appearance of the involved bone. (d) The non-specific but typical findings of metaphyseal lucent lines (arrows) are demonstrated in the radiographs of the knees. MRI imaging illustrates the so-called flip-flop sign: diffuse infiltration of the bone marrow by the tumor causing. (e) Decreased signal within the marrow on T1 (normally bright) and (f) Increased signal on T2 (normally dark).

Table 1.10.3 Hypertrophic osteoarthropathy in childhood

Primary	
With pachyderma	Pachydermoperiostosis (OMIM 167100(4))
Without pachyderma	Primary hypertrophic osteoarthropathy without pachyderma (OMIM 119900(4))
Secondary	
Pulmonary	Cystic fibrosis, infections, fibrosis
Endocrine	Hyperthyroidism, hypothyroidism, hyperparathyroidism
Cardiovascular	SBE[a], cyanotic congenital heart disease
Gastrointestinal	Inflammatory bowel disease, cirrhosis of the liver, bacterial or parasitic infections
Malignancy	Leukaemia, lymphoma, neuroblastoma, medulloblastoma, sarcoma, others

[a]SBE: subacute bacterial endocarditis.

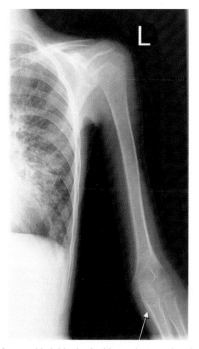

Fig. 1.10.4 A 9-year-old child who had been diagnosed with cystic fibrosis at age 4 developed severe pain in his arms and legs over a 2-month period. Physical examination of all joints was normal but he had exquisite tenderness over the shafts of the long bones. Radiograph confirmed the suspicion of hypertrophic osteoarthropathy, demonstrating periostitis with periosteal new bone formation (arrow). The lungs are hyperinflated with diffuse bronchiectases, typical of severe cystic fibrosis. (Courtesy of Dr Y. Kimura.)

Chapter 2.7). Although coeliac disease may coexist with JIA, enteropathic arthralgia/arthritis may be a manifestation of unrecognized celiac disease and disappear following institution of a gluten-free diet [10]. Gluten enteropathy is frequently unrecognized and any child presenting with undifferentiated musculoskeletal complaints, even when gastrointestinal symptoms are minimal, should have appropriate screen for coeliac disease.

Blood disorders

Introduction

A joint effusion may be caused by bleeding into the joint, either from trauma or occurring spontaneously in a child with a bleeding

Table 1.10.4 Causes of skeletal pain in the haemoglobinopathies

Avascular necrosis
Bone infarction due to oxygen desaturation
Bone marrow infarction
Gout
Non-inflammatory joint effusion
Osteomyelitis
Periostitis
Synovial, joint capsule, or tendon infarction

diathesis; joint swelling may be the first manifestation of disease. Musculoskeletal pain, arthralgia, or avascular necrosis may occur in conditions associated with hypoxia or with infarcts of bone, such as sickle-cell disease.

Sickle-cell anemia

Musculoskeletal pain, including the intense pain known as sickle-cell crisis, is common in homozygous sickle-cell (SS) disease [11] and also occurs in patients with other haemoglobinopathies (e.g. SC disease) (Table 1.10.4). Reduced blood flow and oxygen desaturation in terminal blood vessels predispose to thrombosis and infarction of bone. It was recently reported that the decreased bioavailability of nitric oxide which occurs in patients with sickle-cell anaemia may be a primary event in initiating the cascade of reactions leading to ischemia and musculoskeletal pain [12]. Haemoglobin is a potent scavenger of nitric oxide and excess free haemoglobin, released by destruction of the sickling red cell, leads to increased consumption of nitric oxide. Nitric oxide, produced by the vascular endothelium is a primary regulator of blood flow; high levels of nitric oxide relax the vascular tone whereas low levels cause constriction of blood vessels and decreased flow of oxygen and nutrients to tissues.

Individuals with SS disease are also prone to infection, in particular to Salmonella species, and bone infarcts may become infected, causing osteomyelitis (see also Part 1, Chapter 1.5). Pyomyositis has also been reported with increased frequency in these children. It may be difficult to distinguish between uncomplicated bone infarcts and osteomyelitis; technetium, gallium, and MRI scans may be helpful in this differentiation (see Part 1, Chapter 1.3, Algorthim 1.3.1 and Table 1.3.1). Migratory polyarthritis is a typical feature of sickle-cell crisis. When the child is anaemic and has fever and a heart murmur, it may be difficult to distinguish these episodes from acute rheumatic fever (Part 1, Chapter 1.4). Synovitis of the hip secondary to avascular necrosis of the head of the femur is another manifestation of SS disease. Although bone necrosis is most common in SS disease, sludging may occur in all haemoglobinopathies depending on oxygen saturation and the concentration of less soluble hemoglobin.

During the second half of the first year of life, as the percentage of protective fetal haemoglobin declines, sickling may be accentuated in the most distal bones of the body, resulting in sickle-cell dactylitis (Figure 1.10.5); the hand and foot syndrome of sickle-cell anaemia. Swelling of the hands and feet with exquisite pain is followed in several weeks by characteristic radiographic changes, including periosteal elevation, subperiosteal new-bone formation, and a moth-eaten appearance of bone. This syndrome is rarely seen after the toddler age, presumably because the red marrow of the distal bones by then has been replaced by fibrous tissue that has lower oxygen requirements and fewer blood vessels susceptible to infarction.

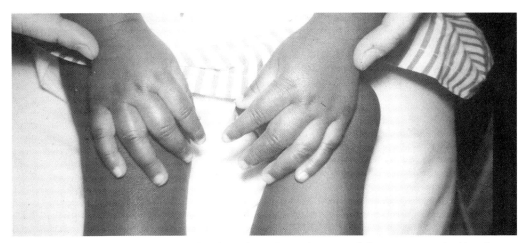

Fig. 1.10.5 Fever and painful swelling of the proximal digits with radiographic evidence of periostitis led to recognition of sickle-cell anaemia in this toddler. (From J. Jacobs)

Thalassaemia

The thalassaemias are a heterogeneous group of hereditary disorders affecting either the α-chain or the β-chain of the hemoglobin molecule. Symptoms develop early in individuals with the severe, homozygous form. Because of the profound anaemia, the bone marrow expands massively, leading to skeletal deformities and thin bones that are prone to fractures. Individuals with β-thalassaemia minor, associated with mild anaemia, have been reported to develop arthralgias and short, recurrent episodes of arthritis [13].

Haemophilia

The most common causes of haemorrhage into the joints are trauma and bleeding disorders (Table 1.10.5). Severe classic haemophilia (plasma factor levels <1 U/dl), while a cause of severe disabling arthropathy, is usually diagnosed prior to the first episode of hemarthrosis, which frequently occurs without trauma. However, moderate (1–5 U/dl) or mild hemophilia (5–30 U/dl) and other more subtle factor deficiencies may present as traumatic haemarthrosis. Since there is a high incidence of de novo mutations it is important to suspect haemophilia even in the absence of a family history. Patients usually come to medical attention with a single knee effusion and a history of trauma. Except in child abuse, bleeding into joints is generally intracapsular and unaccompanied by visible bruising. Arthrocentesis reveals bloody fluid. The presence of blood in the joint is associated with damage to cartilage and bone (Figure 1.10.6). The mechanism is not completely understood but it is likely that the deposition of haemosiderin leads to synovial hypertrophy and inflammation; and the release of free iron may induce the production of toxic oxygen metabolites that directly damage the cartilage [14].

More than 80% of the episodes of haemorrhage in children with severe haemophilia occur into joints or muscle. Chronic arthropathy is directly related to repetitive episodes of articular haemorrhage. Haemorrhage in the iliopsoas muscle must also be considered in the differential diagnosis of hip pain in a child with haemophilia. Detailed coagulation studies are necessary to establish the diagnosis in the patient with suspected haemophilia. Management of haemophila is aimed at the prevention of haemarthrosis by regular infusions of clotting factors, and favorable long-term outcome is critically dependent on the early institution of prophylactic treatment [15]. The arthropathy of haemarthrosis can develop over a short period of time

Table 1.10.5 Causes of haemarthrosis

Trauma
Coagulation factor deficiency
Von Willebrand disease
Anti-coagulation therapy
Circulating inhibitor of specific coagulation-factor
Ehlers–Danlos syndrome vascular type IV
Pigmented villonodular synovitis
Platelet disorders
Scurvy, vitamin C deficiency
Synovial haemangioma and other venous malformations

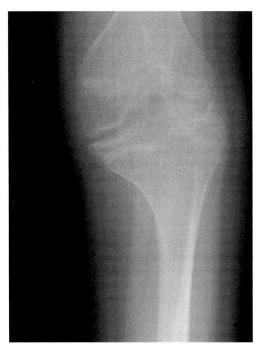

Fig. 1.10.6 This 17-year-old with haemophilia A developed antibodies to factor VIII which complicated his treatment with factor concentrate. Radiograph of the knee shows widening of the intercondylar notch, overgrowth of the epiphyses, erosions, and osteoporosis.

(months to a year) and synovectomy is often recommended to prevent further joint damage [16]. The use of intra-articular corticosteroids in to affected joints remains controversial.

Thrombasthenia

Bleeding associated with platelet disorders is usually in the superficial microcirculation resulting in recurrent bruises, epistaxis, menorrhagia, and bleeding after dental extraction. The few patients reported to have bled into the joints often have had a single haemorrhage into the knee [17]. Diagnosis is suggested by a prolonged bleeding time and confirmed with special platelet studies.

Other less common causes of bloody joint fluid include synovial haemangioma, and congenital and acquired disorders of connective tissue. Scurvy (vitamin C deficiency) is an example of an acquired metabolic disorder in which hemarthrosis may be a manifestation. Patients with scurvy also develop bone pain secondary to subperiostal bleeding. Ehlers-Danlos syndrome (Part 1, Chapter 1.11) is an example of a connective tissue disorder where abnormal structural integrity of the connective tissue, fragile blood vessels, or platelet dysfunction may contribute to a bleeding tendency that may result in synovial haemorrhage after normal activities or minor trauma. Some children who receive chronic anti-coagulation therapy following heart valve replacement or for other reasons, are at risk for bleeding, including haemarthrosis.

Haemochromatosis

Primary haemochromatosis (OMIM 235200 [4]) is a relatively common disorder but it is rarely encountered in the paediatric population. Clinical onset is usually between 20 and 30 years of age with arthritis alone or in association with amenorrhoea, cardiac abnormalities, or a triad of skin pigmentation, diabetes, and cirrhosis. The disease is caused by a genetically controlled error in iron metabolism resulting in increased intracellular storage of iron. Homozygotes for the haemochromatosis - mutation develop severe disease; heterozygotes have a wide spectrum of clinical or subclinical disorders.

The arthritis of haemochromatosis is progressive, starting in the small joints of the hands and later involves the wrists, elbows, hips, knees, and ankles. Patients have severe anemia that is well compensated and helps differentiate this disorder from Rheumatoid Factor Positive Polyarthritis, that has a similar symmetric distribution. Serum transferrin saturation values are elevated. Patients with transfusion induced haemosiderosis may have similar arthritis with iron deposition in the synovium.

Kashin–Beck and Mselini joint disease

These are endemic forms of osteoarthritis thought to result from selenium deficiency associated with ingestion of bread, grain, fungi, soil, or water. Because selenium is involved in thyroid hormone metabolism, iodine deficiency is a risk factor for Kashin–Beck disease (78). Kashin-Beck disease occurs in children living in remote mountainous areas of southeastern Siberia, northeastern China and Korea [18]; the disease is not reported in children fed imported bread and in children moved to a new home in an unaffected area. The affected child develops progressive joint disease characterized by pain, contractures, and

enlargement of involved joints. Interphalangeal, wrist, knee, and ankle joints are symmetrically thickened with progressive limitation of motion. There are no effusions or laboratory signs of inflammation until late in the disease when these are presumably secondary to osteoarthritis. Many patients ultimately develop a dwarfed appearance suggestive of a storage disease or a bone dysplasia with short, stubby fingers.

Mselini joint disease is a similar disorder that is endemic in remote parts of Zululand and affects a large proportion of the population. The large joints of the lower extremities are primarily involved [19].

Endocrine disorders

There is evidence of endocrine control of the synthesis and degradation of connective-tissue molecules, so it is not surprising that musculoskeletal symptoms may be associated with endocrine disorders.

Diabetes

Diabetic cheiroarthropathy or limited joint mobility of the fingers (Figure 1.10.7 (a) and (b)) is a painless complication of diabetes (occurring in both type I and II diabetes) that may be the result of accelerated glycosylation of collagen, causing increased collagen-crosslinking with subsequent thickening and stiffness of periarticular structures [20]. The fingers typically become involved first but as the syndrome progresses other joints may also lose motion resulting in asymptomatic and mild

(a)

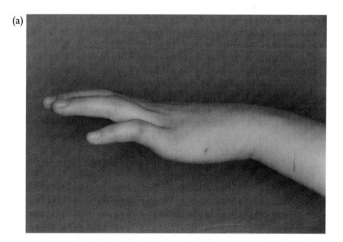

(b)

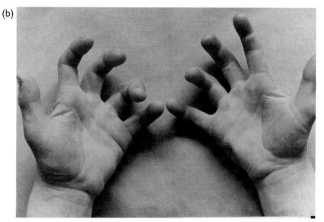

Fig. 1.10.7 Diabetic cheiroarthropathy: (a) early stage and (b) late stage. (Courtesy of Dr A. Benedetti.)

flexion contractures of the wrists, knees, neck, elbows, and hips. Radiographic evaluation of the affected joints shows that the bone and cartilage are not involved. There is generally no pain, although occasional patients may have paresthesias and hyperesthesias, probably from associated diabetic neuropathy or from nerve-entrapment secondary to being bound in connective tissue with abnormal collagen.

Although diabetic cheiroarthropathy is rare in adults, surveys of diabetic children suggest that it is a common feature in adolescents who had the onset of diabetes in infancy and early childhood especially if control of hyperglycaemia had been difficult and/or inadequate. The presence of diabetic cheiroarthropathy is associated with an increased risk (approximately 3-fold) of retinopathy and nephropathy [21].

Thyroid disease

Hypothyroidism

Joint effusions were reported in myxoedema 100 years ago and have been noted in the knees and metacarpo- and metatarsophalangeal joints in many adults with hypothyroid disease [22]. Despite synovial thickening and stiffness, patients report little pain. Thyroid replacement therapy completely relieves the arthritis. The skin disease of myxoedema usually presents as pretibial swelling and biopsy demonstrates mucin deposition in the dermis. Arthralgia [23] and inflammatory polyarthritis [24] have been reported in Hashimoto (autoimmune) thyroditis in the absence of hypothyroidism and do not respond to thyroid replacement therapy. Generalized myalgia is common in patients with overt hypothyroid disease.

Hyperthyroidism

Hyperthyroidism in adults has been associated with a distinctive form of arthritis, termed thyroid acropachy. The main features are swelling of the subcutaneous tissues, "fluffy" subperiosteal new-bone formation in the hands, and clubbing of the fingers and toes. Unlike other forms of hypertrophic osteoarthropathy, no heat or pain is documented in these joints. Hyperthyroidism is usually present for many years before acropachy develops; it is a rare condition in adults, and an extraordinarily rare form of arthritis in childhood.

Muscle-weakness is a characteristic clinical finding in active hyperthyroid disease, probably secondary to the metabolic changes.

Arthralgias/arthritis and skin lesions including leukocytoclastic vasculitis, purpura, erythema multiforme, and erythema nodosum-like lesions have been associated with treatment of hyperthyroidism with propylthiouracil and represent an adverse drug reaction rather than a feature of hypothyroidism [25]. Other rare manifestations of this drug reaction are haematuria or proteinuria, fever, pulmonary haemorrhage, and serositis. The propylthiouracil-induced vasculitis is characterized by a positive ANCA with high titres of anti-myeloperoxidase antibodies. Approximately 20% of patients treated with propylthiouracil are ANCA positive, however, only a small percentage of these individuals develop vasculitis. The ANA test is frequently positive in autoimmune thyroid disease and is not a specific marker of propylthiouracil-induced vasculitis. Discontinuation of propylthiouracil leads to slow resolution of the symptoms, however, recurrence of vasculitis has been reported months after the drug was stopped. Some patients with severe symptoms require therapy with corticosteroids and other immunosuppressive drugs.

Table 1.10.6 Differential diagnosis of hypercalcaemia in childhood

Adrenal insufficiency
Hyperparathyroidism
Hyperthyroidism
Hypophosphataemia
Immobilization with fractures
Leukaemia, neuroblastoma, and other malignancies
Sarcoidosis
Vitamin D intoxication

Hyperparathyroidism

Primary hyperparathyroidism is an exceedingly rare condition in childhood, but hyperparathyroidism secondary to renal disease is not uncommon. In addition to bone pain, symptoms include those due to hypercalcaemia with weakness, hypotonic muscles, anorexia, nausea, mental changes, and joint laxity. The latter is believed to be due to increased collagenase activity caused by the elevated levels of parathyroid hormone. Deposits of calcium in soft tissues, such as ligaments, cartilage, and periarticular structures lead to musculoskeletal symptoms and occasionally to joint effusions. In addition, increased urinary excretion of calcium causes polyuria, polydipsia, calculi, and renal stones.

Bone pain is often the complaint that brings the patient to the doctor. Radiographs show demineralization with thinning of the cortex of the bones. Cyst-like areas of rarefaction with a moth-eaten appearance of the skull and osteoblastic (brown) tumours appear later (osteitis fibrosa). Diagnosis may be apparent radiographically but is documented by appropriate chemical studies that demonstrate high levels of parathyroid hormone, elevated serum calcium, and low serum phosphorus. Peculiar discolouration of permanent teeth, eye findings as well as nail changes that resemble ochronosis have been reported in these children. The differential diagnosis of hypercalcaemia in childhood is shown in Table 1.10.6.

Cushing syndrome and Addison disease

Individuals with Cushing syndrome often have bone pain as a result of osteoporosis and avascular necrosis at multiple sites. Addison disease is accompanied by myalgias, but occasionally joint stiffness may simulate a rheumatic condition. Addison disease may be a presenting manifestation or feature of SLE and the anticardiolipin syndrome (Part 1, Chapter 1.6); some cases are due to thromboembolism of adrenal blood vessels [26].

Metabolic bone disease

Bone is a dynamic organ undergoing constant turnover. It serves as the major reservoir of the divalent minerals, calcium, phosphate, and magnesium. Linear growth is dependent on calcification of metaphyseal cartilage, and extracellular concentrations of calcium and phosphate are major factors in the regulation of bone growth. The vitamin D system and parathyroid hormone are key regulators of the calcium/phosphate homeostasis, and disorders affecting these systems frequently cause growth abnormalities and musculoskeletal symptoms (Table 1.10.7) [27]. Several additional hormones including growth hormone, thyroid hormones, insulin, and oestrogen/androgens act to promote the growth of bone whereas excess amount of corticosteroids impair the growth of bone.

Table 1.10.7 Osteopenic metabolic bone disease in children

Bone disease	Mechanism/cause	Serum laboratory characteristics					
		Ca	PO$_4$	PTH	25(OH)D	1,25(OH)$_2$D	ALP
Hypocalcaemic rickets[a]							
Environmental	Lack of sun exposure	low/nl	low	high	low	nl	high
Nutritional vitamin D deficiency	Exclusive breastfeeding, strict vegetarian diet	low/nl	low	high	low	nl	high
Impaired intestinal absorption of Ca	Dietary deficiency, bowel disease	low/nl	low	high	low	nl	high
Malabsorption of vitamin D in liver disease	Low production of bile salts	low/nl	low	high	low	nl	high
Vitamin D-dependent rickets: type I	Deficiency of renal 1α-hydroxylase	low	low	high	nl	low	high
type II	Target organ: defect in receptor binding of 1,25(OH)$_2$D	low	low	high	nl	high	high
Chronic anticonvulsant therapy[b]	Augmented metabolism of 25(OH)D to inactive metabolite	low/nl	low	high	low	nl	high
Hypophosphataemic rickets							
Proximal renal tubular acidosis	Renal loss of phosphate	nl	low	nl		nl	high
Fanconi syndromes[c]	Renal loss of phosphate	nl	low	nl		nl	high
X-linked dominant, vitamin D resistant	Impaired re-absorption of PO$_4$; mutation in PHEX	nl	low	nl		low/nl	high
Autosomal dominant, vitamin D resistant	Impaired re-absorption of PO$_4$; mutation in FGF-23	nl	low	nl		low/nl	high
Oncogenous rickets with phosphaturia	Secretion by tumor of FGF-23	nl	low	nl		low	high
Medications	Dietary depletion from prolonged use of aluminum containing antacids	nl	low	nl			high

Abbreviations: PTH: parathyroid hormone; 25(OH)D: 25-OH-vitamin D; 1,25(OH)$_2$D: 1,25(OH)$_2$ -vitamin D; FGF-23: fibroblast growth factor 23; *PHEX*: Phosphate regulating gene with homologies to endopeptidases on the X-chromosome; Ca: calcium; ALP: alkaline phosphatase; nl: normal.

[a] Primary hypocalcaemia causes increase of PTH leading to increase of serum Ca (which frequently is low to normal when measured) and renal excretion of phosphate.

[b] Therapy with phenytoin and phenobarbital cause a predisposition to rickets that may be clinically apparent in a child exposed to additional risk factors, such as for example, immobility.

[c] Causes: inborn errors of metabolism (cystinosis, tyrosinosis, Lowe syndrome), acquired forms (exposure to environmental toxins, drugs), and idiopathic forms.

Osteopenia may result in a limp with pain in the knees and ankles, presumably as a result of subclinical compression fractures in weight-bearing metaphyses. Fractures of long bones after minimal trauma and collapse of vertebral bodies may also occur. The osteopenic group of conditions has been divided into those seen primarily as defects in the turnover of bone matrix (osteoporosis) and those that are a result of defective mineralization of bone (osteomalacia). The differentiation is often difficult or impossible but may be accomplished with X-rays, chemical and metabolic studies, or bone biopsy. Idiopathic juvenile osteoporosis is a rare, self-limited condition that often heals spontaneously with the onset of puberty (Part 1, Chapter 1.8).

Rickets

The term rickets indicates failure in mineralization of growing bone. Bone pain, bowing of legs, and poor growth are characteristic of rickets. Myopathy and muscle cramps are characteristics of the calcium-deficient forms of rickets, if serum calcium is sufficiently low, but are not encountered in the primary hypophosphataemic forms.

Hypocalcaemic rickets (Table 1.10.7)

Nutritional deficiency of vitamin D is rare in developed societies but when it occurs it can lead to severe rickets with typical radiographic findings (Figure 1.10.8). Another cause of vitamin D deficient rickets is the lack of exposure to sunlight; in humans 7-dehydrocholesterol in the skin is converted to cholecalciferol (vitamin D$_3$) by ultraviolet

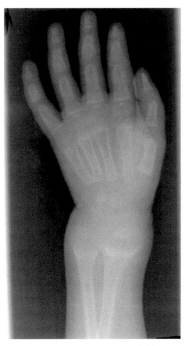

Fig. 1.10.8 Rickets in a 2-year-old who had been fed a diet consisting of breast milk, raisins, and fish. Radiograph of the wrist demonstrates a wide growth plate with fraying and splaying of the distal metaphyses.

light and constitutes a major source of the previtamin. Additional conversion of D_3 and D_2 (ergocalciferol, a synthetic analogue of D_3) take place in the liver to 25-(OH)-vitamin D (calcidiol) and in the kidney to 1,25(OH)$_2$-vitamin D (calcitriol, the active form). Liver disease, malabsorption and anticonvulsant therapy are other causes of vitamin D deficiency that may be associated with rickets (Table 1.10.7).

Genetic causes of hypocalcaemic rickets include vitamin D-dependent rickets type I (OMIM 264700 [4]) and II (OMIM 277420 [4]) caused by a defect in 1-α-hydroxylase that converts 25(OH)-vitamin D to 1,25(OH)$_2$-vitamin D in the kidney, and by a defect in the receptor for 1,25(OH)$_2$-vitamin D, respectively.

Hypophosphataemic rickets (Table 1.10.7)

Children with familial hypophosphataemic forms of rickets present early in life with bowing of the legs, bone pain, and poor growth. Large amounts of phosphate are excreted in the urine. The X-linked dominant form (OMIM 307800 [4]) affects both males and females and is caused by a mutation in PHEX, encoding a phosphate regulating endopeptidase. An autsomal dominant form of hypophosphataemic rickets (OMIM 193100 [4]) has also been identified and is associated with a mutation in the gene encoding fibroblast growth factor 23 (FGF 23) [28]; the mutation stabilizes FGF 23 against proteolysis thus prolonging its half-life. Other forms of hypophosphataemic rickets including one with autosomal recessive inheritance (OMIM 241520 [4]) has been described in individual families. A phosphate-deficient form of rickets occurs in association with some tumours of mesenchymal origin. These tumours are usually benign and may not become apparent until long after the development of rickets. It has been demonstrated that such tumours may secrete excessive amounts of FGF 23 thereby mimicking the pathogenesis of the hereditary disease. A thorough search for skeletal or mesenchymal tumours is essential in all patients with unexplained acquired rickets.

Hypophosphataemia and phosphaturia are associated with conditions, such as renal tubular acidosis and Fanconi syndrome and clinical characteristics of these disorders include rickets and growth failure.

Excess intake of vitamins

Most vitamin poisoning is caused by the excessive use of vitamins to treat acne or other conditions or in the belief that vitamins can only be beneficial.

Vitamin D poisoning

Excess intake of vitamin D may produce bone pain from demineralization just as in hyperparathyroidism. However, the major presenting manifestations are usually secondary to soft-tissue deposit of calcium, especially in the kidney, resulting in obstructive uropathy from stones; in the eyes resulting in band keratopathy; or in the periarticular structures, resulting in limitation of motion of the joints. A biochemical profile will identify hypercalcaemia, low levels of parathyroid hormone and very high levels of calcidiol (25-OH)D and calcitriol (25(OH)$_2$)D.

Vitamin A poisoning

Chronic excess ingestion of vitamin A affects bone metabolism and leads to increased bone resorption and periosteal new bone formation

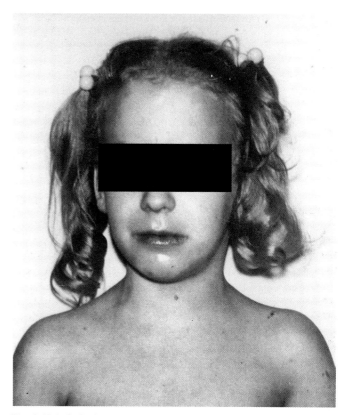

Fig. 1.10.9 Arthralgias and bone pain were the presenting manifestations in this child, who was noted to have frontal bossing, alopecia, an excoriated rash and papilloedema typical of vitamin A poisoning. The sicker she got, the more vitamin A the mother gave her! (from J. Jacobs)

[29] (Figure 1.10.9). Synthetic retinoids prescribed for icthyosis, psoriasis, or other skin diseases, may cause a similar picture. Pain in the bones and joints is often the most troublesome symptom in hypervitaminosis A and the symptom that brings the patient to the doctor. Occasionally, hypercalcaemia is also a consequence of vitamin A poisoning, and calcification of ligaments and tendons may occur. Other symptoms include painful muscular stiffness, fatigue after exercise, anorexia, alopecia, generalized pruritus, and dry, scaling, eczematous skin with yellow palms. If ingestion continues, increased intracranial pressure (pseudotumor cerebri) may develop [29]. The entire clinical picture may simulate connective-tissue disease [30]. Diagnosis can be confirmed with determination of high serum levels of vitamin A and, particularly in early cases, retinal esters. During the early stages of intoxication, vitamin A is deposited in the liver and serum levels are not as high as they become after the liver is saturated. All of the symptoms disappear over a period of months after withdrawal of vitamin A.

Fluorosis

Endemic fluorosis as a cause of chronic rheumatic symptoms occurs in certain areas of the world where especially high natural levels of fluoride in the water supply are found for example, in parts of India. Industrial and environmental poisoning by fluoride pollution may also occur. Excessive intake of fluoride primarily affects the teeth and the skeleton. The first clue to diagnosis is often mottling of the enamel of the permanent teeth. Severe manifestations of skeletal involvement include calcified spinal ligaments and intervetebral discs with a narrowed spinal canal and cord compression from bony overgrowth and generalized calcification of the entheses [31]. Osteoarthritis of the knees may be a characteristic feature of less severe skeletal disease [32]. The most frequent early complaints in children are vague pains in the knees, spine, and small joints of the hands and feet that simulate JIA, particularly the Enthesitis Related Arthritis (ERA see Part 2, Chapter 2.7). Radiographs at an early stage may be normal or may show only increased density of bone; abnormalities are usually first noted in the spinal column and pelvis. Later, all the bones may become dense, and metastatic calcifications may also be seen. The diagnosis is confirmed by measuring the serum fluoride level.

The severe manifestations result from ingestion of large amounts of fluoride (20–80 mg daily) over a period of many years. There is no evidence that controlled fluorination of low-fluoride public water supplies cause any adverse effects. However, levels only twice those that effectively prevent dental caries cause dental mottling; proper care must be exercised in the use of fluoride-containing dental preparations, vitamins, and supplements [33].

Gout

Gout is a frequent cause of arthritis in adults but paediatric gout is extraordinarily rare, probably because of increased renal clearance of uric acid that occurs in children. In reports of childhood-onset gout, the clinical picture has been identical to adult gout with recurring attacks of severe acute arthritis, affecting in particular the first metatarsophalangeal joint. However, when a child presents with 1st MTP arthritis, the more likely cause is JIA not gout. The suspicion of gout should be raised in an older child with acute monoarticular arthritis, in whom the synovial fluid is aseptic but contains numerous neutrophils (with phagocytosed urate crystals). The demonstration of urate crystals (negatively birefringent on polarized light microscopy) confirms the diagnosis.

Gout is a clinical disorder caused by hyperuricaemia and triggered by urate crystals that initiate an inflammatory response. Monoarticular gout may progress to a chronic polyarticular disease with bone destruction, terminal phalangeal bone resorption, growth disturbances, osteoporosis, and flexion deformities. In long-standing disease, soft-tissue deposition of urate crystals (tophi), renal parenchymal disease and uric acid urolithiasis (radiolucent stones) may also be present. However, most individuals with hyperuricaemia do not develop gout and a variety of other factors contribute to the clinical manifestations of the disease. Hyperuricaemia in children is defined as serum uric acid levels >5 mg/dl whereas in adults levels >7 mg/dl constitute hyperuricemia (>2SD above the mean). The limit of solubility of monosodium urate in extracellular fluid is 7 mg/dl and thus levels above 7 pose a risk of gouty arthritis or renal stones.

Hyperuricemia occurs in conditions of increased production of uric acid or decrease in its renal excretion; frequently the underlying cause cannot be identified [34]. However, when elevated uric acid levels are documented in a child, leukaemia should be ruled out first.

Primary causes of hyperuricemia

Complete deficiency of HPRT, a key enzyme in the purine nucleotide salvage pathway (Figure 1.10.10), results in the X-linked, recessive Lesch–Nyhan disease with its characteristic features of hyperuricaemia, gout, developmental delay, neurological symptoms, and a self-mutilating behaviour. The presence of orange (urate) crystals in the diapers is

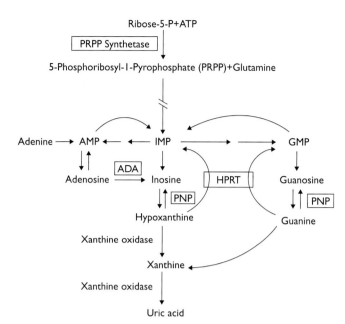

Fig. 1.10.10 Diagram of purine metabolism. PRPP: 5-phosphoribosyl-1-pyrophosphate; HPRT: hypoxanthine-guanine phosphoribosyltransferase; ADA: adenosine deaminase; PNP: purine nucleoside phosphorylase.

sometimes the first sign of the disease. Partial deficiency of HPRT (residual enzyme levels >8%) presents with hyperuricaemia and gout in an otherwise normal child or adolescent [35]. Diagnosis requires analysis of HPRT-activity in blood or cultured fibroblasts. Hyperactivity of PRPP, the initial, rate-limiting enzyme in purine biosynthesis (Figure 1.10.10), is another recognized cause of familial hyperuricaemia.

Allopurinol which inhibits the enzyme xanthine oxidase is very effective in reducing serum levels of uric acid, however, radiolucent xanthine stones may develop as the levels of xanthine increase in the urine.

Secondary causes of hyperuricaemia

Individuals with glycogen storage disease type I (glucose-6-phosphatase-deficiency) develop hyperuricaemia secondary to accelerated degradation of ATP in the liver and decreased renal excretion caused by lactic acidemia [36]. The development of hyperuricaemia in the "muscle glycogenoses" that is, glycogen storage disease type III (amylo-1,6-glycosidase deficiency), type V (myophosphorylase deficiency), and type VII (muscle phosphofructokinase deficiency) has a different mechanism and is related to excessive degradation of muscle purine nucleotides during muscular exertion [37]. Additional clues to the clinical recognition of the myogenic hyperuricaemias are the progressive muscle weakness that occurs in type III glycogenosis and the exercise intolerance that characterizes type V and type VII glycogenosis, respectively [38].

Malignancy, in particular lymphoproliferative disorders, are associated with increased turnover of nucleic acid and increased production of uric acid. The tumour lysis syndrome is associated with rapid increase in serum uric acid (along with potassium and phosphate) and may present with acute joint pain and swelling. The state of chronic compensated hemolysis that occurs for example, in children with sickle-cell anaemia, can lead to hyperuricaemia and development of gout. Individuals with Down syndrome frequently have elevated serum uric acid, believed to be secondary to decreased excretion of urate. It is interesting to note, however, that children with Down syndrome rarely, if ever, develop gout.

Alcaptonuria (OMIM 203500 [4])

Teenagers with this rare (autosomal recessive) deficiency of the enzyme homogentisic acid oxidase may excrete urine that turns black on standing and may begin to deposit visible black pigment in the sclerae, ear, and nasal cartilages (ochronosis). However, the degenerative arthritis that results from deposition of this material in articular cartilage does not occur until middle age. As in all other forms of degenerative arthritis, there may be periods of acute inflammation that may suggest JIA.

Lowe oculocerebrorenal syndrome (OMIM 309000 [4])

This is an X-linked disorder caused by a mutation in a gene encoding a lipid phosphatase [39]. Clinical characteristics include congenital cataracts, renal tubular dysfunction, and mental delay. Affected individuals may develop arthritis and tenosynovitis in the second decade of life. The arthritis is noninflammatory and characterized by a thick, rubbery synovium containing large amounts of fibrous tissue [40].

Type II Hyperlipoproteinaemia (familial hypercholesterolaemia; OMIM 143890 [4])

This is an autosomal dominant disease exhibiting a gene dosage effect. Achilles tendinitis and migratory tenosynovitis are the most common musculoskeletal manifestations in the heterozygote [41] and may resemble ERA (Part 2, Chapter 2.7). The episodes are generally gradual in onset, last 3–12 days, and subside spontaneously. Diagnosis is confirmed by demonstrating significant elevation in plasma cholesterol and low-density lipoproteins with normal levels of triglycerides. The "rheumatic" symptoms may antedate the development of cutaneous xanthomas. Homozygous type II hyperlipoproteinaemia is characterized by the early (often present at birth) development of xanthomas and marked hypercholesterolaemia. Homozygous individuals often have episodes of migratory polyarthritis-simulating acute rheumatic fever; persistent arthritis for periods as long as a month may occur.

Type IV Hyperlipoproteinaemia (OMIM 1446000 [4]) characterized by high levels of triglycerides and normal cholesterol, has been associated with the development of bilateral, asymmetrical arthritis of the lower extremities during the fifth decade of life [42]. This syndrome has not yet been reported in children.

Metabolic storage disorders

The metabolic storage disorders are inherited errors of metabolism that include a large number of conditions that impair various aspects of intracellular metabolism. Most are apparent during the first year of life when abnormal metabolites start accumulating in the cells of different tissues causing symptoms in many organs including the CNS. Selenal storage disorders have predominant effects on the musculoskeletal system with accumulation of metabolites in the synovium and other tissues in and around the joints causing pain, enlargement of the joints, and/or contractures simulating JIA. They are distinguished from JIA by the typical absence of effusions and laboratory signs of inflammation and often by the presence of extra-articular abnormalities, such as hepatosplenomegaly or an associated osteochondrodysplasia (see Part I, Chapter 1.11).

Gaucher disease

Musculoskeletal pain, especially hip, knee, and thigh pain, which is sometimes accompanied by fever and simulates osteomyelitis ("bone crisis") is often the earliest sign of Gaucher disease [43]. Hip lesions may be confused with Legg–Calve–Perthes disease (see Part 1, Chapter 1.8, Figure 1.8.2). This is the most prevalent lysosomal storage disorder and different clinical subtypes have been identified (OMIM 230800, 230900, 231000 [4]). All are caused by deficiency of lysosomal glucocerebrosidase and inherited as autosomal recessive disorders. The enzyme deficiency leads to accumulation of glucosylceramide primarily in the lysosomes of reticuloendothelial cells. In the bone and bone marrow this leads to "blood sludge", bone infarction, and avascular necrosis. Diagnosis may be suspected when musculoskeletal pain is associated with unexplained hepatosplenomegaly or because of the radiographic "Erlenmeyer flask" appearance of the distal femur (Figure 1.10.11). Serum acid phosphatase is usually elevated. Bone marrow examination reveals lipid-laden macrophages (Gaucher cells) and the diagnosis is confirmed by specific enzyme analysis. Enzyme replacement therapy (alglucerase) is now available as the specific treatment for Gaucher disease.

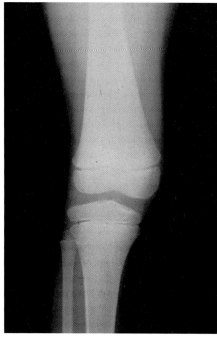

Fig. 1.10.11 Radiograph in a child diagnosed with Gaucher disease demonstrates the characteristic Erlenmyer-flask appearance of the distal femur.

Farber disease

Arthritis is a major manifestation of this rare disorder of lipid metabolism caused by deficiency of lysosomal acid ceramidase and tissue accumulation of ceramide (OMIM 228000 [4]). Inheritance is autosomal recessive. Clinical characteristics include painful swelling of joints, a hoarse voice, subcutaneous nodules predominantly occurring near the joints or at pressure points, and joint contractures (Figure 1.10.12). General malaise with irritability, poor growth and development, and sometimes fever, are other characteristics of the disease. Granulomas of the epiglottis and larynx cause recurrent pneumonia and death in the severely affected child, most commonly during the second year of life. However, a few milder cases have survived. Diagnosis requires specific enzyme analysis in leukocytes or cultured fibroblasts.

Fabry disease

This X-linked recessive deficiency of α-galactosidase leads to systemic deposition of glycosphingolipids (OMIM 3015000 [4]). The disease may present with episodes of polyarthritis, fever, and elevated ESR in adolescent boys. Excruciating burning pain in the fingers and toes may be intolerable. The recurrent episodes tend to last a few days. Limitation of motion is apparent in the fingers and sometimes in the elbows, shoulders, and spine. Confusion with JIA is not unusual. The best clue to the correct diagnosis is recognition of the characteristic skin manifestations, angiokeratoma which usually appear during childhood (Figure 1.10.13): hundreds of tiny red or blue-black flat spots (angiectasias) or papules concentrated between the umbilicus and the knees with a predilection for the lower back, buttocks, and scrotum. Corneal opacities are also early findings (female carriers frequently have corneal abnormalities identified by slit-lamp microscopy) whereas cardiac, neurologic, and severe renal impairment occur later and may result in shortened lifespan. Diagnosis is confirmed by analysis of specific enzyme activity in leukocytes or plasma.

Sitosterolemia

Recurrent brief attacks of arthritis are usually part of this rare autosomal recessive disease in which patients exhibit hypercholesterolaemia, premature arteriosclerosis, and xanthomata of the tendons, accompanied by increased intestinal absorption of dietary sterols. The arthritis responds to treatment with cholestyramine and a low-sterol diet [44]. The underlying defect has been mapped to genes that encode members of the ATP-binding cassette (ABC) transporter family [45] suggesting that these transporters normally limit intestinal uptake of plant sterols and promote their excretion.

Multicentric reticulohistiocytosis

This entity mainly affects the skin and the synovium. Complaints of pruritis followed by the appearance of brownish, wart-like nodules on the face, ears, and dorsum of the hands often heralds the development of arthritis, which may be mistaken for JIA and is typically erosive [46,47]. Nodules may also be found in other locations, such as over elbows and knees. The histiocytic cells found in the nodules have been characterized by immunohistochemistry and stain positive for CD68 (macrophage-marker) and negative for S100 protein [48], among other markers. A familial form has been described; these children also

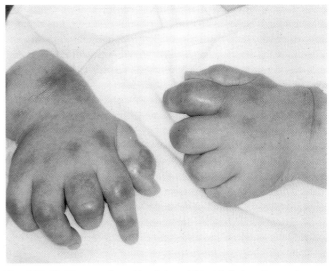

Fig. 1.10.12 Close-up view of hands in a child with Farber disease shows the nodular swelling and erythema around the wrists and phalangeal joints. Note the accentuation of the process over the medial aspects of the wrists about the biopsy scar. (Courtesy of K. Abul-Haj.)

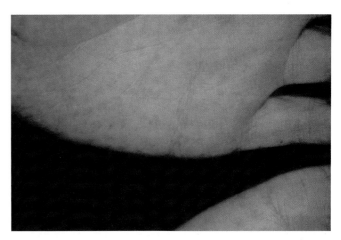

Fig. 1.10.13 Skin lesions of Fabry disease showing angiokeratoma of the ventral aspects of the hand. (From the National Library of Dermatologic Teaching Slides.)

had severe ocular disease including uveitis, cataracts, and glaucoma. Significant association with malignancy has been reported in adults with multicentric reticulohistiocytosis.

Immunodeficiency disorders

An underlying immunodeficiency is not often suspected when a child presents with a swollen joint mimicking JIA or with thrombocytopenia leading to a diagnosis of ITP. An increased risk of autoimmunity is, however, associated with many of the immunodeficiency syndromes and may be the first or the only sign of the underlying condition. The diagnosis of immune-deficiency would usually exclude JIA. Common variable immunodeficiency (CVID) and selective IgA deficiency are the two disorders most frequently associated with autoimmunity. For example, up to 20% of individuals with

CVID have features of autoimmunity [49,50]. The most common autoimmune manifestations are arthritis, and autoimmune hematologic disorders. Other disorders where autoimmunity appears frequently are the complement deficiencies, Wiskott–Aldrich syndrome, and the autoimmune lymphoproliferative syndrome (ALPS). The mechanism underlying the association between immunodeficiency and autoimmunity is complex and not were understood. An inherited immunodeficiency is the result of a mutation that affects one step in a pathway involved in innate or adaptive immune response; many of these pathways intersect and a single defect often affects more than one cellular function. The classification of the immunodeficiencies is traditionally based on the cell type that is primarily affected (Table 1.10.8). A child who presents with an autoimmune disorder of unclear etiology should have laboratory evaluation to screen for the possibility of an underlying immunodeficiency (Table 1.10.9), with individual tests selected based on the clinical history.

Bruton agammaglobulinemia

This is a rare X-linked recessive disorder that, in contrast to partial deficiency of immunoglobulin is quite unlikely to be complicated by autoimmune phenomena. Instead, septic arthritis is the most common cause of a swollen joint in affected children, who usually have been diagnosed with immunodeficiency early in life. Mycoplasma and ureaplasma induced septic arthritis are overrepresented. In addition, there is an unusual sensitivity to enteroviral and echoviral infections, and viral arthritis has been described. An association between these viral infections and meningoencephalitis has been well documented and includes a dermatomyositis like disease (Part 1, chapter 1.6), [51]. Children present in the first year of life with bacterial infections and decrease of all immunoglobulin isotypes. IgG levels are typically <100 mg/dl. Peripheral B cells (CD19 positive) are absent and on physical examination typically B cell-rich lymphoid tissues including tonsils and lymph nodes, are absent.

Common variable immunodeficiency

Diagnosis of Common variable immunodeficiency (CVID) (IgG typically 150–400 mg/dl) requires decrease (>2SD) of two immunoglobulin isotypes (measured at two different times) and deficient antibody response to vaccination with protein or carbohydrate antigens. The incidence of CVID may be as high as 1 : 50,000 with most individuals presenting with symptoms of immunodeficiency in the second decade of life. CVID is a heterogeneous disorder probably reflecting different genetic defects; approximately half of the patients have an associated T cell deficiency. Circulating B and T cell numbers are usually within normal levels; tonsils and lymph nodes are either normal or enlarged and splenomegaly may be present.

Table 1.10.8 Primary immunodeficiency disorders and most common autoimmune associations

Classification	Defect/cause	Autoimmune associations
Lymphocyte disorders		
Primarily B cell defects		
Bruton agammaglobulinema	Tyrosine kinase (btk)	Dermatomyositis-like illness, arthritis
Common variable immunodeficiency	* a	Arthritis, ITP, AHA, vasculitis
Selective IgA deficiency	Not identified	Oligoarthritis, SLE, vasculitis, thyroiditis, IBD, coeliac disease
Primarily T cell defects		
DiGeorge syndrome	22q11.2 deletion	AHA, ITP, arthritis
Hyper IgM immunodeficiency	CD40-ligand	arthritis
Combined B and T cell defects		
Severe combined immunodeficiency	Many genetic defects identified	None reported
Wiskott–Aldrich syndrome (WAS)	WAS-protein	Vasculitis, arthritis, IC-disease, AHA
Phagocyte disorders		
Chronic granulomatous disease (CGD)	Defective NADPH oxidase	DLE, SLE[b]
X-linked carriers of CGD		DLE, SLE[b]
Complement deficiency	C1q,C1r, or C1s deficiency	SLE (C1q: > 99%), urticarial vasculitis
	C2 homozygous deficiency	SLE (33%)
	C2 heterozygous deficiency	SLE (5%)
	C4 deficiency	SLE
	C3 deficiency	Bacterial infections, GN, SLE[c]
	C5–C9 deficiencies	Bacterial infections, SLE[c]
	Deficiency of C1inhibitor	Angioedema, SLE
Abnormalities of apoptosis		
Autoimmune lymphoproliferative syndrome (ALPS)	Fas, Fas ligand, caspase 10	AHA, ITP, neutropaenia

[a] Some individuals with common variable immunodeficiency have a defect in the inducible T cell co-stimulator (ICOS) receptor which regulates T cell activation in the immune response (78). [b] The association between DLE and the carrier-state of CGD appears to be the strongest (75); case reports describe the occurrence of SLE or DLE in patients with CGD (76, 77). [c] rare; case reports.

Abbreviations: AHA: autoimmune haemolytic anaemia, DLE: discoid lupus erythematosus, GN: glomerulonephritis (membranoproliferative), IBD: inflammatory bowel disease, IC: immune complex, ITP: idiopathic thrombocytopenia purpura, SLE: systemic lupus erythematousus.

Table 1.10.9 Laboratory evaluation of suspected immunodeficiency

Step 1
CBC and differential cell count[a]
Quantitative immunoglobulins (IgA, IgG, IgM)
Complement system: CH50
HIV
Any prior blood cultures or X-rays

Step 2
Individual complement components (if CH50 is low)
Antibody response to immunization with protein- and carbohydrate- antigens (pre- and post- immunization titres)
Peripheral blood leukocyte subsets: T (CD3, CD4, CD8), B (CD19), NK (CD56), monocytes (CD16)
Skin test for delayed type hypersensitivity (should include at least 3 different antigens)[b], or *In vitro* tests for T cell
  function: mitogen and/or antigen stimulation
IgG subclasses
Evaluation of phagocytic function[c]
Leukocyte adhesion defect 1(CD18)

Step 3
Specialized tests for phagocytic function: chemotaxis, bactericidal activity
Complement pathway function including alternate pathway
Cytokine production, cytokine receptors, signalling pathways[d]

[a]Lymphopaenia is associated with immunodeficiency disorders, autoimmunity, viral disease, hematopoetic malignancies, and malnutrition. An absolute lymphocyte count <1500 warrants further evaluation.

[b]At ages <1 year the DTH reaction is not reliable (may be falsely negative) for detection of cellular defect.

[c]The NBT-assay, which analyses the ability of the normal phagocyte to reduce the dye nitro blue tetrazolium (NBT) to a purple compound and the failure to do so in phagocytes obtained from individuals with CGD, is still widely used. However, the DHR (dihydrorhodamine) 123 assay, which uses flow cytometry to measure the fluorescence of rhodamine 123 in normal, activated phagocytes is increasingly replacing the NBT test because of its sensitivity and higher reproducibility; stimulated neutrophils are incubated with DHR 123 which is converted to the fluorescent rhodamine 123 if the neutrophil contains an intact NADPH oxidase complex that generates superoxide radicals.

[d]These tests are for the most part only available on a research basis.

The cause of arthritis in CVID is multifactorial and includes both common and uncommon bacterial infections and autoimmunity. Several large, longitudinal studies of arthritis in patients with CVID indicate that they are particularly susceptible to synovial infection with different strains of mycoplasma and ureaplasma [52]. The low immunoglobulin levels appear to predispose to mucosal colonization, with these bacteria leading to increased risk of dissemination to other sites, such as the joint. The differential from reactive or autoimmune arthritis is not as easy as in the case of septic arthritis caused by encapsulated bacteria; PCR-based analysis to detect these organisms in the joint fluid should be considered when cultures are negative. In all individuals with CVID who develop arthritis the first therapeutic modality in addition to antibiotics should be intravenous immunoglobulin (IVIG) to ensure steady state levels above 700 mg/dl. A 3-month course of doxycyclin has been recommended for treatment-resistant arthritis in patients with CVID [52] (see also Part 1, Chapter 1.5). In most patients the arthritis resolves with this treatment. Sometimes antibiotic treatment is not sufficient and it is this group of individuals that has true autoimmune arthritis as compared with those who may suffer from reactive arthritis precipitated by recurrent infection (see also Part 1, Chapter 1.4). Standard anti-inflammatory or immunosuppressive therapy may be indicated but with caution so as to not worsen an already compromised immune status.

Autoimmune haemolytic disorders, gastrointestinal disease (e.g. coeliac disease) and chronic pulmonary disease sometimes with the formation of granuloma are other problems encountered with increased frequency in individuals with CVID [52].

Selective IgA deficiency

This is the most common of all immunodeficiency disorders (IgA <5–10 mg/dl), affecting as many as 1:300–1:500 children depending on the population studied. Approximately half of all affected individuals are asymptomatic, the rest have recurrent infections of the respiratory, gastrointestinal, or urinary tract. IgG2 and/or IgG4 subclass deficiency is found in approximately 15% of individuals with IgA deficiency and increase the risk of overt clinical symptoms. Individuals with IgA deficiency may go on to develop CVID and in some families the two disorders coexist. Autoimmunity occurs frequently (ranging between 7 and 36% in different studies) and includes a spectrum of different disorders (Table 1.10.8) with arthritis and SLE most commonly described.

In patients with JIA the frequency of IgA deficiency is 2–4%, with the majority having Oligoarthritis [53]; however, polyarticular disease and erosions develop in as many as 25% of affected children.

Individuals with IgA-deficiency are at risk of developing anaphylactic reactions to IgA if re-exposed to blood or serum products containing IgA [54]. Peripheral B cell numbers are normal.

DiGeorge syndrome/Velocardiofacial syndrome

The extent of immunodeficiency in patients with DiGeorge syndrome is highly variable and does not correlate with any other phenotypic features. It is caused by the absence or impaired formation of thymic epithelium (the thymic shadow is characteristically absent on chest radiographs) which leads to decreased production of immunocompetent T cells. CD4 and CD8 positive cells are decreased or absent and there is defective response to mitogen and antigen stimulation in the severely affected individual. Immune cytopenias and arthritis have been reported in patients with DiGeorge syndrome and appear to be significantly increased over normal [55].

Velocardiofacial syndrome, a closely related 1q22 deletion syndrome, is also associated with increased prevalence of JIA [56].

Wiskott–Aldrich syndrome (WAS)

Wiskott–Aldrich syndrome is characterized by eczema (Figure 1.10.14), thrombocytopenia (and small platelets), and recurrent infections. Inheritance is X-linked recessive. Often, the affected child presents in infancy with bloody diarrhoea due to thrombocytopenia. Patients have increased susceptibility to pyogenic infections and opportunistic infections. Antibody formation, particularly to carbohydrate antigens, is defective and isohaemagglutinins are typically not present; IgG levels are generally within normal range. T cells respond poorly to *in vitro* stimulation. The defective protein, WASP, is located in the cytoplasm and probably exerts its normal function through interactions with actin and other proteins of the cytoskeleton. The immunodeficiency is believed to result from an inability of the T cell to reorganize its cytoskeleton in the normal response to signals generated through interactions with antigen presenting cells; however, this mechanism only explains some of the immune-related problems encountered in these patients. WASP is mainly expressed in white blood cells and megakaryocytes.

Autoimmune phenomena in the form of Coombs positive haemolytic anaemia, vasculitis, and arthritis are relatively common. Immune complex disease and allergy also appear to be increased [57]. The arthritis associated with WAS is frequently migratory or transient and affects approximately 20% of patients [58]. Rarely described complications include a necrotizing vasculitis affecting medium- and small-size vessels and formation of aneurysms that may lead to life-threatening haemorrhage. Peripheral B and T cell numbers are initially normal but after 6 years of age T cells start to decline and B cells may undergo a general polyclonal expansion [57].

Autoimmune lymphoproliferative syndrome (ALPS)

Autoimmune lymphoproliferative syndrome is characterized by splenomegaly, lymphadenopathy, increased susceptibility to infection, and frequent autoimmunity [59], in particular autoimmune cytopenias. An urticarial rash has also been described. Inheritance is autosomal dominant and clinical heterogeneity expressed even within families is common. The underlying problem is a defect in Fas-mediated apopto-

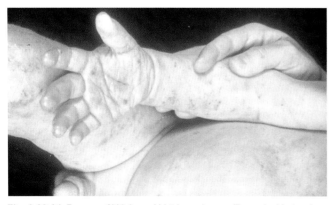

Fig. 1.10.14 Eczema of Wiskott–Aldrich syndrome. (From the National Library of Dermatologic Teaching Slides.)

sis or programmed cell death. Exposure to antigen normally results in massive expansion of activated lymphocytes; most of these cells undergo apoptosis once the infection is cleared and the effector cell is no longer needed. Children with a defect in the apoptotic pathway may develop dramatic lymphadenopathy following infections (Figure 1.10.15 (a), (b)). Slow spontaneous resolution of the lymphadenopathy usually occurs and may be hastened by short-term use of corticosteroids. Apoptosis is also an important mechanism in the regulation of intrathymic maturation of T cells; affected patients release increased numbers of immature, double-negative (DN) T cells (CD3$^+$4$^-$ 8$^-$) into the circulation. An increased number of (DN) T cells in peripheral blood is highly suggestive of ALPS. (DN) T cells normally comprise less than 2% of circulating T cells.

Streaking leukocyte factor

The first case, reported by Jacobs [60], was, a 2-year-old boy with massive monarticular joint effusion and later pyoderma gangrenosum following minor trauma (Figure 1.10.16 (a), (b)). The major early handicap was repetitive, erroneous diagnosis of septic arthritis with unnecessary

(a)

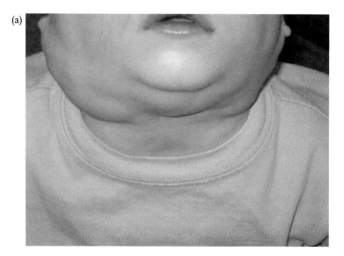

(b)

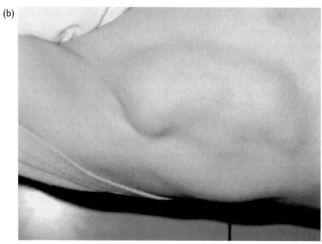

Fig. 1.10.15 This 3½-year-old male presented in the neonatal period with haemolytic anaemia, thrombocytopaenia, and lymphadenopathy. The diagnosis of autoimmune lymphoproliferative syndrome was confirmed by identification of a mutation in Fas receptor (CD95); the same mutation was also found in the patient's mother and sister. He developed massive (a) cervical and (b) axillary lymphadenopathy after an upper respiratory infection.

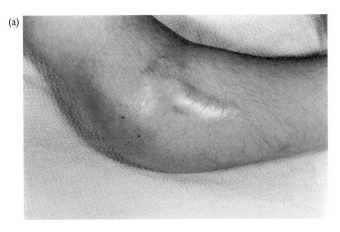

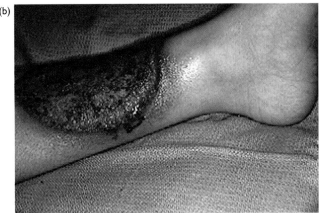

Fig. 1.10.16 (a) Clinical appearance of effused elbow in a boy with "streaking leukocyte factor". Aspiration yielded purulent but sterile fluid (WBC > 100,000/mm³). (b) Giant leg ulcer typical of those that recurred in this patient. Local treatment and grafting were unsuccessful but the ulcers healed promptly when large doses of steroids were administered.

long hospitalizations, surgery, and antibiotic therapy. The episodes of arthritis were ultimately self-limited or could be controlled by corticosteroids. Corticosteroids and later FK506 were required to control the scarring pyoderma lesions. A second patient presenting with pyoderma gangrenosum at the site of DPT injection and subsequently at sites of minor trauma was also identified by Jacobs. These children may have PAPA syndrome (see Part 1, Chapter 1.7).

Dialysis-related arthritis

Beta-2-microglobulin amyloidosis

Amyloid formation with beta-2-microglobulin deposition occurs in approximately 10% of adults receiving long-term haemo- or peritoneal dialysis [61]. The amyloidosis is associated with both articular and periarticular symptoms that include the carpal tunnel syndrome, arthralgia, bone cysts, and destructive arthritis.

Calcific periarthritis

Pseudogout, an acute inflammatory syndrome in elderly patients with chondrocalcinosis is caused by precipitation of calcium pyrophosphate crystals in the synovial space. No such situation has been seen in children. Children with chronic renal failure and receiving dialysis,

may however, develop recurrent attacks of periarticular pain and tenosynovitis caused by precipitation of calcium pyrophosphate crystals in tendons and periarticular tissues. There are usually no detectable microcrystals in the joint fluid [62]. The syndrome is related to the hyperphosphataemia of chronic renal failure and may be prevented by more frequent dialysis, limiting phosphate intake, and the administration of aluminum hydroxide gel to bind phosphates in the gastrointestinal tract and prevent their absorption.

Primary tumours of the bones and joints (Table 1.10.10)

Primary bone tumours are not rare in childhood and may occasionally mimic a rheumatic disorder.

Malignant bone tumors produce pain that increases over a period of weeks; night pain in the adolescent is particularly worrisome. Bony and soft tissue tenderness is often present during palpation of the affected area. Diagnosis is frequently apparent on plain radiographs. Malignant tumours adjacent to the sacroiliac joint may not be visible on plain X-rays but may show up as "hot spots" on bone scan. CT scan is helpful in demonstrating these lesions.

Benign tumours of bone are often asymptomatic and coincidentally noted on X-rays obtained for other reasons but may present with pain, including night pain.

Benign tumours of bone and cartilage

Benign fibrous lesions (fibrous dysplasia, fibrocortical defects, nonossifying fibroma, and ossifying fibroma).

Fibrous dysplasia is a developmental defect of bone that most commonly appears as a single lesion in late childhood particularly of a rib. Expansion and bone deformity with pathologic fractures may develop and internal fixation of the bone may be required. The radiographic appearance of fibrous dysplasia can vary from a discrete lucency to a patchy and sclerotic lesion; there is usually a well-defined sclerotic margin. Periostitis and pain are not reported. Fibrous dysplasia has a

Table 1.10.10 Primary tumours of bone and of tissues in and around the joint

Benign	Malignant
Tumours of bone and cartilage	
Benign fibrous lesions	Ewing sarcoma
Bone cyst	Osteosarcoma
Chondroma/enchondroma	
Eosinophilic granuloma	
Osteoblastoma	
Osteochondroma	
Osteoid osteoma	
Tumours of tissues in and around the joint	
Ganglion	Chondrosarcoma
Lipoma	Clear-cell sarcoma
Neurofibroma	Epithelioid sarcoma
Pigmented villonodular synovitis	Fibrosarcoma
Synovial chondromatosis	Rhabdomyosarcoma
Synovial haemangioma	Synovial sarcoma
Xanthoma	

predilection for the pelvis, proximal femur, ribs, and skull. In the McCune–Albright syndrome patients develop polyostotic fibrous dysplasia (Figure 1.10.17), skin hyperpigmentation (café au lait spots), and endocrine dysfunction. Due to multiple bony lesions, affected individuals develop bone pain, deformity, and recurrent fractures. Biphosphonate therapy diminishes bone pain and increases mobility [63].

Fibrocortical defects produce no symptoms and resolve spontaneously; they occur as an incidental finding on radiographs. A

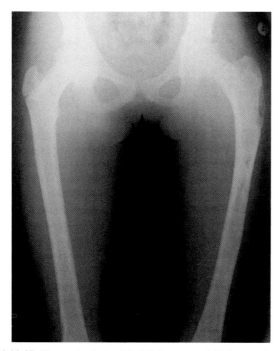

Fig. 1.10.17 Fibrous dysplasia of the left femur in a child diagnosed with McCune–Albright syndrome.

nonossifying fibroma is a large fibrocortical defect (> 2 cm) and has been reported in up to 20% of children. It is usually asymptomatic, heals with sclerosis, and disappears over time. The lesion is typically located in the metaphyseal cortex of the long bones with the characteristic radiograph showing a thin sclerotic border that is scalloped and slightly expansile; there is no associated periostitis or tenderness to palpation. The radiographic diagnosis of nonossifying fibroma is usually sufficient for its correct identification [64] (Figure 1.10.18). Rarely, a pathological fracture occurs requiring excision or internal reinforcement. An ossifying fibroma is a rare fibro-osseous tumour that mainly occurs in the craniofacial region. It is benign but expands locally causing deformity. Complete removal is required to prevent recurrence.

Bone cyst

A simple bone cyst (unicameral bone cyst) occurs commonly in the metaphysis of the proximal humerus or the proximal femur. It is usually asymptomatic but may be complicated by a pathologic fracture (Figure 1.10.19). It has a characteristic radiographic appearance; the lesion is central in location in the affected bone and has well-defined margins and little surrounding reaction. Current treatment includes steroid-injection into the lesion, curettage, and bone grafting. The prognosis is excellent; some bone cysts heal spontaneously.

Chondroma/enchondroma

This is a cartilage tumor that grows within the bone and occurs most often in the small bones of the hands and feet (Figure 1.10.20). It may present as a single painless mass and may be mistaken for arthritis by causing limitations in range of motion. When the tumour is completely confined within the bone it constitutes an enchondroma. Ollier disease (OMIM 166000 [4]) is characterized by multiple enchondromas of the hands and feet; manifesting with stiff joints and limitation in range of motion thus simulating arthritis of the hands. In Maffucci

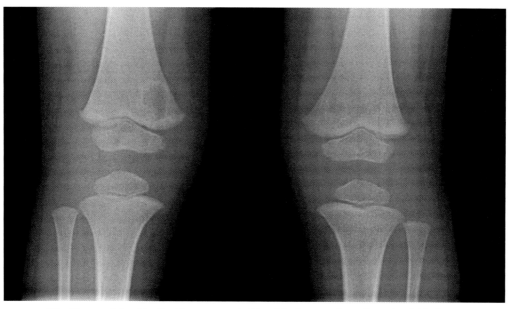

Fig. 1.10.18 A large non-ossifying fibroma of the right distal femur was an incidental finding on radiographs in this child who presented with cellulites of the right thigh and suspected osteomyelitis necessitating radiographic evaluation. A smaller non-ossifying fibroma is also present in the left distal femur.

syndrome (OMIM 166000 [4]), multiple enchondromas coexist with multiple cavernous haemangiomas. In patients with multiple enchondromas, in particular those with Maffucis syndrome, there is a potential for malignant transformation of an enchondroma to a chondrosarcoma or other sarcomas. The chondrosarcoma is usually associated with bone pain. Case reports have described malignant transformation of solitary enchondromas.

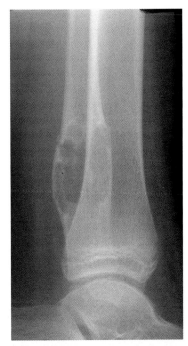

Fig. 1.10.19 Bone cyst of the fibula with secondary fracture in a child who presented with sudden ankle pain.

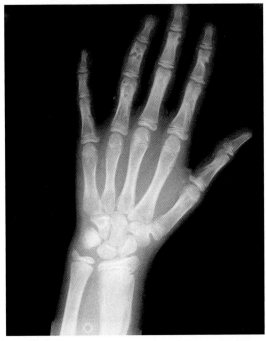

Fig. 1.10.20 Radiograph showing multiple enchondroma in a child who complained of stiffness of the hands.

Eosinophilic granuloma

Langerhans cell histiocytosis includes a diverse group of proliferative disorders originating from cells of the monocyte-macrophage lineage. The clinical spectrum ranges from fatal disseminated disease to a benign lesion of the bone, called eosinophilic granuloma. Bone lesions may be single or multiple and are commonly located in the skull (Figure 1.10.21(a)). A solitary bone lesion may also develop in the bones of the pelvis or femur and present with hip/back pain or a painless limp (Figure 1.10.21(b)). Pathological fractures may occur through an eosinophilic granuloma including compression fractures of the spine. Location in the cervical spine may cause neck pain or torticollis, suggestive of JIA. The solitary form is usually found in children over two years of age. Radiographs are not diagnostic; they demonstrate a lytic or blastic lesion that can be either well or ill defined [64]. Definite diagnosis requires a biopsy with identification of the typical Langerhans cell that stains positive for the S100 protein on immunohistochemistry.

Osteoid osteoma

This relatively common benign tumor of bone produces a characteristic localized aching or boring bone pain, worse at night and at rest or with elevation. The pain is usually responsive to nonsteroidal anti-inflammatory treatment. Half of the reported cases occurred between the ages of 11 and 20 years, with a male predominance; 75% of the reported lesions were in the femur or the tibia. Synovitis, sympathetic effusions, demineralization, and muscle atrophy occur and may be apparent long before the lesion itself is demonstrable radiographically (Figure 1.10.22), which may take up to 2 years. Pain from these tumours may be referred to adjacent joints. When the tumour is in the vertebrae, painful scoliosis or radicular pain down the arm or leg may be the major complaint, sometimes with muscle atrophy. Histologically, this tumour consists of a tiny nidus of osteoid and new bone within highly vascularized osteogenic connective tissue. Radiographically, a reactive layer of sclerotic bone is seen around the lucent or calcified nidus; cortical thickening is a characteristic finding but periosteal new-bone formation is rare and would usually suggest a malignant process. CT scan and technetium bone scan are more sensitive diagnostic

(a)   (b)

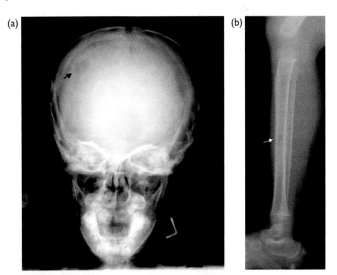

Fig. 1.10.21 Eosinophilic granuloma (lesions indicated by arrows) of the (a) skull and (b) leg in a 2-year-old who presented to the emergency room with a lump on the head after an accidental fall. History obtained in the emergency room revealed prior complaints of leg pain.

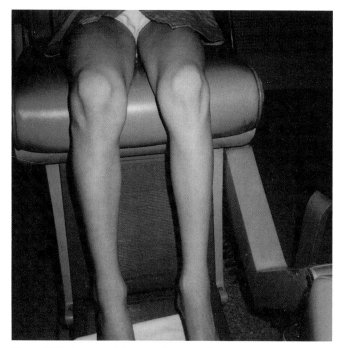

Fig. 1.10.22 Atrophy of the entire leg caused by an unrecognized osteoid osteoma in the foot.

tools than X-rays (Figure 1.10.23 (a), (b)). Depending on the accessibility of the tumour, treatment includes surgical removal and replacement with autologous bone graft, CT-guided core excision or percutaneous radiofrequency (thermal) ablation [65]. In untreated cases the pain may disappear over time and a sclerotic "scar" may be all that remains visible radiographically.

Osteoblastoma

This is a rare lesion that may have the appearance of a giant osteoid osteoma with an osteolytic component >1 cm. The lesion is clinically similar to an osteoid osteoma but is usually more destructive. There are reports of locally invasive osteoblastomas that do not metastasize.

Another radiographic appearance of an osteoblastoma resembles that of an aneurysmal bone cyst with a well-defined, expansile lytic lesion [64].

Osteochondroma

This is the most common benign bone tumour. It arises by enchondral ossification under a layer of cartilage and usually presents as a painless mass that may become painful if traumatized. An osteochondroma may grow to a large size; it is removed only if symptomatic. The radiograph is characteristic, showing a pedunculated or sessile lesion. Osteochondromas are most commonly found in the proximal humerus or in the metaphyses on either side of the joint. Malignant transformation to chondrosarcoma occurs rarely (1%). Multiple osteochondromas (multiple cartilaginous exostoses) occur in some children as an autosomal dominant trait (Figure 1.10.24). This condition is often complicated by deformities of the involved bone or limb-shortening. [66].

Malignant tumours of bone and cartilage

Osteosarcoma

This is the most common malignant bone tumor in children with a peak incidence during the adolescent growth spurt [67]. The tumour often occurs in the metaphysis of rapidly growing bone with typical

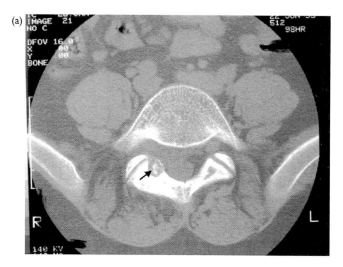

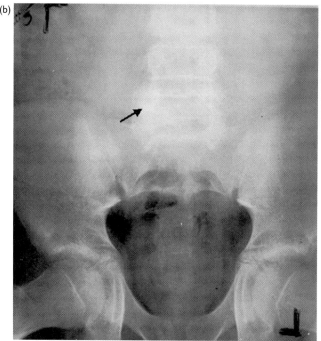

Fig. 1.10.23 (a) CT of the spine in a child who complained of back pain demonstrates an osteoid osteoma with a lytic nidus and surrounding sclerosis. (b) Radiographs of the spine in the same child only showed the reactive sclerosis.

location to the distal femur, proximal tibia, or proximal humerus. It frequently causes an osteoblastic response and a large soft tissue mass adjacent to the primary tumour. A persistent deep bone pain is characteristic. Radiographs commonly identify a destructive and sclerotic lesion with periosteal new-bone formation (Figure 1.10.25); rarely the lesion is entirely lytic [64]. Biopsy is required for diagnosis. Metastatic disease in the lungs (90%) or bone (10%) is present in approximately 20% of individuals at the time of diagnosis [67]. Children with hereditary retinoblastoma, the Li-Fraumeni syndrome (p53 mutation), or enchondromatosis have increased risk of developing osteosarcoma. Prior exposure to ionizing radiation may also increase the risk.

Ewing sarcoma

This is the second most common bone tumour in children with peak incidence during the second decade of life. Its typical location is in the

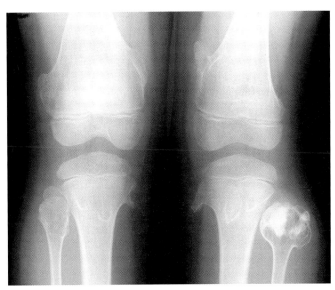

Fig. 1.10.24 Multiple osteochondromas in a child who presented with knee pain and swelling. There was a positive family history of "bumps" around the joints

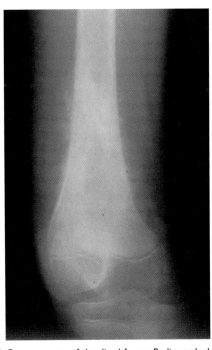

Fig. 1.10.25 Osteosarcoma of the distal femur. Radiograph shows a mixed lytic and sclerotic lesion with an aggressive sunburst periostitis.

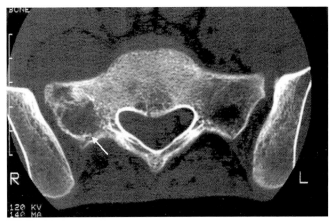

Fig. 1.10.26 Plain radiographs were normal in this child who presented with right-sided hip- and buttock-pain. CT scan demonstrated the lytic lesion of a Ewing sarcoma and disruption of the cortex (arrow).

evaluate the extent of the primary disease and bone scan and bone marrow biopsy are important to demonstrate the presence of metastases. Metastatic disease to the lungs or bones is present in approximately 20% of patients at time of diagnosis. Ewing sarcoma of the spine may present with gait abnormalities and leg pain (Figure 1.10.27).

Benign tumours of tissues in and around the joint

Ganglion

Ganglions are cyst-like, often tense, outpouchings of tendon sheaths or joint capsules and occur commonly in children. They are called Baker's cysts when located in the popliteal space, usually disappear spontaneously over time and tend to recur if surgically removed. Popliteal cysts sometimes dissect and rupture into the calf and simulate venous thrombosis, or rarely may dissect into the anterior leg or the thigh. Ganglions are thought to be a response to local irritation, resulting in increased production of joint fluid and causing the narrow neck between joint and bursa to act as a ball valve, preventing the fluid from re-entering the joint. No treatment is necessary but wrapping the calf with an elastic bandage is helpful.

Synovial outpouchings of the wrists and knees occur frequently in JIA and are usually soft, bilateral, and easily distinguishable from ordinary ganglions because of their size and location. Such cysts contain turbid low-viscosity inflammatory joint fluid, unlike the clear jelly of the simple ganglion. Occasionally, what seems like a ganglion (or Baker cyst) is the first sign of JIA. This is so infrequent, however, that children with ganglions and without arthritis who have undergone a thorough physical examination of their musculoskeletal system and slit-lamp examination of their eyes require no additional studies to exclude JIA.

Neurofibroma

Neurofibromatosis type 1 is a common hereditary disorder with an incidence around 1 in 3000 births. The disease is characterized by café au lait spots, neurofibromas, mental deficiency, and skeletal deformities. Spinal misalignment and scoliosis are the most common skeletal abnormalities. One child presented with monoarthritis of the knee caused by a neurofibroma that involved the vastus lateralis muscle and extended to the level of the knee joint [68]; MRI identified the correct diagnosis.

flat bones or the diaphysis of the long bones but it may also originate in the soft tissues. Patients typically complain of pain and swelling of the involved area often with fever and other systemic symptoms, such as weight loss and elevated ESR. The symptoms may be chronic or intermittent, sometimes leading to a delay in diagnosis. Radiographs demonstrate an aggressive, typically lytic tumour often with adjacent soft tissue mass and occasionally the lesion is predominantly sclerotic or mixed lytic and sclerotic (Figure 1.10.26). Amorphous and sunburst periostitis is a characteristic associated finding. MRI is used to

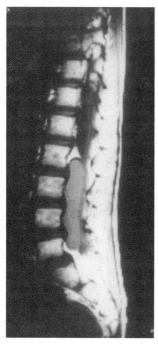

Fig. 1.10.27 MRI revealing non-osseus Ewing sarcoma invading the spinal cord in a young child who presented with polyarthralgias and an unusual gait thought to initially have JIA. (Courtesy of M. Klein-Gitelman.)

Synovial hemangiomas

These blood-vessel tumors (malformations) may occur as part of a more generalized disorder, such as Mafficci syndrome or Von Hippel-Lindau syndrome (visceral angiomatosis) or may be limited to the joints and periarticular tissues. One or multiple joints may be affected. Symptoms generally begin in childhood, but the correct diagnosis is rarely confirmed before young adulthood [69]. The patients have episodic attacks of excruciating pain after mild trauma, sometimes with only minimal swelling and discolouration of overlying skin. Aspiration yields grossly bloody fluid. The knee is most frequently involved, but elbow and ankle haemangiomas have also been reported. A mass may be palpated adjacent to the joint. Recurrent brief attacks of joint pain with effusion are characteristic. MRI has become the preferred diagnostic modality for synovial soft tissue tumours [70]. Surgical removal is often indicated but it may be impossible to completely remove diffuse lesions, and recurrences are common.

Pigmented villonodular synovitis (PVNS)

Teenagers and adults may develop pigmented villonodular synovitis, a unique diffuse chronic synovitis almost always limited to a single knee. PVNS is clinically suggested by the finding of chocolate-brown synovial fluid at arthrocenthesis. The disease is rarely seen in children younger than 10 years [71]. The synovial involvement may be localized to a well-defined mass or it may diffuse; mixed forms are also seen. MRI characteristically demonstrates the intra-articular lesion with areas of low signal (T1- and T2- weighted images) due to hemosiderin deposits within the lesion. Synovial biopsy shows a dense cellular infiltrate without lining-cell hyperplasia but with numerous microscopic villi and hemosiderin-pigment-loaded stromal cells. PVNS may extend into surrounding tissues, such as the tendons, ligaments, muscle, bone, and skin. Invasion of bone is reflected by the radiographic appearance of cystic lesions on both sides of the joint space. The etiology of this uncommon disease is unknown and the course is uncertain;

some patients may be adequately managed with nonsteroidal anti-inflammatory drugs, and the disease may remit without surgery. The localized form is usually amenable to surgical excision but the diffuse form is more difficult to treat and has a high rate of recurrence. Adjuvant post-synovectomy radiotherapy may improve the outcome of the initial surgical resection [72].

Synovial chondromatosis

These patients develop intrasynovial cartilaginous nodules that ultimately project above the surface and may calcify. Some shed into the joint space as loose bodies, producing pain, swelling, and mechanical limitations. The condition is rare; malignant transformation has been reported but is unusual. The male knee is most commonly affected, occasionally bilaterally. The youngest reported patient was 14 years of age. Unless the lesions calcify and are apparent on X-ray, the diagnosis cannot be made clinically but might be confirmed by arthroscopy. Therapy has consisted of removal of the loose bodies and the affected synovium [73], occasional patients have spontaneous regression of the tumour.

Malignant tumours of tissues in and around the joint

Synovial sarcoma

Synovial, epithelioid, and clear-cell sarcomas have all been reported in children but they are extremely rare in this age group. Synovial sarcoma is the most common and, although most cases occur between 15 and 30 years of age, the youngest reported patient was only 13 months old at the time of diagnosis. These tumours are usually located in the soft tissues outside the joints and it is for this reason that joint biopsies generally are not necessary; most reported patients have presented with obvious extra-articular soft-tissue masses that demanded biopsy. A common clinical presentation is a firm or elastic soft-tissue lump that is often painless. Anatomic continuity with a joint or surrounding tissues is rare, and even when the lesions are contiguous with a joint capsule, the joint itself is rarely invaded, although there may be a sympathetic joint effusion. A balanced, pathognomonic translocation: t(X;18) (p11;q11), is found in 90% of synovial sarcomas [74].

Epithelioid sarcomas arise from fascia, tendon sheath, and periosteum. Although related to synovial sarcomas, they are morphologically distinctive with a characteristic nodular pattern that, with low-power microscopy, can be confused with an inflammatory granuloma. This is the most common soft-tissue sarcoma of the hand and presents as a painless mass over the fingers, hand, or wrist; it is rare elsewhere. A similar tumour over the ankle, heel, or plantar region of the foot, said to most resemble an epithelial neoplasm, has been termed clear-cell sarcoma.

Rhabdomyosarcoma

This is the most common paediatric soft tissue sarcoma and accounts for 5–8% of childhood malignancies. While rhabdomyosarcoma may occur in almost any location it has a predilection for the head and neck, and 20% originate in the extremities [67]. Symptoms and prognosis are both site dependent. The most common presentation is a painless mass that may cause musculoskeletal symptoms if located in proximity to the bones and joints (Figure 1.10.28). Metastatic spread occurs to regional lymph-nodes, lungs, bone, and bone marrow. MRI and CT are useful in the initial evaluation of a soft tissue mass and should include draining lymph nodes.

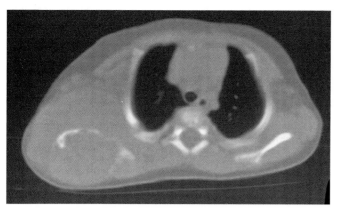

Fig. 1.10.28 CT scan obtained in a 3-year-old who presented with decreased range of motion of the shoulder demonstrates a large tumour identified to be a rhabdomyosarcoma.

Any child suspected to have a malignant tumour should be promptly referred to a paediatric cancer center for complete evaluation and treatment.

Acknowledgment

The author wishes to thank Carrie Ruzal-Shapiro, MD for her invaluable assistance in selecting appropriate images from the teaching file collection of the Department of Pediatrics and Radiology, Columbia University, New York.

References

1. Schaller, J. Arthritis as a presenting manifestation of malignancy in children. *J Pediatr* 1972;81:793–7.

2. Cabral, D.A. and Tucker, L.B. Malignancies in children who initially present with rheumatic complaints. *J Pediatr* 1999;134:53–7.

3. Rogalsky, R.J., Black, G.B., and Reed, M.H. Orthopedic manifestations of leukemia in children. *J Bone Joint Surg Am* 1986;68:494–501.

4. McKusick, V. Online Mendelian Inheritance in Man. Johns Hopkins University. *www.ncbi.nlm.nih.gov/entrez/omim.*

5. Dixey, J., Redington, A.N., Butler, R.C., Smith, M.J., Batchelor, J.R., Woodrow, D.F., Hodson, M.E., Batten, J.C., and Brewerton, D.A. The arthropathy of cystic fibrosis. *Ann Rheum Dis* 1988;47:218–23.

6. Finnegan, M.J., Hinchcliffe, J., Russell-Jones, D., Neill, S., Sheffield, E., Jayne, D., Wise, A., and Hodson, M.E. Vasculitis complicating cystic fibrosis. *Q J Med* 1989;72:609–21.

7. Sagransky, D.M., Greenwald, R.A., and Gorvoy, J.D. Seropositive rheumatoid arthritis in a patient with cystic fibrosis. *Am J Dis Child* 1980;134:319–20.

8. Parasa, R.B. and Maffulli, N. Musculoskeletal involvement in cystic fibrosis. *Bull Hosp Jt Dis* 1999;58:37–44.

9. Lubrano, E., Ciacci, C., Ames, P.R., Mazzacca, G., Oriente, P., and Scarpa, R. The arthritis of coeliac disease: prevalence and pattern in 200 adult patients. *Br J Rheumatol* 1996;35:1314–18.

10. Falcini, F., Ferrari, R., Simonini, G., Calabri, G.B., Pazzaglia, A., and Lionetti, P. Recurrent monoarthritis in an 11-year-old boy with occult coeliac disease. Successful and stable remission after gluten-free diet. *Clin Exp Rheumatol* 1999;17:509–11.

11. Diggs, L.W. Bone and joint lesions in sickle-cell disease. *Clin Orthop* 1967;52:119–43.

12. Reiter, C.D., Wang, X., Tanus-Santos, J.E., Hogg, N., Cannon, R.O., Schechter, A.N., and Gladwin, M.T. Cell-free hemoglobin limits nitric oxide bioavailability in sickle-cell disease. *Nat Med* 2002;8:1383–9.

13. Gerster, J.C., Dardel, R., and Guggi, S. Recurrent episodes of arthritis in thalassemia minor. *J Rheumatol* 1984;11:352–4.

14. Roosendaal, G., Vianen, M.E., Marx, J.J., van den Berg, H.M., Lafeber, F.P., and Bijlsma, J.W. Blood-induced joint damage: a human in vitro study. *Arthritis Rheum* 1999;42:1025–32.

15. Fischer, K., van der Bom, J.G., Mauser-Bunschoten, E.P., Roosendaal, G., Prejs, R., de Kleijn, P., Grobbee, D.E., and van den Berg, M. The effects of postponing prophylactic treatment on long-term outcome in patients with severe hemophilia. *Blood* 2002;99:2337–41.

16. Hilgartner, M.W. Current treatment of hemophilic arthropathy. *Curr Opin Pediatr* 2002;14:46–9.

17. Klofkorn, R.W. and Lightsey, A.L. Hemarthrosis associated with Glanzmann's thrombasthenia. *Arthritis Rheum* 1979;22:1390–93.

18. Sokoloff, L. Kashin-Beck disease. *Rheum Dis Clin North Am* 1987;13:101–4.

19. Solomon, L., McLaren, P., Irwig, L., Gear, J.S., Schnitzler, C.M., Gear, A., and Mann, D. Distinct types of hip disorder in Mseleni joint disease. *S Afr Med J* 1986;69:15–17.

20. Verrotti, A., Chiarelli, F., and Morgese, G. Limited joint mobility in children with type 1 diabetes mellitus. A critical review. *J Pediatr Endocrinol Metab* 1996;9:3–8.

21. Silverstein, J.H., Gordon, G., Pollock, B.H., and Rosenbloom, A.L. Long-term glycemic control influences the onset of limited joint mobility in type 1 diabetes. *J Pediatr* 1998;132:944–7.

22. Bland, J.H. and Frymoyer, J.W. Rheumatic syndromes of myxedema. *N Engl J Med* 1970;282:1171–4.

23. Hunter, T., Chalmers, I.M., Dube, W.J., and Schroeder, M.L. Episodic polyarthralgia associated with Hashimoto's thyroiditis. *Arthritis Rheum* 1988;31:303.

24. LeRiche, N.G. and Bell, D.A. Hashimoto's thyroiditis and polyarthritis: a possible subset of seronegative polyarthritis. *Ann Rheum Dis* 1984;43:594–8.

25. Case records of the Massachusetts General Hospital. Weekly clinicopathological exercises. Case 21–2002. A 21-year-old man with arthritis during treatment for hyperthyroidism. *N Engl J Med* 2002;347:122–30.

26. Levy, E.N., Ramsey-Goldman, R., and Kahl, L.E. Adrenal insufficiency in two women with anticardiolipin antibodies. Cause and effect? *Arthritis Rheum* 1990;33:1842–6.

27. Chesney, R.W. Metabolic bone diseases. *Pediatr in Review* 1984;5:227–37.

28. Autosomal dominant hypophosphataemic rickets is associated with mutations in FGF23. The ADHR Consortium. *Nat Genet* 2000;26:345–8.

29. Hathcock, J.N., Hattan, D.G., Jenkins, M.Y., McDonald, J.T., Sundaresan, P.R., and Wilkening, V.L. Evaluation of vitamin A toxicity. *Am J Clin Nutr* 1990;52:183–202.

30. Lippe, B., Hensen, L., Mendoza, G., Finerman, M., and Welch, M. Chronic vitamin A intoxication. A multisystem disease that could reach epidemic proportions. *Am J Dis Child* 1981;135:634–6.

31. Fisher, R.L., Medcalf, T.W., and Henderson, M.C. Endemic fluorosis with spinal cord compression. A case report and review. *Arch Intern Med* 1989;149:697–700.

32. Savas, S., Cetin, M., Akdogan, M., and Heybeli, N. Endemic fluorosis in Turkish patients: relationship with knee osteoarthritis. *Rheumatol Int* 2001;21:30–5.

33. Mason, J.O. From the Assistant Secretary for Health, US Public Health Service. *JAMA* 1991;265:2939.

34. Wilcox, W.D. Abnormal serum uric acid levels in children. *J Pediatr* 1996;128:731–41.

35. Sege-Peterson, K., Chambers, J., Page, T., Jones, O.W., and Nyhan, W.L. Characterization of mutations in phenotypic variants of hypoxanthine phosphoribosyltransferase deficiency. *Hum Mol Genet* 1992;1:427–32.

36. Greene, H.L., Wilson, F.A., Hefferan, P., Terry, A.B., Moran, J.R., Slonim, A.E., Claus, T.H., and Burr, I.M. ATP depletion, a possible role in the pathogenesis of hyperuricemia in glycogen storage disease type I. *J Clin Invest* 1978;62:321–8.

37. Mineo, I., Kono, N., Hara, N., Shimizu, T., Yamada, Y., Kawachi, M., Kiyokawa, H., Wang, Y.L., and Tarui, S. Myogenic hyperuricemia. A

common pathophysiologic feature of glycogenosis types III, V, and VII. *N Engl J Med* 1987;317:75–80.

38. DiMauro, S. and Lamperti, C. Muscle glycogenoses. *Muscle Nerve* 2001;24:984–99.

39. Suchy, S.F., Olivos-Glander, I.M., and Nussabaum, R.L. Lowe syndrome, a deficiency of phosphatidylinositol 4, 5-bisphosphate 5- phosphatase in the Golgi apparatus. *Hum Mol Genet* 1995;4:2245–50.

40. Athreya, B.H., Schumacher, H.R., Getz, H.D., Norman, M.E., Borden, S.t., and Witzleben, C.L. Arthropathy of Lowe's (oculocerebrorenal) syndrome. *Arthritis Rheum* 1983;26:728–35.

41. Shapiro, J.R., Fallat, R.W., Tsang, R.C., and Glueck, C.J. Achilles tendinitis and tenosynovitis. A diagnostic manifestation of familial type II hyperlipoproteinemia in children. *Am J Dis Child* 1974;128:486–90.

42. Buckingham, R.B., Bole, G.G., and Bassett, D.R. Polyarthritis associated with type IV hyperlipoproteinemia. *Arch Intern Med* 1975;135:286–90.

43. Tauber, C. and Tauber, T. Gaucher disease—the orthopaedic aspect. Report of seven cases. *Arch Orthop Trauma Surg* 1995;114:179–82.

44. Belamarich, P.F., Deckelbaum, R.J., Starc, T.J., Dobrin, B.E., Tint, G.S., and Salen, G. Response to diet and cholestyramine in a patient with sitosterolemia. *Pediatrics* 1990;86:977–81.

45. Berge, K.E., Tian, H., Graf, G.A., Yu, L., Grishin, N.V., Schultz, J., Kwiterovich, P., Shan, B., Barnes, R., and Hobbs, H.H. Accumulation of dietary cholesterol in sitosterolemia caused by mutations in adjacent ABC transporters. *Science* 2000;290:1771–5.

46. Raphael, S.A., Cowdery, S.L., Faerber, E.N., Lischner, H.W., Schumacher, H.R., and Tourtellotte, C.D. Multicentric reticulohistiocytosis in a child. *J Pediatr* 1989;114:266–9.

47. Candell Chalom, E., Elenitsas, R., Rosenstein, E.D., and Kramer, N. A case of multicentric reticulohistiocytosis in a 6-year-old child. *J Rheumatol* 1998;25:794–7.

48. Luz, F.B., Gaspar, T.A.P., Kalil-Gaspar, N., and Ramos-e-Silva, M. Multicentric reticulohistiocytosis. *J Eur Acad Dermatol Venereol* 2001;15:524–31.

49. Cunningham-Rundles, C. and Bodian, C. Common variable immunodeficiency: clinical and immunological features of 248 patients. *Clin Immunol* 1999;92:34–48.

50. Conley, M.E., Park, C.L., and Douglas, S.D. Childhood common variable immunodeficiency with autoimmune disease. *J Pediatr* 1986;108:915–22.

51. Wilfert, C.M., Buckley, R.H., Mohanakumar, T., *et al.* Persistent and fatal central-nervous-system ECHO virus infections in patients with agammaglobulinemia. *N Engl J Med* 1977;296:1485–9.

52. Webster, A.D.B. Common Variable Immunodeficiency. *Immunology Allergy Clinics North America* 2001;21:1–22.

53. Barkley, D.O., Hohermuth, H.J., Howard, A., Webster, D.B., and Ansell, B.M. IgA deficiency in juvenile chronic polyarthritis. *J Rheumatol* 1979;6:219–24.

54. Burks, A.W., Sampson, H.A., and Buckley, R.H. Anaphylactic reactions after gamma globulin administration in patients with hypogammaglobulinemia. Detection of IgE antibodies to IgA. *N Engl J Med* 1986;314:560–4.

55. Jawad, A.F., McDonald-Mcginn, D.M., Zackai, E., and Sullivan, K.E. Immunologic features of chromosome 22q11.2 deletion syndrome (DiGeorge syndrome/velocardiofacial syndrome). *J Pediatr* 2001;139:715–23.

56. Davies, K., Stiehm, E.R., Woo, P., and Murray, K.J. Juvenile idiopathic polyarticular arthritis and IgA deficiency in the 22q11 deletion syndrome. *J Rheumatol* 2001;28:2326–34.

57. Geha, R. *Case Studies in Immunology*. New York: Garland Publishing, 2001.

58. Akman, I.O., Ostrov, B.E., and Neudorf, S. Autoimmune manifestations of the Wiskott-Aldrich syndrome. *Semin Arthritis Rheum* 1998;27:218–25.

59. Drappa, J., Vaishnaw, A.K., Sullivan, K.E., Chu, J.L., and Elkon, K.B. Fas gene mutations in the Canale-Smith syndrome, an inherited lymphoproliferative disorder associated with autoimmunity. *N Engl J Med* 1996;335:1643–9.

60. Jacobs, J.C. and Goetzl, E.J. "Streaking leukocyte factor," arthritis, and pyoderma gangrenosum. *Pediatrics* 1975;56:570–8.

61. Cornelis, F., Bardin, T., Faller, B., *et al.* Rheumatic syndromes and beta 2-microglobulin amyloidosis in patients receiving long-term peritoneal dialysis. *Arthritis Rheum* 1989;32:785–8.

62. Mirahmadi, K.S., Coburn, J.W., and Bluestone, R. Calcific periarthritis and hemodialysis. *JAMA* 1973;223:548–9.

63. Zacharin, M. and O'Sullivan, M. Intravenous pamidronate treatment of polyostotic fibrous dysplasia associated with the McCune-Albright syndrome. *J Pediatr* 2000;137:403–9.

64. Helms, C. *Fundamentals of Skeletal Radiology*. Philadelphia: WB Saunders Company, 1995.

65. Torriani, M. and Rosenthal, D.I. Percutaneous radiofrequency treatment of osteoid osteoma. *Pediatr Radiol* 2002;32:615–18.

66. Pierz, K.A., Stieber, J.R., Kusumi, K., and Dormans, J.P. Hereditary multiple exostoses: one center's experience and review of etiology. *Clin Orthop* Aug: 2002;49–59.

67. Arndt, C.A. and Crist, W.M. Common musculoskeletal tumors of childhood and adolescence. *N Engl J Med* 1999;341:342–52.

68. Till, S.H. and Amos, R.S. Neurofibromatosis masquerading as monoarticular juvenile arthritis. *Br J Rheumatol* 1997;36:286–8.

69. Price, N.J. and Cundy, P.J. Synovial hemangioma of the knee. *J Pediatr Orthop* 1997;17:74–77.

70. Narvaez, J.A., Narvaez, J., Aguilera, C., De Lama, E., and Portabella, F. MR imaging of synovial tumors and tumor-like lesions. *Eur Radiol* 2001;11:2549–60.

71. Flandry, F. and Hughston, J.C. Pigmented villonodular synovitis. *J Bone Joint Surg Am* 1987;69:942–9.

72. Shabat, S., Kollender, Y., Merimsky, O., Isakov, J., Flusser, G., Nyska, M., and Meller, I. The use of surgery and yttrium 90 in the management of extensive and diffuse pigmented villonodular synovitis of large joints. *Rheumatology (Oxford)* 2002;41:1113–18.

73. Gilbert, S.R. and Lachiewicz, P.F. Primary synovial osteochondromatosis of the hip: report of two cases with long-term follow-up after synovectomy and a review of the literature. *Am J Orthop* 1997;26:555–60.

74. Kawai, A., Woodruff, J., Healey, J.H., Brennan, M.F., Antonescu, C.R., and Ladanyi, M. SYT-SSX gene fusion as a determinant of morphology and prognosis in synovial sarcoma. *N Engl J Med* 1998;338:153–60.

75. Brandrup, F., Koch, C., Petri, M., Schiodt, M., and Johansen, K.S. Discoid lupus erythematosus-like lesions and stomatitis in female carriers of X-linked chronic granulomatous disease. *Br J Dermatol* 1981;104:495–505.

76. Cobeta-Garcia, J.C., Domingo-Morera, J.A., Monteagudo-Saez, I., and Lopez-Longo, F.J. Autosomal chronic granulomatous disease and systemic lupus erythematosus with fatal outcome. *Br J Rheumatol* 1998;37:109–111.

77. Manzi, S., Urbach, A.H., McCune, A.B., Altman, H.A., Kaplan, S.S., Medsger, T.A., Jr, and Ramsey-Goldman, R. Systemic lupus erythematosus in a boy with chronic granulomatous disease: case report and review of the literature. *Arthritis Rheum* 1991;34:101–5.

78. Moreno-Reyes, R., Sutens, C., Mathieu, F. Kashin-Beck Osteoarthropathy in rural Tibet in relation to selenium and Iodine Status. *NEJM* 1983;339:1112–20.

1.11 Disorders of bone and connective tissue

Karin S. Peterson

Aim

The aim of this chapter is to provide an extensive review of the congenital and inherited diseases of bones and connective tissues that may present with musculoskeletal symptoms and may be potentially confused with Juvenile Idiopathic Arthritis.

Structure

- Congenital and familial syndromes associated with joint laxity
  - Marfan syndrome (OMIM 154700 [6])
  - Ehlers–Danlos syndrome (EDS)
  - Cutis laxa
  - Familial joint laxity (OMIM 147900 [6])
  - Larsen syndrome
- Congenital and familial disorders associated with stiff joints or joint contractures
  - Athrogryposis multiplex congenita
    - Distal arthrogryposis
  - Fetal alcohol syndrome
  - Nail patella syndrome (OMIM 161200 [6])
  - Congenital contractural arachnodactyly (Beal syndrome; OMIM 121020 [6])
  - Clinodactyly
  - Camptodactyly
  - Camptodactyly–Arthropathy–Coxa Vara–Pericarditis Syndrome (CAPS) (Arthropathy–Camptodactyly Syndrome; OMIM 208250 [6])
  - Leri pleonosteosis (OMIM 151200 [6])
  - Williams syndrome (Williams–Beuren syndrome; OMIM 194050 [6])
  - Emery–Dreifus muscular dystrophy
  - Infantile systemic hyalinosis (OMIM 236490 [6])
  - Fibrodysplasia ossificans progressiva (FOP) (OMIM 135100 [6])
  - The Weill–Marchesani syndrome (OMIM 277600 [6])
  - Homocystinura (OMIM 236200 [6])
  - The mucopolysaccharidoses and mucolipidoses
    - Scheie and Hurler MPS
    - Morquio syndrome (MPS IV)
    - Pseudo-Hurler polydystrophy (ML III; OMIM 252600 [6])
- Osteochondrodysplasias: disorders of chondro-osseous development that frequently are associated with disproportionate short stature and either joint contractures or laxity
  - Achondroplasia
  - Hypochondroplasia (OMIM 146000 [6])
  - Spondyloepiphyseal dysplasias (SED)
  - Spondyloepiphyseal dysplasias congenita (SEDC) (OMIM 183900 [6])
  - Spondyloepiphyseal dysplasias tarda (OMIM 313400 [6])
  - Spondyloepiphyseal dysplasias tarda with progressive arthropathy (pseudorheumatoid arthritis of childhood; OMIM 208230 [6])
  - Schimke immuno-osseous dysplasia (OMIM 242900 [6])
  - Stickler dysplasia
  - Kniest dysplasia (OMIM 156550 [6])
  - Epiphyseal dysplasia
    - Multiple epiphyseal dysplasia
    - Pseudoachondroplasia (OMIM 177150 [6])
    - Other forms of MED
  - Metaphyseal dysplasia
    - Adenosine deaminase deficiency (OMIM 102700 [6])
    - Schwachmann–Diamond syndrome (OMIM 240400 [6])
    - Cartilage–hair hypoplasia (OMIM 250250 [6])
    - Schmid type (OMIM 156500 [6])
    - Jansen type (OMIM 156400 [6])
    - Blomstrand type (OMIM 215045 [6])
  - Mesomelic dysplasia
    - Leri–Weill syndrome (OMIM 127300 [6])
    - Langer mesomelic dwarfism (OMIM 249700 [6])
  - Acro/acro-mesomelic dysplasia
    - Trichorhinophalangeal dysplasia I (OMIM 190350 [6])
    - Langer–Gideon syndrome (TRPS II, OMIM 150230)
  - Chondrodysplasia punctata
    - Conradi–Hunermann syndrome (OMIM 302960 [6])
    - Rhizomelic chondrodysplasia punctata (OMIM 215100 [6])
    - Autosomal-dominant chondrodysplasia punctata (OMIM 118650 [6])
  - Osteochondrodysplasias with decreased bone density
    - Osteogenesis imperfecta (OI)

- Osteochondrodysplasia with increased bone density
  - Osteopetrosis
  - Melorheostosis (OMIM 155950 [6])
  - Camurati–Engelman syndrome (OMIM 131300 [6])
- Idiopathic osteolysis
  - Carpal–tarsal osteolysis
  - Winchester syndrome (OMIM 277950 [6])
  - Familial expansile osteolysis (OMIM 174810 [6])

Introduction

The clinical presentation of inherited and congenital disorders of bone and connective tissue is varied ranging from the fairly typical features of an adolescent with Marfan syndrome to the diagnostic challenge of a child afflicted by a mild form of osteochondrodysplasia where subtle disproportionate short stature may be noticed during the evaluation for arthritis. Musculoskeletal complaints bring these children to the rheumatologist and from this perspective it is useful to divide them into those with joint laxity primarily and those with joint stiffness or contractures. Autoimmune, inflammatory arthritis is rarely present in this group of patients, making it important to correctly diagnose the underlying cause of joint pain to avoid unnecessary treatment with immunosuppressive and potentially toxic therapy. The musculoskeletal pain associated with the bone and connective tissue disorders is, however, often difficult to treat with few beneficial treatment options available.

Many of these syndromes are complex, involving symptoms from musculoskeletal and other organs, sometimes with incomplete phenotypic penetrance. The estimated incidence, when available, of most individual bone and connective tissue disorders is in the order of 1–10 per 10^6 in contrast to the estimated incidence of JIA which is approximately 10 per 10^5 [1]. However, as a group, these disorders are prevalent enough to constitute a diagnostic challenge. Clinical characteristics and typical findings in radiographs are the mainstay of diagnosis. Biochemical and genetic testing is likely to facilitate diagnosis in the future as we continue to learn more about the underlying genetic defects.

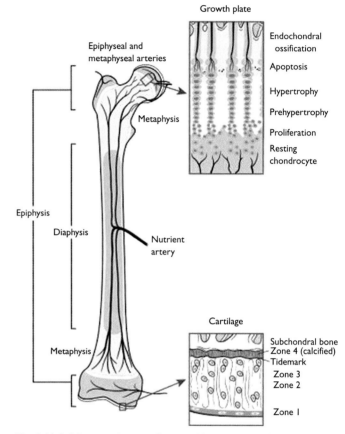

Fig. 1.11.1 Schematic drawing of a normal bone prior to closure of the growth plates. Details of the components of the growth plate and the avascular cartilage are shown in the enlarged views.

Table 1.11.1 Components of normal bone and cartilage

Cells[a]	Cartilage	Bone
	Chondrocytes	Osteoblasts
		Osteoclasts
		Vascular elements, nerves, lymphatics
Exracellular matrix	Collagen type II	Collagen type I
	Collagen types VI, IX, X, XI[b]	Collagen types III, V, XII, XIV[c]
Proteoglycans[d]	Aggrecan,[e] hyaluronan biglycan, decorin	Aggrecan, hyaluronan, biglycan, decorin
Glycoproteins	COMP, matrilin	Osteocalcin, osteopontin
	Matrix GLA protein, link protein	Osteonectin, fibronectin
	Enzymes, Growth factors,	Enzymes, growth factors
	Hormones	Hormones
Minerals		Hydroxyapatite ($Ca_{10}(PO_4)_6(OH)_2$)

[a] The cellular component of bone constitutes approximately 1% of the total tissue, the extracellular matrix component around 29%, and the mineral component around 70%. Chondrocytes occupy 2–10% of cartilage volume.

[b] All minor constituents in cartilage.

[c] All minor constituents in bone.

[d] Space does not permit a comprehensive list of all proteoglycans and glycoproteins that have been identified in bone and cartilage, only a select number of the major constituents are listed in the table. For a review see Kuettner *et al.* [59] and Cassidy and Petty [60].

[e] Aggrecan is the predominant proteoglycan in articular cartilage; it is present in small amounts in bone.

Many of the congenital dysmorphic syndromes, usually readily identified because of unusual facies or developmental delay, include joint laxity or stiffness in their phenotype. For a comprehensive review of these syndromes the reader is referred to Smith's *Recognizable Patterns of Human Malformation* [2] and to the review by Chalom *et al.* [3].

Recent discoveries of specific genetic abnormalities in individual bone and connective tissue disorders have advanced our understanding of normal bone and cartilage development [4]. The development of the normal skeleton follows a tightly controlled pattern of chondrocyte differentiation, growth plate maturation, and ordered closure with ossification of all cartilage except articular cartilage (Figure 1.11.1). Cartilage and bone differ not only in their mineral content but also in the composition of their extracellular matrix (Table 1.11.1). Endochondral bone formation describes the conversion of an initial cartilage template into bone and is the mechanism by which most bones of the skeleton are formed; the exception being the flat bones of the skull, which are formed by mesenchymal precursor cells that differentiate directly into bone forming osteoblasts (intramembranous ossification).

Congenital and familial syndromes associated with joint laxity (Table 1.11.2)

A number of disorders that affect the musculoskeletal system are associated with joint hypermobility, which may cause arthralgias, effusions, and increased risk of joint- and soft-tissue injury including traumatic synovitis, tenosynovitis, torn ligaments, or muscle and joint capsular tears. Hypermobility has been associated with "growing pains" (Part 1, Chapter 1.7) and with idiopathic adolescent scoliosis [5]. Benign hypermobility (Part 1, Chapter 1.7) rarely causes significant problems although some youngsters may have recurrent joint pain and effusion following strenuous exercise. The differential between the upper end of normal mobility or benign hypermobility and mild familial forms of hypermobility is quite difficult or nearly impossible.

Marfan syndrome (OMIM 154700 [6])

Long thin extremities (Marfan used the term dolichostenomelia), (Table 1.11.3) with proportionately more lengthening of the distal extremities (arachnodactyly) result in a tall individual with a low upper-to-lower segment ratio and an arm span greater than the total height (Figure 1.11.2). A decreased upper-to-lower ratio (Table 1.11.4) of <0.85 in Marfan syndrome contrasts to the normal adult ratio of approximately 0.93 [7]; the arm span to height ratio is typically >1.05 in affected individuals. Clinical signs of arachnodactyly are the thumb sign where the entire nail of the thumb extends beyond the ulnar border of the hand when the hand is clenched and the wrist sign where the thumb overlaps the distal phalanx of the fifth finger when grasping the other wrist. Other skeletal characteristics include pectus deformities of the chest, scoliosis, high arched palate, and great toes elongated out of proportion to the others. Ocular manifestations include high myopia and ectopia lentis, with characteristic upward dislocation of the lens, as contrasted with the downward ectopia lentis of homocystinuria and the Weill–Marchesani Syndrome. Cardiac abnormalities include mitral valve prolapse and mitral insufficiency.

Weakness of the tunica media of the aorta results in dilatation of the aortic ring with aortic insufficiency followed by ascending thoracic and sometimes descending abdominal aortic aneurysms, ultimately with possible rupture and death. Most of these deaths can be prevented by the combined use of medications to lower arterial pressure, regular aortic imaging, and elective aortic repair. Occasional patients have considerable myopathy. The presence of dural ectasia or spinal arachnoid cysts is best diagnosed by magnetic resonance imaging (MRI); dural ectasia is a specific diagnostic marker of the disease [8]. The ligamentous laxity associated with Marfan syndrome may be associated with pronounced flat feet (rocker bottoms), genu recurvatum, and frequent joint dislocations. The musculoskeletal symptoms of Marfan syndrome (a result of hypermobility) are the least of the patient's problems and usually present no diagnostic difficulty.

Marfan syndrome has an estimated prevalence of 1 : 5000–10,000. The diagnosis depends mainly on clinical evaluation and is based on a combination of manifestations from the different organ systems that are involved (Table 1.11.5). The diagnostic criteria for Marfan syndrome were revised in 1996 [9] and now include more stringent requirements for diagnosis in relatives of an index patient and inclusion of multiple skeletal abnormalities as a major criterion (Table 1.11.5). The older criteria [10] were developed before the genetic information on the cause of Marfan syndrome was available and may have led to over-diagnosis of the disorder in the mildly affected individual. Marfan syndrome exhibits autosomal dominant inheritance but its phenotypic expression varies widely. The genetic abnormality has been mapped to FBN1, encoding fibrillin I on chromosome 15. Mutation analysis is usually not required for diagnosis.

Other conditions may clinically resemble Marfan syndrome: children with homocystinuria have a marfanoid habitus but their joints tend to be restricted rather than hyperextensible. Homocystinuria is, however, clinically very similar to Marfan syndrome and any child evaluated for the latter should have plasma amino acids analyzed to screen for the presence of homocystinuria. In addition, children with congenital contractural arachnodactyly (Beal syndrome) develop a phenotype that may clinically resemble Marfan syndrome.

Ehlers–Danlos syndrome (EDS)

This is a heterogeneous group of genetic disorders involving either the structure or the synthesis of collagen or other components of the extracellular matrix and affects as many as 1 in 5000 individuals. The phenotype is characterized by the triad of joint hypermobility (Figure 1.11.3(a)), hyperelastic skin (Figure 1.11.3(b)), and fragile tissues. Components of the diagnostic triad are always present but may vary considerably between individuals and the different types of Ehlers–Danlos syndrome. Musculoskeletal pain is a major problem in those patients with significant hypermobility and joint effusions are common in those with recurrent dislocations or instability especially in the ankles and knees. Bleeding diathesis is also common and mainly due to abnormal blood vessels and vessel rupture but platelet dysfunction and other abnormalities of coagulation have been reported in association with EDS [11,12]. In one study of children, referred for the evaluation of unexplained bleeding tendency (i.e. in the setting of normal hemostatic function tests), it was demonstrated that the majority had hyperflexibility of the thumb [13], suggesting an underlying problem of connective tissue and vascular fragility. In some patients with EDS the skin splits apart in minor trauma and may result

Table 1.11.2 Congenital and familial syndromes associated with joint contractures or laxity

Classification	Identified		Joints		Other clinical characteristics	Cognitive,	Dysmorphic
	At birth	After birth	Lax	Stiff		impairment[a]	features[a]
Benign hypermobility		+	+		Joint pain exacerbated by exercise, effusions	−	−
Marfan syndrome		+	+		Tall stature, arachnodactyly, scoliosis, high myopia, ectopia lentis, dilated aortic root, mitral valve prolapse (MVP)	−	−
Homocystinuria		+		+	Marfanoid habitus, ectopia lentis, thrombosis, osteoporosis, livedo reticularis	+	−
EDS (several types)		+	+		Hyperelastic skin, atrophic scarring, vascular fragility, recurrent joint dislocations, musculoskeletal pain (Table 1.10.6)	−	−
Familial joint laxity		+	+		Recurrent joint dislocations, musculoskeletal pain	−	−
Larsen syndrome(s)	+		+		Multiple joint dislocations, pes cavus, spinal anomalies including scoliosis, atlanto-axial instability (rare), extra ossification center in calcaneus	−	+
Down syndrome	+		+		Hypotonia, cardiac defects, short hands with clinodactyly and single crease, wide gap between first and second toes, short neck	+	+
Arthrogryposis multiplex congenital	+			+	Flexion contractures of wrists, hips, knees, abnormal hand and foot creases, abnormal dimples, hypotonia	+	+
Fetal alcohol syndrome	+			+	Short stature, cardiac septal defects	+	+
Nail patella syndrome	+			+	Absent/laterally placed patella, hypoplastic nails, scoliosis, clinodactyly, renal disease	(+)	−
Congenital contractural arachnodactyly (Beal syndrome)	+			+	Tall stature, arachnodactyly, "crumpled" ears, kyphoscoliosis, MVP	−	−
CAPS syndrome	+			+	Camptodactyly, joint effusions in wrists, knees, and ankles, constrictive pericarditis	−	−
Leri pleonosteosis		+		+	Short stature, short spade-like hands, carpal tunnel syndrome	−	(+)
Williams syndrome		+	(+)[b]	+	Outgoing personality, transient hypercalcemia, supravalvular aortic stenosis	+	+
EDMD		+		+	Mild muscular weakness, cardiac conduction defects	−	−
Infantile systemic hyalinosis		+		+	Painful contractures, papular or macular rash, gingival hypertrophy failure to thrive (FTT), diarrhoea, osteoporosis	−	−
Fibrodysplasia ossificans progressiva	+[c]	+		+	Short, broad hallux, localized swelling/pain of subcutaneous tissues followed by calcification	−	−
Weill–Marchesani syndrome		+		+	Short stature, brachydactyly, ectopia lentis, carpal tunnel syndrome	−	−
MPS-I, Scheie type		+		+	Short stature, broad short hands and feet, claw-hand, hernia, corneal clouding, cardiac disease, occasional hepatosplenomegaly [2]	−	−
MPS-I, Hurler type		+		+	Same as above but more severe phenotype Hepatosplenomegaly, deafness [2]	+	+
MPS-II, Hunter		+		+	Short stature, claw-hand, deafness, hernia, hepatosplenomegaly, clear corneas, X-linked [2]	+[d]	+

Table 1.11.2 (*Continued*)

Classification	Identified		Joints		Other clinical characteristics	Cognitive, impairment[a]	Dysmorphic features[a]
	At birth	After birth	Lax	Stiff			
MPS-III (A-C), Sanfilippo		+		+	Short stature, mild skeletal abnormalities, variable hepatomegaly, clear corneas [2]	+	+
MPS-IV, Morquio[e]		+		+	Short stature, platyspondyly, odontoid hypoplasia, kyphoscoliosis, short hands, effusons in large joints, knock-knee, corneal clouding, hepatomegaly, hernia, deafness [2]	−	+
MPS-VI, Maroteaux-Lamy[e]		+		+	Short stature, metaphyseal and epiphyseal irregularities, platyspondyly, and odontoid hypoplasia, fine corneal opacities, hernia, thick and tight skin, hepatosplenomegaly, cardiac disease [2]	−	+
MPS-VII, Sly		+		+	Short stature, widening of ribs, acetabular dysplasia, thoracolumbar gibbus, occasional odontoid hypoplasia, corneal clouding, hernia, hepatosplenomegaly [2]	+	+
ML-III, pseudo-Hurler		+		+	Short stature, mild platyspondyly, flattening of femoral epiphyses, aortic valve disease, hernia, mild corneal opacities, no hepatosplenomegaly [2]	+	+

Abbreviation: MVP: mitral valve prolapse.

[a] A + indicates presence in most but not all affected individuals. A sign in parenthesis indicates that occurrence is rare or not well defined.

[b] Joint laxity may be present in early childhood.

[c] The syndrome may be recognized at birth by the presence of a short broad first toe.

[d] The clinical phenotype may vary from mild to severe. A late onset type with mild to normal intelligence has been described.

[e] Two clinical subtypes exist: a severe and a mild type.

Table 1.11.3 Glossary

Acromelic: refers to distal portion of a limb

Arachnodactyly: long thin hands, fingers, feet, and toes

Arthrogryposis: prenatal onset of joint contractures

Brachydactyly: short finger

Camptodactyly: flexion contractures at the interphalangeal joints; usually at the proximal IP joints

Clinodactyly: curved finger, most commonly affecting the fifth finger; results from hypoplasia of middle phalanx. Occurs as an isolated finding in 2.5% of normal individuals

Dolichostenomelia: long limbs

Dysostosis: defective bone formation

Hyperostosis: thickening of cortical bone from deposit of osseous tissues along periostal and/or endosetal surfaces

Mesomelic: refers to middle segment of a limb

Melorheostosis: "bone flowing in limb"

Osteopoikilosis: describes condition of pathchy sclerosis in bone

Osteosclerosis: increased density of trabecular (spongy) bone

Platyspondyly: flat vertebrae

Rhizomelic: refers to proximal portion of a limb

Synostosis: bony fusion of two bones

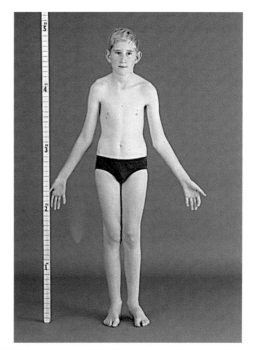

Fig. 1.11.2 Teenage boy with Marfan syndrome. (Courtesy of T.R. Southwood.)

Table 1.11.4 Practical points

Upper to lower segment ratio
  Lower segment: measured from the upper border of the symphysis pubis
  to the floor in a patient standing against a wall
  Upper segment: obtained by subtracting the lower segment from the
  standing height
  The resulting (U/L) segment ratio is compared with normal values for age
  and gender[a]

Arm span
  Distance between fingertips of the middle fingers of each hand, when the
  arms are stretched out horizontally from the body

[a] The normal U/L segment ratio decreases from a value around 1.7 at birth, 1.4 at 2
years, 1.2 at 4 years, 1.1 at 6 years to approximately 0.95 at 16 years for both
females and men [7].

Table 1.11.5 Clinical diagnosis of Marfan syndrome[a]

Major criteria	Minor criteria
Skeletal system[b]	**Skeletal system**
Pectus carniatum; severe pectus excavatum	Pectus excavatum; hypermobility, highly arched palate, facial appearance
Reduced U/L ratio or arm span-to-height ratio >1.05	
Wrist and thumb sign; scoliosis >20%	
Reduced extension of elbow; medial displacement of the medial malleolus; protrusio acetabulae	
Ocular system	**Ocular system**
Ectopia lentis	Flat cornea; increased axial length of globe; hypoplastic iris or hypoplastic ciliary muscle
Cardiovascular system	**Cardiovascular system**
Dilatation or dissection of ascending aorta	Mitral valve prolapse; dilatation of the main pulmonary artery
Lumbosacral dural ectasia	**Pulmonary system**
	Spontaneous pneumothorax; apical blebs
Family/genetic history	**Skin and integument**
First degree relative who meets clinical criteria	Striae; hernia
Presence of mutation in FBN1	
Presence of haplotype containing FBN1-mutation known to have caused Marfan syndrome in a relative	

Abbreviations: *FBN1*: gene encoding fibrillin I; U/L: upper to lower segment ratio.

Note: A positive diagnosis in an index patient requires the presence of two major criteria and involvement of at least one other system. For a relative of an index case, one major criterion and involvement of a second organ system is required. The classification distinguishes between a major criterion being present in a system and the system "being involved" as detailed in Reference 9. For example, for the skeletal system to "be involved" 2/8 components of the major criteria or one major criteria component and two minor criteria must be present.

[a] Adapted from Reference 9.
[b] Presence of at least four of eight manifestations is required for the skeletal system to constitute a major criterion.

in the typical "cigarette paper" scars from minor injury to the forehead and shins (Figure 1.11.3(c)).

Diagnosis is based on typical clinical findings [14] combined with biochemical studies and the identification of genetic defects in those types of EDS where this is known. The classification of the different forms of EDS has been revised (Table 1.11.6) to better reflect the current understanding of the disorder [14]. However, the molecular defects identified to date do not explain all clinical forms of the disease.

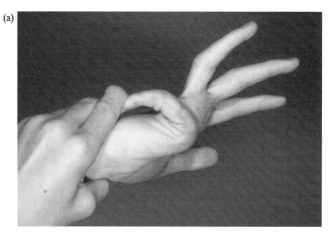

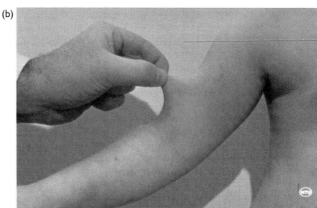

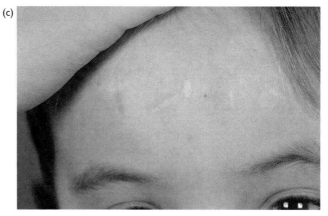

Fig. 1.11.3 (a) Hypermobility of the fifth finger in a child diagnosed with EDS (Courtesy of T. R. Southwood.) (b) Hyperelastic skin typical of EDS (From the National Library of Dermatologic Teaching Slides.) (c) Scar of the forehead after minor trauma in a girl diagnosed with EDS. (Courtesy of T. R. Southwood.)

Table 1.11.6 Classification of EDS

EDS type[a]		Joint laxity	Elastic skin	Rupture of internal organs (arteries, bowel, other)	Other characteristics	Genetic defect	Inheritance
Classic	(I/II)	++++	++++		Atrophic scars, bruising	COL5A1, COL5A2	AD
Hypermobility	(III)	++++	+/−		Musculoskeletal pain	Undefined	AD
Vascular	(IV)	+/−	+/−	+++	Thin skin, bruising	COL3A	AD
Kyphoscoliosis	(VI)	++	++		Congenital scoliosis hypotonia, ocular fragility	Lysyl-hydroxylase	AR
Arthrocalasia	(VII a, b)	++++	+		Scoliosis, bruising	COL1A1, COL1A2	AD
Dermatosparaxis	(VII c)	++	++++		Bruising	Procollagen N-peptidase	AR

[a] Ref: EDSs: revised nosology. Villefranche, 1997 [14]. The corresponding old classification is given in parentheses; I: gravis, II: mitis, III: hypermobile, IV: arterial, VI: ocular-scoliotic, VII a, b: arthrocalasis multiplex congenital, VII c: human dermatosparaxis. EDS type V (X-linked), type VIII (AD; peridontitis), and type X (AR? abnormal platelet aggregation) are grouped under "other rare forms of the EDS" according to the new classification, reflecting their less well-defined aetiology. Entries that were removed from the revised classification include: EDS IX: now called "occipital horn syndrome," is X-linked and allelic to Menke syndrome. EDS XI now called familial articular hypermobility syndrome (OMIM 147900 [6]) resembles the hypermobility form of the EDS but lacks skin involvement.

A newly identified autosomal recessive type (not yet included in the classification) is caused by mutations in the gene encoding tenascin X [15], a large extracellular matrix protein normally synthesized in skin, tendons, muscle, and blood vessels. Manifestations of tenascin X deficiency include hypermobility, hyperelasticity of the skin, and easy bruising without atrophic scarring.

Musculoskeletal pain may be severe especially in those with the hypermobile form of EDS (formerly type III) and often occurs in the absence of radiographic abnormalities causing frustration for the patient and a delay in the recognition of the problem [5,16]. Unusually strenuous physical activity may precipitate or aggravate the pain. Dislocations most commonly occur in the shoulders, elbows, patellae, and fingers. Joint instability may cause problems during regular daily activities such as running or typing. Treatment may require pain control with combination of medications; supervision by a specialist in pain management should be sought. Conventional physical therapy often exacerbates the pain and should be avoided, however, an evaluation by a therapist and modification of physical activity to minimize spontaneous dislocations and other triggers of pain, is a valuable adjunct to the therapeutic approach. Joint effusions are related to activity and bursae may develop in association with tendons or joint capsules. Development of premature osteoarthritis may be associated with hypermobility and the extent of repetitive trauma to which the joint has been exposed.

Cutis laxa

Ehlers–Danlos syndrome should be differentiated from cutis laxa, a disorder characterized by lax rather than hyperelastic skin (Figure 1.11.4). Cutis laxa is characterized by loose, redundant skin that hangs down in folds, similar to skin changes associated with old age. Cutis laxa is a prominent feature of several genetic syndromes (e.g. found in the posterior neck of children born with Turner syndrome) but it may not be clinically apparent until well beyond the neonatal period. Mutations in the elastin gene (OMIM 123700 [6]), and in the copper-transporting ATPase (OMIM 304150 [6]) have also been associated with cutis laxa.

Familial joint laxity (OMIM 147900 [6])

This autosomal dominant condition, also termed familial articular hypermobility syndrome [5], was included in the previous classification

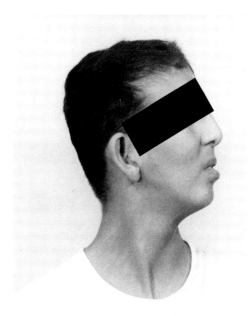

Fig. 1.11.4 Although cutis laxa is sometimes confused with EDS, these individuals do not have hypermobile joints and their skin is lax rater than hyperelastic. The typical drooping facies, illustrated here, is characterized by sagging facial skin and accentuation of the nasolabial and other folds. The child appears older than his or her stated age.

of EDS (Table 1.11.6). Several pedigrees clinically characterized by articular hypermobility and recurrent dislocation of joints, in particular the shoulders and patellae have been identified. Familial joint laxity is sometimes localized to a single anatomic site [5]. The genetic defect has not yet been identified. Familial articular hypermobility resembles the hypermobility form of the EDS but lacks skin involvement.

Larsen syndrome

Extraordinary laxity of the joints with recurrent dislocations, flat facies, widely spaced eyes, abnormal feet, and malformed fingers with a spatulate thumb and short nails characterize this unusual congenital syndrome. Autosomal dominant (OMIM 150250[6]) and autosomal recessive (OMIM 245600[6]) inheritance have been described, however, phenotypic differences have not been clearly delineated between the two. Radiographic demonstration of an extra ossification center in the calcaneus may be a diagnostic clue. Many patients start walking late but with aggressive orthopedic management the overall prognosis is positive. Potential complications include osteoarthritis of large joints and progressive kyphoscoliosis.

Spondyloepiphyseal dysplasias and other osteochondroplasias may also include joint laxity and are discussed later.

Congenital and familial disorders associated with stiff joints or joint contractures (Table 1.11.2)

Many of the syndromes characterized by stiff joints are not apparent at birth and manifest during the first few months or years of life. This group contains a relatively large number of phenotypes for a rather small number of affected individuals.

Athrogryposis multiplex congenita

The common denominator for most patients born with arthrogryposis is the limitation of fetal joint mobility early in intrauterine life [17]. This can be the result of neurologic or musculoskeletal abnormalities in the fetus or caused by physical restraints of the uterine environment. Joint development starts at about 5 weeks of fetal life and by 8 weeks there is movement of the limbs. Unrestricted motion is essential for normal development of the joints and surrounding structures. Arthrogryposis therefore includes a heterogeneous group of disorders, many of unknown origin and usually not hereditary. Although not progressive, there may be considerable disability and long bones may be fractured during delivery. Arthrogryposis is often a part of a multiple defect syndrome including the chromosomal abnormalities of trisomy 18 and 13q-deletion syndrome.

Clues to the early fetal onset of joint contractures include findings on physical examination of absent or abnormal hand and foot creases (indicating abnormal early function) and aberrant dimples (reflecting early fetal cutaneous–osseous approximation leading to abnormal development of subcutaneous tissues) [2]. The clinical picture of arthrogryposis is characterized by (1) flexion of the wrists, (2) extended elbows, (3) partly contracted hips and severely contracted knees and ankles. Muscular hypotonia, congenital dislocation of the hips, and talipes equinovarus (clubfoot) are frequently present.

Distal arthrogryposis

The distal arthrogryposes are a group of disorders characterized by congenital contractures of the distal limbs. Nine different types, all with autosomal dominant inheritance have been identified and classified according to Hall *et al.* [18].

Fetal alcohol syndrome

Alcohol ingestion during pregnancy often results in mental retardation, impaired linear growth, cardiac septal defects, and craniofacial and skeletal defects with abnormalities of joint mobility [2,19]. The skeletal abnormalities include camptodactyly, clinodactyly, inability to completely flex the metacarpophalangeal joints, and inability to completely

extend the elbows. Craniofacial characteristics include mild microcephaly, short palpebral fissures, maxillary hypoplasia, short nose, a smooth philtrum with thin upper lip, together resulting in a characteristic appearance.

Nail patella syndrome (OMIM 161200 [6])

A small, laterally placed or absent patella is often the chief complaint that brings the child to the doctor. This congenital syndrome is also characterized by restricted elbow extension due to posterior dislocation of the radial head, hypoplastic nails with vertical ridging or splitting, poorly formed lunate, hypoplasia of the lateral femoral condyle, and small head of fibula. The dorsal distal IP joints may be missing causing limitations in flexion. A pathognomonic feature is the finding of posterior iliac horns that may be palpable, occur in approximately 80% of patients, and can be identified by bone scan [20]. Inheritance is autosomal dominant and the disease is caused by mutations in the LMX1B transcription factor [21]. LMX1B appears to regulate the synthesis of type IV collagen (α-chains), a major constituent of glomerular basement membrane. This may explain why approximately 40% of affected individuals also develop progressive renal disease.

Congenital contractural arachnodactyly (Beal syndrome; OMIM 121020 [6])

Children born with this autosomal dominant syndrome, present with flexion contractures of the fingers, elbows, and knees that, tend to improve with age. Typically, affected individuals also have abnormal (crumpled) ear crura, progressive kyphoscoliosis, and a marfanoid habitus with long slim limbs and arachnodactyly. Mitral valve prolapse is present in many patients but aortic root dilatation and ectopia lentis have been only rarely described. The genetic defect is in the gene encoding fibrillin II on chromosome 5.

Clinodactyly

Isolated clinodactyly (curved finger) is a common finding occurring in as many as 2.5% of all individuals. It most often affects the fifth finger and results from hypoplasia of the middle phalanx of the digit. Most children have a similarly affected family member. Clinodactyly is also part of several other syndromes.

Camptodactyly

The term camptodactyly refers to a permanent flexion contracture of the interphalangeal joint(s), usually at the proximal interphalangeal joint. It is most commonly found in the fifth finger but may be present in any or all fingers and usually occurs bilaterally. Camptodactyly may occur as an isolated phenomenon or as part of a syndrome; more than 40 such syndromes have been reported [22].

Camptodactyly–Arthropathy–Coxa Vara–Pericarditis Syndrome (CAPS) (Arthropathy–Camptodactyly Syndrome; OMIM 208250 [6])

This disorder appears to be genetically homogenous with autosomal recessive inheritance and genetic linkage to chromosome 1q25–31 and the Camptodactyly–Arthropathy–Coxa Vara–Pericarditis (CACP) gene, although there is some clinical variation among affected individuals. The CACP-encoded proteoglycan is synthesized by synoviocytes and chondrocytes and appears to be a major joint lubricant (recently named Lubricin) [23]. Abnormalities in its structure or production may lead to friction-induced scarring of periarticular tissues; the CACP-transcript is also expressed by non-skeletal tissue including liver and pericardium. Jacobs and Downey first identified this syndrome (initially called familial hypertrophic synovitis) in a family of nine children [24], five of whom had a unique arthropathy characterized by camptodactyly of the fingers (trigger fingers) apparent during the first few months of life and noninflammatory joint effusions (Figure 1.11.5 (a) and (b)). The same authors subsequently reported a second family with three of five affected children. Later a third family with three of five affected children was recognized by Athreya [25]. Large symmetrical effusions in the knees, ankles, and wrists are also characteristic. Contractures of large joints may appear during the course of the disease, particularly in the hips; radiographs may show flattening of the femoral ossification centres (Figure 1.11.6). There is little or no pain, systemic symptoms are absent and laboratory studies remain normal. The synovial pathology is unique and characterized by a striking noninflammatory synovial hyperplasia (Figure 1.11.7 (a) and (b)). Constrictive pericarditis occurs in approximately 40% of affected individuals and biopsy of the pericardium shows thickening and fibrosis without inflammatory changes. Noninflammatory pericardial or plerural effusions have been found in some patients.

Leri pleonosteosis (OMIM 151200 [6])

This apparently autosomal dominant condition was initially described in four generations of one family; affected individuals had short stature, and developed progressive generalized limitation of joint movement. Additional characteristics include broad spadelike hands and thumbs, genu recurvatum, and thickening of the palmar and forearm fasciae. Fibrous hyperplasia may lead to carpal tunnel syndrome and Morton metatarsalgia from compression of the digital nerves of the feet.

Williams syndrome (Williams–Beuren syndrome; OMIM 194050 [6])

Stiff gait and flexion contractures of proximal and distal interphalangeal joints, wrists, elbows, knees, and ankles occur in 50% of children with Williams syndrome. In early childhood, hypermobility rather than stiffness may be present. In addition to the characteristic facies and a friendly personality, this syndrome is associated with both intellectual dysfunction and often a musical talent, supravalvular aortic and peripheral pulmonary stenosis, and transient hypercalcemia in infancy. In most affected individuals, a hemizygous contiguous gene deletion at chromosome 7q11.23 (deleted segment may include up to 17 different genes) has been demonstrated [26]. Fluorescent *in situ* hybridization (FISH) may aid in the diagnosis of a microdeletion syndrome when conventional chromosome analysis is normal [27].

Emery–Dreifus muscular dystrophy

Emery–Dreifus muscular dystrophy (EDMD) manifests during childhood with slowly progressive muscle weakness, in a humeroperoneal distribution, and contractures of the Achilles, neck, and elbow tendons [28]. The child may present with a contracture of an elbow as

might occur in Juvenile Idiopathic Arthritis (JIA); however, it would be unusual for JIA to present with isolated elbow inflammation. These individuals also have cardiac conduction defects that can cause sudden cardiac arrest; regular cardiac evaluation is imperative. Placement of cardiac pacemaker may be lifesaving. Female carriers of the X-linked form are also at risk for cardiac arrhythmias. Two modes of inheritance

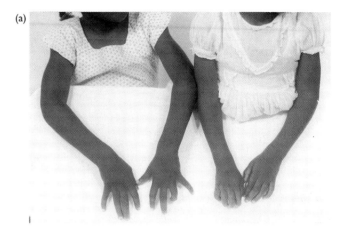

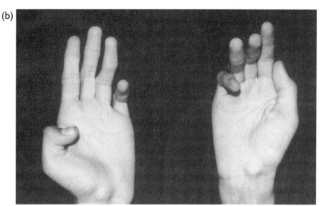

Fig. 1.11.5 (a) Trigger fingers and large-joint effusions in two of six siblings with CAPS syndrome and (b) in one of three affected siblings in another family. The bent thumb appeared soon after birth in both pedigrees and was a first clue to the diagnoses in many affected family members.

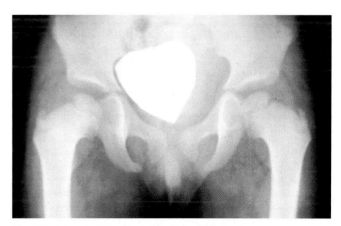

Fig. 1.11.6 Proximal flattening of the femoral ossification centres suggesting tendon contractures analogous to trigger fingers in a child with CAPC syndrome. Similar radiographic findings were also demonstrated in a second child with the same syndrome.

(a)

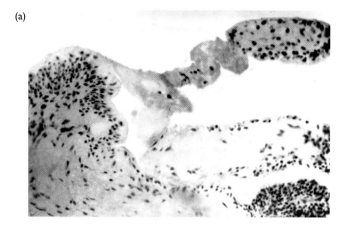

(b)

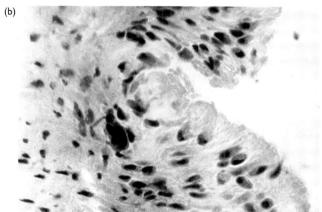

Fig. 1.11.7 Synovial biopsy of affected tissue in CACP syndrome demonstrates (a) large hypertrophic avascular villi and giant cells but no inflammatory infiltrate. (b) The hypertrophy is due solely to extraordinary hyperplasia of the lining cells.

result in a similar EDMD phenotype: X-linked (OMIM 310300 [6]) and autosomal dominant (OMIM 181350 [6]). Both genetic types exhibit variable penetrance; the severity of the disease varies even within families. The gene defects have been mapped to genes encoding components of the nuclear lamina, emerin (X-linked), and lamin A/C (chromosome 1q21). Definitive diagnosis at present depends on mutation analysis.

Infantile systemic hyalinosis (OMIM 236490 [6])

This rare syndrome presents in the neonatal period with painful joint contractures; the infant appears to experience severe pain when tended and held. There is often a skin rash that may either nodular or macular, appearing as a dark red or erythematous discoloration. On palpation, the involved skin is thickened and indurated. Other characteristics include gingival hypertrophy, persistent diarrhoea, failure to thrive, periostitis in the long bones, and osteoporosis. Pathologic examination shows widespread deposits of hyaline material in skin, skeletal muscle, gastrointestinal tract, endocrine glands, and other locations. There is no effective therapy except to control the pain; most affected infants do not survive beyond the first years of life. There is some overlap in clinical features with Winchester syndrome, and with infantile multisystem inflammatory disease (CINCA/NOMID, see Part 1, Chapter 1.7). The disorder is distinct from juvenile systemic hyalinosis, which is considered the same as juvenile hyaline fibromatosis (OMIM 228600 [6]).

Fibrodysplasia ossificans progressiva (FOP) (OMIM 135100 [6])

Affected children have localized, recurrent inflammation of subcutaneous tissue, tendon or fascia that typically presents as rapidly forming lumps (Figure 1.11.8), sometimes associated with pain, fever, and an elevated ESR [29]. Some lumps disappear within a few days and others calcify and ossify over a period of 3–4 weeks. As the name implies these lumps actually develop from heterotopic ossification rather than calcinosis. The lesions characteristically occur in the head and neck (sternocleidomastoid muscle), shoulders, proximal

(a)

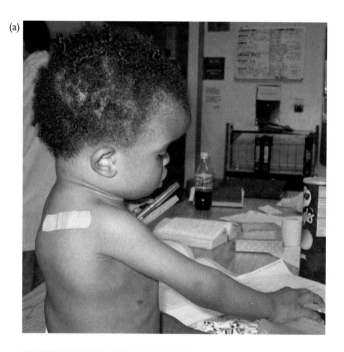

(b)

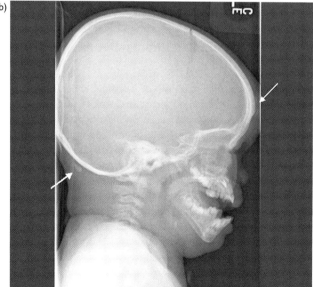

Fig. 1.11.8 (a) A 20-month-old child presented with "lumps" on his forehead and shoulder prompting admission for evaluation of suspected child abuse; however, lesions continued to form while in the hospital. (b) Radiograph of the skull shows swelling of subcutaneous tissue and an area with a small calcification in the posterior neck (arrows).

limbs, and dorsal trunk and affected individuals develop progressive and significantly restricted mobility of arms, neck, and chest. Fibrodysplasia ossificans progressiva (FOP) is the most severe disorder of heterotopic ossification in humans. Symptoms may begin at any age. The infant with FOP characteristically presents with torticollis; when symptoms begin at a later age, FOP may be confused with dermatomyositis (Part 1, Chapter 1.6) or with Weber–Christian disease (Part 1, Chapter 1.7).

Fibrodysplasia ossificans progressiva may be recognized at birth by the presence of a small, broad great toe (Figure 1.11.9(a)), or occasionally a short thumb, sometimes also present in a parent. Radiographs show synostosis of the phalanges of the great toe or a dysplastic or absent proximal first phalanx (Figure 1.11.9(b)). Occasionally, fifth finger clinodactyly is also present. Although most cases are sporadic, the disorder is probably inherited as an autosomal dominant with variable penetrance; linkage to chromosome 4q has been demonstrated. Histopathologic analysis of non-ossified affected tissues demonstrates early infiltration by lymphocytes followed by the appearance of highly vascular fibroproliferative tissue [29]. Trauma or minor procedures such as intramuscular injections may precipitate the formation of new lesions and biopsy of an already formed, early lesion will exacerbate the local ossification and should be avoided. Intramuscular injections are therefore also to be avoided and childhood vaccinations should, if possible, be given by subcutaneous injection [30]. Recognition of the pathognomonic combination of clinical features that is, monophalangic great toes and soft-tissue swelling with progressive calcification in predicted anatomical locations should prompt the diagnosis without the need for biopsy.

The pathologic mechanisms underlying FOP are not known but *in vitro* studies of lesional cells have demonstrated an increased production of bone morphogenic protein 4, an inducer of osteogenesis [29]. Currently, no effective therapy is available but several trials are underway including the use of NSAIDs and leukotrine-inhibitors [30].

The Weill–Marchesani syndrome (OMIM 277600 [6])

Short stature with short hands and feet (brachydactyly; the antithesis of Marfan syndrome), downward ectopia lentis, glaucoma, and immobile, flexed, thick fingers, and stiff joints particularly of the hands, are found in these children. Carpal tunnel nerve compression may develop. Intelligence is usually normal and this rare syndrome is compatible with a long life. Both autosomal recessive and autosomal dominant modes of inheritance have been described.

Homocystinura (OMIM 236200 [6])

This is an inborn error of amino acid metabolism where a defect in the enzyme cystathionin synthase leads to accumulation of homocystine; inheritance is autosomal recessive. Clinical characteristics include a marfanoid habitus, stiff joints, severe osteoporosis, and ocular problems with ectopia lentis being the most characteristic finding. In addition, affected children have a tendency to develop arterial and venous thromboses and thromboembolic disease is a common cause of death. Coagulation studies are normal in these individuals and the exact mechanism through which elevated levels of homocystine promote thrombosis has not been determined. Livedo reticularis and cold extremities are common findings on physical examination. Developmental delay is present in some patients.

The mucopolysaccharidoses and mucolipidoses

These lysosomal storage disorders have many similar features including joint stiffness, short stature, and a characteristic constellation of skeletal abnormalities sometimes referred to as dysostosis multiplex [31]; the exception is Morquio syndrome in which the skeletal abnormalities are specific to the disorder. Because of the associated skeletal findings, these disorders have also been classified as osteochondrodysplasias, however, they are unique among the osteochodrodysplasias because they are also storage disorders.

The mucopolysaccharidoses (MPS) are due to deficiency of specific lysosomal enzymes, required for the degradation of mucopolysaccharides (glycosaminoglycans) whereas mucolipodoses (ML) II and III are the result of a generalized lysosomal enzyme deficiency caused by an inability of the enzymes to reach their location in the lysosomal compartment of the cell. The genetic abnormality in ML lies in an

(a)

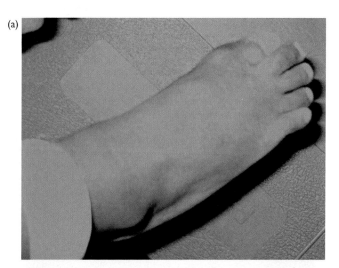

(b)

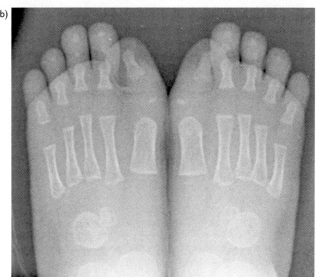

Fig. 1.11.9 (a) The big toes of the child in Figure 1.11.8 were short compared to the rest of the toes and (b) radiographs of his feet demonstrated hypoplastic first proximal phalanges in both feet. The patient's mother (deceased) was recalled as having had abnormally short big toes.

enzyme (a phosphotransferase) that modifies a carbohydrate chain present on all lysosomal enzymes and enables them to be targeted for transport to the lysosomal compartment. In the absence of this targeting signal, lysosomal enzymes are secreted into the extracellular space. Enzyme assays using fibroblasts, leukocytes, or serum are available for the diagnosis of MPS; increased excretion of glycosaminoglycans can also be measured in urine of affected individuals. In ML the diagnosis can be made biochemically by measuring serum lysosomal enzyme levels or by specific enzyme assay of cultured fibroblasts.

Affected children are normal at birth and develop progressive degenerative disease of multiple organs during the first years of life. Clinically, there is a wide spectrum of severity even within each disorder. Limitation of motion with flexion contractures of the fingers is a typical finding in patients with MPS and ML type III (pseudo-Hurler polydystrophy) and the broad, claw-shaped hand is a pathognomonic finding on examination. Multiple skeletal abnormalities may be identified on radiographic evaluation (Figure 1.11.10) in all but MPS IV (Morquio) where the findings resemble those associated with spondyloepiphyseal dysplasia.

Scheie and Hurler MPS

Scheie syndrome (MPS I-S; OMIM 252800 [6]) is an allelic variant of the more severe Hurler syndrome (MPS I-H; OMIM 252800 [6]). The defective enzyme is α-L-iduronidase. Children with Scheie syndrome have normal intelligence, mild skeletal disease, and progressive noninflammatory stiffening of joints that is initially frequently misdiagnosed as arthritis.

Morquio syndrome (MPS IV)

Deficiency of either galactosamine-6-sulfatase (MPS IVa; OMIM 253000) or beta-galactosidase (MPS IVb; OMIM 253010) gives rise to similar phenotypes characterized by short-trunked dwarfism, normal head size, and normal intelligence. By age 3–4 years the joints appear enlarged and an effusion may be present in a large joint raising a concern regarding JIA. Progressive stiffness occurs but hyperextensibility particularly of the wrists with ulnar deviation may also be present. The radiographic findings include platyspondyly, with the vertebral bodies becoming more flat and rectangular as the child grows, posterior displacement of L1 causing a gibbus and frequently absent or hypoplastic odontoid process of C2. The latter may lead to spinal compression secondary to atlantoaxial subluxation and is a cause of death in these patients.

Pseudo-Hurler polydystrophy (ML III; OMIM 252600 [6])

The affected child typically presents with stiff or painful joints (hands and shoulders) after 2 years of age and this may be the first sign of disease, almost invariably leading to an initial diagnosis of JIA. Joint stiffness is progressive during childhood and may involve most joints but in particular those of the hands. The initial joint pain often disappears later. Short stature and scoliosis are usually present by 4–6 years of age and there may be mild corneal opacities, mild coarseness of facial features, and thickening of the skin. Radiographic findings of dysostosis multiplex are mild to moderate in severity; in addition there may be characteristic flattening of proximal femoral epiphyses with valgus deformity of the femoral neck in this disorder. Approximately half of the patients have a learning disability or developmental delay.

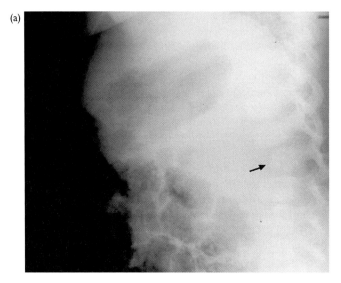
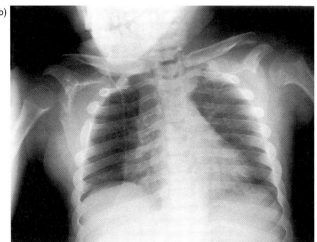
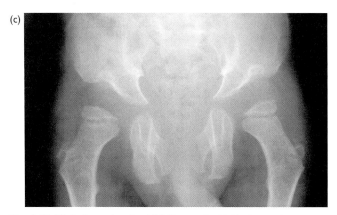

Fig. 1.11.10 Radiographs of a child diagnosed with Hurler syndrome demonstrate some of the characteristic findings associated with dysostosis multiplex: (a) shows a hypoplastic, beaked vertebra (arrow), (b) chest radiograph demonstrates widened "spatula" ribs and the radiograph of the hips, (c) shows the overtabulation of the iliac component of the acetabulum. (Courtesy of C. Ruzal-Shapiro.)

Osteochondrodysplasias: disorders of chondro-osseous development that frequently are associated with disproportionate short stature and either joint contractures or laxity (Table 1.11.7)

The heterogeneous group of osteochondrodysplasis is primarily characterized by abnormal formation of cartilage and/or bone. More than 150 different forms have been identified and the list is still not complete; syndromes that have been identified in only one family are not included in the current classification which is based mainly on radiographic criteria [32]. Affected individuals often present to the clinician with musculoskeletal symptoms that may raise the question of JIA. In this section only those conditions that most resemble JIA, are discussed.

Suspicion regarding an underlying bone or connective tissue disorder rather than JIA should always be raised when there is a family history of early symmetrical joint problems or premature osteoarthritis especially of weight-bearing joints. Disproportionate short stature (sometimes subtle) is a common finding and routine laboratory evaluation is characteristically normal without elevation of inflammatory indices. However, diagnosis may be very difficult in mildly severely affected individuals.

The systematic evaluation of a child with suspected skeletal dysplasia should include an assessment of the upper-to-lower body segment (U/L) ratio (Table 1.11.4). A bone age should also be included in the routine evaluation of short stature. A delayed bone age indicates that the associated short stature may resolve with time or with treatment whereas a normal bone age in a short child is strongly suggestive of a short final stature, and is the characteristic finding in the child with a skeletal dysplasia. The U/L body ratio indicates whether the short stature is proportionate or not. Proportionate short stature is caused by, for example, an endocrine disorder, such as, growth hormone (GH) deficiency or a chronic illness; however, not all skeletal dysplasias affect the final height or the development of the trunk and lower extremities. The complete evaluation of a child with a suspected osteochondrodysplasia must also include appropriate radiographs. Radiodiagnostic criteria have been identified for most osteochondrodysplasias; however, the radiographic abnormalities are usually not present early in life and may disappear or change character once skeletal growth is completed.

Achondroplasia

Classic dwarfism or achondroplasia (OMIM 100.800[6]) was the first disorder where a mutation in the gene encoding fibroblast growth factor receptor 3 (FGFR3) was shown to be the underlying cause; as many as 90% of cases are the result of a de novo mutation. Following this discovery several additional disorders associated with severe skeletal malformations were shown to be the result of mutations in one of the FGFR genes [33]. Four different FGFRs have been identified and they interact with varying specificity with at least nine different members of the FGF family. The expression of FGFRs is highly regulated during development. FGFR3 is mainly expressed in the cartilage growth plates of the long bones during endochondral ossification (Figure 1.11.1).

Hypochondroplasia (OMIM 146000 [6])

The hypochondroplasias include a clinical spectrum of disproportionate short stature ranging from slightly decreased height with normal body proportions to a more severe skeletal dysplasia resembling achondroplasia, but the head is not affected as it is in classic dwarfism. The hypochondroplasias are probably not rare and mild variants remain an unrecognized cause of short stature [34,35]. In affected individuals, the spinal canal is relatively narrow in its caudal portion but is less severely affected than in classic achondroplasia and the neurologic complications of achondroplasia including leg pain secondary to cord compression are usually absent. Other musculoskeletal complications that occur less frequently in patients with hypochondroplasia than in those with achondroplasia are tibial bowing, degenerative lumbar disease, and disc herniation. The diagnosis of hypochondroplasia is confirmed by radiographs of the lumbar spine showing a lack of increase in the interpedicular distance between vertebrae L1 and L5, with short pedicles, in the absence of other radiographic abnormalities. A decrease in the interpedicular distance is found in patients with achondroplasia (Figure 1.11.11). A mutation in the FGFR3 gene has been identified in most individuals with hypochondroplasia suggesting that it may be part of a phenotypic spectrum with achondroplasia as the most severe form.

Spondyloepiphyseal dysplasias (SED)

The spondyloepiphyseal dysplasias primarily affect development of the spine and the epiphyses causing radiographic flattening of the vertebral bodies with hump-shaped central and posterior portions and irregularities of the epiphyses (Figure 1.11.12). The epiphyseal abnormalites often lead to premature osteoarthritis of the weight-bearing joints such as the hips and knees. Impaired growth of the axial skeleton causes disproportionate short stature with short trunk and neck.

Spondyloepiphyseal dysplasias congenita (SEDC) (OMIM 183900 [6])

This severe autosomal dominant form of SED, unlike other SEDs, may be recognized early, even at birth. The newborn may present with rhizomelic shortening of limbs and pes equinovarus. The spine and juxtatruncal epiphysis are primarily involved. There is marked delay in mineralization with restricted growth of long bones and spine. Vitreous degeneration of the eyes and deafness are associated features. The genetic defect has been mapped to COL2A1, encoding the α-1 chain of collagen type II.

Spondyloepiphyseal dysplasias tarda (OMIM 313400 [6])

This is an X-linked recessive disorder with clinically apparent onset around age 10–14 years at which time growth of the spine seems to stop while the limbs continue to lengthen. This leads to disproportionatly short stature with short trunk and neck. Premature osteoarthritis caused by a mild to moderate epiphyseal dysplasia is characteristic and typically affects the hips. Obligate female carriers are clinically and radiographically normal. The gene causing SED tarda (SEDL) maps to Xp22 and encodes a protein that is predicted to function in endoplasmic reticulum-to-Golgi vesicular transport [36]. The SEDL gene-product is widely expressed and it is intriguing that abnormalities in SEDL give rise to a phenotype restricted to the skeleton. An apparent

Table 1.11.7 An approach to the diagnostic evaluation of the osteochondrodysplasias

Clinical characteristics				Radiographs[a]	Classification
Skeletal	Joints		Other		
	lax	stiff			
Achondroplasia (classic dwarfism) and genetically related syndromes					
Short limbs, bowing of legs, large head, lumbar lordosis. Present at birth	+[b]	+	Spinal stenosis. Normal intelligence unless complications from hydrocephalus	Lumbar spine: decrease in interpedicular from above downward. Limbs: rhizomelic shortening. Pelvis: short and wide	Achondroplasia
Disproportionate short stature, normal head, no lumbar lordosis	+/−	+/−		Lumbar spine: unchanged (compared to the normally increased distance) interpedicular distance from above downward	Hypochondroplasia
SED: short stature with short neck and trunk					
				Platyspondyly, delayed mineralization of epiphyses with flattening and irregular shape	
Rhizomelic shortening of limbs, cleft palate, pes equinovarus, hypoplastic C2 odontoid process, marked delay in mineralization		+	Ophthalmopathy, deafness, dysmorphic facies, cognitive dysfunction, hernia	Spine, pelvis, extremities	SED congenita
Early (10–14 years) onset of degenerative arthritis in hips and knees		+		Lumbar spine, epiphyses of affected joints	SED tarda (X-linked)
Painful joint contractures (small and large joints), bony enlargement of joints, osteopenia		+	Muscle weakness, waddling gait	Spine, involved tubular bones	SED tarda with progressive arthropathy (PRAC)
Variable severity of short stature		+	Immunodeficiency, anemia, renal disease, hypertension, multiple lentigines of skin	Spine and epiphyses of affected joints	Schimke immuno-osseous SED
Short-limbed short stature, brachydactyly, Pseudoachondroplasia scoliosis	+		Clinically resembles multiple epiphyseal dysplasia 1 (MED1)	Spine (anterior beaking of vertebrae), long bones and hands	
Epiphyseal dysplasia: short-limbed short stature					
				Delayed mineralization of epiphyses, flattening and fragmentation of mature epiphyses, early osteoarthritis	
Clinically variable. Joint pain with predominant involvement of hips, knees, and ankles; brachydactyly; premature osteoarthritis		+	Waddling gait, AVN of the hips	Hips, knees, ankles, hands. Changes in distal tibia may be diagnostic	MED1
Same		+	Same. Mild proximal myopathy		MED3
Same		+	Waddling gait, AVN of the hips		MED5
Same but brachydactyly may be mild		+	Same	Mainly knees	MED2
Same but brachydactyly is not present		+	Same	Flat femoral heads, normal hands	MED4
Metaphyseal dysplasia: short-limbed short stature					
				Early: poor mineralization with splaying of metaphyses Late: bone fills in; metaphyseal ends are wide	
Mild to moderate short stature			SCID	Ribs: splaying of costochondral ends	ADA deficiency
Mild to moderate short stature, coxa vara			Pancreatic insufficiency, neutropenia, anaemia	Hips, mild splaying of costo-chondral ends	Schwachman–Diamond syndrome
Moderate to severe short stature with delayed growth from birth. Flexion contractures of elbows, loose-jointed fingers			Immunodeficiency, anaemia, sparse hair. Hirschsprung disease	Large joints and hands. Metaphyseal abnormalities improve on radiographs after the growth period is over	Cartilage–hair dysplasia
Mild to moderate short stature, bowing of legs, stiffness of fingers			"Idiopathic" coax vara. Waddling gait, may clinically resemble vitamin D resistant rickets	Hips knees, upper extremities	Schmid metaphyseal dysplasia

Table 1.11.7 (*Continued*)

Clinical characteristics			Radiographs[a]	Classification
Skeletal	**Joints**	**Other**		
	lax stiff			
Metaphyseal dysplasia: short-limbed short stature (cont)				
Severe (rhizomelic) short stature present early in life	+	Hypercalcaemia, hypercaliuria	Spine, pelvis, lower extremities, hands	Jansen metaphyseal dysplasia
Severe short stature		Fetal death is common	Advanced endochondral bone maturation	Blomstrand metaphyseal dysplasia
Stickler–Kniest dysplasias: disproportionate short stature				
			Mild platyspondyly, small and flat epiphyses, and enlarged metaphyses of tubular bones	
Disproportionate short stature. Bony enlargement of knees, ankles, and wrists, premature osteoarthritis	+	Ophthalmopathy with high myopia, deafness, MVP, Pierre–Robin sequence, Legg–Calve–Perthes disease	Spine, hips, knees, ankles	Stickler dysplasia I
Same as above	+	Same as above but minimal ocular disease	Same as above	Stickler dysplasia II
Same as above	+	Same as above but no ocular disease	Same as above	Stickler dysplasia III
Same but in general more severe phenotype. Hands and feet are involved. Lumbar lordosis,	+	Same as above including ophthalmopathy and high myopia, macrocephaly, flat nasal bridge, cleft palate	Same and hands/feet	Kniest dysplasia
Mesomelic dysplasia: short stature with short forelegs				
Short stature with short legs, bowing of forearm		Females more severe by affected than males	Short tibia relative to the fibula. Madelung deformity of the forearm	Leri–Weill syndrome
Severely short stature		Micrognathia	Same as above but more severe phenotype. Hypoplasia or aplasia of ulna and fibula	Langer type
Acro/acro-mesomelic dysplasias				
Large IP joints, mild to moderately short stature		Sparse hair, large, pear-shaped nose, AVN of hips, hypotonia in infancy	Cone-shaped epiphyses of middle phalanges of hands, abnormal PIP joints, short metacarpals and metatarsals, small capital femoral epiphyses	Trichorinophalangeal dysplasia I (TRPS I)
Same as above and multiple cartilaginous exostoses	+	Sparse hair, large protruding ears, broad nasal bridge, cutis laxa, hypotonia, cognitive dysfunction	Same as above. Multiple exostoses of long tubular and other bones	Trichorinophalangeal dysplasia II (TRPS II)
Bone dysplasias with increased bone density				
Unilateral pain and swelling of one bone or joint	+	Oedema and rash or atrophic changes over bony lesion	Cortical hyperostosis, "dripping candle wax" pattern	Melorheostosis
Pain in limb brought on by activity. Presents in early childhood or at birth	+	Gait abnormalities, muscle weakness of involved limb	Hyperostosis of diaphysis of long bone	Camurati–Engelmann syndrome
Frontal bossing, pathologic fractures	+	Neurologic complications due to nerve compression by bone	Osteosclerosis, "bone-within-bone"	Infantile osteopetrosis
Stippled epiphyses: disproportionate short stature				
			Stippled calcification of cartilage	
Asymmetric shortening of limbs, joint contractures often noted at birth, scoliosis	+	Ichtyosiform rash, cataracts	Vertebral bodies, epiphyses of large joints, "stippling" may regress with time	Conradi–Hunermann syndrome
Multiple joint contractures at birth, rhizomelic short limbs	+	Mental retardation, cataracts, ichtyosiform rash, early death	Spine, epiphyses throughout. Coronal clefts in spine	Rhizomelic chondrodysplasia punctata
Disproportionate short stature	+	Ichtyosiform rash, hair abnormalities, hypoplasia of nose	Spine, epiphyses. Coronal clefts in spine. Short second and third metacarpals, short tibiae	Autosomal dominant chodrodysplasia punctata

Table 1.11.7 (*Continued*)

Clinical characteristics			Radiographs[a]	Classification
Skeletal	**Joints**	**Other**		
	lax **stiff**			
Disorganized development of cartilage[c]				
			Cartilaginous skeletal growths	
Pain around joint that may simulate arthritis, limited growth of affected bones	+	Onset between 10 and 30 years	Metaphyses of femur, tibia, fibula, and humerus	Multiple cartilaginous exostoses
Stiffness of fingers that may be mistaken for arthritis, limited growth of affected bones	+	Increased risk fractures. Low risk of malignant transformation of enchondroma	Hands and other involved bones	Enchondromatosis (Ollier)
Same as above	+	Same as above. Haemangioma	Same as above	Enchondromatosis with haemangiomata (Maffuci)
Idiopathic osteolysis				
			Lytic bone lesions often preceded by demineralization and leading to deformities of bone	
Pain, swelling, and warmth of wrists	+		Hand and wrist	Carpal–tarsal osteolysis
Same	+	Nephropathy, hypertension	Same	Osteolysis with nephropathy
Same	+	Nodulosis, arthropathy	Same	Nodulosis–arthropathy–osteolysis syndrome
Pain and swelling of multiple joints, starts in infancy. Short stature, osteoporosis	+	Dysmorphic features, corneal opacities	Skeletal survey	Winchester syndrome
Osteolytic lesions of long bones develop during early childhood	+		Long bones	Familial expansile osteolysis

Abbreviations: MVP: mitral valve prolapse. AVN: avascular necrosis.

[a] Radiographic characteristics of each group are listed in the heading. Specific radiographic features and/or bones that are typically involved in each disorder are listed separately for each disease. Clinical variation is common within the osteochondrodysplasias and the individual patient may not exhibit all (or have additional) radiographic findings on evaluation.

[b] Hypermobility is common in most joints except the elbows where limitation of movement is the typical finding.

[c] This group of disorders is discussed in Part 1, Chapter 1.10.

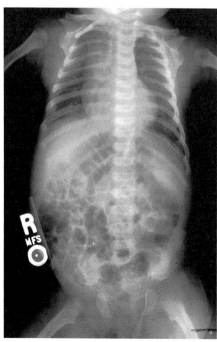

Fig. 1.11.11 Neonate diagnosed with achondroplasia. Radiograph of the spine demonstrates the narrowing of the interpedicular distance from L1 downwards.(Courtesy of C. Ruzal-Shapiro.)

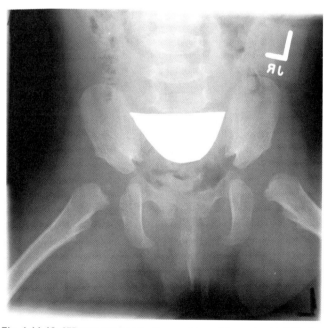

Fig. 1.11.12 SED was incidentally diagnosed in an 18-month-old child who presented with gait-disturbance. Radiograph demonstrates flattening of the vertebral bodies (platyspondyly) and delayed ossification of the epiphyses. The gait-disturbance resolved spontaneously and was later ascribed to a behavioural reaction to a new sibling. (Courtesy of C. Ruzal-Shapiro.)

autosomal dominant form of SED tarda (OMIM 184100 [6]) producing severely short stature has been described in several families.

Spondyloepiphyseal dysplasias tarda with progressive arthropathy (pseudorheumatoid arthritis of childhood; OMIM 208230 [6])

This autosomal recessive disorder is frequently misdiagnosed as JIA. Affected individuals are asymptomatic until early childhood when muscle weakness, walking difficulties (a waddling gait), and progressive, painful joint contractures develop. Neurological examination is normal but manual muscle testing reveals weakness. The interphalangeal and other joints are often enlarged without soft-tissue swelling; synovial biopsy is normal. Radiographically, the thickened joints show distended bony ends. Radiographs also demonstrate platyspondyly with irregular ossification of vertebral bodies, widened epiphyses of long and short tubular bones, narrow joint-spaces with loss of articular cartilage, and generalized osteopenia; bony erosions are not a feature. Functional disability and painful joint contractures necessitate joint replacement surgery in the third or fourth decade of life. The disease has a relentless progression; inflammatory indices are normal and no effective treatment is available. The gene causing this disorder, *WISP3*, encodes a protein that belongs to the CCN family of cystein-rich proteins implicated in cell growth and differentiation [37].

Schimke immuno-osseous dysplasia (OMIM 242900 [6])

This rare autosomal recessive disorder is characterized by short stature, SED, renal dysfunction (focal glomerulosclerosis), and a T cell immunodeficiency [38]. Anaemia, lymphopenia, or pancytopenia may be present in some individuals and autoimmune phenomena may also occur, suggesting an autoimmune illness. The gene defect has been localized to SMARCAL1 encoding an intracellular protein implicated in the regulation of chromatin remodeling [39]. The clinical spectrum ranges from severe to mild disease and the phenotype appears to correlate with the residual activity of the altered protein.

Stickler dysplasia

Stickler dysplasia I (vitreous type; OMIM 108300 [6]) with autosomal dominant inheritance is one of the most common connective tissue dysplasias worldwide with an estimated prevalence of 1 : 10,000. Noninflammatory bony enlargement of the knees, ankles, and wrists often visible early in life are the chief clinical/skeletal features that should lead to a consideration of Stickler syndrome. Hip pain is also common; in a study of more than 50 patients with Stickler, two-thirds had chronic hip pain [40]. Stickler syndrome may be mistaken for JIA. Premature degenerative arthritis is typical. The arthropathy is associated with joint hypermobility (Figure 1.11.13), a characteristic facial appearance, a marfanoid, slender body habitus, and pain after overuse of affected joints. Characteristic radiographic findings include small flat epiphyses, particularly of hips and ankles, enlarged (dumb-bell-shaped) metaphyses of tubular bones and mild platyspondyly. A wide short (valgus) femoral neck is typical but not diagnostic. Skeletal abnormalities may be minimal in some patients. An ocular symptom complex, starting in the first decade of life, of high-grade myopia, cataracts, and retinal disease, sometimes causing blindness, is found in association with Stickler dysplasia. High-grade myopia (>6 diopters

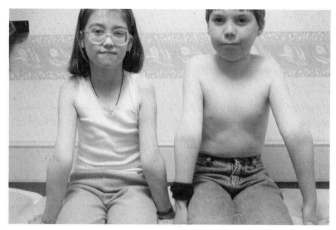

Fig. 1.11.13 Two siblings affected by Stickler dysplasia type I. Note the hypermobility of the elbows in both children and the myopia requiring correction with glasses in the girl. (Courtesy of T. R. Southwood.)

refractive error) in a child is highly associated with ocular and systemic abnormalities and should always initiate a search for associated disorders [41]. Deafness, mitral valve prolapse, depressed nasal bridge, and history of a Pierre–Robin sequence at birth are additional clinical characteristics as is a "family history of Legg–Calve–Perthes disease." The familial occurrence of arthropathy and ocular disease suggests the diagnosis.

The genetic defect in Stickler syndrome type I has been mapped to the gene encoding collagen II (COL2A1). Collagen II is the dominant type of collagen found in cartilage (Table 1.11.1) and is also present in the vitreous, spine (nucleus pulposus), and the inner ear. Stickler syndrome is, however, genetically heterogeneous and Stickler syndrome II ("beaded vitreous type"; OMIM 604841 [6]) is caused by mutations in COL11A1 encoding the α1-chain of collagen type XI (a minor component of cartilage; Table 1.11.1). Individuals with Stickler syndrome III (nonocular type; OMIM 184840 [6]) have mutations in the α2-chain of collagen XI (*COL11A2* gene). A fourth type of Stickler syndrome has been predicted from linkage studies.

Kniest dysplasia (OMIM 156550 [6])

Similar to Stickler type I, Kniest syndrome is the result of a mutation in collagen II and the two disorders share both clinical and radiographic features, although Kniest syndrome is typically associated with a more severe phenotype.

Kniest dysplasia is characterized by short limbs and trunk, macrocephaly, a depressed nasal bridge, and widely spaced eyes. Ocular disease with high myopia, retinal detachment, deafness, and cleft palate represent associated clinical features. Radiographs demonstrate platyspondyly with anterior wedging of vertebral bodies, epiphyseal deformities, and flared metaphyses. Often there are small femoral epiphyses and large epiphyses at the knee, to conform to the flared metaphyses. Both Stickler and Kniest syndromes share certain features with SED, such as, spine involvement but unlike SED, the hands and feet are also affected in Kniest syndrome. Joint involvement is most pronounced at the hips, knees, and hands. Joint contractures and pain are common and occur during the early years of life.

It is interesting that mutations in type II collagen also cause SED congenita. It is possible that the known phenotypic manifestations of defects involving type II collagen, including Stickler I, Kniest, SED congenita, and other, for example, primary osteoarthritis [42] corre-late with as yet undetermined residual functional features of collagen II and represent a genotypic spectrum of "type II collagenopathies." Another clinical example of the relationship between the disorders affecting type II collagen is a case report of the mother with a mild form of Stickler dysplasia who gave birth to a daughter with Kniest syndrome and a more severe phenotype. It was demonstrated that the mother was a mosaic for a somatic mutation in COL2A that she had transmitted in the germline to her child [43].

Epiphyseal dysplasia

These are classified according to the pattern of epiphyseal involvement and are primarily characterized by delayed ossification centres and irregularities of the involved epiphyses, resulting in deformity and delayed growth of the bone (Figure 1.11.14).

Multiple epiphyseal dysplasia

The multiple epiphyseal dysplasias (MEDs) constitute a genetically and phenotypically heterogeneous group of conditions with the clini-cal spectrum ranging from mild to severe. The main characteristics include short-limbed short stature and premature osteoarthritis. Patients come for clinical evaluation because of poor growth, difficul-ties with walking, and/or joint pain; the symptoms rarely manifest prior to 2 years of age. Hips, knees, and ankles are most commonly

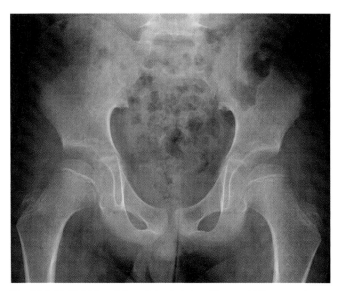

Fig. 1.11.14 Multiple epiphyseal dysplasia in a 10-year-old Korean male who was well until age 7 years when he developed pain in his knees, ankles, and feet, with intermittent limping and inability to run normally. The pain was worse with exercise and there was no morning stiffness. The family history was significant for a mother with arthritis in her knees starting at 17 years and a maternal grandmother who had arthritis of her knees; several other relatives on the maternal side also had arthritis of the knees. The patient's height and weight were at the 75th percentile; he had no dysmorphic features. The knees were large, but not swollen, and they were mildly tender with normal mobility. The ankles were also mildly tender, and there was pain with extension. The feet were pronated and flat, but flexible. Radiographs revealed multiple epiphyseal irregularities of all bones and abnormal carpal and tarsal bones that were small and irregular in shape. The spine and skull were normal. Shown in the figure are the characteristic, flattened epiphyses of the hip joints. (Courtesy of Y. Kimura.)

involved; brachydactyly is characteristically present. Avascular necro-sis of the hip is over-represented in patients with MED.

Genotype analyses have demonstrated mutations in different cartilage-related proteins (Table 1.11.1) and led to the identification of at least five different types of MEDs (MED1-5). MED1 (OMIM 132400 [6]) with autosomal dominant inheritance is caused by muta-tions in the gene encoding cartilage oligomeric matrix protein (COMP) and has in the past been broadly categorized into the more severe Fairbank type and the milder Ribbing type.

Pseudoachondroplasia (OMIM 177150 [6])

Pseudoachondroplasia, classified as a SED, is also the result of muta-tions in the gene encoding COMP and exhibits clinical similarities to MED1. Pseudoachondroplasia is characterized by short stature, brachydactyly, ligamentous laxity, and scoliosis; radiographs show abnormalities of epiphyses and metaphyses of the hands and long bones and anterior beaking of the vertebrae. This is in contrast to patients diagnosed with MED where the spine usually is normal.

Other forms of MED

Mutations in one of the collagen IX alpha chains (a component of normal cartilage) have been identified in other types of MEDs: MED2 (COL9A2; OMIM 600204) and MED3 (COL9A3; OMIM 600969), both with autosomal domiant inheritance. Patients with MED3 often have a mild proximal myopathy in addition to joint stiffness. An autosomal recessive type, MED4 (OMIM 226900) is the result of mutations in a sulfate transporter present in chondrocytes (and in other tissues), SLC26A2. MED4 differs from the autosomal dominant MED by the radiographic presence of flat femoral heads and absence of brachydactyly; normal adult height has been reported in a patient with MED4. MED5 (OMIM 602109) is caused by muta-tions in matrilin-3, an extracellular matrix protein found in carti-lage. One patient diagnosed with MED5 had resolution of joint symptoms as well as radiographic abnormalities with advancing age. Other individuals with MED5 have required hip or knee replacement surgery.

Metaphyseal dysplasia

Metaphyseal dysplasias affect the metaphyses of ribs and long bones with typical radiographic findings demonstrating delayed mineraliza-tion and splaying of the metaphyses. Initially, the metaphyses are widened, cupped, and resembles rickets; later they fill in with foci of irregular calcification of different size and radiographically look almost like normal bone; however, the metaphyses remain wide (Figure 1.11.15). The metaphyseal dysplasias lead to abnormal growth of affected bones, frequently causing short-limbed short stature. Prominent joint contractures are common. Differential diagnosis in early life includes hypophosphatemia and hyperparathyroidism.

Adenosine deaminase deficiency (OMIM 102700 [6])

These children present with severe combined immunodeficiency (SCID) during the first 6 months of life and the skeletal findings are rarely a major problem. In individuals with partial ADA-deficiency in whom the immunodeficiency is less severe, the correct diagnosis may be delayed. The radiographic and skeletal findings include splaying of the ends of the ribs; similar to the findings seen in children with rick-ets ("rachitic rosary"). Case reports have described children with other

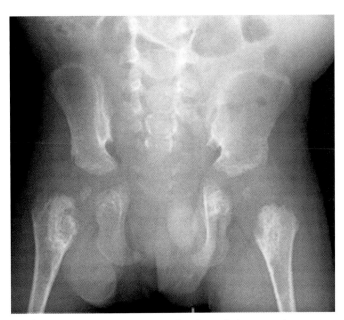

Fig. 1.11.15 Metaphyseal dysplasia with radiograph demonstrating irregularly mineralized femoral metaphyses. (Courtesy of C. Ruzal-Shapiro.)

types of immunodeficiency (including SCID) that are associated with skeletal dysplasias [44].

Schwachmann–Diamond syndrome (OMIM 240400 [6])

In these individuals a metaphyseal dysplasia is associated with pancreatic exocrine insufficiency and chronic, sometimes cyclic, neutropenia frequently with anaemia. Radiographs are most abnormal in the upper ends of the femur and associated with a coxa vara defect; other sites such as the costochondral junctions are often only mildly involved and tend to improve with age. Affected children may complain of joint pain in the lower extremities. Growth hormone deficiency has been reported in association with the Schwachmann–Diamond syndrome in several patients [45].

Cartilage–hair hypoplasia (OMIM 250250 [6])

This autosomal recessive metaphyseal dysplasia is characterized by disproportionate short-limbed short stature, normal head, sparse hair, and impaired cellular immunity; the latter being a consistent manifestation of the disorder. Defects in humoral immunity may also be present [46]. Anaemia is common and there is an increased incidence of Hirschsprung disease. Skeletal growth is delayed from birth and often results in an adult height of 110–140 cm; the hands and feet are short and pudgy. However, the severity of skeletal involvement has a variable expression even within affected families. Radiographs are not diagnostic in adults; the metaphyseal irregularities are predominantly present during the growth period. Ligamentous laxity is typical and is associated with limited extension of the elbows. A mutation in the gene *RMRP*, encoding an endoribonuclease (RNase RMP) co-segregates with the disease [47].

Schmid type (OMIM 156500 [6])

This is an autosomal-dominant metaphyseal dysplasia that results in mild to moderate short-limbed short stature (adult height 130–160 cm) associated with bowing of the legs and a waddling gait. Schmid dysplasia is the most commonly identified metaphyseal

dysplasia. The major long bones are most affected; many cases of "idiopathic" coxa vara defect may in fact be a Schmidt type metaphyseal dysplasia. Clinically, Schmid dysplasia may also be confused with vitamin D resistant rickets but does not display the biochemical abnormalities of rickets (Part 1, Chapter 1.10, Table 1.10.7). The gene defect has been localized to COL10A1 encoding collagen type X α1-chain. Type X collagen is normally restricted in its expression to the zone of hypertrophic cartilage in the growth plate (Figure 1.11.1).

Jansen type (OMIM 156400 [6])

This rare autosomal-dominant metaphyseal dysplasia leads to very short stature (adult height is about 125 cm) with predominantly rhizomelic shortening of the limbs. Growth-retardation becomes apparent during the first few years of life. Associated findings include asymptomatic hypercalcaemia with hypercalciuria. The underlying genetic defect causes an activation mutation of the parathyroid hormone receptor (PTHR) [48]. Radiographs demonstrate extreme disorganization of metaphyses of long bones, metacarpals and metatarsals which appear widely separated from the almost normally appearing epiphyses. The spine and pelvis are also affected.

Blomstrand type (OMIM 215045 [6])

This metaphyseal dysplasia is caused by a mutation in the gene encoding the PTH receptor/PTH-related peptide (PTHrP) receptor leading to functional absence of receptors for both PTH and PTHrP [49] (the mirror image of the defect in Jansen type). This causes a metaphyseal dysplasia characterized by advanced endochondral bone maturation and typically, fetal death.

Mesomelic dysplasia

Leri–Weill syndrome (OMIM 127300 [6])

Affected individuals have short stature caused predominantly by shortening of the lower legs. A marked shortening of the tibia relative to the femur is highly suggestive of a mesomelic dysplasia. Expression is variable, the syndrome is often more severe in females. A Madelung deformity of the forearm with bowing of the radius and dorsal dislocation of the distal ulna is frequently present; the radiographic findings are unique. The Madelung deformity may also be associated with Turner syndrome, occur as an isolated phenomenon, or be secondary to trauma or osteomyelitis. If the patient's height is above the 25th percentile, the presence of a Madelung deformity is unlikely to be a manifestation of a mesomelic dysplasia. A mutation in the short stature homeobox-containing gene, *SHOX* causes Leri–Weill syndrome [50]; inheritance is autosomal-dominant. A mutation in *SHOX* has also been implicated in some forms of "idiopathic" growth retardation.

Langer mesomelic dwarfism (OMIM 249700 [6])

This syndrome is caused by homozygous mutations in the *SHOX* gene causing severely short stature and hypoplasia or aplasia of the ulna and fibula with a Madelung deformity.

Acro/acro-mesomelic dysplasia

Trichorhinophalangeal dysplasia I (OMIM 190350 [6])

Trichorhinophalangeal dysplasia (TRPS I) is an autosomal-dominant disorder that causes asymptomatic enlargement of the interphalangeal joints, and is often mistaken for JIA. Patients with TRPS I are also recognized by their large pear-shaped nose, thin upper lip, sparse, slow-growing hair, and moderately short stature. The hand deformities develop during the second-half of the first decade. Radiographs show cone-shaped epiphyses of the middle phalanges and abnormal proximal interphalgeal joints. The capital femoral epiphyses are small and, as in the epiphyseal dysplasias, avascular necrosis of the hip occurs with increased frequency. Some authors advocate obtaining hand films in all children with bilateral Legg–Perthes' disease to exclude TRPS I. A mutation in a zinc-finger transcription factor causes TRPS I [51].

Langer–Gideon syndrome (TRPS II, OMIM 150230)

Patients exhibit similar skeletal findings to TRPS I but, in addition, have cognitive dysfunction and multiple exostoses. The exact gene defect has not been identified but available data indicate that TRPS II is caused by a contiguous gene syndrome that includes the loss of the *TRPS I* gene.

Chondrodysplasia punctata

Chondrodysplasia punctata or "stippled epiphyses" includes many different conditions; some are sporadic and others are part of syndromes such as forms of Zellweger syndrome (see OMIM 214100 [6]), where chondral calcification often is most marked in the patellae. Abnormal calcification of cartilage may also be present in children with warfarin embryopathy, the fetal alcohol syndrome, and the CHILD syndrome (OMIM 308050 [6]).

Conradi–Hunermann syndrome (OMIM 302960 [6])

This X-linked dominant condition is presumably lethal in males and leads to joint contractures seen at birth in as many as one quarter of affected individuals. There may be asymmetric shortening of the limbs secondary to areas of punctate mineralization of the epiphyses (Figure 1.11.16). Scoliosis is common and related to areas of punctate mineralization as well. Intelligence is normal. Skin abnormalities occur in one-third of patients: ichtyosis is present in early life and later replaced by atrophic changes. Cataracts, often asymmetric and unilateral, are present in up to 20% of patients. Radiographs demonstrate stippled calcification of the vertebral bodies and epiphyses of the extremities, the calcium deposits tend to regress with time and may not be demonstrable in adults. Mutations in the *EBP* gene encoding a sterol-Δ^8 isomerase-binding protein [52] cause this form of stippled epiphyses. The involved enzyme catalyses an intermediate step in cholesterol synthesis, suggesting an important role for sterols in cartilage and bone development.

Rhizomelic chondrodysplasia punctata (OMIM 215100 [6])

Most children affected by the autosomal recessive, rhizomelic chondrodysplasia punctata are born with multiple joint contractures. Associated findings include mental retardation, symmetric, proximal shortening of the limbs, metaphyseal splaying, and multiple foci of epiphyseal calcifications in early infancy. Cataracts are common and are often symmetric and bilateral. Skin changes are of similar type and frequency as in the Conradi–Hunerman syndrome. The rhizomelic type is often fatal during the first year of life. The gene defect has been mapped to PEX7, encoding a peroxisomal (type 2) targeting receptor [53].

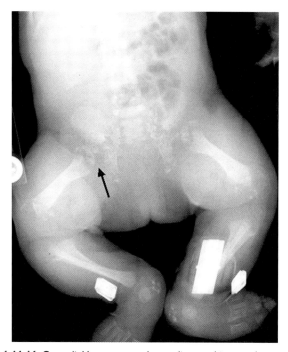

Fig. 1.11.16 Conradi–Hunerman syndrome diagnosed in a newborn. Several areas of stippled calcification (one is indicated by an arrow) of the epiphyses were identified on radiographic evaluation. (Courtesy of C. Ruzal-Shapiro.)

Autosomal-dominant chondrodysplasia punctata (OMIM 118650 [6])

Maternal ingestion of warfarin may lead to a phenotype that is very similar to autosomal-dominant chondrodysplasia punctata, characterized by hypoplasia of the nose, short tibiae, short second and third metacarpals and stippled epiphyses. Ichtyosis and abnormalities of the hair are present in the inherited form but are not associated with warfarin embryopathy; this finding differentiates the two disorders.

Osteochondrodysplasias with decreased bone density

Osteogenesis imperfecta (OI)

Four principal types of osteogenesis imperfecta (OI) have been identified, (Table 1.11.8); all resulting from abnormalities of collagen type I, the main collagen found in bone a significant number of patients with OI cannot be readily classified into any of the four types. OI has an overall prevalence of 1 : 5000 to 1 : 10,000 and is characterized by increased bone fractures, occurring after minimal trauma. Additional features include blue sclerae, hearing loss, scoliosis, progressive limb deformity, musculoskeletal pain, and difficulties with ambulation. Complications from spinal compression and other fractures contribute to the clinical severity of the disease. The joints are hypermobile. Individuals with type I OI (OMIM 166200 [6]) are normal at birth and develop frequent fractures during childhood. Kyphosis, scoliosis, and deformities of the lower legs are common. Type II OI (OMIM 166210 [6]), frequently lethal, is the only form that is easily recognized radiographically demonstrating "ribbon bones" and fractures that are too numerous to count; birth weight and body length are low. In type III OI (OMIM 259420 [6]) the bones are twisted, bowed, and fragile; this is a progressive form of OI with defects that are more pronounced than in type I. Type IV (OMIM 166200 [6]) is characterized by osteoporosis with or without a history of fractures and the skeletal abnormalities are variable.

Osteochondrodysplasia with increased bone density

Osteopetrosis

Different forms of osteopetrosis have been identified and are characterized by increased bone density. In the infantile or precocious form (OMIM 259700 [6]), a majority of patients have a mutation in an osteoclast-specific protein, indicating that functional abnormalities of bone turnover lead to the disease [54]. Radiographic examination shows patterns of osteosclerosis, with a bone-within-bone appearance. Affected children may present at birth with frontal bossing and are prone to pathologic fractures and neurologic complications secondary to compression of cranial or other nerves in canals narrowed by increased bone deposition.

Melorheostosis (OMIM 155950 [6])

This is a rare disorder of cortical hyperostosis that typically affects only one side of the bone on one side of the body. The most common location is the lower limb but the lesion may also occur in the skull, spine, rib, pelvis, or the facial bone. A somatic mutation may be responsible for this localized lesion. Pain, swelling, and stiffness of the involved area are characteristic and often the overlying skin shows abnormalities such as an erythematous shiny rash that later may become atrophic. Linear scleroderma has occurred in association with melorheostosis. Radiographs demonstrate cortical hyperostosis of the affected area, described as "dripping candle wax" (see also Part 1, Chapter 1.6).

Camurati–Engelman syndrome (OMIM 131300 [6])

Camurati–Engelman syndrome is an autosomal-dominant progressive diaphyseal dysplasia characterized by hyperostosis and sclerosis of the diaphyses of the long bones. The disease has been present at birth in some individuals but the usual age of presentation is late childhood. The child develops an asymptomatic contracture of a limb that may become painful after exaggerated activity, if the lesion affects the lower extremities. Muscle weakness and gait abnormalities are frequent. Radiographs show hyperostosis of the diaphyseal cortex which tend to increase with time; bone scintigraphy or CT may aid in the diagnosis. Mutations affecting TGFβ1 have been linked to the disease [55].

Idiopathic osteolysis

This group includes multicentric and monocentric osteolytic syndromes, some of which show dominant or recessive inheritance, while others appear to be sporadic. Lytic bone lesions may also occur secondary to infections (Figure 1.11.17) or be found in patients with a metabolic storage disorder (Table 1.11.9). Radiologic examination initially demonstrates intramedullary and subcortical, ill-defined lucent areas that later expand with progressive loss of density. Reactive bone formation is characteristically not present. Sometimes the distinction between a defect in bone development versus destruction of bone is difficult on radiographic evaluation and, for example, Hajdu–Cheney acroosteolysis (OMIM 102500 [6]), is now considered an osteodysplasia rather than an osteolytic syndrome.

Carpal–tarsal osteolysis

There are many different, poorly understood syndromes that begin in childhood with crippling and progressive osteolysis of the wrists and ankles. Initially, the preschool child is thought to have JIA with heat, tenderness, swelling, and flexion contractures of the wrists. Within a few years, generalized demineralization of the carpal and tarsal bones becomes apparent on radiographs. This is followed by localized destruction of carpal and tarsal bones and then complete resorption

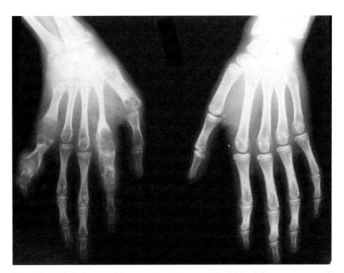

Fig. 1.11.17 A 9-year-old recent immigrant to the United States presented to the emergency room with multiple joint contractures and a brown, wax-like rash involving one earlobe and part of the nose. The patient had had a gradual development of the joint and skin symptoms over more than 6 years. Radiographs demonstrated multiple lytic lesions of all involved bone, as exemplified by the radiographs of her hands. A biopsy of the rash identified growth of the vaccine strain of BCG, which the patient had received as a newborn. Although not proven in this particular child, her unusual sensitivity to BCG may have been caused by an abnormality in the interferon-γ or IL-12 signalling pathway, as has been described in several unrelated pedigrees. The lungs were clear and bone and skin were the only affected organs. (Courtesy of M. Garzon.)

Table 1.11.8 Osteogenesis imperfecta: classification and characteristics

Classification	Clinical characteristics	Type I collagen abnormality
Type I	Fractures, osteopenia, blue sclerae, deafness	Null αl allele; reduced amounts of structurally normal collagen
Type II	Perinatal lethal form; fractures *in utero*, soft cranium, short limbs	Structural mutation in one of the collagen chains; abnormal collagen
Type III	Progressive deforming; fractures, limb deformity, scoliosis, growth retardation	Same as for type II
Type IV	Similar to type III, but less severe	Same as for type II

Table 1.11.9 Differential diagnosis of osteolysis

Multicentric osteolysis[a]	Infectious, granulomatous
Carpal–tarsal osteolysis	Sarcoidosis
Osteolysis with nephropathy[OMIM166300]	Tuberculosis
Nodulosis–arthropathy– osteolysis[OMIM 605156]	Sepsis
	Metabolic disorders
Familial expansile osteolysis[OMIM 174810]	Farber disease[OMIM228000]
Winchester syndrome[OMIM277950]	Pseudo-Hurler dystrophy[OMIM252600]
Other	Tumours

[a]This encompasses a large group of familial or sporadic osteolytic disorders.

and disappearance. The early childhood symptomatic phase is usually followed in adolescence by a relatively pain-free period, during which the bones are disappearing. There is no synovial inflammation. Later in life, deformity may become pronounced.

An autosomal dominant form of carpal–tarsal osteolysis, idiopathic multicentric osteolysis, is associated with hypertension and nephropathy (OMIM 166300 [6]). Another type is characterized by nodulosis, arthropathy, and osteolysis (OMIM 605156 [6]) [56] and is caused by mutations in the gene encoding MMP2 [57].

Winchester syndrome (OMIM 277950 [6])

This autosomal recessive form of multicentric osteolysis manifests during the first months of life. Symmetric swelling of the fingers, hands, wrists, and ankles are accompanied by pain and contractures of the hips and elbows. Osteolysis of the carpal–tarsal bones results in arthritis mutilans (the opera-glass hand). Other features include short stature, corneal opacities, coarse facial features, and generalized osteoporosis. The basic defect has not been identified but studies in cultured fibroblasts and abnormalities detected by electron microscopy have suggested that it may be a metabolic storage disorder.

Familial expansile osteolysis (OMIM 174810 [6])

Autosomal-dominant inheritance characterizes this disorder in which osteolytic lesions of the long bones develop during early adulthood. The genetic defect was recently identified and involves an activating mutation of the gene *TNFRSF11A* encoding RANK (receptor activator of nuclear factor-kappa B), which is essential for osteoclast development, suggesting an underlying mechanism of increased bone resorption [58].

References

1. Andersson Gare, B. Juvenile arthritis—who gets it, where and when? A review of current data on incidence and prevalence. *Clin Exp Rheumatol* 1999;17:367–74.

2. Jones, K.L. and Smith, D.W. *Smith's Recognizable Patterns of Human Malformation*. Philadelphia, PA: Saunders, 1997, xviii, 857 pp.

3. Chalom, E.C., Ross, J., and Athreya, B.H. Syndromes and arthritis. *Rheum Dis Clin North Am* 1997;23:709–27.

4. Schinke, T., McKee, M.D., and Karsenty, G. Extracellular matrix calcification: where is the action? *Nat Genet* 1999;21:150–1.

5. Beighton, P., Grahame, R., and Bird, H.A. *Hypermobility of Joints*. London; New York: Springer, 1999, ix, 182 pp.

6. McKusick, V. *Online Mendelian Inheritance in Man*. Johns Hopkins University. www.ncbi.nlm.nih.gov/entrez/omim.

7. Hall, J.G., Froster-Iskenius, U.G., and Allanson, J.E. *Handbook of Normal Physical Measurements*. Oxford; New York: Oxford University Press, 1989;504 pp.

8. Fattori, R., Nienaber, C.A., Descovich, B., Ambrosetto, P., Reggiani, L.B., Pepe, G., Kaufmann, U., Negrini, E., von Kodolitsch, Y., and Gensini, G.F. Importance of dural ectasia in phenotypic assessment of Marfan's syndrome. *Lancet* 1999;354:910–13.

9. De Paepe, A., Devereux, R.B., Dietz, H.C., Hennekam, R.C., and Pyeritz, R.E. Revised diagnostic criteria for the Marfan syndrome. *Am J Med Genet* 1996;62:417–26.

10. Beighton, P., de Paepe, A., Danks, D., Finidori, G., Gedde-Dahl, T., Goodman, R., Hall, J.G., Hollister, D.W., Horton, W., McKusick, V.A., et al. International nosology of heritable disorders of connective tissue, Berlin, 1986. *Am J Med Genet* 1988;29:581–94.

11. Estes, J.W. Platelet size and function in the heritable disorders of connective tissue. *Ann Intern Med* 1968;68:1237–49.

12. Anstey, A., Mayne, K., Winter, M., Van de Pette, J., and Pope, F.M. Platelet and coagulation studies in Ehlers–Danlos syndrome. *Br J Dermatol* 1991;125:155–63.

13. Kaplinsky, C., Kenet, G., Seligsohn, U., and Rechavi, G. Association between hyperflexibility of the thumb and an unexplained bleeding tendency: is it a rule of thumb? *Br J Haematol* 1998;101:260–3.

14. Beighton, P., De Paepe, A., Steinmann, B., Tsipouras, P., and Wenstrup, R.J. Ehlers–Danlos syndromes: revised nosology, Villefranche, 1997. Ehlers–Danlos National Foundation (USA) and Ehlers–Danlos Support Group (UK). *Am J Med Genet* 1998;77:31–7.

15. Schalkwijk, J., Zweers, M.C., Steijlen, P.M., Dean, W.B., Taylor, G., van Vlijmen, I.M., van Haren, B., Miller, W.L., and Bristow, J. A recessive form of the Ehlers–Danlos syndrome caused by tenascin-X deficiency. *N Engl J Med* 2001;345:1167–75.

16. Sacheti, A., Szemere, J., Bernstein, B., Tafas, T., Schechter, N., and Tsipouras, P. Chronic pain is a manifestation of the Ehlers–Danlos syndrome. *J Pain Sympt Manage* 1997;14:88–93.

17. Gordon, N. Arthrogryposis multiplex congenita. *Brain Dev* 1998;20:507–11.

18. Hall, J.G., Reed, S.D., and Greene, G. The distal arthrogryposes: delineation of new entities—review and nosologic discussion. *Am J Med Genet* 1982;11:185–239.

19. Moore, E.S., Ward, R.E., Jamison, P.L., Morris, C.A., Bader, P.I., and Hall, B.D. The subtle facial signs of prenatal exposure to alcohol: an anthropometric approach. *J Pediatr* 2001;139:215–19.

20. Goshen, E., Schwartz, A., Zilka, L.R., and Zwas, S.T. Bilateral accessory iliac horns: pathognomonic findings in nail-patella syndrome. Scintigraphic evidence on bone scan. *Clin Nucl Med* 2000;25:476–7.

21. Dreyer, S.D., Morello, R., German, M.S., Zabel, B., Winterpacht, A., Lunstrum, G.P., Horton, W.A., Oberg, K.C., and Lee, B. LMX1B transactivation and expression in nail-patella syndrome. *Hum Mol Genet* 2000;9:1067–74.

22. Rozin, M.M., Hertz, M., and Goodman, R.M. A new syndrome with camptodactyly, joint contractures, facial anomalies, and skeletal defects: a case report and review of syndromes with camptodactyly. *Clin Genet* 1984;26:342–55.

23. Marcelino, J., Carpten, J.D., Suwairi, W.M., Gutierrez, O.M., Schwartz, S., Robbins, C., Sood, R., Makalowska, I., Baxevanis, A., Johnstone, B., et al. CACP, encoding a secreted proteoglycan, is mutated in camptodactyly–arthropathy–coxa vara–pericarditis syndrome. *Nat Genet* 1999;23:319–22.

24. Jacobs, J.C. and Downey, J.A. Juvenile rheumatoid arthritis. In J.A. Downey and J.L. Low (ed.), *The Child with Disabling Illness*. Philadelphia, PA: Saunders, 1974;pp. 5–24.

25. Athreya, B.H. and Schumacher, H.R. Pathologic features of a familial arthropathy associated with congenital flexion contractures of fingers. *Arthritis Rheum* 1978;21:429–37.

26. Morris, C.A. and Mervis, C.B. Williams syndrome and related disorders. *Annu Rev Genomics Hum Genet* 2000;1:461–84.

27. Iqbal, M.A., Ulmer, C., and Sakati, N. Use of FISH technique in the diagnosis of chromosomal syndromes. *East Mediterr Health J* 1999;5:1218–24.

28. Bonne, G., Mercuri, E., Muchir, A., Urtizberea, A., Becane, H.M., Recan, D., Merlini, L., Wehnert, M., Boor, R., Reuner, U., *et al.* Clinical and molecular genetic spectrum of autosomal dominant Emery–Dreifuss muscular dystrophy due to mutations of the lamin A/C gene. *Ann Neurol* 2000;48:170–80.

29. Shafritz, A.B., Shore, E.M., Gannon, F.H., Zasloff, M.A., Taub, R., Muenke, M., and Kaplan, F.S. Overexpression of an osteogenic morphogen in fibrodysplasia ossificans progressiva. *N Engl J Med* 1996;335:555–61.

30. Kaplan, F.S. International Fibrodysplasia Ossificans Progressiva Assoc. (IFOPA). website: www.ifopa.org.

31. Scriver, C.R., Beaudet, A.L., Sly, W.S., *et al.* (ed.) *The Metabolic and Molecular Basis of Inherited Disease.* New York: McGraw-Hill. 6th ed. 1989;1590–2.

32. Spranger, J. International classification of osteochondrodysplasias. The International Working Group on Constitutional Diseases of Bone. *Eur J Pediatr* 1992;151:407–15.

33. Burke, D., Wilkes, D., Blundell, T.L., and Malcolm, S. Fibroblast growth factor receptors: lessons from the genes. *Trends Biochem Sci* 1998;23:59–62.

34. Hall, J.G. A bone is not a bone is not a bone. *J Pediatr* 1998;133:5–6.

35. Ramaswami, U., Rumsby, G., Hindmarsh, P.C., and Brook, C.G. Genotype and phenotype in hypochondroplasia. *J Pediatr* 1998;133:99–102.

36. Gedeon, A.K., Colley, A., Jamieson, R., Thompson, E.M., Rogers, J., Sillence, D., Tiller, G.E., Mulley, J.C., and Gecz, J. Identification of the gene (SEDL) causing X-linked spondyloepiphyseal dysplasia tarda. *Nat Genet* 1999;22:400–4.

37. Hurvitz, J.R., Suwairi, W.M., Van Hul, W., El-Shanti, H., Superti-Furga, A., Roudier, J., Holderbaum, D., Pauli, R.M., Herd, J.K., Van Hul, E.V., *et al.* Mutations in the CCN gene family member WISP3 cause progressive pseudorheumatoid dysplasia. *Nat Genet* 1999;23:94–8.

38. Boerkoel, C.F., O'Neill, S., Andre, J.L., Benke, P.J., Bogdanovic, R., Bulla, M., Burguet, A., Cockfield, S., Cordeiro, I., Ehrich, J.H., *et al.* Manifestations and treatment of Schimke immuno-osseous dysplasia: 14 new cases and a review of the literature. *Eur J Pediatr* 2000;159:1–7.

39. Boerkoel, C.F., Takashima, H., John, J., Yan, J., Stankiewicz, P., Rosenbarker, L., Andre, J.L., Bogdanovic, R., Burguet, A., Cockfield, S., *et al.* Mutant chromatin remodeling protein SMARCAL1 causes Schimke immuno-osseous dysplasia. *Nat Genet* 2002;30:215–20.

40. Rose, P.S., Ahn, N.U., Levy, H.P., Magid, D., Davis, J., Liberfarb, R.M., Sponseller, P.D., and Francomano, C.A. The hip in Stickler syndrome. *J Pediatr Orthop* 2001;21:657–63.

41. Marr, J.E., Halliwell-Ewen, J., Fisher, B., Soler, L., and Ainsworth, J.R. Associations of high myopia in childhood. *Eye* 2001;15:70–4.

42. Knowlton, R.G., Katzenstein, P.L., Moskowitz, R.W., Weaver, E.J., Malemud, C.J., Pathria, M.N., Jimenez, S.A., and Prockop, D.J. Genetic linkage of a polymorphism in the type II procollagen gene (COL2A1) to primary osteoarthritis associated with mild chondrodysplasia. *N Engl J Med* 1990;322:526–30.

43. Winterpacht, A., Hilbert, M., Schwarze, U., Mundlos, S., Spranger, J., and Zabel, B.U. Kniest and Stickler dysplasia phenotypes caused by collagen type II gene (COL2A1) defect. *Nat Genet* 1993;3:323–6.

44. Atkinson, A. Humoral immunodeficiencies associated with bone dysplasias. *Immunol Allergy Clinics N Am* 2001;21:113–27.

45. Marseglia, G.L., Bozzola, M., Marchi, A., Ricci, A., and Touraine, J.L. Response to long-term hGH therapy in two children with Schwachman–Diamond syndrome associated with GH deficiency. *Horm Res* 1998;50: 42–5.

46. Makitie, O., Kaitila, I., and Savilahti, E. Deficiency of humoral immunity in cartilage-hair hypoplasia. *J Pediatr* 2000;137:487–92.

47. Ridanpaa, M., van Eenennaam, H., Pelin, K., Chadwick, R., Johnson, C., Yuan, B., vanVenrooij, W., Pruijn, G., Salmela, R., Rockas, S., *et al.* Mutations in the RNA component of RNase MRP cause a pleiotropic human disease, cartilage-hair hypoplasia. *Cell* 2001;104:195–203.

48. Schipani, E., Langman, C.B., Parfitt, A.M., Jensen, G.S., Kikuchi, S., Kooh, S.W., Cole, W.G., and Juppner, H. Constitutively activated receptors for parathyroid hormone and parathyroid hormone-related peptide in Jansen's metaphyseal chondrodysplasia. *N Engl J Med* 1996;335:708–14.

49. Jobert, A.S., Zhang, P., Couvineau, A., Bonaventure, J., Roume, J., Le Merrer, M., and Silve, C. Absence of functional receptors for parathyroid hormone and parathyroid hormone-related peptide in Blomstrand chondrodysplasia. *J Clin Invest* 1998;102:34–40.

50. Shears, D.J., Vassal, H.J., Goodman, F.R., Palmer, R.W., Reardon, W., Superti-Furga, A., Scambler, P.J., and Winter, R.M. Mutation and deletion of the pseudoautosomal gene SHOX cause Leri–Weill dyschondrosteosis. *Nat Genet* 1998;19:70–3.

51. Momeni, P., Glockner, G., Schmidt, O., von Holtum, D., Albrecht, B., Gillessen-Kaesbach, G., Hennekam, R., Meinecke, P., Zabel, B., Rosenthal, A., *et al.* Mutations in a new gene, encoding a zinc-finger protein, cause tricho-rhino-phalangeal syndrome type I. *Nat Genet* 2000;24:71–4.

52. Braverman, N., Lin, P., Moebius, F.F., Obie, C., Moser, A., Glossmann, H., Wilcox, W.R., Rimoin, D.L., Smith, M., Kratz, L., *et al.* Mutations in the gene encoding 3 beta-hydroxysteroid-delta 8, delta 7-isomerase cause X-linked dominant Conradi–Hunermann syndrome. *Nat Genet* 1999; 22:291–4.

53. Braverman, N., Steel, G., Obie, C., Moser, A., Moser, H., Gould, S.J., and Valle, D. Human PEX7 encodes the peroxisomal PTS2 receptor and is responsible for rhizomelic chondrodysplasia punctata. *Nat Genet* 1997;15:369–76.

54. Frattini, A., Orchard, P.J., Sobacchi, C., Giliani, S., Abinun, M., Mattsson, J.P., Keeling, D.J., Andersson, A.K., Wallbrandt, P., Zecca, L., *et al.* Defects in TCIRG1 subunit of the vacuolar proton pump are responsible for a subset of human autosomal recessive osteopetrosis. *Nat Genet* 2000;25:343–6.

55. Kinoshita, A., Saito, T., Tomita, H., Makita, Y., Yoshida, K., Ghadami, M., Yamada, K., Kondo, S., Ikegawa, S., Nishimura, G., *et al.* Domain-specific mutations in TGFB1 result in Camurati–Engelmann disease. *Nat Genet* 2000;26:19–20.

56. Al-Mayouf, S.M., Majeed, M., Hugosson, C., and Bahabri, S. New form of idiopathic osteolysis: nodulosis, arthropathy and osteolysis (NAO) syndrome. *Am J Med Genet* 2000;93:5–10.

57. Martignetti, J.A., Aqeel, A.A., Sewairi, W.A., Boumah, C.E., Kambouris, M., Mayouf, S.A., Sheth, K.V., Eid, W.A., Dowling, O., Harris, J., *et al.* Mutation of the matrix metalloproteinase 2 gene (MMP2) causes a multicentric osteolysis and arthritis syndrome. *Nat Genet* 2001;28:261–5.

58. Hughes, A.E., Ralston, S.H., Marken, J., Bell, C., MacPherson, H., Wallace, R.G., van Hul, W., Whyte, M.P., Nakatsuka, K., Hovy, L., *et al.* Mutations in TNFRSF11A, affecting the signal peptide of RANK, cause familial expansile osteolysis. *Nat Genet* 2000;24:45–8.

59. Kuettner, K.E., Aydelotte, M.B., and Thonar, E.J.-M.A. Articular cartilage matrix and structure: a minireview. *J Rheumatol* 1991;18:46-8.

60. Cassidy, J.T., and Petty, R.E. Anatomy and physiology of the musculoskeletal system. In *Textbook of Pediatric Rheumatology.* J.T. Cassidy, and R.E. Petty, (eds) Philadelphia: W.B. Saunders 2001;9–29.

2

Juvenile Idiopathic Arthritis in children and adolescents

2.1 Classification of childhood arthritis
Taunton R. Southwood

2.2 Systemic Arthritis
*Anne-Marie Prieur, Peter N. Malleson, and
Yukiko Kimura*

2.3 Oligoarthritis
John J. Miller and Peter N. Malleson

2.4 Rheumatoid Factor Positive Polyarthritis
Janet Gardner-Medwin

2.5 Rheumatoid Factor Negative Polyarthritis
Alberto Martini

2.6 Psoriatic Arthritis
David A. Cabral

2.7 Enthesitis Related Arthritis
Ross E. Petty

2.8 Undifferentiated Arthritis
Taunton R. Southwood and Yukiko Kimura

2.9 Immunopathology of the joint in Juvenile
Idiopathic Arthritis
*Lucy R. Wedderburn, Kiran Nistala, and
Taunton R. Southwood*

2.10 Genetic and cytokine associations in Juvenile
Idiopathic Arthritis
Wendy Thomson, Patricia Woo, and Rachelle Donn

2.11 Environmental factors in the pathogenesis
of Juvenile Idiopathic Arthritis
Berent J. Prakken, Salvatore Albani, and Wietse Kuis

2.1 Classification of childhood arthritis

Taunton R. Southwood

Aims

The aims of this chapter are to discuss the historical and philosophical background giving rise to the ILAR classification of Juvenile Idiopathic Arthritis (JIA) and to outline the classification itself. The future evaluation of the classification is also discussed.

Structure

- Overview
- A history of the classification of arthritis in children
- The future of the classification
- The ILAR classification of JIA (2nd revision)
  - Systemic Arthritis
  - Oligoarthritis
  - Rheumatoid Factor Negative Polyarthritis
  - Rheumatoid Factor Positive Polyarthritis
  - Psoriatic Arthritis
  - Enthesitis Related Arthritis
  - Undifferentiated Arthritis
  - Exclusion criteria
  - Glossary of terms

Overview

Juvenile Idiopathic Arthritis (JIA) is a diagnosis of exclusion (see Part 1, Chapter 1.3). JIA refers to those forms of arthritis which begin before the 16th birthday, are persistent for longer than 6 weeks, and for which no cause is currently known [1]. Part 1 of this book gives an overview of the multitude of conditions which may be confused with JIA. Part 2, this section, is concerned with the group of conditions covered by the umbrella term of JIA, except for treatment, which is covered in the third and final section. Underpinning this section, and indeed the whole book, is the proposed ILAR (International League of Associations for Rheumatology) classification of JIA, now at the end of its first decade of existence [2].

The purpose of disease classification is to separate subjects with a disease from those without [3], particularly to improve the understanding of those conditions. This can be extended to identify subjects with a particular form of disease separately from patients without that form of disease and from normal subjects. In general, classification is an ongoing process, as "new diseases do not suddenly present themselves ready labelled in a new patient. They emerge slowly from the collection and interpretation of clinical observations and physiological measurements"[4]. Classification criteria may highlight the presence of a particular disease or specific subsets of that disease, but they are rarely perfect and some patients are likely to be misclassified. Such classification criteria are more suited to the study of groups of patients than the evaluation of individuals [5]. Indeed, one could argue that the greater the scientific precision of disease classification, the less reliable the clinical predictions about that disease (after Heisenberg's Uncertainty Principle 1926).

The core principles of the proposed ILAR classification underlie the philosophy of Part 2; that is each subtype of JIA is a clinically distinct entity and exclusive of the main features of every other subtype, apart from arthritis, which is an essential component of each. This is reflected in the subsequent seven chapters of the section; comprising descriptions of the subtypes of JIA, including discussion of the epidemiology, clinical features, complications, and prognosis of each. Each chapter has used the published literature on that particular ILAR subtype [6,7], and its counterpart under the classification of juvenile chronic arthritis (JCA) or juvenile rheumatoid arthritis (JRA). We have attempted to lessen the subsequent confusion in terminology by capitalizing only the ILAR terms in this textbook (i.e., "Rheumatoid Factor Negative Polyarthritis" as opposed to "polyarticular JRA" or "acute polyarthritis").

The key assumption underlying the proposed ILAR classification is that the clinical similarity of each subtype is likely to reflect an underlying biological or pathophysiological homogeneity. In other words, the classification was originally aimed at facilitating international research efforts to improve the understanding of JIA, rather than providing a clinically validated classification. One could question the sense of using a research classification as the basis for our textbook 'clinical descriptions of the various idiopathic arthritides of childhood.' In the decade since the classification was first published, however, JIA has become widely used internationally in clinical paediatric rheumatology practice, albeit not as extensively as JRA in North America. The final three chapters of the section have used the ILAR classification as it was originally intended, in the context of underlying aetiology and pathogenesis of JIA, covering the immunohistopathology of the inflamed synovium, the inherited predisposition to the disease, and environmental factors which may be involved in triggering the chronic inflammatory process. The aim of this part is to discuss the scientific evidence underlying the process of chronic inflammation in JIA and thereby enable the reader to examine whether the subtypes of JIA reflect biologically different disease states, and eventually to better inform patients, families, and the general public about the disease. A relatively brief history of the classification will serve to illustrate the conundra that gave rise to the organization of current knowledge about arthritis in children.

A history of the classification of arthritis in children

The group of conditions covered by JIA is an excellent example of the evolutionary process of classification. Unfortunately, pathognomonic features of JIA have yet to be discovered and diagnosis depends on typical patterns of articular and extra-articular clinical features together with supportive laboratory and radiographic data.

There have been many attempts at standardizing a set of definitions for different types of arthritis in children [8]. References to the occurrence of swollen and poorly functioning joints in children can be found in portraits and literature for at least the last 500 years. Thomas Phaire, in 1545, referred to a group of conditions characterized by 'stifnes or starckenes of limmes' in the first English language textbook of paediatrics [9].

By the turn of the nineteenth century, Diament-Berger (1891) had reviewed 38 case reports of chronic arthritis which began in childhood. He recognized that the childhood form of arthritis was distinct from adult arthritis (and carried a better prognosis), and he also attempted the first classification into acute, slow, and partial groups. Sir George Frederic Still published the first personal review of chronic joint disease in children 5 years later in 1896 [11]. He suggested that there were likely to be important differences in pathology between his 22 cases and cases of rheumatoid arthritis in adults on the basis of his clinical observations. He particularly described 'chronic progressive enlargement of the joints, associated with general enlargement of the glands and enlargement of the spleen—occasionally with pyrexia and rigors', a disease with which his name became eponymous. He also noted pericarditis, anaemia and growth failure, but not the typical evanescent erythematous rash. In 1897, Still wrote to Dr L. Emmett Holt (the founder of paediatrics in North America, who was in the process of publishing his textbook *The Diseases of Infants and Children*) requesting that a section on arthritis in children be included. It is interesting to speculate that, had Dr Holt done so, none of the transatlantic debate that has raged about the classification of arthritis in children may have occurred.

Publications over the next 50 years revealed a greater understanding of the range of arthritis in children and the associated extra-articular features. Chronic iridocyclitis and its occurrence in association with large joint monoarthritis was recognized [12,13] and the first systematic attempts at classification were made [14]. In 1946, Coss and Boots published a series of 56 cases from New York, and coined the term 'juvenile rheumatoid arthritis' (JRA), a term which became popular in North America [15]. The first formal study of criteria for the classification of JRA was published in 1963 and this was followed up in 1972 with a 9-year retrospective analysis by a committee of American Rheumatism Association paediatric rheumatologists [16]. The resultant JRA criteria were published in 1977 [17].

Coincident with the emerging North America terminology and classification, the Taplow criteria for the diagnosis of Still's Disease were evaluated in a 15-year follow-up study [18]. These were modified and formed the basis of the classification of juvenile chronic arthritis

(JCA), proposed by the European League against Rheumatism [19]. Both classifications have been evaluated prospectively [20,21], but a number of important differences between the two classifications have prevented interchangeable use, and hindered comparative international research for many years (Table 2.1.1). More recently, the diverse nature of the childhood arthritides has been recognized. The syndrome of seronegative enthesitis and arthritis (SEA syndrome) was defined [22], and outcome studies suggested that this combination of clinical features predicted the onset of spondyloarthritis during the adult years [23]. An association between psoriasis and arthritis was also recognized [24] and criteria proposed [25].

A consensus classification was suggested, to promote international research efforts in understanding the heterogeneous group of arthritic diseases in children [8]. In 1994, the International League of Associations for Rheumatology (ILAR) convened an international classification task force of paediatric rheumatologists [2]. The overall aim was to delineate, for research purposes, a classification based on homogeneous groups of patients sharing predominant clinical and laboratory features. It was recognized that such a classification would be unlikely to cover all of the childhood arthritides. A classification framework was proposed, which was to be evaluated internationally, prospectively, and in a variety of ethnic backgrounds [2]. It was hoped that the classification would stimulate research efforts to investigate and improve subgroup homogeneity. The end product would be a classification which would provide a common language between paediatric rheumatologists, scientists, paediatricians, and rheumatologists. It would enable accurate comparisons between research studies emanating from different centres and different countries and assist the

Table 2.1.1 Comparison of classification criteria for chronic arthritis in childhood

Name	ARA (Juvenile Rheumatoid Arthritis)	EULAR (Juvenile Chronic Arthritis)	ILAR (Juvenile Idiopathic Arthritis)
Abbreviation	JRA	JCA	JIA
Age at onset	< 16 years	< 16 years	< 16 years
Minimum arthritis duration	6 weeks	3 months	6 weeks
Onset subtypes	Pauciarticular Polyarticular Systemic	Pauciarticular Polyarticular Systemic	Oligoarthritis Extended Oligoarthritis Systemic Arthritis Psoriatic Arthritis Enthesitis Related Arthritis: ERA Polyarthritis (RF negative)
Rheumatoid factor (RF) +ve	No change in name	Called JRA	Polyarthritis (RF positive)
Undifferentiated option	No	No	Undifferentiated Arthritis
Include spondyloarthro-pathies[a]	No	Yes	Yes (ERA)

[a] 'Spondyloarthropathies' include juvenile ankylosing spondylitis, juvenile psoriatic arthritis, and Reiter's syndrome.

understanding of the aetiology, pathogenesis, response to treatment, and prognosis of childhood arthritis. The World Health Organization endorsed the proposed classification in 1999.

The umbrella term Juvenile Idiopathic Arthritis is defined as definite arthritis of unknown aetiology that begins before the 16th birthday and persists for at least 6 weeks. The classification of JIA is determined by the pattern of disease 6 months after onset of the arthritis, as it is widely recognized that the clinical features commonly evolve during this time [20,21]. During the period between 6 weeks and 6 months after the onset of the disease, many patients with JIA remain undifferentiated, particularly those with joint disease in the absence of extra-articular features of Systemic Arthritis, Psoriasis, or Enthesitis Related Arthritis. Seven categories of JIA are recognized at 6 months, including Oligoarthritis (Persistent and Extended), Rheumatoid Factor Negative Polyarthritis, Rheumatoid Factor Positive Polyarthritis, Systemic Arthritis, Enthesitis Related Arthritis, Psoriatic Arthritis, and Undifferentiated Arthritis. Each category must fulfil the umbrella definition, and is further defined by category specific inclusion criteria and exclusion criteria.

The principle of the classification is that all subtypes of JIA are mutually exclusive, and this is reflected in the list of exclusions for each category. For example, in Enthesitis Related Arthritis, the 'inclusion' criteria of enthesitis, sacroiliac joint tenderness, low back pain, HLA-B27, and a family history of ankylosing spondylitis or related diseases are also 'exclusion' criteria for all the other categories of JIA. In the same way, the presence of psoriasis or other psoriatic inclusion criteria are exclusion criteria for Enthesitis-Related Arthritis. It has been acknowledged that the principle of mutual exclusivity may result in a large number of JIA patients being placed in the 'Undifferentiated Arthritis' category.

Additionally, a number of 'descriptors' have been proposed to gather further information on the pattern of the clinical picture. These include age at onset, further description of the arthritis (large joints, small joints, symmetry, upper or lower limb predominance, and individual joint involvement), disease course (number of joints), presence of ANA, chronic anterior uveitis or acute anterior uveitis, and HLA allelic associations. The descriptors do not form part of the classification of JIA, but may allow reclassification in the future.

The future of the classification

Many challenges remain. There is no doubt that the ILAR classification, now into its second revision, is still a work in progress [6,7] and is likely to continue to require alteration. It has many shortcomings, including the difficulty in defining Oligoarthritis as anything other than a 'time-limited' classification subtype, as the subsequent addition of further inflamed joints (Extended Oligoarthritis), enthesitis (Enthesitis Related Arthritis), or the rash of psoriasis (Psoriatic Arthritis) will change the subtype irrevocably. The use of classification criteria which are relatively common in the non-JIA population, such as a family history of psoriasis, may prevent accurate classification (see Chapter 8, Undifferentiated Arthritis). The term 'juvenile' may have little biological relevance, and the ultimate success of the classification may render the word 'idiopathic' redundant. As it stands, however, the classification still has considerable merit as a consensus opinion which crosses international boundaries and facilitates communication between paediatric rheumatologists worldwide. In summary, the original purpose of the proposed ILAR classification of JIA was to

facilitate international research efforts. The classification consists of seven distinct disease subtypes under the umbrella term JIA, covering idiopathic arthritis beginning before 16 years of age. A number of clinical features (affected joint number, psoriasis, enthesitis, and family history of psoriasis or B27-related disease) and two laboratory features (rheumatoid factor, HLA B27) are used as discriminating factors between JIA subtypes. Prospective evaluation of the JIA classification is needed. The data should be collected at specified time points (e.g. at diagnosis, 6 months, and yearly thereafter) and should include information on all inclusion and exclusion criteria, as well as descriptors used in the current ILAR classification.

The ILAR classification of JIA second revision (1)

Systemic Arthritis

Definition

Arthritis with, or preceded by, daily fever of at least 2 weeks' duration, that is documented to be quotidian for at least 3 days, and accompanied by one or more of the following:

1. Evanescent, non-fixed, erythematous rash.

2. Generalized lymph node enlargement.

3. Hepatomegaly and/or splenomegaly.

4. Serositis.

Exclusions: a, b, c, d (see below).

Oligoarthritis

Definition

Arthritis affecting 1–4 joints during the first 6 months of disease. Two subcategories are recognized:

1. Persistent Oligoarthritis—Affects no more than four joints throughout the disease course.

2. Extended Oligoarthritis—Affects a total of more than four joints after the first 6 months of disease

Exclusions: a, b, c, d, e (see below)

Polyarthritis (RF Negative)

Definition

Arthritis affecting five or more joints during the first 6 months of disease: tests for RF are negative.

Exclusions: a, b, c, d, e (see below)

Polyarthritis (RF Positive)

Definition

Arthritis affecting five or more joints during the first 6 months of disease; tests for RF are positive

Exclusions: a, b, c, e (see below)

Psoriatic Arthritis

Definitions

1. Arthritis and psoriasis or

2. Arthritis and at least 2 of the following

A Dactylitis

B Nail pitting or onycholysis

C Psoriasis in a first degree relative

Exclusions: b, c, d, e (see below)

Enthesitis Related Arthritis

Definitions

1. Arthritis and enthesitis

2. Arthritis or enthesitis with at least 2 of the following:

   A Sacroiliac joint tenderness and/or inflammatory lumbosacral pain

   B Presence of HLA B27

   C Onset of arthritis in a male after age 6 years

   D Ankylosing spondylitis, Enthesitis Related Arthritis, sacroiliitis with inflammatory bowel disease, Reiter's syndrome or acute anterior uveitis in a first-degree relative.

Exclusions: a, d, e (see below)

Undifferentiated Arthritis

Definitions

Arthritis that does not fulfil inclusion criteria for any category, or is excluded by fulfilling criteria for more than one category.

Exclusion criteria for the classification of JIA

a. Psoriasis in the patient or a first-degree relative

b. Arthritis in an HLA B27 positive male with arthritis onset after 6 years of age

c. Ankylosing spondylitis, enthesitis-related arthritis, sacroiliitis with inflammatory bowel disease, Reiter syndrome, acute anterior uveitis in a first degree relative

d. Presence of IgM rheumatoid factor on at least two occasions more than 3 months apart

e. Presence of Systemic Arthritis

Glossary of terms

Arthritis: Swelling within a joint, or limitation in the range of joint movement with joint pain or tenderness, which persists for at least 6 weeks, is observed by a physician and which is not due to primarily mechanical disorders

Dactylitis: Swelling of one or more digits, usually in an asymmetric distribution, which extends beyond the joint margin

Enthesitis: Tenderness at the insertion of a tendon, ligament, joint capsule, or fascia into bone

Inflammatory spinal pain: Pain in the spine at rest, with morning stiffness in the spine that improves on movement

Nail pitting: A minimum of 2 pits on one or more nails at any time

Number of affected joints: Joints able to be individually evaluated clinically to be counted as separate joints

Positive test for rheumatoid factor: At least 2 positive results (as routinely defined in a laboratory using the WHO standard), 3 months apart, during the first 6 months of the disease

Psoriasis: Must be diagnosed by a physician

Quotidian fever: Daily recurrent fever that rises to 39°C or above once a day and returns to 37°C or below between fever peaks

Serositis: Pericarditis, pleuritis, and/or peritonitis

Sacroiliac joint arthritis: Presence of tenderness on direct compression over the sacroiliac joints

Spondyloarthropathy: Inflammation of entheses and joints of the lumbosacral spine

Uveitis: As diagnosed by an ophthalmologist

References

1. Petty, R.E., Southwood, T.R., Manners, P., Baum, J., Glass, D.N., et al. International League of Associations for Rheumatology classification of juvenile idiopathic arthritis: second revision, Edmonton 2001. *J Rheumatol* 2004;31: 390–2.

2. Fink, C.W. et al. for the ILAR Task Force in Paediatric Rheumatology. Proposal for the development of classification criteria for idiopathic arthritides of childhood. *J Rheum* 1995;22: 1566–9.

3. Fries, J.F., Hochberg, M.C., Medsger, T.A. Jr, Hunder, G.G. and Bombardier, C. (1994) Criteria for rheumatic disease. Different types and different functions. The American College of Rheumatology Diagnostic and Therapeutic Criteria Committee. *Arthritis Rheum* 1994;37: 454–62.

4. Claire, O'Brien. *Science* 1996 Jul 5;273(5271):28.

5. Hunder, G.G. The use and misuse of classification and diagnostic criteria for complex diseases. *Annals of Internal Medicine* 1998;129: 417–18.

6. Petty, R.E. Classification of childhood arthritis: a work in progress. *Bailliere's Clinical Rheumatology* 1998;13(2): 181–90.

7. Petty, R.E. Growing Pains: The ILAR Classification of Juvenile Idiopathic Arthritis. *J Rheumatol* 2001;28: 927–8.

8. Southwood, T.R. and Woo, P. Childhood arthritis: the name game. *Br J Rheumatol* 1993;32: 421–3.

9. Phaire, T. (1955, 1545) *The Boke of Chyldren*, pp31–32. Edinburgh: E & S Livingston, 1955.

10. Diamantberger, M.-S. *Du Rheumatisme Noueux (Polyarthrite deformante) chez les enfants*. Paris: Lecrosnier et Babe, 1891. (Reprinted in 1988 by Editions Louis Parente, Paris.)

11. Still, G.F. On a form of chronic joint disease in children. Chirurgical Transactions 80: 47 reprinted in 1978. *Am J Dis Children* 1897;132:195–200.

12. Ohm, J. Bandformige Hornhauttrubung bei einem neunjahrigen Madchem und ihre Behandlung mit subkonjunktivalen Jodkaliumeinspritzungen. *Klinik Monatsbl Augenbeilkd* 1910;48: 243.

13. Sury, B. (1952) Rheumatoid Arthritis in Children. A Clinical Study. Denmark: Munksgaard. , USA National Center for Health Statistics (1985) Health, United States, 1985., DHHS publication 86–132: 170, 1952.

14. Wissler, H. Der Rheumatismus im Kindesalter. Teil 2. In *Die chronische Polyarthritis des Kindes* Dresden and Leipzig, 1942, p. 152.

15. Coss, J.A. and Boots, R.H. Juvenile rheumatoid arthritis. A study of forty six cases with a note on skeletal changes. *J Pediatr* 1946;29: 143–56.

16. Brewer, E.J., Bass, J.C., Cassidy, J.T. et al. Criteria for the classification of Juvenile Rheumatoid Arthritis. *Bull Rheum Dis* 1972;23: 712–19.

17. Brewer, E.J., Bass, J.C., Baum, J. et al. Current proposed revision of JRA criteria. *Arthritis Rheum* 1977;20: 195–99.

18. Bywaters, E.G.L. Diagnostic criteria for Still's Disease (juvenile, RA). In P.H. Bennett, and P.N.H. Wood, eds. *Population Studies of the Rheumatic Diseases, Proceedings of the Third International Symposium*. New York: Excerpta Medica Foundation, 1968, pp. 235–40.

19. Wood, P.H.N. Special Meeting on: nomenclature and classification of arthritis in children. In E. Munthe, ed. *The Care of Rheumatic Children*. Basel: EULAR, 1978, pp. 47–50.

20. Cassidy, J.T., Levinson, J.E., Bass, J.C. *et al.* A study of classification criteria for a diagnosis of juvenile rheumatoid arthritis. *Arthritis Rheum* 1986;29: 274–81.

21. Prieur, A.-M., Ansell, B.M., Bardfield, R. *et al.* Is onset type evaluated during the first 3 months of disease satisfactory for defining the sub-groups of juvenile chronic arthritis? *Clin Experiment Rheumatol* 1990;8: 321–5.

22. Rosenberg, A.M. and Petty, R.E. A syndrome of seronegative enthesopathy and arthropathy in children. *Arthritis Rheum* 1982;25: 1041–46.

23. Cabral, D.A., Oen, K.G., and Petty, R.E. SEA syndrome revisited: a longterm followup of children with a syndrome of seronegative enthesopathy and arthropathy. *J Rheumatol* 1992;19: 1282–5.

24. Shore, A. and Ansell, B.M. Juvenile psoriatic arthritis—an analysis of 60 cases. *J Pediatr* 1982;100: 529–35.

25. Southwood, T.R., Petty, R.E., Malleson, P.N. *et al.* Psoriatic arthritis in children. *Arthritis Rheum* 1989;32: 1007–13.

2.2 Systemic Arthritis

Anne-Marie Prieur, Peter N. Malleson, and Yukiko Kimura

Aims

The aim of this chapter is to discuss the clinical features, investigations, and epidemiology of Systemic Arthritis. The differing clinical courses of this disease and the impact on prognosis, as well as predictors of outcome, are discussed. In addition, there is a discussion of the chief diagnoses that are often confused with Systemic Arthritis.

Structure

- Introduction
- Epidemiology
- Clinical features
  - Diagnosis
  - Features during course of the disease
- Monitoring
- Complications
- Prognosis
- Key Summary Points

Introduction

Systemic Arthritis is classified as belonging in the group of childhood rheumatic diseases gathered together under the umbrella term of Juvenile Idiopathic Arthritis (JIA) [1]. Although all types of JIA have in common arthritis and the risk of joint damage and destruction, it is the extra-articular manifestations of Systemic Arthritis which make it unique. To date, we have used the distinctive clinical features of this disease to make the diagnosis since there is no specific diagnostic test, but this may change with increasing knowledge of disease pathogenesis in the future. This disease occurs in all age groups, including adults. In adults, it is considered a specific entity separate from rheumatoid arthritis and other forms of adult onset arthritis and is called "adult onset Still Disease." Still disease derives its name from George Frederic Still, who described it as a distinct entity in children in 1897 [2] (as did a French doctor in his thesis a few years before) [3]. Still disease has often been the term used to describe this condition in children in the past, although it has now been dropped from the formal classification terminology in favor of the term Systemic Arthritis. It was first reported in adults in 1971, by Eric Bywaters [4].

The aetiology and pathogenesis of Systemic Arthritis are unknown. At onset, the systemic features of fever and rash mimic infection, but no proof of infection has been established. There is relatively limited evidence for a genetic link in this disease (see Chapter 10 "Genetic and Cytokine Associations in JIA"). Inflammatory reactants are highly perturbed, and Systemic Arthritis appears to have a unique cytokine profile compared to other types of JIA [5,6] (see also Part 2, Chapter 2.10).

There is a great variability of outcome, from patients who recover completely without sequelae to those who will remain extremely crippled for life [7–9]. Current treatments are often insufficient, and may lead to serious and sometimes unacceptable side-effects.

Epidemiology

Recent published annual incidence rates for Systemic Arthritis are fairly similar, varying from 0.49 per 100,000 children at risk (95% confidence interval 0.32–0.77) to 1.3 per 100,000 (95% confidence interval 0.3–2.3) [10–12].

The proportion of all children with chronic arthritis having Systemic Arthritis [10–14] varies from a low of 4% [12] to a high of 13.1% [13]. This variation is due to a number of factors, including the classification criteria used in the study, and whether the study is population or clinic based. It is of interest that the most recently published study [12] has the lowest frequency of Systemic Arthritis. This may well be because the overall umbrella term of JIA is more inclusive than are the terms Juvenile Rheumatoid Arthritis (JRA) or Juvenile Chronic Arthritis (JCA), but it raises the interesting possibility that the incidence of Systemic Arthritis is decreasing, as was suggested by Peterson *et al.* [11]; these authors found an incidence of Systemic Arthritis of 1.2 in 1960–9 compared to an incidence of 0 in 1980–93.

There has also been suggestion that the occurrence rate of Systemic Arthritis varies by season with the frequency of new cases being higher than expected from early spring to early autumn, and lower than expected in the winter months [15]. This finding from a single centre in Kansas (USA) raised the possibility of an association with a viral illness. A later study from several centres across Canada [16] showed a seasonal pattern in the Prairie region with peaks in autumn and early spring, but not elsewhere in Canada. As the Prairie region is geographically close to Kansas, this finding might support the possibility that the same seasonal agent, active in the spring and autumn, is responsible for causing Systemic Arthritis in both these areas.

Unlike most other forms of JIA which have a striking female predominance, Systemic Arthritis seems to be as common in boys as girls, with studies either showing no female to male predominance [13], or a very minimal female excess: 1.1 : 1 [10] 1.2 : 1 [14]. The average age of onset is about 5 years [10,13,14], but there is a wide variation with a relatively similar frequency of onset at all age groups [17].

Clinical features

Features at initial evaluation of patients

Extra-articular manifestations

Fever

High spiking daily fever is the most important clinical criterion, as it is almost always present at the onset of the disease. Occasionally, it can start later, after the development of arthritis. According to the Edmonton criteria for JIA, fever must have been present for at least 2 weeks duration, and documented to have a quotidian pattern (a single spike of fever per day) for at least 3 days [1]. Almost always, however, the duration of fevers is much longer, and may stay for several weeks or months if untreated. Typically, there is a single rise occurring in the afternoon or early evening, reaching 39°C or more. The peak is followed by a sharp decrease under 37°C (Figure 2.2.1). The fever swings are correlated with variations in circulating inflammatory cytokines and cytokine inhibitors [5,18]. This pattern may not be present at the beginning of the disease, but it may become more characteristic once treatment with NSAIDs is started. The usual doses of antipyretic drugs used in paediatrics are generally not effective in controlling the fevers, and the child is often unwell, and may have chills or rigors, while the fever is rising.

Rash

The rash represents the second typical extra-articular manifestation, and is present in more than 90% of cases at onset. Physicians who are familiar with these patients and the typical rash are often able to suspect the diagnosis even before the development of arthritis. It is an evanescent, non-fixed, erythematous rash and is easily recognized, appearing as macules that may coalesce (Figure 2.2.2), or be more discrete, occurring in areas of exposure to air or touch (Koebner

phenomenon). The transient presence of even 2 or 3 macules is highly suggestive. The rash occurs typically with the fever spikes, but it may persist when fever has resolved. Sometimes, it can resemble urticaria, and can be quite pruritic.

Organomegaly and lymphadenopathy

Hepatomegaly is often present, but it is usually not tender and mild. Splenomegaly is seen in about 30% of cases, but is usually mild. Massive splenomegaly is unusual and when present deserves further investigation for another diagnosis, particularly a malignancy. Generalized lymph node enlargement is found in about 50% of cases. Enlarged nodes are painless, freely mobile under the skin, and are found in the cervical, axillary, and inguinal areas. Mesenteric lymphadenopathy may cause abdominal pain, sometimes leading to a debate about a possible surgical emergency in an undiagnosed febrile child who has not yet developed arthritis.

Serositis and other visceral manifestations

Pericarditis with or without pleural effusion is a classic feature of Systemic Arthritis. It is generally mild and asymptomatic. An enlarged retropericardal space is often the only feature of pericardial inflammation. Occasionally, however, the pericardial effusion is large (Figure 2.2.3) and symptomatic, requiring corticosteroids to control it. Pericardial tamponade requiring urgent pericardial drainage occurs rarely. Sterile peritonitis can also occur, and may present with abdominal pain.

Myocarditis is rare, and responds well to corticosteroids. Myocardial involvement causing progressive heart failure is a very rare, life-threatening, complication. Endocarditis is very rare.

Other visceral manifestations have been very seldom reported. Eye inflammation, such as anterior uveitis, almost never occurs in Systemic Arthritis. Neurological and psychological abnormalities are generally not due to the disease but are more likely the result of therapeutic complications. Interstitial pneumonitis has been reported, but if present, should lead to an investigation for an infectious aetiology.

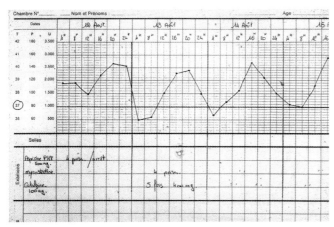

Fig. 2.2.1 Typical fever curve taken 6 times over 24 h showing one peak in the evening and a drop under 37°C in the morning.

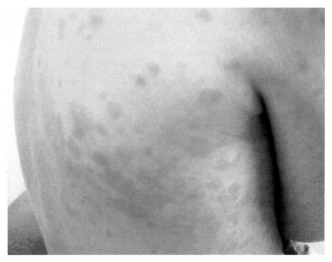

Fig. 2.2.2 Florid Systemic Arthritis rash showing coalescence of urticarial-like lesions.

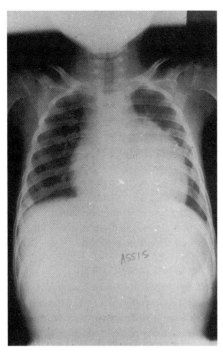

Fig. 2.2.3 Chest radiograph showing an enlarged cardiac silhouette due to a pericardial effusion.

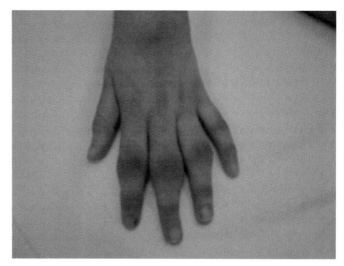

Fig. 2.2.4 Severe PIP joint involvement with sparing of DIP joints.

Musculoskeletal manifestations

Arthritis is absent at onset in about 1/3 of the cases, rendering the diagnosis difficult at times. Even if it is not present at onset, it usually develops within the next few months, but sometimes it can take one or more years. When arthritis occurs, joint involvement is generally symmetrical. Polyarticular involvement (affecting more than four joints) is observed in 1/4 of the cases. The most commonly involved joints are knees, wrists, and ankles. Small joints may also be affected (Figure 2.2.4). The cervical spine is often painful and quite stiff. Hip involvement is common, but usually occurs later, during follow up. The arthritis in Systemic Arthritis can involve any site that contains synovial membrane, including tenosynovial sheaths, vertebral joints, and cricoarytenoid joints. Myalgias are common and often occur during the febrile phase, but there is no elevation in muscle enzymes. Although it can sometimes be extremely painful, the muscle pain completely resolves without sequelae.

Investigations at initial evaluation

In the face of a classical rash, fever, and arthritis, the diagnosis is often clear. However, many childhood illnesses present with a systemically unwell child with fevers, rash, and organomegaly. These children need careful evaluation and investigation, especially to rule out infectious diseases and malignancy (see also Part 1, Chapter 1.3, Algorithm 1.3.1). There are no pathognomonic laboratory tests for Systemic Arthritis, but investigations are helpful in excluding other diagnoses.

Laboratory testing

Chronic anaemia is almost always present, although it can take some time to occur. Haemoglobin levels can become very low in some children, reaching 60 gm/l or even less. The anaemia is related to several causes: chronic inflammation with ineffective erythropoiesis is most common, but gastrointestinal blood loss secondary to medication induced gastritis can occur. Poor nutritional status may also increase the degree of anaemia, which can be very difficult to treat. Oral iron may occasionally be useful, but in severe cases, intravenous iron therapy has been used [19]. There is no endogenous erythropoietin defect, so the role of exogenous erythropoietin therapy is unclear [20,21] (see also Part 3, Chapter 3.11).

Leukocytosis with neutrophilia is a characteristic feature of active Systemic Arthritis. It is such a key feature that if leukocyte counts are normal or low, other diagnoses, such as leukaemia, a viral infection or a complication such as macrophage activation syndrome (MAS) must be considered. This complication is described in more detail below.

Thrombocytosis may reach high levels, (greater than 1,000,000/mm^3), and reflects the extremely inflammatory process. It may correlate with high IL-6 production [22]. There is no risk of thrombosis. This is a consistent feature of active Systemic Arthritis, and so a decreased or normal level of platelets should lead one to consider the possibility of malignancy or MAS. Bone marrow aspiration and biopsy may be necessary to help rule out leukaemia or neuroblastoma.

Systemic Arthritis is the archetypal inflammatory chronic disease, and all acute phase reactants (APR) are typically quite elevated. An elevated erythrocyte sedimentation rate (ESR) is constant, often reaching more than 100 mm/h. High levels of C-reactive protein (CRP) are also characteristic. Some consider the CRP to have a prognostic value with persistently high levels in those who eventually develop amyloidosis [23]. Fibrinogen and serum complement levels also tend to be very high. It is recognized that hyperferritinaemia and decreased relative levels of glycosylated ferritin under 20% are characteristic of adult onset Still disease [24]. In children, ferritin levels are significantly lower than in adults, but are still often quite elevated [25,26]. The diagnostic and/or prognostic value remains to be established in children, but in all ages, extremely elevated ferritin levels are a feature of MAS. A polyclonal immunoglobulin increase, particularly in very active disease, is also frequently observed. Autoantibodies are not generally present. A high ESR without a significant thrombocytosis, or associated with a high lactate dehydrogenase level is highly suggestive of a malignancy mimicking Systemic Arthritis [27].

Imaging

Periarticular soft tissue swelling and joint effusion are common early manifestations. Juxta-articular osteoporosis is also common. The chest X-ray may show an enlarged cardiac silhouette, usually reflecting pericarditis and rarely myocarditis. Echocardiography can be helpful if significant cardiac abnormalities are present, but are not routinely required. The chest X-ray also can be useful to follow rare cases of lung involvement. If there are unusual clinical features, a radionuclide scan such as a bone scan, gallium scan, or a tagged white blood cell (WBC) scan might help to exclude infection or malignancy. In addition, abdominal computerized tomography may help exclude infections, inflammatory bowel disease (IBD), and malignancy.

Diagnosis

The diagnostic criteria have been a matter of long lasting debate. The most recent proposals are those of the ILAR published in 2004 [1]. For Systemic Arthritis, they do not differ much from those previously proposed by the European League Against Rheumatism (EULAR) for JCA or by the American College of Rheumatology (ACR) for JRA, except that the presence of arthritis of unknown origin for a minimum of 6 weeks duration is mandatory to confirm the diagnosis. "Adult Onset Still Disease" has diagnostic criteria known as the Yamagushi criteria [28] but these might not be very specific in children (Table 2.2.1).

The diagnosis can be difficult at onset, particularly when there is only fever, rash, and pain, and the arthritis has not yet developed. The following considerations should be kept in mind:

1. Bacterial infection and malignancy must be ruled out first, since both necessitate urgent therapy. Basic blood tests may be of little value in diagnosis, even in leukaemia, since early on, blasts may not be apparent. If there is any doubt, a bone marrow aspiration and/or biopsy must be performed (see Part 1, Chapter 1.3, Algorithm 1.3.1).

2. During the first year of life, Systemic Arthritis is most often observed after 6 months of age, and only rarely between 3 and 6 months of age. It is observed almost exclusively in girls before the age of 12 months, while the sex ratio is 1:1 male : female after 12 months [29]. In small children, Kawasaki Disease (KD), which manifests with fever, rash, and joint pain, as well as sometimes arthritis, can be confused with Systemic Arthritis [30,31].

3. There are many other causes of unexplained fever in young children that can be considered, including viral infections, other vasculitides besides KD, as well as many other causes of similar symptoms. A list of important diagnoses to consider in a child with possible Systemic Arthritis is given in Table 2.2.2.

Features during the course of the disease

There are three patterns seen in the clinical course of patients with Systemic Arthritis [32].

Monocyclic course

These children present with all the typical features of Systemic Arthritis but eventually remit completely. Generally, the treatment administered at onset can be gradually withdrawn and the symptoms do not recur. In our experience treatment with NSAIDs for several weeks after corticosteroids are stopped is needed because we have seen patients relapse if NSAIDs are rapidly withdrawn. This pattern of disease occurs in about 11% of cases [32].

Polycyclic course

These patients have relapses of disease with intervals of remission. These patients can have very long period of remission, sometimes lasting several years, and may relapse in adulthood. Approximately 34% of children appear to have this pattern of disease [32]. The definition of remission is still controversial, but recently an international workshop agreed on a definition of remission for JIA which included, in addition to being off all medications for 12 months: (a) absence of fever, rash, lymphadenopathy, hepatosplenomegaly, and serositis, (b) no active arthritis, (c) normal ESR and CRP levels, and (d) physician global assessment that was the best possible score for the instrument used [33].

Unremitting course

About 55% of the children with Systemic Arthritis [33] never go into remission, and continue to require anti-inflammatory and anti-arthritis medications indefinitely.

Monitoring

General monitoring

Monitoring guidelines are closely associated with the pharmacological treatment used (see also Part 3, Chapter 3.8). These children do not have to be hospitalized very often. Most monitoring and treatment can be performed in an out-patient setting. However, a regular clinical assessment, in collaboration with the primary care physician, is recommended, in order to assess the control of clinical symptoms and the treatment. We recommend initially a monthly visit with the primary doctor, and at least 2–4 visits per year at the referral centre, but this depends on the health care system in each individual country and whether the arthritis is active or quiescent. Functional assessment tools such as the CHAQ should be performed regularly at these visits.

Laboratory monitoring

Blood testing should be kept at a minimum. However, it is needed to verify whether the inflammation has been controlled, and whether the patient is tolerating the treatment. At onset, blood work is generally performed each month for 6 months. Once the systemic symptoms and arthritis are under better control, the frequency can be reduced to every 6 or 8 weeks.

Imaging

Plain X-rays of affected joints are usually valuable at onset as a baseline, and are sometimes helpful to differentiate Systemic Arthritis from other conditions. If the disease is well controlled, we do not repeat them more than once a year at the most. Joint damage can be classified radiographically as soft tissue swelling (stage I), joint space narrowing (stage II), joint erosions (stage III), and bony anklyosis (stage IV). Several stages can coexist on the same radiograph.

Magnetic Resonance Imaging (MRI), a noninvasive imaging technique, can be extremely useful in assessing soft tissue and bony changes. Contrast with gadolinium allows enhanced imaging of

Table 2.2.1 Comparison between the ILAR classification criteria in children and those proposed for Adult Onset Still Disease

	Systemic Arthritis ILAR [1]	Adult onset Still disease Yamagushi [28]
Characteristics of fever	Quotidian for at least 3 days At least 2 weeks duration	**At least 39°C and at least one week duration
Joint involvement	Arthritis At least 6 weeks duration	**Arthralgia lasting at least 2 weeks
Cutaneous manifestations	* Evanescent non-fixed erythematous rash	**Typical rash (macular nonpruritic salmon pink eruption usually appearing during fever)
Sore throat	NP	Yes
Serositis	*Yes	NP
Lymphadenopathy	*Yes	Yes
Splenomegaly or hepatomegaly	*Yes	Yes (but hepatomegaly not mentioned)
Leucocytosis	NP	**≥10,000/mm3 (with 80% or more granulocytes)
Increased transaminases	NP	Yes
No autoantibodies	NP	Yes
Exclusions	Psoriasis in the patient or a first-degree relative Arthritis in an HLA B27 positive male with arthritis onset after 6 years of age Ankylosing spondylitis, Enthesitis-Related Arthritis, sacroiliitis with inflammatory bowel disease, reactive arthritis, acute anterior uveitis in a first degree relative Presence of IgM rheumatoid factor on at least 2 occasions more than 3 months apart	Infections (especially sepsis and infectious mononucleosis) Malignancies (especially malignant lymphoma) Rheumatic diseases (especially polyarteritis nodosa and rheumatoid vasculitis with extraarticular features)
The diagnosis is likely if:	Arthritis + fever plus at least one other criteria *Defined criteria	At least 5 criteria, with at least 2 major criteria **Major criteria

NP: Not included in criteria.

inflamed areas; the hyaline cartilage can also be visualized, allowing detection of early cartilage erosions. MRI can also help to visualize involvement of tendon sheaths. This expensive technique should be used judiciously, but may be useful particularly when a therapeutic decision is required, such as corticosteroid injection, joint drainage, or synovectomy.

Cervical spine imaging must be performed with a lateral view centered on C1–C2, with dynamic films, at the maximum of flexion and extension. This allows visualization of spine fusion and possible instability above or under the fused area. MRI can also show spine compression (Figure 2.2.5).

Ultrasonography is a noninvasive and inexpensive procedure which can help to discriminate between solid and fluid-filled lesions. It may be useful for assessing deep joints such as hips and shoulders, periarticular cysts, and fluid collection such as pericarditis. In association with Doppler technology, it allows evaluation of vascular flow disturbances which may help determine the degree of active inflammation in the joint.

Dual-energy X-ray absorptiometry (DEXA) allows assessment of bone density and mineral content, and is an appropriate technique for children with acceptably low radiation exposure. The whole body scan assesses total bone mineral content, and fat and lean body mass can also be evaluated. Site-specific mineral content, such as of the distal radius, lumbar vertebral bodies, femoral neck, and the greater trochanteric area of the femur can also be measured. The bone mineral density is measured with the bone mineral content partially corrected for bone size. This technique is extremely valuable for the evaluation of the level of demineralization due to the disease itself or to corticosteroid therapy. It is also useful in following changes in bone density when a therapy to improve bone mineralization has been instituted.

Other techniques such as computerized tomography, scintigraphy, arthrography, and thermography are not commonly used. They do not add more valuable information than the above techniques. However, radionuclide techniques using serum amyloid protein is useful to follow treatment for secondary amyloidosis if this should develop (see p217 below).

Table 2.2.2 Differential diagnosis of Systemic Arthritis (also see Part 1, Chapter 1.3. Algorithm 1.3.1)

Systemic arthritis can occur at any age including in adults, but it almost never occurs before 3 months of age. It is observed almost exclusively in girls before 12 months of age. In boys of this age, other diagnosis of fever of unknown origin must be first considered

CHILDREN LESS THAN 5 YEARS OF AGE

Common diseases

Bacterial infections

Repeated blood cultures, search for an infection. The diagnosis might be difficult if the child has received antibiotics. Bone scan and other imaging studies should be done as indicated to exclude occult infections. In case of severe repeated infection, consider immune deficiency, particularly in boys. (see Part 1, Chapter 1.5)

Malignancy

Splenomegaly, lymphadenopathy, bruising tendency, and bone pain are often clues to this diagnosis. Note that blood counts and differential may be normal, and there should be a low threshold for bone marrow aspiration. Bone scan can be positive at bone malignant sites. If done, MRI may show bone marrow anomalies. Two malignancies that commonly present this way in this age group are leukemia and neuroblastoma. (see Part 1, Chapter 1.8)

Viral infections

These are usually of short duration. The WBC and platelet counts are normal or low, but may be difficult to differentiate from MAS.

Less common diseases

Kawasaki Disease

The diagnosis can be difficult in atypical forms. Cardiac ultrasound looking for coronary aneurysms should be performed if suspected, but absence of findings does not rule out Kawasaki Disease. (see Part 1, Chapter 1.4)

Chronic Inflammatory Neurological Cutaneous and Articular (CINCA) syndrome or Neonatal Onset Multisystem Inflammatory Disease (NOMID) (see Part 1, Chapter 1.7)

Typically, the rash is present within the first days of life which would be unusual for Systemic Arthritis, the fever is often lower and not as periodic as in Systemic Arthritis, joint involvement is initially mild but with time leads to typical metaphyseal deformities. In 60% of the cases, the disease can be confirmed by the presence of a mutation on exon 3 of the *CIAS1* gene. (see Part 1, Chapter 1.7)

Hyper IgD syndrome (HIDS)

The IgD level may be normal in young patients. Raised levels of urinary mevalonic acid may be found during a fever flare. Diagnosis is made by measuring mevalonate kinase activity in leucocytes, and by looking for mutations in the *MVK* gene, which are found in 50% of the cases. (see Part 1, Chapter 1.7)

Blau syndrome

This is sometimes referred as familial sarcoidosis. This genetic disease can resemble Systemic Arthritis, with bouts of fever, rash, and diffuse boggy synovitis. Uveitis is a typical feature of Blau syndrome, not observed in Systemic Arthritis. Synovial biopsy can reveal the typical giant cells and an inflammatory infiltrate. 50% of the cases have mutations in *CARD15* gene. (see Part 1, Chapter 1.7)

Sweet syndrome

This syndrome is characterized by fever, leukocytosis, and inflammatory cutaneous plaques. The skin biopsy shows infiltration with polymorphonuclear cells.

Periodic Fever Aphthous stomatitis Pharyngitis Adenopathy (PFAPA) syndrome. This is characterized by regularly occurring bouts of quotidian fevers lasting 3–7 days. Laboratory testing shows leucokytosis and thrombocytosis, high ESR and CRP levels during the flares. Between flares, the child is perfectly healthy, and laboratory abnormalities return to normal. (see Part 1, Chapter 1.7)

CHILDREN MORE THAN 5 YEARS OF AGE

Note that all the diseases described above can also present in older age groups, but other diseases seen more commonly in older children are described below.

Rheumatic fever

This has become rare in the developed world, but it remains a real problem in developing countries. It should particularly be considered in children from poor socioeconomic groups, living in crowded environments in which streptococcal infections can spread rapidly, but it can also occur rarely in affluent communities as well. The modified Jones criteria help in making the diagnosis. (see Part 1, Chapter 1.4)

Familial Mediterranean Fever (FMF)

FMF is usually clinically distinct from Systemic Arthritis because of the periodic nature of the fever episodes. It usually occurs in predisposed ethnic groups, and is an autosomal recessive disease due to mutations of the *MEFV* gene in 80% of cases. (see Part 1, Chapter 1.7)

Behçet disease

This is a hereditary disease observed in a population whose genetic roots are from the "Silk Road" from Japan to the Mediterranean. The diagnosis is made clinically, with the most common feature being severe, recurrent, oral, and sometimes genital ulcerations, but fever, nodular and pustular skin lesions, uveitis, arthritis, and CNS manifestations may occur. (see Part 1, Chapter 1.6)

Muckle Wells syndrome

This disease manifests as bouts of fever, urticarial rash, and joint symptoms. It is autosomal dominant and other cases are often identified in the family. It is often caused by mutations on exon3 of the *CIAS1* gene, as is CINCA/NOMID, and represents a phenotypical variant of this condition. (see Part 1, Chapter 1.7)

Table 2.2.2 (*Continued*)

Cutaneous polyarteritis

This may be confused with Systemic Arthritis because of high fever and pain, sometimes with arthritis, along with skin lesions. The skin lesions are different from the rash of Systemic Arthritis, with transient nodules. Biopsy of these lesions typically show inflammation of medium size arteries. In this form, there is no visceral involvement. Laboratory findings are similar to those of Systemic Arthritis. (see Part 1, Chapter 1.6)

Castelman disease

This is a rare disease in which there are one or more lymph nodes producing large amounts of inflammatory cytokines. Signs and symptoms include bouts of fever, inflammatory anemia, high ESR, and increased CRP levels. The diagnosis can be difficult, as the responsible lymph node is often in the retroperitoneal area. In children, the most frequent form is monocentric, leading to definite cure after surgical removal.

Inflammatory bowel disease

This diagnosis should be considered even if gastrointestinal manifestations are not predominant. Frequently these children present with fever, weight loss, or growth failure, and sometimes arthritis. Rash may be present in the form of erythema nodosum or pustular skin lesions.

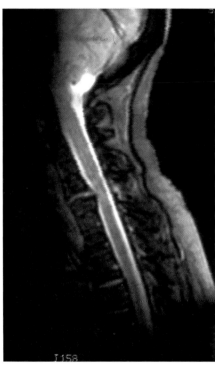

Fig. 2.2.5 MRI of cervical spine showing cord compression in a child with neurological long tract symptoms.

Complications

Systemic complications

Macrophage Activation Syndrome (MAS)

MAS is a haematophagocytic syndrome which is a rare but acute and life-threatening complication of Systemic Arthritis. It has been recognized since at least the early 1980s [34–36], but the term Macrophage Activation Syndrome was first used by Stephan *et al.* in 1993 [37]. The hallmark of this syndrome is the finding on bone marrow aspiration of numerous non-malignant macrophages actively phagocytosing haematopoietic elements [35]. Its clinical features are shown in Table 2.2.3. It can be triggered by abrupt changes in drugs (such as NSAIDs, particularly aspirin) and viral intracellular infections [34,35,38,39]. However, not infrequently no trigger can be

identified. The cause of this syndrome is unclear, but a dysregulation of macrophage-lymphocyte interactions with uncontrolled proliferation of activated macrophages appears to be central to its pathogenesis [40]. It also seems probable that tumor necrosis factor (TNF) is centrally involved in the process, as a marked increase in soluble TNF receptor levels have been found [41], supporting the rationale for the use of anti-TNF therapy in this condition [40]. Mutations in the perforin gene are often the cause of familial haemophagocytic lymphohistiocytosis, a condition with many clinical similarities to MAS occurring in Systemic Arthritis [42]. Defective perforin function has been described in children with Systemic Arthritis, though it appears to be caused by the disease, rather than being a cause of Systemic Arthritis, as the deficiency resolves when the disease remits [43]. It has therefore been suggested that perforin deficiency may lead to a failure to suppress lymphocyte activation leading to secondary macrophage activation.

MAS is characterized by fever, hepatosplenomegaly (sometimes with jaundice), bruising, and coagulopathy, as well as features of encephalopathy such as dizziness, lethargy, and disorientation. Paradoxically, arthritis may improve as MAS develops. Laboratory tests show anaemia, leukopenia (this may manifest as a "normal" WBC count in a child with Systemic Arthritis who usually has leukocytosis), normal or decreased platelet counts, a rapidly dropping ESR due presumably to low fibrinogen levels, high triglycerides, high transaminases, and low vitamin K-dependant clotting factors. Features of consumptive coagulopathy are present, with elevated fibrin split products and D-dimers. Characteristically, the ferritin level are extremely elevated. If a bone marrow aspiration is done, haemophagocytosis is characteristically observed. This is a life-threatening condition and it is important not to be fooled by the apparently improving ESR and WBC. Treatment consists of immediate hospitalization, stopping the possible triggering agent if possible, and institution of high dose intravenous corticosteroids and often cyclosporin. Usually, clinical symptoms resolve rapidly if treated early, but the laboratory anomalies can persist for several weeks. Some patients develop the laboratory findings suggestive of MAS without developing the typical clinical symptoms and signs. These children should be treated with institution of or an increase in corticosteroids and watched carefully for potential evolution of the syndrome (see also Part 3, Chapter 3.14).

Table 2.2.3 Features of MAS

Main triggers

　Abrupt change in treatment
　Introduction of specific medications: NSAIDs (especially aspirin),
　　sulphasalazine, gold, D-penicillamine
　Intercurrent infection, especially viruses and intracellular organisms

Clinical symptoms

　Fever, neurologic abnormalities (dizziness, lethargy, disorientation)
　Bruising, hepatosplenomegaly, jaundice
　Paradoxical improvement in arthritis

Laboratory Features

　Normal or decreased WBC
　Normal or decreased platelets
　Falling or normal ESR
　Increased triglycerides and transaminases
　Extremely high ferritin levels
　Haemophagocytosis in bone marrow

Treatment

　Stop triggering agent if possible
　Emergent hospitalization
　Rapid "aggressive" treatment with high dose corticosteroids and possibly
　　cyclosporin

Infection

Infections are not uncommon, due mainly to the chronic immuno-suppressive treatment that many of these patients require. Therefore there should be high index of suspicion for this complication, and if suspected, rapid appropriate antibiotic therapy should be instituted [44,45].

Secondary amyloidosis

Secondary amyloidosis is due to deposition of the fibrillar protein Serum Amyloid A. It is not specific to Systemic Arthritis, since it can also be seen in chronic infections, and is due to chronic inflammation. This is now a very rare complication since more aggressive therapy has been used in Systemic Arthritis. When it occurs, the deposits particularly affect the kidneys, (inducing proteinuria and nephrotic syndrome), and the digestive tract (causing diarrhea, malabsorption, and hepatomegaly). Amyloidosis can be preceded by high CRP levels [23]. It is diagnosed by examining tissue sections under polarizing microscopy, or stained with Congo Red dye. Radionuclide imaging with radio-labelled autologous serum amyloid P can demonstrate visceral amyloid infiltration [46]. This is a life-threatening complication, which is resistant to most therapies. It may be most responsive to chlorambucil. In a retrospective study of amyloidosis present for a mean of 10 years from diagnosis in 79 children with JIA, 80% treated with chlorambucil were alive compared to only 23.5% not treated with this agent [47]. Renal failure was the cause of death in 82.3% and infection in 11.7%. Toxicity was common in chlorambucil-treated patients and was potentially severe with leukaemia, infertility, and infection being substantial risks of treatment. Other studies have found similar effectiveness and toxicity [48].

Musculoskeletal complications

Joint destruction

Like all other forms of JIA, Systemic Arthritis can be associated with severe joint damage, particularly in those children in whom the inflammation is hard to suppress. As Systemic Arthritis is persistent without remission or even partial disease control in a significant number of children [7,9], quite a large proportion of patients develop progressive joint destruction. Loss of joint space and subsequent erosion reflects progressive cartilage destruction. Any and all joints can be affected in Systemic Arthritis. In the hand, joint destruction can cause loss of carpal bones, epiphyseal changes, and widening of phalanges with osteoporosis (Figure 2.2.6). In other cases, carpal joint fusion may occur (Figure 2.2.7). In the knee, joint widening and overgrowth with squaring of the epiphyses are common. Cartilage loss and bony erosions are observed in severe cases (Figure 2.2.8). Bony ankylosis is rare in the knee. In the hip, local growth disturbances can lead to femoral head overgrowth (Figure 2.2.9) or to joint destruction (Figure 2.2.10). Cervical spine fusion is common, most commonly at C2-3, but widespread ankylosis may develop (Figure 2.2.11) with instability above and below the fused segment, leading to increased risk of spinal cord compression (Figure 2.2.5). A recent radiographic follow up study showed that in Systemic Arthritis joint space narrowing and erosions occurred frequently (38% and 63%, respectively), in children followed for a mean of greater than 6 years from disease onset to time of recent radiographs, and often occurred early in the disease course [49]. This frequent and early radiographic joint damage is mirrored by a poor functional outcome in a high percentage of children and a very high probability of joints requiring arthroplasty (reported as being 57% after 10 years of follow-up in one recent study [9]).

Lymphoedema and synovial cysts

Lymphoedema can be seen occasionally, and generally affects lower limbs (Figure 2.2.12). Its mechanism is unclear. Lymphography if performed suggests the possibility of obstruction of normal superficial lymphatic vessels in the affected limb. The lymphoedema may be cosmetically unsightly, but is rarely of great functional significance, although it may cause difficulty with shoe wear.

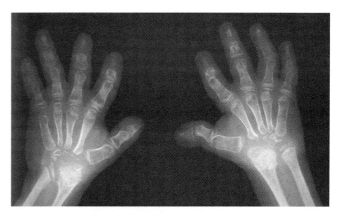

Fig. 2.2.6 Radiograph of hands showing severe destruction of the carpi and damage to the epiphyses of the fingers.

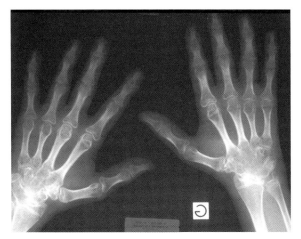

Fig. 2.2.7 Radiograph of hands showing bony ankylosis of the carpi.

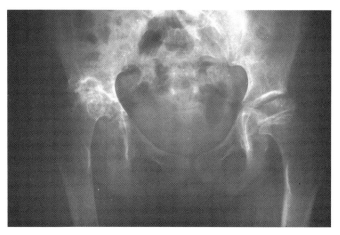

Fig. 2.2.10 Radiograph of the hips showing a severely damaged right hip joint with lesser changes to the left hip.

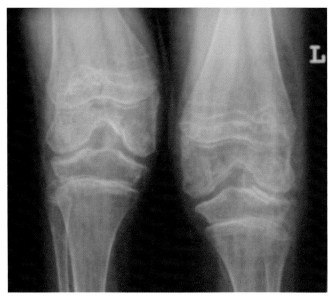

Fig. 2.2.8 Radiograph of the knees showing severe osteopenia, and abnormal epiphyseal growth.

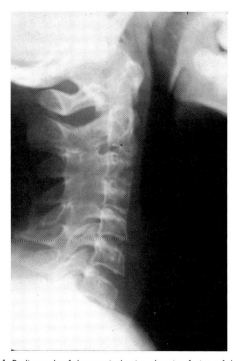

Fig. 2.2.11 Radiograph of the cervical spine showing fusion of the posterior elements from C2 to C6.

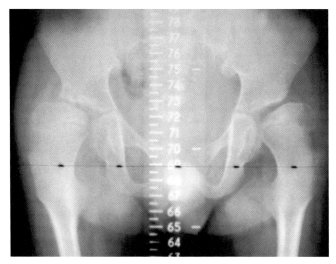

Fig. 2.2.9 Radiograph of the hips showing abnormal femoral head growth and subluxation.

Synovial cysts, seem to occur most frequently and more dramatically than in other forms of JIA. These usually affect the upper limb (Figure 2.2.13). The most common is an inflammatory synovitis in the bicipital tendon sheath often containing rice bodies, but a similar swelling may also be observed at the popliteal fossa (Baker cyst) and may extend quite far down the calf (Figure 2.2.14). When this collection increases greatly in size, disruption of normal venous circulation can result in painful leg swelling resembling thrombophlebitis. Ultrasonography establishes the correct diagnosis.

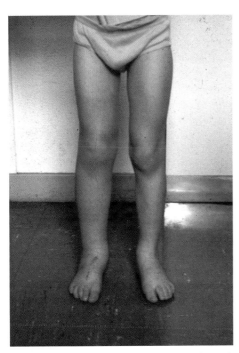

Fig. 2.2.12 Non-tender soft tissue swelling of the right lower limb due to lymphoedema.

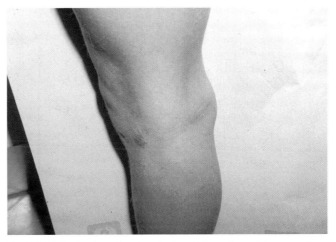

Fig. 2.2.14 Popliteal swelling that developed after a flare of the systemic disease.

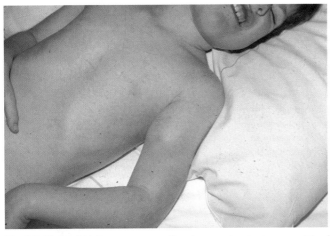

Fig. 2.2.13 Painful left upper arm swelling due to extensive tenosynovitis of the biceps tendon sheath which was found to contain rice bodies.

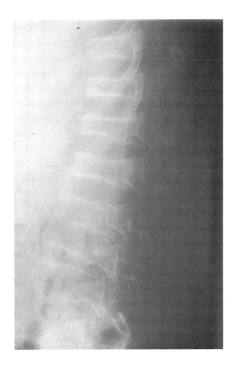

Fig. 2.2.15 Radiograph showing severe osteoporosis of the thoracid and lumbar vertebrae with decreased vertebral body height due to severe disease and corticosteroid therapy.

Osteoporosis

Osteoporosis is often present in Systemic Arthritis, and is secondary to a combination of many factors, including chronic inflammation, reduced activity, poor nutrition, and corticosteroid therapy. Complications due to osteoporosis such as vertebral collapse (Figure 2.2.15), or fractures impact adversely on the child's life, and make management even more difficult. Interestingly, a study from Norway of early onset JIA (mean age of onset 2.8 years) assessed at a mean of 14.2 years after disease onset, found a low total-body bone mineral content in only 2 of 15 (13%) children with Systemic Arthritis, a considerably lower frequency than for Polyarthritis: 9 of 16 (56%) or Oligoarthritis: 31 of 72 (43%) [50]. The reason for this unexpected finding is unclear [50].

Growth retardation

Generalized growth retardation is very commonly associated with Systemic Arthritis, and is due to many factors [51–54]. The severe chronic inflammation itself can induce growth retardation, as it was observed in these children before the corticosteroid era [51]. Poor appetite due to chronic inflammation or adverse medication effects may lead to malnutrition reducing growth. Chronic corticosteroid use, however, is the most important reason for delayed growth as shown in Figure 2.2.16. Loss of height for chronological age is positively correlated with duration of prednisone therapy [54]. The mean

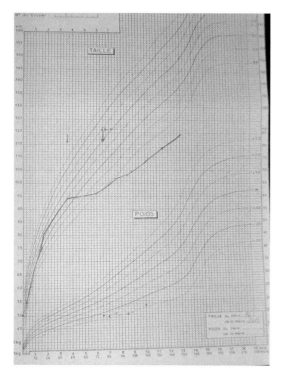

Fig. 2.2.16 Growth chart showing severely diminished height increase in a child following introduction of corticosteroids at 3.5 years of age.

Table 2.2.4 Functional prognosis of Systemic Arthritis depending on disease pattern

Steinbrocker Class	Monocyclic N = 9 (%)	Polycyclic N = 27 (%)	Persistent N = 44 (%)
Class I	9 (100)	18 (67)	16 (36)
Class II	0	3 (11)	11 (25)
Class III	0	6 (22)	14 (32)
Class IV	0	0	3 (7)

Source: Adapted from Wallace *et al.* [33]

Table 2.2.5 Early predictors of poor functional outcome in Systemic Arthritis (at the 6 month visit)

Study Centres	Canadian Halifax, Ottawa, Toronto [8]	European Madrid, London, Paris [58]
General population data		
Number of subjects (M/F)	111 (51/60)	91 (43/48)
Mean age at onset	6.1	5.6
Mean follow up (years)	7.7	8.6
Outcome		
Moderate-to severe outcome	24 (23%)	53 (58%)
Tool for assessing outcome	CHAQ score ≥ 0.75	Joint index
Predictive variables (logistic regression analysis) at the 6 month visit		
Onset before 5	Yes	Yes
Early use of DMARDs	Yes	ND
Persistence of fever	Yes	No
Use of corticosteroids	Yes	No
Thrombocytosis	Yes	Yes
Lymphadenopathy	No	Yes
Polyarticular pattern	No	Yes
Hip involvement	??	Yes
Neck involvement	??	Yes
Low haemoglobin	No	Yes
High ESR	No	Yes
High CRP level	No	Yes

final height is below the expected height in about 90% of patients with Systemic Arthritis. The final height seems to be closely dependent both on the severity of growth retardation during the active phase of the disease and on the duration of linear growth after remission when corticosteroids have been discontinued. Although several studies have shown benefits of short-term growth hormone therapy, these benefits appear limited, particularly if the child has to remain on moderate doses of corticosteroids [55–57] (see also Part 3, Chapter 3.11).

Prognosis

The outcome of children with Systemic Arthritis has been reported in a number of studies and up to one-third or more develop significant permanent disability (depending in part on how disability was measured) [7–9,32,58]. Patients with polycyclic, and especially those with unremitting, disease courses are particularly at risk of an extremely poor outcome [32]. In a retrospective study of 80 consecutive children with Systemic Arthritis followed for a mean of 10 years from Italy, the functional outcome using the Steinbrocker classification was evaluated by the disease pattern (Table 2.2.4) [32]. All nine children who had a monocyclic course were in Steinbrocker Class I, having normal function with the ability to carry on all usual activities normally. Of the 27 patients with a polycyclic course, 18 (67%) were in Class I; 3 (11%) were in Class II having adequate function for normal activities despite having some disability; and 6 (22%) were in Class III, with function limited to no or only few activities of normal living, or having limited ability for self-care. Of the 44 patients with an unremitting disease course, 14 (32%) were in Class III and 3 (7%) were in Class IV (almost totally incapacitated).

Two studies have recently looked for predictors of poor outcome during the first 6 months of disease [8,58]. This data is shown in Table 2.2.5. Although data was collected from 6 different centres (3 in Canada [8] and 3 in Europe [58]), the patient demographics were comparable.

In the Canadian study, 111 patients were followed for a mean follow-up of 7.7 years. High risk factors defined in a previous study [59] were the presence of both: 1. persistent fever or use of corticosteroids, and 2. a platelet count ≥600 × 10⁹/litre. Twenty-two percent of patients were in the high risk group at the 6-month time period. A poor outcome, defined as a CHAQ (Childhood Health Assessment Questionnaire) score ≥0.75 or death, occurred in 26 (2 deaths) (23%) patients. There was also a non-statistically significant trend for those diagnosed before 5 years of age to have a worse outcome than those diagnosed later. In the European study, 91 patients followed for at least 3 years were studied. Two different "clusters" of clinical data were found to be the best indicators of a bad articular outcome: (1) the presence of generalized lymphadenopathy, age less than 8 years, and an articular index score >62, and (2) the presence of a polyarticular pattern of disease at onset plus hip involvement. Interestingly, a poor outcome was twice as frequent in the European study as in the North American one. This discrepancy may be due to the tool used for final assessment. The most reliable functional tool is the CHAQ, a tool which was not validated at the time of the study in European countries, and therefore not used; the European study used a joint count measure only. In both studies, onset before 5 years of age appeared to be associated with a poor outcome. Among markers of inflammation, only thrombocytosis at onset was found in both studies to be a predictor of poor outcome. Death is still an issue, as mentioned in the Canadian series, being more frequent in patients with Systemic Arthritis than in other forms of JIA. The cause of death is most commonly a complication such as MAS, infection, or secondary amyloidosis. Rare cases of "sudden" death have been reported [60]. Some but not all of these cases may have represented unrecognized MAS.

Key summary points

1. Systemic Arthritis is distinct from other forms of JIA, having fever and rash as major manifestations of disease.

2. Systemic Arthritis occurs in about 5–10% of all cases of JIA.

3. Three patterns of disease course are generally recognized: monocyclic, recurrent or polycyclic, and persistent.

4. The long-term outcome of Systemic Arthritis is poor in about 25% of cases.

5. Risk factors for a bad prognosis present at 6 months of disease are high platelet count, and persistent systemic features. Younger age of onset may also be a bad prognostic feature. These risk factors are found in about 25% of patients.

6. Death may occur in this form of JIA, most commonly due to MAS, infection, or amyloidosis (though this latter cause seems to be increasingly uncommon).

7. MAS should be suspected in any child with Systemic Arthritis who becomes unwell with a falling platelet count, and/or WBC, and/or ESR.

References

1. Petty, R.E., Southwood, T.R, Manners, P., Baum, J., Glass, DN., Goldenberg, J., and He, X. International League of Associations for Rheumatology classification of Juvenile Idiopathic Arthritis: Second revision, Edmonton, 2001. *J Rheumatol* 2004;31(2):390–392.

2. Still, G.F. On a form of chronic joint disease in children. *Med Chir Trans* 1897;80:47.

3. Diamantberger, M.S. *Du rhumatisme noueux (polyarthrite deformante) chez les enfants.* Medical Thesis Lecrosnier et Babe, 1891.

4. Bywaters, E.G.L. Still's disease in the adult. *Ann Rheum Dis* 1971;30:121–33.

5. Prieur, A.M., Roux-Lombard, P., and Dayer, J.M. Dynamics of fever and the cytokine network in systemic juvenile arthritis. *Rev Rhum* (Engl Ed), 1996;63:153–70.

6. DeBenedetti, F., Pignatti, P., Gerloni, V., Massa, M., Sartirana, P., Carporali, R. et al. Differences in synovial fluid cytokine levels between juvenile and adult rheumatoid arthritis. *J Rheumatol* 1997;24:1403–9.

7. Svantesson, H., Akesson, A., Eberhardt, K., and Elborgh, R. Prognosis in juvenile rheumatoid arthritis with systemic onset: A follow-up study. *Scand J Rheumatol* 1983;12:139–44.

8. Spiegel, L.R., Schneider, R., Lang, B.A., Silverman E.D., Laxer, R.M., and Stephens, D. Early predictors of poor functional outcome in systemic-onset juvenile rheumatoid arthritis: a multicenter cohort study. *Arthritis Rheum* 2000;43:2402–9.

9. Oen, K., Malleson, P.N., Cabral, D.A., Rosenberg, A.M., Petty R.E., and Cheang M. Disease course and outcome of juvenile rheumatoid arthritis in a multicenter cohort. *J Rheumatol* 2002;29:1989–99.

10. Malleson, P.N., Fung M.Y., and Rosenberg, A.M. for the Canadian Pediatric Rheumatology Association, The incidence of pediatric rheumatic diseases: Results from the Candadian Pediatric Rheumatology Association Disease Registry. *J Rheumatol* 1996;23:1981–7.

11. Peterson, L.S. Mason, T., Nelson, A.M., O'Fallon, W.M., and Gabriel, S.E. Juvenile Rheumatoid Arthritis in Rochester, Minnesota, 1960–1993. Is the epidemiology changing? *Arthritis Rheum* 1996;39:1385–90.

12. Berntson, L., Gäre, B.A., Fasth, A., Herlin, T., Kristinsson, J., Lahdenne, P. et al. Incidence of Juvenile Idiopathic Arthritis in the Nordic countries. A population based study with special reference to the validity of the ILAR and EULAR criteria. *J Rheumatol* 2003;30:2275–82.

13. Bowyer, S. and Roettcher, P. and the members of the Pediatric Rheumatology Database Research Group. Pediatric rheumatology clinic populations in the United States: Results of a 3 year survey. *J Rheumatol* 1996;23:1968–74.

14. Symmons, D.P.M., Jones, M., Osborne, J., Sills, J., Southwood, T.R., and Woo, P. Pediatric rheumatology in the United Kingdom: Data from the British Pediatric Rheumatology Group National Diagnostic Register. *J Rheumatol* 1996;23:1978–74.

15. Lindsley, C. Seasonal variation in systemic-onset juvenile rheumatoid arthritis. *Arthritis Rheum* 1987;30:838–9.

16. Feldman, B.M., Birdi, N., Boone, J.E., Dent, P.B., Duffy, C.M., Ellsworth, J.E. et al. Seasonal onset of systemic-onset juvenile rheumatoid arthritis. *J Pediatr* 1996;129:513–8.

17. Sullivan, D.B., Cassidy, J.T., and Petty, R.E. Pathogenic implications of age of onset in juvenile rheumatoid arthritis. *Arthritis Rheum* 1975;18:251–5.

18. Keul, R., Heinrich, P.C., Muller-Newen, G., Muller, K., and Woo, P., A possible role for soluble IL-6 receptor in the pathogenesis of systemic onset juvenile chronic arthritis. *Cytokine* 1998;10:729–34.

19. Martini, A., Ravelli, A., Di Fuccia G., Rosti, V., Cazzola, M., and Barosi, G. Intravenous iron therapy for severe anaemia in systemic-onset juvenile chornic arthritis. *Lancet* 1994;15:1052–4.

20. Cazzola, M., Ponchio, L., De Benedetti, F., Ravelli, A., Rosti, V., Beguin, Y., Invernizzi, R., Barosi, G., and Martini, A. Defective iron supply or erythropoiesis and adequate endogenous errthropoietin reproduction in the anemia assicated with systemi-onset juvenile chronic arthritis. *Blood* 1996;87:4824–30.

21. Fantini, F., Gattinara, M., Gerloni, V., Bergomi, P., and Cirla, E. Severe anemia associated with active systemic-onset juvenile rheumatoid arthritis successfully treated with recombinant human erythropoietin: A pilot study. *Arthritis Rheum* 1994;35(724–6).

22. DeBenedetti, F. and Martini, A. Is systemic juvenile rheumatoid arthritis an interleukin 6 mediated disease? *J Rheumatol* 1998;25:203–7.

23. Gwyther, M., Schwarz, H., Howard, A., and Ansell, B.M. C-reactive protein in juvenile chronic arthritis: an indicator of disease activity and possible amyloidosis. *Ann Rheum Dis* 1982;41:259–62.

24. Fautrel, B. Ferritin levels in adult Still's disease: Any sugar? *Joint Bone Spine* 2002;69:355–7.

25. Ostrov, B.E. Systemic onset juvenile rheumatoid arthritis and adult-onset Still's disease: Comparison of clinical presentation at a single university center. *Arthritis Rheum* 2002;46:S326.

26. Fujikawa, S. and Okuni, M. Clinical analysis of 570 cases with juvenile rheumatoid arthritis: Results of a nationwide retrospective survey in Japan. *Acta Paediatr Jpn* 1997;39:245–9.

27. Cabral, D.A. and Tucker, L.B. Malignancies in children who initially present with rheumatic complaints. *J Pediatr* 1999;134(53–7).

28. Yamagushi, M., Ohta, A., and Tsuenmatsu, T. *et al.* Preliminary criteria for classification of adult Still's disease. *J Rheumatol* 1992;43:2402–9.

29. Prieur, A.M. and Griscelli, C. Nosologic aspects of systemic forms of very-early-onset juvenile rheumatoid arthritis. Apropos of 17 cases. *Sem Hop* 1984;60:163–7.

30. Kawasaki, T., Kosaki, F., Okawa, S., Shigematsu, I., and Yanagawa, H. A new infantile acute febrile mucocutaneous lymph node syndrome (MLNS) prevailing in Japan. *Pediatrics* 1974;54:271–6.

31. Joffe, A., Kabani, A., and Jadavji, T. Atypical and complicated Kawasaki disease in infants. Do we need criteria? *West J Med* 1995;162:322–7.

32. Lomater, C., Gerloni, V., Gattinara, M., Mazzotti, J., Cimaz, R., and Fantini, F. Systemic onset juvenile rheumatoid arthritis: A retrospective study of 80 consecutive patients followed for 10 years. *J Rheumatol* 2000;27:491–6.

33. Wallace, C.A., Ruperto, N., and Giannini, E. Childhood Arthritis and Rheumatology Research Alliance; Pediatric Rheumatology International Trials Organization: Pediatric Rheumatology Collaborative Study Group. Preliminary criteria for clinical remission for select categories of juvenile idiopathic arthritis. *J Rheumatol* 2004;31:2290–4.

34. Silverman, E.D., Miller III, J.J., Bernstein, B., and Shafai, T. Consumption coagulopathy associated with systemic juvenile rheumatoid arthritis. *J Pediatr* 1983;103:872–6.

35. Hadchouel, M., Prieur A.-M., and Griscelli, C. Acute hemorrhagic, hepatic, and neurologic manifestations in juvenile rheumatoid arthritis: Possible relationship to drugs or infection. *J Pediatr* 1985;106:561–6.

36. Morris, J.A., Adamson, A.R., Holt, P.J., and Davson, J. Still's disease and the virus-associated haemophagocytic syndrome. *Ann Rheum Dis* 1985;44:349–53.

37. Stephan, J.L., Zeller, J., Hubert, P.H., Herbelin, C., Dayer, J.M., and Prieur, A.M. Macrophage activation syndrome and rheumatic disease in childhood: A report of four new cases. *Clin Exp Rheumatol* 1993;11:451–6.

38. Ramanan, A.V. and Schneider, R. Macrophage activation syndrome following initiation of etanercept in a child with systemic onset juvenile rheumatoid arthritis. *J Rheumatol* 2003;30:401–3.

39. Davies, S.V., Dean, J.D., Wardrop, C.A., Jones, J.H. Epstein-Barr virus-associated haemophagocytic syndrome in a patient with juvenile chronic arthritis. *Br J Rheumatol* 1994;33:495–7.

40. Prahalad, S., Bove, K.E., Dickens, D., Lovell, D.J., and Grom A.A. Etanercept in the treatment of macrophage activation syndrome. *J Rheumatol* 2001;28:2120–4.

41. deBenedetti, F., Pignatti, P., Massa, M., Sartirana, P., Ravelli, A., Cassani G.C.A. *et al.* Soluble tumour necrosis factor receptor levels reflect coagulation abnormalities in systemic juvenile chronic arthritis. *Br J Rheumatol* 1997;36:581–8.

42. Stepp, S.E., Dufourcq-Lagelouse, R., Le Deist, F., Bhawan, S., Certain, S., Mathew, P.A. *et al.* Perforin gene defects in familial hemophagocytic lymphohistiocytosis. *Science* 1999;286:1957–9.

43. Wulffraat, N.M., Rijkers, G.T., Elst, E., Brooimans, R., and Kuis, W. Reduced perforin expression in systemic juvenile idiopathic arthritis is restored by autologous stem-cell transplantation. *Rheumatology* 2003;42:375–9.

44. Ansell, B.M. Problems of corticosteroid therapy in the young. *Proc Roy Soc Med* 1968;61:281–2.

45. Ansell, B.M., and Wood, P.N. Prognosis in juvenile chronic polyarthritis. *Clin Rheumatic Dis* 1976;2:397–412.

46. Hawkins, P.N., Richardson, S., Vigushin, D.M., David, J., Kelsey, C.R., Gray, K.E. *et al.* Serum amyloid P component scintigraphy and turnover studies for diagnosis and quantitative monitoring of AA amyloidosis in juvenile rheumatoid arthritis. *Arthritis Rheum* 1993;35:842–51.

47. David, J., Vouyiouka, O., Ansell, B.M., Hall, A., and Woo, P. Amyloidosis in juvenile chronic arthritis: A morbidity and mortality study. *Clin Exp Rheumatol* 1993;11:85–90.

48. Savolainen, H.A. Chlorambucil in severe juvenile chronic arthritis: Longterm followup with special reference to amyloidosis. *J Rheumatol* 1999;26:898–903.

49. Oen, K., Reed, M., Malleson, P.N., Cabral, D.A., Petty, R.E., Rosenberg, A.M., and Cheang, M. Radiologic outcome and its relationship to functional disability in juvenile rheumatoid arthritis. *J Rheumatol* 2003;30:832–40.

50. Lien, G., Flato, B., Haugen, M., Vinje, O., Sorskaar, D., Dale, K., Johnston, V., Egeland, T., and Forre, O. Frequency of osteopenia in adolescents with early-onset juvenile idiopathic arthritis: A long-term outcome study of one hundred five patients. *Arthritis Rheum* 2003;48:2214–23.

51. Ansell, B.M., and Bywaters, E.G.L. Growth in Still's disease. *Ann Rheum Dis* 1956;15:295–319.

52. Falcini, F., Tacetti, G., Trapan, i. S., Tafi, L., and Volpi, M. Growth retardation in juvenile chronic arthritis patients treated with steroids. *Clin Exp Rheumatol* 1991;9(Suppl 6):37–40.

53. Polito, C., Strano, C.G., Olivieri, A.N., Alessio, M., Iammarrone, C.S., Todisco, N., and Papale, M.R. Growth retardation in non-steroid treated juvenile rheumatoid arthritis. *Scand J Rheumatol* 1997;26:99–103.

54. Simon, D., Fernando, C., Czernikow, P., and Prieur, A.M. Linear growth and final height in patients with systemic juvenile idiopathic arthritis treated with long term glucocorticoids. *J Rheumatol* 2002;29:1296–1300.

55. Davies, U.M., Rooney, M., Preece, M.A., Ansell, B.M., and Woo, P. Treatment of growth retardation in juvenile chronic arthritis with recombinant human growth hormone. *J Rheumatol* 1994.21:1583–8.

56. Touati, G., Prieur, A.M., Ruiz, J.C., Noel, M., and Czernichow, P. Beneficial effects of one-year growth hormone administration to children with juvenile chronic arthritis on chronic steroid therapy. I. Effects on growth velocity and body composition. *J Clin Endocrinol Metab* 1998;83:403–9.

57. Davies, U.M., Jones, J., Reeve, J., Camacho-Hubner, C., Charlett, A., Ansell, B.M., Preece, M.A., and Woo, P.M. Juvenile rheumatoid arthritis. Effects of disease activity and recombinant human growth hormone on insulin-like growth factor 1, insulin-like growth factor binding proteins 1 and 3, and osteocalcin. *Arthritis Rheum* 1997;40:332–40.

58. Modesto, C., Woo, P., Garica-Consuegra, J., Merino, R., Garcia-Granero M., Arnal, C., and Prieur, A.M. Systemic onset juvenile chronic arthritis: Polyarticular pattern and hip involvement as markers for a bad prognosis. *Clin Exp Rheumatol* 2001;19:211–7.

59. Schneider, R., Lang, B.A., Reilly, B.J., Laxer, R.M., Silverman, E.D., Ibanez, D. *et al.* Prognostic indicators of joint damage in systemic onset juvenile rheumatoid arthritis. *J Pediatr* 1992;120:200–5.

60. Jacobs, J. Sudden death in arthritic children receiving large doses of indomethacin. *JAMA* 1967;199:932–4.

2.3 Oligoarthritis

John J. Miller and Peter N. Malleson

Aims

The aims of this chapter are to discuss the clinical features, investigations, immunopathology, and genetics of Oligoarthritis. Both Persistent Oligoarthritis (which remains oligoarticular throughout its disease course), and Extended Oligoarthritis (which becomes polyarticular), will be discussed in separate sections of the chapter. As uveitis is common in this form of JIA, this condition will also be discussed here.

Structure

- Introduction
- Persistent Oligoarthritis
- Extended Oligoarthritis
- Uveitis
- Key Point Summary

Introduction

Within the current classification of Juvenile Idiopathic Arthritis (JIA) of the International League of Associations for Rheumatology (ILAR) there are two categories of Oligoarthritis [1]. "Persistent Oligoarthritis," is defined as a disease which starts in four or fewer joints and never involves more than four joints. The second category "Extended Oligoarthritis" is a form in which the arthritis is oligoarticular for at least the first 6 months, but then extends to involve more than four joints at some time in the follow up period.

The term Oligoarthritis is almost synonymous with "pauciarticular arthritis" in the earlier American Rheumatism Association (ARA) [2] or European League against Rheumatism (EULAR) [3] definitions. Since Systemic Arthritis, Psoriatic Arthritis, and Enthesitis Related Arthritis may present initially with arthritis in only a small number of joints, a number of exclusions must be applied to classify a child as having Oligoarthritis [1], and only time will determine if the child has Persistent or Extended Oligoarthritis.

The two categories of Oligoarthritis are discussed separately below. It should be recognized, however, that some of the information included under one category may be germane to the other category also.

Persistent Oligoarthritis

Epidemiology

Oligoarthritis is the most common form of JIA [4,5]. However, it is probably not one disease in respect to epidemiology or pathogenesis. Most of our knowledge is about patients characterized by an age of onset less than 6 years, a female predominance, and a relatively high incidence of complicating uveitis. This syndrome has also been called "EOPA" (early-onset pauciarticular arthritis) [6], or pauciarticular type I [7], and is the most common form seen in Europe and North American Caucasians. However, this disease with these particular associations is rare in Asian, Arab, African, North American Indian [8] and in African American children [9]. The variance is probably due to different genetics related to ethnicity, but geographic, environmental, or social factors may also be involved. For instance the incidence of early onset Oligoarthritis with uveitis is very low in Costa Rica [10], which has a predominately Andalusian ethnicity with little indigenous Indian admixture.

In North America and Europe, a male child with arthritis in only a few joints who is older than 6 years at onset is more likely to have progression to some other form of arthritis or rheumatic disease. The most likely of these would be Enthesitis Related Arthritis associated with the HLA B27 antigen. Arthritis affecting only a few joints may also be the manner of presentation of Psoriatic Arthritis, although these children are more likely to have dactylitis, small finger joint, or wrist disease early after onset than are those children with Oligoarthritis [11]. The athletic adolescent engaged in repetitive activity may present with knee effusions as part of the patellofemoral pain syndrome (chondromalacia patellae syndrome) [12]. In those parts of the world where the early onset type of Oligoarthritis is rare, arthritis affecting only a few joints with a later age of onset but not progressing to other diseases is said to be common, but this disease has not yet been as well studied or characterized [13]. The most important diseases to differentiate at onset of Oligoarthritis (before it is clear that the child has JIA) are septic arthritis, osteomyelitis adjacent to the joint, neoplasia, and acute rheumatic fever. Lyme arthritis is also an important consideration in endemic areas. Some distinguishing features between these conditions are shown in Table 2.3.1.

Little is known as yet about what epidemiological differences, if any, exist between Persistent and Extended Oligoarthritis. The age of

Table 2.3.1 Distinguishing features of diseases presenting with oligoarticular arthritis

Disease	Pain/ tenderness	Local erythema	Fever	Exanthem	High WBC	ESR	Other common features
Oligoarthritis	+	−	−	−	−	+/−	Uveitis
Systemic Arthritis	++	+	++++	Still rash (Part 1, Figure 1.3.2)	++++	++++	Quotidian fever Pericarditis Organomegaly
Septic arthritis	++++	++++	++++	−	++++	++++	Severe LOM of joint
Adjacent osteomyelitis	++++	++	+++	−	++++	++++	Bony point tenderness Refusal to weight bear
Acute Rheumatic Fever	+++	++	++	Erythema Marginatum (rare-Part 1 Figure 1.4.2)	+/−	++++	Arthritis has a migratory pattern Carditis may be present
Enthesitis Related Arthritis	++	−	−	−	−	+	HLA B27 May be +
Reactive arthritis	++	+	+/−	Keratoderma Blennorrhagicum (rare)	+	++	History of antecedent infection
Leukaemia	++++	−	+/−	−	Variable	Variable	Pt may refuse to weight bear
Psoriatic arthritis	++	−	−	Psoriasis or nail changes may be present (variable-see Part 2, Chapter 2.6)	−	+	Uveitis
Lyme arthritis	+	−	−	− (may have had previous Erythema Migrans rash (see Part 1, Figure 1.5.24)	−	++	May have had previous episodes of arthritis

onset and sex ratios of these diseases are the same [5]. Progression to Extended Oligoarthritis has been reported to occur in 20% to 50% of children with Oligoarthritis in different reported series [5,14–19]. Extension beyond four joints usually occurs within 2 years of onset, but the incidence increases until a plateau is reached by about 5 years after onset [14].

Early clinical features

The onset of Oligoarthritis is usually quite insidious. The child does not always verbalize complaints of pain and sometimes is not brought to a physician until advanced changes are present. The parents are most likely to have noticed a limp or seen a swollen joint. A very young child may simply stop walking or standing, or be fussy or unhappy when doing so, especially first thing in the morning after awakening (indicating morning stiffness) with improvement later in the day. These symptoms indicate pain is present even though the child may

not have specifically complained of pain. On examination there will be joint effusion(s), swollen synovial tissue, and local warmth, but only mild or moderate tenderness, and the child will probably not object to gentle palpation of the joint. However, there will be pain on the extremes of range of motion, limitation of range of motion, and pain on weight-bearing or resisted movement. An antalgic gait is likely. The most common joints involved at presentation (Table 2.3.2) are knee (Figure 2.3.1) and ankle (Figures 2.3.2 and 2.3.3); the small joints of the hands and feet are involved in 10% or less [14,15]. Wrists and elbows are not usually involved initially but when present may predict extension to polyarticular disease in the longer term [14]. Hips are rarely involved, and arthritis isolated to one or both hips is virtually always due to some other disease such as Enthesitis Related Arthritis. Temporomandibular joints and the cervical spine, frequently involved in Polyarthritis and Systemic Arthritis, are not commonly involved *at presentation* in Oligoarthritis, but often become involved later in the course of the disease. An acute onset, particularly in association

Table 2.3.2 Distribution of joint involvement at presentation in 357 children with Oligoarthritis [15]

Joint	Percentage of patients with Oligoarthritis
Knee	56
Ankle	20
Wrist	4
Elbow	2
Small joints (hands)	10
Small joints (feet)	6

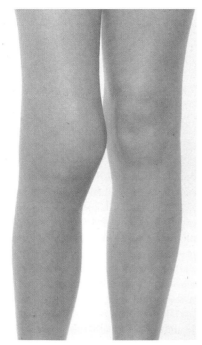

Fig. 2.3.1 Photograph of a girl with Oligoarthritis showing an effusion, bony overgrowth and flexion contracture of the right knee. (Courtesy of C. A. J. Ryder.)

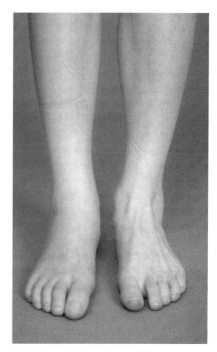

Fig. 2.3.2 Anterior views of Oligoarthritis of the right ankle in a boy showing loss of bony and tendon landmarks. The swelling of the ankle is sometimes much more easily appreciated from behind. (Courtesy of C. A. J. Ryder.)

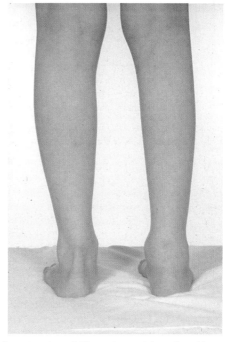

Fig. 2.3.3 Posterior view of Oligoarthritis of the right ankle in a boy showing loss of bony and tendon landmarks. (Courtesy of T. R. Southwood)

with marked tenderness, redness, fever, or severe pain and refusal to weight bear requires care to exclude infection or neoplasm, most often leukaemia. A history of a tick bite or rash preceding the onset of arthritis, or intermittent episodes of arthritis, especially in the knee, in patients who have been in an endemic area, suggests possible Lyme Disease.

Predictors of the development of Extended Oligoarthritis are involvement of wrists or other joints of the upper extremities in the first 6 months, erythrocyte sedimentation rates (ESR) greater than 20 mm/h, and symmetrical joint involvement in the first 6 months [14,17]. The incidence of remission is lower and the potential degree of disability is greater than in patients with Persistent Oligoarthritis [5,14–19].

Clinical features later in the disease are discussed in more detail under "Monitoring" and "Complications."

Investigations

The laboratory data obtained in Oligoarthritis are usually normal. This is important in the differential diagnosis relative to the other causes of Oligoarthritis (Tables 2.3.1 and 2.3.3). Complete blood counts should be normal, but may show moderate increases in white blood cell (WBC) counts or mild anaemia. The ESR may be normal and is not usually greater than 30 mm/h, and higher values may predict progression to polyarthritis [14]. Blood chemistries and urinalyses are

Table 2.3.3 Investigations in the diagnosis of Oligoarthritis

Test	Rationale
Complete Blood Count	May show mild anaemia and thrombocytosis High neutrophil count should raise suspicion of infection or Systemic Arthritis Severe anaemia and thrombocytopenia raises possibility of leukaemia
ESR or CRP	Usually normal or only mildly elevated Very raised values are suggestive of infection or malignancy A high ESR with a normal or low platelet count is very suggestive of leukaemia.
Radiographs	In early Oligoarthritis, should show only soft tissue swelling around the joint and or an effusion Juxta-articular osteopenia may occur Other changes should raise suspicion of other pathology (infection, malignancy, skeletal dysplasia).
Magnetic Resonance Imaging	Not usually needed in diagnosis of Oligoarthritis. Gadolinium enhancement of synovium is "gold-standard" for diagnosis of synovitis (but does not distinguish septic arthritis from Oligoarthritis) Useful in evaluating monarthritis that is in any way atypical (to diagnose conditions such as Osteochondritis dissecans and rarities such as Pigmented Villonodular Synovitis)
Joint fluid analysis and culture	Should be performed in any child with a monarthritis and systemic features compatible with infection. Not required for the great majority of children with oligoarthritis.
TB skin test Lyme serology Other infectious serologies	TB arthritis can present as insidious oligoarticular arthritis. Lyme disease should be considered in children living or traveling from an endemic area Although many infections are associated with arthritis these are rarely truly oligoarticular.
Antinuclear Antibody and Rheumatoid Factor	Not useful diagnostically for Oligoarthritis ANA may have some limited value as prognostic factor for development of uveitis Rheumatoid Factor is an exclusion criterion for Oligoarthritis (if present it augurs early erosive arthritis)

typically normal. Among commonly obtained serological tests, a positive rheumatoid factor (RF) is an exclusion for the classification of Oligoarthritis [1]. However, there is an occasional child with an oligoarticular onset of arthritis who has a persistently positive RF [4,20], and these patients have the poorer prognosis associated with RF Positive Polyarthritis. Antinuclear antibodies (ANA) are present in up to 70–80% of the young girls with Oligoarthritis [21,22]. The presence of ANA in Oligoarthritis has long been considered a risk factor for uveitis [21–23], but this has recently been questioned [14].

Radiographic examination of the involved joints should be obtained on the first visit. Radiographs are usually normal and cannot make a diagnosis of Oligoarthritis, but are necessary to rule out other diagnoses. Early findings should only include evidence of soft tissue swelling or effusion with no bony abnormality except perhaps juxta-articular

osteoporosis. Magnetic resonance imaging (MRI) may show synovial hypertrophy in addition to effusion and gadolinium enhancement of the synovium, but this test is unnecessary unless there is suspicion of another diagnosis.

Most children with Oligoarthritis, even if they present with a monoarthritis, do not need a joint aspiration for cytology and culture. However, there should be a very low threshold for performing this investigation if there is any question that joint sepsis could be present (See Table 2.3.1 and Part 1, Chapter 1.3 "Acute and Chronic Infections of Bones and Joints"). A negative culture from a red, tender joint, particularly in a febrile child who is not bearing weight, does not rule out osteomyelitis adjacent to the joint, because osteomyelitis can cause sterile sympathetic effusions. If this is suspected a radionuclide bone scan and/or MRI should be done. Tuberculosis (TB) of the joint can be very insidious, and it is probably sensible to obtain a TB skin test in all children with a history of TB exposure, monarthritis, or when the population has a high incidence of TB.

Laboratory markers of inflammation are usually either normal or only mildly abnormal in Persistent Oligoarthritis. The incidence of positive antinuclear antibodies and of uveitis is not different between those with Persistent and Extended Oligoarthritis [19], although the presence of ANA may correlate with a longer duration of active joint inflammation [24].

Genetics

We know more about the genetics and immunopathology of early onset Persistent Oligoarthritis than of any of the other arthritides of childhood (see also Part 2, Chapter 2.10). However, most of our knowledge is descriptive, and we do not yet have a clear enough picture of the pathophysiology to be able to mount specific preventive or therapeutic treatment.

Early onset Oligoarthritis is associated with inheritance of a number of histocompatibility (HLA) antigens. The most significant of these are the Class I antigen HLA A2 and the Class II antigens DR 8 (DRB1*0801), DR 5 (DRB1*1104), DR6 (DRB1*1301), DPw2 (DRB1*0201), and DQw4 (DQB1*0401 and DQB1*0402) [6,25]. These antigens are present in children with Oligoarthritis usually about twice as frequently as in normal children, but the absolute proportions vary with ethnic background; for example, in Italy the percentage of children with Oligoarthritis with HLA DR5 is 74% compared to 47% in the general population [26] while in Norway the same proportions are 21% and 9%, respectively [27]. DR6 (DRB1*1301) is not present in some populations [28], and its presence appears to protect against progression to Extended Oligoarthritis [29]. A study from England demonstrated that heterozygosity for DR5 and DR8 was associated with a greater risk for uveitis than homozygosity with either [30]. Since HLA cell surface antigens present foreign peptides to T and B cells, these associations strengthen the long-held theory that this form of arthritis is due to an aberrant immunologic response to an infection.

Immunopathology

The presence of ANA in Oligoarthritis has been recognized for a long time [21,22] (Table 2.3.3), but it has been difficult to determine the specificity of the nuclear antigens. All patterns of ANA may be seen, but reactions with DNA are rare [23]. Antibodies to both histone [31–33] and non-histone nuclear proteins [34–36] have been found.

Indeed, Persistent Oligoarthritis is characterized by a large repertoire of auto-antibodies, and evidence of B cell activation. This is exemplified by increased expression of the V_H4–34 gene [37] which codes a section of immunoglobulin heavy chain normally found on the surface of 7–10% of normal B cells and almost all B-cell lymphoma cells [38], but not usually found in the serum as a circulating immunoglobulin. It is, however, found in the serum of about half of the patients with Persistent Oligoarthritis [37], but not in the serum of children with RF Positive Polyarthritis. The anti-DEK antibody was found to be associated with uveitis and the HLA A2 antigen [39]. Anti-lipid A antibodies are found in higher titre in Persistent Oligoarthritis compared to Polyarthritis and in reduced titre in Systemic Arthritis [40]. Titres correlate with complement activation products in plasma [40]; the titres are higher in synovial fluid than in serum and correlate with joint counts over long periods of time [41]. The complement system is activated in Persistent Oligoarthritis [40,42], consistent with, but not proof of, a role for antibodies in the pathogenesis of this disease. None of the auto-antibodies are specific for Persistent Oligoarthritis, but the repertoire is.

The participation of T cells in Oligoarthritis is also clear (See also Part 2, Chapter 2.9). Studies of T cell receptors demonstrated that there is an oligoclonal expansion of T cells in involved joints [43]. Oligoclonality has been confirmed by studies using DNA hybridization techniques, which show that not only do the clones persist over time, but that in a given child the same clones are present in all involved joints [44]. T cell clones from different children do not show the same hybridization patterns. The clones found to be expanded in the joint tissues are present in very small amounts in peripheral blood, meaning that there is highly selective migration and proliferation in the inflamed joints. The pattern of cytokine expression by cells in the synovium is that of the Th1 type [45].

The specificity of T cell reactivity in Persistent Oligoarthritis is not as well studied as the antibody repertoire, but also seems to include a number of distinct but nonspecific antigens, non-specific in the sense that reactivity to these antigens is found in other forms of arthritis or eye disease. These include soluble retinal protein [46], human [47], and Escherishia coli [48] heat-shock proteins, and lipid A (unpublished). Increased reactivity to heat shock protein is associated with remission of Oligoarthritis, and may represent a protective mechanism [47].

Monitoring

The child with Oligoarthritis must be watched for the severity and sites of inflammation, the effectiveness of medical therapy, and for the development of complications. Physicians often find more extensive disease than parents appreciate, either because the child is too young to express the degree of pain or disability, or perhaps because the arthritis may be insidious and less painful than in other forms of arthritis. Thus the physical examination of these children is important, with emphasis on joints and eyes at intervals appropriate to the degree of disease activity.

Joints are examined for persistence or reappearance of thickened synovium and effusions (see also Part 1, Chapter 1.1). Warmth of joints in Oligoarthritis is usually mild or moderate, and erythema is not usually present except sometimes in the small joints of the hands or feet. A hot, red joint, particularly associated with increased tenderness or systemic fever, indicates a need to reexamine the immediate

diagnosis (Table 2.3.1). The range of motion of joints is important to measure, both to pick up past disease which may not have been recognized, and to determine the need for physical means of treatment, including active or passive exercise and splinting (Fig 2.3.4) (see also Part 3, Chapter 3.9).

One of the characteristics of Oligoarthritis is asymmetrical growth and muscle atrophy, particularly in the legs. The involved joints grow faster in length, width, and bony maturation, (Fig 2.3.5 and 2.3.6). Leg length differences should be monitored by direct measurement during physical examinations, but it is sometimes also helpful to use a radiological measurement such as CT scans. A particular problem at the knee is the development of an increased valgus angle of the lower leg, with or without contractures (Figure 2.3.5).

As the disease progresses children with Oligoarthritis may develop jaw involvement [49]. Unlike the jaw involvement in Polyarthritis, this is usually unilateral, and also usually asymptomatic. In fact, if there is jaw pain it usually emanates from the normal uninvolved TMJ,

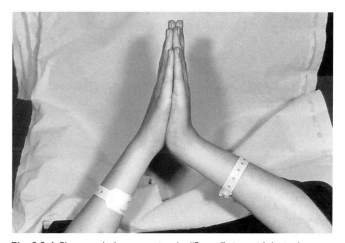

Fig. 2.3.4 Photograph demonstrating the "Prayer" sign, with limited dorsiflexion at both wrists in a girl with Oligoarthritis of several months duration pre-treatment. (Courtesy of C. A.J. Ryder.)

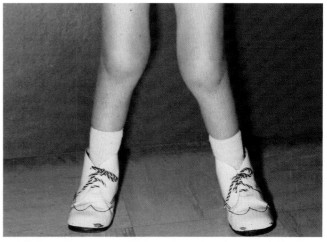

Fig. 2.3.5 Photograph of late complications of Oligoarthritis affecting both knees, which developed at different times and to different degrees, in a 5-year-old girl with Extended Oligoarthritis. There are contractures, increased valgus angles at the knees, muscle atrophy, and different leg lengths.

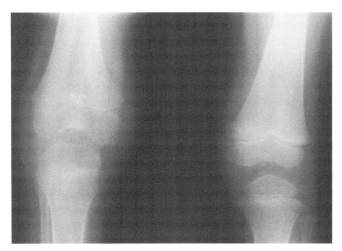

Fig. 2.3.6 Radiograph of the knees of a child with Oligoarthritis affecting one knee showing the advanced growth and maturation of the bone growth centers and epiphysial plates. Part of the appearance of size difference is due to the fact that there was a contracture which kept the affected knee from lying flat on the table so that projection from X-ray source to film was different.

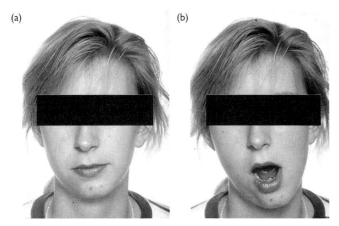

Fig. 2.3.7 An adolescent girl with longstanding Oligoarthritis and left-sided TMJ involvement demonstrating decreased growth of the left side of the mandible, deviation of the jaw to the left with opening of the mouth, and decreased oral aperture on that side. (Courtesy of T. R. Southwood.)

presumably on a "mechanical" basis, as it is having to move abnormally to accommodate decreased movement from the affected temporo-mandibular joint (TMJ). Examination of the child with Oligoarthritis should include feeling for the mandibular condyle and its movement on jaw opening, the presence or absence of deviation of the lower jaw towards the affected side on mouth opening (Figure 2.3.7) and undergrowth of the jaw on the affected side (often best seen from below when the child extends her neck).

Most children with Oligoarthritis do well in respect to psychosocial development [50], but there are always exceptions. In a fairly extensive examination of factors predicting psychosocial dysfunction, the most important predictors for poor outcomes were not the disease *per se*, but the child's social milieu [51]. Specifically, the most significant correlate of poor outcome was maternal depression, and of good outcome, maternal sense of mastery [52]. The mother's psychological state is thus an important part of the child's psychosocial prognosis. In addition,

the impact of the child's illness on the family may have deleterious effects on siblings, so the entire family may require attention.

Complications

One of the most important functional complications of Oligoarthritis is muscle atrophy on both sides of the affected joint. This is particularly obvious as quadriceps atrophy when knees are involved (Figure 2.3.5). The atrophy appears very quickly and is long in recovery. Although it is usually assumed to be due to disuse secondary to pain, it is so persistent a feature and so resistant to therapeutic active or resistive exercise, that it often seems to be a direct rather than indirect part of the disease.

Overgrowth of bone and cartilage of affected joints is a virtually constant complication (Figure 2.3.6). The cause is usually ascribed to increased blood flow to the synovium and the contiguous growth plates, but this may be a simplistic explanation. Since the growth centers mature more rapidly than in unaffected joints, the epiphysial plates may fuse earlier, allowing unaffected joints to "catch up," but differences in length and width may persist after remission has occurred.

An increased valgus angle of the lower leg results from arthritis of the knees (Figure 2.3.5). This is sometimes ascribed to tightening of the iliotibial fascial band as a result of inflammation in the knee preventing varus movement, but in the more extreme cases it is clear that there is an asymmetrically increased growth rate on the medial versus lateral tibial epiphysis.

The destruction of the cartilaginous surfaces in this form of arthritis is generally believed to be slower than in most other forms of JIA [53]. However, there are as yet no studies which specifically measure this. The fact that the characteristic child is young with developing ossification centers makes measurement of cartilage thickness difficult by standard radiographs, but MRI should make this possible.

One of the most important complications of Oligoarthritis is uveitis, which is discussed later in this chapter.

Prognosis

It has been long assumed that children with Oligoarthritis have a generally good chance for remission with little functional residual by the time they reach adulthood. However, this assumption has not been supported by careful metanalysis of published series [53] or by studies using modern assessment tools [5,14,16–19,54]. Approximately 50% of children with Oligoarthritis at onset will have ongoing disease or functional joint problems 10 or more years after onset [5,16–19]. For a few children, the presence of long-term psychological effects is also a potential cause of poor social functioning, although most studies show a surprising resilience in these children [54].

Extended Oligoarthritis
Epidemiology

The age of onset and sex ratios of the children who develop Extended Oligoarthritis are initially the same as those who have Persistent Oligoarthritis [5]. As mentioned earlier, extension to more than four joints usually occurs within the first 5 years or so of onset of the disease [14]. Whether there are population differences in the frequency of Oligoarthritis becoming extended is unknown. Some authors have pointed out the similarities between Extended Oligoarthritis and Rheumatoid Factor Negative Polyarthritis (see Part 2, Chapter 2.5).

Clinical characteristics

Predictors of developing Extended Oligoarthritis are involvement of wrists or other joints of the upper extremities in the first 6 months, sedimentation rates greater than 20 mm/h, and symmetrical joint involvement in the first 6 months [14,17]. The incidence of remission is lower and the potential degree of disability is greater than in patients with Persistent Oligoarthritis [5,14–19].

Investigations

Laboratory patterns of inflammation, such as the ESR, tend to be somewhat more abnormal than in Persistent Oligoarthritis, having more in common with Polyarthritis. Levels of complement activation are the same during the course of Extended Oligoarthritis as in RF Negative Polyarthritis and are different than Persistent Oligoarthritis [40,42].

Genetics

The principal differences between children with Extended Oligoarthritis and those with Persistent Oligoarthritis are genetic. None of the children with Extended Oligoarthritis have the HLA antigen DR6 (DRB1*1301), although this antigen has a positive genetic association with Oligoarthritis in general [28]. Conversely there is an association of Extended Oligoarthritis with DR1 (DRB1*0101), which is predictive of progression to more joints, and to joint erosions, in children with an oligoarticular onset [16].

Course and prognosis

The distinction between Persistent Oligoarthritis and Extended Oligoarthritis is only recent, so there are only a few studies which specifically address the long-term course and prognosis of Extended Oligoarthritis. In a 5-year study, a higher proportion of children with a polyarticular course after an oligoarticular onset (Extended Oligoarthritis), had received intra-articular corticosteroids, oral corticosteroids, and second-line agents than children with an oligoarticular course (Persistent Oligoarthritis) [18]. Joint erosions and destruction increase with increasing numbers of joints involved [14]. In England, adults who had had Extended Oligoarthritis had more complications from uveitis, more joint replacement operations, and worse scores on the Health Assessment Questionnaire than those who had had Persistent Oligoarthritis after a follow-up of almost 30 years [19]. On the positive side, children with Extended Oligoarthritis are apparently more likely to respond well to treatment with methotrexate than are children with other forms of JIA [55]. Anecdotally, lymphoedema of the lower limits has been reported in both Oligoarthritis and Extended Oligoarthritis.

Uveitis

Introduction

The most serious complication for all children with Oligoarthritis is the potential blindness caused by uveitis. The incidence of uveitis in Oligoarthritis seems to have varied with time [56] but is currently expected in about 30% of these patients [57]. Uveitis may also occur in RF Negative Polyarthritis, Enthesitis Related Arthritis, and Psoriatic Arthritis or as part of the presentation of sarcoidosis or Behçet

Table 2.3.4 Characteristics of uveitis in rheumatic diseases of children (modified from [60])

Disease	Site	Onset	Pain
Oligoarthritis	Anterior	Insidious	+/−
Enthesitis Related Arthritis	Anterior	Acute	++++
Psoriatic Arthritis	Anterior and/or Posterior	Insidious	+/−
Sarcoidosis	Anterior and/or Posterior	Variable	++
Behçet disease	Pan-uveitis	Acute	+++
Isolated Idiopathic Uveitis	Anterior or Posterior	Insidious	+/−

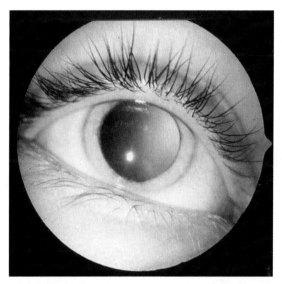

Fig. 2.3.8 A 5-year-old girl who developed anterior uveitis 6 months after diagnosis of Oligoarthritis. The photograph shows keratic precipitates (seen as dark "spots" floating in the lower portion of anterior chamber). The uveitis responded well to topical steroids. (Courtesy of A. McCormick.)

disease in childhood. It may also occur as an isolated phenomenon not associated with arthritis [58] (see Table 2.3.4).

Clinical characteristics

The uveitis associated with Oligoarthritis is insidious in onset and relatively painless. It usually presents in one eye but may be or may become bilateral. This is in contrast to the painful, acute uveitis associated with Enthesitis Related Arthritis. On examination, dilatation of the blood vessels immediately adjacent to the cornea in a red ring is a classical but uncommon sign, but some children will have had enough irritation to have rubbed the eye and to have produced a generalized reddening of the conjunctivae. In most children the conjunctival changes are minimal. The earliest changes are only visible by a slit lamp, so examination by an ophthalmologist should be performed on all children with Oligoarthritis, and preferably repeated at

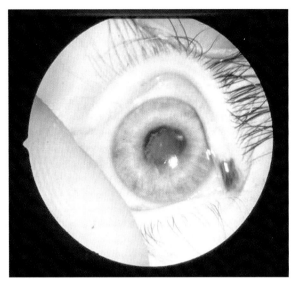

Fig. 2.3.9 A 4-year-old girl presented with Oligoarthritis of her right knee of 2 months' duration. Although she had no symptoms, slit lamp examination revealed advanced changes of uveitis with synechiae fixing parts of the iris to the lens. (Courtesy of A. McCormick.)

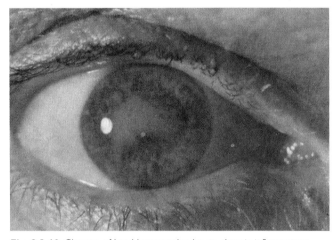

Fig. 2.3.10 Changes of band keratopathy due to chronic inflammatory changes in the anterior chamber in another patient with severe chronic uveitis due to Oligoarthritis. (Courtesy of A. McCormick.)

3 month intervals [59]. The eyes should also be examined with a regular ophthalmoscope on every visit to any physician, looking for evidence of inflammation, which would include pericorneal vascular dilatation, keratic (cellular) precipitates in the anterior chamber (Figure 2.3.8), synechiae (Figure 2.3.9) or band keratopathy (Figure 2.3.10). However, these are all late findings, and for early diagnosis, frequent slit lamp examination by an ophthalmologist is essential.

Pathology

The disease is primarily in the iris and ciliary body. The first abnormality is an exudate of serum protein and WBCs into the anterior chamber. The cells may be seen with a slit lamp prior to any other change, and therapy is usually based on the degree of "flare" caused by these abnormalities. The protein and cells collect between the iris and lens to cause synechiae (Figure 2.3.9), gradual immobility of the iris, and opaqueness in a band across the cornea and over the anterior surface of the lens (band keratopathy) (Figure 2.3.10). Drainage of the anterior chamber is impeded and glaucoma results, leading to cataracts [60].

Course and prognosis

The course of uveitis in these children is variable, from self-limited and mild to relapsing or persistent inflammation with progression to blindness. Outcome appears to be worse than for the uveitis associated with other rheumatic diseases of childhood, and is worse in Extended Oligoarthritis than in Persistent Oligoarthritis [19]. Complications as a consequence of uveitis occur in about 20% [60]. Predictors for a poor outcome are advanced disease at presentation, an extended course, male sex, and older age at onset [61]. Good prognostic features are absence of uveitis at onset of arthritis and a prolonged gap between onset of arthritis and onset of uveitis [61].

Treatment with local administration of corticosteroids and mydriatics controls most cases, but an ophthalmologist is required to judge effect. Some children do not respond to topical medication, or are dependent on topical treatment (which can also cause complications), and therefore require subconjunctival injection, systemic steroids, or systemic immunomodulating drugs for control.

A final caveat

The classification process is an ongoing work, and it is clear that Oligoarthritis is no more a single disease than is JIA in general. The nomenclature and criteria will undoubted change as more is learned about pathogenesis. Already a study of children in Italy showed that greater homogeneity of demographic data (age of onset and sex ratio) and of the course and outcome of joint disease was obtained by dividing patients into those with or without antinuclear antibodies, irrespective of whether they had Persistent Oligoarthritis, Extended Oligoarthritis, or RF Negative Polyarthritis [62].

Key point summary

1. Oligoarthritis is a common form of JIA. Its frequency probably varies between different ethnic groups.

2. The ILAR classification criteria recognize two forms of Oligoarthritis, a form in which the cumulative joint count never exceeds four affected joints (Persistent Oligoarthritis), and an form in which five or more joints become affected after 6 or more months of disease (Extended Oligoarthritis).

3. Although Oligoarthritis may have less joint involvement than some other forms of JIA, individual joints can become seriously damaged. Bony overgrowth or undergrowth of the limbs and jaw can lead to significant disability, particularly if treatment is not adequately aggressive.

4. Uveitis, which is usually asymptomatic, is a common complication of both forms of Oligoarthritis, and if unrecognized or is resistant to treatment, can lead to blindness.

5. For a significant minority of children, Oligoarthritis is a life-long condition. Although most children cope well with the disease, it can have profound effects on long-term physical, psychological, and social wellbeing.

References

1. Petty, R.E., Southwood, T.R., Manners, P. *et al.* International League of Associations for Rheumatology Classification of Juvenile Idiopathic Arthritis: Second Revision, Edmonton, 2001. *J Rheumatol* 2004;31:390–2.

2. Brewer, E.J., Bass, J.C., Baum, J. *et al.* Current proposed revision of JRA criteria. *Arthritis Rheum* 1977;20 (Suppl):195–9.

3. European League Against Rheumatism (EULAR) Bulletin 4. Nomenclature and classification of arthritis in children. Basel: National Zeitung AG, 1977.

4. Cassidy, J.T., Levinson, J.E., Bass, J.C. *et al.* A study of classification criteria for a diagnosis of juvenile rheumatoid arthritis. *Arthritis Rheum* 1986;29:274–81.

5. Hofer, M.F., Mouy, R., Prieur, A.-M. Juvenile idiopathic arthritides evaluated prospectively in a single center according to the Durban criteria. *J Rheumatol* 2001;28:1083–90.

6. Glass, D.N. and Giannini, E.H. Juvenile rheumatoid arthritis as a complex genetic trait. *Arthritis Rheum* 1999;42:2261–8.

7. Schaller, J.G. Chronic arthritis in children. Juvenile rheumatoid arthritis. *Clin Orthop* 1984;182:79–84.

8. Graham, T.B. and Glass, D.N. Juvenile rheumatoid arthritis: Ethnic differences in diagnostic types. *J Rheumatol* 1997;24:1677–9.

9. Schwartz, M.M., Simpson, P., Kerr, K.L., and Jarvis, J.N. Juvenile rheumatoid arthritis in African Americans. *J Rheumatol* 1997;24:1826–9.

10. Arguedas, O., Fasth, A., Andersson-Gare, B., and Porros, O. Juvenile chronic arthritis in urban San Jose, Costa Rica: A 2 year prospective study. *J Rheumatol* 1998;25:1844–50.

11. Huemer, C., Malleson, P.N., Cabral, D.A. *et al.* Patterns of joint involvement at onset differentiate oligoarticular juvenile psoriatic arthritis from pauciarticular juvenile rheumatoid arthritis. *J Rheumatol* 2002;29:1531–5.

12. Tria, A.J., Palumbo, R.C., and Alicea, J.A. Conservative care for patellofemoral pain. *Orthop Clin North Am* 1992;23:545–54.

13. Arguedas, O., Fasth, A., and Andersson-Gare. A prospective population based study on outcome of juvenile chronic arthritis in Costa Rica. *J Rheumatol* 2002;29:174–83.

14. Guillaume, S., Prieur, A.-M., Coste, J., and Job-Deslandre, C. Long-term outcome and prognosis in oligoarticular-onset juvenile idiopathic arthritis. *Arthritis Rheum* 2000;43:1858–65.

15. Sharma, S. and Sherry, D.D. Joint distribution at presentation in children with pauciarticular arthritis. *J Pediatr* 1999;134:642–3.

16. Flato, B., Lien, G., Smerdal, A. *et al.* Prognostic factors in juvenile rheumatoid arthritis: A case-control study revealing early predictors and outcome after 14.9 years. *J Rheumatol* 2003;30:386–93.

17. Al-Matar, M.J., Petty, R.E., Tucker, L.B., Malleson, P.N., Schroeder, M.L., and Cabral, D.A. The early pattern of joint involvement predicts disease progression in children with oligoarticular (pauciarticular) juvenile rheumatoid arthritis. *Arthritis Rheum* 2002;46:2708–15.

18. Bowyer, S.L., Roettcher, P.A., Higgins, G.C. *et al.* Health status of patients with juvenile rheumatoid arthritis at 1 and 5 years after diagnosis. *J Rheumatol* 2003;30:394–400.

19. Packham, J.C. and Hall, M.A. Long-term follow-up of 246 adults with juvenile idiopathic arthritis: functional outcome. *Rheumatology* 2002;41:1428–35.

20. Sailer, M., Cabral, D., Petty, R.E., and Malleson, P.N. Rheumatoid factor positive, oligoarticular onset juvenile rheumatoid arthritis. *J Rheumatol* 1997;24:586–8.

21. Petty, R.E., Cassidy, J.T., and Sullivan, D.B. Clinical correlates of antinuclear antibodies in juvenile rheumatoid arthritis. *J Pediatr* 1973;83:386–9.

22. Schaller, J.G., Johnson, G.D., Holborow, E.J., Ansell, B.M., and Smiley, W.K. The association of antinuclear antibodies with the chronic iridocyclitis of juvenile rheumatoid arthritis (Still's Disease). *Arthritis Rheum* 1974;17:409–16.

23. Alspaugh, M.A. and Miller, J.J. A study of specificities of antinuclear antibodies in juvenile rheumatoid arthritis. *J Pediatr* 1977;90:391–5.

24. Oen, K., Malleson, P.N., Cabral, D.A. et al. Early predictors of long-term outcome in patients with juvenile rheumatoid arthritis: subset-specific correlations. J Rheumatol 2003;30:585–93.

25. Woo, P. Genetic aspects of juvenile chronic arthritis. *Clin Orthop* 1990;259:11–17.

26. Fantini, F., Gerloni, V., Murelli, M. *et al.* HLA phenotypes in Italian children affected with juvenile chronic arthritis. *Clin Exp Rheumatol* 1987;51 (Suppl) 2:17.

27. Forre, O., Dobloug, J.H., Hoyeraal, H.M., and Thorsby, E. HLA antigens in juvenile arthritis: Genetic basis for the different subtypes. *Arthritis Rheum* 1983;26:35–8.

28. Cerna, M., Vavrincova, P., Havelka, S., Isakova, E., and Stastny, P. Class II alleles in juvenile arthritis in Czech children. *J Rheumatol* 1994;21:159–64.

29. Fernandez-Vina, M., Fink, C.W., and Stastny, P. HLA associations in juvenile arthritis. *Clin Exp Rheumatol* 1994;12:205–14.

30. Hall, P.J., Burman, S.J., Laurent, M.R. *et al.* Genetic susceptibility to early onset pauciarticular juvenile chronic arthritis: a study of HLA and complement markers in 158 British patients. *Ann Rheum Dis* 1986;45:464–74.

31. Malleson, P., Petty, R.E., Fung, M., and Candido, E.P.M. Reactivity of antinuclear antibodies with histones and other antigens in juvenile rheumatoid arthritis. *Arthritis Rheum* 1989;32:919–23.

32. Ostensen, M., Fredriksen, K., Kass, E., and Rekvig, O.-P. Identification of antihistone antibodies in subsets of juvenile chronic arthritis. *Ann Rheum Dis* 1989;48:114–17.

33. Pauls, J.D., Silverman, E.D., Laxer, R.M., and Frilzler, A.J. Antibodies to histones H1 and H5 in sera of patients with juvenile rheumatoid arthritis. *Arthritis Rheum* 1989;32:877–83.

34. Burlingame, R.W., Rubin, R.L., and Rosenberg, A.M. Antibodies to chromatin components in juvenile rheumatoid arthritis. *Arthritis Rheum* 1993;36:836–41.

35. Jung, F., Neuer, G., and Bautz, F.A. Antibodies against a peptide sequence located in the linker region of the HMG-1/2 box domains in sera from patients with juvenile rheumatoid arthritis. *Arthritis Rheum* 1997;40:1803–9.

36. Szer, I.S., Sierakowski, H., and Szer, W. A novel autoantibody to the putative oncoprotein DEK in pauciarticular onset juvenile rheumatoid arthritis. *J Rheumatol* 1994;21:2136–42.

37. Miller, J.J., Bieber, M.M., Levinson, J.E., Zhu, S., Tsoo, E., and Teng NNH. $V_H4\text{-}34$ ($V_H4.21$) gene expression in the chronic arthritides of childhood: Studies of associations with anti-lipid A antibodies, HLA antigens, and clinical features. *J Rheumatol* 1996;23:2132–9.

38. Stevenson, F.K., Spellerberg, M.B., Treasure, J. *et al.* Differential usage of an Ig heavy chain variable region gene by human B cell tumors. *Blood* 1993;82:224–30.

39. Murray, K.J., Szer, W., Gromm, A.A. *et al.* Antibodies to the 45 kD DEK nuclear antigen in pauciarticular onset juvenile rheumatoid arthritis and iridocyclitis: Selective association with an MHC gene. *J Rheumatol* 1997;24:560–7.

40. Olds, L.C. and Miller, J.J. C3 activation products correlate with antibodies to lipid A in pauciarticular juvenile arthritis. *Arthritis Rheum* 1990;33:520–4.

41. Miller, J.J. and Olds, L.C. Antibodies to lipid A in pauciarticular arthritis: Clinical studies. *J Rheumatol* 1992;19:959–63.

42. Miller, J.J., Olds, L.C., Silverman, E.D., Milgrom, H., and Curd, J.G. Different patterns of C3 and C4 activation in the varied types of juvenile arthritis. *Pediatr Res* 1986;20:1332–7.

43. Grom, A.A., Thompson, S.D., Luyrink, L., Passo, M., Choi, E., and Glass, D.N. Dominant T cell receptor beta chain variable region V beta 14 clones in juvenile rheumatoid arthritis. *Proc Natl Acad Sci USA* 1993;90:11104–8.

44. Wedderburn, L.R., Maini, M.K., Patel, A., Beverly, P.C., and Woo, P. Molecular finger printing reveals non-overlapping T cell oligoclonality between an inflamed site and peripheral blood. *Int Immunol* 1999;11:535–43.

45. Wedderburn, L.R., Robinson, N., Patel, A., Varsani, H., and Woo, P. Selective recruitment of polarized T cells expressing CCR5 and CXCR3 to the inflamed joints of children with juvenile idiopathic arthritis. *Arthritis Rheum* 2000;43:765–74.

46. Petty, R.E., Hunt, D.W., Rollins, D.F., Schroeder, M.L., and Puterman, M.L. Immunity to soluble retinal antigen in patients with uveitis accompanying juvenile rheumatoid arthritis. *Arthritis Rheum* 1987;30:287–93.

47. Prakken, A.B., van Eden, W., Rijkers, G.T. *et al*. Autoreactivity to human heat-shock protein 60 predicts disease remission in oligoarticular juvenile rheumatoid arthritis. *Arthritis Rheum* 1996;39:1826–32.

48. Albani, S., Ravelli, A., Massa, M. *et al*. Immune responses to the Escherichia coli dnaJ heat shock protein in juvenile rheumatoid arthritis and their correlation with disease activity. *J Pediatr* 1994;124:561–5.

49. Karhulahti, T., Ylijoki, H., and Ronning, O. Mandibular condyle lesions related to age at onset and subtypes of juvenile rheumatoid arthritis in 15-year-old children. *Scand J Dent Res* 1993;101:332–8.

50. Miller, J.J. Psychosocial factors related to rheumatic diseases in childhood. *J Rheumatol* 1993;20 (Suppl) 38:1–11.

51. Timko, C., Stovel, K., Moos, R.H., and Miller, J.J. A longitudinal study of risk and resistance factors among children with juvenile rheumatic disease. *J Clin Child Psychol* 1992;21:132–42.

52. Daniels, D., Miller, J.J., Billings, and Moos, R.H. Psychosocial functioning of siblings of children with rheumatic disease. *J Pediatr* 1986;109:379–83.

53. Wallace, C.A. and Levinson, J.E. Juvenile rheumatoid arthritis: Outcome and treatment for the 1990s. *Rheum Dis Clin North Am* 1991;17:891–905.

54. Miller, J.J., Spitz, P., Simpson, U., and Williams, G. The social functions of young adults who had arthritis in childhood. *J Pediatr* 1982; 100:378–82.

55. Ravelli, A., Viola, S., Migliavacca, D., Ruperto, N., Pistorio, A., and Martini, A. The extended oligoarticular subtype is the best predictor of methotrexate efficacy in juvenile idiopathic arthritis. *J Pediatr* 1999;135:316–20.

56. Sherry, D.D., Mellins, E.D., and Wedgwood, R.J. Decreasing severity of chronic uveitis in children with pauciarticular arthritis. *A J Dis Child* 1991;145:1026–8.

57. Petty, R.E., Smith, J.R., and Rosenbaum, J.T. Arthritis and uveitis in children. A pediatric rheumatology perspective. *Am J Ophthalmol* 2003;135:879–84.

58. Kanski, J.J. and Shun-Shin, A. Systemic uveitis syndromes in childhood: An analysis of 340 cases. *Ophthalmology* 1984;91:1247–52.

59. Yancey, C., White, P., Magilavy, D. *et al*. Guidelines for ophthalmologic examinations in children with juvenile rheumatoid arthritis. *Pediatrics* 1993;92:295–6.

60. Rosenberg, A.M. Uveitis associated with childhood rheumatic diseases. *Curr Opin Rheumatol* 2002;14:542–7.

61. Edelsten, C., Lee, V., Bentley, C.R., Kanski, J.J., and Graham, E.M. An evaluation of baseline risk factors predicting severity in juvenile idiopathic arthritis associated uveitis and other chronic anterior uveitis in early childhood. *Br J Ophthalmol* 2002;86:51–6.

62. Magni-Manzoni, S., Felici, E., Novarini, C. *et al*. Patients with antinuclear antibody positive juvenile idiopathic arthritis constitute a homogenous subgroup irrespective of the course of articular involvement. (abstract) *Arthritis Rheum* 2003;48 (Suppl.):S96.

2.4 Rheumatoid Factor Positive Polyarthritis

Janet Gardner-Medwin

Aims

The aims of this chapter are to discuss the clinical features, investigations, and complications of Rheumatoid Factor (RF) Positive Polyarthritis, which is similar to but is somewhat distinct from rheumatoid arthritis in adults. This chapter also contains a discussion of RF, the presence of which is a requirement in the diagnosis of RF Positive Polyarthritis.

Structure

- Introduction and classification
- Epidemiology
- Clinical features
- Investigations
- Monitoring
- Complications
- Prognosis
- Key point summary

Introduction and classification

Rheumatoid Factor (RF) Positive Polyarthritis is the smallest category of Juvenile Idiopathic Arthritis (JIA), making up about 5% of cases. It is most common in teenage girls, and is associated with a poor prognosis. RF Positive Polyarthritis may be considered the youngest end of the distribution of rheumatoid arthritis (RA), but the impact of the disease in a young person or child who is still growing and developing warrants a clear distinction from the adult disease, and critical differences between the adult and paediatric classifications do not allow direct comparison. RF is usually present early in the disease

course, and almost always at a high titre unlikely to be seen in healthy children. There is a distinctive pattern of joint involvement, which is that of a symmetrical polyarthritis of the small and large joints, often involving the wrists, metacarpophalangeal (MCP), and proximal interphalangeal (PIP) joints. The disease may develop rapidly, and erosive change may be seen on radiographs as early as 6 months after onset. Rheumatoid nodules are often palpable at or just distal to the elbow or in other areas of friction. Acute or chronic uveitis is unusual compared to other forms of JIA, but other types of eye involvement such as keratitis and the dry eyes of Sjögren syndrome are occasionally present.

The revised International League of Associations for Rheumatology (ILAR) classification of RF Positive Polyarthritis from 2001 is given in Table 2.4.1 [1]. RF Positive Polyarthritis is the only subgroup of JIA which cannot fulfil classification criteria through clinical features alone, but requires the presence of a positive laboratory test (RF). The relationship between RA and RF Positive Polyarthritis is tacit in the ILAR classification. However, the currently accepted classification of RA identifies a broader cohort of patients from RF Positive Polyarthritis (Table 2.4.2) [2]. In this classification, although a positive RF is included in the classification for RA, it is not a requirement for diagnosis, and clinical characteristics of the disease are given equal importance. Examination of the features of JIA in a mathematical model found the importance of the pattern of joint involvement to be more discriminatory than the presence of RF [3], and it will be interesting to see how the classification system of JIA continues to evolve. Since there is no age restriction in the classification of RA, a 13-year-old seeing an adult rheumatologist fulfilling criteria 1 through 4 (without a positive RF) would be classified as having RA. In contrast, the same patient seeing a paediatric rheumatologist would be classified as having RF Negative Polyarthritis.

The older classifications still dominate the published literature, and can cause confusion (Table 2.4.3). In North America, the term

Table 2.4.1 ILAR classification of RF Positive Polyarthritis (2001) [1]

Criteria 1–4 must all be fulfilled for classification as RF Positive Polyarthritis	
1. Polyarthritis	Arthritis affecting five or more joints during the first 6 months of disease
2. Positive RF	At least two positive RF tests (as routinely defined in a laboratory using the WHO standard) at least 3 months apart during the first 6 months of observation
3. Age	Under 16 years at onset of arthritis
4. Minimum duration of arthritis	6 weeks
5. Descriptors	Immunogenetic characteristics comparable to adult populations with RA.

Table 2.4.2 The 1987 ARA criteria for RA [2]

At least four criteria must be fulfilled for classification as RA; patients with two clinical diagnoses are not excluded	
1. Morning stiffness	Morning stiffness in and around the joints, lasting at least 1 h before maximal improvement
2. Arthritis in three or more joint areas[a]	Soft-tissue swelling or fluid (not bony overgrowth) observed by a physician, present simultaneously for at least 6 weeks
3. Arthritis of hand joints	Swelling of wrist, MCP, or PIP joints for at least 6 weeks
4. Symmetric arthritis	Simultaneous involvement of the same joint areas (defined in 2) on both sides of the body (bilateral involvement of PIP, MCP, or MTP joints is acceptable without absolute symmetry) for at least 6 weeks
5. Rheumatoid nodules	Subcutaneous nodules over bony prominences, extensor surfaces, or in juxta-articular regions observed by a physician
6. RF	Detected by a method positive in less han 5% of normal controls
7. Radiographic changes	Typical of RA on postero-anterior hand and wrist radiographs; it must include erosions or unequivocal bony decalcification localized in or most marked adjacent to the involved joints (OA changes alone do not qualify)

[a] Possible areas: right or left PIP, MCP, wrist, elbow, knee, ankle, MTP.

Table 2.4.3 Differences between the classifications and nomenclature of polyarthritis

Characteristic	JIA (ILAR)[1]	JRA (ACR)[4]	JCA (EULAR 1977) [5]	Adult RA
Age at onset	<16 years	<16 years	<16 years	All ages
Minimum duration of arthritis	6 weeks	6 weeks	3 months	6 weeks
Nomenclature depending on RF status	RF Negative Polyarthritis	Polyarticular JRA (RF does not alter classification)	Polyarticular JCA	Polyarthritis including RF negative RA
	RF Positive Polyarthritis		JRA	RA associated with a positive RF

'juvenile rheumatoid arthritis' (JRA) is still often used [4] to refer to patients with various forms of chronic childhood arthritis, not only RF Positive Polyarthritis. Confusingly, the European League Against Rheumatism (EULAR) classification of 'juvenile chronic arthritis' (JCA) [5] reserved the term "juvenile rheumatoid arthritis" only for those with polyarthritis associated with a positive RF.

Epidemiology

There are no population-based surveys identifying the community-based epidemiology of juvenile arthritis. Hospital-based surveys from across the world suggest an incidence of 5–18 per 100,000, and a prevalence of 30–150 per 100,000 children [6–9]. There are no specific data on the epidemiology of RF Positive Polyarthritis in isolation, although cases are identified as a subgroup of JCA, and have been identified within JRA in later series. The proportion of RF Positive Polyarthritis is estimated as 5–10% of JCA and JRA in most, predominantly Caucasian, series [9], giving a crudely estimated incidence of 0.25–1.8 per 100,000 (0.4–3 per 100,000 in girls). In comparison, the incidence of RA is estimated at about 24 per 100,000 of Caucasian populations, with a prevalence of 0.5–2% of the population [10]. The age distribution of RA shows the lowest incidence rates in the youngest adults, with a rate of 3/100,000 in males aged 15–24 years, and between 9 and 12.4/100,000 in females of the same age using the American Rheumatism Association (ARA) criteria [10]. Only 26% of these cases of RA were RF positive, a more comparable group to RF Positive Polyarthritis. This suggests the incidence of RF positive RA is of the same order of magnitude as RF Positive Polyarthritis in a comparably aged population. Figure 2.4.1 shows the rising incidence of RA with age.

RF Positive Polyarthritis has a mean age of onset around 9–12 years, which is some 2–4.4 years older than the mean onset of RF Negative Polyarthritis [10–12]. RF Positive Polyarthritis is more common in girls than boys in all reports with ratios between 5.7 and 12.8:1 (F : M) [10–12]. The incidence rates of JIA also vary with ethnicity. In non-Caucasian populations, polyarticular disease, and particularly RF Positive Polyarthritis, is more common [13]. Populations well known to have a high incidence of RA as well as RF Positive Polyarthritis [14–16] include the Native North American [17] and Canadian Aboriginal populations [18]. African American [19], Caribbean [20], Black and Indian South African children [21], and Latin American populations [22] are more likely to develop RF Positive Polyarthritis disease, have an older mean age at onset of polyarticular arthritis and RF Positive Oligoarthritis [19,20,23], and are less likely to be ANA positive [19]. Nodules are more often present in these populations. An increased incidence of RF Positive Polyarthritis is also recognized in Arab [24] and Asian populations [25]. HLA DR4 has the highest frequency in northern Europe [26] and is not associated with polyarthritis in the African American population.

Clinical features

RF Positive Polyarthritis is characterized by a symmetrical polyarthritis affecting large and small joints, often associated with rheumatoid nodules. There can be tenosynovitis associated with the

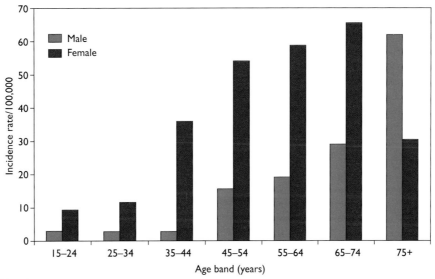

Fig. 2.4.1 The incidence of RA with age.

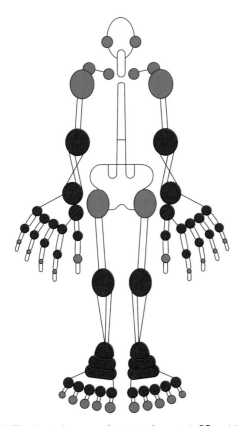

Fig. 2.4.2 The classical pattern of joint involvement in RF positive polyarthritis. Joints marked in red are the most frequently involved, as recognised by the RA classification criteria [1], and clinical paediatric practice.

arthritis, but this should also raise the possibility of other diagnoses, especially systemic lupus erythematosis (SLE) or sarcoid. There may be associated low-grade fever and slight or moderate hepatosplenomegaly and lymphadenopathy. Serositis and small pericardial effusions may be identified on echocardiography but clinically evident effusions are rare. Chronic uveitis is unusual.

Pattern of joint involvement

RF Positive Polyarthritis is typically an aggressive, symmetrical polyarthritis (Figure 2.4.2). Wrists, MCP, and PIP joints are usually affected early, with significant functional impact (Figure 2.4.3). Hip involvement is also critical, as aggressive disease can lead to the need for early, often bilateral, hip replacements (Figure 2.4.4). Erosive changes may occur early in the disease course (Figure 2.4.5). RF Positive Polyarthritis often presents with a large number of affected joints over a short time period. Although palindromic RA is well described in adults, it is not recognized in the paediatric literature. Patients with Oligoarthritis presenting with small joints of the hands and feet may have an increased risk of progressing to polyarticular arthritis [27], and RF may be of value predicting those with more aggressive disease course [28,29].

Rheumatoid nodules

In children, rheumatoid nodules are limited almost exclusively to those with RF Positive Polyarthritis (Figure 2.4.6). Ten per cent of adults with RA develop nodules, and this is strongly associated with HLA DR4, rising to 20–30% in Caucasian patients [30], but directly comparable figures in children are not available. Ten per cent of RF positive children developed nodules in a very small JRA cohort (all disease types) [31]. Many rheumatic diseases can be associated with nodules, however. The differential diagnoses as well as differentiating characteristics of various nodules are shown in Table 2.4.4.

Extra-articular features

Extra-articular features are well described in RA, but are less commonly reported in the paediatric literature. It is not clear if this is because they occur less often, or are less often reported. Since these features are associated with long-standing RA, they may be under-reported in RF Positive Polyarthritis because they occur after patients leave the care of the paediatrician or have (mistakenly) changed their diagnostic label to RA when they became adults.

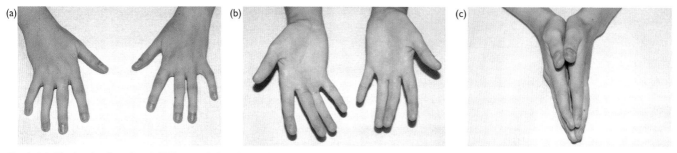

Fig. 2.4.3 The hands of a girl with RF Positive Polyarthritis of 6 years duration showing subluxation and radial deviation at the wrist; ulnar deviation, swan neck, and boutonnière deformities of the fingers, and shortening of two fingers from premature fusion of the epiphyses. There is muscle wasting, and swelling of several DIP joints, and the wrists. Her hands are also small (not obvious in this photograph).

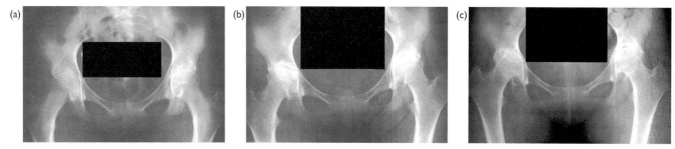

Fig. 2.4.4 A sequence of radiographs in a girl with RF Positive Polyarthritis showing the rapid destruction of the hip joints during the course of the second year of her arthritis. She required bilateral hip replacements at the age of 14 years. The radiographs show (a) loss of joint space and sclerosis, but a normal contour of the femoral head, (b) early osteophyte formation and advanced degenerative change with worsening sclerosis and loss of the normal femoral head contour, (c) subchondral cysts, osteophytes, complete loss of joint space, and protrusio acetabuli which is progressive across the three images.

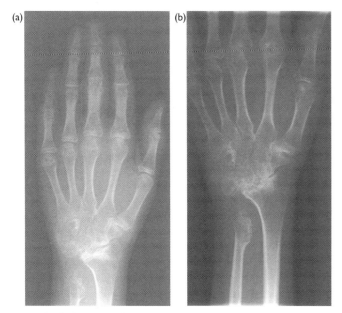

Fig. 2.4.5 Radiographs of the left wrist in a girl with RF Positive polyarthritis of 4 years duration, starting at the age of 11. These films are taken 16 months apart, and show the rapid loss of joint space with fusion of most carpal bones, severe erosive and degenerative change at the radiocarpal joint, and shortened eroded ulna. There are worsening and new erosions affecting the index and middle MCP joints and thumb IP joint.

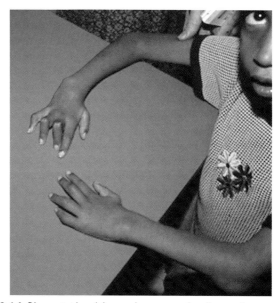

Fig. 2.4.6 Rheumatoid nodules can be seen on the elbows of an unusually young girl with severe RF Positive Polyarthritis. (Courtesy of Y. Kimura)

Table 2.4.4 The differential diagnosis of nodules in a child

Diagnosis	Ref.	Description	Clinical situation	Depth	Duration	Histopathology	Disease
Rheumatoid nodules Figure 2.4.6	[30, 85]	Single, multiple, freely mobile or fixed nodules varying up to several cm in diameter	Extensor surfaces (olecranon, ulna, and Achilles tendon) and sites of mechanical irritation in a patient with polyarthritis. Rarely in visceral organs	Subcutaneous	Chronic	Central necrosis, palisading mononuclear cells, perivascular lymphocytic infiltration	Adult RA and RF Positive Polyarthritis Rarely in Systemic Arthritis
Benign rheumatoid nodules Part 1, Figures 1.3.4 and 1.3.11	[30, 86],	Identical to rheumatoid nodules	Occurs on anterior tibia, feet, or scalp in an otherwise normal patient (without arthritis)	Subcutaneous	Transient but often lasts months	Identical to rheumatoid nodules	No associated disease, RF and ANA negative
Granuloma annulare Part 1, Figure 1.3.4	[30]	Identical to rheumatoid nodules, but more superficial, and often associated with annular, erythematous, raised skin lesions	Same as in benign rheumatoid nodules	Intradermal	Variable	Identical to rheumatoid nodules	No associated disease, RF and ANA negative
Rheumatic fever nodules Part 1, Figures 1.3.10 and 1.4.3		Small pea-like lesions	Bony prominences, including vertebrae in a patient with acute migratory polyarthritis and possibly carditis	Subcutaneous	Transient	Central necrosis but little histiocyctic or lymphocytic infiltration	Acute or recurrent rheumatic fever
Calcinosis Part 1, Figure 1.3.31		Hard calcareous deposits, may discharge from the skin	Extensor surfaces, pressure points, and sites of trauma in a patient with signs and symptoms of dermatomyositis or scleroderma	Intracutaneous, subcutaneous, fascia, or muscle	Chronic	Calcareous deposits which may liquefy	Scleroderma and dermatomyositis
Erythema nodosum Part 1, Figures 1.3.6 and 1.3.8		Tender, red, coin-sized nodules darkening to a bruise, and healing completely	Typically shins, less often thighs or forearms, may be associated with signs and symptoms of other inflammatory conditions	Subcutaneous	Transient	Panniculitis with a lymphocytic infiltrate and haemorrhage at the septa between fat cells	Infections (especially streptococcal, fungal, and tuberculous), sarcoid, drugs, and inflammatory bowel disease
Superficial aneurysms		Tender nodules following the line of arteries	Shin, upper arms, and overlying superficial arteries in a systemically ill patient with pulmonary and/or renal involvement	On arteries	Chronic	Focal, necrotising inflammation through the wall of small- and medium-sized arteries causing disruption of the vessel wall and aneurysm formation	Polyarteritis nodosa
Methotrexate associated nodules	[87]	Identical to rheumatoid nodules	Same as rheumatoid nodules; associated with transient development of RF in a patient with Systemic Arthritis taking methotrexate or accelerated development of multiple nodules in a patient with RF Positive Polyarthritis taking methotrexate	Subcutaneous	Variable	Same as rheumatoid nodules	RP Positive Polyarthritis and Systemic Arthritis patients taking methotrexate

Investigations

Initial evaluation

Investigations in RF Positive Polyarthritis, as in other forms of JIA, are predominantly to exclude other diagnoses, aid in classification, support the clinical findings, and form a baseline for future monitoring. The initial investigation of the child presenting with a widespread polyarthritis should therefore include the following:

1. **Full blood count, differential white cell count and blood film, erythrocyte sedimentation rate (ESR) and C-reactive protein (CRP).** Typically there is a normocytic normochromic anaemia with a raised white cell count, predominantly neutrophilia, and/or platelet count in proportion to the acute phase response (APR). At times, the APR can be surprisingly normal in the face of widespread synovitis, but in such situations noninflammatory diagnoses should be considered such as skeletal dysplasias and mucopolysaccharidoses.

2. **Urinalysis, urea, creatinine and electrolytes, liver function tests.** These should be normal, and are useful as baseline tests prior to commencement of medications.

3. **RF** (discussed in the next section)

4. **ANA, anti-extractable nuclear antigens (ENA), anti-SSA and SSB, anti-double stranded DNA, and quantitative immunoglobulins.** Tests for autoantibodies help distinguish RF Positive Polyarthritis from SLE, mixed connective tissue disease, overlap syndromes, and Sjögren syndrome, all of which can be associated with a positive RF. Quantitative immunoglobulins may also be elevated in these diseases, or if decreased, point to immunodeficiencies.

5. **Radiographs and DEXA.** Radiographs of the joints are usually normal at presentation, but are valuable to exclude other conditions such as skeletal dysplasia and malignancy, and to record a baseline from which to judge the rate of development of erosions and destructive change. A dual-energy X-ray absorptiometry (DEXA) at or near baseline is also useful to assess the rate of change in bone density.

Table 2.4.5 Investigations in RF Positive Polyarthritis

Investigation	Value in RF Positive Polyarthritis	Results typical of RF Positive Polyarthritis	Results atypical for RF Positive Polyarthritis	Other diagnoses to consider when results are atypical
Pubertal status, height, sitting height, and weight	Baseline and serial measurements for assessment of growth, nutritional status, and pubertal development	Poor growth and delayed puberty relating to the severity of disease	Failure to grow in the absence of clinically active disease	CINCA Skeletal dysplasias Other causes of failure to thrive
Full blood count and differential and Acute phase response (ESR and CRP)	To document the extent of disease activity in conjunction with clinical history and examination For drug monitoring Acute phase response assists in determining response to treatment and disease activity	Anaemia of chronic disease proportional to the associated raised acute phase response Normal or mildly raised WBC and platelet counts Elevated acute phase response	Isolated lymphopaenia, leukopenia, thrombocytopenia, ESR raised in face of a normal CRP Pancytopenia, or a low or low normal neutrophil, lymphocyte or platelet count in the face of a high acute phase response	Connective tissue diseases particularly SLE Malignancy, particularly leukaemia
Plain radiographs	The early appearance of radiographic erosions is associated with a poor prognosis, and serial radiographs are valuable in documenting progressive disease damage	Radiographs may only show soft-tissue changes initially Early erosive change and loss of joint space are associated with a poor prognosis	Metaphyseal lucencies and lytic metastatic lesions with pathological fractures may be seen in leukaemia and metastatic neuroblastoma Suspicion of skeletal dysplasia warrants a selective skeletal survey interpreted by a radiologist with particular expertise Note: Radiographs may be misleading in determining bone age because arthritis of the wrist leads to accelerated bone maturation	Skeletal dysplasia Malignancy
Liver function (transaminases, albumin, and total protein), and	Baseline and serial levels valuable for disease and drug monitoring	Normal	Hypoalbuminaemia, persistent anaemia, ± acute phase response out of proportion to clinical findings	Occult inflammatory bowel disease with associated arthritis
Renal function (urea, creatinine, urinalysis and BP)	Renal function monitoring for patients on methotrexate. A number of drugs may cause liver of kidney dysfunction		Haematuria, proteinuria, deranged liver transaminases, a high total protein, or impaired renal function Hypoproteinaemia	SLE Agammaglobulinaemia, or isolated Ig deficiency

Table 2.4.5 summarizes useful investigations, their indications, role in monitoring and pointers to other diagnoses.

Rheumatoid factor

The importance of RF in identifying a subgroup of children with arthritis and a poor outcome has been recognized for more than 30 years [32–34]. However, it is important to be aware of the limitations of the lack of specificity and sensitivity of this test.

Rheumatoid factors are a subset of antiglobulin antibodies directed against the Fc region of IgG. Historically, the presence of IgM antibody has been most commonly reported, measured by agglutination methods which use latex fixation uses particles coated with IgG and agglutinated by IgM RF. The titre represents the highest dilution visibly associated with agglutination. A titre of 1 : 80 is usually considered positive. Other methods for measurement of RF are listed in Table 2.4.6, but the use of enzyme linked immunosorbent assays (ELISA) is becoming increasingly common.

The importance of RF in the definition of arthritis is not as a diagnostic test, but as an aid to classification once a diagnosis of arthritis is made on clinical assessment. For example, a common referral to the paediatric rheumatologist is the child with musculoskeletal pain who is RF positive, but who is not found to have arthritis. This patient would not have RF Positive Polyarthritis, because arthritis should be diagnosed on the basis of clinical features, particularly persistent joint swelling, not simply on the basis of a positive RF.

The majority of people with increased RF are asymptomatic and healthy, and the production of RF may be a part of normal immune responses. An increased concentration of RF can be found in a variety of conditions, which cause B-cell hyperactivity, including infections, other autoimmune diseases, B-cell lymphoproliferative disorders, and following immunization. The incidence of RF in the healthy population is around 1%, and rises with age in the healthy population, as well as in RF Positive Polyarthritis and RA. In the few studies performed, low-titre RF is found in 0.5–4% of healthy children [35–38] and higher proportions of teenagers [37].

The predictive value of a positive RF for developing RA is poor. Even when using a combination of different RF isotypes, which are more specific for RA than IgM alone [39,40], the specificity remains low. In subjects with two or three isotypes persistently raised over 13 years, only 14% (two isotypes) and 40% (three isotypes) developed RA.

Seventy-five to eighty per cent of adults with RA are positive for RF using the older Latex fixation method. The ELISA is more sensitive [41] and increased specificity can be obtained by looking at the titre [42]. In patients with RA who have the most severe disease, have late onset polyarthritis and are predominantly female, RF can be found in 90% of cases [43], and the titre is highest in this group. Higher titres

Table 2.4.6 Different ways to measure RF

Agglutination
Latex fixation test
Sensitized sheep cell agglutination assay
RAHA or Rose–Waaler
Radioimmunoassay
Indirect immunofluorescence
ELISA
Laser nephelometry

of RF identify a similar subgroup of JIA with a worse prognosis. Significant titres of RF also infrequently occur in children with atypical Oligoarthritis and Systemic Arthritis [43], independent of HLA DR4 status and associated with erosive disease [29]. (See Part 2, Chapter 2.8.)

HLA DR4

HLA DR4 has long been associated with adult RA [44]. RF Positive Polyarthritis is strongly associated with HLA DR4, and its subtype DRB*0401 and Dw4 [45], identifying older onset, polyarticular disease [46–48]. Sixty per cent of RF positive children had HLA DR4, versus 29% of children without RF, the same level of HLA DR4 as the Caucasian population [49].

Monitoring

Arthritis

Good disease control is the primary aim of management. The key to monitoring disease control is by regular, meticulous clinical assessment. The presence of active joint inflammation, muscle wasting, progressive joint damage, local growth abnormalities, and loss of joint function needs to be carefully monitored and acted upon. Chronic inflammation has many general effects on growth, nutrition, energy levels, early morning stiffness, and gelling, and these can be used as additional indicators of poor disease control. Investigations identifying persistent inflammation include a raised acute phase response, the anaemia of chronic disease, persistent thrombocytosis, leucocytosis, and a low albumin.

Chronic active disease is associated with the development of many complications and poor prognostic indicators such as osteoporosis, poor growth, erosions, poor functional outcome, and the need for joint replacement. The longer term risks associated with chronic inflammation such as infection, premature cardiovascular disease, and malignancy are becoming more apparent in RA.

Children with RF Positive Polyarthritis are usually on disease modifying anti-rheumatic drugs (DMARDs) such as methotrexate early, and so should have blood tests (blood counts, liver function tests) on a regular basis (usually monthly) for safety monitoring. This is an opportunity to also monitor the acute phase response and other markers of disease activity.

Aggressive disease is associated with the early development of erosions. Serial radiographs may be helpful, but magnetic resonance imaging (MRI) may have a role in identifying erosions before they become apparent on plain radiographs. In a child with poorly controlled disease, 6–12 monthly radiographs may demonstrate progressive erosive damage, but these are required much less often where there is good disease control.

Growth, development, and nutritional status

The monitoring of growth and pubertal development should be fundamental to the care of RF Positive Polyarthritis. Measurement of height, weight, and identification of local growth abnormalities should be a fundamental part of each clinical assessment. Those children with persistently active disease or significant corticosteroids should also be offered regular assessment of bone quality with DEXA scans. There is a paucity of normal paediatric values, and interpretation is complicated by abnormal growth. A baseline scan at presentation, followed by serial scans at 6–24-month intervals, depending on severity, can be very valuable in assessing the rate of accrual of bone quality. Children with polyarticular disease and poor disease control often have associated poor nutritional status despite an increased intake of protein and energy [50].

Psychosocial development

The impact of developing JIA during adolescence on psychosocial development is considerable, and has long-term consequences. It interferes with the normal adolescent development of coping strategies, and anxious and helpless responses are more common in patients whose disease starts during adolescence [51,52]. Awareness and support for these problems on an ongoing basis is important.

Complications
Eye involvement

Uveitis is rare in RF Positive Polyarthritis [53] as it is in RA, and may be associated with vasculitis [54]. In RA, keratoconjunctivitis sicca is the most common ocular feature, occurring in 10–35% of cases, and may be associated with secondary Sjögren syndrome. These are both probably under-recognized in children [7,55]. Episcleritis is less common in RA, but is a more severe complication, correlating with RA activity, causing a red and painful eye, but is unlikely to alter visual acuity. Scleritis is a severe and rare complication of vasculitis in RA. The lack of reports of these features in the JIA literature suggests they are not recognized in children.

Reticuloendothelial system involvement

Felty syndrome (consisting of the triad of RA, splenomegaly, and leukopenia) can be a complication of longstanding, erosive RA, and is associated with an increased risk of infection. It is described in JIA [56–60].

Vasculitis

Although well-described in adult RA, there exist only a few case reports of vasculitis in JIA, and those cases were associated with drugs [61], other types of JIA than RF Positive Polyarthritis, and cerebral involvement [62,63].

Other complications

Atlanto-axial subluxation is critical to recognize in RF Positive Polyarthritis. Neuromuscular complications of RA such as peripheral entrapment syndromes like carpal tunnel syndrome, are not well recognized in children with RF Positive Polyarthritis but do occur. Low-grade pericardial or pleural effusions are rarely reported. Asymptomatic and low-grade impaired lung function can be associated with active disease, but progressive fibrosis and methotrexate-related lung fibrosis has not been reported in children as it is in RA [64,65]. Aortic valve involvement has infrequently been reported in RF Positive Polyarthritis [66,67], but pericarditis, myocarditis, and valvulitis are more common in adult RA and Systemic Arthritis. Lymphoedema may occur in all types of JIA and RA but is not particularly increased in RF Positive Polyarthritis [68].

Prognosis
Functional outcome

RF Positive Polyarthritis has a poor long-term prognosis compared to other categories of JIA. When the prognostic indicators for JIA are identified, it is clear why the outlook of RF positive disease is uniformly poor. Female sex, polyarticular disease, ongoing disease activity, and a positive IgM RF are all identified as poor prognostic indicators in terms of functional outcome (Steinbrocker and CHAQ), and risk of joint surgery [69]. These patients have many involved joints, and disability relates to the extent of arthritis. Hand and wrist involvement, erosions, nodules, an unremitting disease course, or unremitting inflammatory response are all associated with a poor prognosis. Arthritis persisting for 7 or more years is unlikely to go into remission. In a cohort of 392 patients with JRA, only 6% of RF Positive Polyarthritis achieved remission at 10 years, a dramatically poorer rate than other JRA subgroups [70]. In patients with all forms of polyarticular arthritis, 47% had active disease at 26-year follow-up, but 70% of those who were RF positive still had active, erosive disease [71] and were more likely to have had major arthritis-related surgery, a poorer Steinbrocker functional class which had continued to fall with time and to have had systemic steroids. This group also reported the highest incidence of joint replacement, particularly hip replacement, occurring after the shortest disease duration, and continuing need for arthroplasty thereafter, and the highest ongoing disease activity and requirement for ongoing DMARDs [52].

Osteoporosis

The risk of osteoporosis and related fractures is dependent on achieving peak bone mass. The 2–3 years of accelerated growth at puberty are critical in achieving this. Bone mass increases at the fastest rate, 8% a year, during puberty, and although final bone mass is not achieved until the third decade, it may not be repaired through 'catch-up' mineralization [72]. For young people with JIA, failure to achieve the expected pubertal increase in bone mass [73], and the subsequently increased risk of fractures later in life [74] is influenced by the degree and persistence of inflammation, lack of mobility, low body mass, poor intake of calcium and acquisition of vitamin D, delay in the onset of puberty [75], and medication, especially glucocorticoids.

Puberty and fertility

For a disease presenting in young adolescent women, it is important to remember the impact of RF Positive Polyarthritis on emergent sexuality, puberty, and fertility. These teenagers need advice about delayed puberty, which is most pronounced in girls with polyarticular disease, contraception, planned pregnancy, which may not be far in the future, and the need for monitoring. RF Positive Polyarthritis may have an impact on pregnancy and motherhood because of ongoing disease activity or end-organ damage. Young women with RF Positive Polyarthritis are particularly at risk because of ongoing disease activity, high frequency of arthroplasty and the significant impact on adolescence and growth [76,77]. Drug effects on female and male reproduction are important in this group of patients, and they should be offered good advice on contraception and good reproductive care [78].

Mortality

There are few studies, but those that exist suggest that the mortality for JIA is falling, and remains low or nil in most studies [79–81]. Polyarthritis is over represented in these groups but the association with RF is not known [82]. Children with polyarthritis are at increased risk of mortality from cardiac involvement, infections, and rarely amyloidosis (although this is more common in Systemic Arthritis). Even though the decline in the incidence of amyloid has been associated with a fall in the mortality rate [83], it is still nearly four times higher than the death rate in the general population at this age. In adults with JIA, mortality is associated with other autoimmune disease [84].

Key point summary

• RF Positive Polyarthritis is an idiopathic polyarthritis starting before the 16th birthday associated with a persistently raised RF.

• Girls are approximately nine times as likely to develop RF Positive Polyarthritis as boys and the incidence of RF positive polyarthritis rises with age.

• RF Positive Polyarthritis is a symmetrical large- and small-joint arthritis typically involving the wrist, MCP, and PIP joints, and is associated with rheumatoid nodules.

• RF antibodies are antiglobulin antibodies which can be found in normal healthy children, and in other conditions besides RA and RF Positive Polyarthritis.

• RF Positive Polyarthritis has a poor prognosis, with an aggressive, unremitting disease course, early erosive disease, a poor functional outcome, and a high incidence of joint replacement.

References

1. Petty, R.E., Southwood, T.R., Manners, P., et al. International League of Associations for Rheumatology classification of juvenile idiopathic arthritis: second revision, Edmonton, 2001. J Rheumatol 2004;31:390–2.

2. Arnett, F.C., Edworthy, S.M., and Bloch, D.A. et al. The American Rheumatism Association revised criteria for the classification of rheumatoid arthritis. Arthritis Rheum 1988;31(3):315–24.

3. Thomas, E., Barrett, J.H., Donn, R.P., Thomson, W., and Southwood, T.R. Subtyping of juvenile idiopathic arthritis using latent class analysis. British Paediatric Rheumatology Group. Arthritis Rheum 2000;43(7):1496–503.

4. Cassidy, J.T., Levinson, J.E., Bass, J.C., et al. A study of classification criteria for a diagnosis of JRA. Arthritis Rheum 1986;29(2):274–81.

5. European League Against Rheumatism. Nomenclature and Classification of Arthritis in Children. Basel, National Zeitung 1977; Bulletin 4.

6. Cassidy, J. and Petty, R. Textbook of Pediatric Rheumatology, 3rd edn. Philadelphia, PA: W.B. Saunders, 1995.

7. Fink, C.W., Fernandez-Vina, M., and Stastny, P. Clinical and genetic evidence that juvenile arthritis is not a single disease. Pediatr Clin N Am 1995;42(5):1155–69.

8. Kaipiainen-Seppanen, O. and Savolainen, A. Incidence of chronic juvenile rheumatic diseases in Finland during 1980–1990. Clin Exp Rheumatol 1996;14:441–4.

9. Gare, A.B. and Fasth, A. Epidemiology of juvenile chronic arthritis in southwestern Sweden: a 5-year prospective population study. Pediatrics 1992;90(6):950–8.

10. Symmons, D.P., Barrett, E.M., Bankhead, C.R., Scott, D.G., and Silman, A.J. The incidence of rheumatoid arthritis in the United Kingdom: results from the Norfolk Arthritis Register. Br J Rheumatol 1994;33(8):735–9.

11. Bowyer, S. and Roettcher, P. Pediatric rheumatology clinic populations in the United States: results of a 3 year survey. J Rheumatol 1996;23(11):1968–74.

12. Denardo, B.A., Tucker, L.B., Miller, L.C., Szer, I.S., and Schaller, J.G. Demography of a regional pediatric rheumatology patient population. J Rheumatol 1994;21:1553–61.

13. Oen, K. and Cheang, M. Epidemiology of chronic arthritis in childhood. Semin Arthritis Rheum 1996;26(3):575–91.

14. Peschken, C.A. and Esdaile, J.M. Rheumatic diseases in North America's indigenous peoples. Semin Arthritis Rheum 1999;28(6):368–91.

15. Oen, K., Schroeder, M., Jacobson, K., Anderson, S., Wood, S., Cheang, M., et al. Juvenile rheumatoid arthritis in a Canadian First Nations (aboriginal) population: onset subtypes and HLA associations. J Rheumatol 1998;25(4):783–90.

16. Oen, K. Comparative epidemiology of the rheumatic diseases in children. Curr Opin Rheumatol 2000;12(5):410–14.

17. Rosenberg, A.M., Petty, R., Oen, K., and Schroeder, M. Rheumatic diseases in western Canadian children. J Rheumatol 1982;9(4):589–92.

18. Oen, K., Fast, M., and Postl, B. Epidemiology of juvenile rheumatoid arthritis in Manitoba, Canada, 1975–92: cycles in incidence. J Rheumatol 1995;22(4):745–50.

19. Schwartz, M.M., Simpson, P., Kerr, K.L., and Jarvis, J.N. Juvenile rheumatoid arthritis in African Americans. J Rheumatol 1997;24(9):1826–9.

20. Pagan, T.M. and Arroyo, I.L. Juvenile rheumatoid arthritis in Caribbean children: a clinical characterization. Bol Asoc Med P R 1991;83(12):527–9.

21. Haffejee, I.E., Raga, J., and Coovadia, H.M. Juvenile chronic arthritis in black and Indian South African children. S Afr Med J 1984;65(13):510–14.

22. Arguedas, O., Fasth, A., Andersson-Gare, B., and Porras, O. Juvenile chronic arthritis in urban San Jose, Costa Rica: a 2 year prospective study. J Rheumatol 1998;25(9):1844–50.

23. Gare, A.B. Juvenile arthritis—who gets it, where and when? A review of current data on incidence and prevalence. Clin Exp Rheumatol 1999;17:367–74.

24. Khuffash, F.A. and Majeed, H.A. Juvenile rheumatoid arthritis among Arab children. Scand J Rheumatol 1988;17(5):393–5.

25. Aggarwal, A. and Misra, R. Juvenile chronic arthritis in India: is it different from that seen in Western countries? Rheum Int 1994;14(2):53–6.

26. Rittner, C., Zaschke, S., Berghoff, E., Mollenhauer, E., Opferkuch, W., and Baur, M.P. Comparative studies of human C4 phenotypes, their population genetics, and association with HLA-B antigens. Immunobiology 1980;158(1–2):119–28.

27. Naidu, S., Ostrov, B.E., and Pellegrini, V.D. Small hand joint involvement in juvenile rheumatoid arthritis. J Pediatr 2000;136(1):134–5.

28. Al Matar, M.J., Petty, R.E., Tucker, L.B., Malleson, P.N., Schroeder, M.L., and Cabral, D.A. The early pattern of joint involvement predicts disease progression in children with oligoarticular (pauciarticular) juvenile rheumatoid arthritis. Arthritis Rheum 2002;46(10):2708–15.

29. Sailer, M., Cabral, D.A., Petty, R.E., and Malleson, P.N. Rheumatoid factor positive, oligoarticular onset juvenile rheumatoid arthritis. J Rheumatol 1997;24(3):586–8.

30. Veys, E.M. and De Keyser, F. Rheumatoid nodules: differential diagnosis and immunohistological findings. Ann Rheum Dis 1993;52(9):625–6.

31. Muzaffer, M.A., Schneider, R., Cameron, B.J., Silverman, E.D., and Laxer, R.M. Accelerated nodulosis during methotrexate therapy for juvenile rheumatoid arthritis. J Pediatr 1996;128(5 Pt 1):698–700.

32. Ansell, B.M., Holborow, J., Zutshi, D., Reading, A., and Epstein, W.V. Comparison of three serological tests in adult rheumatoid arthritis and Still's disease (juvenile rheumatoid arthritis). Ann N Y Acad Sci 1969;168(1):21–9.

33. Cassidy, J.T. and Valkenberg, H.A. A five year prospective study of rheumatoid factor tests in juvenile rheumatoid arthritis. Arthritis Rheum 1967;10(2):83–90.

34. Hanson, V., Drexler, E., and Kornreich, H. The relationship of rheumatoid factor to age of onset in juvenile rheumatoid arthritis. *Arthritis Rheum* 1969;12(2):82–6.

35. Kasapcopur, O., Ozbakir, F., Arisoy, N., Ingol, H., Yazici, H., and Ozdogan, H. Frequency of antinuclear antibodies and rheumatoid factor in healthy Turkish children. *Turkish J Pediatr* 1999;41(1):67–71.

36. Goel, K.M., Shanks, R.A., Whaley, K., Mason, M., and MacSween, R.N. Autoantibodies in childhood connective tissue diseases and in normal children. *Arch Dis Child* 1975;50(6):419–23.

37. Martini, A., Lorini, R., Zanaboni, D., Ravelli, A., and Burgio, R.G. Frequency of autoantibodies in normal children. *Am J Dis Child* 1989;143(4):493–6.

38. Kanakoudi-Tsakalidou, F., Tzimouli, V., Kapsahili, O., Dadalian, M., and Pardalos, G. Detection of rheumatoid factor and antinuclear antibodies in 1500 healthy and 625 hospitalized children. *Clin Exp Rheumatol* 1995;13:557.

39. Mannik, M. and Nardella, F.A. IgG rheumatoid factors and self-association of these antibodies. *Clin Rheum Dis* 1985;11(3):551–72.

40. Jonsson, T., Thorsteinsson, J., and Valdimarsson, H. Elevation of only one rheumatoid factor isotype is not associated with increased prevalence of rheumatoid arthritis—a population based study. *Scand J Rheumatol* 2000; 29(3):190–1.

41. Aggarwal, A., Dabadghao, S., Naik, S., and Misra, R. Serum IgM rheumatoid factor by enzyme-linked immunosorbent assay (ELISA) delineates a subset of patients with deforming joint disease in seronegative juvenile rheumatoid arthritis. *Rheumatol Int* 1994;14(4):135–8.

42. Lawrence, J.M., III, Moore, T.L., Osborn, T.G., Nesher, G., Madson, K.L., and Kinsella, M.B. Autoantibody studies in juvenile rheumatoid arthritis. *Semin Arthritis Rheum* 1993;22(4):265–74.

43. Walker, S.M., Shaham, B., McCrudy, D.K., Wietting, H., Arora, Y.K., Hanson, V., and Bernstein, B. Prevalence and concentration of IgM rheumatoid factor in polyarticular onset disease as compared to systemic or pauciarticular onset disease in active juvenile rheumatoid arthritis as measured by ELISA. *J Rheumatol* 1990;17(7):936–40.

44. Stastny, P. Association of the B-cell alloantigen DRw4 with rheumatoid arthritis. *New Engl J Med* 1978;298(869):871.

45. Stastny, P. and Fink, C.W. Different HLA-D associations in adult and juvenile rheumatoid arthritis. *J Clin Invest* 1979;63(1):124–30.

46. Nepom, G.T., Mickelson, E., Schaller, J.G., Antonell, P., and Hansen, J.A. Specific HLA-DR4-associated histocompatibility molecules characterize patients with seropositive juvenile rheumatoid arthritis. *J Clin Invest* 1984;74(1):287–91.

47. Glass, D.N. and Giannini, E.H. Juvenile rheumatoid arthritis as a complex genetic trait. *Arthritis Rheum* 1999;42(11):2261–8.

48. Murray, K.J., Moroldo, M.B., Donnelly, P., Prahalad, S., Passo, M.H., Giannini, E.H., *et al*. Age-specific effects of juvenile rheumatoid arthritis-associated HLA alleles. *Arthritis Rheum* 1999;42(9):1843–53.

49. Clemens, L.E., Albert, E., and Ansell, B.M. HLA studies in IgM rheumatoid-factor-positive arthritis of childhood. *Ann Rheum Dis* 1983;42(4):431–4.

50. Haugen, M.A., Hoyeraal, H.M., Larsen, S., Gilboe, I.M., and Trygg, K. Nutrient intake and nutritional status in children with juvenile chronic arthritis. *Scand J Rheumatol* 1992;21(4):165–70.

51. Aasland, A., Flato, B., and Vandvik, I.H. Psychosocial outcome in juvenile chronic arthritis: a nine-year follow-up. *Clin Exp Rheumatol* 1997;15(5):561–8.

52. David, J., Cooper, C., Hickey, L., Dore, C., McCullough, C., and Woo, P. The functional and psychological outcomes of juvenile chronic arthritis in young adulthood. *Br J Rheumatol* 1994;33(9):876–81.

53. Petty, R.E., Smith, J.R., and Rosenbaum, J.T. Arthritis and uveitis in children. A pediatric rheumatology perspective. *Am J Ophthalmol* 2003;135(6):879–84.

54. Klippel, J.H. and Dieppe, P.A. Rheumatology, 2nd edn. London: Mosby, 1998.

55. Jain, V., Singh, S., and Sharma, A. Keratonconjunctivitis sicca is not uncommon in children with juvenile rheumatoid arthritis. *Rheumatol Int* 2001;20(4):159–62.

56. Bloom, B.J., Smith, P., and Alario, A.J. Felty syndrome complicating juvenile rheumatoid arthritis. *J Pediatr Hematol Oncol* 1998;20(5):511–13.

57. Toomey, K. and Hepburn, B. Felty syndrome in juvenile arthritis. *J Pediatr* 1985;106(2):254–5.

58. Rosenberg, A.M., Mitchell, D.M., and Card, R.T. Felty's syndrome in a child. *J Rheumatol* 1984;11(6):835–7.

59. Sienknecht, C.W., Urowitz, M.B., Pruzanski, W., and Stein, H.B. Felty's syndrome. Clinical and serological analysis of 34 cases. *Ann Rheum Dis* 1977;36(6):500–7.

60. Laszlo, J., Jones, R., Silberman, H.R., and Banks, P.M. Splenectomy for Felty's syndrome. Clinicopathological study of 27 patients. *Arch Intern Med* 1978;138(4):597–602.

61. Bresnihan, F.P. and Ansell, B.M. Effect of penicillamine treatment on immune complexes in two cases of seropositive juvenile rheumatoid arthritis. *Ann Rheum Dis* 1975;35(5):463–5.

62. Pedersen, R.C. and Person, D.A. Cerebral vasculitis in an adolescent with juvenile rheumatoid arthritis. *Pediatr Neurol* 1998;19(1):69–73.

63. Sievers, K., Nissila, M., and Sievers, U.-M. Cerebral vasculitis visualized by angiography in juvenile rheumatoid arthritis simulating brain tumor. *Acta Rheum Scand* 1968;14:222–32.

64. Pelucchi, A., Lomater, C., Gerloni, V., Foresi, A., Fantini, F., and Marazzini, L. Lung function and diffusing capacity for carbon monoxide in patients with juvenile chronic arthritis: effect of disease activity and low dose methotrexate therapy. *Clin Exp Rheumatol* 1994;12(6):675–9.

65. Graham, L.D., Myones, B.L., Rivas-Chacon, R.F., and Pachman, L.M. Morbidity associated with long-term methotrexate therapy in juvenile rheumatoid arthritis. *J Pediatr* 1992;120(3):468–73.

66. Delgado, E.A., Petty, R.E., Malleson, P.N., Patterson, M.W., D'Orsogna, L., and LeBlanc, J. Aortic valve insufficiency and coronary artery narrowing in a child with polyarticular juvenile rheumatoid arthritis. *J Rheumatol* 1988;15(1):144–7.

67. Leak, A.M., Millar-Craig, M.W., and Ansell, B.M. Aortic regurgitation in seropositive juvenile arthritis. *Ann Rheum Dis* 1981;40(3):229–34.

68. Bardare, M., Falcini, F., Hertzberger-ten Cate, R., Savolainen, A., and Cimaz, R. Idiopathic limb edema in children with chronic arthritis: a multicenter report of 12 cases. *J Rheumatol* 1997;24(2):384–8.

69. Gare, B.A. and Fasth, A. The natural history of juvenile chronic arthritis: a population based cohort study. II. Outcome. *J Rheumatol* 1995;22(2):308–19.

70. Oen, K., Malleson, P.N., Cabral, D.A., Rosenberg, A.M., Petty, R.E., and Cheang, M. Disease course and outcome of juvenile rheumatoid arthritis in a multicenter cohort. *J Rheumatol* 2002;29(9):1989–99.

71. Zak, M. and Pedersen, F.K. Juvenile chronic arthritis into adulthood: a long-term follow-up study. *Rheumatology* (Oxford) 2000;39(2):198–204.

72. Cassidy, J.T. and Hillman, L.S. Abnormalities in skeletal growth in children with juvenile rheumatoid arthritis. *Rheum Dis Clin N Am* 1997;23(3):499–522.

73. Hopp, R., Degan, J., Gallagher, J.C., and Cassidy, J.T. Estimation of bone mineral density in children with juvenile rheumatoid arthritis. *J Rheumatol* 1991;18(8):1235–9.

74. Riggs, B.L., Nguyen, T.V., Melton, L.J. III, Morrison, N.A., O'Fallon, W.M., Kelly, P.J., *et al*. The contribution of vitamin D receptor gene alleles to the determination of bone mineral density in normal and osteoporotic women. *J Bone Miner Res* 1995;10(6):991–6.

75. Fraser, P.A., Hoch, S., Erlandson, D., Partridge, R., and Jackson, J.M. The timing of menarche in juvenile rheumatoid arthritis. *J Adolesc Health Care* 1988;9(6):483–7.

76. Ostensen, M. Pregnancy in patients with a history of juvenile rheumatoid arthritis. *Arthritis Rheum* 1991;34(7):881–7.

77. Ostensen, M. The effect of pregnancy on ankylosing spondylitis, psoriatic arthritis, and juvenile rheumatoid arthritis. *Am J Reprod Immunol* 1992;28(3–4):235–7.

78. Janssen, N.M. and Genta, M.S. The effects of immunosuppressive and anti-inflammatory medications on fertility, pregnancy, and lactation. *Arch Intern Med* 2000;160(5):610–19.

79. Baum, J. and Gutowaska, G. Death in JRA. *Arthritis Rheum* 1977;20 (Suppl.):253–5.

80. Rennebohm, R. and Correll, J.K. Comprehensive management of juvenile rheumatoid arthritis. *Nurs Clin N Am* 1984;19(4):647–62.

81. Petty, R.E. Prognosis in children with rheumatic diseases: justification for consideration of new therapies. *Rheumatology* (Oxford) 1999;38(8):739–42.

82. De Inocencio, J., and Lovell, D.J. Clinical and functional monitoring; outcome measures and prognosis of JRA. *Bailliere's Clin Paediatrics* 1993;1:769–801.

83. Wallace, C.A. and Levinson, J.E. Juvenile rheumatoid arthritis: outcome and treatment for the 1990s. *Rheum Dis Clin N Am* 1991;17(4):891–905.

84. French, A.R., Mason, T., Nelson, A.M., O'Fallon, W.M., and Gabriel, S.E. Increased mortality in adults with a history of juvenile rheumatoid arthritis: a population-based study. *Arthritis Rheum* 2001;44(3): 523–7.

85. Mellbye, O.J., Forre, O., Mollnes, T.E., and Kvarnes, L. Immunopathology of subcutaneous rheumatoid nodules. *Ann Rheum Dis* 1991;50(12):909–12.

86. Burry, H.C., Caughey, D.E., and Palmer, D.G. Benign rheumatoid nodules. *Aust N Z J Med* 1979;9(6):697–701.

87. Falcini, F., Taccetti, G., Ermini, M., Trapani, S., Calzolari, A., Franchi, A., *et al.* Methotrexate-associated appearance and rapid progression of rheumatoid nodules in systemic-onset juvenile rheumatoid arthritis. *Arthritis Rheum* 1997;40(1):175–8.

2.5   Rheumatoid Factor Negative Polyarthritis

Alberto Martini

Aims

The aim of this chapter is to discuss the clinical characteristics, epidemiology, and HLA associations in Rheumatoid Factor (RF) Negative Polyarthritis. The heterogeneity of this category of Juvenile Idiopathic Arthritis (JIA), as well as similarities between a clinical sub-group of RF-Negative Polyarthritis and Oligoarthritis (both Persistent and Extended) will be emphasized.

Structure

- Introduction and classification
- Epidemiology
- HLA associations
- Clinical features
- Investigations
- Monitoring
- Complications
- Prognosis
- Conclusions
- Key summary points

Introduction and classification

According to the revised International League of Associations for Rheumatology (ILAR) classification criteria [1] (Table 2.5.1), Rheumatoid Factor (RF) Negative Polyarthritis is defined as any form of arthritis which meets criteria for Juvenile Idiopathic Arthritis (JIA) (unknown origin, onset before the 16th birthday, at least 6 week duration), lacks circulating RF, and affects five or more joints during the first 6 months of disease. It is the least defined and possibly the most heterogeneous form of JIA. Patients who meet the criteria for the diagnosis of Systemic Arthritis, RF Positive Polyarthritis, Psoriatic Arthritis, and Enthesitis Related Arthritis are excluded.

The criterion of the number of joints involved with arthritis has been useful to broadly separate those forms of arthritis which tend to affect few large joints (usually in an asymmetrical pattern) from arthritis that tends to affect many small as well as large joints (often in a symmetrical pattern). Although this is useful from a practical point of view, there is nothing magical about the number of five joints. It is therefore conceivable that a patient who presents with four

Table 2.5.1 ILAR revised classification criteria for RF Negative Polyarthritis

Definition
> Arthritis affecting five or more joints during the first 6 months of disease
> A test for RF is negative

Exclusions
> Psoriasis or a history of psoriasis in the patient or first degree relative
> Arthritis in an HLA-B27 positive male beginning after the 6th birthday
> Ankylosing spondylitis, enthesitis related arthritis, sacroiliitis with inflammatory bowel disease, Reiter syndrome, or acute anterior uveitis, or a history of one of these disorders in a first degree relative
> The presence of IgM rheumatoid factor on at least two occasions at least 3 months apart
> The presence of Systemic Arthritis in the patient

or fewer joints initially but develops one or more joints within the first 6 months would be categorized as having RF-Negative Polyarthritis, whereas an identical patient who presents with four or fewer joints initially but then develops arthritis in one or more joints after the first 6 months would be categorized as having Extended Oligoarthritis. Moreover, in addition to being a useful instrument to separate broad categories of arthritis, the number of joints involved may also represent a marker of severity for certain categories of JIA [2]. Lastly, using the number of joints involved to classify various types of JIA runs the risk of misclassifying patients because the experience and skill of the clinician in diagnosing an arthritic joint is variable. This is particularly true in a disease such as JIA, in which pain may not be prominent, as well as when joint involvement is asymmetrical, or when single small joints in the hands or the feet are affected, which can be easily missed. Clinical evaluation of joints, even among experienced paediatric rheumatologists, has indeed been shown to be quite subjective and variable, with low inter-observer agreement [3].

Epidemiology

Prevalence and incidence

Quite consistently, in reports from Europe and the United States, about one quarter of all patients with JIA have polyarticular disease at onset, and the vast majority of them belong to the RF negative subgroup [4]. In the British Paediatric Rheumatology National

Diagnostic Register, RF-negative polyarticular disease accounted for 17% of patients [5]. In a population based cohort study in Sweden, 29% of patients had polyarticular juvenile chronic arthritis (JCA) that was RF-negative [6], while RF negative polyarticular juvenile rheumatoid arthritis (JRA) represented 32% of all JRA patients in a 3-year survey made in 73 US paediatric rheumatology centres [7]. A study of long-term surveillance of a fixed population [8] showed a decline in the incidence of both pauciarticular and systemic JRA with no change in polyarticular JRA; however, the observed decline in some subtypes may reflect improved diagnosis and recognition of other diseases that may have been misclassified previously as JRA (such as Lyme arthritis) rather than a true decreasing incidence.

Age and sex distribution

The mean age at onset of RF-negative polyarticular JCA was 6.5 years in the British Paediatric Rheumatology National Diagnostic Register (311 patients) [5] and 6.9 in the 3-year survey in the United States (666 patients) [7]. Although RF Negative Polyarthritis is found at all ages, two peaks are usually observed, one during the toddler to pre-school age group and the other in the preadolescent age group [9] with about half of patients having disease onset before 5 years of age [10,11,12]. RF negative polyarticular JCA is more common in girls with a female to male ratio of about 3 : 1 [5,7,8].

Ethnic differences

In Caucasians in Europe as well as in North America, Oligoarthritis is by far the most common form of JIA. In contrast, in other parts of the world (such as South Africa, India, and Thailand), as well as among African American and Canadian aboriginal populations, Polyarthritis appears to be the most frequent type [4,13,14]. These data often come from clinical series rather than from epidemiological studies and therefore may be influenced by selection bias toward the more severe cases. Another source of error could be the difficulty in distinguishing patients who have both a polyarticular onset and course (RF Negative Polyarthritis) from those who actually had an oligoarticular onset in the first 6 months of illness but a polyarticular course later on (Extended Oligoarthritis), if patients are not seen early enough in their disease course. In most of these studies, the higher incidence of polyarticular disease in these populations was due in large part to a higher proportion of RF Positive Polyarthritis. Again, the high frequency of RF Positive Polyarthritis may be affected by a selection bias toward more severe cases, but also could be due to genetic differences, such as in the Canadian First Nation (aboriginal) population [14] or to environmental factors such as polyclonal B-cell activation caused by frequent infections.

HLA associations

RF Negative Polyarthritis is probably the most heterogeneous type of JIA. Predictably, this clinical heterogeneity is paralleled by inconsistent results in HLA association studies. On the other hand, studies regarding incidence and disease concordance in affected sib pairs have shown the presence of a genetic component in RF Negative Polyarthritis, although this is probably less so than in Oligoarthritis [15,16].

Several groups [10,11,12,17] have reported an increase in DRB1*0801 (DRw8) in RF Negative Polyarthritis patients. DRB1*0801 is an allele that is also associated with early-onset Oligoarthritis.

Interestingly, an increase in DRw8 tended to also be associated with an early age at onset, ANA (antinuclear antibodies) positivity and the presence of uveitis in patients with Polyarthritis, suggesting that early onset, ANA positive, RF Negative Polyarthritis (see "Clinical Subtypes" below) is related to, or may be the same disease as, early onset Oligoarthritis, with the former representing disease with more rapid spread of arthritis.

In the early 1990s [11], an association was reported between RF-negative polyarticular JRA and DPB1.0301. This association, at variance with the association with DR8, was independent of age at onset and was observed mainly in ANA negative patients. Interestingly, the same group also reported an association between DPB1*0301 and sero (RF) negative rheumatoid arthritis in adults [18].

Clinical features

The onset of RF Negative Polyarthritis may be acute or insidious, with progressive joint involvement. Fever may be mild but is usually absent; persistent, high-spiking fever, as observed in Systemic Arthritis is by definition absent in RF Negative Polyarthritis. Hepatosplenomegaly, lymphadenopathy, and serositis are almost never observed. Arthritis may be symmetric or asymmetric and both large and small joints are often involved. Knees, ankles, wrists, elbows, cervical spine, the small joints of the hands and feet, shoulders, and the temporomandibular joints (TMJ) (Figures 2.5.1a and b may all be progressively affected. Involvement of the hips is not an early feature but often occurs later in patients with persistent disease. At least initially, proximal interphalangeal joints are affected more often than metacarpophalangeal joints (Figure 2.5.2). Tenosynovitis, in particular of the wrists, the ankle, and the flexor tendons of the hands is common (Figures 2.5.3 and 2.5.4). The majority of children show prolific synovitis but, as discussed later, a small subset of patients show little palpable synovial thickening (dry synovitis) (Figure 2.5.6.). The arthritis may not be painful, and therefore a careful general joint examination is always needed in particular in young children, where an apparent lack of joint tenderness or pain on motion is common. Subcutaneous nodules are much rarer than in the RF-Positive Polyarthritis, but may occur in the same usual sites. Chronic anterior uveitis is observed in RF Negative Polyarthritis, with a frequency ranging from 5 up to 20% [9,19,20], and as in Oligoarthritis, is strongly associated with early age at onset, female sex, and ANA positivity.

The heterogeneity of RF Negative Polyarthritis is also confirmed by a study by Thomas et al. [21], who used statistical techniques to identify underlying subtypes of JIA. Information on 572 patients with JIA was summarized by 10 clinical and laboratory categorical variables (age at onset, large joint involvement, small joint involvement, polyarthritis, symmetric arthritis, spinal pain, fever, psoriasis, ANA, and RF). Latent class analysis was used to identify seven underlying ("latent") classes that explained the relationships among the observed variables. When these seven latent classes were compared with the ILAR JIA classification, RF Negative Polyarthritis was the category which was most scattered among the different latent classes. Moreover, more than half of the patients who did not fit any of the latent classes had symmetric polyarthritis involving large and small joints, were ANA and RF negative, had no psoriasis or fever and were classified as RF Negative Polyarthritis by the ILAR criteria. Most of the remainder of the unclassifiable patients had Extended Oligoarthritis.

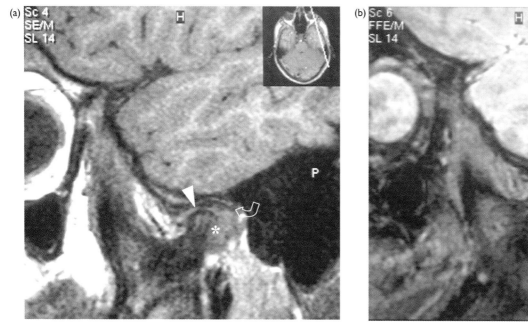

Fig. 2.5.1 MRI of TMJ in a patient with RF Negative Polyarthritis (a: sagittal T1 weighted b: sagittal T2 weighted). The sequence shows a widening of the articular space which is filled by the synovial pannus. White arrow: condyle; bent arrow: joint roof; asterisk: synovial pannus.

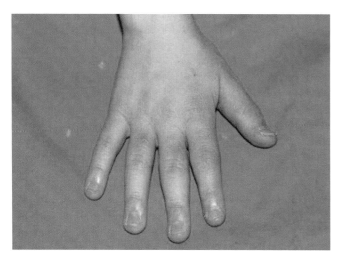

Fig. 2.5.2 The proximal interphalangeal (PIP) joints are often the first joints to become involved, as seen in these hands of a girl with RF Negative Polyarthritis.

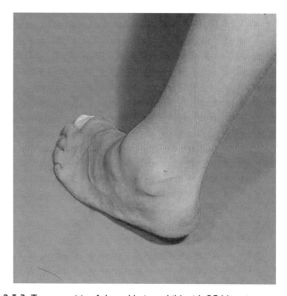

Fig. 2.5.3 Tenosynovitis of the ankle in a child with RF Negative Polyarthritis.

Clinical subgroups

On the basis of current information and according to at least one other author [22], there are at least three subgroups of RF Negative Polyarthritis that can be identified on clinical grounds (Table 2.5.2).

Early-onset, ANA positive polyarthritis

This subgroup, which affects about one-third of patients with RF Negative Polyarthritis, is characterized by the following features: an asymmetric onset arthritis affecting both large and small joints, onset before 6 years of age, ANA positivity, female predominance, and a high

Table 2.5.2 Clinical subgroups in RF Negative Polyarthritis

ANA positive polyarthritis
  Early onset (<6 years), high risk of anterior uveitis, marked female
  predominance, asymmetric arthritis

Prolific symmetric synovitis
  Later onset (7–9 years), symmetric arthritis, low risk of anterior uveitis

Dry synovitis
  Later onset (~7 years), little palpable synovitis, poor response to therapy

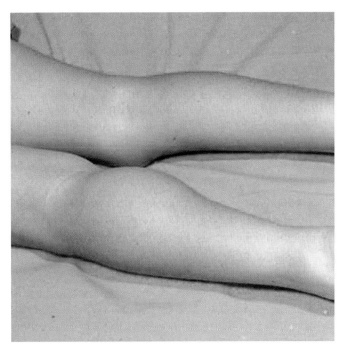

Fig. 2.5.4 A Baker cyst behind the left knee can be seen extending into the calf of a patient with RF Negative Polyarthritis.

risk of developing chronic anterior uveitis. It is in this group of patients that a higher prevalence of HLA-DRB1*0801 (DRw8) has been observed. These features are identical to those observed in the majority of patients with early onset Persistent and Extended Oligoarthritis. This strongly suggests that patients who share these common characteristics, although presently classified as having different types of JIA, may be affected by the same disease, differing only in extent and rapidity of joint involvement [2].

The hypothesis that early-onset ANA-positive RF Negative Polyarthritis and early-onset Oligoarthritis are the same disease is supported by studies on the frequency of the various types of JIA in different ethnic populations. Several studies [4] have indeed shown that early onset, ANA positive, uveitis-associated Oligoarthritis is rare in many countries, including Costa Rica, India, New Zealand and South Africa. In these same countries, RF Negative Polyarthritis is not usually seen in early childhood, is rarely ANA positive and is not associated with chronic anterior uveitis [13,23]. In other words, in those countries in which ANA positive, early onset, uveitis-associated Oligoarthritis is rare, ANA positive, early onset, uveitis-associated RF Negative Polyarthritis is also seldom observed.

In a recent study of 256 patients with ANA positive Oligoarthritis and Polyarthritis, ANA positivity appeared to be much more useful in detecting homogeneous disease categories than the number of joints involved [24]. The ANA-positive patients were comparable for age at disease presentation ($p = 0.11$), female/male ratio ($p = 0.98$), and frequency of symmetric arthritis ($p = 0.10$) and iridocyclitis ($p = 0.97$). The ANA-negative polyarticular cohort had older age at disease presentation ($p < 0.0001$), lower frequency of uveitis ($p = 0.02$), higher frequency of symmetric arthritis ($p = 0.0004$), greater cumulative number of joints affected over time ($p < 0.0001$ at 6, 12, and 24 months), and different pattern of joint disease when compared to the ANA-positive polyarticular patients. The strong

relationship between the presence of ANA and younger age at disease presentation, asymmetric arthritis, and development of uveitis was confirmed by multivariate regression analysis.

Prolific symmetric synovitis

The most classic form of RF Negative Polyarthritis has the following pattern: symmetrical joint involvement affecting large joints as well as the small joints of hands and feet, elevated ESR, negative ANA and age at onset at about 7–9 years (Figure 2.5.2). The relationship between this form of arthritis and the so-called RF- or seronegative rheumatoid arthritis that represents 25% of adults with rheumatoid arthritis is unknown, since no reliable markers exist for either condition. As previously mentioned, Fernandez [11] reported an association between RF negative polyarticular JRA and DPB1.0301; this association, at variance with the association with DR8, was independent from age at onset and was observed mainly in ANA negative patients. Interestingly, the same group also reported an association between DPB1*0301 and RF-negative adult rheumatoid arthritis [18].

Dry synovitis

Ansell [25] recognized a subgroup of patients with RF-Negative Polyarthritis who have little palpable synovial thickening but gradually develop joint contractures in a manner that later leads to marked loss of function (Figure 2.5.6). The children tend to be about 7 or 8 years of age at presentation. There is usually little pain in the affected joints. The disease often follows a destructive course and is poorly responsive to common treatments. The ESR in these patients is often normal or only modestly raised and the ANA is negative. This type of RF Negative Polyarthritis is uncommon, and the peculiarities of the clinical picture with respect to the other forms of JIA raises the

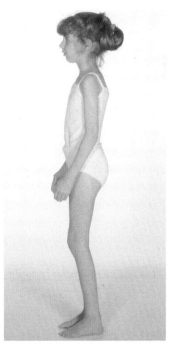

Fig. 2.5.5 A 7-year-old girl with RF Negative Polyarthritis displays the classic pattern of joint involvement, with symmetrical polyarthritis of both small and large joints, which have all developed flexion contractures. (Courtesy of T. R. Southwood)

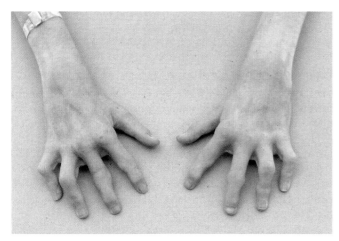

Fig. 2.5.6 The hand of a young patient with the "dry synovitis" clinical sub-type of RF Negative Polyarthritis. Every joint displays swelling, which was all bony, and there are multiple joint contractures. (Courtesy of T. R. Southwood)

suspicion that it might represent some as yet unknown, possibly genetic, disease. Because physical findings are either subtle or absent and the patients do not complain of pain or stiffness, the diagnosis is frequently delayed for years, further contributing to the poor outcome.

Investigations

The acute phase reactants (APR), such as the C-reactive protein (CRP) and ESR, are usually elevated in RF Negative Polyarthritis, although to a variable degree. In a population based cohort study of all types of JIA in Sweden, the correlation between ESR and disease activity was strongest in the polyarticular group, but almost 40% of the patients of this group classified as active or stable had ESR ≤ 10 [6]. Inflammatory anaemia, if present, is usually moderate and microcytosis is much rarer than in Systemic Arthritis. The rheumatoid factor is negative by definition. About 20–40% of patients are ANA positive [10,11,12, 26, 27], and ANA positivity is strongly associated with early age at onset. The specificity against the 45 kD DEK nuclear antigen which has been found in early-onset, ANA positive Oligoarthritis, has also been observed in ANA positive RF Negative Polyarthritis [28]. Patients who are ANA positive are at high risk of developing chronic anterior uveitis and should be submitted to periodic (at least every 3 months) slit lamp examinations. It is advisable to perform a baseline X-ray of affected joints in order to be able to assess disease progression over time.

Monitoring

Monitoring of children with RF Negative Polyarthritis should consist of periodic clinical evaluations to assess the severity and the extent of arthritis. Laboratory examinations, such as the haemoglobin and APR, if abnormal at baseline, help monitor the disease and response to treatment. In addition, most children with RF Negative Polyarthritis are on medications that require relatively frequent monitoring of blood counts, liver, and kidney function. Periodically, assessment of growth velocity, muscular atrophy, nutritional status, and the potential need of psychological support for children and their families

should be performed. It is prudent to perform slit lamp examinations every 6 months in most patients with RF Negative Polyarthritis. Patients with the ANA positive early onset clinical subtype must have this done every 3 months. X-rays of the involved joints should be taken at proper intervals in order to assess disease progression. In particular, in cases where there is wrist involvement, the determination of Poznanski score on a periodic (yearly) basis may allow a good estimation of osteoarticular damage and disease progression [29].

Complications

Linear growth may be retarded, although much less than in patients with Systemic Arthritis [30]. The growth retardation is proportional to the degree and duration of inflammation and appears to be independent of steroid treatment [31]. Low levels of circulating insulin-like growth factor-1 (IGF-1) have been reported in systemic JCA and to a lesser degree in polyarticular JCA patients with active disease [32]. A direct effect of the inflammatory cytokine IL-6 on growth retardation and IGF-1 serum levels has been described [33], and circulating levels of IL-6 in patients with RF Negative Polyarthritis have been reported to be elevated, although much less than in Systemic Arthritis [34].

Decreased bone mineral content and low bone turnover have been reported in RF negative polyarticular JRA, as well as in other forms of JRA [35,36]. The degree of decreased bone loss tends to be related to disease severity [36].

Eye complications, in the patients with ANA positive, RF Negative Polyarthritis appear to be similar or the same as described for Oligoarthritis. However, the risk of uveitis in other clinical subtypes of RF Negative Polyarthritis appears to be much less.

Prognosis

The outcome of RF Negative Polyarthritis is variable, with regression over time of sign and symptoms in some cases and progressive joint damage in others. Joint deformities in RF Negative Polyarthritis do not differ from those observed in other types of JIA. These may include: (a) growth disturbances, which are more frequent if the onset of the disease is precocious and aggressive (knee, hands, and wrists, TMJ, hips in particular) (Figure 2.5.7); (b) subluxation and dislocation secondary to joint destruction and/or anomalous traction (more frequent in the knee, hip, hands, and wrist) (Figure 2.5.8); (c) joint space narrowing and osseous erosions (Figure 2.5.9); (d) bone ankylosis which is more frequent in the carpal bones, the cervical spine (Figure 2.5.10) and in the feet.

As compared to the other subgroups of JIA, the percent of patients with bad outcome varies widely among series [37–39] probably reflecting differing patient selection. Symmetrical arthritis and early hand involvement appears to predict future disability and poorer overall wellbeing [40]. In a multi-centre cohort study of about 400 patients classified according to the ILAR criteria, the probability of remission at 10 years in RF Negative Polyarthritis was 23% [41], and remissions most often occurred within the first 5 years after onset. Several studies have shown that the overall prognosis in RF Negative Polyarthritis is worse than in Oligoarthritis but better than in RF Positive Polyarthritis [41].

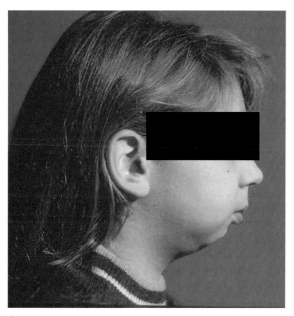

Fig. 2.5.7 Mandibular hypoplasia due to TM joint involvement is common in RF Negative Polyarthritis.

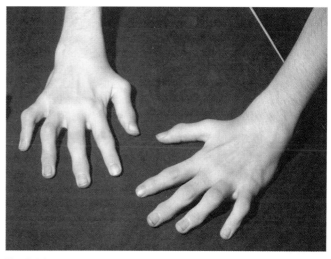

Fig. 2.5.8 Multiple joint contractures can be seen of the PIP joints (as well as synovitis of the MCP, DIP, and wrist joints) in a girl with severe long standing RF Negative Polyarthritis.

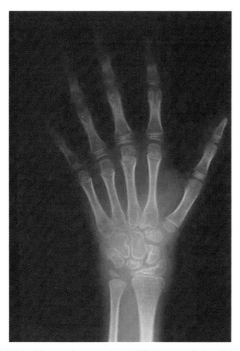

Fig. 2.5.9 Wrist X-rays of a patient with RF Negative Polyarthritis showing joint space narrowing and erosions in the carpal bones.

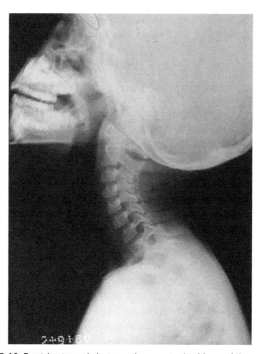

Fig. 2.5.10 Partial spine ankylosis can be seen in this X-ray of the cervical spine in a patient with RF Negative Polyarthritis.

Conclusions

In the context of the ILAR classification, RF Negative Polyarthritis still represents a heterogeneous condition in which different subsets can be recognized. Their identification is important in order to detect patients who are at risk for specific complications, such as anterior uveitis in ANA positive patients. Future studies are needed to better unravel the heterogeneity of RF Negative Polyarthritis

Key summary points

- RF Negative Polyarthritis appears to be one of the least defined subsets of JIA.
- Several clinical subgroups can be seen within this subset of JIA
  - Early onset ANA positive, asymmetric polyarthritis
  - Prolific symmetric polyarthritis
  - Dry synovitis
- The ANA positive polyarthritis subgroup has clinical and genetic similarities to patients with Persistent and Extended Oligoarthritis.
- The overall prognosis of RF Negative Polyarthritis is worse than in Oligoarthritis but better than in RF Positive Polyarthritis.

References

1. Petty, R.E., Southwood, T.R., Manners, P., Baum, J., Glass, D.N., Goldenberg, J., He, X., Maldonado-Cocco, J., Orozco-Alcala, J., Prieur, A.M., Suarez-Almazor, M.E., and Woo, P. International League of Associations for Rheumatology classification of juvenile idiopathic arthritis: second revision, Edmonton, 2001. *J Rheumatol* 2004;31:390–2.

2. Martini, A. Are the number of joints involved or the presence of psoriasis still useful tools to identify homogeneous entities in juvenile idiopathic arthritis? *J Rheumatol* 2003;30:1900–3.

3. Guzman, J., Burgos-Vargas, R., Duarte-Salazar, C., and Gomez-Mora, P. Reliability of the articular examination in children with juvenile rheumatoid arthritis: interobserver agreement and source of disagreement. *J Rheumatol* 1995;22:2331–6.

4. Andersson Gäre, B. Juvenile arthritis. Who gets it, where and when? A review of current data on incidence and prevalence. *Clin Exp Rheumatol* 1999;17:367–74.

5. Symmons, D.P.M., Jones, M., Osborne, J., Sills, J., Southwood, T.R., and Woo, P. Paediatric rheumatology in the United Kingdom: data from the British Paediatric Rheumatology Group National Diagnostic Register. *J Rheumatol* 1996;23:1975–80.

6. Andersson Gäre, B. and Fasth, A. The natural history of juvenile chronic arthritis: a population based cohort study. I. Onset and disease process. *J Rheumatol* 1995;22:295–307.

7. Bowyer, S., Roettcher, P., and the members of the Pediatric Rheumatology Database Research Group. Pediatric rheumatology clinic populations in the United States: results of a 3 year survey. *J Rheumatol* 1996;23:1968–74.

8. Peterson, L.S., Mason, T., Nelson, A.M., O'Fallon, W.M., and Gabriel, S.E. Juvenile rheumatoid arthritis in Rochester, Minnesota 1960–1993. Is the epidemiology changing? *Arthritis Rheum* 1996;39:1385–90.

9. Fink, C.W., Fernandez-Vina, M., and Stastny, P. Clinical and genetic evidence that juvenile arthritis is not a single disease. *Pediatr Clin N Am* 1995;42:1155–69.

10. Hall, P.J., Burman, S.J., Barash, J., Briggs, D.C., and Ansell, B.M. HLA and complement C4 antigens in polyarticular onset seronegative juvenile chronic arthritis: association of early onset with HLA-DRw8. *J Rheumatol* 1989;16:55–9.

11. Fernandez-Vina, M., Fink, C.W., and Stastny, P. HLA antigens in juvenile arthritis. Pauciarticular and polyarticular juvenile arthritis are immunogenetically distinct. *Arthritis Rheum* 1990;33:1787–94.

12. Barron, K.S., Silverman, E.D., Gonzales, J.C., Owebach, D., and Reveille, J.D. DNA analysis of HLA-DR, DQ, and DP alleles in children with polyarticular juvenile rheumatoid arthritis. *J Rheumatol* 1992;19:1611–16.

13. Aggarwal, A. and Misra, R. Juvenile chronic arthritis in India: is it different from that seen in Western countries? *Rheumatol Int* 1994;14:53–56.

14. Oen, K., Schroeder, M., Jacobson, K., Anderson, S., Wood, S., Cheang, M., and Dooley, J. Juvenile rheumatoid arthritis in a Canadian First Nation (aboriginal) population: onset subtypes and HLA associations. *J Rheumatol* 1998;25:783–90.

15. Moroldo, M.B., Tague, B.L., Shear, E.S., Glass, D.N., and Giannini, E.H. Juvenile rheumatoid arthritis in affected sibpairs. *Arthritis Rheum* 1997;40:1962–66.

16. Prahalad, S., Ryan, M.H., Shear, E.S., Thompson, S.D., Giannini, E.H., and Glass, D.N. Juvenile rheumatoid arthritis. Linkage to HLA demonstrated by allele sharing in affected sibpairs. *Arthritis Rheum* 2000; 43:2335–38.

17. Ploski, R., Vinje O: Rønningen, K.S., Spurkland, A., Sørskaar, D., Vartdal, F., and Førreø;. HLA class II alleles and heterogeneity of juvenile rheumatoid arthritis. *Arthritis Rheum* 1993;36:465–72.

18. Gao, X., Fernandez-Vina, M., Olsen, N.J., Pincus, T., and Stastny, P. HLA-DPB1*0301 is a major risk factor for rheumatoid factor-negative adult rheumatoid arthritis. *Arthritis Rheum* 1991;34:1310–12.

19. Chalom, E.C., Goldsmith, D.P., Koehler, M.A., Bittar, B., Rose, C.D., Ostrov, B.E., and Keenan, G.F. Prevalence and outcome of uveitis in a regional cohort of patients with juvenile rheumatoid arthritis. *J Rheumatol* 1997;24:2031–34.

20. Cassidy, J.T. and Petty, R.E. Juvenile rheumatoid arthritis. In J.T. Cassidy and R.E. Petty, eds. *Textbook of Pediatric Rheumatology*. Philadelphia, PA: WB Saunders; 2001, pp. 218–321.

21. Thomas, E., Barrett, J.H., Donn, R.P., Thomson, W., and Southwood, T.R. Subtyping of juvenile idiopathic arthritis using latent class analysis. British Paediatric Rheumatology Group. *Arthritis Rheum* 2000;43:1496–503.

22. Prieur, A.M. Rheumatoid factor-negative polyarthritis in children ("seronegative" polyarthritis). In *Oxford Textbook of Rheumatology*. P.J. Maddison, D.A. Isenberg, P. Woo, and D.N. Glass, (Eds), 1998 pp. 1131–43.

23. Arguedas, O., Fasth, A., Andersson-Gäre, B., and Porras, O. Juvenile chronic arthritis in urban San Josè, Costa Rica: a 2 year prospective study. *J Rheumatol* 1998;25:1844–50.

24. Ravelli, A., Felici, E., Magni-Manzoni, S., Pistorio, A., Novarini, C., Bozzola, E., Viola, S., and Martini, A. Patients with antinuclear antibody-positive juvenile idiopathic arthritis constitute a homogeneous subgroup irrespective of the course of joint disease. *Arthritis Rheum* 2005;52:826–32.

25. Ansell, B.M. Juvenile chronic arthritis. *Scand J Rheumatol* 1987; 66(Suppl):47–50.

26. Cassidy, J.T., Levinson, J.E., Bass, J.C., Baum, J., Brewer, E.J. jr, Fink, C.W., Hanson, V., Jacobs, J.C., Masi, A.T., Schaller, J.G., Fries, J.F., McShane, D., and Young, D. A study of classification criteria for a diagnosis of juvenile rheumatoid arthritis. *Arthritis Rheum* 1986;29:274–81.

27. Andersson-Gäre, B. and Fasth, A. Epidemiology of juvenile chronic arthritis in southwestern Sweden: a 5- year prospective population study. *Pediatrics* 1992;90:950–8.

28. Murray, K.J., Szer, W., Grom, A.A., Donnelly, P., Levinson, J.E., Giannini, E.H., Glass, D.N., and Szer, I.S. Antibodies to the 45 kDa DEK nuclear antigen in pauciarticular onset juvenile rheumatoid arthritis and iridocyclitis: selective association with MHC gene. *J Rheumatol* 1997;24:560–7.

29. Magni-Manzoni, S., Rossi, F., Pistorio, A., Temporini, F., Viola, S., Beluffi, G., Martini, A., and Ravelli, A. Prognostic factors for radiographic progression, radiographic damage, and disability in juvenile idiopathic arthritis. *Arthritis Rheum* 2003;48:3509–17.

30. Bernstein, B.H., Stobie, D., Singsen, B.H., Koster-King, K., Kornreich, H.K., and Hanson, V. Growth retardation in juvenile rheumatoid arthritis. *Arthritis Rheum* 1977;20:212–6.

31. Polito, C., Strano, G.G., Olivieri, A.N., Alessio, M., Iammarrone, C.S., Todisco, N., and Papale, M.R. Growth retardation in non-steroid treated juvenile rheumatoid arthritis. *Scan J Rheumatol* 1997;26:99–103.

32. Allen, R.C., Jimenez, M., and Cowell, C.T. Insulin-like growth factor and growth hormone secretion in juvenile chronic arthritis. *Ann Rheum Dis* 1991;50:602–6.

33. De Benedetti, F., Alonzi, T., Moretta, A., Lazzaro, D., Costa, P., Poli, V., Martini, A., Ciliberto, G., and Fattori, E. Interleukin 6 causes growth impairment in transgenic mice through a decrease in insulin-like growth factor-I. A model for stunted growth in children with chronic inflammation. *J Clin Invest* 1997;99:643–50.

34. De Benedetti, F., Robbioni, P., Massa, M., Viola, S., Albani, S., and Martini, A. Serum interleukin-6 levels and joint involvement in polyarticular and pauciarticular juvenile chronic arthritis. *Clin Exp Rheumatol* 1992;10:493–8.

35. Cassidy, J.T., Langman, C.B., Allen, S.H., and Hillman, L.S. Bone mineral metabolism in children with juvenile rheumatoid arthritis. *Pediatr Clin North Am* 1995;42:1017–33.

36. Pepmueller, P.H., Cassidy, J.T., Allen, S.H., and Hillman, L.S. Bone mineralization and bone mineral metabolism in children with juvenile rheumatoid arthritis. *Arthritis Rheum* 1996;39:746–57.

37. Wallace, C.A. and Levinson, J.E. Juvenile rheumatoid arthritis: outcome and treatment for the 1990s. *Rheum D Clin N Am* 1991;17:891–905.

38. Andersson Gare, B. and Fasth, A. The natural history of juvenile chronic arthritis: a population based cohort study. II. Outcome. *J Rheumatol* 1995;22:308–19.

39. Ruperto, N., Levinson, J., Ravelli, A., Shear, E.S., Tague, B.L., Murray, K., Martini, A., and Giannini, E.H. Longterm health outcomes and quality of life in American and Italian inception cohorts of patients with juvenile rheumatoid arthritis. I. Outcome status. *J Rheumatol* 1997;24:945–51.

40. Ruperto, N., Ravelli, A., Levinson, J., Shear, E.S., Murray, K., Tague, B.L., and Martini, A., Giannini, E.H. Longterm health outcomes and quality of life in American and Italian inception cohorts of patients with juvenile rheumatoid arthritis. II. Early predictors of outcome. *J Rheumatol* 1997;24:952–58.

41. Oen, K., Malleson, P.N., Cabral, D.A., Rosenberg, A.M., Petty, R.E., and Cheang, M. Disease course and outcome of juvenile rheumatoid arthritis in a multicenter cohort. *J Rheumatol* 2002;29:1989–99.

2.6 Psoriatic Arthritis

David A. Cabral

Aims

The aim of this chapter are to discuss the clinical manifestations, investigations, and classification of Psoriatic Arthritis in children. The difficulties inherent in correctly diagnosing and classifying patients with this type of arthritis in particular will be emphasized.

Structure

- Introduction
- Epidemiology
- Pathogenesis
- Clinical Features
- Investigations and Monitoring
- Complications
- Prognosis
- Key Point Summary

Introduction

Psoriatic Arthritis in children has only recently been recognized as a distinct condition among the chronic arthritides of childhood. In many centres, it continues to be under-diagnosed. This chapter will concentrate on the clinical characteristics of childhood Psoriatic Arthritis and point out largely unappreciated differences between this arthritis and the other types of Juvenile Idiopathic Arthritis (JIA).

Historical considerations

The association between psoriasis and arthritis in adults has been known since the nineteenth century [1], but descriptions of Psoriatic Arthritis in children are confined to the last two decades. Juvenile psoriatic arthritis was first defined as a form of chronic arthritis with an onset before the age of 16 years occurring in association with characteristic psoriatic rash or with rash occurring within the subsequent 15 years [2,3]. Because of the recognized delay in the appearance of the psoriatic rash, this condition has been under-diagnosed, and criteria for the diagnosis of juvenile psoriatic arthritis in the child with arthritis who may or may not have a typical psoriatic rash were first proposed in 1989 [4] as the "Vancouver Criteria." The key clinical elements of these classification criteria included arthritis, psoriasis, or a psoriatic-like rash, a family history of psoriasis, and psoriatic nail changes.

In the adult literature in the 1960s, psoriatic arthritis was distinguished from rheumatoid arthritis (RA) clinically, and serologically

Table 2.6.1 Classification of patterns of Psoriatic Arthritis in adults [5]

Onset type	%
Asymmetric oligoarthritis of small or medium sized joints	75
Symmetric Polyarthritis indistinguishable from rheumatoid arthritis	15
Spondyloarthropathy	5
Distal arthritis involving the distal interphalangeal joints	<5
Arthritis mutilans, a destructive, deforming arthritis	<5

by the absence of the rheumatoid factor. Because some patients had sacroiliitis or spondylitis and an association with HLA-B27 antigen, psoriatic arthritis was classified as a seronegative spondyloarthropathy, although several other distinctive patterns of joint involvement at onset are also recognized (Table 2.6.1) [5]. In children, the most common pattern of arthritis is that of asymmetric involvement of both large and small joints; sacroiliitis occurs in a very small minority [6]. In some ways Psoriatic Arthritis is more similar to Oligoarthritis (Part 2, Chapter 2.3) than to Enthesitis Related Arthritis, the ILAR diagnostic category for children who have, or are likely to develop, spondyloarthritis (Part 2, Chapter 2.7). For example, it is far more frequent in girls than boys, it has an onset in early childhood and not in adolescence, and patients are prone to asymptomatic chronic uveitis and not to symptomatic acute uveitis. However, unlike children with Oligoarthritis, those with Psoriatic Arthritis frequently have dactylitis and involvement of both small and large joints (Table 2.6.2) [6]. It is appropriate therefore that Psoriatic Arthritis of childhood has now found a unique home as another chronic arthritis under the umbrella term of JIA.

Criteria and classification

Comparing the "Vancouver Criteria" for juvenile psoriatic arthritis (Table 2.6.3) to the most recently revised "ILAR criteria" for the diagnosis of Psoriatic Arthritis, the common elements are the presence of (a) arthritis and psoriasis and (b) arthritis and at least two of the following. (i) dactylitis, (ii) nail abnormalities (pitting or onycholysis), (iii) family history of psoriasis in a first-degree relative. Under the JIA umbrella, arthritis is defined as swelling within the joint, or limitation in the range of joint movement with joint pain or tenderness that persists for more than 6 weeks, is observed by a physician, and is not due to other disorders. Psoriasis affecting either the patient or a first degree relative needs to be diagnosed with certainty by a physician. Dactylitis, representing the effect of both arthritis and tenosynovitis, represents swelling of one or more digits that extends beyond the joint margin (usually in asymmetric distribution) (Figure 2.6.1). Compared to previous definitions, both of these criteria enable diagnosis in the absence of definite psoriasis [7]. The "Vancouver Criteria" differs from

Table 2.6.2 Comparison of Psoriatic Arthritis with oligoarthritis, ERA and JAS[a]

Clinical Characteristic	Psoriatic Arthritis	Oligoarthritis	Enthesitis related Arthritis	Juvenile Ankylosing Spondylitis
Mean onset age (y)	6	3	10	>10
Male:Female	1:2	1:4	9:1	7:1
Family history	Frequent for psoriasis	Rare	Frequent for HLA-B27 associated disease	Frequent for HLA-B27 associated disease
Enthesitis	Unknown; (criteria allow for the presence of enthesitis in HLA-B27 negative patients exclusively)	Uncommon	Common	Very common
Uveitis	Asymptomatic	Asymptomatic	Symptomatic	Symptomatic
ANA positivity	50%	80%	<10%	<10%
HLA-B27 positivity	15% (HLA B27 positivity is not allowed if patient is a boy >6 yrs of age)	10%	75%	90%

[a] These numbers are extrapolated from studies on SEA syndrome, pauciarticular JRA and juvenile psoriatic arthritis (Vancouver criteria).

Table 2.6.3 Comparison of criteria for diagnosis and classification of psoriatic arthritis in children

Vancouver criteria	ILAR criteria

Definite JPsA
  Arthritis with psoriatic rash,
or
  Arthritis and three of the following minor criteria:
    Nail pitting or onycholysis
    Family history of psoriasis
      in first- or second-degree relative
    Dactylitis
    Psoriasis like rash
 	
Probable JPsA:
  Arthritis and 2 of the minor criteria
	Inclusion criteria
	  Arthritis and Psoriasis
	or
	  Arthritis and two or more of
	    dactylitis
	    nail pitting or onycholysis
	    FH of psoriasis in a first-degree relative
	
	Exclusion criteria
	  Arthritis in HLA-B27 positive male beginning after the sixth birthday
	  Ankylosing spondylitis, Enthesitis Related Arthritis, sacroiliitis with
	    inflammatory bowel disease, reactive arthritis syndrome, or acute anterior
	    uveitis, or history of one of these disorders, in a first-degree relative
	  The presence of IgM rheumatoid factor on at least two occasions
	    at least 3 months apart
	  The presence of Systemic Arthritis in the patient

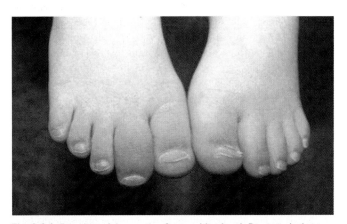

Fig. 2.6.1 Dactylitis of the toe in a 2-year-old girl with Psoriatic Arthritis. Note the bony overgrowth of the entire toe in addition to the obvious swelling. These were initially the only joints affected by arthritis. (Courtesy of Y. Kimura.)

the ILAR criteria in that it allows diagnosis of "probable" juvenile psoriatic arthritis. The ILAR criteria, in an attempt to define mutually exclusive diagnostic subsets, philosophically allow no such uncertainty. Therefore, patients with features of Psoriatic Arthritis will be classified as having Undifferentiated Arthritis if criteria are incomplete (Part 2, Chapter 2.8), or if they have features of another category of JIA as defined by specific exclusion criteria (Table 2.6.2).

Epidemiology

The concept of Psoriatic Arthritis as a unique entity is not universally accepted [8,9]. Since both psoriasis and inflammatory arthritis are common conditions, each occurring in about 3% of the general population, their association may be coincidental. An alternative explanation is that psoriasis may enhance a susceptibility to arthritis or modify the disease expression [10]. It may be that all hypotheses are true to some degree, and this is reflected in Dr Jerry Jacobs' statement: "all forms of arthritis may occur coincidental with psoriasis, but arthritis that mainly involves the distal interphalangeal joints of the hand is most distinctive and thus usually called 'psoriatic'. Less than half of all children with psoriasis and synovitis have this form of arthritis." Epidemiological evidence supports the notion that Psoriatic Arthritis exists as a distinct disease entity, but it is likely that not all patients with psoriasis and inflammatory arthritis have Psoriatic Arthritis. Whereas the prevalence of arthritis in the general population is estimated at 3%, the prevalence of arthritis in adults with psoriasis is 6–42% [8]. Similarly, the prevalence of psoriasis among adult patients with seronegative arthritis is about 20% [1]. In adults, psoriatic arthritis is distinguished from rheumatoid arthritis, but its subsequent classification as a seronegative, HLA-B27 associated spondyloarthropathy may also be simplistic. The likely heterogeneity of this disease is reflected in the different patterns of psoriatic arthritis in adults, originally described by Moll and Wright and recognized by others (Table 2.6.1). Although most patients are seronegative, the majority of patients have either asymmetric oligoarticular or polyarticular patterns (depending on the definitions used), but at the most only 40% have sacroiliitis [11]. As described in a preceding paragraph on historical considerations, children with Psoriatic Arthritis are even less likely to have sacroliitis or spondylitis. This may also partly reflect the natural history of ERA occurring later in childhood; and children with early onset Psoriatic Arthritis are unlikely to have ERA-like pattern of disease. The ILAR diagnostic criteria for Psoriatic Arthritis in children may well define a homogeneous population, but the heterogeneity of the disease will be reflected in the category of JIA that is described as Undifferentiated Arthritis (Part 2, Chapter 2.8). Preliminary studies of this classification system have found a preponderance of patients categorized as having Undifferentiated Arthritis who have diagnostic features of both Psoriatic Arthritis and other forms of JIA, particularly Enthesitis Related Arthritis [12].

Estimates of incidence and prevalence of Psoriatic Arthritis vary tremendously and reflect the problems of using varied diagnostic criteria, whether or not the studies were population based or referral center based, and/or collected from a spectrum of geographic locations. The figures likely underestimate true incidence, as half of the children ultimately diagnosed with Psoriatic Arthritis develop arthritis long before psoriasis; this interval may be longer than 15 years. The annual incidence of Psoriatic Arthritis from relatively recent studies is in the order of 0.23 to 0.4 per 100,000 children with a prevalence of 10–16 per 100,000 [13–15]. Children with Psoriatic Arthritis represent 2–15% of all children with JIA [13,14,16–18]. Using the Vancouver criteria, girls are affected twice as frequently as boys, and the mean age of onset of arthritis is about 6 years. It should be noted that children as young as 1 year of age may be affected [15]. Interestingly, in an earlier reported series that used traditional criteria for diagnosis (requiring both a psoriatic rash and arthritis) this sex ratio was almost completely reversed and the mean age of onset was 11 years [19]. These divergent results are reflected in the former study, where age of onset of Psoriatic Arthritis was bi-modally distributed with preschool and late childhood peaks and the median age of onset for girls was 4.5 years and for boys 10 years. That the majority of children with Psoriatic Arthritis develop psoriasis years after arthritis explains the later age of onset using traditional diagnostic criteria.

Pathogenesis

In studies of adults with arthritis and psoriasis, a genetic predisposition is evident from family studies, from associations identified with antigens of the histocompatibility system [20], and with the identification of susceptibility loci on several chromosomes [21–23]. None of this has been well studied in children. However, a family history of psoriasis in a first or second degree relative was noted in about half of the children with juvenile psoriatic arthritis compared to 21% of children with other forms of arthritis [15]. Studies of HLA associations in children with JIA in the United Kingdom support the notion that the ILAR classification system does define genetically distinctive subgroups [24]; whereas within the heterogeneous population of adults with Psoriatic Arthritis, the HLA associations are multiple and correlate with differing clinical manifestations [20].

Studies of immunological mechanisms principally in adults with psoriatic arthritis have identified humoral and other local factors that differ between psoriatic arthritis and rheumatoid arthritis [25–28]; they have also demonstrated cellular mechanisms that suggest a predilection for inflammation being confined to the skin and the synovium [29].

While the role of environmental factors such as trauma [30,31] and streptococcal infections [31,32] in precipitating flares of psoriasis (and sometimes arthritis) have been well described, the role of infectious agents and trauma in triggering the onset of the disease is more speculative.

Any aetiological explanation must account for the predilection for inflammation being confined mainly to the skin and the synovium; the exact pathogenetic mechanisms may be more likely elucidated when investigation is focused on more homogeneous clinical subsets.

Clinical features

Arthritis

The patterns of arthritis in children with traditionally defined psoriatic arthritis [33] are much the same as those described by Moll and Wright [5], (Table 2.6.1). These subdivisions, however, may not be particularly helpful; there is considerable overlap between the subtypes, and the relative frequencies in children versus adults differ considerably particularly if children with psoriatic arthritis and no rash (as defined by the Vancouver criteria) are included. At the onset of disease, in a group of 63 children with juvenile psoriatic arthritis defined by the Vancouver criteria, the majority (73%) had oligoarticular disease (<5 joints), the knees were the most commonly involved joints (65%), but arthritis of the small joints of hands (21%) or feet (19%) and dactylitis (19%) were also common [6]. Arthritis of the distal interphalangeal joints was uncommon. In the same study population followed for 5 years or more, the overall pattern was of persistent, low-grade asymmetrical arthritis involving three to five joints at any one time over many years, with 33% of patients continuing with an oligoarticular pattern of arthritis. The knee continued to be the most commonly affected joint (84%), followed by the ankle (60%), and arthritis affecting one or more of the small joints of the hands or feet also became increasingly common (62% and 56%, respectively). Dactylitis occurred in 35%, more commonly in the feet than in the hands and most frequently in the second digits

(Figure 2.6.1). Sacroiliac and lumbosacral spine joints were infrequently affected at any time.

There is limited literature thus far on disease pattern and disease course for children with Psoriatic Arthritis as a defined subset of JIA using the ILAR criteria. It should be noted that within that classification system, by definition, no patients with Psoriatic Arthritis have enthesitis, sacroiliitis, or spondylitis. The disease most closely resembles Oligoarthritis within JIA, but the ILAR definition distinguishes between them by psoriatic rash, nail changes, and family history. Not only is dactylitis a characteristic pattern of Psoriatic Arthritis compared to Oligoarthritis, but arthritis of the small joints of hands and feet, and wrist involvement are also more common [34]. The onset of arthritis may sometimes be quite sudden with acute pain and swelling. Chronic recurrent multifocal osteomyelitis (Part 1, Chapter 1.5) that may be accompanied by pustulosis palmar plantaris, may need to be distinguished from Psoriatic Arthritis. Patients with chilblains may be confused as having "dactylitis". During the acute phase, chilblains are readily distinguishable by the presence of characteristic papular nodules on the lateral and medial aspects of the distal digit (not on the tip). During recovery the nodules may be less apparent but the finger may still be ruddy, diffusely swollen, and tender. The clinical context, with a history of cold exposure and the absence of other findings suggestive of Psoriatic Arthritis may help establish the diagnosis.

Enthesitis

Enthesitis is inflammation of the entheses, which are the sites of attachment of tendons, ligaments, or fascia to bone. By definition, children with the Psoriatic Arthritis do not have enthesitis. Within this ILAR classification system, children with psoriasis, arthritis, and enthesitis will be described as Undifferentiated Arthritis. This group of children probably accounts for about 5% of children with psoriasis and arthritis, and this group probably represents the predominant pattern of psoriatic arthritis in adults, in which spondylitis is a relatively predominant pattern. In adult psoriatic arthritis, enthesitis has been proposed as a unifying feature. In children, enthesitis is a defining characteristic of ERA under the JIA umbrella; children with ERA would previously have been described as having seronegative enthesopathy and arthropathy (SEA) syndrome, HLA-B27-associated enthesopathy and arthropathy syndrome, and type II pauciarticuar onset juvenile rheumatoid arthritis.

Psoriasis

All forms of psoriasis have been described in children, but the predominant pattern in children who have arthritis is that of psoriasis vulgaris (Figures 2.6.2 and 2.6.3). This obvious pattern is characterized by well demarcated, scaly erythematous lesions occurring predominantly over the extensor surfaces of the elbows, forearms, knees, and interphalangeal joints. A more subtle presentation requires careful examination for rash in the hairline, behind the ears (Figure 2.6.4), in the navel (Figure 2.6.5), the groin, and the natal cleft. The onset of psoriasis and the onset of arthritis are rarely simultaneous. In several studies, arthritis precedes the onset of psoriasis in 33–67% of cases; this is in contrast to adult studies where arthritis precedes the rash in only 20% of patients. Among children diagnosed with Psoriatic Arthritis in the absence of skin rash, about 25% develop a psoriatic rash within 2 years [6].

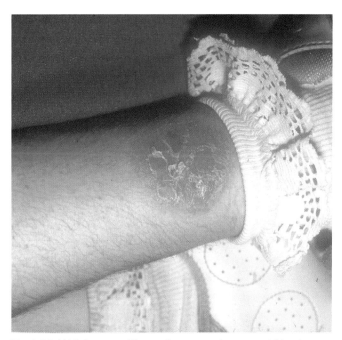

Fig. 2.6.2 Well demarcated lesion of psoriasis vulgaris in a child with Psoriatic Arthritis. (Courtesy of B. Cunningham.)

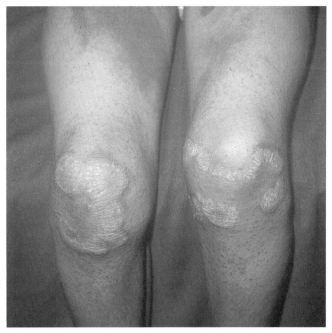

Fig. 2.6.3 Scaly erythematous plaques over extensor surfaces of both knees, typical of psoriasis. (Courtesy of B. Cunningham.)

The nail lesions associated with arthritis include pitting (Figure 2.6.6), onycholysis and subungual hyperkeratosis (Figure 2.6.7). The nail changes, together with family history of psoriasis are often the defining features of Psoriatic Arthritis prior to the development of a rash. Nail pits, usually shallow and no bigger than 1 mm in diameter, are best seen with a light shone tangentially across the nail surface. Although characteristic of psoriasis, nail pitting is not unique to psoriasis and may also be seen in association with eczema, trauma, and in healthy individuals.

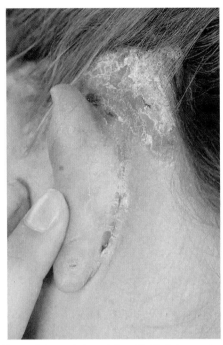

Fig. 2.6.4 More subtle psoriatic rash found behind the ears in a child with Psoriatic Arthritis. (Courtesy of T. R. Southwood.)

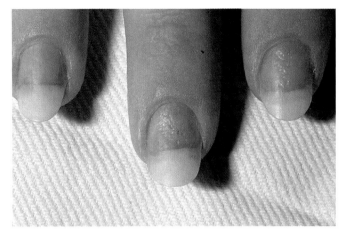

Fig. 2.6.6 Typical nail pitting seen in an adult with Psoriatic Arthritis. (Courtesy of T. R. Southwood.)

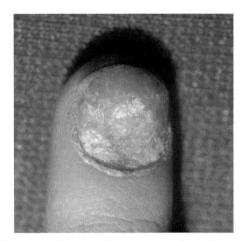

Fig. 2.6.7 Severe onycholysis and hyperkeratosis of the nail in a patient with Psoriatic Arthritis. (Courtesy of B. Cunningham.)

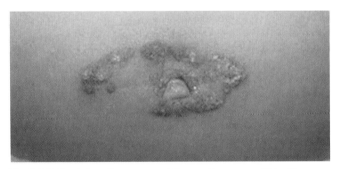

Fig. 2.6.5 Psoriatic rash seen around the navel in a young child with arthritis; the rash was not seen elsewhere and the paediatrician initially thought it was secondary to irritation or infection caused by drainage from a possible urachal sinus. (Courtesy of Y. Kimura.)

Investigations and monitoring

Laboratory tests

There are no diagnostic laboratory tests for Psoriatic Arthritis. Laboratory tests may be valuable in following the course of inflammatory disease, monitoring for side-effects of treatments, and excluding other diseases. About two-thirds of patients have some laboratory evidence of acute-phase inflammatory response such as elevations of erythrocyte sedimentation rate (ESR), C-reactive protein (CRP), platelet count or anaemia of chronic inflammation. Absence of these findings does not exclude the diagnosis. According to the ILAR system of classification, Psoriatic Arthritis is diagnosed on the basis of clinical findings and/or family history (Table 2.6.2); some laboratory test results confirm that the patient does not have features of more than one JIA, that is, the absence of rheumatoid factor and HLA-B27 antigen. A proportion of patients also have positive ANA, but this is of no diagnostic value for any of the JIA subcategories and may be found in healthy children.

Radiographs

Radiographic changes within the first few weeks, and sometimes first few months of disease, will generally be indistinguishable from other forms of chronic arthritis in children. Soft tissue swelling around the affected joints may be the only abnormality. Periarticular osteopenia may occur within a few months after onset, and periosteal new bone formation may occur especially in the digits affected by dactylitis. Periostitis, likely due to enthesitis, is characteristic of adult psoriatic arthritis and is uncommon in children; this likely contributes to the "pencil in cup" appearance of the DIP joint that is also rare in children. Children diagnosed with Psoriatic Arthritis, by ILAR definition, do not have enthesitis, and it is not known whether periostitis and pencil in cup changes occur at all. These changes may of course be found in children described as having Undifferentiated Arthritis because they have arthritis, psoriasis, and enthesitis.

Complications

Uveitis

While uveitis, traditionally described as being of the acute and symptomatic type associated with the spondyloarthropathies, occurs in 5–10% of adults with psoriatic arthritis [35,36]. More recent studies importantly underscore that the uveitis associated with psoriatic arthritis is much more insidious in onset, relatively asymptomatic, posterior, and often bilateral [37,38]. In children, uveitis is frequent, occurring in up to 20% of patients [15] and the pattern is very similar to that seen in Oligoarthritis (Part 2, Chapter 2.3): almost always insidious in onset, asymptomatic, chronic and anterior, found in the younger child, usually a girl in association with positive antinuclear antibodies (ANA) [15]. As such, all children with Psoriatic Arthritis should have regular ophthalmologic screening with a slit-lamp, every 3 months, to detect either protein flare or the presence of cells in the anterior chamber that occur often in the absence of symptoms (the same recommendation is made for children with Oligoarthritis). As in Oligoarthritis, unrecognized, persistent, or untreated uveitis may lead to visual impairment or blindness as a consequence of synechiae, band keratopathy, cataracts, or glaucoma (Part 2, Chapter 2.3, Figures 2.3.10–2.3.12). Early detection and treatment is essential, as there is some evidence that chronic anterior uveitis associated with Psoriatic Arthritis is more resistant to treatment [39] than that associated with Oligoarthritis.

Prognosis

Using traditional criteria for diagnosis, in a retrospective review of 60 children with juvenile psoriatic arthritis followed for a mean of 10.8 years, 40% were asymptomatic at follow up [19]. However, 25% had severe persistent arthritis, 10% were severely functionally limited, and 6% required bilateral hip replacements; 4% needed this surgery within only 5 years of onset. Nearly half of these patients developed radiological abnormalities of the sacroiliac joints; these individuals would now not be described as having Psoriatic Arthritis, so it is difficult to universally assign the poor prognosis to currently diagnosed patients. In a retrospective review of 63 patients diagnosed with juvenile psoriatic arthritis using the "Vancouver Criteria" followed for a mean of 7 years (6 months to 20 years), 40% had persisting active disease, the majority progressed to polyarthritis, 8% were severely functionally limited (class IV ACR criteria [40] and 3 patients had joint replacement surgery [6]). While the "Vancouver Criteria" more closely resemble the ILAR criteria than traditional criteria, it does not exclude patients with HLA-B27 antigen or with enthesitis. For children with psoriasis, arthritis, and overlapping features that preclude a diagnosis of Psoriatic Arthritis (ILAR), the long-term outcome will be determined with long-term follow-up of children diagnosed with Undifferentiated Arthritis of JIA.

Key point summary

- Psoriatic Arthritis, a recently defined distinct chronic arthritis of childhood (Vancouver criteria), now falls under the umbrella of JIA (ILAR criteria).

- Children with Psoriatic Arthritis represent 2–15% of all children with JIA.

- The diagnosis of Psoriatic Arthritis can be made in a patient without a psoriatic rash if in addition to arthritis the patient has two of the following: dactylitis, psoriatic nail changes, or a family history of psoriasis in a first degree relative.

- Even if a patient has both arthritis and psoriasis, their disease may not be defined as Psoriatic Arthritis if they have features overlapping with other JIA categories, and commonly, for example, if onset is in a boy over 6 years of age with HLA-B27, or if they have enthesitis.

- Uveitis, seen in up to 20% of children with Psoriatic Arthritis is identical to the pattern seen in Oligoarthritis affecting younger girls who are ANA positive and they should be similarly screened for asymptomatic inflammation.

- The onset of psoriasis and the onset of arthritis are uncommonly simultaneous.

- After years of follow up, 40% have persisting active disease and the majority progress to polyarthritis.

References

1. O'Neill, T. and Silman, A.J. Psoriatic arthritis. Historical background and epidemiology. *Baillieres Clin Rheumatol* 1994;8(2):245–61.

2. Lambert, J.R., Ansell, B.M., and Stephenson, E. Psoriatic arthritis in childhood. *Clin Rheum Dis* 1976;2:339–52.

3. Shore, A. and Ansell, B.M. Juvenile psoriatic arthritis—an analysis of 60 cases. *J Pediatr* 1982;100:529–35.

4. Southwood, T.R., Petty, R.E., Malleson, P.N., Delgado E.A., Hunt, D.W.C., Wood, B. *et al.* Psoriatic arthritis in children. *Arthritis Rheum* 1989;32:1007–13.

5. Moll, J.M. and Wright, V. Psoriatic arthritis. *Semin Arthritis Rheum* 1973;3:55.

6. Roberton, D.M., Cabral, D.A., Malleson, P., and Petty, R.E. Juvenile psoriatic arthritis: Followup and evaluation of diagnostic criteria. *J Rheumatol* 1996;23:166–170.

7. Fink, C.W. Proposal for the development of classification criteria for idiopathic arthritides of childhood [see comments] [published erratum appears in J Rheumatol 1995 Nov;22(11):2195]. *J Rheumatol* 1995;22(8):1566–69.

8. Gladman, D.D. Psoriatic arthritis. *Baillieres Clin Rheumatol* 1995;9(2):319–29.

9. Bruce, I.N. and Silman, A.J. The aetiology of psoriatic arthritis. *Rheumatology* (Oxford) 2001;40(4):363–6.

10. Martini, A. Are the number of joints involved or the presence of psoriasis still useful tools to identify homogeneous disease entities in juvenile idiopathic arthritis? *J Rheumatol* 2003;30(9):1900–3.

11. Lambert, J.R. and Wright, V. Psoriatic spondylitis: A clinical and radiological description of the spine in psoriatic arthritis. *Q J Med* 1977;46(184): 411–25.

12. Hofer, M.F., Mouy, R., and Prieur, A.M. Juvenile idiopathic arthritides evaluated prospectively in a single center according to the Durban criteria. *J Rheumatol* 2001;28(5):1083–90.

13. Berntson, L., Andersson, G.B., Fasth, A. *et al.* Incidence of juvenile idiopathic arthritis in the Nordic countries. A population based study with special reference to the validity of the ILAR and EULAR criteria. *J Rheumatol* 2003;30(10):2275–82.

14. Gare, B.A. and Fasth A. Epidemiology of juvenile chronic arthritis in southwestern Sweden: A 5-year prospective population study. *Pediatrics* 1992;90(6):950–8.

15. Southwood, T.R., Petty, R.E., Malleson, P.N. *et al.* Psoriatic arthritis in children. *Arthritis Rheum* 1989;32:1007–13.

16. Bowyer, S. and Roettcher, P. Pediatric rheumatology clinic populations in the United States: Results of a 3 year survey. Pediatric Rheumatology Database Research Group. *J Rheumatol* 1996;23(11):1968–74.

17. Malleson, P.N., Fung, M.Y., and Rosenberg, A.M. The incidence of pediatric rheumatic diseases: Results from the Canadian Pediatric Rheumatology Association Disease Registry. *J Rheumatol* 1996;23(11):1981–87.

18. Symmons, D.P., Jones, M., Osborne, J., Sills, J., Southwood, T.R., and Woo, P. Pediatric rheumatology in the United Kingdom: Data from the British Pediatric Rheumatology Group National Diagnostic Register. *J Rheumatol* 1996;23(11):1975–80.

19. Shore, A. and Ansell, B.M. Juvenile psoriatic arthritis—an analysis of 60 cases. *J Pediatr* 1982;100:529–35.

20. Gladman, D.D. and Farewell, V.T. HLA studies in psoriatic arthritis: Current situation and future needs. *J. Rheumatol* 2003;30(1):4–6.

21. Bhalerao, J. and Bowcock, A.M. The genetics of psoriasis: A complex disorder of the skin and immune system. *Hum Mol Genet* 1998;7(10):1537–45.

22. Karason, A., Gudjonsson, J.E., Upmanyu, R. *et al.* A susceptibility gene for psoriatic arthritis maps to chromosome 16q: Evidence for imprinting. *Am J Hum Genet* 2003;72(1):125–31.

23. Rahman, P., Bartlett, S., Siannis, F. *et al.* CARD15: A pleiotropic autoimmune gene that confers susceptibility to psoriatic arthritis. *Am J Hum Genet* 2003;73(3):677–81.

24. Thomson, W., Barrett, J.H., Donn, R. *et al.* Juvenile idiopathic arthritis classified by the ILAR criteria: HLA associations in UK patients. *Rheumatology* (Oxford) 2002;41(10):1183–89.

25. Ritchlin, C., Haas-Smith, S.A., Hicks, D., Cappuccio, J., Osterland, C.K., and Looney, R.J. Patterns of cytokine production in psoriatic synovium. *J Rheumatol* 1998;25(8):1544–52.

26. Spadaro, A., Rinaldi, T., Riccieri, V., Valesini, G., and Taccari, E. Interleukin 13 in synovial fluid and serum of patients with psoriatic arthritis. *Ann Rheum Dis* 2002;61(2):174–6.

27. Fearon, U., Griosios, K., Fraser, A. *et al.* Angiopoietins, growth factors, and vascular morphology in early arthritis. *J Rheumatol* 2003;30(2):260–8.

28. Fraser, A., Fearon, U., Reece, R., Emery, P., and Veale, D.J. Matrix metalloproteinase 9, apoptosis, and vascular morphology in early arthritis. *Arthritis Rheum* 2001;44(9):2024–28.

29. Borgato, L., Puccetti, A., Beri, R. *et al.* The T cell receptor repertoire in psoriatic synovitis is restricted and T lymphocytes expressing the same TCR are present in joint and skin lesions. *J Rheumatol* 2002;29(9):1914–19.

30. Scarpa, R., Del Puente, A., di Girolamo, C., della, V.G., Lubrano, E., and Oriente, P. Interplay between environmental factors, articular involvement, and HLA-B27 in patients with psoriatic arthritis. *Ann Rheum Dis* 1992;51(1):78–9.

31. Punzi, L. Pianon, M. Bertazzolo, N. *et al.* Clinical, laboratory and immunogenetic aspects of post-traumatic psoriatic arthritis: A study of 25 patients. *Clin Exp Rheumatol* 1998;16(3):277–81.

32. Telfer, N.R., Chalmers, R.J., Whale, K., and Colman, G. The role of streptococcal infection in the initiation of guttate psoriasis. *Arch Dermatol* 1992;128(1):39–42.

33. Lambert, J.R., Ansell, B.M., and Stephenson, E. Psoriatic arthritis in childhood. *Clin Rheum Dis* 1976;2:339–52.

34. Huemer, C., Malleson, P.N., Cabral, D.A. *et al.* Patterns of joint involvement at onset differentiate oligoarticular juvenile psoriatic arthritis from pauciarticular juvenile rheumatoid arthritis. *J Rheumatol* 2002;29(7):1531–5.

35. Lambert, J.R. and Wright, V. Eye inflammation in psoriatic arthritis. *Ann Rheum Dis* 1976;35(4):354–6.

36. Gladman, D.D., Shuckett, R., Russell, M.L., Thorne, J.C., and Schachter R.K. Psoriatic arthritis (PSA)—an analysis of 220 patients. *Q J Med* 1987;62(238):127–41.

37. Queiro, R., Torre, J.C., Belzunegui, J. *et al.* Clinical features and predictive factors in psoriatic arthritis-related uveitis. *Semin Arthritis Rheum* 2002;31(4):264–70.

38. Paiva, E.S., Macaluso, D.C., Edwards, A., and Rosenbaum, J.T. Characterisation of uveitis in patients with psoriatic arthritis. *Ann Rheum Dis* 2000;59(1):67–70.

39. Cabral, D.A., Petty, R.E., Malleson, P.N., Ensworth, S., McCormick, A.Q., and Shroeder, M.L. Visual prognosis in children with chronic anterior uveitis and arthritis. *J Rheumatol* 1994;21:2370–75.

40. Hochberg, M.C., Chang, R.W., Dwosh, I., Lindsey, S., Pincus, T., and Wolfe, F. The American College of Rheumatology 1991 revised criteria for the classification of global functional status in rheumatoid arthritis. *Arthritis Rheum* 1992;35(5):498–502.

2.7 Enthesitis Related Arthritis

Ross E. Petty

Aims

The aims of this chapter are to describe the epidemiology, clinical features and complications of Enthesitis Related Arthritis (ERA). Similarities between ERA and seronegative enthesitis arthritis (SEA) syndrome and juvenile ankylosing spondylitis (JAS) are also discussed.

Structure

- Introduction and classification
- Epidemiology
- Aetiology and pathogenesis
- Clinical features
- Investigations
- Monitoring
- Complications
- Prognosis
- Key point summary

Introduction and classification

The term Enthesitis Related Arthritis (ERA) was introduced in 1995 as a category in the International League of Associations for Rheumatology (ILAR) classification of childhood arthritis [1] to designate a type of Juvenile Idiopathic Arthritis (JIA) that had previously been called juvenile ankylosing spondylitis (JAS) [2], seronegative enthesitis arthritis (SEA) syndrome [3], or in more general terms, spondylarthropathy or seronegative spondylarthropathy (Table 2.7.1). Each of these terms has similar but different definitions.

In the 2001 Edmonton revision of the ILAR criteria, ERA is defined as arthritis with enthesitis, or arthritis *or* enthesitis with at least two of the following: sacroiliac joint tenderness and/or inflammatory spinal pain; the presence of HLAB27; a family history in at least one first degree relative of medically confirmed HLAB27 associated disease; acute (symptomatic) anterior uveitis; or the onset of arthritis after the age of 6 years. Patients with rheumatoid factor on at least two occasions at least 3 months apart, those with psoriasis or a first degree relative with psoriasis, those with a first degree relative with an HLAB27 related disease, and those with Systemic Arthritis are excluded. (Table 2.7.2)

Epidemiology

Although ERA undoubtedly contributes substantially to the population of children and adolescents with chronic arthritis, there are no data specifically describing the epidemiology of this recently defined entity. As a result, we must rely on studies of closely related diseases, the SEA syndrome and JAS (Table 2.7.3). Follow-up studies [4] have demonstrated that SEA syndrome most often eventually evolves into ankylosing spondylitis as defined by, among other things, the presence of radiographic evidence of bilateral sacroiliitis. It is presumed, although not yet proven, that the ILAR category of ERA describes children who have or will have what is considered to be the prototype of this group of diseases: inflammation of entheses and of the sacroiliac joints and lumbosacral spine.

SEA syndrome and JAS are much more frequent in males than females (7:1 to 9:1). They are most frequent in older children and adolescents, and are very uncommon before the age of 7 or 8 years. They are strongly associated with the HLA antigen B27 [3].

There is considerable variation in the frequency with which SEA syndrome and JAS are recognized throughout the world. In some

Table 2.7.1 Terms and their origins

Terms	Reference	Disorders included
Spondylarthritis	Wright and Moll [26]	Ankylosing spondylitis Psoriatic arthritis Reiter disease Arthritis with inflammatory bowel disease Juvenile chronic arthritis Whipple disease Behçet disease Reactive arthritis Acute anterior uveitis
Spondylarthropathy	Dougados *et al.* [27]	Ankylosing spondylitis Psoriatic arthritis Reactive arthritis Arthritis with Inflammatory bowel disease Unclassified spondylarthropathy
Ankylosing spondylitis	Bennett and Wood [2]	Ankylosing spondylitis (Does not exclude other diagnoses)
SEA Syndrome	Rosenberg and Petty [3]	Ankylosing spondylitis (some) Reactive arthritis (some) Psoriatic arthritis (some) Arthritis with IBD (some) Idiopathic SEA syndrome
Enthesitis Related Arthritis	Petty *et al.* [1]	Ankylosing spondylitis (some) Arthritis with IBD (some) SEA syndrome (some)

Table 2.7.2 Enthesitis Related Arthritis: classification criteria

Arthritis and enthesitis or Arthritis *or* enthesitis plus at least two of:

- Presence of or history of sacroiliac joint tenderness or inflammatory spinal pain
- Presence of HLAB27 antigen
- Family history of HLAB27-associated disease
- Acute anterior uveitis
- Onset of arthritis in a male after the 6th birthday

Exclusions

If any of the following are present, the patient is excluded from the category of ERA

- Presence of rheumatoid factor on two occasions at least 3 months apart
- Presence of Systemic Arthritis
- Psoriasis or a history of psoriasis in patient or first degree relative

Table 2.7.3 Epidemiology of ERA

Sex ratio	Up to 9 males to 1 female
Age at onset	Usually in late childhood and adolescence
Genetics	Strongly associated with HLAB27
Frequency	Accounts for 4–15% of children <16 years of age with arthritis

reports JAS and spondyloarthropathies accounted for 4% [5] to 39% [6] of children with chronic arthritis. Part of this variation reflects differences in the application of diagnostic criteria; many patients may be included under the term juvenile chronic arthritis (JCA), and not otherwise differentiated, others are identified as having late onset oligoarticular juvenile rheumatoid arthritis (JRA). In addition, part of the variation undoubtedly reflects differences in the frequency of the predisposing genes in the populations studied. The strong association with HLAB27 means that ERA is found more frequently in populations with a higher incidence of this gene. In adults, ankylosing spondylitis (AS) has an estimated frequency of 129 per 100,000 in an American population of north European origin [7]. Childhood onset of the disease occurs in approximately 11% of cases [8].

Aetiology and pathogenesis

The aetiology of ERA is unknown, but its clinical and genetic relationship to bacterially induced reactive arthritis suggests the possibility of extra-articular infection as an initiating event. While the understanding of the role of infection is limited, the importance of the histocompatibility antigen HLAB27 is clear. The high frequency of this antigen in children with JAS (~90%) [9] and SEA syndrome (~70%) [3] is likely to be reflected by those with ERA, although there are no reported studies to verify this. From studies in adults with AS it is likely that other genetic polymorphisms may also play an important role in predisposing the child to ERA. These include a polymorphism in the promoter region of the *TNF-α* [10] gene, and a polymorphism in the interleukin 1 receptor antagonist gene [11]. It is likely that the products of many genes contribute to the pathogenesis of ERA by modifying the expression of pro

Table 2.7.4 Clinical characteristics of ERA

Oligo or polyarthritis predominantly in the lower extremities

Enthesitis particularly around the knee and foot

Lumbosacral spine symptoms or signs may be present or absent

Few systemic symptoms or signs

Onset most commonly in pre-adolescent or adolescent boys

and anti-inflammatory cytokines, and, perhaps, by influencing antigen processing and presentation. Bacterial invasion of cells that express HLAB27 has been found to be abnormal in some studies [12] but not in others [13]. Killing of bacteria has been shown to be impaired in cells that express HLAB27, thereby permitting the infective organisms to persist [14]. Further discussion of these factors is found in Chapters 2.10 and 2.11 of this section ("Genetic and cytokine associations in JIA" and "Environmental factors in the pathogenesis of JIA").

Clinical features

Children and adolescents with ERA have insidious or abrupt onset of signs of inflammation in one or more joints or entheses. Precipitating factors are not known, although prior gastrointestinal infection with species of salmonella, shigella, campylobacter, or yersinia, or genitourinary tract infection with chlamydia trachomatis may be important in some patients. Symptoms suggestive of sacroiliac or lumobosacral spine inflammation are sometimes present at onset, but more common during the disease course. The most important clinical characteristic is the presence of enthesitis. (Table 2.7.4)

Enthesitis

Enthesitis is inflammation of the site of attachment of a ligament, tendon, joint capsule, or fascia to bone [15]. Symptomatic enthesitis usually occurs around the foot and knee, and less commonly, the pelvis. Entheses that are typically inflamed in ERA [3] are at the calcaneal insertions of the Achilles tendon and plantar fascia, and the plantar fascia attachments to the base of the fifth metatarsal and the heads of the first through fifth metatarsals. At the knee the typical locations of enthesitis are the patellar ligament attachments to the tibia, and the inferior pole of the patella, and at the insertions of the quadriceps muscle at 10 o'clock and 2 o'clock on the patella. [3] Much less commonly affected are the attachment of the adductor magnus at the ischial tuberosity, and the attachment of sartorius to the superior anterior iliac spine. Rarely other sites in the lower or upper extremities are affected. The sites may not be symptomatic, but tenderness elicited by pressure over the inflamed entheses may be quite severe. Pain at the attachments of the plantar fascia may occur with weight-bearing. At the Achilles insertion, retrocalcaneal bursitis may also be present, causing swelling just above the enthesis.

Arthritis

Arthritis most commonly affects the joints of the lower extremities, including the hip. The disease may be oligoarticular or polyarticular, symmetrical or asymmetrical, and may affect large or small joints. Joints of the upper extremities are sometimes involved, but seldom in the absence of lower extremity disease. Symptoms include morning stiffness and sometimes night pain. The affected joints are swollen, warm and tender, and are painful when moved. Symptoms affecting the spine, although quite uncommon at disease onset [3], probably supervene at some time during the disease course, and restriction of range of motion of the lumbosacral spine as determined by Schober's measurement, is a hallmark of the disease. Cervical spine inflammation can also occur, occasionally causing instability of C1 and C2 [16]. Spinal joint symptoms are those of any inflammatory arthritis: morning stiffness with pain on motion. Tenderness can sometimes be elicited by direct pressure over the sacroiliac joints, and by distraction of the sacroiliac joints (Patrick test), but these signs are often absent. Sacroiliac joint involvement may be unilateral initally, but eventually progresses to involve both joints.

Early ERA infrequently causes symptoms or signs in the spine, although in one study, Mexican patients with JAS had early lumbosacral spine involvement [17]. It is interesting that progression of SEA syndrome in the same population was much more rapid than in a Canadian population [18]. Whether this indicates that Mexican children and youth have a more severe form of the disease, or whether detection is later in that population is unclear.

Although measurements of lumbosacral spine mobility are of limited use as individual measurements, a trend toward decreasing mobility of the lumbosacral spine may be reflected by the Schober measurement which is important in monitoring patients with ERA. One application of the Schober measurement [19] notes the increase in distance between 5 cm below and 10 cm above the dimples of Venus caused by forward flexion. A normal measurement is at least 21 cm, and varies surprisingly little with age and gender [20]. Loss of range of motion of the lumbosacral spine is often insidious and may occur in the absence of symptoms of pain or morning stiffness. It is also important to evaluate the contour of the lumbosacral spine in the upright and forward flexed positions (Figure 2.7.1). Loss of the normal

lordosis in the upright position, and of a smooth convex contour in the flexed position may indicate inflammation of the spinal and sacroiliac joints, even if the Schober measurement is normal. Loss of hyperextension, lateral flexion, and rotation of the spine may also be observed. Chest expansion may be diminished, although the findings are inconsistent [21].

Systemic manifestations

Systemic illness is not usually a prominent feature of ERA, although occasionally low grade fever, weight loss, and fatigue are noted. Loss of muscle mass around affected joints may be dramatic. Visceromegaly and lymphadenopathy do not occur. Rashes are not present unless ERA occurs as part of a reactive arthritis with Reiter syndrome (arthritis, conjunctivitis, and urethritis, sometimes with keratoderma blennorrhagicum).

Investigations

In order to document the presence and extent of inflammation, the erythrocyte sedimentation rate (ESR), or C-reactive protein (CRP), white blood cell count (WBC) and differential, and platelet count should be recorded. Usually the ESR is elevated, sometimes strikingly. The WBC count is usually normal or moderately increased. Anaemia is usually mild, but can be quite severe, in which case underlying inflammatory bowel disease (IBD) should be suspected. Tests for antinuclear antibodies (ANA) and rheumatoid factor (RF) are negative (Table 2.7.5).

In evaluating HLA antigens, it should be recalled that while HLAB27 occurs in approximately 90% of children with ERA, it also occurs in 8–10% of the healthy north European Caucasian population, and that its presence does not indicate the presence of disease. Nonetheless, the presence of B27 is one of the criteria used in the diagnosis of ERA, and screening should be performed for this reason.

Synovial fluid analysis indicates the presence of an inflammatory reaction within the joint, but does not differentiate ERA from other types of chronic inflammatory joint disease. The WBC count is elevated and consists predominantly of macrophages and neutrophils. Synovial biopsy is seldom indicated, but if obtained shows nonspecific synovitis with lymphocytic and macrophage infiltration of hypertrophic synovium.

Plain anterior–posterior radiographs of the sacroiliac joints should be obtained, although early in the disease, they are likely to be normal. With progression of the disease, however, sclerosis and erosions,

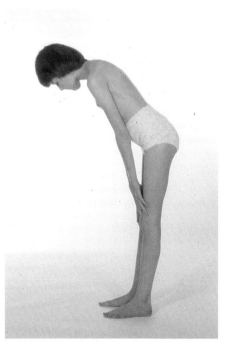

Fig. 2.7.1 A pre-adolescent girl with ERA demonstrating a very straight lumbar profile with anterior flexion of the spine. (Courtesy of T.R. Southwood.)

Table 2.7.5 Investigation of a patient with suspected ERA

Assessment of the acute inflammatory response (ESR, CRP, WBC, platelets)

Determination of HLAB27 antigen positivity

Demonstration of ANA and RF negativity

Radiographic evaluation
    Plain radiographs of the affected peripheral joints, and the sacroiliac joints
    CT or MRI of sacroiliac joints if plain radiographs are normal
    Lateral views of the calcanei if enthesitis at Achilles' insertion or plantar
      fascia insertion to calcaneus is suspected

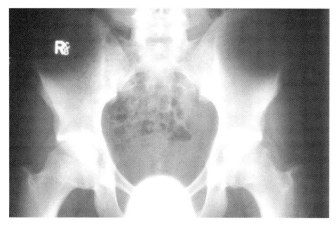

Fig. 2.7.2 AP radiograph of the pelvis demonstrating sclerosis of the left sacroiliac joint, especially noticeable on the iliac side of the joint.

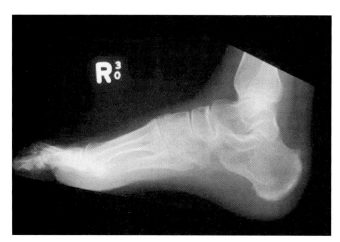

Fig. 2.7.3 Lateral view of the calcaneus and foot illustrating the development of osteophytes at the insertion of the plantar fascia to the calcaneus and the Achilles tendon to the calcaneus.

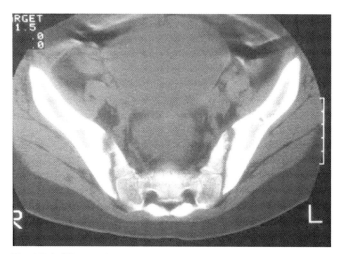

Fig. 2.7.4 CT view of the sacroiliac joints, illustrating the presence of erosions.

predominantly on the iliac side of the joint, and much later, fusion of the sacroiliac joint occur (Figure 2.7.2). Radiographic evaluation of the entheses may demonstrate erosions or spur formation, particularly at the Achilles tendon insertion to the calcaneus and the origin of the plantar fascia at the calcaneus (Figure 2.7.3). When plain radiographs of the sacroiliac joint are normal, and further documentation of involvement of the sacroiliac joint is required, computed axial tomography (CT) should be obtained (Figure 2.7.4). Radionuclide scans of the sacroiliac joints are seldom useful in this age group, and increased uptake may be overinterpreted as indicating disease when in fact it represents the normal metabolic activity of growing bones, or asymmetric weight-bearing. Experience with magnetic resonance imaging (MRI) of the sacroiliac joint of children and adolescents is very limited, but this technique may demonstrate changes that are not revealed by other methods [22].

Monitoring

The patient should be monitored at regular intervals for the development of complications of disease or therapy. Annual slit-lamp screening examinations to detect anterior uveitis are recommended, although ocular inflammation in ERA is usually symptomatic.

The inflammatory activity of patients with ERA varies considerably over time, and may disappear entirely for period of months or years. Routine follow-up at 3–4 month intervals is appropriate, although the intervals between visits can be increased when the disease is quiet. Because of the often insidious nature of the range loss, however, monitoring should occur not less frequently than 6 monthly. Monitoring for drug-induced toxicity as well as for abnormalities in indicators of inflammation should occur in a similar fashion. Radiographic follow-up should be dictated by the clinical signs and symptoms.

Complications

A number of characteristic, but uncommon complications can occur in children with HLAB27 related diseases, such as ERA (Table 2.7.6).

Spinal fusion

Spinal fusion that results in significant loss of range of motion or function is uncommon in childhood and adolescence, although there are exceptions to this generalization (Figure 2.7.5) [18]. In adulthood, however, fusion of the sacroiliac joints and the joints of the lumbosacral spine may result in severe disability.

Table 2.7.6 Complications of ERA

Musculoskeletal
  Spinal fusion
  Sacroiliac joint fusion
  Peripheral joint ankylosis

Systemic
  Acute anterior uveitis
  Aortic valve insufficiency
  Association with inflammatory bowel disease
  Association with reactive arthritis syndrome

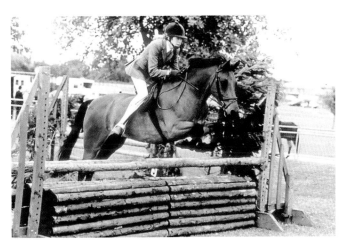

Fig. 2.7.5 A girl with ERA and spinal fusion who used her straight back to her advantage in competitive horseback riding. (Courtesy of T.R. Southwood.)

Aortic valve insufficiency

Aortic valve disease is rare in children or adolescents with ERA, [23] but it may increase in frequency through the adult years, [24] and it may be a source of severe morbidity. It is usually detected by routine auscultation and confirmed by echocardiography.

Acute anterior uveitis

Acute anterior uveitis is a significant complication of ERA. It differs from that seen in Oligoarthritis in that it is symptomatic: the eye is red and painful, and photophobia is often present. It is often unilateral, and often recurrent. Its frequency is approximately 10–15%, although the cumulative frequency in adulthood may be much higher [9,25]. Possibly because the symptomatic nature of the iritis brings it to early medical attention, the visual outcome is usually very good. Synechiae, band keratopathy, and other manifestations of complicated chronic uveitis are uncommon in children with ERA.

Associated conditions: ulcerative colitis, regional enteritis, reactive arthritis

Children with ERA may have evidence of either Crohn disease or ulcerative colitis. (see Part 1, Chapter 1.4) In such patients, symptoms of gastrointestinal inflammation (abdominal pain, weight loss, hematochesia, fever, erythema nodosum, and pyoderma gangrenosum) may occur. Reactive arthritis (arthritis, conjunctivitis, and urethritis) occasionally occurs, even in young children, following enteric or genitourinary tract infection with specific organisms.

Prognosis

Children and adolescents with ERA probably have the same outcome as those with SEA syndrome evolving to JAS. In childhood, the prognosis is quite good, although Burgos Vargas et al. have demonstrated the evolution of disease in patients with SEA syndrome at quite a rapid rate [18], and have documented the occurrence of severe JAS involving the sacroiliac joints and lumbosacral spine in childhood [17]. More commonly, however, at least in North America, the evolution of the disease appears to be much slower.

The disease course is often marked by periods of apparent remission of inflammatory disease. Although extensive peripheral joint involvement can occur, approximately half of children with ERA have four or fewer joints affected. Changes in the joints of the axial skeleton are often subtle, and insidious restriction of range of motion of the spine may not occur until a decade or more after disease onset. Long-term outcome data are still fragmentary, but careful long-term observation of patients with ERA appears to be essential.

Key point summary

- The terms SEA syndrome, JAS and ERA describe similar, but not identical clinical syndromes that probably describe elements of the same disease.
- ERA is strongly associated with HLAB27
- Enthesitis is most common around the foot and knee, arthritis is predominantly in the lower extremity, and back signs or symptoms are usually absent at onset
- Systemic complications include acute iritis and aortic valve insufficiency and may be associated with IBD.
- Radiographs may show erosions or spurs at entheses, soft tissue, and bony changes at peripheral joints, but seldom changes in the sacroiliac joints or axial skeleton early in the disease course

References

1. Petty, R.E., Southwood, T.R., Manners, P., et al. International League of Associations for Rheumatology classification of juvenile idiopathic arthritis; Second Revision, Edmonton, 2001. J Rheumatol 2004;31:390–2.
2. Bennett, P.H. and Wood, P.H.N (eds). Population studies in the rheumatic diseases. New York, Excerpta Medica 1968;456–7.
3. Rosenberg, A.M. and Petty, R.E. A syndrome of seronegativity, enthesopathy and arthropathy in children. Arthritis Rheum 1982;25:1041–7.
4. Cabral, D.A., Oen, K.G., and Petty, R.E. SEA syndrome revisited: a longterm followup of children with a syndrome of seronegative enthesopathy and arthropathy. J Rheumatol 1992;19:1282–5.
5. Andersson-Gare, Fasth A., Andersson J., et al. Incidence and prevalence of juvenile chronic arthritis: a population survey. Ann Rheum Dis 1987;46:277–81.
6. Malleson, P.N., Fung, M.Y., Rosenberg, A.M., for the Canadian Pediatric Rheumatology Association. The incidence of pediatric rheumatic diseases: results from the Canadian Pediatric Rheumatology Association Disease Registry. J Rheumatol 1996;11:1981–7.
7. Carter, E.T., McKenna, C.H., Brian, D.D., and Kurland, L.T. Epidemiology of ankylosing spondylitis in Rochester, Minnesota, 1935–1973. Arthritis Rheum 1979;22:365–70.
8. Gomez, K.S., Raza, K., Jones, S.D., et al. Juvenile onset ankylosing spondylitis—more girls than we thought? J Rheumatol 1997;24:735–7.
9. Hafner, R. Die juvenile Spondarthritis. Retrospektive Untersuchung an 71 Patienten. Monatsschr Kinderheilkd 1987;135:41–6.
10. McGarry, F., Walker, R., Sturrock, R., and Field, M. The -308.1 polymorphism in the promoter region of the tumor necrosis factor gene is associated with ankylosing spondylitis independent of HLA-B27. J Rheumatol 1999;26:1110–6.
11. McGarry, F., Neilly, J., Anderson, N., et al. A polymorphism within the interleukin 1 receptor antagonist (L1Ra) gene is associated with ankylosing spondylitis. Rheumatology (Oxford) 2001;40:1359–64.

12. Kapasi, K. and Inman, R.D. HLA B-27 expression modulates gram-negative bacterial invasion into transfected L cells. *J Immunol* 1992;148:3554–9.

13. Ortiz-Alvarez, O., Yu, D., Petty, R.E., and Finlay, B.B. HLA-B27 does not affect invasion of arthritogenic bacteria into human cells. *J Rheumatol* 1998;25:1765–71.

14. Granfors, K. Host-microbe interaction in HLA-B27 associated diseases. *Ann Med* 1997;29:153–7.

15. Ball, J. The enthesopathy of ankylosing spondylitis. *Br J Rheumatol* 1983;22 (Suppl. 2):25–8.

16. Foster, H.E., Cairns, R.A., Burnell, R.H., *et al.* Atlantoaxial subluxation in children with seronegative enthesopathy and arthropathy syndrome: 2 case reports and a review of the literature. *J Rheumatol* 1995;22:548–51.

17. Burgos-Vargas, R., Vazquez-Mellado, J., Cassis, N., *et al.* Genuine ankylosing spondylitis in children: a case-control study of patients with early definite disease according to adult onset criteria. *J Rheumatol* 1996;23:2140–7.

18. Burgos-Vargas and Clark, P. Axial involvement in the seronegative enthesopathy and arthropathy syndrome and its progression to ankylosing spondylitis. *J Rheumatol* 1989;16:192–7.

19. Macrae I.F. and Wright, V. Measurement of back movement. *Ann Rheum Dis* 1969; 28:584–9.

20. Moran, H.M., Hall, M.A., Barr, A., and Ansell, B.M. Spinal mobility in the adolescent. *Rheumatol Rehabil* 1979;18:181–5.

21. Burgos-Vargas, R., Castelazo-Duarte, G., Orozco, J.A., *et al.* Chest expansion in healthy adolescents and patients with the seronegative enthesopathy and arthropathy syndrome or juvenile ankylosing spondyltis. *J Rheumatol* 1993;20:1957–60.

22. Bollow, M., Braun, J., Biedermann, T., *et al.* Use of contrast-enhanced MR imaging to detect sacroiliitis in children. *Skeletal Radiol* 1998;27:606–16.

23. Stamato, T., Laxer, R.M., de Freitas, C., *et al.* Prevalence of cardiac manifestations of juvenile ankylosing spondylitis. *Am J Cardiol* 1995; 75:744–6.

24. O'Neill, T.W., King, G., Graham, I.M., *et al.* Echocardiographic abnormalties in ankylosing spondylitis. *Ann Rheum Dis* 1992;51:652–4.

25. Ansell, B.M. Juvenile spondylitis and related disorders. In J.M.H. Moll, ed. *Ankylosing Spondylitis.* Edinburgh: Churchill Livingstone, 1980, pp. 120–36.

26. Wright, V. and Moll, J.M.H. *Seronegative Polyarthritis.* Amsterdam: North Holland, 1976.

27. Dougados, M. van der Linden, S., Juhlin, R., *et al.* The European Spondylarthropathy Study Group preliminary criteria for the classification of spondylarthropathy. *Arthritis Rheum* 1991;34:1218–27.

2.8   Undifferentiated Arthritis

Taunton R. Southwood and Yukiko Kimura

Aim

The aim of this chapter is to discuss the clinical features of the variety of arthritides classified under the heading of Undifferentiated Arthritis. The differing clinical courses of this disease and the impact on prognosis, as well as predictors of outcome, are discussed.

Structure

- Introduction
- Definition
- Epidemiology
- Clinical patterns
- Moving towards a classification which is more useful in the clinical situation
- Changes proposed for the classification
- Key summary points

Introduction

One of the greatest challenges in clinical medicine is to discern relevant disease patterns in a morass of clinical and laboratory features. It becomes even more difficult if recognition of new patterns requires a shift away from traditional diagnostic or classification paradigms. The 'Undifferentiated Arthritis' subtype of JIA is undoubtedly the most problematic and controversial area of the proposed International League Against Rheumation (ILAR) classification. The recognition of this subtype is unique to the proposed ILAR Juvenile Idiopathic Arthritis (JIA) classification; there is no equivalent category in either the American Rheumatism Association (ARA) (now ACR) classification of Juvenile Rheumatoid Arthritis (JRA) or the European League Against Rheumatism (EULAR) classification of Juvenile Chronic Arthritis (JCA) [reviewed in 1]. In fact, the presence of patients in the Undifferentiated Arthritis subtype of JIA is often viewed as a failing of the new classification, particularly from a clinical perspective. Clinicians, patients, and their families find it difficult enough to come to terms with the uncertainty of the umbrella term JIA, let alone the further confusion that a relatively undifferentiated clinical pattern seems to imply. A particular concern is that the classification criteria that have created the need for this subgroup are seen as somewhat arbitrary, lacking in objectivity and are possibly biologically irrelevant. From the point of view of understanding disease, however, it is likely that further study of the Undifferentiated Arthritis subgroup will

yield additional disease subtypes and even important insights into the aetiology of JIA as a whole. At the very least, the controversy has stimulated a great deal of international discussion [2]. It remains to be seen whether this energy sheds light on the area, or merely generates heat.

Definition

Juvenile Idiopathic Arthritis refers to those forms of arthritis which begin before the 16th birthday, are persistent for longer than 6 weeks, and for which no cause is currently known [3]. In this context, Undifferentiated Arthritis is defined as arthritis that does not fulfil sufficient inclusion criteria for any category, or is excluded by fulfilling criteria for more than one category (Table 2.8.1). It is likely that there are a multitude of different types of JIA in this subtype, including those 'overlapping' forms manifesting a variety of extra-articular manifestations. Undifferentiated Arthritis will also include any form of arthritis in which one or more of the prerequisite classifying features are unknown. Examples include lack of, or inability to obtain, knowledge about a family history of psoriasis or eye disease, and the absence of laboratory investigation results such as rheumatoid factor (RF) or HLA B27 [4]. It follows that the proportion of patients classified as having Undifferentiated Arthritis is likely to be increased in retrospective studies of JIA patients from whom standardized prospective data collection has not occurred.

Epidemiology

In series published to date, between 2% and 56% of patients have been assigned to the Undifferentiated Arthritis category (Table 2.8.2), [4–15, 24]. A meta-analysis of 343 patients with Undifferentiated Arthritis indicated that the proportion of patients having insufficient criteria for

Table 2.8.1 Rank order of exclusion criteria most frequently resulting in assignation of patients to the 'Undifferentiated Arthritis' JIA subtype

1. Family history of psoriasis in a first-degree relative
2. Family history of ankylosing spondylitis, enthesitis related arthritis, sacroiliitis with inflammatory bowel disease, Reiter syndrome, acute anterior uveitis in a first degree relative
3. HLAB27 positivity
4. IgM rheumatoid factor positivity
5. Presence of features of Systemic Arthritis

Table 2.8.2 Distribution of the patients in the Undifferentiated Arthritis category

Authors	Total number of patients	Patients with Undifferentiated Arthritis (%)	Patients who did not meet criteria (%)	Patients who fulfilled criteria for more than one category (%)
Ramsey	69	11	10	1
Cleary	57	23	11	12
Fantini	683	23	14	9
Foeldvari	97	12	8	4
Thomas	572	2	NA	NA
Hofer	194	20	9	11
Langkammerer	172	16	9	7
Merino	125	15	5	10
Berntson (2003)	321	22	16	6
Hayata	152	9	NA	NA
Manners	50	28	27	1

Source: Adapted from Reference 1.

subtyping was 60% (207 patients), whereas 40% (136 patients) had enough criteria to fit into more than one subtype [1]. It should be recognized, however, that even the placement of a patient in one or other of these subcategories ('insufficient criteria' or 'overlapping criteria') may be difficult. For example, a child with RF Negative Polyarthritis and a family history of psoriasis, but no other features of psoriasis, has insufficient criteria for subtyping as Psoriatic Arthritis, but overlapping criteria for both Polyarthritis and Psoriatic Arthritis subtypes. Of course, this distinction may be quite unimportant from a treatment perspective.

There are potentially a very large number of combinations of classification criteria which require a child's disease to be placed in the Undifferentiated Arthritis category. As yet, there have been no published formal, prospective, epidemiologically based studies to determine the frequency of each possible configuration of criteria. In clinical practice, and from such data as has been published, the most frequently observed combination of features is the overlap between Oligoarthritis and Psoriatic Arthritis, due to a positive family history for psoriasis in the absence of other criteria to fulfil the definition of Psoriatic Arthritis. Other relatively commonly observed patterns included a positive family history for either psoriasis or HLA-B27 related diseases in combination with Polyarthritis and, less commonly, Systemic Arthritis [15]. The presence of a positive RF without polyarthritis was another relatively commonly observed reason for placing a patient in the Undifferentiated Arthritis category.

Clinical patterns

Systemic arthritis

Children with Systemic Arthritis are rarely classified as Undifferentiated Arthritis, although this might be expected more frequently due to the potential overlap with psoriasis. In a large study of 521 patients classified in the Systemic Arthritis category by ILAR criteria, all were also

considered as systemic by both EULAR and the ACR classifications [14]. However, since objective evidence of arthritis is required to place a patient in the Systemic Arthritis category, patients with systemic features 'sine arthritis' cannot be classified as Systemic Arthritis until arthritis appears. Additionally, Hofer et al. (2000) described seven children with typical quotidian systemic fever patterns and arthritis who were classified in either the Oligoarthritis or RF Negative Polyarthritis categories because other criteria for Systemic Arthritis (e.g. serositis, lymphadenopathy, organomegaly, or typical rash) were missing [9]. More accurately, these patients should have been placed in the Undifferentiated Arthritis category, because they fulfilled criteria for more than one category. In addition, there are patients with clinical features of Systemic Arthritis who carry RF [16]; these patients should be classified as having Undifferentiated Arthritis.

Oligoarthritis

Although the majority of children with Oligoarthritis do not fit any other category, there are many patients who are excluded due to one of the following exclusion criteria: a positive family history for psoriasis, a positive family history for HLAB27 related diseases, or a positive RF. There are reports of positive RF tests in patients with oligoarticular arthritis [16,17]. All such patients should be categorized as having Undifferentiated Arthritis: they would be excluded from Oligoarthritis by the presence of RF, but would not fulfil criteria for RF Positive Polyarthritis in the absence of polyarthritis. Whether these patients ultimately develop RF Positive Polyarthritis or rheumatoid arthritis as adults is not yet clear, but there are reports of early erosive disease in such patients [16] (see RF Positive Polyarthritis below).

Manners et al. studied 50 children with oligoarticular arthritis, and found that more than half (56%) did not fulfil criteria for any category of JIA and therefore were categorized as having Undifferentiated Arthritis [4]. Most of these patients (18 of 28) were deemed not to have sufficient criteria for any category because of lack of knowledge about, or inability to obtain, sufficient family history of psoriasis or of an HLAB27 related disease (e.g. because one parent was adopted). If lack of family history was not used as a reason to exclude patients, only 10 patients remained in the Undifferentiated Arthritis category, and all but one of these patients were found to have insufficient criteria to fulfil any category.

Of course, this example further emphasizes the disparity between the clinical perspective on arbitrary classification boundaries, and the principal aim of the ILAR classification; to categorize patients into homogeneous subgroups for the purposes of research. The key question is; 'would the inclusion, in the Oligoarthritis category, of patients who have four inflamed joints or less, but in whom there is a lack of knowledge about the exclusion criteria, be likely to improve the clinical homogeneity of that category?' If this is not the case, the patients should remain grouped within the Undifferentiated Arthritis category.

RF Negative Polyarthritis

The majority of RF Negative Polyarthritis patients classified as Undifferentiated Arthritis fulfilled more than one category because they also had criteria for Enthesitis Related Arthritis (ERA) or Psoriatic Arthritis. Indeed, the RF Negative Polyarthritis category, unlike Oligoarthritis, does not have explicitly listed exclusion criteria for ERA or Psoriatic Arthritis, although the principle of exclusivity is indicated in the text of each classification [3]. The homogeneity of the RF Negative Polyarthritis category has also been challenged by the observations of Langkammerer et al. [9]. Eighteen of the forty-four polyarthritis patients had a symmetrical polyarthritis of more than eight large and small joints, and 26 had asymmetrical arthritis of large joints with high frequency of positive ANA and chronic uveitis. The authors argued that these patients had more in common with

Table 2.8.3 Reasons for classification in the Undifferentiated Arthritis category

Author	Total number	Fits no other category		Fits more than one category	
		number	Reason(s)	number	Reason(s)
Foeldvari	12	8	Oligoarthritis and Family history of psoriasis	4	Oligoarthritis and PsA: 2 Polyarthritis RF- and ERA: 1 Polyarthritis RF- and PsA: 1
Ramsey	8	6	Oligoarthritis Family history of psoriasis: 5 RF +: 1	2	Oligoarthritis and ERA: 1 Polyarthritis RF- and PsA: 1
Cleary (patients with HLA-B27)	13	6	ERA and Family history of psoriasis	7	Polyarthritis RF- and ERA: 7
Fantini	157	98	Oligoarthritis Family history of psoriasis: ++ RF + ERA	59	Not described in detail
Hofer	39	17	Oligoarthritis Family history of psoriasis: 13[a] RF +: 4[a] Family history of HLA-B27: 2[a]	22	Oligoarthritis and ERA: 4 Polyarthritis RF- and ERA: 8 Polyarthritis RF- and PsA: 10
Langkammerer	27	11	Oligoarthritis Family history of psoriasis or Family history of HLA-B27: 8 No reason(s) detailed: 3	16	Oligoarthritis and ERA: 4 Polyarthritis RF- and ERA: 7 Polyarthritis RF- and PsA: 5
Merino	19	13	Oligoarthritis Family history of psoriasis: 12[a] RF +: 1[a] Family history of HLA-B27: 1[a]	6	Polyarthritis RF- and ERA: 5 Polyarthritis RF- and PsA: 1
Berntson	68	48	Oligoarthritis Family history of psoriasis: 35[a] RF +: 8[a] Family history of HLA-B27: 5[a] ERA Family history of psoriasis: 5[a]	20	Oligoarthritis and ERA: 8 Oligoarthritis and PsA: 1 Polyarthritis RF- and ERA: 10 Polyarthritis RF- and PsA: 1
Hayata	13	NA		NA	

[a] Some patients had two different exclusion criteria.

number of patients

Source: Adapted from Reference 1.

Extended Oligoarthritis than with RF Negative Polyarthritis, but the ILAR classification system categorized them as the latter because they had developed more than four joints within the first 6 months of their disease. The biological importance of this observation, in aetiologic, treatment, or prognostic terms, remains unclear.

RF Positive Polyarthritis

Although RF is an inclusion criteria for the RF Positive Polyarthritis category of JIA (the only category in which a laboratory test is a requirement for inclusion), tests for RF are commonly positive in a variety of acute or chronic inflammatory conditions and therefore are not specific for JIA (see Part 2, Chapter 2.4). One study of the prevalence of RF in 68 children with various forms of JRA found that although RF was positive in 16 of 24 children with polyarticular JRA, it was also positive in 7 of 27 with systemic JRA, and 1 of 17 children with pauciarticular onset JRA [16]. In another study, RF was found in two patients with Oligoarthritis who had early erosive disease [17]. Several broader studies of the ILAR classification system also identified children with an oligoarticular pattern of arthritis who also had RF; these were classified in the Undifferentiated Arthritis category (Table 2.8.3). It is unclear if these children represent early adult-type rheumatoid arthritis. The presence of the HLA class II allele *DR4* or other alleles associated with adult rheumatoid arthritis would be an argument in favour of this hypothesis.

Enthesitis Related Arthritis

Two criteria for ERA were largely responsible for patients being placed in the Undifferentiated Arthritis category. First, the classification criteria of 'inflammatory spinal pain' could be interpreted as including cervical arthritis. This has been reported in six patients with either RF Negative Polyarthritis or Systemic Arthritis [9]. Most clinicians, however, differentiate between cervical arthritis and the mainly lumbar inflammatory spinal pain of ERA.

Additionally, a family history of psoriasis excluded some patients from the ERA category and placed them in the Undifferentiated Arthritis category. For example, features of ERA such as sacroilitis and enthesitis can be seen in up to 40% of adult patients classified as having Psoriatic Arthritis [17], and, although axial skeletal disease is less common in the paediatric age group, these features occasionally occur in children with arthritis and psoriasis. In addition, at least 16 patients have been reported who fulfilled criteria for ERA but were classified as having Undifferentiated Arthritis because they also satisfied criteria for Oligoarthritis or RF Negative Polyarthritis [6,10].

Psoriatic Arthritis

Features of psoriasis are among the most contentious criteria in the classification and are responsible for many patients being placed in the Undifferentiated Arthritis category. A positive family history for psoriasis in both the Oligoarthritis and ERA categories led to exclusion of children from these categories (Table 2.8.3). It is also a reason for exclusion from RF Negative Polyarthritis, albeit reported less frequently than in Oligoarthritis. Several children with psoriasis, arthritis, and other features of RF Negative Polyarthritis or Systemic Arthritis have been reported [6]. A family history of psoriasis is very common, as psoriasis itself is a common condition, occurring in as many as 3% of the general population [reviewed in Reference 19]. In addition, Psoriatic Arthritis in adults is known to have several distinct patterns of arthritis, some of which overlap closely with the ERA subtype. Since these patterns can occur in children (see Part 2, Chapter 2.6), this could potentially lead to overlap of features of Psoriatic Arthritis with ERA.

Moving towards a classification which is more useful in the clinical situation

The current second revision of the proposed ILAR classification of JIA has a number of limitations. The criteria are most often based on relatively arbitrary clinical variables, such as the presence of psoriasis, enthesitis, sacroiliac tenderness, or lymphadenopathy, which may be interpreted differently from observer to observer. Even the number of joints in individual patients assessed as having arthritis can vary widely between experienced paediatric rheumatologists [20]. The time points used to define the classification and its criteria are also arbitrary, and the number of inflamed joints may vary markedly with time. For example, there is probably little biological relevance to the time periods of 6 weeks or 16 years used to define JIA.

In order to validate this classification for clinical purposes, three factors need to be taken in to account: the homogeneity of the categories, the precision of the criteria, and the number of unclassified patients. There is an interesting philosophical dilemma which should be borne in mind when considering these points. Consider the question: 'what is the effect of increasing the number and rigour of the classification criteria to improve the clinical homogeneity of each JIA category?'. The answer is clear; more patients will be placed in the Undifferentiated Arthritis category. Every increase in criteria, while likely to improve the level of certainty about the homogeneity of a category, is also likely to limit the numbers of patients who fulfil the criteria for that category. As all researchers in this field appreciate, this is also likely to result in considerable difficulty in recruiting the numbers of patients required to achieve a powerful research study. Additionally, fewer patients in a particular category mean that data resulting from study of those patients becomes more difficult to interpret in the real-life clinical situation. In other words, the Heisenberg Uncertainty Principle could be restated in clinical terms as: the greater the scientific precision of disease definition, the less reliable the clinical predictions about that disease become.

Changes proposed for the classification

Efforts to reduce the number of patients classified in the Undifferentiated Arthritis category is generally regarded as clinically beneficial. From the published literature, it appears that the homogeneity of the different categories is improved in the ILAR classification when compared to the traditional classifications of JCA and JRA [21,22]. The type of changes proposed for the ILAR classification could be divided under two principal headings: modifications to the existing classification, and development of innovative criteria, categories, or an entirely new classification (Table 2.8.4).

Table 2.8.4 Proposed changes in the classification of JIA

Author	Category	Proposed change
Foeldvari	Oligoarthritis	Extend exclusion: family history for psoriasis + nail pitting + dactylitis
Ramsey	Oligoarthritis	Family history for psoriasis: remove from exclusion criterion
Fantini	Oligoarthritis ERA RF Positive Polyarthritis Ranking of the categories	Family history for psoriasis: remve from exclusion criteria Psoriasis: remove from exclusion criterion RF positive symmetrical arthritis Patient fitting two categories should be classified in the category: 　Which is the most severe 　Which is the more differentiated
Hofer	RF Positive Polyarthritis ERA New category	Replace by RF+ arthritis new labelling: inflammatory spinal pain *not limited to the neck* Probable psoriatic arthritis: inclusion criterion: positive family 　history for psoriasis
Langkammerer	New category	Extended Oligoarthritis at onset: 5–8 joints during the first 6 months, and same exclusion criteria as Oligoarthritis

Source: Adapted from Reference 1.

Under the first heading, many of the proposed modifications to improve the internal consistency of the existing ILAR classification, especially those published before the most recent published revision, have already been incorporated. For example, Merino's observation of the inconsistency of psoriatic family history as an inclusion criteria for Psoriatic Arthritis (first-degree relatives) and as an exclusion criteria for other categories (second-degree relatives), has now been rectified [3,13]. Bernston *et al.* recommended clarification of the psoriatic issue [23] and also the number of RF tests, which should be internally consistent for both inclusion and exclusion criteria [6] and this has now been incorporated [3]. Additionally, the age at which possession of the *HLA B27* gene becomes clinically relevant has been resolved to 6 years [24].

Modifications to existing classification criteria may serve to reduce the numbers in the Undifferentiated Arthritis category (Table 2.8.4). Foeldvari *et al.* suggested altering a Psoriatic Arthritis criterion to improve its specificity, for example, the 'presence of dactylitis and nail pitting', whereas Fantini proposed that it should be eliminated altogether [11,14]. In both cases, the change would be likely to decrease the homogeneity of the Oligoarthritis category. It should be recognized that not all of the classification categories are equivalent, and this may be reflected in the composition of the Undifferentiated Arthritis category. Some are 'time-point' categories, such as Oligoarthritis, while others are 'end-point categories', such as Psoriatic Arthritis. A patient will only be classified as Oligoarthritis up to the time point of the most recent clinical review, if the patient has not developed another criterion such as psoriasis or enthesitis. However, once a patient has developed Psoriatic Arthritis, the categorization of that patient is relatively fixed and any additional clinical feature may move the patient into the Undifferentiated Arthritis category.

Fantini proposed modifying existing categories in the ILAR classification. He suggested that the classification of patients into the RF Positive Polyarthritis category should be limited to only those children with symmetrical arthritis. Investigations of the HLA distribution in both RF positive Oligoarthritis and polyarthritis patients may help to determine if they should fit the same category [14].

There have been several suggestions for creating new classification criteria. For example, computer-based statistical techniques such as latent class analysis using different objective variables may define new and more relevant JIA categories [7]. A category proposed from this study was the combination of Oligoarthritis and positive anti-nuclear antibody tests, which is currently not part of the ILAR classification criteria. Similarly, creation of new classification categories could be considered, which could reduce the numbers in the Undifferentiated Arthritis category. For example, Langkammerer *et al.* suggested the introduction of a category termed 'Extended Oligoarthritis at onset', comprising children with 5–8 arthritic joints during the first 6 months in the absence of the exclusion criteria for the Oligoarthritis category [5]. This would deal with the RF Negative Polyarthritis patients who appear clinically to be closer to Extended Oligoarthritis than to other polyarthritis patients.

Finally, wholesale changes to the classification itself have been suggested. Perhaps the most innovative approach has been adopted by Fantini [14] and Manners [4], who have suggested ranking JIA categories according to a hierarchy, with Systemic Arthritis and RF Positive Polyarthritis being the most easily defined. For these two categories at least, the presence of systemic features or RF would outweigh any other criteria. For example, a child with Systemic Arthritis and psoriasis would be categorized as Systemic Arthritis, irrespective of the psoriasis. This concept may be clinically attractive, but it is an example of misunderstanding of the purposes of the proposed ILAR classification. If, by making a change, the defined groups become more homogeneous, then the change would appear to be sensible from a research perspective. If robust research-based data are to drive a clinically useful classification, then untested proposals for change must be resisted. The most positive outcome of the controversy and debate about the Undifferentiated Arthritis category should be increased clinical research activity to inform the debate, and this is to be encouraged.

Apart from Undifferentiated Arthritis, the face validity of the ILAR proposal has been little questioned, presumably because most paediatric rheumatologists recognize the classification categories such as Extended Oligoarthritis within their clinical practices. Assessments of construct and criterion validity have formed the bulk of the published work to date. Unfortunately, there have been no published classification studies of patients from other than predominantly Caucasian backgrounds. This is a key test of the proposed criteria. Predictive validity is one of the ultimate tests of the classification, but this will only become apparent after long-term follow-up studies. A clinically useful classification will be one based on a combination of unequivocal clinical features and readily available investigations. It will allow accurate predictions about therapeutic response, expected complications, and prognosis. In short, it will reflect the biology and pathophysiology of JIA, and its myriad subtypes. Were such a classification to exist, we could look forward to a nomenclature that no longer needs the rather deflating term 'idiopathic'. Prospective studies of the genetic, immunological, microbiological, and biochemical basis of JIA, based on clinically homogeneous patient populations are still desperately needed.

Key summary points

- Undifferentiated Arthritis is a category of JIA which is not homogeneous.

- Patients with Undifferentiated Arthritis are placed in this category because they either fulfil criteria from more than one category or because they do not fulfil sufficient criteria for one category of JIA.

- As little as two and as many as 56% of patients have been assigned to the Undifferentiated Arthritis category in various published series.

- Many overlapping clinical patterns of arthritis are seen among Undifferentiated Arthritis patients.

- The purpose of the ILAR classification system is to increase the homogeneity of the defined groups for research purposes, but this also increases the number of patients in the Undifferentiated Arthritis category.

- The validity of the classification system will be tested in future studies looking at both clinical usefulness in its ability to predict therapeutic response, complications, and prognosis, as well as its scientific usefulness in reflecting the biology and pathophysiology of the different subtypes of JIA.

References

1. Hofer, M. and Southwood, T.R. Classification of childhood arthritis. *Best Pract Res Clin Rheumatol* 2002;16(3):379.

2. Duffy, C.M., Colbert, R.A., Laxer, R.M., Schanberg, L.E., and Bowyer, S.L. Nomenclature and classification in chronic childhood arthritis: time for a change? *Arthritis Rheum* 2005;52:382–5.

3. Petty, R.E., Southwood, T.R. *et al.* The ILAR criteria for the classification of juvenile idiopathic arthritis: second revision, Edmonton, 2001. *J Rheumatol* 2004;31(2): 390–2.

4. Manners, P., Lesslie, J., Speldewinde, D., and Tunbridge, D. Classification of juvenile idiopathic arthritis: should family history be included in the criteria? *J Rheumatol* 2003;30(8):1857–63.

5. Berntson, L., Andersson Gare, B., Fasth, A., Herlin, T., Kristinsson, J., Lahdenne, P., Marhaug, G., Nielsen, S., Pelkonen, P., and Rygg, M., Nordic Study Group. Incidence of juvenile idiopathic arthritis in the Nordic countries. A population based study with special reference to the validity of the ILAR and EULAR criteria. *J Rheumatol* 2003;30(10):2275–82.

6. Berntson, L., Fasth, A., Andersson-Gare, B. *et al.* Construct validity of ILAR and EULAR criteria in juvenile idiopathic arthritis: a population based incidence study from the Nordic countries. International League of Associations for Rheumatology. European League Against Rheumatism. *J Rheumatol* 2001;28:2727–43.

7. Thomas, E., Barrett, J.H., Donn, R. *et al.* Subtyping of juvenile idiopathic arthritis using latent class analysis. *Arthritis Rheum* 2000;43: 1496–503.

8. Hayata, A.L.S., Kochen, J.A.L., and Goldenstein-Schainberg, C. Comparison of ACR, EULAR and ILAR (Durban) classification criteria for juvenile idiopathic arthritis (JIA) on a cohort of 154 Brazilian children. *Arthritis Rheum* 2001;44(9):S169.

9. Hofer, M.F., Mouy, R., and Prieur, A.-M. Juvenile idiopathic arthritides evaluated prospectively in a single center according to the Durban criteria. *J Rheumatol* 2000;28:1083–90.

10. Krumrey-Langkammerer and Hafner, R. Evaluation of the ILAR criteria for juvenile idiopathic arthritis. *J Rheumatol* 2001;28:2544–7.

11. Foeldvari, I. and Bidde, M. Validation of the proposed ILAR classification criteria for juvenile idiopathic arthritis. *J Rheumatol* 2000;27: 1069–72.

12. Ramsay, S.E., Bolaria, R.K., Cabral, D.A. *et al.* Comparison of criteria for the classification of childhood arthritis. *J Rheumatol* 2000;27: 1283–6.

13. Merino, R., De inocencio, J., and Garcia-Consuegra, J. Evaluation of ILAR classification criteria for juvenile idiopathic arthritis in Spanish children. *J Rheumatol* 2001;12:2731–6.

14. Fantini, F. Classification of chronic arthritides of childhood (juvenile idiopathic arthritis): criticisms and suggestions to improve the efficacy of the Santiago–Durban criteria. *J Rheumatol* 2001;28:456–9.

15. Cleary, A.G., Sills, J.A., Davidson, J.E. Revision of the proposed classification criteria for juvenile idiopathic arthritis: Durban 1977. *J Rheumatol* 2000;27:1568.

16. Walker, S.M., Shaham, B., McCurdy, D.K., Wietting, H., Arora, Y.K., Hanson, V., and Bernstein, B. Prevalence and concentration of IgM rheumatoid factor in polyarticular onset disease as compared to systemic or pauciarticular onset disease in active juvenile rheumatoid arthritis as measured by ELISA. *J Rheumatol* 1990;17:(7):936–40.

17. Sailer, M., Cabral, D., Petty, R.E., and Malleson, P.N. Rheumatoid factor positive, oligoarticular onset juvenile rheumatoid arthritis. *J Rheumatol* 1997;24:586–8.

18. Lambert, J.R. and Wright, V. Psoriatic spondylitis: a clinical and radiological description of the spine in psoriatic arthritis. *Q J Med* 1977;46(184): 411–25.

19. Southwood, T.R., Petty, R.E, Malleson, P.N. *et al.* Psoriatic arthritis in children. *Arthritis Rheum* 1989;32:1007–13.

20. Guzman, J., Burgos-Vargas, R., Duarte-Salazar, C., and Gomez-Mora, P. Reliability of the articular examination in children with juvenile rheumatoid

arthritis: interobserver agreement and sources of disagreement. *J Rheumatol* 1995;12:2331–6.

21. Thomson, W., Barrett, J.H., Donn, R., Pepper, L., Kennedy, L.J., Ollier, W.E., Silman, A.J., Woo, P., and Southwood, T.; British Paediatric Rheumatology Study Group. Juvenile idiopathic arthritis classified by the ILAR criteria: HLA associations in UK patients. *Rheumatology* 2000;41(10):1183–9.

22. Petty, R.E. Exclusivity versus the hierarchy, of fear and loathing of the undefined. *J Rheumatol* 2003;30:1663–4.

23. Berntson, L., Fasth, A., Andersson-Gare, B., Herlin, T., Kristinsson, J. *et al.* The influence of heredity for psoriasis on the ILAR classification of juvenile idiopathic arthritis. *J Rheumatol* 2002;29:2454–8.

24. Murray, K.J., Moroldo, M.B., Donnelly, P., *et al.* Age specific effects of juvenile rheumatoid arthritis-associated HLA alleles. *Arthritis Rheum* 1994;4:1843–53.

2.9 Immunopathology of the joint in Juvenile Idiopathic Arthritis

Lucy R. Wedderburn, Kiran Nistala, and Taunton R. Southwood

Aim

The aim of this chapter is to describe the macroscopic pathology, histopathology, and immunopathology of the inflamed joint in Juvenile Idiopathic Arthritis (JIA). The pivotal and multifaceted role of the T cell in mediating inflammation and joint damage, as well as the complex and multifactorial nature of this process, will be discussed.

Structure

- Introduction
- Appearances of the joint in JIA
- Mediators of joint damage in JIA
- Cytokine imbalance and T cells
- Understanding arthritis—the role of immunoregulation
- The role of other cells in the pathology of JIA
- Conclusions

Introduction

The inflamed joint is central to the clinical manifestations of Juvenile Idiopathic Arthritis (JIA), and understanding the pathological alterations associated with this manifestation is essential to understanding the disease itself. There have been important advances in defining the cell numbers, subpopulations, and cell functions within the synovial tissues, synovial fluid, adjacent cartilage and bone in JIA. The aim of this chapter is to review and interpret these findings in the context of their potential contribution to the aetiology of JIA.

Appearances of the joint in JIA

Macroscopic pathology

The arthroscopic appearance of normal synovial tissue is pale pink and folded. Cartilaginous surfaces are easily distinguishable by their white, smooth, glistening appearance. Bare areas of bone surface may be seen between the edge of the cartilage and the synovial attachment at the margins of the joint; sites. These are vulnerable to destruction as part of the inflammatory process. Macroscopic inspection of the joint in the earliest stages of JIA usually reveals few abnormalities except for hyperaemic synovial tissues. Observations of the pattern and arrangement of superficial synovial vasculature in adults with

various types of arthritis have suggested associations with the clinical subtype of arthritis ("straight" patterns in rheumatoid arthritis, "convoluted" patterns in psoriatic arthritis, possibly secondary to differences in vasoactive cytokine activity [1,2], but these findings have yet to be extended to JIA. With disease progression, the synovium becomes increasingly thickened, eventually forming deep, redundant folds and fronds of tissue which protrude into the joint space and may obstruct the smooth movement of the articular surfaces (Figure 2.9.1).

Histopathology

Normal synovium comprises a cellular intimal layer and a relatively acellular, supporting, subintimal mesh of collagen fibres, blood vessels, adipose tissue, and nerves. The intimal or synovial lining layer is usually 1–3 cells thick and is primarily composed of two cell types: the predominant, fibroblast-like, type B cell, and the macrophage-like, phagocytic, type A cell.

Bywaters provided a classic description of the pathology of inflamed synovium. An inflammatory proliferation of blood vessels precedes increased synovial membrane surface area and villus formation, hypertrophy and hyperplasia of the lining cells [3,4]. In the most florid cases, distinct nodules of lymphocytes with germinal centres around blood vessels may be observed. Interestingly, Bywaters and Ansell noted no correlation between the histological appearance of the synovium and the subsequent disease course. More detailed microscopic evaluation of inflamed synovium shows marked hyperplasia due to accumulation of macrophages and fibroblast like synoviocytes in the lining layer. In the sub-lining layer there is infiltration of T cells, plasma cells, mast cells, and NK cells (Fig 2.9.2(a)) as well as cells of the macrophage/dendritic cell lineage.

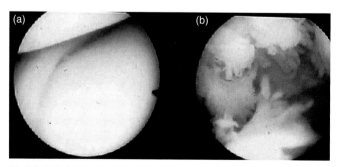

Fig 2.9.1 Arthroscopic views of the knee of a child with JIA. (a) shows the smooth surface of an unaffected area; (b) shows hypertrophied synovium with villi.

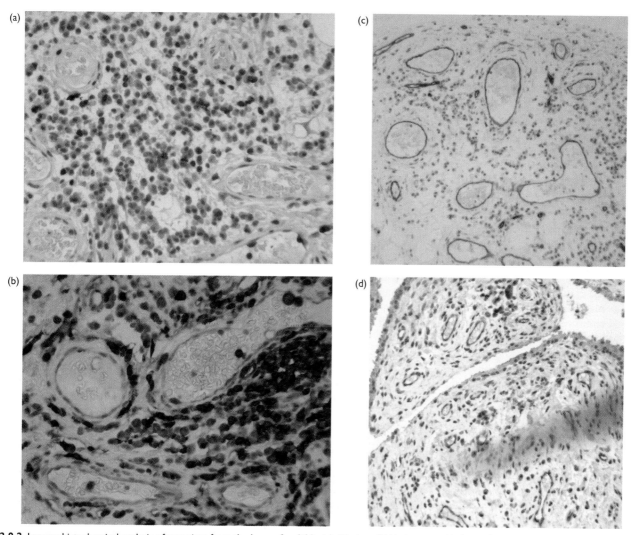

Fig. 2.9.2 Immunohistochemical analysis of synovium from the knee of a child with JIA show highly hypertrophied vascular synovium with dense inflammatory infiltrate. (a) Stained for CD3 (surface protein carried on T lymphocytes); (b) stained for HLA-DR which is highly expressed on the inflammatory cells (activated T cell, B cells and macrophage/ monocytes) as well as on the endothelium. (c) stained for ICAM-1 which is expressed both on the endothelium and a proportion of the infiltrating cells (d) stained for CD34 a protein expressed on vascular endothelium (as well as haematopoetic stem cells).

The hypertrophied synovial layer is highly vascular, with endothelium expressing markers of activation such as HLA-DR and ICAM-1 (Figure 2.9.2(b) and (c)). Recent studies have shed light upon possible mechanisms for the highly vascular synovium in JIA (Figure 2.9.2(d)). Work using synovial tissue explants from patients with JIA into the mouse SCID model showed high expression of the pro-angiogenic factor vascular endothelial growth factor (VEGF) in JIA synovial tissue [5], and two studies of VEGF in serum and synovial fluid showed that levels are raised, in particular in patients with active polyarthritis [6, 7]. A study of gene expression analysis from blood and synovial fluid cells from a JIA patient has confirmed the expression of pro-angiogenic factors, many of them chemokines, in polyarthritis [8]. Levels of the glycoprotein osteopontin are also raised in JIA synovial fluid and tissue and this was shown to correlate closely with new vascularisation [9]

The T cell aggregate in JIA synovium is present very early in the disease and is predominantly activated CD4+ cells, although some clinical subtype-specific alterations in CD4:8 ratios have been observed in JIA. Murray *et al.* observed two patterns of T cell infiltration in synovial tissue specimens from 22 patients with JIA. The predominant pattern seen in the majority of patients with polyarthritis was of intense lymphocytic aggregates, and even follicle formation, dominated by CD4 T cells, usually adjacent to blood vessels. CD8 cells were seen towards the periphery (mantle) of the aggregate. Patients with Oligoarthritis tended to exhibit a milder, more diffuse infiltration of lymphocytic cells in which the ratio of CD4:CD8 cells was relatively even. Activated T cells, particularly of the CD8 phenotype, expressing IL-2R, were more commonly seen in the latter group [10].

The inflammatory infiltrate leads to pannus formation and cartilage and bone destruction via degradative enzymes such as metalloproteinases [11]. As well as this increasing understanding of the destructive processes involved in the synovitis of JIA, there is also emerging interest in the role of regulatory (CD4+ CD25+) T cells in this inflammatory process [12,13].

Key point summary: Histopathology

- Normal synovial membrane is relatively acellular with fibroblast and macrophage type synoviocytes in the lining layer.

- Inflamed synovium in JIA shows hyperplasia of the lining layer, and accumulation of inflammatory cells including T cells, plasma cells, dendritic cells, mast, and NK cells in the sub-lining layer.

- The T cell aggregate is present early in JIA. Its specific cell type and tissue organization shows some correlation with the subtype of arthritis.

- Chronic inflammation leads to the destruction of cartilage and bone by several mechanisms including degradative enzymes such as metalloproteinases, cytokines, and other mediators.

Mediators of joint damage in JIA

Innate immunity and initiation of inflammation

Sibling studies have suggested an important, though incomplete role for genetic factors in the pathogenesis of JIA and many of the implicated genes code for proteins of the immune system (Part 2, Chapter 2.10, "Genetic and Cytokine Associations in JIA"). Environmental agents, and in particular infectious agents, have been sought to explain the initiation and perpetuation of JIA. Infection with enteric bacteria is well known to act as a precipitant for reactive arthritis. Immune responses to bacterial components and molecular evidence of bacterial DNA have been found in JIA synovial fluid and peripheral blood [14, 15]. Bacteria can activate the innate immune system by binding to Toll-like receptors (TLR) which are present on synovial fibroblasts, macrophages, monocytes and dendritic cells (DC). TLR are phylogenetically preserved transmembrane proteins which one word upregulate pro-inflammatory cytokines and chemokine production. Bacterial oligonucleotides have been shown to engage TLR and either cause arthritis directly in rodents or accentuate adjuvant induced arthritis[16]. Preliminary data suggest that TLR4 polymorphisms do not have a particular role in JIA [17]. However, the synovial exudates of patients with Oligoarthritis and Polyarthritis contain a significant population of cells with the features of myeloid-dendritic cells [18] and these have recently been shown to express high levels of TLR including TLR4 (L Wedderburn, personal communication).

Adaptive immune system and the persistence of inflammation

If activation of the innate immune system is indeed the trigger for inflammation, the prominent and early accumulation of T cells in synovium, as well as the strong genetic association of disease with several alleles of the MHC Class I and II loci, [19–21] which code for proteins that present antigens to T cells, suggests a role for these cells in its perpetuation. The synovial T cell population is in a dynamic state of flux between factors that promote T cell recruitment, division, emigration, and death. We will discuss each of these factors before considering why the balance may become dysregulated in JIA leading to persistent inflammation.

T cell recruitment

Recruitment of T cells into the joint requires initial binding to the endothelium before transmigration through the basement membrane. This is dependant on a family of adhesion molecules (including E selectin and ICAM), [22] expressed by endothelial cells in response to cytokines such as IL-1 and tumor necrosis factor (TNF)α. The

degree of systemic inflammation may influence the T cell populations recruited to the synovial compartment, [23] possibly due to upregulation of adhesion molecules on the high endothelial venules of the synovium. In animal models of JIA, upregulation of selectin ligands in T cells increases the accumulation of these cells into synovial tissue, suggesting an important role for chemokines for enhancing T cell recruitment to the synovium [24]. In JIA synovium, levels of ICAM1 and selectin correlate with measures of disease activity; lower levels predict a better response to intra-articular injection [22]. Other integrins, such as the gut mucosa-associated integrin α4β7 and synovial αEβ7, may also be involved in T cell recruitment in JIA [25]. These findings may have therapeutic significance, as blocking adhesion molecules may minimize T cell recruitment and halt inflammation at an early stage. In addition to adhesion molecule expression, increased expression of the pro-inflammatory chemokines IP-10 (CXCL10), RANTES (CCL5), and MIP1α(CCL3) has been demonstrated in JIA [26].

T cell division

T cells within the JIA joint are highly activated, expressing both rapidly upregulated (CD69) and persistent (DR) activation markers [23]. They express a restricted set of TCR specificities as analysed by molecular assays of TCR variability including heteroduplex or spectratyping [27, 28]. Interestingly these TCR defined 'clonotypes' are long lived and the same hierarchy of clones may re-expand during a relapse or flare of disease [27]. The finding that oligoclonality in the intra-articular T cell population was more marked in CD4+ T cells in Oligoarthritis (which is associated with class II, HLA-DR genes) yet more marked in CD8+ T cells in Enthesitis Related Arthritis, (which is associated with the class l allele HLA-B27), supports the concept that recognition of MHC-peptide complexes by T cells plays a role in the pathogenesis of JIA [28]. There is little evidence of large-scale antigen-driven T cell proliferation within the JIA joint [23], and synovial fluid T cells are typically 'hyporesponsive' to signals through the TCR [29], although recent studies suggest that this may be due to the influence of CD25+CD4+ regulatory T cells in the joint [30]. Even in the presence of large clonal expansions compared to the peripheral blood TCR repertoire, antigen specific T cells are likely to be present at low frequencies in the joint (1:100–1:2000 or less). However, specific recognition of self proteins including those of the conserved heat shock protein (hsp) family has been observed in JIA, and has been shown to correlate with a good clinical outcome [31, 32]. In addition some data suggest that the strong genetic associations of certain subtypes of JIA (see Part 2, Chapter 2.10) with HLA-DR alleles could be explained by mimicry by peptides from virus antigens such as Epstein–Barr Virus (EBV) with self peptides [33].

T cell retention

The stimulus to retain T cells within the inflamed joint in JIA is unclear. Chemokines regulate the migration of leukocytes between tissue compartments via specific receptors. Elevated synovial levels of the chemokine SDF-1 and its receptor CXCR4 have been found in RA [34]. CXCR3 and CCR5 are up regulated on infiltrating T cells in JIA [35]. CXCR3 is a cell surface receptor for the pro-inflammatory chemokines IP-10 (CXCL10), and Mig, while the chemokine ligands for CCR5 include RANTES (CCL5) and MIP1α(CCL3) which have been shown to be highly expressed in JIA [26]. It is likely that CXCR3 and CCR5 expression favour accumulation of inflammatory T cell in JIA joints [35]. In contrast, it is interesting that in some JIA patients with mild disease, a population of T cells expressing CCR4, a receptor thought to be expressed on regulatory T cells has been demonstrated [36]. Once in the synovium it would appear that T cells in the inflammatory environment may not require a TCR driven signal in order to survive: however, it has been shown that these cells are highly cytokine responsive, in particular to cytokines such as IL-2 and IL-15 [30].

T cell death

During normal recovery from tissue inflammation, programmed cell death (apoptosis) contributes to the resolution of the cellular infiltrate. In viral infections, apoptosis is mediated by cytokine deprivation [37]. Apoptosis has shown to be disrupted in RA because type 1 interferons prolong T cell survival [38], but this has yet to be demonstrated in JIA. Another mechanism of apoptosis, via the FAS signaling pathway, has been shown to be up regulated in JIA, but this may just be an epiphenomenon of a highly inflammatory state [39, 40]. Indeed, SF T cells may survive despite expressing CD95, a marker for FAS mediated apoptosis [40].

A further insight into defective apoptosis has come from studying patients with Systemic Arthritis, particularly those with macrophage activation syndrome, a haemophagocytic complication. Natural Killer (NK) cells normally play a homeostatic role in inducing apoptosis through perforin/granzyme B—mediated cell wall puncture. NK cells from these patients have reduced activity and low levels of perforin production [41]. Activated T cells are no longer controlled by apoptosis and instead produce high levels of TNFα and interferon (IFN) γ that may lead to macrophage activation. Autologous haemopoetic stem-cell transplantation has been shown to correct this perforin defect [42].

Key point summary: T cell abnormalities in JIA

- There is good evidence to suggest that T cells play an important role in pathogenesis and regulation of inflammation in JIA.

- T cells are recruited to the joint by upregulation of adhesion molecules on synovial endothelium and the corresponding T cell ligands.

- T cells found in synovial fluid are highly activated, oligoclonal, and skewed to a Th1 phenotype

- Synovial T cells are typically hyporesponsive to T cell receptor mediated signals. This maybe due to a subset of T cells (CD4+ CD25+) with an immunoregulatory phenotype which are also present in the joint.

- T cells may be retained within inflamed joints because of high levels of chemokines which normally favour the migration of leucocytes into inflamed tissue compartments.

- Abnormalities of cytotoxic NK have been found in Systemic Arthritis. This may be responsible for defective apoptosis of activated T cells leading to macrophage activation syndrome.

Cytokine imbalance and T cells

Taken together there is convincing evidence that factors controlling T cell dynamics are disordered in arthritis. Is there a common aetiology underlying the demonstrated abnormalities of adhesion molecules, chemokines and apoptosis? All three are influenced by the cytokine microenvironment in the joint. Factors that account for disturbed cytokine production could explain the abnormal T cell persistence found in JIA. One such explanation may be found in recent evidence linking specific cytokine polymorphisms to JIA [43, 44]. In this model, the risk of developing JIA and its severity is partly related to the levels of TNFα (pro-inflammatory) or IL-10 (anti-inflammatory) produced. It is important to note that such polymorphisms may be JIA subtype specific. For example, IL-6 polymorphisms appear to be associated with Systemic Arthritis [45,46]. This supports the possibility that the clinical subtypes may represent distinct forms of disease which have different underlying genetic factors in their aetiology. The clinical associations of polymorphisms in cytokine and other genes are further discussed in Part 2, Chapter 2.10.

T cells secrete as well as respond to cytokines and there is good evidence for a predominantly Th1 or pro-inflammatory pattern that could maintain inflammation in JIA [35, 47]. This pattern has been demonstrated by cultured clones *in vitro* [48], direct *ex vivo* assays on synovial T cells [35] and PCR from synovial tissue [47].

Understanding arthritis—the role of immunoregulation

To discover therapies that are effective in bringing about remission we need to understand not only why chronic inflammation persists but also how it may be regulated and switched off. JIA offers an excellent paradigm for understanding immunoregulation, with several disease subgroups of varying natural history than can offer comparisons between biological findings and clinical outcome. There is mounting evidence that in those children whose disease is oligoarticular and remains mild (Persistent Oligoarthritis), the balance of IFNγ: IL-4 (or IL10) production in the joint is skewed towards IL4 or IL10 production (anti-inflammatory cytokines) [30,35,36] compared to those whose disease progresses to the Extended Oligoarthritis or starts as Polyarthritis. This may reflect genetic differences which can influence the clinical course of JIA, such as the association of a low IL-10 producing haplotype with an increased risk of extension of Oligoarthritis [43].

It has increasingly become recognized that T cells present in both peripheral blood and lymphoid organs play an important regulatory role. To date the most fully characterized of these 'regulatory T cells' are the CD4+CD25+ cells (Treg), which make up approximately 5% of peripheral CD4+ T cells in health [49]. Several lines of evidence suggest that in Persistent Oligoarthritis, mechanisms involving immunoregulation may contribute to the mild clinical picture in this subtype [13]. Thus some children with Oligoarthritis have a population of IL-4 producing T cells within the joint (35), and IL-4 mRNA was previously demonstrated in this group of patients [50]. The observation that a population of CCR4+ cells is increased in the joint of those children with higher IL-4 production is significant given that CCR4 has been shown to be expressed at high levels on regulatory cells [36,51]. Several studies have suggested that self-reactive T cells specific for the heat shock protein hsp60 may be involved in such regulation. A strong T cell response to hsp60 has been suggested to correlate with Persistent Oligoarthritis which remains mild or even self remits, [31] and these T cells have been shown to express CD30 and produce IL-10 [52]. Recent studies have shown that there are a significant number of CD4+CD25+ cells in synovial exudates of children with JIA, and that these have suppressive ability *in vitro*. Depletion of these cells *in vitro* restores the proliferative response of synovial T cells *in vitro* and these synovial CD25+ cells will actively suppress proliferation. Interestingly a significantly higher number of these cells were demonstrated in children with Persistent Oligoarthritis than those with the extended form of disease [30]. These regulatory T cells within the joint expressed foxp3, a transcription factor shown to be associated with the Treg phenotype and function, as well as expressing high levels of CTLA4, GITR, and CCR4, all markers associated with regulatory T cells.

These differences between groups of patients with JIA, whose clinical outcomes are different, may be of fundamental importance to our understanding of the disease process. Thus in the future it may be possible to predict which children will evolve to severe disease, based upon the balance of inflammation and regulation in the joint, early in the disease process. In addition it may be possible to use regulatory pathways, such as that governed by foxp3, to design specific drugs which will tip the balance back towards regulation, in arthritis and other autoimmune diseases.

Key point summary: Cytokine imbalance and the role of immunoregulation

- Within the joint in JIA there are high levels of pro-inflammatory cytokines and the T cell infiltrate is heavily Th1 skewed.

- The ability to produce anti-inflammatory or regulatory cytokines such as IL-10 may be an important factor affecting the degree of joint damage or severity of arthritis

- There is good evidence for a population of regulatory T cells (Treg) within the joint

- The number and functional ability of Treg within the joint may be correlated with clinical outcome, for example in the difference between Persistent Oligoarthritis and Extended Oligoarthritis

The role of other cells in the pathology of JIA

In addition to a role for T cells in the tissue damage of JIA, other cells in the immune system are implicated. Synovial fluid obtained fresh from the inflamed joint also contains B cells, monocyte/macrophages, dendritic cells (DC), and neutrophils; the latter may make up the greatest proportion early in the disease process. Research is beginning to clarify the abnormalities of these cells both in their interaction with T cells and in other mechanisms of inflammation.

A role for the pro-inflammatory proteins of the S100 family, known as MRP8 and MRP14, which are produced predominantly by neutrophils and monocytes, has been suggested by the finding that these proteins are present at high levels in JIA joint fluid, and that serum levels, which are also raised, mirror disease activity and fall with remission [53]. Interestingly, these proteins are also expressed in the rash of active Systemic Arthritis, where they are synthesised both by infiltrating inflammatory cells and also activated keratinocytes [54].

Myeloid- derived and plasmacytoid DC, [18,55,56] have been shown to be present at increased proportions in both synovial fluid and tissue sections. Both of these are potent stimulators of T cells and also producers of pro-inflammatory cytokines. Interestingly myeloid derived DC in the joint express high levels of RANK, a TNFR-family member which is also implicated in the balance of osteoclast/osteoblast regulation in bone [18].

Although B cells are present in synovial fluid, and some patients with JIA have hypergammaglobulinaemia, the role of B cells in the pathogenesis of JIA is unclear. In some patients, lymphoid aggregates and even follicle like structures may be seen within the synovium, as for some adult patients with RA: such children are more likely to have RF Positive Polyarthritis. The presence of particular auto-antibodies, notably the ANA, may be associated with poor prognosis and increased risk of uveitis [57–59]. In Oligoarthritis, levels of the soluble CD23 protein, thought to be shed from activated B cells, and also correlated with ANA status, have been shown to correlate with

Table 2.9.1 Roles of various cell types in the pathogenesis of JIA

Cell type	Possible roles
T cells	T cell and monocytes interact, releasing cytokines that can activate themselves or adjacent cells such as fibroblasts. Pro-inflammatory cytokine release from T cells (TNF α, Inf-γ, IL2, MIF) and monocytes (TNFα, IL1, IL6, IL 8, IL12) pivotal in driving local and systemic inflammation. Immunoregulatory roles that may be disordered in JIA: Release of anti-inflammatory cytokines IL4, IL 10, and TGF β. CD4+CD25+ cells can directly suppress other T cells, B cells, and cells of innate immune system
Monocytes and neutrophils	Produce oxygen free radicals and proteolytic enzymes causing tissue damage Release chemoattractant peptides (defensins) which recruit T cells and monocytes Secrete MRP 8 and 14 (pro-inflammatory proteins which promote further leucocyte recruitment) Express surface Toll-Like receptors important in recognition of bacterial DNA and activation of innate immune system
Dendritic cells	Potent activator of naïve T cells Express high levels of RANK, which activates osteoclasts and causes bone loss.
B cells	Produce auto-antibodies which are deposited in the joint leading to complement activation and results in inflammation (direct evidence for pathogenesis in JIA is limited)
Fibroblasts	Produce cytokines and chemokines (Inf-β, TGF-β, SDF-1, CXCL12) which favour lymphocyte accumulation in joint Release metalloproteinases which contribute to cartilage and bony destruction

disease activity [60]. Clinical aspects relating to autoantibodies including ANA are further discussed in Part 2, Chapter 2.3 ('Oligoarthritis').

Cells of the immune system have been the focus for research into JIA for some time: however, some researchers in the RA field challenge their primacy [61]. Stromal cells, such as fibroblasts, make up a significant component of thickened synovial membrane in JIA [3]. Buckley and Salmon have shown that, in patients with RA, these fibroblasts produce T cell recruiting, pro survival (IFNβ) and retentive factors (SDF-1) and may even be involved in Th class switching [62]. Fibroblast derived cytokines may be responsible for a stromal microenvironment that favours T cell retention and persistent inflammation. Studies of fibroblasts in JIA are beginning to emerge which corroborate this picture. Synovial fibroblasts from JIA, but not other arthritides, produce high levels of pro-inflammatory cytokines and have morphological abnormalities suggestive of deregulated fibroblast proliferation [63].

Key point summary: Other cells in the pathogenesis of JIA

- Monocytes and neutrophils are increasingly recognized as playing an important role in JIA and the inflammatory proteins they produce, such as those of the S100 family, may be useful markers of disease activity (Table 2.9.1).

- Dendritic cells (of both myeloid and lymphoid lineages) are present in the joint and may play a critical role in the balance between pro- and anti-inflammatory factors.

- B cells also have a role in pathogenesis, particularly in Polyarthritis.

- Synovial fibroblasts contribute fundamentally to the synovial microenvironment which allows persistence of inflammation.

Conclusions

Improving the outcome of children with arthritis depends on progress in our scientific understanding of the disease. Disruption of inflammatory cell trafficking, retention and survival within the joint can lead to a chronic inflammatory process. Further research is needed to fully understand the entire pathway leading to childhood arthritis, and how regulation and inflammation are controlled. In the future, the pattern of cell or gene expression within the joint early in disease may provide prognostic clues which aid prediction of severity, disease course, or response to treatment [8,64]. Thus ongoing investigation into the mechanisms of tissue damage at the disease site is an important part of the research effort aimed to improve the care of children with arthritis.

References

1. Reece, R.J., Canete, J.D., Parsons, W.J., Emery, P. and Veale, D.J. Distinct vascular patterns of early synovitis in psoriatic, reactive, and rheumatoid arthritis. *Arthritis Rheum* 1999;42(7):1481–4.

2. Fearon, U. Griosios, K., Fraser, A., Reece, R., Emery, P., Jones, P.F., and Veale, D.J. Angiopoietins, growth factors, and vascular morphology in early arthritis. *J Rheumatol* 2003;30(2):260–8.

3. Bywaters, E.G. Pathologic aspects of juvenile chronic polyarthritis. *Arthritis Rheum* 1977;20(2 Suppl l):271–6.

4. Prahalad, S. and Glass, D.N. Is juvenile rheumatoid arthritis/juvenile idiopathic arthritis different from rheumatoid arthritis? *Arthritis Res* 2002;4(3):303–10.

5. Scola, M.P., Imagawa, T., Boivin, G.P., Giannini, E.H., Glass, D.N., Hirsch, R., and Grom, A.A. Expression of angiogenic factors in juvenile rheumatoid arthritis: correlation with revascularization of human synovium engrafted into SCID mice. *Arthritis Rheum* 2001;44(4): 794–801.

6. Maeno, N., Takei, S., Imanaka, H., Takasaki, I., Kitajima, I., Maruyama, I., Matsuo, K. and Miyata, K. Increased circulating vascular endothelial growth factor is correlated with disease activity in polyarticular juvenile rheumatoid arthritis. *J Rheumatol* 1999;26(10):2244–8.

7. Vignola, S., Picco, P., Falcini, F., Sabatini, F., Buoncompagni, A., and Gattorno, M. Serum and synovial fluid concentration of vascular endothelial growth factor in juvenile idiopathic arthritides. *Rheumatol* 2002;41(6): 691–6.

8. Barnes, M.G., Aronow, B.J., Luyrink, L.K., Moroldo, M.B., Pavlidis, P., Passo, M.H., Grom, A.A., Hirsch, R., Giannini, E.H., Colbert, R., Glass, D.N., and Thompson, S.D. Gene expression in juvenile arthritis and spondyloarthropathy: pro-angiogenic ELR+ chemokine genes relate to course of arthritis. *Rheumatol* 2004;43(8):973–9.

9. Gattorno, M., Gregorio, A., Ferlito, F., Gerloni, V., Parafioriti, A., Felici, E., Sala, E., Gambini, C., Picco, P., and Martini, A. Synovial expression of osteopontin correlates with angiogenesis in juvenile idiopathic arthritis. *Rheumatology* 2004;43(9):1091–6.

10. Murray, K.J., Luyrink, L., Grom, A.A., Passo, M.H., Emery, H., Witte, D. and Glass, D.N. Immunohistological characteristics of T cell infiltrates in different forms of childhood onset chronic arthritis. *J Rheumatol* 1996; 23(12):2116–24.

11. Gattorno, M., Gerloni, V., Morando, A., Comanducci, F., Buoncompagni, A., Picco, P., Fantini, F., Pistoia, V., and Gambini, C. Synovial membrane expression of matrix metalloproteinases and tissue inhibitor 1 in juvenile idiopathic arthritides. *J Rheumatol* 2002;29(8):1774–9.

12. Prakken, B., Kuis, W., van Eden, W., and Albani, S. Heat shock proteins in juvenile idiopathic arthritis: keys for understanding remitting arthritis and candidate antigens for immune therapy. *Curr Rheumatol Rep* 2002;4(6):466–73.

13. Wedderburn, L.R. T Cell Regulation in Juvenile Arthritis. Paediatric Rheumatology Online Journal 2004; May 2004 (http://www.pedrheumonlinejournal.org/).

14. Pacheco-Tena, C., Alvarado De La Barrera, C., Lopez-Vidal, Y., Vazquez-Mellado, J., Richaud-Patin, Y., Amieva, R.I., Llorente, L., Martinez, A., Zuniga, J., Cifuentes-Alvarado, M., and Burgos-Vargas, R. Bacterial DNA in synovial fluid cells of patients with juvenile onset spondyloarthropathies. *Rheumatol* 2001;40(8):920–7.

15. Bibi, F., Rider, C.A.J., Gardner- Medwin, J.M., Sharif, E., Brown, N.L., Kingsley, G., and Southwood, T. Molecular detection of bacterial DNA in synovial fluid and peripheral blood of children with juvenile idiopathic arthritis. *Rheumatol* 2002;41(suppl 1):4.

16. Ronaghy, A., Prakken, B.J., Takabayashi, K., Firestein, G.S., Boyle, D, Zvailfler, N.J., Roord, S.T., Albani, S., Carson, D.A., and Raz, E. Immunostimulatory DNA sequences influence the course of adjuvant arthritis. *J Immunol* 2002;168(1):51–6.

17. Lamb, R., Zeggini, E., Thomson, W., *et al.* Toll-like receptor 4 gene polymorphisms and susceptibility to juvenile idiopathic arthritis. *Lancet* 2005;64:767–9.

18. Varsani, H., Patel, A., van Kooyk, Y., Woo, P., and Wedderburn, L.R. Synovial dendritic cells in juvenile idiopathic arthritis (JIA) express receptor activator of NF-kappaB (RANK). *Rheumatol* 2003;42(4):583–90.

19. Thomas, E., Barrett, J.H., Donn, R.P., Thomson, W., and Southwood, T.R. Subtyping of juvenile idiopathic arthritis using latent class analysis. British Paediatric Rheumatology Group. *Arthritis Rheum* 2000;43(7): 1496–503.

20. Thomson, W., Barrett, J.H., Donn, R., Pepper, L., Kennedy, L.J., Ollier, W.E., Silman, A.J., Woo, P., and Southwood, T. Juvenile idiopathic arthritis classified by the ILAR criteria: HLA associations in UK patients. *Rheumatol* 2002;41(10):1183–9.

21. Donn, R.P. and Ollier, W.E. Juvenile chronic arthritis—a time for change? *Eur J Immunogenet* 1996;23(3):245–60.

22. Bloom, B.J., Nelson, S.M., Alario, A.J., Miller, L.C., and Schaller, J.G. Synovial fluid levels of E-selectin and intercellular adhesion molecule-1: relationship to joint inflammation in children with chronic arthritis. *Rheumatol Int* 2002;22(5):175–7.

23. Black, A.P., Bhayani, H., Ryder, C.A., Gardner-Medwin, J.M., and Southwood, T.R. T-cell activation without proliferation in juvenile idiopathic arthritis. *Arthritis Res* 2002;4(3):177–83.

24. De Benedetti, F., Pignatti, P., Biffi, M., Bono, E., Wahid, S., Ingegnoli, F., Chang, S.Y., Alexander, H., Massa, M., Pistorio, A., Martini, A., Pitzalis, C., Sinigaglia, F., and Rogge, L. Increased expression of alpha(1,3)-fucosyltransferase-VII and P-selectin binding of synovial fluid T cells in juvenile idiopathic arthritis. *J Rheumatol* 2003;30(7):1611–5.

25. Black, A.P., Bhayani, H., Ryder, C.A.J., Gardner- Medwin, J.M., and Southwood, T. An association between the acute phase response and patterns of antigen induced T cell proliferation in juvenile idiopathic arthritis. *Arthritis Res* 2003;5(5):R277–84.

26. Pharoah, D., Tatham, R., Klein, N., and Wedderburn, L.R. Production of CXCR3/CCR5 ligands, RANTES and MIP1a in juvenile arthritis. *Immunology* 2002;107(S1):S87

27. Wedderburn, L.R., Maini, M.K., Patel, A., Beverley, P.C.L., and Woo, P. Molecular fingerprinting reveals non-overlapping T cell oligoclonality between an inflamed site and peripheral blood. *Int Immunol* 1999;11(4):535–43.

28. Wedderburn, L.R., Patel, A, Varsani, H., and Woo, P. Divergence in the degree of clonal expansions in inflammatory T cell subpopulations mirrors HLA-associated risk alleles in genetically and clinically distinct subtypes of childhood arthritis. *Int Immunol* 2001;13(12):1541–50.

29. Patel, A., Varsani, H., and Wedderburn, L.R. The hyporesponsiveness of synovial T cells in JIA is a property of CD4+CD25+ T cells: evidence for regulatory T cells in juvenile arthritis. *Rheumatol* 2003;42(S1):11.

30. de Kleer, I.M., Wedderburn, L.R., Taams, L.S., Patel, A., Varsani, H., Klein, M., de Jager, W., Pugayung, G., Giannoni, F., Rijkers, G., Albani, S., Kuis, W., and Prakken, B. CD4+CD25(bright) regulatory T cells actively regulate inflammation in the joints of patients with the remitting form of juvenile idiopathic arthritis. *J Immunol* 2004;172(10):6435–43.

31. Prakken, A.B., van Eden, W., Rijkers, G.T., Kuis, W., Toebes, E.A., de Graeff-Meeder, E.R., van der Zee, R., and Zegers, B.J. Autoreactivity to human heat-shock protein 60 predicts disease remission in oligoarticular juvenile rheumatoid arthritis. *Arthritis Rheum* 1996;39(11):1826–32.

32. Kamphuis, S., Kuis, W., de Jager, W., *et al.* Tolerogenic immune responses to novel T-cell epitopes from heat-shock protein 60 in juvenile idiopathic arthritis. *Lancet* 2005; 366:50–6.

33. Massa, M., Mazzoli, F., Pignatti, P., De Benedetti, F., Passalia, M., Viola, S., Samodal, R., La Cava, A., Giannoni, F., Ollier, W., Martini, A., and Albani, S. Proinflammatory responses to self HLA epitopes are triggered by molecular mimicry to Epstein-Barr virus proteins in oligoarticular juvenile idiopathic arthritis. *Arthritis Rheum* 2002;46(10): 2721–9.

34. Buckley, C.D., Amft, N., Bradfield, P.F., Pilling, D., Ross, E., Arenzana-Seisdedos, F., Amara, A., Curnow, S.J., Lord, J.M., Scheel-Toellner, D., and Salmon, M. Persistent induction of the chemokine receptor CXCR4 by TGF-beta 1 on synovial T cells contributes to their accumulation within the rheumatoid synovium. *J Immunol* 2000;165(6): 3423–9.

35. Wedderburn, L.R., Robinson, N., Patel, A., Varsani, H., and Woo, P. Selective recruitment of polarized T cells expressing CCR5 and CXCR3 to the inflamed joints of children with juvenile idiopathic arthritis. *Arthritis Rheum* 2000;43(4):765–74.

36. Thompson, S.D., Luyrink, L.K., Graham, T.B., Tsoras, M., Ryan, M., Passo, M.H., and Glass, DN., Chemokine receptor CCR4 on CD4+ T cells in juvenile rheumatoid arthritis synovial fluid defines a subset of cells with increased IL- 4:IFN-gamma mRNA ratios. *J Immunol* 2001;166(11): 6899–906.

37. Soares, MV., Maini, M.K., Beverley, P.C., Salmon, M., and Akbar, A.N., Regulation of apoptosis and replicative senescence in CD8+ T cells from patients with viral infections. *Biochem Soc Trans* 2000;28(2):255–8.

38. Akbar, A.N., and Salmon, M., Cellular environments and apoptosis: tissue microenvironments control activated T-cell death. *Immunol Today* 1997;18(2):72–6.

39. Smolewska, E., Brozik., H., Smolewski, P., Biernacka-Zielinska, M., Darzynkiewicz, Z., and Stanczyk, J., Apoptosis of peripheral blood lymphocytes in patients with juvenile idiopathic arthritis. *Ann Rheum Dis* 2003;62(8):761–3.

40. Knipp, S., Feyen, O., Ndagijimana, J., and Niehues, T., Ex vivo apoptosis, CD95 and CD28 expression in T cells of children with juvenile idiopathic arthritis. *Rheumatol Int* 2003;23(3):112–5.

41. Grom, A.A., Villanueva, J., Lee, S., Goldmuntz, E.A., Passo, M.H., and Filipovich, A., Natural killer cell dysfunction in patients with systemic-onset juvenile rheumatoid arthritis and macrophage activation syndrome. *J Pediatr* 2003;142(3):292–6.

42. Wulffraat, N.M., Rijkers, G.T., Elst, E., Brooimans, R., and Kuis, W., Reduced perforin expression in systemic juvenile idiopathic arthritis is restored by autologous stem-cell transplantation. *Rheumatol* 2003;42(2): 375–9.

43. Crawley, E., Kay, R., Sillibourne, J., Patel, P., Hutchinson, I., and Woo, P., Polymorphic haplotypes of the interleukin-10 5′ flanking region determine variable interleukin-10 transcription and are associated with particular phenotypes of juvenile rheumatoid arthritis. *Arthritis Rheum* 1999; 42(6):1101–118.

44. Zeggini, E., Thomson, W., Kwiatkowski, D., Richardson, A., Ollier, W., and Donn, R. Linkage and association studies of single-nucleotide polymorphism-tagged tumor necrosis factor haplotypes in juvenile oligoarthritis. *Arthritis Rheum* 2002;46(12):3304–11.

45. Fishman, D., Faulds, G., Jeffery, R., Mohamed-Ali, V., Yudkin, J.S., Humphries, S., and Woo, P., The effect of novel polymorphisms in the interleukin-6 (IL-6) gene on IL-6 transcription and plasma IL-6 levels, and an association with systemic-onset juvenile chronic arthritis. *J Clin Invest* 1998;102(7):1369–76.

46. Pignatti, P., Vivarelli, M., Meazza, C., Rizzolo, M.G., Martini, A., and De Benedetti, F., Abnormal regulation of interleukin 6 in systemic juvenile idiopathic arthritis. J., *Rheumatol* 2001;28(7):1670–6.

47. Scola, M.P., Thompson, S.D., Brunner, H.I., Tsoras, M.K., Witte, D., Van Dijk, M.A., Grom, A.A., Passo, M.H., and Glass, D.N., Interferon-gamma: interleukin 4 ratios and associated type 1 cytokine expression in juvenile rheumatoid arthritis synovial tissue. *J Rheumatol* 2002;29(2):369–78.

48. Gattorno, M., Facchetti, P., Ghiotto, F., Vignola, S., Buoncompagni, A., and Prigione, I., Synovial fluid T cell clones from oigoarticular juvenile arthritis patients display a prevalent Th1/Th0 pattern of cytokine secretion irrespective of immunophenotype. *Clin Exp Immunol* 1997;109(4–11).

49. Jonuleit, H., and Schmitt, E., The regulatory T cell family: distinct subsets and their interrelations. *J Immunol* 2003; 171(12): 6323–7.

50. Murray, K.J., Grom, A.A., Thompson, S.D., Lieuwen, D., Passo, M.H., and Glass, D.N., Contrasting cytokine profiles in the synovium of different forms of juvenile rheumatoid arthritis and juvenile spondyloarthropathy: prominence of interleukin 4 in restricted disease. *J Rheumatol* 1998;25(7):1388–98.

51. Iellem, A., Mariani, M., Lang, R., Recalde, H., Panina-Bordignon, P., Sinigaglia, F., and D'Ambrosio, D., Unique chemotactic response profile and specific expression of chemokine receptors CCR4 and CCR8 by CD4(+)CD25(+) regulatory T cells. *J Exp Med* 2001;194(6): 847–53.

52. de Kleer, I.M., Kamphuis, S.M., Rijkers, G.T., Scholtens, L., Gordon, G., De Jager, W., Hafner, R., van de Zee, R., van Eden, W., Kuis, W., and Prakken, B.J. The spontaneous remission of juvenile idiopathic arthritis is characterized by CD30+ T cells directed to human heat-shock protein 60 capable of producing the regulatory cytokine interleukin-10. *Arthritis Rheum* 2003;48(7):2001–10.

53. Wulffraat, N.M., Haas, P.J., Frosch, M., De Kleer, I.M., Vogl, T., Brinkman, D.M., Quartier, P., Roth, J., and Kuis, W., Myeloid related protein 8 and 14 secretion reflects phagocyte activation and correlates with disease activity in juvenile idiopathic arthritis treated with autologous stem cell transplantation. *Ann Rheum Dis* 2003;62(3):236–41.

54. Frosch, M., Vogl, T., Seeliger, S., Wulffraat, N., Kuis, W., Viemann, D., Foell, D., Sorg, C., Sunderkotter, C., and Roth, J. Expression of myeloid-related proteins 8 and 14 in systemic-onset juvenile rheumatoid arthritis. *Arthritis Rheum* 2003;48(9):2622–6.

55. Harding, B., and Knight, S.C., The distribution of dendritic cells in the synovial fluids of patients with arthritis. *Clin Exp Immunol* 1986;63(3):594–600.

56. Gattorno, M., Chicha, L., Gregorio, A., Ferlito, F., Viola, S., Ravelli, A., Mantz, M., and Martini, A., Enrichment of plasmacytoid dendritic cells in synovial fluid of juvenile idiopathic arthritis. *Arthritis Rheum* 2003;48 (9, Suppl. 1):S101.

57. Oen, K., Malleson, P.N., Cabral, D.A., Rosenberg, A.M., Petty, R.E., Reed, M., Schroeder, M.L., and Cheang, M., Early predictors of longterm outcome in patients with juvenile rheumatoid arthritis: subset-specific correlations. *J Rheumatol* 2003;30(3):585–93.

58. Cassidy, J.T., Sullivan, D.B., and Petty, R.E., Clinical patterns of chronic iridocyclitis in children with juvenile rheumatoid arthritis. *Arthritis Rheum* 1977;20(2, Supp. l):224–7.

59. Kanski, J.J. Uveitis in juvenile chronic arthritis. *Clin Exp Rheumatol* 1990;8(5):499–503.

60. Massa, M., Pignatti, P., Oliveri, M., De Amici, M., De Benedetti, F., and Martini, A., Serum soluble CD23 levels and CD23 expression on peripheral blood mononuclear cells in juvenile chronic arthritis. *Clin Exp Rheumatol* 1998;16(5):611–6.

61. Firestein, G.S., and Zvaifler, N.J., How important are T cells in chronic rheumatoid synovitis?: II. T cell-independent mechanisms from beginning to end. *Arthritis Rheum* 2002;46(2):298–308.

62. Buckley, C.D., Pilling, D., Lord, J.M., Akbar, A.N., Scheel-Toellner, D., and Salmon, M., Fibroblasts regulate the switch from acute resolving to chronic persistent inflammation. *Trends Immunol* 2001;22(4): 199–204.

63. Fawcett, L.B., Fawcett, P.T., Vinette, K.M.B., Stetson, T., Rose, C., and Jefferson, T., Culture and charateristics of synovial fibroblast like cells from samples of synovial fluid obtained from pateitns with juvneile arthritis. *Arthritis Rheum* 2003;48(9, Suppl):S101.

64. Jarvis, J., Dozmorov, I., Jiang, K., Frank, M., Szodaray, P., Alex, P., and Centola, M., Novel approaches to gene expression analysis of active polyarticular juvenile rheumatoid arthritis. *Arthritis Res Ther* 2004;6(1): R15–R32.

2.10 Genetic and cytokine associations in Juvenile Idiopathic Arthritis

Wendy Thomson, Patricia Woo, and Rachelle Donn

Aim

Juvenile idiopathic arthritis (JIA) is a heterogeneous condition of unknown aetiology but both environmental and genetic factors are believed to play a role. The aim of this chapter is to review the evidence that supports a genetic basis to JIA and to detail our current understanding of the genes involved in JIA susceptibility.

Structure

- The evidence for a genetic component to JIA
- Methods for investigating the genetic basis of JIA
- Genes involved in susceptibility to JIA
- Conclusions

The evidence for a genetic component to JIA

Evidence for a genetic component to a disease can come from a variety of sources, such as twin studies, family studies, or association studies. The degree of disease concordance in monozygotic (MZ) twins gives an indication of the level of involvement of genetic factors within a given disease. An alternative estimate of the genetic component of a disease can be obtained from family studies using the sibling recurrence risk or lambda s (λs). Lambda s is calculated as the prevalence of the disease in sibs of affected individuals divided by the prevalence of the disease in the general population.

Unfortunately, for a disease with low population prevalence such as JIA, accounts of twin- and family-based studies are quite limited. Some reports do exist and these are summarized below. From these it is possible to infer that there is a sizeable genetic component to JIA.

Twin studies

Meyerowitz reported [1] on eight sets of twins discordant for rheumatoid arthritis (RA), three of which had a juvenile onset (one seropositive, the other two pauciarticular). Ansell *et al.* reported 11 twin pairs (5 MZ and 6 dizygotic (DZ) [2]. Two pairs, both MZ, were concordant for disease. This study was later extended to include a total of 24 twin pairs (12 MZ and 12 DZ) in which 6 MZ pairs, but no DZ pairs, were concordant for disease [3]. Baum and Fink described a set of female MZ twins concordant for seronegative erosive arthritis [4]. Kapusta detailed concordance of juvenile rheumatoid arthritis (JRA) in a mother and her two identical twin sons, and Husby described a set of twins concordant for clinical features, including iritis, but discordant for amyloidosis and monoclonal gammopathy [5,6]. The largest study comes from the National Institute of Arthritis and Musculoskeletal and Skin Diseases (NIAMS) sponsored Research Registry for JRA Affected Sibling Pairs (ASPs). Of 118 ASPs on the register in 2000, there were 14 pairs of twins where both twins have arthritis [7]. One pair comprises a girl with polyarticular JRA and a boy with pauciarticular JRA. The other 13 pairs (11 MZ, 2 DZ, and 2 of unknown zygosity) were concordant for gender (9 female, 4 male), disease onset (10 pauciarticular, 3 polyarticular), and disease course (8 pauciarticular, 5 polyarticular).

Finally, in a recent Finnish study of JIA multicase families, eight sets of twins were identified, two of which were concordant for arthritis. A concordance rate of 25% for a disease with a population prevalence of 1 per 1000 implies a relative risk of JIA of 250 for an MZ twin.

Affected Sibling Pairs (ASP) studies

There have been only a few reports of multicase families in the literature and, to date, only three ASP series have been described. Clemens *et al.* identified 12 ASPs with seronegative juvenile chronic arthritis from the United Kingdom and Germany [8]. Ten out of twelve of these pairs were concordant for pauciarticular onset.

As mentioned above, the largest series of ASPs comes from the NIAMS sponsored registry for JRA ASPs in the United States. In 1997, the registry contained a series of 71 ASPs, 63% were concordant for gender and 76% for onset type, higher than expected based on comparisons with non-ASP populations. This study provided, for the first time, an estimate of the λs for JRA; this was around 15, a value similar to that seen in insulin-dependent diabetes mellitus (IDDM) and multiple sclerosis (MS). However, it also provided evidence that this value is likely to differ between subtypes [9,10]. The registry now contains 183 ASPs from 164 families, 19 of which are twin pairs [11]. There is a relatively high degree of disease onset type concordance between the ASPs, 53% concordant for pauciarticular onset and 19% for polyarticular onset, except for those with systemic disease. In addition, the clinical manifestations seen within ASPs are similar to those in a simplex population, the only exception being a higher number of affected joints in simplex polyarticular patients.

In Finland, 49 ASPs from 37 families were identified from a population of approximately 2000 JIA cases. Within the ASPs there was little difference found for either onset type (57% concordance in ASPs), or disease course (61% concordance in ASPs) when compared with a population-based JIA series. Given a population prevalence of JIA of around 1 per 1000, this study suggests that the λs for JIA is around 25, again supporting the idea of a substantial genetic component in the aetiology of JIA [12].

Key point summary

- There is a strong genetic component to JIA.

- Family studies suggest that the λs for JIA as a whole is between 15 and 25. This may vary between the different JIA subtypes.

- Twin and family studies support the idea of JIA being a complex oligogenic disease.

Methods for investigating the genetic basis of JIA

Two types of study design are widely employed to determine whether nucleotide variations within a gene contribute to the expression of a complex genetic disease, such as JIA. These are linkage- and association-based studies. Linkage and association studies are distinct approaches, each with advantages and limitations in the context of studying JIA and are best viewed as complementary methods.

Association studies

The commonest form of association analysis is a case-control study. Here assessment is made as to whether the frequency of a particular allele (i.e. difference in DNA sequence in or near the gene of interest), genotype (the set of alleles on both chromosomes in an individual), or haplotype (a series of alleles on one chromosome) is enriched in JIA patients compared with that observed in unaffected controls. The controls should be individuals that are not related to the cases, but are of the same genetic ancestry (Caucasian, Asian, or Mongoloid). Genetic markers are usually, but not necessarily, polymorphic sites within a gene of interest. Much recent interest has focussed on single nucleotide polymorphisms (SNPs). Allelic enrichment (or association) implies that:

(1) the marker is causally involved in disease susceptibility or severity; or

(2) the pathogenic gene(s) is in *linkage disequilibrium* (LD) (i.e. non-randomly mixed during meiosis) with alleles of the associated marker

Polymorphic changes conferring only a marginal increase in disease risk (defined as *neither necessary nor sufficient for disease to manifest*) can be identified by association studies. Cumulatively, or individually, these changes may have functional consequences that cause the disease, or alter the disease severity and course.

Association studies are advantageous in terms of 'statistical power' as each affected case and control subject is utilized in the analysis, leading to high sensitivity in the test. However, they are plagued by the concern of 'population stratification'. This occurs where cases and controls differ, not only with respect to the expressed phenotype (i.e. observed clinical outcome) and its underlying genetic risk components, but also with respect to their overall population genetic ancestry. This can occur despite efforts of researchers to 'genetically match' cases and controls. As a result, many genetic markers can spuriously appear to be associated with disease. To circumvent this problem, case-control studies have to be replicated in different populations, or confirmed by the transmission disequilibrium test.

Linkage studies

Linkage studies employ the use of *family* material, such as affected sibling pairs and multicase families. Linkage compares the segregation pattern of genetic markers across the genome and the disease state. Since stretches of DNA that are physically close to each other are less likely to be separated during meiotic recombination than distantly spaced sequences, markers that co-segregate with the disease (in family studies) are close to the chromosomal localization of the underlying disease gene. For a positive result from linkage analysis the mathematics dictates that the mutations/polymorphism under investigation must be strong predictors of the disease (*actually necessary and sufficient for the expression of the disease to occur*). The comparison of different alleles of the tested markers in different families can provide cumulative evidence for positive linkage to disease.

To ensure linkage studies have adequate statistical power to identify the susceptibility loci, sufficient numbers of either multicase families or affected sibling pairs with JIA must be studied. Unfortunately, this is largely an unfeasible undertaking, since multicase families are exceedingly rare and sibling pairs uncommon. A popular alternative is the transmission disequilibrium test (TDT). The advantage of the TDT for JIA is that it requires only one affected (child) and one, or both, of their parents (simplex or TDT-families). The analysis is dependant on the genotype information from a parent heterozygous for the marker locus. It considers whether one allele is preferentially transmitted to the affected child more often than would be expected by chance. If a heterozygous parent has one copy of a marker allele then there would be a 50:50 chance that they would transmit it to a child. However, if a marker is both linked to and associated with a disease gene, then the total number of transmissions of this allele as compared to the non-associated allele in a cohort of simplex families, will be greater than 50:50. Usually, a large cohort of simplex families is needed to have sufficient statistical power to assess this distortion in transmission. A distinct advantage of the TDT method is that even if only one parent is available the test can be informative. It does, however, depend on that parent being a heterozygote. Hence, the usefulness of the TDT is maximised when using genetic markers with high heterozygosity.

Clinical and biological homogeneity is important

Juvenile Idiopathic Arthritis is a group of heterogeneous diseases in terms of both pathology and clinical course. This clinical heterogeneity implies genetic heterogeneity. Therefore, there are at least two hypotheses that can be explored. The first is that there are gene(s) contributing to JIA as a whole, and that different phenotypes are the result of modifying environmental influences. The second is that each clinical subgroup is a separate disease, each with a potentially diverse genetic base. These questions are central to the design and subsequent analysis of data generated from studies looking for disease susceptibility and severity genes. There is no doubt that the more clinically homogeneous the disease group studied, the greater the possibility of detecting true genetic effects.

Power

Central to all the genetic studies undertaken for JIA, or any disease, is the issue of statistical power. If, as is the case for a rare condition such as JIA, only a limited pool of cases are available for study, the important question is 'how likely is it that a statistically significant effect of a given magnitude can be identified among this patient group?'. Several packages exist for calculating power. Quanto (http://hydra.usc.edu/gxe) is one which is particularly user-friendly and can be used to generate power calculations for both case-control (association) and TDT studies [13,14].

Replication studies

With any positive association found in a case-control study, *replication* is critical. This can be done by:

1. Looking at the same factors in a JIA population of different genetic ancestry.

2. Studying JIA in one population, but taking an initial result from an association study and attempting to confirm the result by linkage analysis, or vice-versa.

Through international collaborations this process should become an achievable goal. This will enhance the quality of the genetic findings reported for JIA and help to focus researchers' attentions to the most promising loci for additional investigation.

Key point summary

- There are two main types of studies used to investigate the genetic component of a complex disease such as JIA. These are association and linkage studies. The TDT analysis, which determines linkage in the presence of association, is particularly useful for studying JIA.

- Large panels of JIA TDT families have been collected in both the United States and the United Kingdom and will enhance the genetic studies being undertaken.

- Genetic studies require replication.

- Genetic studies should be performed in clinically homogeneous groups.

Genes involved in susceptibility to JIA

The various types of arthritides in children (collectively known as JIA) differ in their clinical manifestations, severity, clinical disease course, and immunopathology. In the rest of this chapter, positive disease associations are described for a number of candidate genes. The rationale for the choice of candidate genes by investigators has often been based on the information for disease pathogenesis in adult RA, although this disease (RF Positive Polyarthritis—see Part 2, Chapter 2.4) is rare in children. More recently, as the pathology has become better described in the different types of JIA, candidate genes have been proposed from results of studies on disease mechanisms found in the different types of JIA.

For example, Systemic Arthritis is a syndrome with a characteristic quotidian fever pattern that parallels the rise and fall of serum interleukin (IL)-6 levels [15]. IL-6 has been found to be associated with disease activity in Systemic Arthritis, but not in Polyarthritis or Oligoarthritis [16]. The latter two types of arthritides have a different disease course and severity profile. Polarised Type 1 T cell responses in the blood and synovial fluid have been demonstrated for Polyarthritis and Oligoarthritis but this is not found in children with Systemic Arthritis [17] (see also Part 2, Chapter 2.9, 'Immunopathology of the joint in JIA'). Furthermore, the synovial tissues from Persistent Oligoarthritis patients show different proportions of type 1 and regulatory T cells, compared with that observed in Polyarthritis [18,19]. In the absence of any identifiable agent found within the joint, genetic imbalance of the cytokine network, as well as disturbances of the MHC/peptide/T cell complex, have been postulated to be causal and/or contributory to the diseases and candidate genes in these areas have been analysed for disease association.

Some arthritides are more erosive than others (e.g. RF Positive Polyarthritis and Systemic Arthritis, compared with Enthesitis Related Arthritis or Oligoarthritis), suggesting differing pathological processes. Genetic differences in bone turnover and repair may be important. Neuroendocrine control of the stress response may also be relevant if data in RA are extrapolated to some types of JIA. Candidate genes in these areas have also been studied and will be briefly reviewed.

Finally, the data from the first whole genome scan in JIA has recently been published and will also be reviewed.

HLA and JIA

Much of the genetic work in the past three decades has centred around HLA genes. HLA genes are found in a region of the genome called the Major Histocompatibility Complex, located on chromosome 6p21.3. HLA molecules can be divided into class I (HLA-A, HLA-B, and HLA-C) and class II (HLA-DR, DQ, and DPB) depending upon their function. In brief, HLA class I molecules are expressed on the surface of all nucleated cells and are involved in the presentation of endogenous antigens to CD8+ cytotoxic T cells, whereas, class II molecules are only expressed on the surface of cells involved in the immune response (e.g. macrophages, dendritic cells, B cells, and endothelial cells) and present exogenous antigens to CD4+ helper T cells. The fact that HLA molecules play a central role in the immune system has led to HLA genes being considered as candidates in association studies in many diseases, particularly those thought to have an immune basis such as JIA.

Most of the previous studies of HLA and JIA have been in children classified according to either the European League Against Rheumatism (EULAR) or American College of Rheumatology (ACR) criteria. Further subdivision of pauciarticular JRA/JCA (juvenile chronic arthritis) according to the age at disease onset and polyarticular JRA according to rheumatoid factor status has often been included.

HLA class I associations

The earliest report for HLA class I was of an association between HLA-B27 and older, particularly male, children with pauciarticular JRA [20]. This has since been confirmed in a number of studies [21,22]. Many of these children also develop sacroiliitis, and would be classified as Enthesitis Related Arthritis (ERA) by the current ILAR classification. In a recent study of UK cases classified according to the ILAR criteria, 76% of ERA patients were found to be HLA-B27 positive [23] compared with a population frequency of around 10%.

A second well-documented HLA class I association is, that of HLA-A2 with Oligoarthritis patients. HLA-A2 was first reported to be associated with female Oligoarthritis patients [24]. The association between HLA-A2 and Oligoarthritis has since been confirmed and has also been demonstrated to be particularly strong in children with an early disease onset (22,25–27).

HLA class II associations

The first studies looking at HLA class II associations demonstrated an increase in HLA-DR5 and DR8 in early onset Oligoarthritis patients [28,29] (see also Part 2, Chapter 2.3). Since then there have been numerous studies of HLA class II associations. Many of the early studies were reviewed by Donn and Ollier [22] and Albert and Scholtz [30]. A brief description of the associations found with each of the different subgroup is given below.

The largest number of studies has focused on the association of HLA class II genes with Oligoarthritis. The majority have confirmed the original finding of an increase in HLA-DRB1*11 (a subtype of HLA-DR5) and HLA-DRB1*08 (26,27,31–35). In addition, many studies have also shown a significant decrease in both HLA-DRB1*04 and HLA-DRB1*07(27,33,34,36). These associations are particularly strong in children with an early disease onset (27,35,37). Some studies also report an increase in HLA-DRB1*13, particularly in ANA positive children [38].

HLA DPB1*0201 has also been consistently shown to be associated with Oligoarthritis and, again, this is strongest in females with an early disease onset [30,38].

In a recent study of ILAR classified UK cases, the haplotypes DRB1*0801-DQA1*0401-DQB1*0402 and DRB1*11-DQA1*05-DQB1*03 were increased and DRB1*0401-DQA1*03-DQB1*03 and DRB1*0701-DQA1*0201-DQB1*0201 decreased in both Persistent and Extended Oligoarthritis. In addition, DRB1*13-DQA1*01-DQB1*06 was associated with an increased risk of Persistent Oligoarthritis. HLA-DPB1*0201 was also increased in both groups [23].

RF Negative Polyarthritis in children is less well studied and the HLA associations less well defined. Associations have been reported with HLA-DR8 (32,33,39,40) and HLA-DQ4 (DQA1*0401/DQB1*0402) [32,40]. An increase in HLA-DP3 (DPB1*0301) has also been found in some studies (32,33,40). Within the United Kingdom the association with HLA-DRB1*08 has been confirmed recently in ILAR classified children [23].

Children with RF Positive Polyarthritis are generally considered to be immunogenetically similar to adult RA. Early studies of children with RF Positive Polyarthritis demonstrated an increase in HLA-DR4 [28]. This similarity with adult RA has since been confirmed in many studies (32,33,41). In a Japanese population HLA-DRB1*0405 was shown to be increased in both RF Positive Polyarthritis and RF positive adult RA cases [42]. Within a UK cohort the association with HLA-DR4 has also been confirmed [23]. In contrast to previous studies, a recent study of a small number of children with RF Positive Polyarthritis in the Cree and Ojibway populations in Canada found no association with HLA-DR4 or any other shared epitope positive allele, but did find an increase in HLA-DRB1*0901 [43].

Systemic Arthritis consistently shows the weakest and most limited HLA associations. Some studies have reported an increase in HLA-DR5 and HLA-DR8 (38,39,44). Other studies have shown an increase in HLA-DR4 in Systemic Arthritis patients [45–49]. A more recent study of 108 French children with Systemic Arthritis found no association with HLA-DR4 [50] and a Greek study of JIA cases, classified according to the ILAR criteria, also found no HLA associations with this subgroup of patients [51]. In a recent study of 502 UK cases, classified according to the ILAR criteria, we reported an increase in HLA-DRB1*11 (a subset of HLA-DR5) in children with Systemic Arthritis [23].

To date there has only been one study which included ERA and Psoriatic Arthritis. In this study, a UK cohort, there was an increase in the haplotype DRB1*01-DQA1*0101-DQB1*0501. This association appears to be independent of HLA-B27 [23].

HLA linkage in JIA

Despite there being multiple case-control studies showing an association between HLA and JIA susceptibility, it is still possible that these findings are spurious and simply due to population stratification. A number of recent studies have been able to confirm the association by establishing linkage. Moroldo et al. showed linkage to both HLA class I and class II using the TDT in pauciarticular-onset JRA patients [52]. HLA-A2, HLA-B27 and B35, and HLA-DR5 and DR8 all showed excess transmission, whereas HLA-DR4 was under transmitted. A second study confirmed linkage using the TDT in a UK cohort of Oligoarthritis [53]. Here HLA-A2, HLA-DRB1*08, and DRB1*11 were over-transmitted and HLA-A3 and HLA-DRB1*04 and 07 under-transmitted. This study was able to demonstrate that the effects at these two loci are independent. Finally, linkage analysis utilising the ASPs within the NIAMS sponsored registry for JRA, has confirmed linkage between pauciarticular JRA and HLA-DR and established linkage between polyarticular JRA and HLA-DR [54]. This report estimated that the λs_{HLA} is 2.5, indicating that HLA accounts for only 17% of total genetic component of pauciarticular JRA. Hence, other non-HLA genes must play a role in susceptibility.

Key point summary

- There are both HLA class I and class II associations with JIA.

- Some HLA associations are common to all JIA and others subgroup specific.

- Non-HLA genes also play a role in JIA susceptibility.

Cytokine genes in JIA

Cytokines and T cell polarisation

After exposure to an antigen precursor, helper T cells differentiate predominantly into two major types with respect to their function and the range of cytokines they produce [40]. The degree of polarization and heterogeneity of T cells may reflect the nature of the antigenic and environmental stimuli to which the cells have been exposed. This is particularly true of responses to persistent infections with microbes, such as Leishmania, Listeria, mycobacteria (Th1), and helminths (Th2). The cytokines produced by Th1 T cells include IL-2, -3, interferon (IFN)γ, granulocyte–macrophage colony stimulating factor (GM-CSF), and tumour necrosis factor (TNF)α and β. Th2 cells secrete IL-3, 4, 5, 6, 10, GM-CSF, and TNFα. These two major pathways of T cell differentiation are mutually antagonistic. Two other 'regulatory' or 'anti-inflammatory' CD4+ T cell subtypes have been described: Th3 cells that are characterized by secretion of transforming growth factor (TGF)β, and 'regulatory' T cells that are characterised by the secretion of IL-10 (see Part 2, Chapter 2.9 'Immunopathology of the joint in JIA').

Differentiation into these types of cells occurs mainly under the influence of two cytokines, IL-12 and IL-4. IL-12 is produced by monocytic antigen presenting cells, including dendritic cells. In conjunction with co-stimulatory molecules, IL-12 promotes differentiation of potential T helper cells (Th0) to an IFNγ secreting Th1 phenotype, which is responsible for cell-mediated immunity. IL-4 is the cytokine with an autocrine function that promotes T cells to differentiate into the Th2 phenotype, responsible for T cell help in antibody response.

Predominantly, Th1 type T cells are found in certain autoimmune diseases (e.g. IDDM, RA, MS [55–57] and Oligoarthritis [58], and a Th2 polarisation is seen in systemic lupus erythematosus (SLE). Thus, persistent polarisation into either Th1 or 2 can lead to pathology [59]. There is some evidence that the pro-inflammatory element is mediated by T memory cells with the Th1 phenotype which secrete IL-17. The question of whether this is antigen-driven or genetically driven is still open. Recent work on T cell receptor usage to characterize oligoclonality in synovial fluid cells has shown multiple oligoclonalities in Oligoarthritis and Polyarthritis [60] (also see Part 2, Chapter 2.9 'Immunopathology of the joint in JIA'). These findings, coupled with the effect of TNFα on cell signaling [61], suggest a non-antigenic driven event that can be pathogenic. One hypothesis is a genetically deregulated immune response, allowing the network to 'settle' in a polarized manner upon stimulation independent of a specific antigenic drive.

Balance within the cytokine network in inflammation

Cytokines are small proteins and polypeptides that mediate cell growth, differentiation, and cell-to-cell interactions. They have been recognised as critical mediators within the immune system and the inflammatory response. The generic term also encompasses the chemokines, which are mediators of cell traffic [62]. These mediators interact with each other in a complex network. There are hierarchical cascades, positive and negative feedback loops (Figure 2.10.1), which lead to some redundancy and pleiotropism of each cytokine. This is important in a biological system in order to allow a degree of inertia to an external stimulus, but also rapid response and recovery. The network has 'nodal' or key players, whose effects are more influential. A few have been identified. For example, IL-1 and TNFα are two major pro-inflammatory cytokines, each with the ability to initiate a cascade of other pro-inflammatory cytokines and chemokines and also have direct effects on cell function. TNF has anti-apoptotic

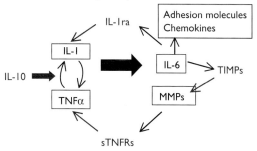

Figure 2.10.1 An example of the interactions of some of the 'key cytokines' and their inhibitors. Pro-inflammatory cytokines are in white, and the inhibitors are in red. IL-6 is interesting in that it induces the cellular inflammatory reaction, but also induces inhibitors of the pro-inflammatory cytokines such as IL-1ra and sTNFR. IL-1, 6, 10 = interleukin 1, 6, 10; IL-1ra = interleukin 1 receptor antagonist; TNFα = Tumour necrosis factor alpha; sTNFRs = soluble TNF receptors, which serve as inhibitors of TNF signalling; MMP = metalloproteinases; TIMP = metalloproteinase inhibitors.

effects and affects T cell receptor signalling, while IL-1 can stimulate proteinases that degrade cartilage and matrix. IL-6 is another potent pro-inflammatory cytokine, leading to chemokine release and accumulation of inflammatory cell types, such as granulocytes. It also has the ability to stimulate a number of cytokine antagonists, such as IL-1RA, sTNFR, and inhibitors of metalloproteinases, thus occupying a unique position as a 'nodal' member in several networks. A potent anti-inflammatory cytokine is IL-10, which suppresses the synthesis of the above three key pro-inflammatory cytokines. It is also the mediator that is secreted by regulatory T and B cells. With respect to the differentiation and polarization of type 1 and type 2 T helper cells, IL-4 and IFNγ are mutually inhibitory, and IL-10, secreted by regulatory T cells, have an additional effect on both types of cells.

Cytokine gene polymorphisms

The coding sequences of cytokine and cytokine receptor genes are generally highly conserved. Mutations usually lead to alteration in the function of the protein and subsequent pathology. More recently, Single nucleotide polymorphisms (SNPs) in the 5′ flanking regions of cytokine receptor genes, such as IL-4R and IFNγR1, have been described. Whether they affect the expression of the receptors remains to be determined. Cytokine genes are highly polymorphic in the 5′ and, to a lesser extent, the 3′ and intronic regions. Studies of the polymorphic variants of cytokine and cytokine receptor genes have shown *in vitro* and *in vivo* variations in gene expression (e.g. TNFα [63,64] TNFβ [65], IL-1 gene cluster [66,67], IL-6 [68,69], IL-10 [70,71], MIF (see below), IFNγ [72], IFNγR1 [73], and TGFβ [74]). Many of these variations are SNPs in the 5′ flanking regions of the gene, causing variation in gene transcription. They may represent candidate alleles for disease susceptibility, or severity, as well as responders and non-responders to drug therapies.

Cytokine and cytokine receptor genes as candidates for susceptibility to inflammatory and autoimmune diseases have been studied by case control association methods in the majority of cases [62]. One of the first genetic associations of JIA with an inflammatory cytokine was described by McDowell *et al.* [75]. This study showed that an IL-1A2 polymorphism in JIA is associated with a higher risk for developing uveitis in Norwegian Oligoarthritis, but Donn *et al.* [76] failed to confirm this association in a UK cohort. This association will need confirmation by the TDT in Norwegian families to see if the IL-1 locus has an influence on the phenotype of Oligoarthritis and, in particular, uveitis. Furthermore, this is likely to be in linkage disequilibrium with other SNPs and haplotype analysis is needed across the whole IL-1 region. The function of this SNP is also unknown at present and, again, functional haplotype analysis is required. Another key pro-inflammatory cytokine is TNFα. There are many reports of positive and also negative disease associations with a few TNFα SNPs. Until recently, the TNFα literature has been difficult to follow. This has been partly because of contradictory reports, underpowered studies, and authors ignoring the linkage/interaction with other genes in the major histocompatibility region of chromosome 6. However, haplotype analyses of a control population and a population of Oligoarthritis have revealed that there are HLA-independent TNF haplotypes that are significantly associated with JIA [77]. What these haplotypes do still needs to be characterized.

There have been many studies of the anti-inflammatory gene IL-10 and the allelic associations with inflammatory rheumatic diseases. Although there have been reports of raised levels of inflammatory cytokines in the synovial fluid and plasma of children with JIA, it has been difficult to demonstrate imbalance on a molecular basis. This is mainly due to the instability of some inflammatory cytokines and the differing sensitivity of the method of detection of the individual cytokines and their antagonists. The hypothesis that the expression of the general anti-inflammatory cytokine IL-10 is genetically lower in the more severe JIA subtype was tested by a combination of a case-control genetic association study of children with Persistent Oligoarthritis versus Extended Oligoarthritis and a study of IL-10 protein production in blood cultures from parents of children with either phenotype. The production of IL-10 was lower in the parents of children with Persistent Oligoarthritis and these parents had a significantly increased frequency of the 'ATA' IL-10 haplotype [70]. The children with the more severe disease (Extended Oligoarthritis) also had a significantly increased frequency of the IL-10 ATA haplotype. In asthma, the ATA allele of IL-10 was also significantly raised in the more severe cases of a case-control study [78], thus providing further evidence for the probability that the IL-10 ATA allele is at least a disease severity gene in inflammatory diseases. More recent work has identified a large number of SNPs further upstream of these haplotypes as well as two variable microsatellites, Further work is therefore needed to determine which haplotypic variants are functionally important in the regulation of the expression of IL-10, and whether a disease susceptibility/severity haplotype exists.

A positive association between a polymorphism in the 3′UTR of the interferon regulatory factor (IRF)-1 gene, which maps to a 'cytokine gene cluster' on the long arm of chromosome 5 (5q31), has been found to be significantly associated with JIA as a whole [79]. IRF-1 is an important transcription factor for Type 1 T cell cytokines and the function of this genetic variant has yet to be established.

There are two genes that have proven to be disease susceptibility genes in JIA: IL-6 and macrophage inhibitory factor. The case for Systemic Arthritis being an IL-6 mediated disease has been proposed by Woo [80] and well argued in an editorial by De Benedetti and Martini [81]. Many of the clinical features are typical of excessive IL-6 production (e.g. fever, hypergamma globulinaemia, thrombocytosis, anaemia, and stunted growth). A SNP (-174) in the regulatory region of the IL-6 gene, that determines transcriptional response of the IL-6 gene to IL-1 and LPS, was identified. The GG genotype has significantly higher serum IL-6 levels than CC. There was a significant lack of the protective genotype (CC: low producer of IL-6 on stimulation by IL-1/LPS) in children that develop Systemic Arthritis [68]. A multi-centre TDT study confirmed that IL-6 G allele is a susceptibility gene for Systemic Arthritis [82]. Further SNPs upstream of this variant have been found and analyses of haplotypes suggest a more complex genetic regulation of IL-6. Therefore, identification of functional haplotypes and re-examination of these disease cohorts will be necessary to assess the relative risk conferred by IL-6 in this particular disease.

Macrophage inhibitory factor is a unique molecule that has pro-inflammatory, hormonal, and enzymatic properties [83]. A novel polymorphism in the 5′ flanking region (-173) of the macrophage migration inhibitory factor (MIF) gene was reported to be associated, initially with UK Systemic Arthritis [84], and subsequently with susceptibility to all JIA irrelevant of subgroup [85]. The mutant allele of this SNP (MIF-173*C) results in higher endogenous MIF production in the serum of healthy individuals and in higher MIF production in both the serum and synovial fluids of JIA cases. Furthermore, this same promoter polymorphism of MIF (MIF-173*C) has also been shown to be predictive of disease outcome in patients with Systemic Arthritis [86]. More specifically, De Benedetti et al. found that carriage of the MIF-173*C polymorphism was correlated with raised serum and synovial fluid levels of MIF protein and predictive of the duration of response to intra-articular injection of triamcinolone hexacetonide (TXA). Those individuals with a mutant allele at -173 (MIF-173*C) relapsed more quickly than individuals with the MIF-173 GG wild type genotype [86]. This effect has now been demonstrated for the response to intra-articular TXA injection in patients with Oligoarthritis. Again, the duration of clinical response to the steroid treatment (months with no clinical evidence of synovitis) was significantly shorter in patients carrying a MIF-173*C allele (median 6 months; range 1–39) than in the MIF-173*GG homozygotes (median 9 months, range 2–62) (87).

Donn et al. replicated their initial association study of MIF and JIA using the TDT test. This work revealed that a particular promoter haplotype of the MIF gene (CATT$_7$-MIF-173*C) is both linked and associated with an increased risk of JIA susceptibility [88]. Further studies have shown this promoter haplotype to also confer increased risk to adult inflammatory polyarthritis [89] and to psoriasis [90].

Key point summary

- Studying the polymorphisms in cytokine genes and their functional significance will give a clearer indication as to which cytokines are important in the pathogenesis of JIA.

- Association studies should attempt to consider all the possible variants within the gene locus and disease associations and functional analysis of gene regulation should be with haplotypes.

- While several positive associations have been described for cytokine gene polymorphisms and JIA susceptibility, only a limited number of these have been replicated.

- Determining the association with, and the functional significance of cytokine gene polymorphisms could offer novel therapeutic targets for the management of JIA patients.

Other genes and JIA

In common with other chronic inflammatory diseases, the genetic basis to JIA is complex. In particular, genes that have actions specific to the type of arthritis, or certain clinical aspects, may be more difficult to identify. Our current selection of candidate genes for investigation in JIA is based simply on our perceptions of the underlying pathological processes thought to be occurring, either locally within an inflamed joint, or systemically. In addition to the cytokine gene polymorphisms discussed above, several researchers have studied other genetic loci. A number of positive associations have been described for genes within the Major histocompatibility complex (MHC) region, other than HLA molecules. However, the possibility of these 'positive' findings being the result of linkage disequilibrium with HLA alleles has not always been fully investigated. These non-HLA MHC loci may represent additional susceptibility genes and, as such, further studies would be of interest.

Positive associations with non-HLA MHC genes and JIA

Pryhuber et al. have found a particular genotype of the proteasome LMP2 gene (LMP2BB) is associated with children who have a late age of disease onset (≥6 years) and less than five joints at initial presentation. This genotype was also increased in patients with Polyarthritis at initial presentation and in individuals who progressed from <5 joints to having ≥5 joints involved. Pryhuber also found the effect of the BB genotype not to be due to linkage disequilibrium with HLA-B27 [91].

Ploski et al. looked at polymorphisms of the transporters associated with antigen processing genes (TAP1 and TAP2) and found TAP1B to be associated with juvenile arthritis patients (of mixed phenotypes) [92]. This association was independent of the known HLA class II associations with TAP genes.

Donn et al. also looked at the TAP genes and found an association, this time with the TAP2B allele and early onset Oligoarthritis (age at onset ≤ 6 yrs, ≤ 4 joints at presentation). This was found to be independent of the known linkage disequilibrium described between TAP2B and HLA-DRB1 [93].

Other genes within the extended MHC may also play a role in JIA. Linkage and association of multiple markers across the MHC have been assessed in Oligoarthritis using the TDT [53]. This study suggested that in addition to HLA-A and HLA-DRB1 there could be as many as three other JIA susceptibility regions, the strongest evidence being in the region of marker D6S265, which lies approximately 100 kb centromeric of HLA-A. The association with D6S265 has since been replicated in two Norwegian studies. The first was only in HLA-DR8 positive individuals [94], but this was later extended to include other haplotypes [95]. Further studies will be required in order to identify the actual genes involved.

Non-MHC genes

Outside of the MHC region, very few non-cytokine susceptibility genes have been considered in JIA. Several neuroendocrine genes (corticotrophin releasing hormone, corticotrophin binding globulin, cytochrome p450 family 19, oestrogen receptor, and prolactin) were studied in a large panel of UK JIA patients and controls, but no positive associations observed [96].

A study of juvenile arthritis patients and controls from Latvia found an association with a particular microsatellite marker and a functional polymorphism in the natural resistance associated macrophage protein (NRAMP1) gene [97]. This has not yet been replicated in a different population of JIA patients.

Preliminary data from Taubert et al. showed an increased occurrence of the Pro/Pro haplotypes for codon 73 of the proto-oncogene p53 in juvenile arthritis [98]. Strikingly few genetic associations have been described for specific features of JIA. An exception to this is the identification of a polymorphic site 5′ to the serum amyloid P component gene. An 8.8 kb Restriction fragment length polymorphism (RFLP) band has been shown to be associated specifically with the secondary amyloidosis occurring in juvenile arthritic patients by Woo et al. [99]. This RFLP did not serve as a genetic marker for the development of secondary amyloidosis in adult rheumatoid arthritis [100].

Whole genome scans

In all of the above studies, a predetermined susceptibility locus has been selected and allele and genotype frequencies assessed in the relevant group of JIA patients and compared to those found in a suitable control panel. Such studies form the basis of genetic observations recorded for JIA. In a different approach, Wise et al. report a potential genomic region of interest for further investigation in JIA [101]. They studied a three generation family in which nine members had received the diagnosis of JIA. All the affected individuals had very early onset disease and episodic inflammation. Although several features were in common with JIA, some were distinct and the individuals included in this study were said to have 'familial recurrent arthritis'. A genome wide scan with polymorphic markers has defined a candidate region for further investigation on chromosome 15q22–23.

More recently, the results of the first whole genome scan, based on 247 JRA cases (patients fulfilling the ACR criteria) from 121 families, have been published [102]. In addition to the HLA region, this study identified five putative JRA regions (1p36, 1q31,15q21, 19p13, and 20q13) as well as several regions related to specific JIA phenotypes (1p13, 1q31, 2p25, 4q24, 5p13, 6q16–22, 7q11, 10q21, 12q24, 17q25, 19p13, Xp11). Interestingly, of the five regions identified for JRA, four show overlap with other autoimmune diseases and only the region on chromosome 15 appears to be JRA specific. All of these regions will now require fine mapping in order to identify the actual genes involved in JIA susceptibility.

Whole genome scans have recently identified a gene (PTPN22) which may be common to a number of different autoimmune phenotypes, including type 1 diabetes mellitus, adult rheumatoid arthritis, systemic lupus erythematosus and autoimmune thyroid disease. The gene, coding for the protein tyrosine phosphatase, appears to be a negative regulator for T cell and B cell activation. A recent study has also found an association between the PTPN22 gene and JIA in a large population of JIA patients in the UK [103].

Key point summary

- Several positive associations for non-HLA genes within the MHC region have been described.

- The full extent of linkage disequilibrium with neighbouring genes always needs to be addressed for any positive genetic associations that are described.

- Emerging loci will help identify JIA and phenotype-specific effects.

Conclusions

To date, the focus of the genetic research into JIA has centred around finding susceptibility loci. Future directions include the replication of key loci and the extrapolation into functional studies. While the genetic basis of susceptibility is important, so too is the assessment of outcome. What better than to be able to predict, at initial consultation, the disease course and optimal treatment regime for any given JIA patient? The genetic basis of such determinants would enhance JIA patient management and welfare. To explore such criteria, large, well-designed, prospective studies of children presenting with inflammatory arthritis need to be undertaken. From such prospectively conducted studies, serial samples may become available allowing for genetic determinants at critical disease phases to be understood.

Finally, through a unified (ILAR) classification and international collaborations of different research groups, the possibility for enhanced power and ease of replication for any genetic findings will be certain. From such an understanding, the advancement of JIA genetics can only continue to strengthen and accelerate. Such collaborative efforts are critical to realizing our goals of applying genomic tests for JIA patients for the prediction of disease progression and drug response.

References

1. Meyerowitz, S., Jacox, R.F., and Hess, D.W. Monozygotic twins discordant for rheumatoid arthritis: a genetic, clinical and psychological study of 8 sets. *Arthritis Rheum* 1968;11:1–21.

2. Ansell, B.M., Bywaters, E.G.L., and Lawrence, J.S. Familial aggregation and twin studies in Still's disease: juvenile chronic polyarthritis. *Rheumatology* (Oxford) 1969;2:37–61.

3. Ansell, B.M. Chronic arthritis in childhood. *Ann Rheum Dis* 1978; 37:107–20.

4. Baum, J., and Fink, C. Juvenile rheumatoid arthritis in monozygotic twins: a case report and review of the literature. *Arthritis Rheum* 1968; 11:33–6.

5. Kapusta, M.A., Metrakos, J.D., Pinsky, L., Shugar, J.L., and Naimark, A.P. Juvenile rheumatoid arthritis in a mother and her identical twin sons. *Arthritis Rheum* 1969;12:411–3.

6. Husby, G., Williams-R.C.J., Tung, K.S., Smith, F.E., Cronin, R.J., Sletten, K., *et al.* Immunologic studies in identical twins concordant for juvenile rheumatoid arthritis but discordant for monoclonal gammopathy and amyloidosis. *J Lab Clin Med* 1988;111:307–14.

7. Prahalad, S., Ryan, M.H., Shear, E.S., Thompson, S.D., Glass, D.N., and Giannini, E.H. Twins concordant for juvenile rheumatoid arthritis. *Arthritis Rheum* 2000;43:2611–2.

8. Clemens, L.E., Albert, E., and Ansell, B.M. Sibling pairs affected by chronic arthritis of childhood: evidence for a genetic predisposition. *J Rheumatol* 1985;12:108–13.

9. Moroldo, M.B., Tague, B.L., Shear, E.S., Glass, D.N., and Giannini, E.H. Juvenile rheumatoid arthritis in affected sibpairs. *Arthritis Rheum* 1997;40:1962–6.

10. Glass, D.N. and Giannini, E.H. Juvenile rheumatoid arthritis as a complex genetic trait. *Arthritis Rheum* 1999;42:2261–8.

11. Moroldo, M.B., Chaudhari, M., Shear, E., Thompson, S.D., Glass, D.N., and Giannini, E.H. Juvenile rheumatoid arthritis affected sibpairs: extent of clinical phenotype concordance. *Arthritis Rheum* 2004;50:1928–34.

12. Saila, H.M., Savolainen, H.A., Kotaniemi, K.M., Kaipiainen-Seppanen, O.A., Leirisalo-Repo, M.T., and Aho, K.V. Juvenile idiopathic arthritis in multicase families. *Clin Exp Rheumatol* 2001;19:218–20.

13. Gauderman, W.J. Sample size requirements for association studies of gene–gene interaction. *Am J Epidemiol* 2002;155:478–84.

14. Gauderman, W.J. Sample size requirements for matched case-control studies of gene–environment interaction. *Stat Med* 2002;21:35–50.

15. Prieur, A.M., Roux-Lombard, P., and Dayer, J.M. Dynamics of fever and the cytokine network in systemic juvenile arthritis. *Rev Rhum Engl Ed* 1996;63:163–70.

16. De Benedetti, F., Pignatti, P., Gerloni, V., Massa, M., Sartirana, P., Caporali, R. *et al.* Differences in synovial fluid cytokine levels between juvenile and adult rheumatoid arthritis. *J Rheumatol* 1997;24:1403–9.

17. Wedderburn, L.R. and Woo, P. Type 1 and type 2 immune responses in children: their relevance in juvenile arthritis. *Springer Semin Immunopathol* 1999;21:361–74.

18. Murray, K.J., Grom, A.A., Thompson, S.D., Lieuwen, D., Passo, M.H., and Glass, D.N. Contrasting cytokine profiles in the synovium of different forms of juvenile rheumatoid arthritis and juvenile spondyloarthropathy: prominence of interleukin 4 in restricted disease. *J Rheumatol* 1998; 25:1388–98.

19. de Kleer, I.M., Wedderburn, L.R., Taams, L.S., Patel, A., Varsani, H., Klein, M. *et al.* CD4+CD25 bright regulatory T cells actively regulate inflammation in the joints of patients with the remitting form of juvenile idiopathic arthritis. *J Immunol* 2004;172:6435–43.

20. Rachelefsky, G.S., Terasaki, P.I., Katz, R., and Stiehm, E.R. Increased prevalence of W27 in juvenile rheumatoid arthritis. *N Engl J Med* 1974; 290:892–3.

21. Friis, J., Morling, N., Pedersen, F.K., Heilmann, C., Jorgensen, B., Svejgaard A, *et al.* HLA-B27 in juvenile chronic arthritis. *J Rheumatol* 1985;12:119–22.

22. Donn, R.P. and Ollier, W.E.R. Juvenile chronic arthritis: a time for change. *Eur J Immunogenet* 1996;23:245–60.

23. Thomson, W., Barrett, J.H., Donn, R., Pepper, L., Kennedy, L.J., Ollier, W.E., *et al.* Juvenile idiopathic arthritis classified by the ILAR criteria: HLA associations in UK patients. *Rheumatology* (Oxford) 2002;41:1183–9.

24. Oen, K., Petty, R.E., and Schroeder, M.L. An association between HLA-A2 and juvenile rheumatoid arthritis in girls. *J Rheumatol* 1982;9:916–20.

25. Brunner, H.I., Ivaskova, E., Haas, J.P., Andreas, A., Keller, E., Hoza, J., *et al.* Class I associations and frequencies of class II HLA-DRB alleles by RFLP analysis in children with rheumatoid-factor-negative juvenile chronic arthritis. *Rheumatol Int* 1993;13:83–8.

26. Paul, C., Schoenwald, U., Truckenbrodt, H., Bettinotti, M.P., Brunnler, G., Keller, E., *et al.* HLA-DP/DR interaction in early onset pauciarticular juvenile chronic arthritis. *Immunogenetics* 1993;37:442–8.

27. Murray, K.J., Moroldo, M.B., Donnelly, P., Prahalad, S., Passo, M.H., Giannini, E.H., *et al.* Age-specific effects of juvenile rheumatoid arthritis-associated HLA alleles. *Arthritis Rheum* 1999;42:1843–53.

28. Stastny, P. and Fink, C.W. Different HLA-D associations in adult and juvenile rheumatoid arthritis. *J Clin Invest* 1979;63:124–30.

29. Glass, D., Litvin, D., Wallace, K., Chylack, L., Garovoy, M., Carpenter, C.B., *et al.* Early-onset pauciarticular juvenile rheumatoid arthritis associated with human leukocyte antigen-DRw5, iritis, and antinuclear antibody. *J Clin Invest* 1980;66:426–9.

30. Albert, E.D. and Scholz, S. Juvenile arthritis: genetic update. *Baillieres Clin Rheumatol* 1998;12:209–18.

31. Hall, P.J., Burman, S.J., Laurent, M.R., Briggs, D.C., Venning, H.E., Leak, A.M., *et al.* Genetic susceptibility to early onset pauciarticular juvenile chronic arthritis: a study of HLA and complement markers in 158 British patients. *Ann Rheum Dis* 1986;45:464–74.

32. Ploski, R., Vinje, O., Ronningen, K.S., Spurkland, A., Sorskaar, D., Vartdal, F., *et al.* HLA class II alleles and heterogeneity of juvenile rheumatoid arthritis: DRB1*0101 may define a novel subset of the disease. *Arthritis Rheum* 1993;36:465–72.

33. Fernandez-Vina, M.A., Fink, C.W., and Stastny, P. HLA antigens in juvenile arthritis: pauciarticular and polyarticular juvenile arthritis are immunogenetically distinct. *Arthritis Rheum* 1990;33:1787–94.

34. Haas, J.P., Nevinny-Stickel, C., Schoenwald, U., Truckenbrodt, H., Suschke, J., and Albert, E.D. Susceptible and protective major histocompatibility complex class II alleles in early-onset pauciarticular juvenile chronic arthritis. *Hum Immunol* 1994;41:225–33.

35. Haas, J.P., Truckenbrodt, H., Paul, C., Hoza, J., Scholz, S., and Albert, E.D. Subtypes of HLA-DRB1*03, *08, *11, *12, *13 and *14 in early onset pauciarticular juvenile chronic arthritis (EOPA) with and without iridocyclitis. *Clin Exp Rheumatol* 1994;12 (Suppl. 10):S7–14.

36. De Inocencio, J., Giannini, E.H., and Glass, D.N. Can genetic markers contribute to the classification of juvenile rheumatoid arthritis? *J Rheumatol* 1993;40 Suppl.:12–8.

37. Fantini, F., Gerloni, V., Murelli, M., Gattinara, M., Negro, A., Sciascia, T., *et al.* HLA phenotypes in subsets of pauciarticular onset juvenile chronic arthritis (JCA). *Eur J Pediatr* 1987;146:338.

38. Donn, R.P., Thomson, W., Pepper, L., Carthy, D., Farhan, A., Ryder, C., *et al.* Antinuclear antibodies in early onset pauciarticular juvenile chronic arthritis (JCA) are associated with HLA-DQB1*0603: a possible JCA-associated human leucocyte antigen haplotype. *Br J Rheumatol* 1995; 34:461–5.

39. Morling, N., Friis, J., Heilmann, C., Hellesen, C., Jakobsen, B.K., Jorgensen, B., *et al.* HLA antigen frequencies in juvenile chronic arthritis. *Scand J Rheumatol* 1985;14:209–16.

40. Barron, K.S., Silverman, E.D. Gonzales, J.C. Owerbach, D., and Reveille, J.D. DNA analysis of HLA-DR, DQ, and DP alleles in children with polyarticular juvenile rheumatoid arthritis. *J Rheumatol* 1992;19:1611–6.

41. Vehe, R.K. Begovich, A.B., and Nepom, B.S. HLA susceptibility genes in rheumatoid factor positive juvenile rheumatoid arthritis. *J Rheumatol* 1990;26 Suppl.:11–5.

42. Okubo, H., Itou, K., Tanaka, S., Watanabe, N., Kashiwagi, N., and Obata, F. Analysis of the HLA-DR gene frequencies in Japanese cases of juveniles rheumatoid arthritis and rheumatoid arthritis by oligonucleotide DNA typing. *Rheumatol Int* 1993;13:65–9.

43. Oen, K., El Gabalawy, H.S., Canvin, J.M., Hitchon, C., Chalmers, I.M., Schroeder M *et al*. HLA associations of seropositive rheumatoid arthritis in a Cree and Ojibway population. *J Rheumatol* 1998;25:2319–23.

44. Forre, O., Dobloug, J.H., Hoyeraal, H.M., and Thorsby, E. HLA antigens in juvenile arthritis: genetic basis for the different subtypes. *Arthritis Rheum* 1983;26:35–8.

45. Glass, D.N. and Litvin DA. Heterogeneity of HLA associations in systemic onset juvenile rheumatoid arthritis. *Arthritis Rheum* 1980;23:796–9.

46. Miller, M.L., Aaron, S., Jackson, J., Fraser, P., Cairns, L., Hoch, S. *et al*. HLA gene frequencies in children and adults with systemic onset juvenile rheumatoid arthritis. *Arthritis Rheum* 1985;28:146–50.

47. Singh, G., Mehra, N.K., Taneja, V., Seth, V., Malaviya, A.N., and Ghai, O.P. Histocompatibility antigens in systemic-onset juvenile rheumatoid arthritis [letter]. *Arthritis Rheum* 1989;32:1492–3.

48. Bedford, P.A., Ansell, B.M., Hall, P.J., and Woo, P. Increased frequency of DR4 in systemic onset juvenile chronic arthritis. *Clin Exp Rheumatol* 1992;10:189–93.

49. Date, Y., Seki, N., Kamizono, S., Higuchi, T., Hirata, T., Miyata, K. *et al*. Identification of a genetic risk factor for systemic juvenile rheumatoid arthritis in the 5′-flanking region of the TNFalpha gene and HLA genes. *Arthritis Rheum* 1999;42:2577–82.

50. Desaymard, C., Kaplan, C., Fournier, C., Manigne, P., Hayem, F., Kahn, M.F. *et al*. Major histocompatibility complex markers and disease heterogeneity in one hundred eight patients with systemic onset juvenile chronic arthritis. *Rev Rheum Engl Ed* 1996;63:9–16.

51. Pratsidou-Gertsi, P., Kanakoudi-Tsakalidou, F., Spyropoulou, M., Germenis, A., Adam, K., Taparkou A *et al*. Nationwide collaborative study of HLA class II associations with distinct types of juvenile chronic arthritis (JCA) in Greece. *Eur J Immunogenet* 1999;26:299–310.

52. Moroldo, M.B., Donnelly, P., Saunders, J., Glass, D.N., and Giannini, E.H. Transmission disequilibrium as a test of linkage and association between HLA alleles and pauciarticular-onset juvenile rheumatoid arthritis. *Arthritis Rheum* 1998;41:1620–4.

53. Zeggini, E., Donn, R.P., Ollier WER, The BPRG Study Group, and Thomson, W. Genetic dissection of the major histocompatibility complex in juvenile oligoarthritis. *Arthritis Rheum* 2002;46: S272.

54. Prahalad, S., Ryan, M.H., Shear, E.S., Thompson, S.D., Giannini, E.H., and Glass, D.N. Juvenile rheumatoid arthritis: linkage to HLA demonstrated by allele sharing in affected sibpairs. *Arthritis Rheum* 2000;43: 2335–8.

55. Katz, J.D., Benoist, C., and Mathis, D. T helper cell subsets in insulin-dependent diabetes. *Science* 1995;268:1185–8.

56. Miller, S.D., McRae, B.L., Vanderlugt, C.L., Nikcevich, K.M., Pope, J.G., Pope, L. *et al*. Evolution of the T-cell repertoire during the course of experimental immune-mediated demyelinating diseases. *Immunol Rev* 1995;144:225–44.

57. Schulze-Koops, H., Lipsky, P.E., Kavanaugh, A.F., and Davis, L.S. Elevated Th1- or Th0-like cytokine mRNA in peripheral circulation of patients with rheumatoid arthritis. Modulation by treatment with anti- ICAM-1 correlates with clinical benefit. *J Immunol* 1995;155:5029–37.

58. Wedderburn, L.R., Robinson, N., Patel, A., Varsani, H., and Woo, P. Selective recruitment of polarized T cells expressing CCR5 and CXCR3 to the inflamed joints of children with juvenile idiopathic arthritis. *Arthritis Rheum* 2000;43:765–74.

59. Abbas, A.K., Murphy, K.M., and Sher, A. Functional diversity of helper T lymphocytes. *Nature* 1996;383:787–93.

60. Wedderburn, L.R., Patel, A., Varsani, H., and Woo, P. Divergence in the degree of clonal expansions in inflammatory T cell subpopulations mirrors HLA-associated risk alleles in genetically and clinically distinct subtypes of childhood arthritis. *Int Immunol* 2001;13:1541–50.

61. Cope, A.P., Liblau, R.S., Yang, X.D., Congia, M., Laudanna, C., Schreiber, R.D. *et al*. Chronic tumor necrosis factor alters T cell responses by attenuating T cell receptor signalling. *J Exp Med* 1997;185:1573–84.

62. Woo P. Cytokine polymorphisms and inflammation. *Clin Exp Rheumatol* 2000;18:767–71.

63. Wilson, A.G., Symons, J.A., McDowell, T.L., McDevitt, H.O., and Duff, G.W. Effects of a polymorphism in the human tumor necrosis factor alpha promoter on transcriptional activation. *Proc Natl Acad Sci USA* 1997; 94:3195–9.

64. Skoog, T., van't Hooft, F.M., Kallin, B., Jovinge, S., Boquist, S., Nilsson, J. *et al*. A common functional polymorphism (C— > A substitution at position -863) in the promoter region of the tumour necrosis factor-alpha (TNF-alpha) gene associated with reduced circulating levels of TNF-alpha. *Hum Mol Genet* 1999;8:1443–9.

65. Messer, G., Spengler, U., Jung, M.C., Honold, G., Blomer, K., Pape, G.R. *et al*. Polymorphic structure of the tumor necrosis factor (TNF) locus: an NcoI polymorphism in the first intron of the human TNF-beta gene correlates with a variant amino acid in position 26 and a reduced level of TNF- beta production. *J Exp Med* 1991;173:209–19.

66. Pociot, F., Molvig, J., Wogensen, L., Worsaae, H., and Nerup, J. A TaqI polymorphism in the human interleukin-1 beta (IL-1 beta) gene correlates with IL-1 beta secretion in vitro. *Eur J Clin Invest* 1992;22:396–402.

67. Tarlow, J.K., Blakemore, A.I., Lennard, A., Solari, R., Hughes, H.N., Steinkasserer, A. *et al*. Polymorphism in human IL-1 receptor antagonist gene intron 2 is caused by variable numbers of an 86-bp tandem repeat. *Hum Genet* 1993;91:403–4.

68. Fishman, D., Faulds, G., Jeffery, R., Mohamed-Ali, V., Yudkin, J.S., Humphries, S. *et al*. The effect of novel polymorphisms in the interleukin-6 (IL-6) gene on IL-6 transcription and plasma IL-6 levels, and an association with systemic-onset juvenile chronic arthritis. *J Clin Invest* 1998;102:1369–76.

69. Terry, C.F., Loukaci, V., and Green, F.R. Cooperative influence of genetic polymorphisms on interleukin 6 transcriptional regulation. *J Biol Chem* 2000;275:18138–44.

70. Crawley, E., Kay, R., Sillibourne, J., Patel, P., Hutchinson, I., and Woo, P. Polymorphic haplotypes of the interleukin-10 5′ flanking region determine variable interleukin-10 transcription and are associated with particular phenotypes of juvenile rheumatoid arthritis. *Arthritis Rheum* 1999;42:1101–8.

71. Eskdale, J., Gallagher, G., Verweij, C.L., Keijsers, V., Westendorp, R.G., and Huizinga, T.W. Interleukin 10 secretion in relation to human IL-10 locus haplotypes. *Proc Natl Acad Sci USA* 1998;95:9465–70.

72. Pravica, V., Asderakis, A., Perrey, C., Hajeer, A., Sinnott, P.J., and Hutchinson, I.V. In vitro production of IFN-gamma correlates with CA repeat polymorphism in the human IFN-gamma gene. *Eur J Immunogenet* 1999;26:1–3.

73. Rosenzweig, S.D., Schaffer, A.A., Ding, L., Sullivan, R., Enyedi, B., Yim, J.J. *et al*. Interferon-gamma receptor 1 promoter polymorphisms: population distribution and functional implications. *Clin Immunol* 2004;112:113–9.

74. Awad, M.R., El Gamel, A., Hasleton, P., Turner, D.M., Sinnott, P.J., and Hutchinson, IV. Genotypic variation in the transforming growth factor-beta1 gene: association with transforming growth factor-beta1 production, fibrotic lung disease, and graft fibrosis after lung transplantation. *Transplantation* 1998;66:1014–20.

75. McDowell, T.L., Symons, J.A., Ploski, R., Forre, O., and Duff, G.W. A genetic association between juvenile rheumatoid arthritis and a novel interleukin-1 alpha polymorphism. *Arthritis Rheum* 1995;38:221–8.

76. Donn, R.P., Farhan, A.J., Barrett, J.H., Thomson, W., Worthington, J., and Ollier, W.E. Absence of association between interleukin 1 alpha and oligoarticular juvenile chronic arthritis in UK patients. *Rheumatology* (Oxford) 1999;38:171–5.

77. Zeggini, E., Thomson, W., Kwiatkowski, D., Richardson, A., Ollier, W., and Donn, R. Linkage and association studies of single-nucleotide polymorphism-tagged tumor necrosis factor haplotypes in juvenile oligoarthritis. *Arthritis Rheum* 2002;46:3304–11.

78. Lim, S., Crawley, E., Woo, P., and Barnes, P.J. Haplotype associated with low interleukin-10 production in patients with severe asthma. *Lancet* 1998;352:113.

79. Donn, R.P., Barrett, J.H., British Paediatric Rheumatology Study Group, Farhan, A., Stopford, A., and Pepper, L. *et al.* Cytokine gene polymorphisms and susceptibility to juvenile idiopathic arthritis. *Arthritis Rheum* 2001;44:802–10.

80. Woo, P. Cytokines in childhood rheumatic diseases. *Arch Dis Child* 1993;69:547–9.

81. De Benedetti, F. and Martini A. Is systemic juvenile rheumatoid arthritis an interleukin 6 mediated disease? *J Rheumatol* 1998;25:203–7.

82. Ogilvie, E.M., Fife, M.S., Thompson, S.D., Twine, N., Tsoras, M., Moroldo, M. *et al.* The -174G allele of the interleukin-6 gene confers susceptibility to systemic arthritis in children: a multicenter study using simplex and multiplex juvenile idiopathic arthritis families. *Arthritis Rheum* 2003;48:3202–6.

83. Donn, R.P. and Ray, D.W. Macrophage migration inhibitory factor: molecular, cellular and genetic aspects of a key neuroendocrine molecule. *J Endocrinol* 2004;182:1–9.

84. Donn, R.P., Shelley, E., Ollier, W.E., and Thomson, W. A novel 5′-flanking region polymorphism of macrophage migration inhibitory factor is associated with systemic-onset juvenile idiopathic arthritis. *Arthritis Rheum* 2001;44:1782–5.

85. Donn, R., Alourfi, Z., De Benedetti, F., Meazza, C., Zeggini, E., Lunt, M. *et al.* Mutation screening of the macrophage migration inhibitory factor gene: positive association of a functional polymorphism of macrophage migration inhibitory factor with juvenile idiopathic arthritis. *Arthritis Rheum* 2002;46:2402–9.

86. De Benedetti, F., Meazza, C., Vivarelli, M., Rossi, F., Pistorio, A., Lamb, R. *et al.* Functional and prognostic relevance of the -173 polymorphism of the macrophage migration inhibitory factor gene in systemic-onset juvenile idiopathic arthritis. *Arthritis Rheum* 2003;48:1398–407.

87. De Benedetti, F., Vivarelli, M., Lamb, R., Meazza, C., Muratori, F., Cioschi, S. *et al.* Association of the -173 SNP of the macrophage migration inhibitory factor (MIF) gene with response to intraarticular glucocorticoids in oligoarticular JIA. *Arthritis Rheum* 2003;48:S254.

88. Donn, R.P., Alourfi, Z., Zeggini, E., Lamb, R., Jury, F., Lunt, M. *et al.* A functional promoter haplotype of macrophage migration inhibitory factor (MIF) is linked and associated with juvenile idiopathic arthritis. *Arthritis Rheum* 2004;50:1604–10.

89. Barton, A., Lamb, R., Symmons, D., Silman, A., Thomson, W., Worthington, J. *et al.* Macrophage migration inhibitory factor (MIF) gene polymorphism is associated with susceptibility to but not severity of inflammatory polyarthritis. *Genes Immun* 2003;4:487–91.

90. Donn, R.P., Plant, D., Jury, F., Richards, H.L., Worthington, J., Ray DW *et al.* Macrophage migration inhibitory factor gene polymorphism is associated with psoriasis. *J Invest Dermatol* 2004;123:484–7.

91. Pryhuber, K.G., Murray, K.J., Donnelly, P., Passo, M.H., Maksymowych, W.P., Glass, D.N. *et al.* Polymorphism in the LMP2 gene influences disease susceptibility and severity in HLA-B27 associated juvenile rheumatoid arthritis. *J Rheumatol* 1996;23:747–52.

92. Ploski, R., Undlien, D.E., Vinje, O., Forre, O., Thorsby, E., and Ronningen KS. Polymorphism of human major histocompatibility complex-encoded transporter associated with antigen processing (TAP) genes and susceptibility to juvenile rheumatoid arthritis. *Hum Immunol* 1994;39:54–60.

93. Donn, R.P., Davies, E.J., Holt, P.L., Thomson, W., and Ollier W. Increased frequency of TAP2B in early onset pauciarticular juvenile chronic arthritis. *Ann Rheum Dis* 1994;53:261–4.

94. Smerdel, A., Lie, B.A., Ploski, R., Koeleman, B.P., Forre, O., Thorsby, E. *et al.* A gene in the telomeric HLA complex distinct from HLA-A is involved in predisposition to juvenile idiopathic arthritis. *Arthritis Rheum* 2002;46:1614–9.

95. Smerdel, A., Lie, B.A., Finholt, C., Ploski, R., Forre, O., Undlien, D.E. *et al.* An additional susceptibility gene for juvenile idiopathic arthritis in the HLA class I region on several DR-DQ haplotypes. *Tissue Antigens* 2003; 61:80–4.

96. Donn, R.P., Farhan, A., Stevans, A., Ramanan, A., Ollier, W.E., and Thomson, W. Neuroendocrine gene polymorphisms and susceptibility to juvenile idiopathic arthritis. *Rheumatology* (Oxford) 2002;41:930–6.

97. Sanjeevi, C.B., Miller, E.N., Dabadghao, P., Rumba, I., Shtauvere, A., Denisova, A. *et al.* Polymorphism at NRAMP1 and D2S1471 loci associated with juvenile rheumatoid arthritis. *Arthritis Rheum* 2000;43: 1397–404.

98. Taubert, H., Thamm, B., Meye, A., Bartel, F., Rost, A.K., Heidenreich, D. *et al.* The p53 status in juvenile chronic arthritis and rheumatoid arthritis. *Clin Exp Immunol* 2000;122:264–9.

99. Woo, P., O'Brien, J., Robson, M., and Ansell, B.M. A genetic marker for systemic amyloidosis in juvenile arthritis. *Lancet* 1987;2:767–9.

100. Grateau, G., Baudis, M., and Delpech, M. Study of a restriction fragment length polymorphism for serum amyloid P gene in rheumatoid arthritis with amyloidosis. *J Rheumatol* 1991;18:994–6.

101. Wise, C.A., Bennett, L.B., Pascual, V., Gillum, J.D., and Bowcock, A.M. Localization of a gene for familial recurrent arthritis. *Arthritis Rheum* 2000;43:2041–5.

102. Thompson, S.D., Moroldo, M.B., Guyer, L., Ryan, M., Tombragel, E.M., Shear, E.S. *et al.* A genome-wide scan for juvenile rheumatoid arthritis in affected sibpair families provides evidence of linkage. *Arthritis Rheum* 2004;50:2920–30.

103. Hinks, A., Barton, A., John, S., Bruce, I., Hawkins, C., *et al.* Association between the PTPN22 gene and rheumatoid arthritis and juvenile idiopathic arthritis in a U.K. population: Further support that PTPN22 is an autoimmunity gene. *Arthritis Rheum* 2005;52:1694–9.

2.11 Environmental factors in the pathogenesis of Juvenile Idiopathic Arthritis

Berent J. Prakken, Salvatore Albani, and Wietse Kuis

Aim

The aim of this chapter is to provide an overview of the importance of the environment (especially the microbial environment) and its interaction with the immune system in immunopathogenesis and disease susceptibility in Juvenile Idiopathic Arthritis (JIA).

Structure

- Introduction
- The environment in JIA: socioeconomic factors, climate, and nutrition
- Mechanisms of autoimmunity: interactions between the microbial environment and the immune system
- Microbial environment and immune mediated diseases: the Hygiene Hypothesis
- The influence of the microbial environment on JIA

Introduction

Juvenile Idiopathic Arthritis (JIA) consists of a complex of diseases with a multi-factorial pathogenesis [1]. Although genetic predisposition does play a role in disease susceptibility, JIA is not a monogenetic disease [2–4] (See Part 2, Chapter 2.10 "Genetic and Cytokine Associations in JIA"). Aside from genetic susceptibilities, environmental factors play an additional role in the pathogenesis of the disease.

Many environmental factors may influence both the induction of JIA and the course of disease. Those factors include geographical and socioeconomic factors, climate, air pollution (including cigarette smoking), breastfeeding, nutrition, trauma, infections, and immunizations. JIA is a chronic disease of childhood with a gradual onset and it is tempting to speculate that environmental factors, such as infections and immunizations, might provoke the onset of arthritis. Trauma, vaccinations, and infections are, however, common, normal events in early childhood that may simply coincide with the onset of JIA, and there may not be a causal relationship. Thus far, the role of environmental factors in the pathogenesis of JIA has not been confirmed or excluded in proper epidemiological studies, and many unsubstantiated myths and beliefs may still exist in the minds of doctors, patients, and parents.

The environment in JIA: socioeconomic factors, climate, and nutrition

Socioeconomic variables are among the most influential of the factors that determine the child's environment. Parental income and housing are important factors that directly or indirectly have an impact on disease severity and disease outcome. A study on the socioeconomic background of children in Denmark diagnosed with JIA between 1988 and 1991 identified three socioeconomic variables that act as independent risk factors for the development of JIA: high parental income, absence of siblings, and living in a flat [5]. Although the identified socioeconomic factors were clearly correlated with an increased risk, several questions remained unsolved by this study. For example, although being an only child increased the risk, the age or number of siblings did not seem to matter. The study thus failed to reveal a relationship between environment and risk for JIA unlike the "hygiene hypothesis" for atopic diseases (see p293).

The role of air-borne pollution in the pathogenesis of chronic arthritis stems from studies on cigarette smoking in rheumatoid arthritis (RA). The effects of smoking on RA are complex. The evaluation of the risks attributed to smoking is hampered by other factors such as psychosocial factors and other diseases related to smoking. However, it is clear that either directly or indirectly, smoking is a risk factor for RA. Several studies have shown consistently that smokers are more likely to be rheumatoid factor (RF) positive, and that smokers are more likely to develop extra-articular complications such as rheumatoid nodules, interstitial lung diseases, and vasculitis [6–8]. One recent study suggested that fetal exposure to tobacco smoke increases the risk of JIA in girls [8]. The risks associated with smoking should be taken into account when providing information on guidelines for a healthy lifestyle for adolescent patients with JIA, as well as counselling on the risks of passive smoking for young children with JIA.

The role of nutrition as an environmental factor influencing the pathogenesis and course of JIA is not clear. Although initial reports suggested a protective effect of breastfeeding on the risk of development of JIA [9], this relationship could not be confirmed in subsequent studies [10]. In addition, in rare cases food intolerance may play a role in aggravating joint symptoms in patients with JIA [11]. However, taken together, no clear associations exist between nutrition and JIA that can be translated into evidence-based dietary advice for patients with JIA.

The environmental factors that are most consistently suggested as being involved in the pathogenesis of the disease are immunizations and microbial agents [12]. This chapter will therefore focus primarily on the influence of the interaction between the host immune system and the microbial environment on the pathogenesis of JIA.

Key summary points

- There is no convincing evidence that socioeconomic or nutritional factors are directly related to JIA.

- Smoking is a risk factor for RA, and thus smoking (passive or active) may influence the onset and course of JIA.

Mechanisms of autoimmunity: interactions between the microbial environment and the immune system

Microbial agents interact with cells from the immune system non-stop, and this continuous cross-talk between microbes and immune competent cells, without a doubt, forms the most important environmental factor that influences the course of immune-mediated diseases. Four general mechanisms can be distinguished through which the microbial environment may influence the course of arthritis: persisting antigen, bystander activation, molecular mimicry, and bystander suppression (Table 2.11.1) [13].

The persistence of a microbial antigen triggering a pro-inflammatory response is obviously the most straightforward explanation. This is the case in Lyme arthritis, reactive arthritis, or a chronic viral infection that directly induces arthritis [14]. However, in most cases of JIA, no persisting microbial agent can be found. Molecular mimicry is a most appealing possibility: it assumes that an epitope present on a microbial antigen is structurally similar to one on a self (host) antigen, leading to the expansion of cross-reactive autoimmune cells. However, to date, only a few examples of molecular mimicry have been convincingly demonstrated in human arthritis [13,15,16]. In JIA, an example of possible molecular mimicry is the relationship between Epstein–Barr Virus (EBV) proteins and self-HLA in patients

with Oligoarthritis [17]. Bystander activation is here defined as the expansion and activation of pro-inflammatory immune competent cells at the site of initial inflammation. It includes enhanced antigen presentation, epitope spreading, and the attraction of other pro-inflammatory cells and mediators. These processes are not mutually exclusive and probably all take place at the same time in inflamed synovial tissue from patients with JIA [18–21]. Non-specific pro-inflammatory pathways are certainly important in later stages of disease, and may perpetuate the inflammatory state in the synovium. At late phases of inflammation, the presence of a microbial antigen may not be necessary any longer, but evidence is mounting that bacterial DNA present in or around the synovial tissue may play a role at maintaining a pro-inflammatory environment [22]. The last and perhaps most intriguing possibility of interaction between microbes and the immune system is bystander suppression through the induction of regulatory T cells, as a result of interaction with the environmental microbial flora in the gut. This possibility has gained more interest thanks to the "hygiene hypothesis" and can be substantiated by data from both animal models and patients with JIA [23,24]. Since part of our understanding of those mechanisms stems from studies in animal models with a direct relation to JIA and RA, those models will also be briefly discussed.

Persisting microbial antigens and JIA: evidence from epidemiological studies

Little or no evidence exists that a microbial agent directly causes JIA, although the discovery of *Borrelia Burgdorferi* as the cause of Lyme arthritis raises the expectation that more microbial agents will be discovered. One of the most common explanations for the disease is that an infection sets off the disease in a genetically susceptible individual [3,4]. This is supported by the initial clinical features of JIA that can be very similar to those of an infection and the fact that several viral infections, such as parvovirus B19 and rubella virus, can induce arthritis [25,26]. In cross-sectional studies, evidence for persisting parvovirus B19 infections in synovial fluid of several patients with JIA was found, even prompting treatment trials with gamma globulin in a small group of patients [27–29]. The role of parvovirus B19 in the pathogenesis and course still remains unclear, since prospective studies in large cohorts of patients are lacking. Systemic Arthritis at onset closely mimics an infection with characteristic features such as fever, rash, and lymphadenopathy. Indeed, case reports have appeared in literature relating the onset of individual cases of Systemic Arthritis to mumps, Coxsackievirus, rubella, and adenovirus [30,31]. Since infections can vary according to seasonal changes, epidemiological surveys have been performed to determine whether there is a characteristic seasonal pattern to the onset of Systemic Arthritis. An initial study showed a higher incidence of new cases of Systemic Arthritis from early spring to early autumn, and a lower frequency then expected number of cases during the winter months. Such a pattern suggests a role for a virus (possibly an enterovirus) initiating the disease. Another study, performed in a regional center in Canada, suggested cycles of increased incidence of Oligoarthritis, Polyarthritis, and Systemic Arthritis concurrent with increases in the frequency of *Mycoplasma pneumoniae* infections [32]. However, a larger study that included all major paediatric rheumatology centres in Canada between 1980 and 1992 did not reveal any seasonal pattern to the onset of Systemic Arthritis or a correlation between onset and the incidence of *M. pneumoniae*

Table 2.11.1 Possible mechanisms of interaction between the immune system and the environment in arthritis pathogenesis

Mechanism	Possible examples
Persisting antigen	Lyme arthritis Reactive arthritis
Molecular mimicry	Shared and Self-HLA epitopes in JIA Lyme arthritis Rheumatic fever
Bystander activation	CpG-arthritis S Arthritis following immunization
Bystander suppression	Induction of Regulatory T cells (through interaction with gut microbial flora) via the "hygiene hypothesis"

infections [33]. Interestingly enough, the same study did show a significant seasonal pattern in the prairie region with peak onset months in early fall and fewer then expected cases in the winter. This is again suggestive of an infectious agent playing a role in the onset of Systemic Arthritis at least in this specific region. A multi-centre study performed in Israel between 1982 and 1997 did not reveal a seasonal pattern of onset of Systemic Arthritis, but suggested that the onset of disease in patients with more severe chronic relapsing disease tended to be more common in winter [34]. This underlines the complexity of this issue. It is conceivable that within the whole group of children with Systemic Arthritis, subgroups will be identified with different mechanisms of disease pathogenesis, ranging from inherited regulatory defects [35] to ultimately environmental disease-causing pathogens.

Bystander activation: persisting microbial DNA

The continuous presence of bacterial DNA in or around synovial tissue has been recently identified as a possible target for microbial-induced activation of the immune system. Most of the attention has focused on the role of immune-stimulatory DNA sequences [36,37]. Immune-stimulatory DNA sequences (ISS), or CpG motifs, are palindromic sequences of unmethylated CpG dinucleotides that are present in bacterial DNA but not in mammalian DNA [38]. ISS form molecular patterns that are readily recognized by the innate immune system, resulting in activation of first line defenses against bacterial infections. They can stimulate the expression of co-stimulatory molecules and the production of cytokines such as IL-12, TNFα, and interferons (IFN) by macrophages, dendritic cells, B cells, and NK cells [38], and are capable of skewing an immune response toward a strong and prolonged Th1 type of immunity [36]. Interestingly, joint damage in a model of septic arthritis is linked to the same CpG motifs [39]: an injection of bacterial DNA or oligonucleotides containing ISS in the joint leads to the clinical picture of septic arthritis, whereas injection of mammalian DNA did not induce arthritis. An influx of monocytes and macrophages and only a small number of CD4 positive T-lymphocytes characterizes the resulting arthritis, and locally in the arthritic joint, increased mRNA expression of TNFα, IL-1β, IL-12 and the chemokines RANTES and MCP-1 is found [40]. This indicates that bacterial DNA containing unmethylated CpG motifs play a pivotal role in the pathogenesis of acute arthritis and raises the question whether ISS also play a role in the pathogenesis of chronic autoimmune arthritis [40]. Indeed, in Adjuvant Arthritis (AA), a model of immune-mediated arthritis that will be discussed below, the severity of arthritis induced by intracutaneous injection with heat killed *Mycobacterium tuberculosis* appears completely dependent on the presence of ISS in *M tuberculosis* [41]. The arthritis-promoting capacity of ISS in combination with DNase treated CFA correlated with the *in vitro* production of IFNγ and RANK-ligand in response to mycobacterial antigens. Strikingly, following injection with CFA, mycobacterial DNA can be detected at sites distant from the site of immunization, such as the bone marrow and spleen but not in the synovium. It has been described that, following intradermal DNA immunization, DNA can be transported beyond regional lymph nodes to distant sites of inflammation [40]. The demonstration of mycobacterial DNA at distant sites after immunization with heat-killed *M tuberculosis* may well be contributing to the same mechanisms. The persisting presence of bacterial DNA in the bone marrow can lead to an environment that promotes the invasion of mesenchymal cells from the bone marrow

into the inflamed synovium. Thus, after an initial T cell mediated antigen-specific phase, the presence of ISS may form the second hit and determine the severity and possibly also the chronicity of the inflammation in the joint. The increasing number of reports on the presence of bacterial DNA in the synovial fluid of patients with RA and JIA suggests that similar mechanisms may play a role in the perpetuation of inflammation in human autoimmune arthritis [20,42–44].

Molecular mimicry in JIA

As stated before, molecular mimicry is an appealing explanation for the induction of an autoimmune disease by microbial agents. This is supported by the fact that the interaction between the T cell receptor (TCR) and an antigen presented by the MHC complex on an antigen presenting cell is far less specific then was thought earlier. The plasticity of the interaction allows the possibility that the same TCR may respond to structurally different peptide epitopes. However, the evidence that such mechanism may actually cause autoimmune arthritis is still lacking. The most prominent examples for molecular mimicry in childhood arthritis are found in Lyme arthritis and Oligoarthritis. In Lyme arthritis, the immune dominant epitope of the outer surface protein A (OspA) of *B. Burgdorferi* is HLA DR4-restricted and has a structural homology with a peptide derived from human LFA-1α. This led to the following possible immunopathogenic model of molecular mimicry in Lyme arthritis. Following infection with *B. Burgdorferi*, the immune system mounts a pro-inflammatory response toward the immune dominant epitope from the OspA of *B. Burgdorferi*. [45,46]. At the site of synovial inflammation, synoviocytes and other immune competent cells express increased amounts of LFA-1, leading to the enhanced presentation of self peptides derived from LFA-1, which could subsequently function as a secondary cross-reactive target for OspA-induced pro-inflammatory T cells [45]. Definitive proof for this attractive scenario, however, is still lacking [15,47]. Another interesting possibility of molecular mimicry in JIA is described in Oligoarthritis involving EBV proteins and self-HLA. Sequence homologies have been identified between two EBV proteins (Bolf1 and Balf2) and the HLA-DRB1*1101, DRB1*0801 and DPB1*0201 alleles associated with Oligoarthritis [17]. Strikingly, patients with Oligoarthritis, but not controls matched for the mentioned DR and DP alleles, have cytotoxic T cell responses to self HLA-derived peptides that contain sequence homologies with the two EBV proteins. This self-reactivity could be the consequence of the activation of cross-reactive T cells through the homologous EBV proteins. This mechanism may be one of the examples through which molecular mimicry at the level of the TCR leads to the initiation of a general pro-inflammatory pathway.

Molecular mimicry: potential risks and benefits of immunizations

It is still highly controversial whether immunizations may play a direct or indirect role in the onset of autoimmune diseases either through antigenic mimicry or through general activation of the immune system [48–50]. As discussed below, recent studies in allergic diseases suggest that vaccination may be connected to immune-mediated diseases through an indirect mechanism: a reduced infectious load in childhood in the industrialized Western countries may lead to an immune environment that lacks healthy regulatory T cells responses [51]. Apart from this, immunizations may directly contribute to autoimmune phenomena in a susceptible individual. For example, immunization with Bacillus Camette-Guerin (BCG) for the treatment of bladder carcinoma can induce a severe polyarthritis that has many similarities with AA an animal model of experimental arthritis. The pathogenesis of this BCG-induced reactive arthritis in human is still largely unknown, but the disease appears T cell driven, with presumably an important pathogenetic role for both CD4 and CD8 positive lymphocytes [52]. In children, mumps and rubella vaccination are most commonly associated with reports of joint symptoms, depending on the type and strain of the vaccine used [53]. A large study in the United Kingdom between 1989 and 1990 showed that 6 weeks following measles, mumps, and rubella (MMR) vaccination children have increased risk of episodes of joint and limb complaints [54]. The authors concluded that the rubella component of the vaccine most likely was to blame for the joint complaints. However, the risk of developing clinical arthritis after immunization with MMR was far less then following a natural rubella infection. The question whether immunization may influence the course of an already established chronic arthritis is more difficult to answer. A study in Canada with regard to influenza vaccination did not yield any evidence of increased risks of flares in patients with JIA [55]. With the advent of more severely immune-suppressive treatment regimens in JIA, the risks and benefits of vaccination in increasingly immunocompromised hosts have to be considered. Using the experience of vaccination in immuno-compromised or immunodeficient children with other diseases may be very helpful.

The concept that immune-mediated diseases may be strongly influenced by the environment has gained more support, thanks to several striking observations in the epidemiology of allergic diseases. These observations and subsequent immunological studies have led to the 'hygiene hypothesis,' which may also relate to autoimmune diseases such as JIA.

Key point summary

- No evidence exists for a single infectious agent causing JIA.
- Persistent bacterial DNA can be found in synovial tissue from patients with JIA and RA.
- Possible mechanisms of interaction between microbes and the immune system that could be operating in JIA include:
  - Persisting antigen
  - Bystander activation
  - Molecular mimicry
  - Bystander suppression
- Epidemiological studies have not provided a link between immunizations and JIA

Microbial environment and immune-mediated diseases: the hygiene hypothesis

The prevalence of atopic diseases, such as asthma, atopic dermatitis, and hay fever, has increased dramatically in Western industrialized countries over the last two decades. This rapid increase has not been seen in developing countries, thereby calling attention to the role of the environment in this increased prevalence. According to the so-called 'hygiene hypothesis' this increased prevalence is due to reduced exposure to infections in childhood, a consequence of the improved hygiene and immunizations in industrialized Western countries [51]. The hygiene hypothesis assumes that an increased exposure to infections leads to a Th1 like environment and thus, in the case of allergic disease, inhibits the occurrence of detrimental Th2 like responses. Indeed circumstantial evidence from epidemiological studies suggests that there may be such a relationship. For instance, an inverse relationship is found between family size and the risk of developing asthma, while other studies revealed that early placement in day care centers, and exposure to farm animals and raw milk appears to reduce the risk of developing asthma or other allergic conditions [51,56].

The specific immunological mechanisms that may contribute to these associations are still largely unknown. However, animal studies revealed that some of the mechanisms behind such associations might be more complex then just influencing the Th1/Th2 balance. A good example for the latter is the association between hepatitis A virus and allergic disease. Hepatitis A virus is correlated with protection against the development of asthma, and it has been assumed that this relationship was merely a reflection of the correlation between poor hygiene favoring a Th1 bias and the risk of allergy development. However, it turns out to not be that simple. Recently, an allergy susceptibility gene was identified, called *Tim1*. Polymorphisms in *Tim1* are associated with the development of and protection from airway hyper-reactivity in certain mice strains. Moreover, *Tim1* is expressed on CD4 T cells and is associated with the development of Th2 like responses. The human homologue of *Tim1*, located at human chromosome 5q33.2, codes for the cellular receptor of hepatitis A virus [57]. Although the relationship between hepatitis A virus, its cellular receptor *Tim1*, and the development of atopic diseases still has to be elucidated, this shows that a very specific molecular mechanism can be the basis of a descriptive epidemiological correlation between environment and an immune-mediated disease.

It is conceivable that the relation between an increased incidence of atopic diseases and the environment is far more complex than the hygiene hypothesis suggests [56]. An environment with more infections may not just prime an individual to develop a Th1-biased immune system and so be protected from allergic diseases. In Western industrialized countries, not only is the prevalence of Th2-mediated atopic diseases increasing, but so is the prevalence of Th1-mediated autoimmune diseases such as type I diabetes. Moreover, an inverse relationship has been found between helminth infections, potent inducers of a Th2-biased immune response, and atopic diseases. This is at first sight puzzling given the strong induction of Th2 responses by parasites. However, helminth infections induce regulatory T cells capable of down regulating both Th1 and Th2 cells [58]. Several types of regulatory T cells (Treg) have now been identified, among which are CD4+CD25+ double positive cells and Th3 cells (induced via mucosal tolerance). Regulatory T cells have been found to suppress both Th1 and Th2-mediated responses, with a crucial role of IL-10. The microbial flora interacts with the mucosal immune system to trigger the induction of several subtypes of regulatory T cells. The presence of such strong regulatory T cells may be necessary for the inhibition of the development of both Th2 and Th1 mediated diseases.

That similar mechanisms may indeed play a role in arthritis is highlighted by data in animal models of arthritis that suggest that the presence of a normal gut mucosal bacterial flora is essential for protection from arthritis. In the context of the hygiene hypothesis, a protective role of intestinal colonization with Lactobacilli on disease susceptibility has been suggested, which has led to clinical trials using probiotics. Taken together, it can be concluded that the microbial environment is indeed crucial for disease susceptibility. Evidence for a similar important role for the microbial flora in arthritis is increasing rapidly.

Key point summary

- The hygiene hypothesis assumes that the increased prevalence of allergic diseases in the Western world is related to a reduced exposure to infections.

- A similar relationship may play a role in the increased prevalence of autoimmunity in the Western world.

- The induction of regulatory T cells by the microbial environment appears to be instrumental in suppressing both Th1 and Th2 mediated diseases.

The influence of the microbial environment on JIA

Evidence from animal models

The understanding of the influence that the microbial environment has on chronic arthritis has increased significantly, thanks to studies performed in animal models of chronic arthritis. One of the most widely used models of experimental arthritis is the model of adjuvant arthritis (AA). AA is induced in susceptible animals (mostly rats) by intracutaneous injection of Complete Freund's Adjuvant (CFA: heat-killed mycobacteria in Incomplete Freund's Adjuvant). Following immunization with CFA, animals develop a polyarthritis with accompanying systemic features such as weight loss and uveitis. The disease is self-remitting, and following the initial phase of arthritis, animals are protected from subsequent induction of arthritis. AA is commonly regarded as an excellent model of RA, and, indeed, the histopathological changes in the synovial tissue closely resemble those found in both RA and JIA. However, for several reasons, it can be argued that this model fits better with reactive arthritis or JIA. First, an infectious agent induces the disease. Second, AA is a self-limiting and naturally self-remitting disease, which also can be one of the most striking features of JIA. Third, uveitis, and other systemic features that can be seen in JIA also accompany. Lastly, many remarkable similarities can be found in AA immune pathogenesis. In the early stages of AA, the histopathological abnormalities are characterized by the infiltration of mononuclear cells into the synovial tissue. This cellular infiltrate consists primarily of lymphocytes, but plasma cells and at later stages neutrophils are also present. Lymphocytes play a central role in triggering AA [59]. The complete clinical picture of AA can be adoptively transferred with primed lymph node cells or thoracic duct lymphocytes from diseased animals into recipient rats without co-immunization with mycobacteria or any other triggering antigen [60]. The induction

of the disease is completely T cell driven, since a T cell clone, called A2b, directed at an epitope of heat shock protein (hsp) 65 of *M tuberculosis*, is capable of transferring AA to irradiated recipient rats [61]. The fact that a T cell line raised against a noninfectious (heat-killed) microorganism is able to induce the complete clinical picture of AA gave support to the "hit and run" hypothesis: a microbial agent pulls the trigger to initiate a self-perpetuating autoimmune process in a susceptible individual [62]. However, T cell responses directed against the same hsp appears to play an equally important role in the remittance of the disease, which has led to a wide spread study on the role of immune reactivity toward microbial heat shock proteins in arthritis.

Microbial heat shock proteins as key environmental regulators of arthritis

Heat shock proteins (hsp), or stress proteins, are highly conserved cellular proteins. Hsp play an important role in protein folding and assembly in the cell, as so called molecular chaperones [63,64]. Hsp are considered to be immunologically important proteins for several reasons. Hsp are called stress proteins because they are increasingly produced when a cell is confronted with an environmental stressor [63,65,66]. Because of this, self-hsp expression is upregulated at sites of cell stress, such as in damaged or inflamed tissue, irrespective of the cause of damage. Second, hsp are remarkably conserved during evolution [65]. Third, despite the high degree of homology among hsp of different species, hsp have been found to be strong immunogens [67,68]. Bacterial hsp are easily recognized by the immune system, which in turn can lead to cross-recognition of self-hsp and provide a link between an immune response to infection and autoimmunity [69,70]. In the healthy immune system, this does not seem to occur, perhaps as a consequence of the overwhelming presence of bacterial hsp on the mucosal surfaces of the gastrointestinal tract. Autoreactive responses against self-hsp may be held in check by an idiotypic network in the normal immune system. The finding that the arthritogenic T cell clone A2b responded to a mycobacterial hsp65 (Mhsp65) sequence gave rise to the suspicion that the pathogenesis of AA may be a textbook case of antigenic mimicry. In that view, the immunization with heat-killed mycobacteria within CFA induces a primary immune response toward an epitope derived from Mhsp65, which subsequently leads to a cross-reactive T cell response directed at the homologous self-hsp60 sequence. However, the mapped T cell epitope from A2b turned out not to be a part of a conserved region of Mhsp65, but of a non-conserved part of the molecule, which decreases the chances of antigenic mimicry [71]. Later studies confirmed that the self cross-reactive antigen of A2b is not a self-hsp but instead a structure derived from cartilage proteoglycan [72,73]. In fact, pre-immunization with Mhsp65 protects rats against subsequent induction of arthritis, not only in AA, but also in virtually all other experimental arthritis models such as collagen type II induced arthritis, avridine arthritis, pristane arthritis and streptococcal cell wall induced arthritis [74–76]. This led to the assumption that immunization with Mhsp65 activates a more general anti-inflammatory pathway. The subsequent identification of T cell epitopes of Mhsp65 showed that only peptides containing conserved epitopes with a high degree of homology with the homologous rat peptide and capable of inducing T cell responses to "self"-rat hsp60 can be protective not only in AA, but also in other experimental non-microbial induced arthritis models [77]. The specific mechanism through which these self-hsp60 cross-reactive T cells protect is still largely unknown, although recent studies suggest that this is an active cell-mediated process involving the induction of functional regulatory T cells [78,79].

Conserved microbial antigens as target for immune regulation in JIA

Another issue with important clinical implications is whether immunological mechanisms that determine a normal regulatory immune response in chronic inflammation in an animal model can also be applied to the human situation, and if so, whether it would be possible to apply the same mechanistic principle to the treatment of human arthritis. Studies in patients with JIA suggest that this indeed may be the case. T and B cell responses to several classes of microbial hsp can be found in patients with JIA [80–83]. These studies at first glance seem to implicate a role for the microbial gut environment in the induction of the disease [12]. Later studies revealed that most T cell responses to hsp are found in Oligoarthritis, the subtype of JIA with the best prognosis [84,85]. This includes the induction of actual self-hsp reactive cells that have the full characteristics of regulatory T cells, and are capable of producing IL-10 and TGF-β [86]. Thus, a picture arises that is remarkably similar to the concept of the hygiene hypothesis: namely a protective role of the microbial environment in the gut that steers the immune system toward a regulatory T cell response. This concept is further strengthened by additional studies on the role of the gut flora in AA.

The gut microbial environment and arthritis susceptibility

It is conceivable that the presence of bacterial hsp epitopes in the gut is the very reason that regulatory T cells are induced, on the basis of similar mechanisms as found in experimentally induced mucosal tolerance [87,88]. Fisher rats, in contrast to Lewis rats, are resistant to the induction of AA. However, germ-free Fisher rats are susceptible to the induction of AA. The reconstitution of the gut flora with *E. coli* re-establishes resistance to arthritis [89]. Apparently, the conventional microbial gut environment in Fisher rats induces a T cell mediated protection against arthritis. Naïve, non-immunized Fisher rats raised in a normal microbial environment develop T cell responses to Mhsp65, whereas Fisher rats raised in a barrier facility fail to do so [90]. These Mhsp65 specific T cell responses are responsible for the reduced incidence and severity of arthritis in Fisher rats. The priming for Mhsp65 specific T cells is explained by molecular mimicry between Mhsp65 and homologues in the normal microbial environment of the rats, mainly the gut microbial flora.

Key point summary

- AA is an experimental animal model of T cell mediated arthritis with a close resemblance to JIA, and is an excellent model to study the interaction between the microbial environment and the immune system in arthritis.

- Hsp are highly conserved immune dominant proteins, which are up-regulated during cellular stress, and are seen in the

synovial tissue of animals with arthritis, as well as JIA and RA patients.

- Hsp appear to induce a regulatory T cell response in patients with JIA and this response appears to be correlated with remittance of disease in Oligoarthritis.

- In experimental arthritis, the microbial environment, and regulatory T cells responding to microbial hsp, determines disease susceptibility. Similar mechanisms appear to be in place in JIA.

Conclusion

Although many issues still have to be resolved, it is clear that the environment plays an important role in disease susceptibility in patients with JIA. This role may not just be in initiating disease through persisting antigens, bystander activation, and molecular mimicry in promoting and maintaining the ongoing inflammatory response. In addition to this, the microbial environment of an individual may also be instrumental in initiating a secondary regulatory immune response.

References

1. Woo, P. and Wedderburn, L.R. Juvenile chronic arthritis. *Lancet* 1998;351:969–73.
2. Prahalad, S., Ryan, M.H, Shear, E.S., Thompson, S.D., Giannini, E.H., and Glass, D.N. Juvenile rheumatoid arthritis: linkage to HLA demonstrated by allele sharing in affected sib pairs. *Arthritis Rheum.* 2000; 43:2335–8.
3. Glass, D.N. and Giannini, E.H. Juvenile rheumatoid arthritis as a complex genetic trait. *Arthritis Rheum.* 1999;42:2261–8.
4. Murray, K., Thompson, S.D., and Glass D.N. Pathogenesis of juvenile chronic arthritis: genetic and environmental factors. *Arch Dis Child* 1997; 77:530–4.
5. Nielsen, H.E., Dorup, J., Herlin, T., Larsen, K., Nielsen, S., and Pedersen, F.K. Epidemiology of juvenile chronic arthritis: risk dependent on sibship, parental income, and housing. *J Rheumatol.* 1999;26:1600–5.
6. Mattey, D.L., Dawes, P.T., Clarke, S., Fisher, J., Brownfield, A., Thomson, W. *et al.* Relationship among the HLA-DRB1 shared epitope, smoking, and rheumatoid factor production in rheumatoid arthritis. *Arthritis Rheum.* 2002;47:403–7.
7. Hutchinson, D., O'Leary, C., Nixon, N.B., and Mattey, D.L. Serum complexes of immunoglobulin A-alpha1 proteinase inhibitor in rheumatoid arthritis: association with current cigarette smoking and disease activity. *Clin Exp Rheumatol* 2002;20:387–91.
8. Jaakkola, J.J., and Gissler, M. Maternal smoking in pregnancy as a determinant of rheumatoid arthritis and other inflammatory polyarthritis during the first 7 years of life. *Int J. Epidemiology* 2005;34:664–71.
9. Mason, T., Rabinovich, C.E., Fredrickson, D.D., Amoroso, K., Reed, A.M., Stein, L.D. *et al.* Breast feeding and the development of juvenile rheumatoid arthritis. *J Rheumatol* 1995;22:1166–70.
10. Rosenberg, A.M., Evaluation of associations between breast feeding and subsequent development of juvenile rheumatoid arthritis. *J Rheumatol* 1996;23:1080–2.
11. Schrander, J.J., Marcelis, C., de Vries, M.P., and Santen-Hoeufft, H.M. Does food intolerance play a role in juvenile chronic arthritis? *Br J Rheumatol* 1997;36:905–8.
12. Pugh, M.T., Southwood, T., and Hill Gaston, J.S. The role of infection in Juvenile Chronic Arthritis. *Br J Rheumatol* 1993;32:838–44.

13. Wucherpfennig, K.W. Mechanisms for the induction of autoimmunity by infectious agents. *J Clin Invest* 2001;108:1097–104.

14. Sibilia, J. and Limbach, F.X. Reactive arthritis or chronic infectious arthritis? *Ann Rheum Dis.* 2002;61:580–7.

15. Benoist, C. and Mathis, D. Autoimmunity provoked by infection: how good is the case for T cell epitope mimicry? *Nat Immunol* 2001;2:797–801.

16. Rose, N.R. and Mackay, I.R. Molecular mimicry: a critical look at exemplary instances in human diseases. *Cell Mol Life Sci* 2000;57:542–51.

17. Massa, M., Mazzoli, F., Pignatti, P., De Benedetti, F., Passalia, M., Viola, S. et al. Proinflammatory responses to self HLA epitopes are triggered by molecular mimicry to Epstein-Barr virus proteins in oligoarticular juvenile idiopathic arthritis. *Arthritis Rheum* 2002;46:2721–9.

18. Wedderburn, L.R., Patel, A., Varsani, H., and Woo, P. Divergence in the degree of clonal expansions in inflammatory T cell subpopulations mirrors HLA-associated risk alleles in genetically and clinically distinct subtypes of childhood arthritis. *Int Immunol* 2001;13:1541–50.

19. Wedderburn, L.R., Robinson, N., Patel, A., Varsani, H., and Woo, P. Selective recruitment of polarized T cells expressing CCR5 and CXCR3 to the inflamed joints of children with juvenile idiopathic arthritis. *Arthritis Rheum* 2000;43:765–74.

20. Black, A.P., Bhayani, H., Ryder, C.A., Gardner-Medwin, J.M, Southwood, T.R. T-cell activation without proliferation in juvenile idiopathic arthritis. *Arthritis Res* 2002;4:177–83.

21. Murray, K.J., Grom, A.A., Thompson, S.D., Lieuwen, D., Passo, M.H., and Glass, D.N. Contrasting cytokine profiles in the synovium of different forms of juvenile rheumatoid arthritis and juvenile spondyloarthropathy: prominence of interleukin 4 in restricted disease. *J Rheumatol* 1998;25:1388–98.

22. van dH, I., Wilbrink, B., Tchetverikov, I., Schrijver, I.A., Schouls, L.M., Hazenberg, M.P. et al. Presence of bacterial DNA and bacterial peptidoglycans in joints of patients with rheumatoid arthritis and other arthritides. *Arthritis Rheum* 2000;43 (3):593–8.

23. Prakken, B., Kuis, W., Van Eden, W., Albani, S. Heat shock proteins in juvenile idiopathic arthritis: keys for understanding remitting arthritis and candidate antigens for immune therapy. *Curr Rheumatol Rep* 2002;4(6):466–73.

24. Van Eden, W., van der Zee, R., Paul, A.G.A., Prakken, B.J., Wendling, U., Anderton, S.M. et al. Do heat shock proteins control the balance of T-cell regulation in inflammatory diseases? *Immunol Today* 1998;19:303–7.

25. Hyrich, K.L. and Inman, R.D. Infectious agents in chronic rheumatic diseases. *Curr Opin Rheumatol* 2001;13:300–4.

26. Moore, T.L., Parvovirus-associated arthritis. *Curr Opin Rheumatol* 2000;12:289–94.

27. Lehmann, H.W., Plentz, A., Von Landenberg, P., Muller-Godeffroy E, and Modrow, S. Intravenous immunoglobulin treatment of four patients with juvenile polyarticular arthritis associated with persistent parvovirus B19 infection and antiphospholipid antibodies. *Arthritis Res Ther* 2004;6:R1–R6.

28. Lehmann, H.W., Knoll, A., Kuster, R.M., and Modrow, S. Frequent infection with a viral pathogen, parvovirus B19, in rheumatic diseases of childhood. *Arthritis Rheum* 2003;48:1631–8.

29. Oguz, F., Akdeniz, C., Unuvar E, Kucukbasmaci, O., and Sidal M. Parvovirus B19 in the acute arthropathies and juvenile rheumatoid arthritis. *J Paediatr Child Health* 2002;38:358–62.

30. Rahal, J.J., Millian, S.J., and Noriega, E.R. Coxsackievirus and adenovirus infection. Association with acute febrile and juvenile rheumatoid arthritis. *JAMA* 1976;235:2496–501.

31. Gordon, S.C. and Lauter, C.B. Mumps arthritis: a review of the literature. *Rev Infect Dis* 1984;6:338–44.

32. Oen, K., Fast, M., and Postl, B. Epidemiology of juvenile rheumatoid arthritis in Manitoba, Canada, 1975–92: cycles in incidence. *J Rheumatol* 1995;22:745–50.

33. Feldman, B.M., Birdi, N., Boone, J.E., Dent, P.B., Duffy, C.M., Ellsworth, J.E. et al. Seasonal onset of systemic-onset juvenile rheumatoid arthritis. *J Pediatr* 1996;129:513–8.

34. Uziel, Y., Pomeranz, A., Brik R, Navon, P., Mukamel M, Press, J. et al. Seasonal variation in systemic onset juvenile rheumatoid arthritis in Israel. *J Rheumatol* 1999;26:1187–9.

35. Wulffraat, N.M., Rijkers, G.T., Elst, E., Brooimans, R., and Kuis, W. Reduced perforin expression in systemic juvenile idiopathic arthritis is restored by autologous stem-cell transplantation. *Rheumatology* (Oxford) 2003;42:375–9.

36. Kyburz, D., Rethage, J., Seibl, R., Lauener, R., Gay, R.E., Carson, D.A. et al. Bacterial peptidoglycans but not CpG oligodeoxynucleotides activate synovial fibroblasts by toll-like receptor signaling. *Arthritis Rheum.* 2003;48:642–50.

37. Tolusso, B., Fabris, M., Di Poi, E., Assaloni, R., Tomietto, P., and Ferraccioli, G.F. Response of mononuclear cells to lipopolysaccharide and CpG oligonucleotide stimulation: possible additive effect in rheumatoid inflammation. *Ann Rheum Dis* 2003;62:284–5.

38. Krieg, A.M., The role of CpG motifs in innate immunity. *Curr Opin Immunol* 2000;12(1):35–43.

39. Deng, G.M., Nilsson, I.M., Verdrengh, M., Collins, L.V., Tarkowski, A. Intra-articularly localized bacterial DNA containing CpG motifs induces arthritis. *Nat Med* 1999;5(6):702–5.

40. Deng, G.M., Tarkowski, A. The features of arthritis induced by CpG motifs in bacterial DNA. *Arthritis Rheum* 2000;43(2):356–64.

41. Ronaghy, A., Prakken, B.J., Takabayashi, K., Roord, S.T.A, Firestein, G.S., Albani, S. et al. Immunostimulatory DNA sequences influence the course of adjuvant arthritis. *J Immunol* 2002;168:51–6.

42. Sigal, L.H. Synovial fluid-polymerase chain reaction detection of pathogens: what does it really mean? *Arthritis Rheum* 2001;44:2463–6.

43. Pacheco-Tena, C., Alvarado, D.L.B., Lopez-Vidal, Y., Vazquez-Mellado, J., Richaud-Patin, Y., Amieva, R.I. et al. Bacterial DNA in synovial fluid cells of patients with juvenile onset spondyloarthropathies. *Rheumatology* (Oxford) 2001;40:920–7.

44. Schnarr, S., Putschky, N., Jendro, M.C., Zeidler, H., Hammer, M., Kuipers, J.G. et al. Chlamydia and Borrelia DNA in synovial fluid of patients with early undifferentiated oligoarthritis: results of a prospective study. *Arthritis Rheum* 2001;44:2679–85.

45. Trollmo, C., Meyer, A.L., Steere, A.C., Hafler, D.A., Huber, B.T. Molecular mimicry in Lyme arthritis demonstrated at the single cell level: LFA-1 alpha L is a partial agonist for outer surface protein A-reactive T cells. *J Immunol* 2001;166:5286–91.

46. Hemmer, B., Gran, B., Zhao, Y., Marques, A., Pascal, J., Tzou, A. et al. Identification of candidate T-cell epitopes and molecular mimics in chronic Lyme disease. *Nat Med* 1999;5:1375–82.

47. Huppertz, H.I. Lyme disease in children. *Curr Opin Rheumatol* 2001;13:434–40.

48. Borchers, A.T., Keen, C.L., Shoenfeld, Y., and Silva, J., Jr., Gershwin, M.E. Vaccines, viruses, and voodoo. *J Investig Allergol Clin Immunol* 2002;12:155–68.

49. Shoenfeld, Y. and Aron-Maor A. Vaccination and autoimmunity- "vaccinosis": a dangerous liaison? *J Autoimmun* 2000;14:1–10.

50. Wraith, D.C., Goldman, M., and Lambert, P.H. Vaccination and autoimmune disease: what is the evidence? *Lancet* 2003;362: 1659–66.

51. Wills-Karp, M., Santeliz, J., and Karp C.L. The germless theory of allergic disease: revisiting the hygiene hypothesis. *Nat Rev Immunol* 2001; 1:69–75.

52. Bartolome Pacheco, M.J., Martinez-Taboada, V.M., Blanco, R., Rodriguez-Valverde, V., Valle, J.I., and Lopez-Hoyos, M. Reactive arthritis after BCG immunotherapy: T cell analysis in peripheral blood and synovial fluid. *Rheumatology* (Oxford) 2002;41:1119–25.

53. Benjamin, C.M. and Silman, A.J. Adverse reactions and mumps, measles and rubella vaccine. *J Public Health Med* 1991;13:32–4.

54. Benjamin, C.M., Chew, G.C., and Silman, A.J. Joint and limb symptoms in children after immunisation with measles, mumps, and rubella vaccine. *BMJ* 1992;304:1075–8.

55. Malleson, P.N., Tekano, J.L., Scheifele, D.W., Weber, JM. Influenza immunization in children with chronic arthritis: a prospective study. *J Rheumatol* 1993;20:1769–73.

56. Umetsu, D.T., McIntire, J.J., Akbari, O., Macaubas, C. DeKruyff, R.H. Asthma: an epidemic of dysregulated immunity. *Nat Immunol* 2002; 3:715–20.

57. McIntire, J.J., Umetsu, S.E., Akbari, O., Potter, M., Kuchroo, V.K., Barsh, G.S. *et al.* Identification of Tapr (an airway hyperreactivity regulatory locus) and the linked Tim gene family. *Nat Immunol* 2001;2:1109–16.

58. Yazdanbakhsh, M., van den, B.A., and Maizels, R.M. Th2 responses without atopy: immunoregulation in chronic helminth infections and reduced allergic disease. *Trends Immunol* 2001;22:372–7.

59. Prakken, B.J., Roord, S., Ronaghy, A., Wauben, M., Albani, S., and Van Eden, W. Heat shock protein 60 and adjuvant arthritis: a model for T cell regulation in human arthritis. Springer *Semin Immunopathol* 2003; 25:47–63.

60. Whitehouse, D.J., Whitehouse, M.W., and Pearson, C.M. Passive transfer of adjuvant-induced arthritis and allergic encephalomyelitis in rats using thoracic duct lymphocytes. *Nature.* 1969;224:1322–6.

61. Holoshitz, J., Naparstek, Y., Ben-Nun A, and Cohen, I.R. Lines of T lymphocytes induce or vaccinate against autoimmune arthritis. *Science* 1983;219:56–8.

62. Cohen, I.R., Holoshitz, J., Van Eden, W., and Frenkel, A. T lymphocyte clones illuminate pathogenesis and affect therapy of experimental arthritis. *Arthritis Rheum* 1985;28:841–5.

63. Welch, W. How cells respond to stress. *Sci Am* 1993;268:56–64.

64. Glick, B.S. Can hsp70 proteins act as force-generating motors? *Cell* 1995;80:11–4.

65. Young, R.A. Stress proteins and immunology. *Ann Rev Immunol* 1990;8:401–20.

66. Collins, P.L., Hightower, L.E. Newcastle virus stimulates the cellular accumulation of stress (heat shock) mRNA's and proteins. *J Virol* 1982; 44:703–7.

67. Young, D.R., Lathigra, R., Hendrix, R., Sweetser, D., Young, R.A. Stress proteins are immune targets in leprosy and tuberculosis. *Proc Natl Acad Sci USA* 1988;85:4267–70.

68. Kauffmann, S.H.E. Heat shock proteins and the immune response. *Immunol Today* 1990;11:129–36.

69. Lamb, J.R., Mendez-Samperio, P., Mehlert, A., So A, Rothbard, J., Jindal, S. *et al.* Stress proteins may provide a link between the immune response to infection and autoimmunity. *Int Immunol* 1989;1:191–6.

70. Young, R.A., and Elliot, T.J. Stress proteins, infection and immune surveillance. *Cell* 1989;59:5–8.

71. Van Eden, W., Thole, J.E.R., van der Zee, R., Noordzij, A., van Embden, J.D.A., Hensen, E.J. *et al.* Cloning of the mycobacterial epitope recognized by T lymphocytes in adjuvant arthritis. *Nature* 1988;331:171–3.

72. Wilbrink, B., Holewijn, M., Bijlsma, J.W.J., van Roy, J.L.A.M., van der Zee, R., Boog, C.J.P. *et al.* Antigen-activated T cells inhibit cartilage proteoglycan synthesis idependently of T-cell proliferation. *Scand J Immunol* 1992; 36:733–43.

73. Van Bilsen, J.H., Wagenaar-Hilbers, J.P., Boot, E.P., Van Eden, W., and Wauben, M.H. Searching for the cartilage-associated mimicry epitope in adjuvant arthritis. *Autoimmunity* 2002;35:201–10.

74. van de Broek, M.F., Hogervorst, E.J.M., van Bruggen, M.C.J., Van Eden, W., van der Zee, R., van den Berg, W. Protection against streptococcal cell wall-induced arthritis by pretreatment with the 65-kD mycobacterial heat shock protein. *J Exp Med* 1989;170:449–66.

75. Billingham, M.E.J., Carney, S., Butler R, Colston, M.J. A mycobacterial 65-kD heat shock protein induces antigen specific suppression of adjuvant arthritis, but is not itself arthritogenic. *J Exp Med* 1990;171:339–44.

76. Beech, J.T., Khai Siew, L., Ghoraishian, M., Stasiuk, L.M., Elson, C.J., and Thompson, S.J. CD4+T cells specific for mycobacterial 65-kilodalton heat shock protein protect against pristane induced arthritis. *J Immunol* 1997;159:3692–7.

77. Anderton, S.M., van der Zee, R., Prakken, A.B.J., Noordzij, A., Van Eden W. Activation of T-cells recognizing self 60 kDa heat shock protein can protect against experimental arthritis. *J Exp Med* 1995;181:943–52.

78. Paul, A.G., van Der, Z.R., Taams, L.S., and Van Eden, W. A self-hsp60 peptide acts as a partial agonist inducing expression of B7–2 on mycobacterial hsp60-specific T cells: a possible mechanism for inhibitory T cell regulation of adjuvant arthritis? *Int Immunol* 2000;12:1041–50.

79. Paul, A.G., van Kooten, P.J., Van Eden, W., van Der, Z.R. Highly autoproliferative T cells specific for 60-kDa heat shock protein produce IL-4/IL-10 and IFN-gamma and are protective in adjuvant arthritis. *J Immunol* 2000;165:7270–7.

80. de Graeff-Meeder, E.R., Zee, R., Rijkers, G.T., Schuurman, H-J, Kuis, W., Bjlsman, J.W.J. *et al.* Recognition of human 60 kD heat shock protein by mononuclear cells from patients with juvenile chronic arthritis. *Lancet* 1991;337:1368–72.

81. de Graeff-Meeder, E.R., Voorhorst, M., Van Eden, W., Schuurman, H-J, Huber, J., Barkley, D. *et al.* Antibodies to the mycobacterial 65-kD heat shock protein are reactive with synovial tissue of adjuvant arthritic rats and patients with rheumatoid arthritis and osteoarthritis. *Am J Path* 1990;137:1013–7.

82. Albani, S., Ravelli, A., Massa, M., De Benedetti, F., Andree, G., Roudier, J. *et al.* Immune responses to the Escherichia coli dnaJ heat shock protein in juvenile rheumatoid arthritis and their correlation with disease activity. *J Pediatr* 1994;124:561–5.

83. Life, P., Hassel, A., Williams, K., Young, S., Bacon, P., Southwood, T. *et al.* Responses to gram negative enteric bacterial antigens by synovial T cells from patients with Juvenile Chronic Arthritis: recognition of heat shock protein hsp60. *J Rheumatol* 1993;20:1388–96.

84. de Graeff-Meeder, E.R., Van Eden, W., Rijkers, G.T., Prakken, A.B.J., Kuis, W., Voorhorst-Ogink, M.M. *et al.* Juvenile Chronic Arthritis: T Cell Reactivity to Human HSP60 in Patients with a Favourable Course of Arthritis. *J Clin Invest* 1995;95:934–40.

85. Prakken, A.B.J., van Hoeij, M.J., Kuis, W., Kavelaars, A., Heijnen, C.J., Scholtens, E., *et al.* T-cell reactivity to human hsp60 in oligoarticular juvenile chronic arthritis is associated with a favorable prognosis and the generation of regulatory cytokines in the inflamed joint. *Immunol Lett* 1997;57:139–42.

86. de Kleer, I.M., Kamphuis, S.M., Rijkers, G.T., Scholtens, L., Gordon, G., de Jager, W. *et al.* The spontaneous remission of juvenile idiopathic arthritis is characterized by CD30+T cells directed to human heat-shock protein

60 capable of producing the regulatory cytokine interleukin-10. *Arthritis Rheum* 2003;48:2001–10.

87. Weiner, H.L. Oral tolerance: immune mechanisms and the generation of Th3-type TGF-beta-secreting regulatory cells. *Microbes Infect* 2001;3: 947–54.

88. Van Eden, W., Wendling, U., Paul, A.G., Prakken, B., van Kooten, P., van der Zee, R. Arthritis protective regulatory potential of self-hsp cross-reactive T cells. *Cell, Stress, Chaperones* 2000;5:452–7.

89. Kohashi, O., Kohashi, Y., Ozawa, A., Shigematsu, N. Suppressive effect of E. coli on adjuvant-induced arthritis in germ free rats. *Arthritis Rheum* 1986;29:547.

90. Moudgil, K.D., Kim, E., Yun, O.J., Chi, H.H., Brahn, E., and Sercarz, E.E. Environmental modulation of autoimmune arthritis involves the spontaneous microbial induction of T cell responses to regulatory determinants within heat shock protein 65. *J Immunol* 2001;166: 4237–43.

3

The approach to treating Juvenile Idiopathic Arthritis

3.1   Introduction
      Peter N. Malleson

3.2   Patient-centred care and the team approach
      Ciarán Duffy

3.3   Adolescent rheumatology services
      Janet E. McDonagh and Patience White

3.4   Disease evaluation
      Lori B. Tucker

3.5   Educational issues
      Laurie Ebner-Lyon and Joy Brown

3.6   Psychosocial aspects
      Karen Shaw

3.7   Pain assessment and management
      David D. Sherry, James W. Varni, and Michael A. Rapoff

3.8   Pharmacological treatment of early or established arthritis
      Peter N. Malleson

3.9   Physiotherapy and occupational therapy
      Gay Kuchta and Iris Davidson

3.10 Nutrition
      Deborah Rothman

3.11 Adjunctive therapies
      Marisa Klein-Gitelman

3.12 Surgical interventions
      Ann Hall

3.13 Clinical trials
      Brian Feldman

3.14 Pharmacological treatment: Approach to the management of refractory arthritis
      Nico M. Wulffraat and Berent J. Prakken

      Appendix: Intra-articular corticosteroid injections
      Clive A.J. Ryder, Taunton R. Southwood, and Peter N. Malleson

3.1　Introduction

Peter N. Malleson

Introduction

Juvenile Idiopathic Arthritis (JIA) is a difficult condition to treat for a number of reasons. As has been discussed in the previous section JIA is not a single disease, but several conditions linked by the presence of a chronic arthritis affecting one or more joints in a child. A child with Oligoarthritis who has one inflamed knee is going to require a different management approach to a child who has Systemic Arthritis associated with severe daily fevers and pericarditis. Even within any particular subtype, the management may vary substantially for different individuals. For example, a young child who is just learning to walk, and who develops a swollen knee will have different functional problems than a school-aged child with a monoarthritis of a wrist who must write a lot. We are increasingly aware that children with JIA have a very high probability of continuing with active arthritis for many years, and that even if the arthritis remits, it may recur after many years for no apparent reason. At present, although we are able to make some general statements about the likelihood of remission for individual subsets of JIA, we are unable to tell an individual child and her parents whether or not the arthritis will remit, whether it will stay in remission, or what medications are going to be required to control the disease.

The basic tenet underlying this section is that the management of JIA requires a multidisciplinary approach, as no single individual can effectively cope with all the facets of the disease. Not only must the management be multidisciplinary, but it must also be interdisciplinary. In other words, the optimal treatment of JIA with its uncertain and variable disease course, requires close collaboration between a number of different experts (including the parents and child) working together as a team. Given the need for a team approach, it follows that all children with JIA should ideally be cared for by a paediatric rheumatology service, working closely with family physicians, and paediatricians. However, because of the paucity of paediatric rheumatology programs, even in the developed world, we recognize that this ideal is not always achievable, and that general paediatricians with an interest in childhood arthritis, and adult-trained rheumatologists may often have to provide much, or all, of the child's care. Hopefully, the various chapters in this section will be of help in guiding physicians and other health care professionals in their interactions with children with JIA.

To help the reader understand how treatment decisions are arrived at, and why and when the treatment is modified, we have asked the contributing authors, where appropriate, to divide the disease course into three stages; early, established, and refractory. These divisions are of course somewhat arbitrary because JIA is such a variable chronic disease, and the definitions we have used are certainly open to criticism; nevertheless, we believe that they are a valuable way of thinking about how to manage a child with chronic arthritis. However, as the contributors make clear, treatment decisions have to be made based not only on the disease course, but on other very critical factors, that are often difficult to define or quantify, such as the disease severity, the extent of the child's pain, the apparent effect of the disease on the child's quality of life, the child's and parent's own belief systems, and the child's developmental level.

Listed below are some definitions of the terms we use in this section. Although they are arbitrary, (except for the criteria for remission, which were developed through a consensus conference), and would not be universally accepted, these definitions probably approximate how paediatric rheumatologists approach these diseases from a practical point of view.

Active arthritis. Swelling within a joint, or limitation in range of joint movement with joint pain or tenderness.

Remission (as defined in the Preliminary criteria for inactive disease and clinical remission in JIA) (1)

Inactive disease

1. No joints with active arthritis[a,b]

2. No fever, rash, serositis, splenomegaly, or generalized lymphadenopathy attributable to JIA

3. No active uveitis (to be defined)

4. Normal ESR or CRP (if both are tested, both must be normal)

5. Physician's global assessment of disease activity indicates no disease activity (i.e., best score attainable on the scale used)

Clinical remission

Clinical remission on medication. The criteria for inactive disease must be met for a minimum of 6 continuous months while the patient is on medication in order for the patient to be considered to be in a state of clinical remission on medication.

Clinical remission off medication. The criteria for inactive disease must be met for a minimum of 12 continuous months while off all

---

[a] The ACR defines a joint with active arthritis as a joint with swelling not due to bony enlargement or, if no swelling is present, limitation of motion accompanied by either pain on motion and/or tenderness.
[b] An isolated finding of pain on motion, tenderness, or limitation of motion on joint examination may be present only if explained by either prior damage attributable to arthritis that is now considered inactive, or non-rheumatological reasons such as trauma.

anti-arthritis and anti-uveitis medications in order for the patient to be considered to be in a state of clinical remission off medication.

Flare. Any increase in disease activity in a child with previous or current arthritis which requires an increase in treatment. Although a flare of disease does not necessarily lead to a change in treatment, any clinically significant flare probably should.

Early disease. Active arthritis within first 6 months of onset of arthritis in a child with no previous history of arthritis. There is nothing 'magic' about the 6-month time span, but is long enough to:

1. Allow for the 6 weeks needed to establish that the child does indeed have a chronic arthritis, and fulfils classification criteria for JIA.
2. Enable classification of the type of JIA.
3. Allow for many weeks of initial treatment before the disease is considered as 'established'; occasionally children do have complete resolution of arthritis within a number of weeks.
4. Enable the family and child accept that they are going to have to live with a chronic disease.

Established disease. Persistence of arthritis in one or more joints despite appropriate treatment can be considered established disease. The acceptance that the child has established arthritis, means that, if not already prescribed, the child requires treatment with second-line agents, may require modifications to family and school life, and needs regular ongoing clinic follow-up over many years.

Refractory disease. Persistently active arthritis in one or more joints despite a prolonged period (perhaps 2 years or more) of consistent therapy with at least non-steroidal anti-inflammatory drugs (NSAIDs), intra-articular corticosteroid injections and methotrexate, or/and sulfasalazine could be considered refractory disease. A child with refractory disease should certainly be considered a candidate for anti-(tumour necrosis factor) TNF therapy. Increasingly, paediatric rheumatologists are using anti-TNF drugs earlier on in the disease course, and would not consider the child as having refractory disease until treatment with these class of drugs has failed to establish a drug-maintained remission. However, anti-TNF drugs and other biologics should probably still be considered somewhat experimental, as data about long-term efficacy, and importantly, safety are not yet available. Once a child is accepted as having refractory disease, more experimental therapies are increasingly likely to be options considered by the physician and the child and family. Also the child and family will need to re-evaluate their life goals, and review whether or not their long-term plans are appropriate given the child's disease severity.

Disease activity

Mild disease

Active arthritis which:

1. Does not interfere with a child's normal activities of daily living.

2. Is not associated with any evidence of disease progression (either clinically or radiographically) over a 6-month period.

Moderate disease

Active arthritis which:

1. Interferes with a child's normal activities to some extent, but does not prevent participation in most school activities including Physical Education, or equivalent activities if the child is of pre-school age.
2. Apparently mild disease, but associated with disease progression (either clinically or radiographically).

Severe disease

1. Active arthritis which severely inhibits normal activities of daily living.
2. Active arthritis associated with the development of erosions and/or ankylosis

Disease damage

Damage refers to any change in the anatomy or function of an individual joint as a consequence of current or previous active arthritis that is considered likely to be permanent even if the arthritis is in remission.

Mild damage

1. Loss of joint range of movement of less than 10%
2. Radiographic changes that demonstrate some bony overgrowth only.

Moderate damage

1. Loss of joint range of movement of greater than 10% but less than 25%
2. Radiographic changes that demonstrate joint space narrowing, but no bony erosions or ankylosis.

Severe damage

1. Loss of joint range of movement of greater than 25%
2. Radiographic changes that demonstrate erosions or ankylosis.

References

1. Wallace, C.A., Ruperto, N., Giannini, E.H., *et al.* Preliminary criteria for clinical remission for select categories of Juvenile Idiopathic Arthritis. *J Rheumatol* 2004;31:2290–4.

3.2 Patient-centred care and the team approach

Ciarán Duffy

Aim

The aim of this chapter is to describe how an ideal paediatric rheumatology clinic might be structured, recognizing that such an ideal is not always obtainable. The rationale for a paediatric team and the important concept of making the patient a central component of the team is discussed.

Structure

- Introduction
- The concept of patient-centred care
- The importance of the team approach
- The importance of communication
- Overall objectives of delivery of care
- The paedatric rheumatology team
- Consultants to the paedatric rheumatology team
- Team dynamics (interaction/team meetings)
- School issues
- Delivery of a comprehensive clinical service
- The team approach to the child with JIA at various stages
- Incorporating academic responsibilities into the clinic setting
- Other issues
- Summary and conclusions

Introduction

The delivery of health care to the population at large is an incredibly complex task that has become increasingly more difficult over these past few decades. Amazing technological advances, groundbreaking new discoveries, new treatments, evidence-based approaches, outcomes research, 'managed care', and easy access to information via the Internet are some of the factors that have contributed to this complexity. While these advances should lead to enhanced patient outcomes, they can also make delivery of optimal patient care more difficult. This 'modernization' has resulted in an exponential increase in costs. For this reason, it is incumbent upon everyone involved in health care delivery to ensure that we do our utmost to use our resources wisely and efficiently in ensuring appropriate care for our patients. Although in many countries government and/or private insurance schemes dictate the global distribution of health care delivery, individual health care providers can still influence how health care is effectively provided to individual patients.

The provision of health care to children with chronic disabling diseases such as the rheumatic diseases is a particular challenge. Their health care costs are proportionately higher than adults, and this is largely due to the need to provide a more intricate approach that is largely team-based as opposed to the mainly solitary caregiver delivery system of adult medicine.

Children with Juvenile Idiopathic Arthritis (JIA) and other rheumatic diseases have particular needs that must be emphasized. This chapter describes a team approach that has evolved over a number of years, and that works well, we believe, in providing high-quality care. It is not a fixed template, as different systems will require modifications of this approach. Nevertheless, the general outline is applicable to most situations. Individuals working with children with JIA and other rheumatic diseases need to try and incorporate most of these ideas if the children are to receive optimal care. Although this book's focus is on chronic arthritis, the paediatric rheumatology team looks after children with a wide variety of musculoskeletal, and systemic diseases, and so this chapter describes the whole range of issues that have to be addressed, and discusses all the resources needed to provide a complete paediatric rheumatology programme.

The concept of patient-centred care

Patient-centred care is a powerful concept. It not only implies that the whole focus of the delivery of care should be on the patient (and in the case of children this automatically also means on the family), but it further implies that the patient and their family should be active participants in decisions regarding management. Given the broad heterogeneity of society in terms of cultural differences, and family structure, in addition to the heterogeneity of the rheumatic diseases themselves and the broad age range of affected children, this presents a significant challenge. It is extremely important to ensure that patients and their families have a clear understanding of the disease and the rationale for its treatment. A lack of understanding on the part of the family is associated with poor adherence to the treatment regimen [1]. Incorporating the wishes of the child and family into the treatment regimen, as long as these are not contrary to the overall philosophy of the programme, is associated with better adherence [2].

The importance of the team approach

Most treatment situations in medicine are based on the concept of the single patient–single physician relationship. Even though this still represents an important aspect of successful management in all situations, completely successful delivery of care to children with rheumatic diseases depends, in addition, on a highly functional, interactive, and committed, specialized team. This is important because management is multi-faceted and, therefore, no one individual can oversee all aspects of care. Smooth team interactions with an absence of overtly hierarchical structures is of paramount importance; each team member has an important role to play and at any one time the needs of the patient may require more or less input from a particular team member. Nevertheless, the leadership role provided by the paediatric rheumatologist must be emphasized. Regular team meetings enable ease of transfer of important information, thereby ensuring that all team members are up to date on all patients. Such meetings help ensure consistency in the delivery of care for individual patients in the responses from team members to questions from the patient and their family. A consistent message to the child and family is associated with better adherence to the treatment regimen [2].

The importance of communication

Successful outcomes depend on maintenance of good communication. Team members are helped in this regard by frequent interactions and team meetings. Generally speaking, it is the responsibility of the patient's paediatric rheumatologist to communicate with the patient and family regarding the diagnosis, disease status, objectives for treatment, treatment regimen, and treatment side effects. The paediatric rheumatologist must also communicate both verbally and in writing with the patient's primary care physician, and other physicians involved in the child's care. The paediatric rheumatology nurse will generally reinforce what the paediatric rheumatologist has conveyed to the patient and can, by acting as a liaison, ensure that information passes back and forth between the patient and the team as needed between clinic visits. Usually patients prefer to communicate on an ongoing basis with one individual as specific needs arise and in most situations the team nurse takes on this role [3,4]. However, at different times and with different individuals and families different team members may become the contact person for the family. The team nurse may also liaise with community-based institutions such as the child's school or local health centre.

Overall objectives of delivery of care

The overall objectives of delivery of care are listed below (Table 3.2.1) [2]. For the most part, since these diseases are not curable, the major focus is on controlling the disease and reducing the risk of poor outcomes. Initially, the focus is on relieving pain and discomfort, controlling inflammation, maintaining function, and preventing deformities. Over the long term the aim is to promote normal growth and development while minimizing systemic side-effects of the disease and its treatment. Whatever the severity of the child's disease, it is critical to ensure access to a full education if the child is going to grow into a functionally independent adult.

The impact of the rheumatic disease on children, their psychosocial development, family and school life have been studied to some extent [5–9] (see also Part 3, Chapter 3.6). Children with arthritis generally

Table 3.2.1 Overall objectives of the delivery of care

Early disease
  Relieve pain and discomfort
  Control inflammation
  Maintain physical functioning
  Prevent early development of deformities
  Maintain psychological functioning

Established and/or recalcitrant disease
  Minimize the systemic effects of the disease
  Minimize the side-effects of treatment
  Maintain physical functioning
  Prevent permanent deformities and damage
  Maintain psychological functioning
  Ensure ongoing education
  Promote good nutrition
  Promote and permit normal growth and development

function well as adults. Many go on to lead full lives, completing their education and having families of their own [10,11], but appropriate preparation is usually required for this to occur [12] (Part 3, Chapter 3.3). A Federal commission in the United States in the late 1980s, stated that optimal care for children with chronic diseases should be child- and family-centred, community-based, and coordinated [13,14]. The paediatric rheumatology team in most centres has adopted this approach.

The paediatric rheumatology team

The paediatric rheumatology team is multidisciplined (Figure 3.2.1). It is usually centred in an academically based tertiary care centre although this is not always the case. In order to function appropriately the main team must consist of, at the very least, the following members—a paediatric rheumatologist, a paediatric rheumatology nurse specialist, a paediatric rheumatology physical therapist, a paediatric rheumatology occupational therapist and a social worker. Almost all patients with JIA will require input from these team members on an ongoing basis.

Paediatric rheumatologist(s)

Usually the team leader is a paediatric rheumatologist, that is, a physician who has trained and is certified in paediatrics with further training and certification in paediatric rheumatology. In situations where there is no paediatric rheumatologist, a paediatrician or an "adult" rheumatologist who, while not certified in paediatric rheumatology, has further training and an interest in the specialty might assume this role. Ideally, this situation should be uncommon in developed countries but still does occur in the United States, Canada, and European Union countries. It is even more likely to occur in less developed countries. If at all possible, communication should take place with a paediatric rheumatologist regarding the patient at some point. To be effective, such communication should take place as early as possible after diagnosis and from time to time over the course of the disease.

The responsibilities of the paediatric rheumatologist are listed below (Table 3.2.2). Although the paediatric rheumatologist is usually the team leader, other members of the team have to be able to function largely independently of the paediatric rheumatologist.

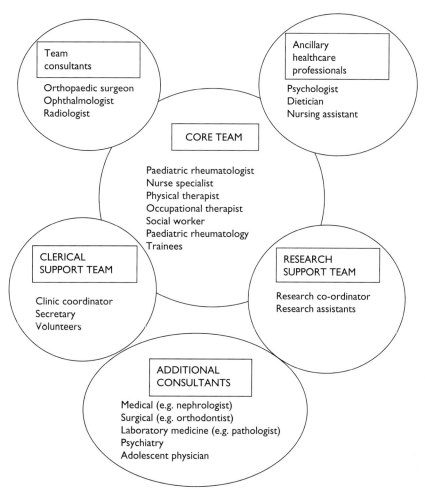

Fig. 3.2.1 The paediatric rheumatology team.

Table 3.2.2 The role of the paediatric rheumatologist

Evaluates the patient

Makes and confirms the diagnosis

Initiates the treatment plan

Educates the patient/family regarding the diagnosis, treatment, side effects of treatment, and prognosis

Communicates the plan to other team members

Communicates the diagnosis and plan to the primary care physician

Responds appropriately to questions arising from the diagnosis and treatment plan from all sources

Promotes a positive approach to management

Table 3.2.3 The role of the paediatric rheumatology nurse

Reinforces issues regarding the diagnosis and treatment plan with the patient/family and other team members

Evaluates the effects of the diagnosis and treatment plan

Explores in greater depth the psychosocial situation for the family and their beliefs about the disease and its treatment

Evaluates the competency of the family in adhering to the treatment plan

Serves as an educational resource for the patient/family

Explores available community resources and promotes appropriate implementation

Liaises with the school

Maintains ongoing communication with the patient/family between clinic visits

Functions as the team coordinator and keeps team members informed appropriately on developments

Paediatric rheumatology nurse

The paediatric rheumatology nurse plays a pivotal role in coordination of care and in team functioning and in many respects is the most important member of the team. Data show that the incorporation of a nurse specialist for a whole variety of areas in the paediatric domain is cost-effective [15]. The nurse usually functions as the coordinator of most team activities and serves to keep everybody up to date with individual patient problems. The nurse also plays an important direct role in patient management and education, a role that is critical to

ensuring appropriate understanding of the patient and his/her family of the disease and its management. The team nurse's main responsibilities are listed above (Table 3.2.3).

The individual assuming this position must be highly competent, astute, a good observer, and possess a great amount of 'common sense' since team dynamics depend on it. Some centres are fortunate to have more than one nurse specialist. Where there is more than one, it is important that the roles of each are clearly defined. Ultimately, it is preferable to have one assume the role of overall coordinator.

Physical therapist

Physical therapy is a fundamental component of the treatment of all patients with chronic forms of arthritis. It is also important for many patients with other rheumatic diseases. It is important that the team physical therapist be sufficiently experienced in treating patients with inflammatory diseases and understands the incredible variability that occurs between different patients with apparently similar diseases, as well as the variation that occurs within an individual child over time. Furthermore, the therapist must be fully cognizant of the developmental stage of the child and its variability. Such issues must be taken into consideration both in prescribing an initial program and in monitoring its effectiveness. Generally speaking, patients need to be seen by the physical therapist more frequently early in the course of the disease to consolidate the physical therapy program and to ensure adherence (Table 3.2.4). (see Part 3, Chapter 3.9)

Occupational therapist

Occupational therapy is also a fundamental component of the treatment of patients with rheumatic diseases. All of the points made above in relation to the team physical therapist are equally applicable to the team occupational therapist. In addition to the initiation of a therapy programme, the occupational therapist is usually involved in the manufacture of orthotics (wrist, knee, foot, and finger splints) and in monitoring their use. As the child gets older, this therapist also plays an important role in suggesting and improving the ability of the child to participate in age-appropriate activities, with an emphasis on activities of daily living (Table 3.2.4). The occupational therapist and physiotherapist need to work closely together, often seeing the patient at the same time to optimize treatment interventions (see Part 3, Chapter 3.9).

Table 3.2.4 The role of the paediatric rheumatology physical and occupational therapists

Evaluate the extent of the functional limitations of the child in an age-appropriate manner

Initiate a rehabilitation programme for home use that is developmentally appropriate

Emphasize range of motion exercises and maintenance of a good functional joint position in the early stages of the disease, and continue to maintain this during long-term follow-up

Emphasize strengthening exercises when the initial acute inflammatory stage of the disease has started to abate

Promote strategies to avoid development of deformities

Monitor progress continuously and promote adherence with the therapeutic regimen

Evaluate the need for and prescribe functional aids (orthotics, walking aids, etc.) when appropriate

Additional members of the team—ancillary health care professionals, social worker, psychologist, and dietician

Given the complexity of JIA and the other rheumatic diseases, and their potential to have profound negative psychosocial effects and effects on normal growth and development, there is a need to have input from a variety of ancillary health care professionals including a social worker, psychologist, and dietician. Some centres also have a parent liaison. Ideally, each of these individuals should be an integral member of the team but lack of resources often does not permit this.

The families of children with these diseases may induce significant financial hardship, as a result of costs of medications, orthotics, travel to appointments, and days lost from school and work. Therefore, the social worker has an important role to play in ensuring that appropriate community and other resources are in place and utilized [16,17] (Table 3.2.5).

The multiple problems associated with a chronic painful disease can have significant negative psychological effects on the child and the child's family, with tremendous potential to impact negatively on school performance, peer relationships, and to induce family discord [9–11]. Input from a psychologist is often required to address these effects (Table 3.2.5). (See Part 3, Chapter 3.6.)

The added financial burden, effects of disease on growth and development, and the side effects of medications such as corticosteroids, may all affect nutritional status, so advice from a dietician/nutritionist is often required [18,19] (Table 3.2.5). In situations where these health professionals are not available for team meetings, it is important for the team coordinator to obtain appropriate input from them prior to team meetings, and to provide feedback to them after these meetings. When they are not available at all some other member of the team has to assume their role, a task often assumed by the team nurse.

Paediatric rheumatology trainees

Several centres train paediatricians in the art and science of paediatric rheumatology. In such centres, trainees play an integral part in team functioning. They are often the point of first physician contact for patients and continue to provide ongoing care for a large number of patients. As their experience increases they often assume a significant team role, taking on some of the responsibilities of the paediatric rheumatologist, under his or her supervision.

Medical students and trainees in paediatrics, immunology, and adult rheumatology may transiently be involved with the team but

Table 3.2.5 The role of other allied health professionals

Evaluate socio-familial factors likely to influence adherence with suggested therapeutic regimen
family structure, ethnicity, cultural mores, finances, support systems

Ensure establishment of a liaison with community resources

Evaluate psychosocial factors likely to impact on the child and family with particular emphasis on family functioning, peer relationships, and school performance

Evaluate growth and development with a particular emphasis on nutritional status

Provide education in advocacy and school-related issues

Table 3.2.6 Consultants to the team

Paediatric surgical/diagnostic consultants
    Ophthalmologist
    Orthopaedic surgeon
    Orthodontist/oral surgeon
    Pathologist
    Musculoskeletal radiologist

Paediatric medical consultants
    Cardiologist
    Dermatologist
    Gastroenterologist
    Immunologist
    Nephrologist
    Neurologist
    Psychiatrist

their role during this time is usually minor and must be under the careful supervision of the paediatric rheumatologist.

Consultants to the paediatric rheumatology team

There are a variety of physician consultants who provide important input on individual patient status (Table 3.2.6).

Ophthalmologist

The role of the ophthalmologist is a critical one for patients with JIA as they have an increased risk of developing uveitis, as well as being at risk from ocular toxicities associated with corticosteroids and anti-malarial drugs. Close coordination of care between the ophthalmologist and the paediatric rheumatologist is associated with a better outcome for eye disease [20].

Orthopaedic surgeon

While the paediatric rheumatologist conducts most intra-articular injections in most settings, occasionally an orthopaedic surgeon might be required to undertake some. This is apt to occur in situations where the child requires general anaesthesia or when assisted imaging is required. Additionally, children with rheumatic diseases often develop deformities requiring input from an orthopaedic surgeon. Specific surgical interventions, including tendon-lengthening procedures for hip flexion contractures and joint replacements, may be required for some patients. It is imperative to involve the orthopaedic surgeon early in the disease course so that an appropriate baseline assessment can be conducted and thus intervention can be undertaken in a timely fashion. To facilitate interaction between the paediatric rheumatologist and the orthopaedic surgeon, a combined clinic with both in attendance is very helpful if this can be arranged.

Orthodontist/oral surgeon/oral hygienist

Many patients with JIA develop micrognathia due to bilateral temporomandibular joint involvement with resultant overbite. Others may develop asymmetric jaw growth due to unilateral temporomandibular involvement. Such patients may benefit from input from an orthodontist and/or an oral surgeon. Additionally, proper oral hygiene is of paramount importance as poor dental hygiene may lead to an increased risk of infection [21], especially in an era in which there is an increase in the use of immunomodulating agents.

Paediatric radiologist

It is essential to have a highly experienced paediatric musculoskeletal radiologist as a consultant to the team. It is extremely valuable to have weekly meetings for the radiologist to review all imaging studies performed in the preceding week. It is also often very important to review radiographs performed at outside institutions, as the reports by adult radiologists may be incorrect. Regular radiology sessions provide a tremendous opportunity not only to make diagnoses but also to evaluate changes in patients over time. This clearly impacts on decision-making regarding patient management, but also provides an important learning opportunity for the paediatric rheumatologists and the trainees.

It is critical that a paediatric rheumatology centre has access to all the modern imaging technologies, if an optimal service is to be provided.

Other medical consultants

A number of medical consultants might be called upon to provide input regarding the evaluation and management of children with rheumatic diseases. These include specialists in cardiology, dermatology, gastroenterology, immunology, nephrology, and neurology. Input from these and other medical consultants may be required for individual patients, particularly during an inpatient hospitalization. Additionally, some of these consultants might attend a clinic specifically designated for a particular disease. For example, to set up a systemic lupus erythematosus (SLE) clinic together with a paediatric nephrologist has distinct practical benefits when there is a sufficiently large SLE cohort to justify such a clinic.

The number and breadth of consultants needed for an optimal paediatric rheumatology service makes it very difficult to run an appropriate service outside of a tertiary/quaternary care paediatric facility.

Team dynamics (interaction/team meetings)

The team should meet formally on a regular basis, preferably once a week, although individual team members might interact much more often to discuss specific issues. Patients seen in the preceding interval are discussed. Those with major problems should be discussed in detail. Such meetings serve as a forum for information sharing and are of vital importance for team functioning. It is common for one member to divulge important patient information of which other members might be unaware. Such meetings also provide a forum for discussion of new data and new interventions. They also assure consistency in delivery of care and in particular of the message that one wishes to convey to patients and their families.

While it is important to have input from all present it is also important to have a designated individual to run the meetings and to ensure that the meeting proceeds and concludes in a timely fashion. Furthermore, it is also necessary to ensure that required information such as laboratory results and consultation reports are available at the meeting to ensure appropriate decision-making. The nurse coordinator will usually assume this role but clearly it is a role that can be performed by others. Having good secretarial/clerical support further facilitates having appropriate information.

It is also important to ensure that issues that come up between meetings and clinic visits of specific patients are noted and shared among team members. This role is invariably assumed by the nurse coordinator. This individual is usually the point of first contact for patients who generally prefer to deal with one person to deliver new information [3].

School issues

Children with rheumatic diseases must attend school regularly. The team works to ensure that as little school as possible is missed. Furthermore, the team has a responsibility to communicate with the school should specific services be required to ensure that the child can attend school on a regular basis. Frequently, physical education teachers lack the knowledge and understanding required to provide an appropriate programme for these children. Communication with these teachers, in particular, is required. Children are often penalized because of their inability to carry out tasks in physical education or to complete tests requiring handwriting. These incidents occur all too frequently and can be avoided if there is appropriate communication from the team to the school [22]. A careful evaluation of each child with a rheumatic disease should be undertaken by the school in communication with the team coordinator to devise an appropriate programme specific to that child.

Delivery of a comprehensive clinical service

Inpatient service

Inpatient facilities

Some paediatric rheumatology centres are large enough to require specifically designated beds, the number of designated beds dependent upon the likelihood of occupancy within a given time period. This permits consistency regarding delivery of care and facilitates ease of training of ward personnel regarding the specific needs of these patients. However, few centres have this facility and most admit to general paediatric beds. Ideally, when it is necessary to admit patients it is preferable for all of them to be admitted to the same inpatient unit to enable inpatient staff expertise to be developed. When this fails to occur repetitive in-house training of ward personnel becomes the norm, a process that is quite inefficient. In such circumstances, the team nurse has a critical role to play in educating and liaising with the ward nurses to ensure that quality of patient care is not compromised.

Inpatient consultations

In addition to providing comprehensive inpatient care to rheumatology inpatients, it is also necessary to provide a consultation service to patients admitted to other services, or to patients who present to the emergency department. The type of patient for whom consultations are requested varies considerably, comprising acute and chronic conditions with a variety of symptoms from fever to bone and joint pain (see Algorithms, Part 1, Chapter 1.3). Some patients will be felt to have conditions that fall under the purvey of a paediatric rheumatologist, such as Systemic Arthritis, others not. A significant number of such patients will require ongoing follow-up by a paediatric rheumatologist following discharge from hospital to ensure that their acute problem has resolved or to watch for the evolution of a rheumatic disease.

Rheumatology inpatients

A number of children with rheumatic diseases require admission to hospital. These include children with significant systemic diseases not yet diagnosed, requiring intensive investigations, or children with exacerbations of diseases such as Systemic Arthritis, SLE, juvenile dermatomyositis, and others. Occasionally, children with Polyarthritis require hospitalization for intensive rehabilitation. Patients with pain syndromes such as reflex neurovascular dystrophy also may require hospitalization for intensive therapy. A number of patients require short hospital stays for intravenous therapies that cannot for practical reasons be administered as outpatients, although most centers now have specified outpatient infusion capabilities. As treatments have improved, and better organization of outpatient facilities has evolved fewer and fewer patients require hospital inpatient stays, with most care being provided in the ambulatory setting.

Outpatient service

Clinic coordination and clinic personnel

For most paediatric rheumatology centers, it is the outpatient service that represents the vast majority of clinical activity. Organization in this area is, therefore, of paramount importance in ensuring delivery of an appropriate service. Often visits to the rheumatology clinic for many of these patients coincide with visits to other clinics (ophthalmology, gastroenterology) and services (physiotherapy). Additionally, patients require blood procurement for laboratory investigations and frequently require imaging and other studies. Therefore, it is imperative that a system be put in place to allow for appropriate coordination and evaluation of these patients while maintaining efficiency in the delivery of care. The need for the patient to have to return at another time, for anything other than a new consultation with another service or for a more advanced imaging study, such as magnetic resonance imaging (MRI), should be avoided if at all possible. This exemplifies the notion of patient-centred care.

It is not possible for all of this to be done without a designated clerical clinic coordinator, trained in the specific issues pertinent to the delivery of care to this complex group of patients (Table 3.2.7). Aside from the booking and coordination of visits, the coordinator may also confirm visits with the patient's caregiver prior to the visit. This significantly reduces 'no shows' and permits a smoother transition of care. In performing this task, the coordinator may also field calls from patients and direct them appropriately. The coordinator may also serve as the clinic receptionist, thus ensuring ongoing coordination and overall efficiency. Centralized booking, and the use of a standardized software system, may assist this process but is not an

Table 3.2.7 Functions of the clerical clinic coordinator

Books rheumatology clinic appointments
Coordinates appointments with other services
Confirms all appointments with patient's caregiver prior to clinic visit
Fields calls from patient's caregiver
Functions as clinic receptionist

adequate substitute for a responsible, specifically designated, clerical clinic coordinator.

While the team nurse might attend all clinics, her role is quite broad, as previously described, and clearly not confined to the clinic. Thus, most clinics require the presence of a nursing assistant to document vital signs and growth parameters.

The clinic facilities

The layout and requirements of the ideal clinic set up for children with rheumatic diseases are listed below (Table 3.2.8). It is imperative that the space is child-friendly and inviting, being appropriately colourful with adequate distractions for small children. Also, as a large proportion of paediatric rheumatology patients are adolescents; it is very important that their specific needs and sensitivities are taken into consideration in the design of the clinic area.

A reception area separating the waiting room area from the examination area is important to ensure adequate flow through the clinic. A waiting room area, of adequate size and with sufficient and appropriate seating for children, parents, and siblings is essential. It should also be large enough to accommodate ambulatory aids. The addition of a small play facility for younger children is desirable. In addition, the provision of a bulletin board in this area is very useful, permitting ready transfer of new information, notices regarding ongoing studies, and the posting of a newsletter.

Examination rooms of adequate size to accommodate everything mentioned above, and sufficiently large to assess gait, as well as being appropriately equipped are also important. An examination table that can be readily moved to permit an appropriate musculoskeletal examination is desirable. The number of examining rooms clearly depends on the number of patients to be seen by a certain number of physicians in a given time frame. This will be discussed further below.

Additionally, it is important to have a private conferencing area that will permit discussion of cases with trainees and others, while allowing for adequate review of patient imaging studies. Such a

Table 3.2.8 The clinic requirements

Appropriate reception area to permit the private transfer of patient information

Appropriately designed waiting area specific to the needs of the child with a musculoskeletal problem

Bulletin board in the waiting area for general information, research studies, newsletter

Space that is tastefully designed in appropriate colouring to suit a broad age spectrum

Adequate number of examination rooms appropriate to the number of patients and personnel who will attend the clinic

Adequate room size to permit appropriate musculoskeletal examination including assessment of gait

Adequate conference/education room

Adequate space to accommodate nurse, therapists, and trainees

Appropriately located viewing boxes to evaluate sequential imaging studies

Private space to record patients' vital statistics including height and weight

Appropriate technical aids—dictation system, phones, computer for access to laboratory data and literature searching

space is important both to ensure that appropriate and full discussion of the cases can be undertaken, so that 'sensitive' issues can be discussed in private, and to facilitate the education of trainees. A computer link to permit access to laboratory results facilitates this process. It can also facilitate a rapid search of the literature for pertinent clinical information. This area might also be used for dictation of clinic notes and letters; having an appropriate dictation system located there, or in another private area within the clinic, is important as it facilitates communication with community-based health care providers.

New outpatient consultations

A considerable number and variety of patients may be referred for evaluation to the rheumatology clinics. The incidence of a variety of conditions presenting to paediatric rheumatologists has been described in three distinct geographic locations in the mid 1990s—the United Kingdom, the United States, and Canada [23–25]. There is surprising similarity among the three studies.

Such referrals may arise from a variety of sources. They may emanate from within one's own institution or from outside. Some children indeed may be referred from considerable distances (Figure 3.2.2). Such referrals must be pre-screened to ascertain the appropriateness of the referral and its relative urgency. The receipt of a concise referral letter from the referring physician aids this process. When this is not forthcoming a one-page summary sheet with focused questions can be faxed to the source of referral with a request for it to be returned (Figure 3.2.3). All of this can be done by the clerical clinic coordinator who can then consult with the team nurse or paediatric rheumatologist regarding the appropriateness of the referral and ascertain the time within which the patient must be seen. A time for the appointment can then be set while advising the referring physician to contact the paediatric rheumatologist, directly, if there is a perception of more urgent need. Additionally, suggestions can be given to the referring physician regarding the interim management of the patient. If a patient needs to be seen on an urgent basis outside of a regular scheduled visit then a facility to permit this must be available since not all services have clinic space designated for their exclusive use.

Some centres have completely separate screening clinics where only new referrals are seen. Others see such patients in general rheumatology clinics, that is, in clinics that do not have a specific disease dedication. Newly referred patients should probably never be seen in clinics with a specific disease dedication even if the likelihood of that specific disease is high. The first visit can be overwhelming for such patients and families whose many questions need to be addressed, and who frequently require support to help deal with the fact that their child has just been diagnosed with a significant condition. Also, it is best not conducted in a setting with a large number of patients with established disease, some of whom might have severe debilitating disease. Additionally, the focus in such clinics should be on patients with established disease whose considerable needs must be met by the clinic team.

One advantage of a screening clinic for new referrals is that it more readily permits appropriate allocation of time and resources for the consultation. If pre-screening occurs appropriately, it is easier to determine the precise number of patients that might be seen in each screening clinic and to allocate time accordingly. It also facilitates alerting other team members to the potential for a new patient with a certain diagnosis thereby, improving efficiency. One disadvantage of a

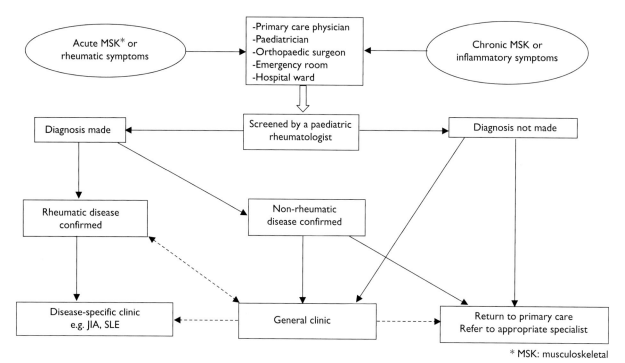

Fig. 3.2.2 Sources of referrals for evaluation to the rheumatology clinics.

Figure 3.2.3 Paediatric Rheumatology Clinic Screening Form

Date:

Referring Physician's Name: _____

Phone #: _____   Fax #: _____

Patients' Name: _____   Patient's DOB: _____

Home Phone #: _____   Hospital ID #: _____

Brief History: _____
_____
_____
_____

Examination: _____
_____
_____
_____

Investigations Done:

  Labwork _____
(Append Reports)_____

  *Imaging _____
(Append Reports)_____

Working Diagnosis: _____
_____

Specific question(s): _____
_____

(*Please ensure that originals or copies of imaging studies accompany patient to the visit)

screening clinic is that the proportion of 'no shows' is often higher. This may occur if the problem for which the patient has been referred has already resolved by the time of the appointment or that the family did not fully understand the need for the consultation. The latter is compounded by the fact that a relationship has yet to be established with the patient and family, unlike with follow-up patients. This might prove to be a significant issue in certain locations. Finally, some centres may not see a sufficiently large number, or indeed might see too large a number, of new referrals to make having a screening clinic practical. The ideal number of new referrals, based on our experience, is approximately 4–5 per paediatric rheumatologist per week to justify running a weekly half-day screening clinic. This is based on a 20–25% likelihood of a significant rheumatologic diagnosis. Clearly, some physicians may choose to see more patients than this, while others may see less.

Once patients have been screened, a diagnosis may or may not be established. Nonetheless, a treatment and follow-up plan must be put in place. This plan must be communicated to the referring physician in a timely fashion. Patients whose diagnosis does not require that they be followed in a rheumatology clinic, for example, growing pains, anterior patellar syndrome, slipped capital femoral epiphysis, and many other conditions, may be returned to the referring physician or referred on to a more appropriate specialist, for example, an orthopaedic surgeon.

Outpatients without established rheumatic diseases

A patient whose diagnosis has not yet been established but who has an acute problem not yet resolved, a diagnostic dilemma or an unclear diagnosis but with significant musculoskeletal symptoms, or the possibility of an evolving rheumatic disease probably merits follow-up in a rheumatology clinic. Such a patient might be followed in a general rheumatology clinic (Table 3.2.9). Such patients can be followed in this type of clinic until their problem has resolved, or until a

Table 3.2.9 Examples of diagnostic entities followed in a general rheumatology clinic

Acute arthritides (not yet resolved or of uncertain etiology)
Fever of unknown origin
Periodic fever syndromes
Inflammatory conditions of unclear etiology
Mechanical or noninflammatory conditions of unclear etiology
Nonspecific pain disorders
Miscellaneous others, for example, chronic recurrent multifocal osteomyelitis

Table 3.2.10 Examples of diagnostic entities followed in disease-specific, rheumatology clinics

JIA
Juvenile dermatomyositis and other myositides
SLE
Scleroderma, overlap syndromes, and other connective tissue diseases
Kawasaki disease
Systemic vasculitides
Specific pain disorders such as reflex neurovascular dystrophy or fibromyalgia

Table 3.2.11 Advantages of disease-specific rheumatology clinics

Permits delivery of comprehensive patient care
Facilitates clinic organization and coordination
Reduces clinic waiting times
Permits a standardized set up
Facilitates incorporation of a multidisciplinary approach
Facilitates incorporation of trainees
Guarantees trainees adequate exposure to specific conditions
Facilitates incorporation of standard data forms
Facilitates longitudinal data collection
Facilitates accumulation of clinic statistics and computerization of clinic data
Facilitates patient recruitment for studies

diagnosis is made. At this point, they might be returned to their primary care physician for ongoing care, referred on to a more appropriate specialist, or moved to a clinic designated for that specific disease. Indeed, some of these patients may continue to be seen in a general rheumatology clinic indefinitely, even when a specific diagnosis has been made (Table 3.2.9). Clearly it is not possible or desirable to have clinics specific to each and every conceivable diagnosis.

Scheduling for this type of clinic, however, may be difficult because of the case mix. Some visits may be very brief and others much longer, the latter being the case when patients have symptoms that induce significant anxiety in parents but a diagnosis has not yet been made. Coordination for this type of clinic is a challenge that is compounded by the addition of new referrals. Careful planning of this type of clinic is important in order to avoid prolonged waiting times. In general, 7–8 patients per paediatric rheumatologist per half-day clinic is an appropriate number of patients to see in such a clinic. Again the value of a designated and competent clerical clinic coordinator cannot be overestimated in this context.

Outpatients with established rheumatic diseases

Patients diagnosed with a defined rheumatic disease may best be followed in a clinic dedicated for that specific disease (Table 3.2.10). In most centres that provide care for children with rheumatic diseases it seems prudent to run a separate clinic exclusive to patients with JIA. Indeed some larger centres might have clinics specific to Systemic Arthritis or Enthesitis Related Arthritis for example. Others run clinics specific to SLE or juvenile dermatomyositis (JDM). Most tertiary referral centres have a clinic specific to children with JIA and another for children with connective tissue diseases. Clearly, the need for disease-specific clinics is influenced not only by the number of patients with the specific diagnosis being seen at that centre but also by the particular interests including research interests of the individual physicians.

There are many advantages in establishing these disease-specific clinics (Table 3.2.11). Since patients with the same disease have similar requirements, this type of clinic allows one to organize and coordinate the clinic in a better manner. A standard approach to care can be adopted that includes a multidisciplinary approach and thus facilitates the inclusion of other services and specialists. It also facilitates the incorporation of a standardized chart and the collection of data in a standardized fashion. This permits readily the conduct of longitudinal studies and facilitates the set up a computerized database. In our experience, 5–6 patients per paediatric rheumatologist per half-day clinic is an appropriate number to book for most disease-specific

clinics, but this is influenced by the number of patients with early, established, and recalcitrant disease in each clinic.

Integration of the extended team into the clinic

Ideally, other team members, particularly the therapists, should have the opportunity to be present within the clinic setting. For practical reasons, this often does not work well, mainly due to space limitations. However, if it is possible to design a structure where these individuals have space that is close to the clinic area this is the next best scenario. This facilitates flow of information back and forth and capitalizes on the time the patient spends in the clinic. Planning of clinic space is extremely important. It must take into account not only the number of patients to be seen but also the number of personnel who will be in the clinic at any one time. Unfortunately, most clinics do not take these issues into consideration adequately and chronic lack of space is the norm.

Technical procedures (intra-articular injections and intravenous infusions)

The main technical procedure that paediatric rheumatologists undertake is intra-articular corticosteroid injection. Some of these may be performed in the clinic setting without sedation. Most must be done with sedation or light general anaesthesia. It is essential to have an appropriate space specifically designated for this purpose. Patients also frequently require intravenous infusions (pulse corticosteroids, intravenous immunoglobulins, pulse cyclophosphamide, and biologic agents). These must be undertaken in an appropriate setting where there is adequate monitoring by designated nursing staff. Admission to the hospital should be avoided, if at all possible, for most of these procedures.

The team approach to the child with JIA at various stages

Early disease

As already mentioned, new patients with a specific diagnosis should be screened before being brought to a clinic specific to that disease. Thereafter, they can be followed in a disease-specific clinic. These patients should be seen frequently during the first few months after diagnosis, initially every few weeks, both to ensure appropriate monitoring of the disease, its treatment, and the side-effects thereof, and to ensure that adequate support is provided for the child and family. Some centres have clinics exclusively for patients with early disease but this is not an established practice in most settings. The provision of such support in addition to appropriate education of the family might be associated with better adherence, which in turn might produce better outcomes. However, this has yet to be confirmed.

Established disease

Once the diagnosis has been made and patient follow-up has been established for several months and there are signs that the activity of the disease is coming under control, patients can be followed less frequently, perhaps every 3–4 months, dependent on the specific disease. This is certainly adequate for most patients with JIA. When there are no signs of active inflammation and medications have been weaned or discontinued, patients can be seen less frequently, perhaps every 6–9 months. Such patients merit long-term follow-up because of the risk of recurrence of disease activity. Occasionally, this needs to be emphasized, both to the family and the family physician. Furthermore, the need for ongoing eye examinations, particularly in the high-risk JIA population often requires re-emphasizing. Additionally, complications of previously active disease, such as leg-length discrepancies need to be monitored.

Refractory disease

Some patients, despite the very best efforts, continue to have ongoing active disease often for many months and sometimes for years following initial diagnosis. Such patients represent a major challenge and although they might represent less than 10% of the total population of patients followed in the clinic, they consume a much higher proportion of time.

Scheduling for such patients can be problematic. Problems frequently arise suddenly and the patient may have to be accommodated in any clinic at any time. The visits invariably take a long time. Thus, it is advisable to limit the number of such patients in any given clinic to maintain efficiency. While it might be advisable to run a clinic exclusive to children with JIA and recalcitrant disease this is usually not practical. It is too difficult to coordinate, given the unpredictability of problems and parental work commitment. Furthermore, these patients frequently end up needing to be seen between scheduled clinic visits. It is advisable to maintain phone contact by a team member with these patients between visits to anticipate problems and to offer support.

Incorporating academic responsibilities into the clinic setting

Many paediatric rheumatology centres have a university affiliation and are responsible for the maintenance of an academic programme that includes teaching and research.

Trainee education

Paediatric rheumatology centres are responsible for the education of a whole series of trainees. Several centres train paediatricians in the art and science of paediatric rheumatology. Training periods vary by country. In most countries trainees complete core training in paediatrics in 3–5 years, and follow this with fellowship training in paediatric rheumatology. Fellowship training is a minimum of 2 years in Canada, 3 years in the United States, and more in some other countries. For those intent on pursuing a research career in addition to maintenance of a clinical practice even further training is required. Therefore, such trainees are affiliated with the training centre for a relatively long period of time, 2–4 years. Incorporating them into the clinical milieu and into the paediatric rheumatology team is relatively easy. Once they have adapted to the clinical set up, they can take on a large amount of responsibility under the supervision of a paediatric rheumatologist.

In addition, most centres have other trainees including medical students, and paediatric, immunology, and 'adult' rheumatology trainees who are usually affiliated with the centre for a short period of time, usually 1–2 months. It is not possible for such trainees to assume the same level of responsibility as paediatric rheumatology trainees. However, they can assume different roles commensurate with their level of training.

The number and level of trainees does affect how smoothly and efficiently the clinic runs. Trainees usually do not see patients as quickly or as efficiently as the paediatric rheumatologist. Therefore, clinic appointments have to take this into consideration. When there is more than one paediatric rheumatologist in the clinic one might assume the task of seeing a larger number of patients while the other supervises the trainees. This is one way to maintain clinic times and to avoid excessive patient delays. It also guarantees the educational process by providing a more in-depth opportunity for case review and the discussion and demonstration of clinical skills. Clearly, organization in this area is totally dependent on the size of the service and the number of staff and trainees.

Research

Most paediatric rheumatology centres are engaged in either clinical or basic research or both. Research is facilitated by many of the issues already alluded to in the set up of the clinic structure. In particular, disease-specific clinics facilitate research by guaranteeing a large volume of patients for studies and permitting a standardized approach to data collection (Table 3.2.11). Having the space to permit research personnel within the clinic area is extremely important. This assists with patient recruitment and data collection. All of this facilitates both clinical and fundamental research. Having an appropriate facility for the acquisition and storage of laboratory samples may further facilitate the latter.

Over the years, it has become increasingly important that paediatric rheumatology centres participate in clinical trials. As more and more agents are developed, this will become even more important. Such participation does, however, impact significantly on clinic coordination. These patients must be seen at very specific times and the data to be collected are frequently beyond the usual amount collected during a standard visit. This has to be factored into the clinic-appointment schedule. Occasionally, it may be necessary to set up special times for such patients to be seen. Indeed, some centres set up specific clinics to see these patients, and use research personnel for patient evaluations and data collection. Ideally, all patients should be incorporated into the standard clinic schedule. This ensures that other important aspects of their care are not overlooked. Occasionally, this proves to be impractical.

Other issues

Single-handed physician and small centre practice

Single physicians, some of whom also engage in clinical responsibilities other than just in paediatric rheumatology, run many of the smaller paediatric rheumatology facilities. In fact, many paediatric rheumatology centres are of this type. Thus, some of the issues raised above might not be pertinent to all practices. While the clinic set up may differ in such practices—it may not be practical to run disease-specific clinics, for example—most of the principles should still hold. In particular, the need for a multidisciplinary team approach is still valid. Such a team might be smaller in terms of personnel and scope but the philosophy of team integration should still hold. In addition, the need to have access to other paediatric subspecialty expertise is also valid. Although this may not necessarily be available precisely at the same location, there still should be reasonable access to such expertise. It is incumbent upon the paediatric rheumatologist in such locations to seek out such expertise and to refer patients appropriately.

Some paediatric rheumatology facilities are run exclusively by adult rheumatologists. In such circumstances appropriate referral to a paediatric centre should occur when necessary. As the number of individuals trained in the specialty of paediatric rheumatology increases the need to have adult rheumatologists perform this function should diminish.

Outreach clinics

Many centres do not have a paediatric rheumatologist. In the United States, 45 medical schools do not have a paediatric rheumatologist affiliated with them. Therefore, for many patients, the nearest paediatric rheumatology centre is at a considerable distance. Paediatricians and/or 'adult' rheumatologists usually care for patients in such locations. To improve service to these areas, many paediatric rheumatologists travel to outreach clinics. Such clinics take on many forms but usually consist of a physician travelling to a particular location at a distance from the central location where they may see a large number of patients over the course of 1–2 days. Ideally, such a clinic should be run in conjunction with the patient's paediatrician or 'adult' rheumatologist to maximize communication and education of the local personnel. The latter aspect is extremely important because the local personnel must manage the patient between outreach visits, which might be quite infrequent. This is particularly important regarding monitoring of medication toxicities, and especially the follow-up of laboratory results.

Transition clinics

Transition from early childhood through adolescence is a dynamic process. Physicians and health care teams caring for children with chronic diseases should be cognizant of this. It is incumbent to ensure that patients are progressing naturally through these stages. It is particularly important that when they reach their adolescent years we encourage them to assume an increasing level of responsibility for their own care [12,26]. By the time patients reach their late teen years, they must be capable of assuming full responsibility for their care so that their transfer to an adult facility occurs smoothly. Thus, transition should begin early. To aid in this process, many centres run a separate transition clinic for certain patients (See Part 3, Chapter 3.3).

Adherence

It is wonderful to have potent therapies combined with a comprehensive health care delivery system, encompassing excellence in all domains, but this is all to no avail if the patient is not adherent with the therapeutic regimen. In fact, relatively little is known about patient adherence to the therapeutic regimen [1]. We need to understand more about the factors associated with poor adherence and ascertain which factors are amenable to intervention. Techniques to measure adherence in the clinical setting are rudimentary. While most clinicians may inquire about adherence with the regimen, few make any attempt to measure this in a meaningful or quantifiable way. Much work needs to be undertaken in this extremely important area.

Quality assurance

Delivery of quality service is essential to ensure appropriate management of all of our patients. For this reason, it is important to have some system in place to guarantee good quality of service. To some extent, this can be achieved by having regular team meetings. Problems as they arise can be discussed among the team members and appropriate measures can then be put in place to deal with them. For most issues, this is all that is required. Periodically, it is advisable to have an open forum for discussion so that issues can be readily brought forth. When a more serious problem arises it must be dealt with more formally. Most systems have a formal mechanism to deal with this. For all of these issues, it is ideal to have one person assigned the task of periodic reporting.

Summary and conclusions

In this chapter, an overview of the main factors that are important in ensuring a top-quality paediatric rheumatology service is provided. An emphasis has been placed on guaranteeing a service that is patient-centred and that is based on a team approach. Incorporating the needs and beliefs of the family, when feasible, is emphasized. Such an approach depends on the presence of a strong interactive committed health care team. Regular team meetings are important to permit appropriate communication among the members. This permits a consistent approach to the care of each patient by all the team. The role of the team coordinator, usually the team nurse, is strongly emphasized.

Also described, is an approach to the set up of both an outpatient and inpatient service for paediatric rheumatology that should work in most settings. This emphasizes an appropriate clinic set up with a strong emphasis on appropriate screening of patients and their ultimate placement in clinics that are disease-specific. The precise requirements of the clinic space are also described. The advantages of this approach are delineated. How disease-specific clinics enhance patient care and permit the incorporation of education of trainees and research into the clinic setting is also discussed. The importance of the clerical clinic coordinator and the key role this individual plays in guaranteeing the quality of the paediatric rheumatology service is emphasized.

This chapter briefly alludes to outreach and transition clinics and how they need to be incorporated to enhance the overall quality of the service provided. Their importance should not be underestimated. The need to measure adherence with the treatment regimen and the factors that influence it are discussed. Finally, this chapter mentions the importance of maintenance of quality of care and the necessity of having a system in place to objectively measure it, and to conduct appropriate quality assurance reporting.

References

1. Rapoff, M.A., Lindsley, C.B., and Christophersen, E.R. Parent perception of problems experienced by their children in complying with treatment for juvenile rheumatoid arthritis. *Arch Phys Med Rehabil* 1985;66:427–9.

2. Athreya, B.H. A general approach to management of children with rheumatic diseases. In Cassidy, Petty eds, *Textbook of Pediatric Rheumatology*, 4th edn. Toronto: Saunders, 2001, pp. 189–211.

3. Mervyn, F.A. They get this training but they don't know how you feel. Horsham, England, National Fund for Research into Crippling Diseases, 1975.

4. Athreya, B.H. Regionalized arthritis resources. *Arthritis Rheum* 1977;20 (Suppl.):604–5.

5. McAnarney, E.R., Pless, I.B., Satterwhite B, *et al.* Psychological problems of children with juvenile chronic arthritis. *Pediatrics* 1974;53:523–8.

6. McCormick, M.C., Stemmler, M.M., and Athreya, B.H. The impact of childhood rheumatic diseases on the family. *Arthritis Rheum* 1986;29:872–9.

7. Lovell, D.J., Athreya, B.H., Emery, H.M., *et al.* School attendance and patterns, special services and special needs in paediatric patients with rheumatic diseases. *Arthritis Care Res* 1990;3:196–201.

8. Allaire, S.A., De Nardo, B.S., Szer, I.S., *et al.* The economic impact of juvenile rheumatoid arthritis. *J Rheumatol* 1992;19:952–5.

9. Miller, J.J. Psychosocial factors related to rheumatic diseases in childhood. *J Rheumatol* 1993;20(Suppl.):1–11.

10. Peterson, L.S., Mason, T., and Nelson, A.M. Psychosocial outcomes and health status of adults who have had juvenile rheumatoid arthritis—a controlled population-based study. *Arthritis Rheum* 1997;40:2235–40.

11. Frank, R.G., Hagglund, K.J., Schopp, L.H., *et al.* Disease and family contributors to adaptation in juvenile rheumatoid arthritis and juvenile diabetes. *Arthritis Care Res.* 1998;11:166–76.

12. Rettig, P. and Athreya, B.H. Leaving home-preparing the adolescent with arthritis for coping with independence and the adult rheumatology world. In D., Isenberg and J.J. Miller eds. *Adolescent Rheumatology*. London: Martin Dunitz, 1998.

13. Koop, C.E. Surgeon-General's Report: Children with special health-care needs—Campaign '87—Commitment to family-centred, co-ordinated care for children with special health care needs. Washington DC: US Department of Health and Human Services, Government Printing Office, 1987.

14. Brewer, E.J., McPherson, M., Magrab, P., *et al.* Family-centered, community-based, coordinated care for children with special health-care needs. *Pediatrics* 1989;83:1055–60.

15. Pless, I.B., Feeley, N., Gottlieb, L., Rowat, K., Dougherty, G., and Willard, B. A randomized trial of a nursing intervention to promote the adjustment of children with chronic physical disorders. *Pediatrics* 1994;87:70–5.

16. Cassidy, J.T. and Lindley, C.B. Legal rights of children with musculoskeletal disabilities. *Bull Rheum Dis* 1996;45:1–5.

17. Spencer, C.H., Fife, R.Z., and Rabinovich, E. The school experience of children with arthritis: Coping in the 1990s and transition into adulthood. *Pediatr Clin N Am* 1995;42:1285–98.

18. Bacon, M.C., White, P.H., Raiten, D.J., *et al.* Nutritional status and growth in children with juvenile rheumatoid arthritis. *Semin Arthritis Rheum* 1990;20:96–106.

19. Henderson, C.J. and Lovell, D.J. Nutritional aspects of JRA. *Rheum Dis Clin N Am* 1991;17:403–13.

20. Duffy, C.M., Watanabe Duffy, K.N., Polomeno, R., Gibbon, M., Yang, H., Platt, R., and Flanders, M. Prevalence and severity of uveitis in children with juvenile arthritis. *Arthritis Rheum* 1999;42:S226.

21. Walton, A.G, Welbury, R.R., Foster, H.E., *et al.* Juvenile chronic arthritis: A dental review. *Oral Dis* 1999;5:68–75.

22. Walker, D.K. Care of chronically ill children in schools. *Pediatr Clin N Am* 1984;31:221–33.

23. Symmons, D.P.M., Jones, M., Osborne, J., *et al.* Paediatric rheumatology in the UK: Data from the British Paediatric Rheumatology Group National Diagnostic Register. *J Rheumatol* 1996;23:1975–80.

24. Bowyer, S., Roettcher, P., and the Members of the Pediatric Rheumatology Database Research Group. Pediatric Rheumatology clinic populations in the US: Results of a 3-year survey. *J Rheumatol* 1996;23:1968–74.

25. Malleson, P.N., Fung, M.Y., and Rosenberg, A.M., for the Canadian Pediatric Rheumatology Association. The incidence of pediatric rheumatic diseases: Results from the Canadian Pediatric Rheumatology Association Disease Registry. *J Rheumatol* 1996;23:1981–87.

26. White, P.H. Success on the road to adulthood: Issues and hurdles for adolescents with disabilities. *Rheum Dis Clin N Am* 1997;23:697–707.

3.3   Adolescent rheumatology services

Janet E. McDonagh and Patience White

Aim

The aim of this chapter is to examine the specific issues that are pertinent to the care of adolescents with Juvenile Idiopathic Arthritis (JIA). In particular the importance of transition from childhood to adult rheumatology care is discussed in detail.

Structure

- Introduction
- Transition—raising expectations and the concept
- Why adolescent services are needed
- Health education/promotion
- Exercise
- Nutrition
- Sexuality issues
- Substance abuse
- Confidentiality issues
- Adherence
- School issues
- Work issues
- Self-determination and self-advocacy
- Consulation dynamics
- Advocacy issues for parents
- Transition clinic models
- Summary

Introduction

All adolescents including those with chronic illnesses and/or disabilities have hopes and dreams. They want to be valued as human beings and treated with dignity, obtain education and job training, have opportunities for social experiences, community involvement, recreation and worship, and find meaningful work for reasonable pay. Yet studies show that they are more often unemployed, have lower health status, and are more socially isolated compared to peers without disabilities. Studies have also shown that those who are involved in their care have lower expectations for them in the future. Improving the future of these young people with chronic

illnesses and/or disabilities is the primary goal of successful transition to adulthood.

Transition—Raising expectations and the concept

A major theme for young people with chronic illnesses and/or disabilities is that over 90% survive into adulthood and will move from paediatric-focused systems to adult oriented systems. With reference to JIA, at least one-third will have active inflammation as adults [1] and hence will require care in an adult rheumatology environment. This movement toward adulthood is called transition and has the following major components: early preparation, medical health issues including control of the disease and promotion of growth and development, skill building including communication skills, school and vocational issues, and community support and self-determination/self-advocacy as they move from home to interdependence. Independence is often the stated goal for youth with disabilities moving to adulthood; yet all adults whether with or without disabilities rely on others or have interdependent relationships to attain their desire for a happy productive life. Thus a final step beyond independence is interdependence. This chapter will focus in more detail on the medical transition issues.

Transition in healthcare can be defined as 'a multifaceted, active process that attends to the medical, psychosocial, and educational-vocational needs of adolescents as they move from child-oriented to adult-oriented lifestyles and systems [2]. The ultimate goal of transition is an individual who is an interdependent, confident, fulfilled young adult unrelated to their chronic illness such as JIA. Transition is a process, which ideally begins on the day of diagnosis with a written transition plan established on entry into secondary education at the latest. A transition policy published by The American Academy of Pediatrics recommends the transition plan be completed by 14 years of age [3]. Coordination and planning are integral aspects of transitional care. A survey of service providers in the rehabilitation, education, and medical care of children in the United States showed that lack of planning for transition was second only to inadequate financing as the most common reason for failure to move successfully into an adult-oriented system [4].

The important tasks during adolescence (Table 3.3.1) may be delayed or may remain uncompleted in the context of a chronic illness [5]. To complete these maturational tasks, there are biological, social, and emotional changes, which must occur for the adolescent to be successful. At the same time they need to negotiate the transition from

Table 3.3.1 Tasks of adolescence [4]

- To consolidate his/her identity
- To establish relationships outside the family
- To achieve independence from parents
- To find a vocation

paediatric to adult healthcare and from school to tertiary education or work. These tasks of transition are interdependent and the transitions will not be successful if the tasks are not accomplished.

The aims of medical transition

When medical transition is successful, the adolescent should have:

- received coordinated, uninterrupted healthcare which was age and developmentally appropriate, and comprehensive;
- obtained skills in communication, decision-making, assertiveness, and self-care;
- an enhanced sense of control and independence in healthcare.

One common mistake is to confuse transition with transfer. Transfer implies one *event* within the transition *process* when the young person moves from paediatric into adult care. The timing of a successful transfer depends on many factors such as level of maturity, health status /disease activity, disease severity, co-morbidities, status of preparation of the healthcare professional, young person and family, and not just chronological age. For those patients newly diagnosed with JIA in adolescence, understanding the illness, controlling the disease, and establishing a management plan are the priority. A component of the initial discussion should include an introduction to the concept of transition planning. Expansion of this discussion is undertaken as the disease comes under control and the young person and family become more familiar with the condition. Discussing that the young person will grow up and move to an adult healthcare provider gives the message to the young person and family that the young person is expected, like all young people, to grow up and be an adult with adult responsibilities. If adult rheumatology care is required, transfer of care to an adult healthcare provider should ideally occur during a period of good disease control and only after appropriate preparation of both the young person and their parents. Ideally, it is preferable for the young person and family to be able to choose their adult healthcare provider when the young person is well and not when they are in a crisis and have to accept the healthcare provider who is available. In general, if the young person chooses their provider or feels the provider understands them and their medical condition, they are more apt to be willing to follow the advice given. Young people with refractory disease may have a more protracted period of transition, and often benefit (if feasible) from a shared care arrangement between the paediatric/adult rheumatologist and internist/paediatrician. This arrangement allows a more gradual transfer of responsibility of care in the form of either alternate visits or combined clinics with both a paediatric and adult rheumatology presence.

Why adolescent services are needed

In today's world, adolescents, particularly those with chronic illness and/or disability, can be uncomfortable attendees of family-centred paediatric services where the focus is often on child development and the parents, and less on their growing independence, increasingly adult behaviours and desire for confidentiality[6]. The same young people may also be equally uncomfortable within the adult medical service that, although acknowledging patient autonomy, and reproductive and employment issues, may neglect growth, development and family concerns. The different cultures of paediatric and adult healthcare have been highlighted by several authors [7,8]. High quality transitional care for young people with rheumatic conditions therefore must involve both paediatric and adult rheumatologists. If professionals simply 'pass the buck', young people and their families often encounter difficulties as they attempt to negotiate this gap.

The term 'adolescent' is in itself confusing with no clarity of definition. The onset of adolescence is frequently attributed a biological definition in terms of the onset of puberty. In contrast, adulthood and hence the end of adolescence, in many countries, is determined legally by age. This is reflected in part, in the breadth of more recent definitions of adolescence. For example, WHO criteria suggest ages 10 to 20 years and the American Academy of Pediatrics suggests ages 14 to 21 years [9,10]. If one considers the tasks of adolescence (Table 3.3.1), it is obvious that such definitions are too narrow and fail to encompass the major cultural and psychosocial aspects of adolescence. Whatever the definition, adolescents are not large children nor small adults and their inherent differences need to be appreciated by both paediatric and adult health professionals.

Evidence of need for transitional care services

Advances in the ability to treat and care for children with chronic illnesses and/or disabilities have prolonged life expectancy and improved well being for many including the vast majority of children with JIA. Unfortunately the manner in which we deliver care to these young people once they reach early adulthood has not always kept pace with these medical advances. Studies of physically disabled young people in the United Kingdom have reported that the quality of medical care (as defined by the experiences of young people with chronic illness and/or disability), declines after transfer to adult services [11].

The outcome data of childhood-onset rheumatic diseases also supports the need for continuity of care in the transitional period. As mentioned previously, at least one-third of young people with JIA continue to have active inflammatory disease into their adult years and up to 60% of all patients continue to have some limitation of their activities of daily living [1,12–17]. Furthermore it has been shown that for many young people with JIA in the United Kingdom, unemployment is common and does not correlate with educational achievement or level of disability [13,14,18]. There is evidence that this trend towards unemployment starts in adolescence. In the United States, White reported reduced levels of work readiness and work experience in adolescents with chronic illness and/or disabilities (including JIA) compared to their healthy peers without disabilities, placing the former at a disadvantage in today's competitive job market [19].

JIA has been reported to impact on the quality of life of children with the condition, and this impact may persist into adulthood. Raised levels of depression, anxiety [12], and isolation [20] in young adults with JIA have been reported. Petersen reported in a 25-year follow-up study that young adults with JIA reported more bodily pain, poorer health perception, and decreased physical functioning [16]. A lack of serious relationships with young people of the opposite sex has been reported in significant proportions of selected JIA populations [21–24].

Indirect evidence for the need for transitional care services comes from the impact of adolescence on chronic illness itself. Adolescence is a critical time period that may be disrupted by a chronic illness. The reciprocal influences of a chronic illness and adolescent development need to be anticipated and addressed by multidisciplinary rheumatology teams. JIA can adversely influence physical development causing both growth retardation and delayed puberty. This is particularly true for those patients with refractory active disease. The stage of physical development can influence the outcome of the youth's growth. For example, puberty is associated with potentially greater corticosteroid-induced growth retardation. Chronic illness can influence the cognitive development of young people by a number of mechanisms including drug side-effects, school absence, pain, depression, and fatigue. The stage of cognitive development will influence such aspects of care as communication and disease education. Finally, a chronic illness like JIA can influence psychosocial development through the development of an adolescent's self-concept, the family interactions, peer relationships, sexual identity; conversely their psychosocial development may influence such aspects of healthcare as adherence to therapy, and risk-taking behaviours.

There is growing evidence to support the benefits of coordinated transitional care programmes in several chronic illnesses with both improved disease control [25], and improved quality of life [26, 27]. There is only one reported study of transitional care in JIA, which showed improved follow-up in a US tertiary referral hospital-based population [28].

Medical transition—key areas and hurdles to consider

For young people with JIA, the medical management of disease in transition is similar no matter what the age of the person and include disease control, pain management, and prevention of deformity. The implementation of strategies to deal with such issues need to be age and developmentally appropriate acknowledging the evolving roles of the young person and their parent/guardian.

There are key areas to consider in the transitional care of young people with chronic rheumatic diseases. Health professionals involved in the care of these young people with JIA must identify one person who will ensure all of the transition issues are being addressed as they can impact on the youth with chronic illness, whether it is by primary or secondary healthcare professionals. For whoever becomes the guide for the transition process, there are several potential hurdles to successful transition, many of which are attitudinal and are amenable to positive change. These are summarized in Table 3.3.2.

Health education/promotion

Health education and promotion is influenced by the cognitive development of children and young people. Not all 'chronological' adolescents will have the same intellectual ability to understand their illness. Berry et al. reported that many adolescents with JIA answered questions on arthritis at the concrete operational stage of cognitive development, more characteristic of younger children and unlike that

Table 3.3.2 Hurdles to successful transition

The young person	Lack of familiarity with adult clinic and team
	Reluctance to leave paediatric team especially after long disease duration
	Immaturity
	Dependence on parents
	Non-adherence
	Not yet independent in their own healthcare
The parents	Lack of familiarity with adult clinic and/or team
	Dislike of individual approach of adult care
	Over-protectiveness
	Negative preconceptions of adult care
	Awareness of lack of confidence of paediatric team in adult service
The paediatric health professional	Reluctance to let go of long-term patients
	Lack of confidence in adult team
	No paediatric-adult interface
	Research interests
The adult rheumatology health professional	Lack of confidence in paediatric team
	Lack of training in adolescent healthcare
	Individual rather than family-centred approach
	Negative attitudes of paternalistic style and paediatric care
The delivery system	Lack of planning
	Lack of preparation of young person, their family and the adult team
	Suitable clinic space
	Administrative transfer of patient notes and x-rays
	Consensus regarding management guidelines between paediatric and adult rheumatology services
Time and money	Lack of available time for the full spectrum of transitional care
	Lack of funding

of adults [29]. At this stage, children and young people are capable of limited logical thought processes, and can only see relationships and classifications, as long as concrete materials are available. According to Piaget's theory of cognitive development, logical and abstract reasoning, enabling function at the formal operational level (the level that reflects adult levels of understanding and thinking), only develops in adolescence [30]. This therefore highlights potential differences between adolescents and adults in the ways they interpret, understand, and respond to their arthritis and their treatment. Another finding from this study was that adolescents with arthritis had significant levels of inaccuracies and misunderstandings about causes of arthritis and its symptoms despite the fact that many were long-time clinic attendees [29]. This may reflect that much of the initial disease education was directed to the parents if the youth was a child at disease onset, and/or that it was not delivered in age and developmentally appropriate formats as the young person matured.

All adolescents have common concerns such as 'Am I normal? Do I fit in? Am I good looking? Can I be sexy? How can I be safe?' Young people with JIA have these concerns as well. In a study of adolescents with chronic illness, more age-related concerns such as alcohol and drug issues, menstrual periods, sexual health, and worry about height and weight, were reported compared to their healthy peers [31].

Many adult health-promoting (or health-damaging) behaviours become established during adolescence. Hence, adolescence is a key time to establish good health behaviours, especially when chronic rheumatic conditions and their therapies will be affected by such behaviours. The need to integrate comprehensive adolescent preventive services such as those developed by the American Medical Association called GAPS—(Guidelines for Adolescent Preventive Services) into routine medical care has been highlighted in the literature [32]. Though preventive care is often integrated into primary care settings, subspecialists have lagged behind. For example, a survey of adolescent rheumatology service provision in the United Kingdom identified a demand for patient information resources specifically aimed at adolescents [33]. Provision of resources regarding other generic health issues such as substance abuse, alcohol, sex education were only addressed specifically by 2 of the 9 clinics identified in the UK survey [28] but are considered important in the development of any adolescent healthcare service [32]. For young people with vasculitis and/or those on long-term corticosteroid therapy, the risk of premature atheroslerosis should be considered and preventive measures instituted such as non-smoking, decreased fat intake, and blood pressure monitoring and control.

To assist the paediatric and adult rheumatologist who may be less familiar with the preventive issues that need to be discussed, a mnemonic is presented called HEADS (Table 3.3.3). The HEADS mneumonic is a useful aide-memoire to help the professional remember the issues to address with adolescence in routine clinical practice.

Exercise

Encouraging general exercise for all young people, with or without chronic illness, remains an important area of health promotion, especially in this increasingly computer dominated society. Greater levels of exercise are associated with wellbeing and long-term functioning in patients with a number of chronic conditions [34]. Klepper *et al.*

Table 3.3.3 Aide-memorie for adolescent issues

Getting into Adolescent HEADS

H	Home (e.g. relationships, social support, household chores)
E	Education—(e.g. school, exams, work experience, career) Exercise
A	Activities—(e.g: peer network, time away from home) Ambitions Affect
D	Drugs, cigarettes, alcohol Diet—(e.g. calcium, vitamin D, weight, caffeine, cola-based drinks) Dental care Driving—(e.g. learning, use of public transportation)
S	Sex—(e.g. concerns, periods, contraception, sexual health, puberty) Sleep

Source: Adapted from Goldenring, J.M. and Cohen, E. Getting into adolescent heads. *Contemp pediatr* 1988;July:75–80 [71].

reported reduced fitness in children with polyarticular JIA compared to controls, though lack of fitness was not associated with the activity of arthritis [35]. In a case-control study, young adults with JIA had a lower level of general exercise, lower levels of physical functioning, lower health perception, and higher levels of fatigue compared to healthy peers [16]. As well as addressing specific muscle strengthening exercises and aerobic fitness, rheumatology healthcare professionals need to remember the importance of weight-bearing exercise in chronic rheumatic conditions like JIA in view of the risk of premature osteoporosis [36]. This age group of young people often demand a creative approach to physical exercise such as going to gyms and group exercise classes as they quickly lose interest in regimented and often boring home exercise programmes.

Nutrition

Physical growth is a key area for consideration during adolescence and transition. The psychological implications of growth retardation during adolescence can often be significant in terms of body image and peer acceptance. Bullying as a negative consequence of growth retardation must be borne in mind [37].

The general nutritional status of the adolescent with chronic disease is similarly important. Protein–energy malnutrition has been reported in 10–50% of adolescents with arthritis [38]. Reduced lean body mass in JIA patients has been reported in association with low versus normal total body bone mass content [39] and may reflect a preferential utilization of energy substrate from the use of fat to lean body mass in the presence of chronic inflammation.

The greatest increase in bone mineral content during life occurs during the adolescent years — between 11 and 14 years in girls and between 13 and 17 years in boys and culminates in their attaining peak bone mass in their mid-twenties. Young adults who have higher peak bone mass are likely to be at lower risk of developing osteoporosis in later life although the long-term studies have not been done. Several studies have now reported reduced bone mineral density in JIA [36,39]. It is therefore important for those caring for children and young people, to recognize the important potential window of opportunity for primary preventive strategies earlier in life before peak bone mass is attained. Nutrition is one of several relevant factors amenable to change and has important practical implications. Preoccupation with being thin is common in this age group (especially among females), as is the misconception that all dairy foods are fattening. The findings of the UK National Diet and Nutrition Survey found that 11% of boys and girls aged between 11 and 14 years as well as 16% of boys and 10% of girls aged between 15 and 18 years were deficient in vitamin D [40]. In a US study of healthy adolescents, 89% were found to consume less than the recommended dietary calcium allowance [41]. Of equal concern, only a third of paediatricians surveyed in a recent study knew the recommended daily allowance for calcium in adolescents [42]. Calcium requirements increase with age, being highest in adolescence, and increased intake did improve bone mineral density at the time [43]. Long-term studies of the effects of current US recommended calcium and/or vitamin D intakes (or indeed studies of supplementation) beginning during childhood are as yet unavailable either in healthy populations or in JIA populations. A recent review of available epidemiological data in healthy populations, however, supports the view that maintaining a diet with recommended calcium intakes will increase peak bone mass and lower the incidence of fractures [44]. This is a key area to address in adolescent healthcare.

Sexuality issues

Parents can be reluctant to address sensitive topics such as sexuality with their healthy children and often never discuss these issues with their son/daughter with a chronic illness [45]. Similarly, many health professionals who have cared for a young person with chronic illnesses since early childhood do not tackle these subjects. One rheumatologist in a recent study commented that he did not screen for risk-taking behaviours, as he believed strongly that 'he would be interfering with the parent–child relationship if he engaged in inquiries regarding risky behaviours' [46]. Young people with chronic illnesses and/or disabilities may be seen by adults as less sexual than their peers. In fact, chronically ill adolescents become sexually active at rates comparable to healthy adolescents [47]. Chronic illnesses and/or their therapy may delay puberty. Some of the drugs frequently used in these conditions are teratogenic (e.g. methotrexate) and/or affect fertility (e.g. cyclophosphamide). Cervical cytology screening is also important in sexually active female patients. Cervical atypia has been reported in SLE patients although the exact nature of the relationship to the disease and/or immunosuppressive therapy is still unclear [48].

Care must also be taken by health professionals not to always assume heterosexuality in discussions regarding sexual health; homosexuality issues may need to be considered and addressed in this age-group. Finally, cultural and religious sensitivity in the area of sexual health (and substance abuse) must be remembered at all times and respected by the multidisciplinary team.

Substance use

Substance use is another area at risk of neglect in the adolescent rheumatology clinic. Timko et al. studied substance use in adolescents with JIA and their healthy siblings and reported similar rates at baseline although, after 1 year of disease, patients with JIA were less involved in their use [49]. In another US study of adolescents with JIA who had a mean age 13.9 years, Nash et al. reported 30.7% of patients were drinking alcohol, including 23.5% of who were on methotrexate. The average age of initiation of alcohol use in this population was 13.6 years. Interestingly there was no significant difference in alcohol use between methotrexate and non-methotrexate patients. Also 13.4% of patients reported the use of other illicit substances at some time [41].

Cigarette smoking has both generic and disease/treatment-specific importance. In the aforementioned study of adolescents with JIA, Nash et al. reported that 37% of alcohol users were also smokers [50].

Confidentiality Issues

To consider discussing such subjects as sexual activity and alcohol use in the rheumatology clinic needs preparation of both the patient and their family. Such consultations require settings conducive to confidentiality, patient and physician comfort and a good working knowledge of local resources specifically for young people (such as sexual health clinics, counselling services etc.) Most important of all, the young person needs to have confidence in the health professional and this is optimized by the young person seeing the same professional at each visit. In a UK study of adolescents in primary care, confidentiality was their major priority when asked what were the most important attributes of an adolescent friendly practice [51]. Yet in a US study, paediatric practices were less likely than family medicine to offer confidential services to adolescents [6]. Seeing the young person independently from the parents often makes the visit more conducive to such conversations and confidences (see below). Sometimes the offer of separate visits will not be taken up initially, but only at a later visit when the young person has gained confidence in the professional. Learning problem-solving, negotiating, and communication skills are all part of the transitional process for the young person to take over control of their medical care.

Adherence

Adherence can be defined as an active, responsible process of care, in which the patient works to maintain their health in close collaboration with healthcare personnel. It is now the preferred terminology as the alternative term, compliance, was perceived 'to perpetuate an atmosphere of expectation in which the dictatorial doctor gives orders to the *submissive* patient' [52].

The interpretation of non-adherence can vary between involved parties. Whereas the health professional may consider non-adherence to be the young person's unwillingness to acknowledge the realities of the illness and its treatment, the young person may view it as reflecting their desire to live 'normally', to make independent decisions in the context of an unpredictable disease, and express their autonomy. Frightening the patient with stories of joint damage and replacement surgery is likely to be counterproductive in the management of a non-adherent young person with active JIA. It is therefore important to decriminalize non-adherence and address the underlying issues (see Table 3.3.4).

Adherence in the context of a chronic illness like JIA has some special considerations worthy of highlighting here. Many treatment regimens for JIA are complex, varying from medium to long term duration and have few immediate overt positive consequences. Many require regular monitoring and frequent re-adjustments that can interrupt family, school, and social lives at a time when the young person is seeking relationships and experiences beyond the family. A proactive approach to enhance adherence is more effective than a reactive one. Knowledge is one determinant of adherence but does not ensure adherence. As previously mentioned, education must be age, developmentally and culturally appropriate for each individual patient. The pace, amount, and presentational style needs to be matched to the capabilities of the young person and their family. Discussion of expectations, concerns, or barriers to following treatment plans is important. Repetition of expectations is a key component whether verbal, written, or visual, especially as the young person grows up.

In addition to knowledge, behavioural competency in terms of self-monitoring as well as organizational competency such as appointment

Table 3.3.4 Potential negative influences of adherence in young people with JIA

Demographic factors	
Disease and therapy related factors	Younger age at onset
	Delay of therapeutic effect
	Lack of immediate effect of cessation of therapy
	Need for continuous treatment even when in remission
	Longer duration of therapy
	Increased complexity of regimen
	Toxicity of treatment (anticipated and/or real)
	Pain and discomfort of therapy
	Subjective dissatisfaction with treatment or/and therapists
Educational factors	Lack of information
	Misunderstandings and misconceptions
	Limited cognitive ability
Psychological factors	Depression and hopelessness
	Significant personal costs due to behavioural modification
	Lack of belief in terms of susceptibility, seriousness of illness
	Lack of belief in efficacy of treatment
Family and socio-cultural factors	Family conflict or instability
	Parental over-protection
	Rejection by peers
	Negative impact of health regimens on leisure time, personal freedom, spontaneity
	Negative experience of others with similar disease, for example, role models
Organizational factors	Inconvenient appointment scheduling
	Transport difficulties to access rheumatology services
Economic factors	Cost and/or limited access to therapy

Table 3.3.5 Behaviour modification strategies to promote adherence

- Proactive rather than reactive approach
- Cues or reminders
- Positive feedback
- Steps to minimize discomfort and inconveniences
- Dealing effectively with complaints
- Develop social skills to deal with negative peer responses
- Making therapies interesting/exciting
- Avoid rigidity
- Negotiation of therapy breaks
- Prioritize
- Shared decision-making
- Use of contracts
- Goal setting
- Regular review
- Offer choices—even when limited

scheduling are other determinants to be considered. Above all, demonstrating how the young person can become an active partner in self-management is imperative and strategies such as making contracts between the young person and the team or a team member can facilitate this. Useful behaviour modification strategies in promoting adherence are listed in Table 3.3.5.

Finally it is worth remembering that non-adherence does not correlate with other risk-taking behaviour in adolescence and is not just indicative of a 'difficult teenager'. Non-adherence in adolescent healthcare must be kept in context and not over-emphasized especially as it is estimated that 25–95% of adult out-patients do not take their medications as prescribed [53]. However, the different determinants and consequences as detailed above, need to be acknowledged.

School issues

Today's economy is a knowledge-based economy requiring more, and continuous education for success in the workforce. It is still true that for those with and without disability, ones income is higher the more education one attains. Consistent attendance at school sets a pattern for consistent attendance on the job.

Lovell *et al.* report an average school absence rate for children with arthritis of 12 days per school year compared with a national average of 5 days per year [54]. Maximizing school attendance is vital during adolescence particularly because major examinations are taken at this time. This may have organizational repercussions such as after-school/early evening physician visits being preferable to morning ones. The needs of teachers of such young people must also be addressed, particularly those of the physical education teacher [55]. Channels of communication between schools and the healthcare teams need to be nurtured and a named liaison person in both sectors can facilitate this in addition to advocacy on the part of the young person and their family. An educational checklist can be useful for health professionals to address the impact of a chronic illness and/or disability in specific areas with respect to the school and post secondary experience especially if the young person will be living away from home: education, environmental considerations, medical needs, and activities of daily living all need to be considered [56]. Solutions to these issues should be arrived at in collaboration with the young person. Discussions with the young person and their family should emphasize strengths rather than limitations and aim for inclusion rather than exclusion. Self-advocacy and involvement in decision-making are as important in the school as in the healthcare setting.

Work issues

Young people themselves have identified vocational issues to be the important goal of transition. In several recent surveys of adolescents with chronic illnesses (including JIA), career counselling was identified as an unmet need [57]. In the United States in 1999 [58] and in an audit of adolescent rheumatology services in the United Kingdom provision of information and advice regarding careers was found to be lacking [33].

Despite their keen interest in job readiness skills, cross-sectional studies of young adults with JIA in the UK report an unemployment rate 2–3 times higher than the expected rate calculated from national figures [13,18]. Unemployment however did not correlate with educational achievement or level of disability [13]. Similar results have been found in the United States [16]. The trend towards unemployment is likely to start in adolescence. Healthcare professionals should foster successful career development in young people with chronic illnesses and/or disabilities and consider all aspects of vocational readiness including educational achievement, prior work experience (including household chores); psychological factors such as self-esteem; expectations of both the young person, their family and their teachers, and health professionals; knowledge of availability of resources including career services; and societal attitudes towards chronic illness and/or disability [19].

For those rheumatologists who practice in both adult and paediatric rheumatology clinics, there are many differences in the range of questions used in each clinic setting. This is particularly true for vocational issues. In the paediatric clinic for example, healthcare professionals routinely ask about school, the number of days absent, academic progress to date, any problems identified by the teacher or parent etc. In the adult clinic, the same issues are translated into questions of employment, the number of days absent, any problems encountered in the workplace including a discussion of needed accommodations if appropriate.

However, the context of vocational issues is very different for the adolescent with arthritis compared to the person with arthritis that developed in adulthood.

1.   Adolescents with chronic illnesses may have no memory of a disease-free life. Such young people may well differ from those who developed their disease later, and who do have memories of a disease-free life.

2.   As in the rest of paediatric care, assessment of adolescents must be age, developmental stage and disease appropriate and must also reflect the issues of adolescence.

3.   When considering pre-vocational issues, unlike adults, young people will have had little or no prior work experience and this may influence their attitudes towards and knowledge of work. Also they may have had less opportunity to meet role models.

4.   The role of the family remains important throughout adolescence and the parents and family are key players in the transition period and need guidance as to their role in assisting the young person find a career and work.

Work skills start with taking on responsibilities/tasks in the family. The earliest working experience is in the home with household chores and is even one of the specific questions of the Childhood Health Assessment Questionnaire [59]. Long-term studies of children with disabilities report that early incorporation into household chores/responsibilities is essential for fostering competence and responsibility [60]. This simple aspect of family life is often lost in the presence of JIA with consequent over-protective parenting. This is a key area for all health providers to address both with children as well as with their parents, acknowledging the interesting gender and cultural issues of this area. Health professionals can help by asking the young person with JIA what are their future plans and support those plans, help them identify a passion and skills for a future job, assist them in landing their first job either volunteer or for pay so they can leap to the next more interesting and higher paying job, and last but not least, help them to stay well so they can be a part of the action in life. Working gainfully is a major aspect of adult life, potentially providing status and achievement to an individual and defining who they are to society as well as to themselves. It also provides income, structure, social interaction, an opportunity to learn and practice skills, as well as being a source of self-esteem.

Self-determination and self-advocacy

In the context of a disease such as JIA, characterized by a lack of predictability of disease course and prognosis, nurturing a sense of control and self-efficacy is an important aspect of care, as the young person gradually finds and makes sense of their own identity. Patient empowerment, including disease education, communication, and self-advocacy skills are integral to successful transition. One of the objectives of transition in adolescent healthcare is for the young person to gradually take over the responsibility for their disease management and to become their own advocate. An individualized goal-setting yet flexible policy is appropriate with direct involvement of the young person. Plans for self-medication, self-injection of parenteral therapies, personal copies of blood monitoring forms/result flow sheets, provision of personal copies of clinic letters for the adolescent themselves are some practical examples of enhancing self-advocacy.

An important component of self-advocacy training should be the preparation for and implementation of independent visits including independent use of transportation by the adolescent without their parent. However, in the studies reported to date, the majority of young people are not seen independently in adolescent rheumatology clinics [46,49,50]. This is in contrast to their 'healthy peers'. In primary healthcare, young people in the United Kingdom go to the family physician on their own by age 14–15 years [51,61]. Independent visits can be difficult to contemplate for both the young person with JIA and their parent(s) when there may have been many years when the parent has accompanied the child, and made most of the decisions without perhaps always actively involving the child. Preparation and planning is vital for success with a goal of introducing the idea of independent visits at the age of 11 or 12—'*In a few years time you may feel able to come in to see the doctor on your own*'. By the age of 13–14 both young person and their parents are likely to feel ready to be seen independently for at least part of the consultation. The healthcare professional can set the stage by asking the teenager to think of three questions about their medical situation for the next visit when they will be seen without their parents. In addition, the parent may value the opportunity to talk to a health professional alone. Independent visits are only part of the process of the young person becoming a good self-advocate. It can be useful to emphasize to the anxious parent(s) that the healthcare setting is a safe and often familiar area to practice a range of self-advocacy skills such as communication skills, independent living skills, skills in accessing health services, which are in turn, important for success in independent living and the world of work. Another area to practice self-advocacy and decision-making skills is to discuss with the adolescent the desired characteristics and kinds of adult healthcare professionals they will need and encourage the adolescent to practice obtaining the information and choosing to whom they want to transfer their care.

Anyone who cares for young people should be aware of the legislation governing consent and decision-making in this age-group in their country of practice. Shared decision-making should be encouraged from an early age and when written informed consent is required, age and developmentally appropriate information and consent forms should be used. There is a spectrum of involvement of the young person in the shared decision-making process and their degree of involvement depends on many factors including, in addition to age, capacity to understand the nature of the problem and the decisions to be made, the nature of the medical decision, the seriousness of the consequences of the decision, the relationship between the young person and their parents, legal constraints etc. Informed decision-making requires both age and developmentally appropriate disease education and appropriate communication skills within the healthcare setting.

Consultation dynamics

During adolescence, the goal is to have the young person become more independent and the role of the parent/guardian(s) and family evolves in parallel to allow this to happen successfully. This evolution has an impact on consultation dynamics. The classical paediatric triangular relationship of child–parent–professional ideally moves towards the linear, autonomous young adult–professional therapeutic model. All the participants including health professionals may have difficulties during this process of adaptation. Successful transition requires these difficulties to be anticipated, acknowledged, and addressed. Communication skills needed for a 14-year-old young person with JIA with their parent(s) are markedly different from those required for a 4-year-old child with JIA and their attendant parent. The monosyllabic adolescent with the all too familiar 'grunt phenomenon' and hidden agendas presents a significant communication challenge.

Advocacy issues for parents

One of the main differences between paediatric and adult-centred care is the role of parents. During adolescence and the associated increasing autonomy for the young person, parents need guidance, support, and encouragement to become an advocate for their son/daughter's independence and not be abruptly 'exiled' to the waiting area immediately when their son/daughter turns 16. The goal for the parents is to move from a caregiver role to being a resource for their adolescent when asked. It is useful therefore to consider a parallel transition process for the respective parents/guardians during this period and some of the issues for parents are discussed below.

Expectations of parents for their son/daughter with JIA are important to address. In one study, although parents of non-disabled young people with JIA denied any impact of the disease on their child, they still had lower expectations for their education compared to their healthy siblings. Only 17% of parents expected their non-disabled child with JIA to go to university compared to 73% of their healthy siblings [62]. When 100 adolescents with chronic illness and/or physical disabilities were studied in the United States, their lack of career maturity and paucity of early work experience was related to their parent's view that the mean age for first work experience should be 16 years or older [19]. This is compared to reports of 50% of healthy 13-year olds being involved in work experience

outside their home [63]. Parents therefore need to be supported, made aware of resources available and encouraged to ensure that their son/daughter attains the developmental milestones in the different components of transition equivalent to their healthy peers. The positive, affirming role of the family is essential to engender increasing adolescent independence. Studies have shown that emotional wellbeing in adolescence has been reported to be strongly correlated to 'family connectedness' irrespective of presence or absence of chronic illness [18]. Family connectedness, family role models, family concern for the well-being of the child and autonomy at home are all factors identified that foster resilience in children and should be encouraged particularly in adolescence [64]. However, family connectedness must be balanced to avoid over-protectiveness. One cause of problematic peer acceptance is often parental over-protection with resultant social isolation for the young person.

Planning and preparation of both the young person and the parent/guardian for independent visits while continuing to emphasize the vital role of the supportive parent is another integral part of any transitional care programme. As the young person grows up, it is important to remember that they will not always talk openly in front of their parents regarding medication or risk-taking behaviours. If possible, a multidisciplinary team approach to such visits may be extremely useful particularly when one team member can be seeing the parent/guardian while another is meeting with the young person. This can still be perceived as inclusive and positive for the parent as it can provide an opportunity for the parent to ask questions they may not wish to ask in front of their son/daughter. A good working knowledge of the social history and family dynamics is invaluable particularly in these days when non-nuclear families are becoming the norm. If the young person is living with a step-parent, does the biological parent have informational needs if they are in regular contact? It is important to not forget fathers, who often are not in attendance during hospital visits but still need to be involved. It is also important to establish who has legal responsibility of the young person. Cultural awareness with respect to parental roles during adolescence is a further important consideration for the team.

The relationship between parent and young person as well as with the health professional is dynamic and may vary from visit to visit through adolescence. Managing these interactions requires sensitivity and perception on behalf of the health professional. The educational and informational needs of the parent should be addressed and may include both healthcare-related information as well as basic facts about adolescent development such as how to deal with siblings and knowledge of community resources, and disability legislation.

Transition clinic models

Transitional care should be seen as an essential component of high quality healthcare in any service caring for children and young people with chronic illness and/or disability. Various models have been reported including disease-specific, generic, primary care based, community-based and single-site models [58,65]. There is as yet no reported evidence for their relative efficacy and suitability for different patient and/or disease groups. It is not known whether different models of transitional care produce equivalent medical and psychological outcomes or indeed which patient characteristics (medical, social, psychological) identify those who need which transitional program. Whatever the structure, an identified person (key worker or case manager) within the paediatric and/or adult teams must be responsible for transition arrangements.

The most common model is the *disease-based model*, which can tailor transition to the particular needs of rheumatology patients and clinics. When the receiving adult clinic has large numbers of elderly patients, a young adult rheumatology clinic is an ideal compromise. Having the paediatric and adult services on a single site allows for close collaboration to develop, thereby reducing the administrative hurdles, all too familiar to the other models. It must be emphasized, however, that geographical closeness does not automatically imply collaboration.

Generic adolescent transition medicine programs also can be developed offering transition resources to young people with a variety of chronic illnesses and disabilities. This could avoid the duplication of resources which may occur if small specialties like paediatric rheumatology develop independent programmes. Shared resources such as an adolescent nurse specialist, youth worker can be offered that may be hard to justify in a stand-alone discipline. Some community-based models are also generic [56]. Although primary care involvement in the transition process is vital, there are problems establishing a truly *primary care based transition model* when many young people with chronic illnesses prefer to use the subspecialty services for most of their needs. Which model to use largely depends on local resources available in terms of staff and finance as well as geography.

The key players in adolescent rheumatology services remain the same whatever the model and include first and foremost the young people themselves. Young people should be involved in the development of new services from the outset as well as active participants in developing their own individual transition plan. Peer education is another channel for their involvement as well as youth mentoring programmes. Young adults in the adult service can similarly be used as role models particularly with respect to vocational issues, as contacts for work experience for example. Other key players in transitional care programmes include their parents and family, primary healthcare team, community health services, hospital speciality services both paediatric and adult, education (including vocational training, college and university), social services, and voluntary organizations.

The essentials of a transitional care service

(1) Individualized Transition Plans;

(2) Collaboration of Adult and Paediatric Rheumatology Services;

(3) Administrative support;

(4) Primary care involvement;

(5) Direct involvement of the young people themselves;

Consideration of how an adolescent rheumatology service is set up in terms of process and personnel is also important (Table 3.3.6).

These are all discussed below and summarized in Table 3.3.7.

Individualized transition plans

For all young people, a written individualized transition plan should be developed in conjunction with the young person as early as possible, outlining the anticipated events of transition including medical,

Table 3.3.6 Useful strategies for adolescent rheumatology service development

Personnel
Continuity of personnel
Identify key 'adolescent' team member
Offer professional of preferred gender when feasible
Use of peers in disease education programmes
Use of role models, for example, young adults with JIA in employment
Advisory panel of young people for service developments

Administrative
Encourage the use of a notebook held by the young person, for questions to bring to clinic
Information sheets (disease specific, generic health promotion, careers advice) specifically written with and for young people
Letter to patient reiterating the information exchanged during each clinic visit and suggesting issues that need further discussion/review at the next visit.

Environmental
'Dedicated' space if feasible (e.g. latter half of a general paediatric clinic, corner of general paediatric waiting area etc)
Rooms available for young person and parent to be seen independently
Careful arrangement of consultation room to facilitate eye contact between professional and the young person.

Table 3.3.7 Essentials of a transitional care service

Multidisciplinary involvement—including key coordinator

A policy on timing of transition and transfer
Flexible
Early start
Written policy developed by the team and in agreement with the target
Adult services
Regular review of policy

A preparation period

A disease education programme

Address needs of both young person and their parent(s)/guardians

A co-ordinated transfer process

A committed adult rheumatology service

Administrative support

Primary care involvement

Involvement of young people themselves
In developing their own individualized transition plans
As advisors to service development
As educators of peers and health professionals

Key liaison personnel in paediatric and adult services (if possible)

Regular evaluation and audit

vocational, and psychosocial issues along with the responsibilities that each person and the professionals have in the process. This plan can then be kept under regular review and when necessary, revised through the adolescent years. An example of this is shown in Figures 3.3.1–3.3.3 in the form of a case history and a formulated transition plan for a young person with JIA and her mother.

Aspects of an individualized transition plan include full understanding of disease and therapy, self-medication, independent visits,

Fig. 3.3.1

Case history

Jenny is 16 years old and has had severe polyarticular JIA since the age of 12 years. She has attended the children's hospital since she was diagnosed. She is currently on methotrexate 20 mg subcutaneous once weekly (given by her mother), naproxen 375 mg twice daily, alternate day prednisolone 10 mg, daily calcium and vitamin D supplements and intermittent intra-articular steroids which she refuses unless they are given under conscious sedation. Her mother has recently found several loose calcium and naproxen tablets in the bathroom.

Her disease has recently become very active. Her height is below the 10th centile but her weight is above the 75th centile. The methotrexate is due to be increased but her liver function tests have become abnormal despite previously stable doses for several months. Jenny has missed 5 days off school for the last year. She has also recently stopped going to the local teenage hydrotherapy session which she previously enjoyed.

She always attends clinic with her mother but rarely says anything, preferring to sit frowning. She says she has no real friends but stays out late, refusing to tell her mother where she has been. She hasn't a clue of what she wants to do with her life. She gets upset at the mention of transfer to an adult rheumatology team in a neighbouring hospital.

Fig. 3.3.2 Jenny's individualized transitional care plan.

Start Date: as early as possible and when disease is controlled.

Health

- JIA-specific
  — Maximize medical regimen to improve disease control and limit drug toxicities (e.g. steroid toxicity including osteoporosis and implications to body image from cushingoid appearance)
  — Present information as choices to Jenny and rationale of therapies proposed
  — Introduce concept of eventual injections under local anaesthetic. Always seek parallel consent from Jenny as well as her mother for all procedures
  — Assess current level of knowledge and understanding of disease and determine informational needs
  — Suggest Jenny uses a notebook to write down questions she wants answers to for each hospital visit
  — Reinforce information given at each visit with letter written to Jenny summarizing plan of management and issues for her to think about prior to her next visit
  — Explore reasons for non-adherence with hydrotherapy (?body image)
  — Discuss increase dietary calcium intake if intolerant of supplements
  — Consider once daily NSAID rather than twice daily naproxen
- Generic health and wellness needs [see Table 3.3.3]
  — Discuss dental, diet (calcium), cigarettes, sex
  — Explore possibility of alcohol being cause of abnormal liver function
  — Consider healthy eating concept rather than dieting[!]
  — Explore general exercise options for improved mobility and weight reduction
  — explore opportunities for peer support
- Self-advocacy issues
  — Gradually develop self medication including self-injection of methotrexate if necessary
  — Use peer educators or mentors
  — Gradually develop independent visits. While Jenny is seen, mother can be seen by nurse specialist and then brought in for the end of the consultation when the management plan can be summarized

— Encourage Jenny to make and keep own appointments and phone appropriate healthcare provider with own queries
— Discuss financial implications of healthcare, for example, health insurance, prescription charges, costs of medical equipment

- Transfer to adult rheumatology
  — Delay until disease in remission, able to self-medicate, being seen independently
  — Discuss desired characteristics of adult health care providers required
  — Discuss differences between paediatric and adult care provision
  — Plan provisional visit to adult unit prior to transfer date
  — Create with Jenny a detailed written summary for adult providers
- Educational/vocational
  — Explore reasons why she is missing school—for example need for accommodations, bullying
  — Discuss importance of completion of secondary education for future employment potential
  — Explore involvement in household responsibilities/chores
  — Explore her aspirations for the future
  — Begin career exploration—liaise with school-teachers; role models/mentors
  — Encourage volunteer/paid work experience—keep on developmental milestones like healthy peers
  — Understand implications of disability legislation on education, employment, and disclosure
- Independent living
  — Learn to drive and use public transportation
  — Organize (if necessary) home visit by occupational therapist to ensure maximal independence in activities of daily living and encourage household chores
  — Explore opportunities to experience time away from home, for example, summer camp
  — Encourage independence in use of transportation
- Social/recreation
  — Enquire about what she enjoys doing
  — Enquire about peer activities—with able and disabled peers
  — Explore opportunities for physical activities

Fig. 3.3.3 Individualized Transitional Care Program for Jenny's mother.

Support

— Ensure ongoing support of parents as their role evolves particularly as they learn 'to let go'
— Acknowledge their needs and address their concerns re: transition

Health

- Advocacy
  — Encourage and support self medication program
  — Encourage and support independent visits
- Information needs
  — Assess current level of knowledge and understanding of disease and determine informational needs
  — Understanding of adolescent development and impact of chronic illness during adolescence
- Generic health and wellness (see Table 3.3.3)
  — Encourage behaviours of future health and wellness within family
  — Remind parent that their health is important for themselves as well as their child
  — Contact with other parents of adolescents with same condition

Educational/vocational

— Encourage career exploration

— Understand implications of disability legislation on education, employment, and disclosure

— Encourage exploration of opportunities within parent network of volunteer/ paid work experience keep on developmental milestones like healthy peers

Independent living

— Encourage autonomy in home, for example. involvement in household chores

— Have friends around for meal/to stay

— Information of community resources

the source of symptoms, recognition of disease flares, and functional deterioration, and taking appropriate action, how to seek help and operate within the medical system. Written information for both young person and their parent/guardian are useful adjuncts to this process. A similar individualized plan devised with and for the parent of the young person is also useful. These plans with their regular updates should be communicated to the whole multidisciplinary team with the professionals responsible for specific tasks identified. The role of the healthcare provider is to identify the team member who will fulfil a coordinating role for each individual patient. This mainly entails asking the appropriate questions and assisting the young person and their family in finding the necessary resources. The central theme of such plans is that all those involved with Jenny should have the expectations that she will become a happy, independent, and fulfilled adult.

Collaboration of adult and paediatric rheumatology services

A transition program can only be successful if organized with the active participation and interest of the staff caring for adults with arthritis. A 'transition map' of interested and committed adult rheumatologists, detailing where and how transfer occurs, can be useful for large paediatric services. Once a map has been identified, local guidelines developed by joint working parties of adult and paediatric rheumatologists are potentially useful developments to ensure successful transition. Regular communication at the paediatric–adult interface is ideal both at a local and national level for both future service developments in adolescent rheumatology as well as prospective research into the long-term outcome of JIA and it's therapies.

Administrative support

The administrative costs of transition are often underestimated and must be considered prior to the development of any new service. Detailed multidisciplinary summaries need to be produced, typed, and copied to all involved parties. Copies of previous notes, X-rays may need to be copied. Clinic letters may need to be written to both healthcare professionals as well as the young person themselves. Other professionals need to be informed when the young person is being seen independently so that this can be recognized in any non-rheumatological visits. Secretaries and receptionists may require training in handling young people on the phone as they are encouraged by the team members to learn to use the health system directly rather than via their parents.

Primary care involvement

The primary care team may provide much needed continuity in adolescent healthcare though many young people with chronic illness unfortunately have little involvement with their primary care provider. It is important for hospital-based teams to keep the respective primary care team informed so that they can continue to address the generic issues detailed above.

Direct involvement of the young people themselves

As mentioned previously, this is an essential but often challenging component of any successful transition programme. Apart from being actively involved in their own healthcare, young people can be key players and advisors in the development of any new services and the evaluation and development of any established service. Peer education [57], mentoring programs, and peer support program [58] are also worthy of consideration.

Transition and rheumatic disease characteristics

Just as in the rest of medicine, no two patients are the same and this is true for adolescents. The essence of much of what has been detailed above is flexibility of approach with no rigid age criteria. Physical, cognitive, and psychosocial development varies among all adolescents, with or without JIA. It is worth reflecting on how duration and severity of disease impacts on adolescence and rheumatology management during this period [66,67]. It is important to note that the psychosocial ramifications and perceptions of the young person do not correlate closely with the medical severity of the disease [68–70].

Patients with recent onset disease For young people recently diagnosed the main priority (as for all patients with JIA) is to control the inflammation and pain, limit deformity, and maintain growth and development. Educating the young person and their family about the condition and its therapy is important from disease onset and this often needs to be reiterated during the initial stages of adjusting to such a diagnosis. Providing space for the young person to express their own concerns and ask their own questions is important from the outset, as is their active involvement in decision-making. Preparation for transition should start early and initial written information about the paediatric rheumatology service given to the young person and their family should include details of how the service addresses transition and eventual transfer to adult services. Once the arthritis disease activity is stable, preparation for transition can then start as detailed above.

Patients with established disease For young people with established disease it is important to revisit the extent of their knowledge about their disease and its therapy as misunderstandings and deficits may be revealed even in long-term clinic attendees [24]. Health issues that were not relevant during childhood such as alcohol and sexual activity may also need to be addressed. Preparation for transition for both young person and parent(s) should commence early. Continuity of health personnel becomes increasingly important. The identification of a key person to coordinate the transition process is useful and ideally is the team member in whom the young person has confidence and interacts with best.

Patients with refractory disease These patients are the ones most likely to have the most obvious effects on physical development in terms of pubertal delay, growth retardation, and joint deformity. They are also likely to have parents with the highest level of concern, be the most attached to the paediatric team, and have the most complex therapy regimens. Often the generic health concerns for these young people are hidden by the major overriding concern of the refractoriness of arthritis. Preparation for transition must still take place acknowledging it may be protracted. Transitional care, however, provides an important message for the young person and their family in that the rheumatology team are considering the future in real terms and the present. Initial shared care with adult rheumatology teams can be a great option in late adolescence for such young people.

Cost implications of transitional care

In the current economic climate time and financial constraints are obvious major hurdles to the development of adolescent rheumatology services. Fully supported, dedicated, multidisciplinary services are likely to be a rarity. The paucity and heterogeneity of adolescent rheumatology services in the United Kingdom has been recently highlighted [33]. However, age and developmentally appropriate delivery of care for adolescents within every paediatric rheumatology service remains imperative. Being aware of the need is a simple but major step forward especially when the attitudinal hurdles are acknowledged (Table 3.3.2). Having a key person within each paediatric rheumatology team whose role is to maintain the profile of adolescent issues within the department may be useful. Even if there is no dedicated outpatient area or inpatient ward, a 'space' within a clinic or ward can be made more adolescent-friendly with the help and advice of the young people themselves. Since many of the issues confronting young people with chronic illnesses are generic and not disease-specific resources may be shared between specialties within the same hospital, with shared use of adolescent clinical nurse specialists, youth workers. Interdisciplinary meetings of professionals interested in adolescent healthcare can help to raise and maintain awareness within a large institution.

Summary

Adolescent issues are often as important as rheumatological issues in the care of a young person with JIA and is an area ripe for further research and development. The models of service delivery will vary according to the type of health service provision but the fundamentals remain true to all. Adolescent services should be age-appropriate and developmentally appropriate, involve the young person, their family and a variety of disciplines and agencies, and encompass medical psychosocial and vocational issues. The needs of the parents must also be addressed and the process of transition be at all times inclusive and not exclusive of their needs. Although there are many unknowns, there seems very little doubt that adolescent services, including transition programs, have a beneficial effect in helping children with JIA become physically, and psychologically functioning independent adults with JIA. Results of further research is awaited with interest and anticipation.

References

1. Gare, B.A. and Fasth, A. The natural history of juvenile chronic arthritis. A population based cohort study. II. Outcome. *J Rheumatol* 1995;22:308–19.
2. Blum, R.W., Garell, D., Hadgman, C.H. *et al*. Transition from child-centred to adult health-care systems for adolescents with chronic conditions. A position paper of the Society for Adolescent Medicine. *J Adolesc Health* 1993;14:570–6.
3. American Academy of Pediatrics. A Concensus Statement on Health Care Transitions for young adults with Special Health Care Need. *Pediatrics* 2002;110(Suppl.):1304–6
4. Blum, R.W. and Okinow, N.A. *Teenagers at Risk—A national perspective of state level services for adolescents with chronic illnesses or disabilities*. Minneapolis, USA: National Center for Youth with Disabilities, 1993.
5. Strax, T.E. Psychological issues faced by adolescents and young adults with disabilities. *Pediatr Ann* 1991;20:501–6.
6. Akinbami, L.J., Gandhi, H., and Cheng, T.L. Availability of Adolescent Health Services and Confidentiality in Primary Care Offices. *Pediatrics* 2003; 111: 394–401.
7. Viner, R.M. Transition from paediatric to adult care. Bridging the gaps or passing the buck? *Arch Dis Child* 1999;81:271–5.
8. Rosen, D. Between two worlds: Bridging the cultures of child health and adult medicine. *J Adoles Health* 1995;17:10–16.
9. Society for Adolescent Medicine. A position statement of the Society for Adolescent Medicine. *J Adolesc Health* 1995;16:413.
10. World Health Organization. The health of young people. Geneva, 1993.
11. Florentino, L., Datta. D., Gentle, S., Hall, D.M.B., Harpin, V., Phillips, D., and Walker, A. Transition from school to adult life for physically disabled young people. *Arch Dis Child* 1998;79:306–11.
12. David, J., Cooper, C., Hickey, L., Lloyd, J., Dore, C., McCullough, C., and Woo, P. The functional and psychological outcomes of juvenile chronic arthritis in young adulthood. *Br J Rheumatol* 1994;33:876–81.
13. Martin, K. and Woo, P. Outcome in juvenile chronic arthritis. *Rev Rhum* (Eng Edn) 1997;10:S242.
14. Foster, H.E., Marshall, N., Myers, A., Dunkley, P., and Griffiths, I.D. Outcome in Adults with Juvenile idiopathic Arthritis: a quality of like study. *Arthritis Rheum* 2003; 48:767–75
15. Oen, K., Malleson, P.N., Cabral, D.A., Rosenberg, A.M., Petty, R.E., and Cheang, M. Disease course and outcome of Juvenile rheumatoid arthritis in a multicenter cohort. *J Rheumatol* 2002; 29:1989–99.
16. Petersen, L.S., Mason, T., Nelson, A.M., Fallon, W., and Gabriel, S.E. Psychosocial outcomes and health studies in adults who have had juvenile arthritis: a controlled population based study. *Arthritis Rheum* 1997;40:2235–40.
17. Ruperto, N., Levinson, J.E., Ravelli, A., Shear, E.S., Tague, B.L., Murray, K., Martini, A., and Giannini, E.H. Long-term health outcomes and quality of life in American and Italian inception cohort of patients with juvenile rheumatoid arthritis. I. Outcome status. *J Rheumatol* 1997;24:945–51.
18. Packham, J.C. and Hall, M.A. Long-term outcome of Juvenile Idiopathic Arthritis, Education and Employment status. *Arch Dis Child* 1999;80(Suppl. 1):P22.
19. White, P.H., Gussek, D.G., Fisher, B., *et al*. Career maturity in adolescents with chronic illness. *J Adolesc Health Care* 1990;11:372.
20. Billings, A.G., Moos, P.H., Miller, J.J., and Gottlieb, J.E. Psychosocial adaptation in juvenile rheumatic disease: a controlled evaluation. *Health Psych* 1987;6:343–59.
21. Ungerer, J.A., Horgan, B., Chaitow, J., and Campion, G.D. Psychosocial functioning in children and young adults with juvenile arthritis. *Pediatrics* 1988;81:195–202.
22. Ostensen, M., Almberg K., and Koksvik, H.S. Sex, reproduction and gynecological disease in young adults with a history of juvenile chronic arthritis. *J Rheumatol* 2000; 27: 1783–7.
23. Packham, J.C. and Hall, M.A. Longterm Followup of 246 adults with juvenile idiopathic arthritis: social function, relationships and sexual activity. *Rheumatology* 2002;41:1440–3
24. Packham, J.C. and Hall, M.A. Longterm follow-up of 246 adults with juvenile idiopathic arthritis: education and employment. *Rheumatology* 2002;41:1436–9.

25. Salmi, J., Huuponen, T., Oksa, H., Oksala H., Koivula, T., and Raita, P. Metabolic control in adolescent insulin-dependent diabetics referred from pediatric to adult clinic. *Ann Clin Res* 1986;4:174–80.

26. Sawyer, S.M. The process of transition to adult health care services. In George Werther and John Court, eds. *Diabetes and the Adolescent.* Melbourne: Blackwell, 1998.

27. Nasr, S.Z. Campbell, C., and Howatt, W. Transition program from paediatric to adult care for cystic fibrosis patients. *J Adol Health* 1992;13:682–5.

28. Rettig, P. and Athreya, B.H. Adolescents with chronic disease: transition to adult health care. *Arthritis Care Research* 1991;4:174–80.

29. Berry, S.L., Hayford, J.R., Ross, C.K., Pachman, L.M., and Lavigne, J.V. Conceptions of illness by children with juvenile rheumatoid arthritis: a cognitive developmental approach. *J Pediatr Psychol* 1993;18:83–97.

30. Piaget, J. Intellectual evolution from adolescence to adulthood. *Human Dev* 1972;15:1–12.

31. Carroll, G., Massarelli, E., Opzoomer, A., Pekeles, G., Pedneault, M., Frappier, J.Y., and Onetto, N. Adolescents with chronic disease: are they receiving comprehensive health care? *J Adol Health Care* 1983;17:32–6.

32. Elster, A.B. and Levenberg, P. Integrating comprehensive adolescent preventive services into medicine care. *Ped Clin N America* 1997;44:1365–77.

33. McDonagh, J.E., Foster, H., Hall, M.A., and Chamberlain, M.A. Audit of rheumatology services for adolescents and young adults in the UK. *Rheumatology* 2000;39:596–602.

34. Stewart, A.L., Hays, R.D., Wells, K.B., Rogers, W.H., Spritzer, K.L., and Greenfield, S. Long-term functioning and well-being outcomes associated with physical activity and exercise in patients with chronic conditions in the Medical outcomes study. *J Clin Epidemiol* 1994;47:719–30.

35. Klepper, S., Darbee, J., Effgenr, S.K., and Singsen, B.H. Physical fitness levels in children with polyarticular juvenile rheumatoid arthritis. *Arthritis Care* Res 1992;5:93–100.

36. Kotaniemi, A., Savolainen, A., Kroger, H. *et al.* Weight-bearing physical activity, calcium intake, systemic glucocorticoids, chronic inflammation and body constitution as determinants of lumbar and femoral bone mineral in juvenile chronic arthritis. *Scand J Rheumatol* 1999;28:19–26.

37. Voss, L.D. and Mulligan, J. Bulluing in school: are short pupils at risk? Questionnaire study in a cohort. *BMJ* 2000;320:612–3.

38. Henderson, C.J. and Lovell, D.J. Nutritional aspects of juvenile rheumatoid arthritis. *Rheum Dis Clin North Am* 1991;17:403–13.

39. Henderson, C.J., Specker, B.L., Sierra, R.I. *et al.* Total-body bone mineral content in non-corticosteriod-treated post pubertal females with juvenile rheumatoid arthritis. *Arthritis Rheum* 2000;43:531–40.

40. Gregory, J., Lowe, S., Bates, C.J. *et al.* National Diet and Nutrition survey (NDNS) of people aged 4–18 years, Vol 1. London HMSO, 2000.

41. Harel, Z., Riggs, S., Vaz, R., White, L. and Menzies, G. Adolescents and Calcium: what they do and do not know and how much they consume. *J Adol Health* 1998;22:225–8.

42. Fleming, R. and Patrick, K. Osteoporosis prevention: pediatrician's knowledge, attitudes and counselling practices. *Prev Med* 2002;34:411–21.

43. Johnston, C.C., Miller, J.Z., Slemenda, C.W., *et al.* Calcium supplementation and increases in bone mineral density in children. *N Eng J Med* 1992;327:82–7.

44. National Institutes of Health consensus conference. NIH consensus development panel on optimal calcium intake. *JAMA* 1994;272:1942–8.

45. Zuengler, K.L. and Neubeck, G. Sexuality: developing togetherness. In *Stress and the Family* McCubben H., ed. New York; Bruner/Mazel, 1983:41–3.

46. Britto, M.T., Rosenthal, S.L., Taylor, J., and Passo, M.H. Improving rheumatologists screening for alcohol use and sexual activity. *Arch Pediatr Adolesc Med* 2000;154: 478–83.

47. Choquet, M., Fediaevsky, L.D.P., and Manfredi, R. Sexual behaviour among adolescents reporting chronic conditions: a French national survey. *J Adol Health* 1997;20:62–7.

48. Blumenfeld, Z., Lorber, M., Yoffe, N., and Scharf, Y. Systemic lupus erythematosus: predisposition for uterine cervical dysplasia. *Lupus* 1994;3:59–61.

49. Timko, C., Stovel, K.W., Moos, R.H., and Miller, J.J. Adaptation to juvenile rheumatic disease: a controlled evaluation of functional disability with a one-year follow-up. *Health Psycho* 1992;11:67–76.

50. Nash, A.A., Britto, M.T., Lovell, D.J., Passo, M.H., and Rosenthal, S.L. Substance use among adolescents with JRA. *Arthritis Care Res* 1998;11: 391–6.

51. Jacobson, L. and Owen, P. Study of teenage care in one general practice. *Br J Gen Pract* 1993;43:349.

52. Kroll, T., Barlow, J.H., and Shaw, K. Treatment adherence in Juvenile rheumatoid arthritis—a review. *Scand J Rheumatol* 1999;28:10–18.

53. Stewart, R.B. and Claff, L.E. Review of medication errors and compliance in ambulatory patients. *Clin Pharmacol Ther* 1972;13:463–5.

54. Lovell, D.J., Athreya, B., Emery, H.M., Gibbas, D.L., Levinson, J.E., Lindsley, C.B. *et al.* School attendance and patterns, special services and special needs in paediatric patients with rheumatic diseases. *Arthritis Care Res* 1990;3:196–203.

55. Mukherjee, S., Lightfoot, J., and Sloper, P. Improving communication between health and education for children with chronic illness or physical disability, Social Policy Research Unit, University of York, UK (1999) (see: *www.york.ac.uk/inst/spru/*).

56. Edelman, A., Schuyler, V., and White, P.H. Maximising success for young adults with chronic health related conditions. Transition planning for education after high school. Washington, DC: HEATH Resource Center, American Council on Education, 1998.

57. Beresford, B. and Sloper, T. The information needs of chronically ill or physically disabled children and adolescents. Social Policy Research Unit, University of York, UK (1999) (*www.york.ac.uk/inst/spru/*).

58. Scal, P., Evans, T., Blozis, S., Okinow, N., and Blum, R. Trends in transition from pediatric to adult health care services for young adults with chronic conditions. *J Adolesc Health* 1999;24:259–64.

59. Singh, G., Athreya, B., Fries, J., Goldsmith, D.P., and Ostrov, B.E. Measurement of health status in children with juvenile rheumatoid arthritis. *Arthritis Rheum* 1994;37:1761–9.

60. Werner, E.E. and Smith, R.S. *Overcoming the Odds: High risk children from birth to adulthood.* Cornell University Press, Ithaca, 1992.

61. Balding, J. *Young People into the Nineties. Book 1. Doctor and Dentist.* University of Exeter, Schools Health Education Unit, 1991.

62. McAnarney, E.R., Pless, I.B., Satterwhite, B. Friedman, S.B. Psychological problems of children with chronic juvenile arthritis. *Pediatrics* 1974;53:523–8.

63. Phillips, S. and Sandston, K.L. Parental attitudes toward work. *Youth Soc,* 1990;22:160.

64. Patterson, J. and Blum, R.J. Risk and resilience among children and youth with disabilities. Arch *Pediatr Adolesc-Med* 1996;150:692–8.

65. Chamberlain, M.A. and Rooney, C.M. Young adults with arthritis: meeting their transitional needs. *Br J Rheumatol* 1996;35:84–90.

66. Mellanby, A.R., Phelps, F.A., Crichton, N.J., and Tripp, J.H. School sex education: an experimental programme with educational and medical benefit. *Br Med J* 1995;311:414–7.

67. Olsson, C.A. Sawyer, S.M., and Boyce, M. What are the special needs of chronically ill young people? *Aust Fam Physician* 2000;29: 299–300.

68. Wolman, C., Resnick, M.D., Harris, L.J., and Blum, R.W. Emotional well-being among adolescents with and without chronic conditions. *J Adol Health* 1994;15:199–204.

69. Baildam, E.M., Holt, P.J.L., Conway, S.C., and Morton, M.J.S. The association between physical function and psychological problems in children with juvenile chronic arthritis. *Br J Rheumatol* 1995; 34:470–7.

70. Stevens, S.E., Steele, C.A., Jutai, J.W., Kalnins, IV, Bortolussi, J.A., and Biggar, W.D. Adolescents with Physical disabilities: some psychosocial aspects of health. *J Adol Health* 1996 19:157–64.

71. Goldenring, J.M. and Cohen, E. Getting into adolescent heads. *Contemp Pediatr* 1988:75–80.

Appendix 1

Examples of useful websites in adolescent rheumatology

Health transitions

www.aap.org
Website for the American Academy of Pediatrics. Click on the Medical Home section and then to the Transition section. There is a slide presentation, resources, and references listed.

http://depts.washington.edu/healthtr/Providers/transfer.htm
Deciding to Transfer the Child From Pediatric to Age-appropriate Adult Care from the Adolescent Health Transition Project—Information For Health Care Providers and Educators.

All people are entitled to receive health care in age-appropriate settings which promote autonomy and enrich social growth. Health care providers should advocate self-empowerment and full societal participation for their young adult clients.

School/work transitions

www.after16.org.uk
Family fund Trust (UK charity) website. Choices and challenges for young disabled people after the age of 16

www.skill.org.uk
National UK Bureau for Students with Disabilities

http://interact.uoregon.edu/wrrc/trnfiles/trncontents.htm
The Individuals With Disabilities Education Act Of 1997—Transition Requirements—A Guide for States, Districts, Schools, Universities and Families. A wonderful resource on IDEA plus a bonus: the design of this can be altered/customized for your state! Great info, super checklist.

www.disAbility.gov
A one-stop online access to resources, services and information available throughout the USA Federal Government.

Family/peer support and information

www.fvkasa.org
Family Voices—*Kids As Self-Advocates (KASA)*. KASA is a national, grassroots network of youth with disabilities needs (and our friends), speaking out. We are leaders in our communities, and we help spread helpful, positive information among our peers to increase knowledge around various issues.

http://www.girlpower.gov/girlarea/bodywise/disability/talk/tips.htm
Site developed to help encourage and motivate 9- to 14-year-old girls to make the most of their lives. Girls at 8 or 9 typically have very strong attitudes about their health, so *Girl Power!* seeks to reinforce and sustain these positive values among girls ages 9–14 by targeting health messages to the unique needs, interests, and challenges of girls.

www.familyvoices.org/YourVoiceCounts/AccessToRehabSvcs-ExecSum.pdf
Family voices—*Access to Rehabilitation Services and Technology for Children with Special Health Care Needs: Findings and Recommendations for Families and Providers. 9/01.*

www.cafamily.org.uk
UK based Contact-a-Family charity; useful information re benefits, transition, statementing etc that can be downloaded for parents.

www.rch.unimelb.edu.au/ChIPS/
Website of Chronic Illness Peer Support programme from Melbourne, Australia.

www.faculty.fairfield.edu/fleitas/contents.html
US based website 'Band-aides and Blackboards' aims to provide age appropriate information for all children with chronic illnesses.

Generic transition websites

www.communityinclusion.org
Online guides for students, parents and professionals on education and transition/person-centred planning.

http://chs.state.ky.us/ccshcn/ccshcntransition.htm
Healthy & ready to work—in Kentucky. *Life maps—KY teach Project:Life Maps* are developmentally appropriate transition questionnaires that allow families and young people to identify their own individual needs. The Life Maps cover a range of topics from health promotion and health problem management to independence and work issues. These clinical tools encourage staff to provide family-centred care that focuses on the individual needs of the young person.

http://depts.washington.edu/healthtr
Adolescent health transition project in Washington. Online transition timelines and resources from the adolescent health transition project at the University of Washington.

http://internet.dscc.uic.edu/dsccroot/parents/transition.asp
The Illinois Chapter of the American Academy of Pediatrics (ICAAP) has developed an informational brochure titled '*Preparing for the Future: Transition to Adulthood*' to help teenagers and their families prepare for their future during the transition process to adulthood. The brochure outlines the school, medical, financial and legal issues that should be considered and addressed.

www.hrtw.org
Health & Ready to Work National Center's mission is to create changes in policy, programs and practices that will support Youth with Special Health Care Needs as they transition to adult health care, to work, and to independence.

http://hctransitions.ichp.edu/
US based transition website with resources and annotated bibliography that also includes a Transition Special Interest Group on the web for patients and professionals.

Arthritis and teenagers

www.arc.org.uk
website of the Arthritis Research Campaign in the UK
Leaflet 'Arthritis in teenagers' available online.

www.arthritiscare.org.uk
Website of the UK-based charity Arthritis Care; "The Source" is a help-line for young people under 25 (email:thesource@arthritiscare.org.uk)

www.arthritis.org
US-based national charity 'Arthritis Foundation'—Juvenile Arthritis section with site specifically for teenagers

Other transitional care resources

ONTRAC transition programme
British Columbia Children's Hospital
4480 Oak St
Vancouver BC
Canada 3V4
Tel: (604) 875–3472

Room 2D 20

Parent Training and Information Centre
PACER Center Inc
4826 Chicago Avenue South
Minneapolis MN 55412
USA
Tel: (612) 827–2966

National Center for Youth with Disabilities
University of Minnesota
PO Box 721
420 Delaware St SE
Minneapolis MN 55455
USA
Tel: (612) 626 2931

Adolescent Employment Readiness Centre
Children's National Medical Center
111 Michigan Ave NW
Washington DC 20010–2970
Tel: (202) 884 3203
Fax: (202) 884 3385

Addendum:

Recent key references concerning transition.

(i) Evidence of need for transition in adolescent rheumatology

Shaw, K.L., Southwood, T.R., McDonagh, J.E. Developing a Programme of Transitional Care for Adolescents with Juvenile Idiopathic Arthritis: Results of a Postal Survey. *Rheumatology* 2004;43:211–19.

Shaw, K.L., Southwood, T.R., McDonagh, J.E. Users' perspectives of transitional care for adolescents with juvenile idiopathic arthritis. *Rheumatology* 2004;43:770–8.

McDonagh, J.E., Southwood, T.R., Shaw, K.L. Unmet adolescent health training needs for rheumatology health professionals. *Rheumatology* 2004;43:737–43.

Shaw, K.L., Southwood, T.R., McDonagh, J.E. Transitional care for adolescents with Juvenile Idiopathic Arthritis: Results of a Delphi study. *Rheumatology* 2004;43:1000–6.

Shaw, K.L., Southwood, T.R., and McDonagh, J.E. On behalf of the British Society of Paediatric and Adolescent Rheumatology. Growing up and moving on in Rheumatology: a multicentre cohort of adolescents with juvenile idiopathic arthritis. *Rheumatology* 2005;44:806–12.

(ii) Evidence of positive outcome of a transitional care programme in adolescent rheumatology

McDonagh, J.E., Southwood, T.R., Shaw, K.L. Growing up and moving on in rheumatology: development and preliminary evaluation of a transitional care programme for a multicentre cohort of adolescents with juvenile idiopathic arthritis. *J Child Health Care* 2005 (in press).

Robertson, L.P., McDonagh, J.E., Southwood, T.R., Shaw, K.L. Growing up and moving on. A multicentre UK audit of the transfer of adolescents with Juvenile Idiopathic Arthritis JIA from paediatric to adult centred care. *Ann Rheum Dis* 2006;65: 74–80.

(iii) Miscellaneous

Adam, V., St-Pierre, Y., Fautrel, B., Clarke, A.E., Duffy, C.M., Penrod, J.R. What is the impact of adolescent arthritis and rheumatism? Evidence from a national sample of Canadians. *J Rheumatol* 2005;32:354–61.

Bailey, K.M., McDonagh, J.E., Prieur, A.M. Systemic juvenile idiopathic arthritis presenting in a young child with long-term disability as an adolescent. *Ann Rheum Dis* 2004;63:1544–8.

Tucker, L.B., Cabral, D.A. Transition of the adolescent patient with rheumatic disease: issues to consider. *Pediatr Clin North Am* 2005;52:641–52.

3.4 Disease evaluation
Lori B. Tucker

Aim

The aim of this chapter is to discuss the different components of the disease that must be evaluated in order to determine if a child with JIA is actually improving or not. The chapter details those instruments that are available to measure these different aspects of disease.

Structure

- Introduction
- Measurement of disease activity
- Measurement of disease damage
- Quantifying disease improvement or worsening
- Measurement of health-related quality of life
- Summary

Introduction

In caring for the child with Juvenile Idiopathic Arthritis (JIA), the goals are elimination or decrease of active disease as much as possible, improvement in the disability, or impairment resulting from active disease, and an improved quality of life for the affected child and the family. As our armamentarium of therapies to treat JIA increases, accurate methods for evaluating the effects of our interventions on the natural course of disease are essential.

One of the essential components of quality care for children and adolescents with JIA is accurate, complete, and comprehensive disease evaluation during the course of illness. Disease evaluation is a multifaceted concept, and must include measures of current disease activity, degree of damage from previous and ongoing disease, and impact of disease on quality of life (Table 3.4.1). Using this conceptual framework, one can assess either improvement or worsening of the child's disease over time.

Measurements of disease activity

The measurement of disease activity of JIA should include not only an assessment of the number of active joints and the degree of inflammation, but also degree of pain, laboratory measures as appropriate, and functional status of the child. These "domains" of disease activity are relatively independent as shown by Ravelli *et al.* [1] where correlation between the domains was low. These data confirm the impression that

Table 3.4.1 Domains to measure in evaluation of patients with JIA

Disease process
Disease activity
Examination, laboratory, radiographic
Physician, patient, parent global assessment
Damage
Health related quality of life
Toxicity/adverse effects of therapies

Source: Adapted from OMERACT recommendations [46].

each of these areas are in fact important, but distinct, and that each should be taken into account when arriving at an estimate of overall current disease activity.

Articular measures

There is no universally accepted method of measuring articular disease activity in children with JIA. The active joint count is frequently used by many clinicians, with an "active" joint defined as one with tenderness and/or pain and/or swelling. Joints with limited range of motion may not represent active disease, but may reflect joint contractures as a consequence of previously active disease. Given the subjective nature of tenderness and pain, the objective finding of joint swelling is the most accurate measure of an actively inflamed joint, but this finding is not present in the neck, or hip, and is often not obvious at the shoulder joint. An articular severity index has been described by Giannini *et al.* [2], which requires a 0–3 grading of swelling, pain on motion and/or tenderness, and limitation of motion (0 = none, 1 = mild, 2 = moderate, or 3 = severe) for every joint, and a sum of all the severity ratings to give a final index score. Although this index has been used in some studies, it is too cumbersome to use routinely in the clinical setting.

Pain

Pain is a part of JIA for most children, and may have significant impact on functional status and psychological well-being. Pain may result from active articular disease, or may be a result of joint damage related to prior episodes of active disease. Although the majority of children with JIA report pain in the mild-moderate range, several studies have shown that 25–30% of patients reported moderate-severe pain [3]. In one study, children with JIA reported pain occurring for a mean of 4 h per day [4]. Importantly, pain and disease activity do not appear to be highly correlated [3]. Measurement of pain should be an integral part of overall disease assessment, although in many clinical settings, routine, standardized pain assessments are not carried out. Pain assessment can be done with a simple single question, utilizing a visual analogue scale (VAS), or for young children, simple face pictures depicting states of pain. The Childhood Health Assessment Questionnaire (CHAQ) (see below) has a pain domain using a VAS scale, with a separate pain score. The Juvenile Arthritis Quality of Life Questionnaire (see below) also includes a pain assessment, with a separate score. Pain may also be assessed in a more comprehensive manner using a questionnaire, such as the Varni/Thompson Paediatric Pain Questionnaire [5,6]. The Childhood Arthritis Health Profile (see below) has generic and disease-specific pain questions, with a separate pain scale score (see also Part 3, Chapter 3.7).

Laboratory measures

Laboratory tests play a relatively minor role in determining the degree of disease activity in JIA, and in most cases, have not been proven to be useful in following the course of disease. One major exception to this rule is the presence of a Rheumatoid Factor in a child or adolescent with JIA; this suggests a high likelihood of more severe and long-lasting disease with high risk for early erosive joint damage and functional disability. Other commonly used laboratory tests which indicate inflammation, such as elevated acute phase reactants (erythrocyte sedimentation rate—ESR and C-reactive protien—CRP), anaemia of chronic inflammation, and elevated platelet count, are less valuable in determining disease activity in many children with JIA, although in those with Systemic Arthritis such tests may be useful. Children with active Systemic Arthritis will generally have highly elevated ESR, elevated white blood cell counts, anaemia, very high platelet counts, and mild hypoalbuminemia. Many children with Systemic Arthritis also have elevated d-dimer levels during active disease [7], which return to normal when the disease becomes less active. A very highly elevated ferritin level, together with rapidly decreasing ESR, elevated liver enzymes, increasing d-dimers, and decreasing haematologic values (development of cytopenias) may indicate the onset of the Macrophage Activation Syndrome, a serious and life-threatening complication of active Systemic Arthritis.

A study of children with Oligoarthritis comparing the responsiveness of outcome measures over 3 months found that laboratory measures (ESR, CRP, platelet count, and haemoglobin) had limited responsiveness to clinical change [8]. A long-term follow-up study by Flato and colleagues, looking for clinical factors predictive of poor outcome after many years of disease, did show that a persistently elevated ESR was predictive of later development of joint erosions [9]. In one study of children with Systemic Arthritis, an elevated platelet count (above $600 \times 10^9/L$) which persisted over the first 6 months of disease was associated with a higher risk of later joint destruction [10].

Functional assessment measures

Evaluation of a child or adolescent's functional abilities is another important component of measurement of disease activity at one point in time, as well as providing a basis for comparison to judge any improvement or worsening over time. Standardized questionnaires which ask a parent or child to evaluate the child's functional abilities, and which can be scored to give either a single numerical score or a profile of scores, are becoming a routine component of assessment in the paediatric rheumatology clinic.

Childhood Health Assessment Questionnaire

The Childhood Health Assessment Questionnaire(CHAQ) was modified from the adult Health Assessment Questionnaire by Singh *et al.* [11] to be used for children and adolescents. This questionnaire measures function in eight domains: dressing and grooming, arising, eating, walking, hygiene, reach, grip, and activities. The respondent (parent or child) is asked how much difficulty the child has with each item, whether aids are used, and whether the patient needs the assistance of another person to perform the activity. The total Disability Index score is the average of scores of each individual domain (score can range from 0, or no disability, to 3, or severe disability). There is also a global pain scale which is scored to give a Pain Index score. The CHAQ can be used for children aged 1–19 years, and has been translated into many languages: Spanish–Mexican, Argentine, Spanish–Castilian, Costa Rican, Norweigan, Swedish, and Italian [9,12–17]. The Disability Index of the CHAQ has shown excellent reliability and validity [18].

The CHAQ is easy for patients and families to complete, and easy to score; however, there is a significant ceiling effect with most children with JIA having scores of 0 or less than 0.5. The CHAQ, therefore, may not be highly responsive to clinical change in children with JIA or may be less responsive in certain conditions in the umbrella term of JIA. A small study examining this issue by Ruperto and colleagues showed that CHAQ scores in a group of children with Oligoarthritis were not responsive to clinical change as measured by articular exam and physician global assessment [8]. The authors suggest that these results may reflect a difficulty of using the CHAQ in a younger age group, and in a group in which functional disability due to arthritis is minimal.

Juvenile Arthritis Self-Report Index

The Juvenile Arthritis Self-Report Index (JASI) was developed by Wright *et al.* [19,20] as a self-report questionnaire for children with arthritis aged 8 years and older. It is an extensive tool that specifically addresses functional status, with items in the following domains of function: self-care, mobility, school, and extra-curricular. It is a long questionnaire (100 items) with two sections. Part 1 results in an overall functioning score based on the answers to the 100 items. In Part 2, subjects are asked to select five activities for improvement, and then to prioritize them. Over time, changes in these specific activities can be calculated. The JASI addresses functional aspects only with no measures of pain or impact of disease on quality of life. More recently, a computerized version of the JASI has been developed, which improved the ease of administration and scoring. This questionnaire, particularly in its computerized format, may be particularly useful in situations in which an intensive physiotherapy functional assessment is required.

Juvenile Arthritis Functional Assessment Scale and Report

The Juvenile Arthritis Functional Assessment Scale (JAFAS) and Juvenile Arthritis Functional Assessment Report (JAFAR) were developed by Lovell and colleagues [21,22], and both are functional assessment tools. The JAFAS is administered by a health professional (nurse clinician, therapist) who measures the patient's performance on a set of timed physical tasks. Although reliability and validity are good for the JAFAS, the limitation of requiring standardized equipment and a professional assessor led to the development of the JAFAR, which is a self-report version of this instrument. The JAFAR (JAFAR-P for parents, JAFAR-C for children) asks about the ability to perform 23 standard physical tasks, with scores summed across the items. Small studies have shown very good reliability and validity for the JAFAR; responsiveness has not yet been adequately established. The JAFAR is simple to use and to score, and may be a practical choice for following functional status in the clinical setting. Its use, limited to children over the age of 7 years, is a slight drawback.

Measurements of disease damage

In any of the chronic rheumatic diseases, patients may have problems relating to either active disease or as a result of permanent damage from previous episodes of active disease. In JIA, patients may suffer from joint pain, stiffness, and loss of motion of joints relating to active synovitis, but also may have disability, pain, or limitations due to damage accumulated over time. This concept has been outlined more clearly by adult rheumatologists [23]. Clinical tests used to determine, quantify, and follow disease damage are primarily radiographic. Standard radiographs are helpful in determining the presence of joint erosions or joint space narrowing. The accuracy of standard radiographs is only fair, and the changes they detect are not early changes; magnetic resonance imaging (MRI), or ultrasound imaging may be more sensitive to early changes and may allow better comparison of change over time. However, at this time, there is no good evidence documenting this in JIA; one study examining MRI changes in children with JIA of duration less than 1 year showed synovial hypertrophy and joint effusions by MRI, changes which are usually easily determined by physical examination [24].

One standard method of assessing functional effects of damage due to arthritis is the Steinbrocker classification system [25](Table 3.4.2). This classification system places patients into four classes based on their overall functional disabilities. The Steinbrocker classification was developed for use in adults with rheumatoid arthritis, and although it has been applied to children with JIA, it is an insensitive measure of functional outcome.

Quantifying disease improvement or worsening

An integral part of the ongoing care of a child with JIA is the consideration at each evaluation as to whether a patient has improved, stayed the same, or worsened during the interval since the last evaluation. Clinicians make this assessment in an informal way each time they evaluate a patient, and use this assessment to make decisions regarding necessary changes in the child's therapy. Similarly, physiotherapists follow joint range of motion, strength, and functioning during a course of therapy. However, when one wants to compare the disease course and outcomes across patients seen in different clinical centers or determine the impact of a new therapy, a more standardized approach to determining improvement or worsening is needed. This standardized approach is particularly important when organizing clinical treatment trials, allowing trials with fewer numbers of patients and less statistical error.

Table 3.4.2 Steinbrocker classification of functional impairment

Class	Impairment
I	Complete functional ability to carry on all usual duties without handicap
II	Functional capacity adequate to conduct normal activities despite handicap of discomfort or limited mobility of one or more joints
III	Functional capacity adequate to perform only little or none of the duties of usual occupation or self-care
IV	Largely or wholly incapacitated with patient bedridden or confined to a wheelchair, permitting little or no self-care

Table 3.4.3 Pediatric ACR Score (Core set outcome variables for JIA)

1. Physician global assessment of disease activity [a]
2. Parent/patient global assessment of overall well-being [a]
3. Functional ability
4. Number of joints with active arthritis
5. Number of joints with limited range of motion
6. ESR

Improvement is: three of any six core set variables improved by at least 30%, and no more than one of the remaining variables worsened by more than 30%.
[a] Scored on a 10 cm VAS.

An international group of paediatric rheumatologists, led by E. Giannini and colleagues in Cincinnati and A. Martini and colleagues in Paivia, have developed a standardized set of response criteria for JIA, referred to as the "core set", or the ACR Pediatric Score [26]. The JIA core set was modeled on a similar set of outcome variables that have been developed for adults with rheumatoid arthritis. The process of developing the JIA core set was a scientifically rigorous multistep process, first surveying paediatric rheumatologists for candidate outcome variables and then reaching consensus through a consensus conference. The resulting core set variables and the definition for improvement (Table 3.4.3) has 100% sensitivity and 85% specificity, with high face validity ratings [27].

Although these response criteria are a step in the direction of improved standardized assessments in JIA, they should be viewed as a preliminary step. Clinicians should remember that the core set was developed as a tool for clinical trials and needs further study to understand its utility for following individual patients in the clinic setting. Further research may lead to clarifications of some of the variables; for example, the method of assessment of functional ability is not specified. The inclusion of the ESR as a measure of active inflammation may prove not as useful over time. The inclusion of number of joints with active arthritis (which includes those with limited range of motion), and number of joints with limited range of motion is a redundancy. Although the developers of the core set recognized this problem and suggested that further testing might be helpful in this regard, there has been no further work in this area to date. The core set outcome variables are currently being incorporated as a standard approach to measurement of outcome in new drug trials for children with JIA. For example, a study of the efficacy of etanercept in children with Polyarthritis [26] showed that 74% of patients given Etanercept in an open-label trial fulfilled the standard improvement criteria (30% improvement in three of six variables). The investigators also reported the majority of patients in this study (64%) actually had >50% improvement in three of six core set variables, and a smaller number (36%) even had >70% improvement in three of six variables. In this study, the investigators used this standard definition of improvement to determine which patients responded adequately to the study drug to allow further randomization into a placebo-controlled arm of the trial. This example illustrates the power of using standardized assessment definitions in improving clinical trials in paediatric rheumatology. It should be noted that no formal definition of disease worsening using these core set variables has been established.

Measurement of health-related quality of life

Juvenile Idiopathic Arthritis and the other childhood rheumatic disorders have broad effects on the lives of affected patients and their families. The impact of these disorders goes far beyond the physical symptoms and functional disability, and includes impact on development, mental health, behaviour, self-esteem, the development of normal social roles (peer and family-related, school and work-related), and family functioning. The term "quality of life" has been used to indicate an individual's overall state of well-being, incorporating the integration of all physical, psychological, and social factors which may contribute to this state. The concept of quality of life (QOL) has been derived from the World Health Organization definition of health as "a state of complete physical, mental, and social well-being, and not merely the absence of disease or infirmity." As clinicians, our view of a patient's QOL is related to the medical condition which brings the patient to our attention and care. Therefore, the term "health-related QOL" (HRQOL) is more relevant to our interests.

The information gained from measuring HRQOL (see Table 3.4.4) includes a description of health status, allowing comparison of patients with different diseases, disease subtypes, or stages of disease; assessment of the impact of treatment programs on global well-being as well as functional status; identification of psychological dysfunction or risk factors for future psychological problems; and providing critical information on the effectiveness (or ineffectiveness) of health services and programs. People who have a potential interest in this area include families, paediatric rheumatologists, nurses, social workers, psychologists, hospital administrators, and public policy planners.

Table 3.4.4 Why measure HRQOL?

1. To gain descriptive information about health status

2. To assess the impact of treatment programs/protocols on global well-being as well as functional status

3. To identify potential psychological risk factors or problems which may be subtle

4. To provide important information on the effectiveness of health services and programs in addressing the needs of children and adolescents with rheumatic disease

Although there have been a large number of questionnaires developed and validated for measurement of HRQOL in adults, these generally have poor applicability to children and adolescents. Children and adolescents are in the process of development, and change over time in their behaviour and functional abilities. Their lives involve a completely different set of activities from adults, and these activities also change over time. Therefore, it is critical to use paediatric HRQOL measures, which have been specifically developed for children, and validated in paediatric populations.

Another important issue in measuring HRQOL is parental versus child self-report. Questionnaires to assess the HRQOL of very young children (<5years) from self-report are currently not available, and would have to be administered by interview. The question of how young children might understand some of the concepts of well-being is not clear. In these cases, parent report is generally the only mechanism to obtain HRQOL data. School-aged children may have variable difficulty in reading and understanding the language of questions, and based on their developmental stage, may answer questions in a concrete manner with little ability to interpret general ideas. For example, it may not be possible for an 8-year-old boy or girl to appropriately answer a question which asks about how cheerful he/she has been over the past 4 weeks. Parent-proxy report of HRQOL of school-aged children and adolescents offer more complex interpretation of QOL issues, especially in the areas of family functioning and behavioural impact of illness [28].

Relatively few studies in paediatric rheumatology have compared directly parent and child ratings of HRQOL. Duffy et al. [29] compared level of agreement between children with JIA and their parents for ratings of physical and psychosocial dysfunction. Forty patients with JIA and their parents were interviewed using an extensive item listing, and level of agreement calculated. Although overall there was good agreement on many of the questionnaire items, there were many specific items on which parents and their child did not agree; this appeared more frequently with psychosocial items than with physical functioning or general symptoms. Similarly, in studies comparing child self-report of pain and parent proxy report, there has been poor correlation between children and parents on this issue [4,30,31].

There is no clear answer to date as to which is better or "correct": parent report or child report of HRQOL. Future studies may identify the specific areas in which it is not necessary to obtain parent-report in children old- enough to answer for themselves. However, it seems clear as well that to understand the complete picture of HRQOL of children and adolescents, parent information provides important information. Collecting information from both parents and children may provide the most accurate data.

Health-related QOL measures can be generic or condition-specific (Table 3.4.5). There are benefits to both approaches. The use of a generic instrument allows the comparison of HRQOL across disease categories, allowing one to estimate the relative burden of disease. However, a generic measure may not be sensitive to small clinically important changes for a specific disease. Increasingly, experts in HRQOL research are suggesting that questionnaires which incorporate both generic and disease-specific measures are likely to provide the most helpful information [32].

The field of HRQOL measurement in paediatrics is undergoing great expansion. This discussion provides an overview of the concepts in this area; for more detail concerning concepts, methodology, and measures under development and currently available, the reader is referred to the following references: [28,32–36]. Table 3.4.6 shows a summary of the following HRQOL questionnaires that are available for use in paediatric rheumatology.

The Juvenile Arthritis Quality of Life Questionnaire

The Juvenile Arthritis Quality of Life Questionnaire (JAQQ) was developed by Duffy *et al.* to address both physical and psychosocial function of children with JIA [37]. The JAQQ is a self-report measure, designed for use in children of any age. The questionnaire includes five dimensions: gross motor function, fine motor function, psychosocial function, general symptoms, and pain. There are 74 items in total. Patients select five items in each dimension to score, or add their own items if none seem applicable to them. Difficulty is assessed on a 7-point Likert scale. In each dimension, a mean score is calculated; the total JAQQ score is the mean across the four dimensions (excluding pain).

Table 3.4.5 Generic versus condition specific measurement of HRQOL

Generic measures
  Apply to all children and youth, healthy or ill
  Allow comparisons of health status across patient populations
  Provides information on global well-being and psychological functioning
  May not be very sensitive to change among a specific population
  (children with disease)

Condition-specific measures
  Developed specifically for use in a particular patient population;
    that is children with JIA
  Improves sensitivity to small changes which
    are important in a particular patient population

The developers of the JAQQ have carried out several studies to examine the validity, reliability, and responsiveness of the instrument [3–40]. The JAQQ has very good validity and the ability to discriminate among patients based on physician-assessed degree of change. Excellent responsiveness was shown in one small treatment trial, which implies that the JAQQ is a good measure to accurately reflect small changes in overall function over time. One difficulty with the JAQQ is that each child essentially answers their own individual questionnaire, having chosen items which will be different from another patient. This may make comparisons between patients across a group difficult. However, the responsiveness of the JAQQ may indicate an important role in treatment trials in JIA.

The Childhood Arthritis Health Profile

The Childhood Arthritis Health Profile (CAHP) was developed by Tucker *et al.* to address the broad range of health domains which can be affected by JIA, including physical function, pain, emotional and behavioural function, mental health, self-esteem, morning stiffness impact on function, specific impact of JIA on school and social function, family function, and the impact of JIA on parent emotions and their time for themselves [41]. The CAHP includes both generic- and disease-specific scales. The generic scales of the CAHP are taken from the Child Health Questionnaire (CHQ) [42], and scores from these scales can be compared across other populations of children with illness or healthy children. The JIA-specific scales were developed by a multidisciplinary development team to address issues specifically of concern in JIA, with the aim to improve the sensitivity of the instrument. There is a parent-report CAHP (aged 5–18 years), and a teen-report CAHP (aged 13–18 years). The CAHP provides scores for 12 generic scales and 7 JIA-specific scales, with a total of 100 items.

Table 3.4.6 HRQOL questionnaires currently used in paediatric rheumatology

Questionnaire	Age range	# items	Generic	JIA specific	Scoring	Scales
PedsQL	Parent proxy—2–18 years Child report— 5–18 years	45	Yes	Yes	0–100 scale (higher scores=best QL)	Physical, emotional, social, and school functioning; pain, daily activities, treatment, worry, communication
JAQQ	Child self report	74	No	Yes	Mean of scores for top five items, of each scale	Gross motor, fine motor, and psychosocial function, general, symptoms, pain
CAHP	Parent proxy—5–18 years Child report— 12–18 years	100	Yes	Yes	0–100 scale (higher scores=best QL)	Physical and emotional function, general health perceptions, pain, emotion, and behaviour, self-esteem, mental health, impact on parent time and emotions, impact on family cohesion and activities. Morning stiffness, gross and fine motor function, arthritis pain impact, activity limitations
CHQ	Parent proxy— 5–18 years Child report— 12–18 years	50	Yes	No	0–100 scale (higher scores=best QL)	Physical and emotional function, general health perceptiaons, pain, emotion and behaviour self-esteem, mental health, impact on Parent time and emotions, impact on family cohesion and activities

Initial pilot testing of the CAHP showed very good validity and internal reliability. There was evidence of good discriminatory ability of the JIA-specific scales among children with mild, moderate, and severe disease activity as assessed by physician global assessment [43]. A large multicentre study is underway to assess the CAHP sensitivity to clinical change and discriminatory characteristics in a larger cohort of patients. The CAHP has the benefit of providing information which is not available in other health status instruments, such as wellbeing, behaviour, self-esteem, and impact of JIA on parent and family life. However, the questionnaire is long and the scoring complex, making it less attractive for quick clinical use at present. In addition, self-report is only available for children over 13 years.

The PedsQL (Generic and Rheumatology Modules)

The PedsQL is a HRQOL questionnaire with a well-developed and widely tested generic core module developed by Varni *et al.*, and a recently developed rheumatology module by Szer *et al.* [44,45]. The generic module (23 items) has four scales which measure physical, emotional, social, and school functioning. The rheumatology module (22 items) has five additional scales which measure pain, daily activities, treatment, worry, and communication. There are both child and parent self-report versions for children aged 5–18 years; there is a parent proxy form for children under 5 years. The scoring system for the PedsQL is relatively simple, making it easy to implement.

Varni and colleagues have done a large study in one center showing excellent validity and reliability of the PedsQL in a paediatric rheumatology clinical practice [45]. The PedsQL was reliable and accurate in discriminating between healthy children and those with rheumatic disease. Scores on the PedsQL Generic- and Rheumatology-specific scales, particularly pain, emotional, social, and school functioning, showed that children with fibromyalgia had significantly-worse scores than children with JIA or other rheumatic diseases; therefore the PedsQL may be useful in discriminating HRQOL concerns among different paediatric rheumatic conditions (see also Part 3, Chapter 3.7).

Summary

In this chapter, the components of disease evaluation of JIA have been discussed, including domains of disease activity, functional ability, disease damage, and HRQOL. The standardized method for assessment of disease improvement or worsening, the core set, was described. As clinical treatment trials in paediatric rheumatology become more sophisticated and collaborative, standardized disease evaluation will become a routine part of clinical care for children with JIA.

References

1. Ravelli, A., Viola, S., Ruperto, N., Corsi, B., Ballardini, G., and Martini, A. Correlation between conventional disease activity measures in juvenile chronic arthritis. *Ann Rheum Dis* 2001;56(3):197–200.

2. Giannini, E.H., Brewer, E.J., Kuzmina, N., Shaikov, A., *et al.* Methotrexate in resistant juvenile rheumatoid arthritis. Results of the USA–USSR double-blind, placebo-controlled trial. The Pediatric Rheumatology Collaborative Study Group and The Cooperative Children's Study Group. *New Engl J Med* 1992;326(16):1043–9.

3. Schanberg, L.E., Lefebvre, J.C., Keefe, F.J., Kredich, D.W., and Gil, K.M. Pain coping and the pain experience in children with juvenile chronic arthritis. *Pain* 1997; 73(2):181–9.

4. Benestad, B., Vinje, O., Veierod, M.B., and Vandvik, I.H. Quantitative and qualitative assessments of pain in children with juvenile chronic arthritis based on the Norwegian version of the Pediatric Pain Questionnaire. *Scand J Rheum* 1996;25(5):293–9.

5. Varni, J.W., Thompson, K.L., and Hanson, V., The Varni/Thompson Pediatric Pain Questionnaire. I. Chronic musculoskeletal pain in juvenile rheumatoid arthritis. *Pain* 1987;28(1):27–38.

6. Gragg, R.A., Rapoff, M.A., Danovsky, M.B., Lindsley, C.B., Varni, J.W., Waldman, S.A., *et al.* Assessing chronic musculoskeletal pain associated with rheumatic disease: further validation of the pediatric pain questionnaire. *J Ped Psyche* 1996;21(2):237–50.

7. Bloom, B.J., Tucker, L.B., Miller, L.C., and Schaller, J.G. Fibrin D-dimer as a marker of disease activity in systemic onset juvenile rheumatoid arthritis. *J Rheum* 1998;25(8):1620–5.

8. Ruperto, N., Ravelli, A., Migliavacca, D., *et al.* Responsiveness of clinical measures in children with oligoarticular juvenile chronic arthritis. *J Rheum* 1999; 26(8):1827–30.

9. Flato, B., Sorskaar, D., Vinje, O., *et al.* Measuring disability in early juvenile rheumatoid arthritis: evaluation of a Norwegian version of the childhood Health Assessement Questionnaire. *J Rheum* 1998;25(9):1851–8.

10. Schneider, R., Lang, B.A., Reilly, B.J., *et al.* Prognostic indicators of joint destruction in systemic-onset juvenile rheumatoid arthritis. *J Pediatr* 1992;120:200–5.

11. Singh, G., Athreya, B.H., Fries, J.F., and Goldsmith, D.P. Measurement of health status in children with juvenile rheumatoid arthritis. *Arthritis Rheum* 1994;37(12):1761–9.

12. Andersson Gare, B., Fasth, A., and Wiklund, I. Measurement of functional status in juvenile chronic arthritis: evaluation of a Swedish version of the Childhood Health Assessment Questionnaire. *Clin Exp Rheum* 1993;11(5):569–76.

13. Arguedas, O., Andersson Gare, B., Fasth, A., and Porras, O. Development of a Costa Rican version of the Childhood Health Assessment Questionnaire. *J Rheum* 1997;24(11):2233–41.

14. Fantini, F., Corvaglia, G., Bergomi, P., *et al.* Validation of the Italian version of the Stanford Childhood Health Assessment Questionnaire for measuring functional status in children with chronic arthritis. *Clin Exp Rheum* 1995; 13(6):785–91.

15. Garcia-Garcia, J.J., Gonzalez-Pascual, E., Pou-Fernandez, J., Singh, G., and Jimenez, R. Development of a Spanish (Castillian) version of the Childhood Health Assessment Questionnaire. Measurement of health status in children with juvenile chronic arthritis. *Clin Exp Rheum* 2000;18(1):95–102.

16. Goycochea-Robles, M.V., Garduno-Espinosa, J., Vilchis-Guizar, E., Ortiz-Alvarez, O., and Burgos-Vargas, R. Validation of a Spanish version of the Childhood Health Assessment Questionnaire. *J Rheum* 1997;24(11):2242–5.

17. Moroldo, M.B., De Cunto, C., Hubscher, O., Liberatore, D., Palermo, R., Russo, R., *et al.* Crosscultural adaptation and validation of an Argentine Spanish Version of the Stanford Childhood Health Assessment Questionnaire. *Arthritis Care Res* 1998;11(5):382–90.

18. Singh, G., Brown, B., and Athreya, B.H. Functional status in juvenile rheumatoid arthritis: sensitivity to change of the Childhood Health Assessment Questionnaire. *Arthritis Rheum* 2001;34:S81.

19. Wright, F.V., Kimber, J.L., Law, M., Goldsmith, C.H., Crombie, V., and Dent, P., The Juvenile Arthritis Functional Status Index (JASI): a Validation Study. *J Rheum* 1996;23:1066–79.

20. Wright, F.V., Law, M., Crombie, V., Goldsmith, C.H., and Dent, P., Development of a Self-Report Functional Status Index for Juvenile Rheumatoid Arthritis. *J Rheum* 1994;21:536–44.

21. Howe, S., Levinson, J., Shear, E., *et al.* Development of a disability measurement tool for juvenile rheumatoid arthritis. *Arthritis Rheum* 1991;34(7):873–80.

22. Lovell, D., Howe, S., Shear, E., *et al.* Development of a disability measurement tool for juvenile rheumatoid arthritis: the Juvenile Arthritis Functional Assessment Scale. *Arthritis Rheum* 1989;32:1390–5.

23. Wolfe, F., Lassere, M., van der Heijde, D., *et al.* Preliminary core set of domains and reporting requirements for longitudinal observational studies in rheumatology. *J Rheum* 1999;26(2):484–9.

24. Gylys-Morin, V.M., Graham, T.B., Blebea J.S., *et al.* Knee in early juvenile rheumatoid arthritis: MR imaging findings. *Radiology* 2001;220(3):696–706.

25. Steinbrocker, O., Traeger, C.H, and Batterman, R.C., Therapeutic criteria in rheumatoid arthritis. *J Am Med Assoc* 1949;140:659–62.

26. Giannini, E.H., Ruperto, N., Ravelli, A., *et al.* Preliminary definition of improvement in juvenile arthritis. *Arthritis Rheum* 1997;40(7):1202–9.

27. Lovell, D., Giannini, E.H., Reiff, A., *et al.* Etanercept in children with polyarticular juvenile rheumatoid arthritis. *N Engl J Med* 2000;342:763–9.

28. Eiser, C., Children's quality of life measures. *Arch Dis Child* 2001;77:350–4.

29. Duffy, C.M., Arsenault, L., and Watanabe Duffy, K.N. Level of agreement between parents and children in rating dysfunction in juvenile rheumatoid arthritis and juvenile spondyloarthritides. *J Rheum* 1993;20:2134–9.

30. Doherty, E., Yanni, G., Conroy, R.M., and Bresnihan, B. A comparison of child and parent ratings of disability and pain in juvenile chronic arthritis. *J Rheum* 1993; 20(9):1563–6.

31. Chambers, C.T., Reid, G.J., Craig, K.D., McGrath, P.J., and Finley, G.A., Agreement between child and parent reports of pain. *Clin J Pain* 2001;14(4):336–42.

32. Koot, H.M. Challenges in child and adolescent quality of life research. *Acta Paediatr* 2002;91:265–6.

33. Connolly, M.A. and Johnson, J.A. Measuring quality of life in paediatric patients. *Pharmacoecon* 2001;16(6):605–25.

34. Jenney, M.E.M. and Campbell, S. Measuring quality of life. *Arch Dis Child* 2001;77:347–50.

35. Murray, K.J. and Passo, M.H. Functional measures in children with rheumatic diseases. *Ped Clin N Am* 1995;42(5):1127–53.

36. Tucker, L.B. Outcome measures in childhood rheumatic diseases. *Curr Rheumatol Rep* 2000;2[4]:349–54.

37. Duffy, C.M., Arsenault, L., Watanabe Duffy, K.N., Paquin, J.D., and Strawczynski, H. The Juvenile Arthritis Quality of Life Questionnaire—Development of a new responsive index for juvenile rheumatoid arthritis and juvenile spondyloarthitides. *J Rheum* 1997;24:738–46.

38. Duffy, C.M., Arsenault, L., Watanabe Duffy, K.N., Paquin, J.D., and Strawczynski, H., Validity and sensitivity to change of the Juvenile Arthritis Quality of Life Questionnaire (JAQQ). *Arthritis Rheum* 1993;37:S144.

39. Duffy, C.M., Arsenault, L., Watanabe Duffy, K.N., Paquin, J.D., and Strawczynski, H. Relative sensitivity to change of the Juvenile Arthritis Quality of Life Questionnaire following a new treatment. *Arthritis Rheum* 1994;37:S196.

40. Duffy, C.M., Arsenault, L., Watanabe Duffy, K.N., Paquin, J.D., and Strawczynski, H. Relative sensitivity to change of the Juvenile Arthritis Quality of Life Questionnaire on sequential followup. *Arthritis Rheum* 1995;38:S178.

41. Tucker, L.B., DeNardo, B.A., Abetz, L.N., Landgraf, J.M., and Schaller, J.G. The Childhood Arthritis Health Profile (CAHP): validity and reliability of the condition specific scales. *Arthritis Rheum* 1995;38:S183.

42. Landgraf, J.M., Abetz, L.N., and Ware, J.E., The Childhood Health Questionnaire: a user manual. Boston, MA: New England Medical Center, The Health Institute 1996.

43. Tucker, L.B., DeNardo, B.A., and Schaller, J.G., The Childhood Arthritis Health Profile: correlation of juvenile rheumatoid arthritis specific scales with disease severity and activity. *Arthritis Rheum* 1996;39:S57.

44. Varni, J.W., Seid, M., and Rode, C.A., The PedsQL: measurement model for the pediatric quality of life inventory. *Medical Care* 1999;37(2):126–39.

45. Varni, J.W., Seid, M., Knight, T.S., Burwinkle, T., Brown, J., and Szer, I.S. The PedsQL in Pediatric Rheumatology: reliability, validity, and responsiveness of the Pediatric Quality of Life Inventory. *Arthritis Rheum* 2002;46(3):714–25.

46. Wolfe, F., Lassere, M., van der Heijde, D., *et al.* Preliminary core set of domains and reporting requirements for longitudinal observational studies in rheumatology. *J Rheumat* 1999;26(2):484–9.

3.5 Educational issues

Laurie Ebner-Lyon and Joy Brown

Aim

The aim of this chapter is to discuss the central role of education in helping children with JIA and their families cope with a chronic disease.

Structure

- Importance of education for patient and family
- Issues surrounding education of others involved with the family
- Educational and support organizations
- Advocacy
- Conclusion

Importance of education for patient and family

When a child is diagnosed with a chronic illness the entire family is affected in multiple ways. If family members are properly educated about the illness, it becomes possible for them to form a genuine partnership with the medical team to treat their child's disease, allowing them to feel they have some control over the disease and its management. Knowledge about the disease becomes crucial when a parent is forced to balance the risks of the illness versus the risks of treatment. It is insufficient to expect families to "buy into" treatment because they are given a prescription. A large number of variables influence adherence to a treatment regime, and several strategies may help to improve adherence [1] (Table 3.5.1) However, a study examining adherence-facilitating behaviors of a multidisciplinary paediatric rheumatology staff showed that there was a very low frequency of such behaviours accompanying treatment recommendations [2]. A greater use of techniques, such as discussing patient's beliefs, expectations, fears, and barriers to treatment would potentially lead to improved adherence (see also Part 3, Chapter 3.3).

It has been reported that up to 86% of paediatric arthritis patients have tried complementary and/or alternative medicine (CAM) [3]. In a national survey of 1035 American adults with a 69% response rate, factors influencing use of CAM included a higher education level, poorer health status, a holistic approach to health, being an environmentalist, and having a commitment to spiritual and personal growth [4]. Factors influencing the choice of CAM in children included fear of medication side-effects, having a chronic medical problem, dissatisfaction with conventional medicine, and word-of-mouth. The majority of parents did not tell their physicians their children have used CAM because of: fear of censure, perceived lack of physician interest, fear of being dissuaded, fear of physician refusing to see the child, considered "natural" and not worth mentioning, and embarrassment over cultural practices [4]. Healthcare providers need to be cognizant of, and open-minded to, CAM practices and encourage open communication. Educating families about the rationale for treatment recommendations, the expected effects of treatment, and potential adverse effects are required for them to agree and adhere to a treatment plan for their child. Similarly the families of children with Juvenile Idiopathic Arthritis (JIA) need educating about how to interpret the beneficial claims made for CAM.

While clearly there are basic facts that parents must be given about the disease and medications, parents differ significantly in the amount of technical detail they wish to be provided at any given time. The physician and the other team members should assess the emotional and cognitive level of the parents and present the information appropriately. Medical jargon is often incomprehensible to parents and it is important to "speak the parents' language". No matter how interested they are, however, if given too much information initially, only some of it will be retained. Information presented orally should be specific and relevant with additional written materials provided for perusal at their convenience and readiness [5]. Opportunity for further discussion of this material should be made available and the preferred learning style of the individual (e.g. auditory versus visual) taken into consideration.

In addition to learning the specifics of the disease itself, the families of children with newly diagnosed rheumatic diseases such as JIA must also learn the basics of managing a chronic illness. The administration of medications, the coordination of therapy and doctor appointments, the importance of good recordkeeping, the skills required to advocate for the patient, and techniques to balance the needs of other family members are all part of the knowledge that must be formulated [6]. In most cases, nothing in past experiences has prepared parents for this aspect of raising a child, and the medical team must take care not to just assume these skills will automatically be acquired. In a study examining the needs and preferences of children with JIA and their parents, several unmet educational needs were discovered [7]. The family may not be prepared for self-management of JIA, the time commitment involved, or the fluctuating nature of the disease. Parents wanted to know more about disease management at home, the psychosocial impact of JIA, and to what extent their child's future disease course could be predicted. Children with JIA felt that the education they had received had failed to address how arthritis can affect school life, friendships, and family functioning. Major themes

Table 3.5.1 Adherence

Factors reducing adherence	Strategies to improve adherence
Educational factors	Educational strategies
Lack of information or misunderstanding of disease and treatment	Provide information verbally and in writing, matching pace, volume, and presentational style to family
Limited cognitive ability	Repeat key instructions multiple times
Language barrier	Tailor information to child's age, cultural background, language, cognitive ability, and self-perception of disease and treatment
Different cultural belief system	
Increased severity and chronicity of disease and symptoms	
Need for continuous treatment when asymptomatic or no visible signs of disease	Facilitate education of siblings, extended family, teachers, and friends about disease and treatment
Prolonged duration of treatment	
Toxicity, or perceived toxicity, of treatment	
Increased complexity of treatment	
Young age at onset	
Emotional/behavioural factors	Behavioural strategies
Oppositional defiant behaviour	Provide a safe atmosphere where problems/barriers can be openly discussed
Inadequate behaviour-centered instructions	Discuss fears of adverse effects
Family conflict or dysfunction	Dispel unrealistic fears
Rejection or perceived rejection by peers	Allow active patient/family involvement in treatment planning, goal-setting, self-monitoring, and self-management
Overprotection by parents	
Passive involvement in therapy	
Attempting to regain control	Assist in fitting treatment plan into daily routine
Dissatisfaction with treatment	
Delay of desired effect	Provide positive reinforcement
Economic/organizational factors	Economic/organization strategies
Difficulty with access to transportation to medical facility	Provide information on and access to financial aid organizations
Inconvenient scheduling of appointments	Permit long-range scheduling of appointments
Increased financial burden, directly and indirectly	

Source: Adapted from Kroll [1]

that were identified as issues to be addressed by future psycho educational interventions included: disease identity (symptoms) and disease management (including self-management and medical management), the psychological and social impact of JIA on the child, and social and communication skills, including assertiveness and listening. In another study, parents identified knowledge about the disease, effects of the disease, treatments, and future prognosis as issues that they most wanted to know more about. Siblings were interested in understanding how the child with JIA feels [8]. A summary of unmet educational needs is provided in Table 3.5.2.

The social and emotional impact of the diagnosis (see Chapter 3.5) must also be understood if the family unit is to successfully thrive with the additional complication of a chronic illness. Parents are likely to be "grieving" the loss of their healthy child and their receptiveness to information may vary according to the stage of grieving (shock, denial, sadness and anger, acceptance) [9]. The health care providers should continue to be aware that the stages of grief are not linear and a previous acceptance may be reversed if there is a flare in disease activity.

After the initial diagnosis, the need for education does not abate. For example, changes in medications require the patient to learn about potential new side effects, additional monitoring to be done, and different methods and times of administration to be considered.

Table 3.5.2 Educational needs of families

Parents	Disease information and treatment
	Disease management: medical management, impact on daily life, time commitment
	Fluctuating nature of disease
	Psychosocial impact
	Communication skills: assertiveness training
	Future prognosis
Patient	Disease information and treatment
	Disease management: self-management, medical management
	Impact of JIA on
	School life
	Friendships
	Family functioning
Siblings	Feelings of affected child
	Disease information
	Personal impact

Source: Adapted from Barlow [7] and Konkol [8].

This education should be provided whenever a new treatment is introduced. Decisions on moving to the next level of treatment are more easily made when the patient/parent is aware of the implications of the change. Parents and health professionals alike struggle with the difficult task of weighing the benefits of a new treatment against the risks. Parents need to be well informed, and feel a sense of control and partnership with the physician in making decisions to initiate potentially toxic medications. Families need to fully understand their child's potential prognosis if a medication is not started. For example, if the child with JIA that is unresponsive to nonsteroidal drugs alone, parents must understand something about the degree of risk of joint damage if the inflammation is not suppressed before being able to accept the decision to start methotrexate. Continual reassessment of understanding and knowledge is required throughout the course of the illness. Table 3.5.3 illustrates how educational needs for the patient and family change as the child progresses from the early stages of the disease, to established disease, and then on to refractory disease.

In parallel with parent education, patients and siblings should also be provided with developmentally appropriate education that is continuously modified as they mature. As the patient matures, changes in independence, self-image, and acceptance of the disease may require a more in-depth understanding of what is happening to his or her body. The team must be prepared to recognize and accommodate these changing needs. Health professionals should welcome sibling participation in the office visit and elicit questions and concerns regarding the illness [5]. Children's understanding of illness parallels the developmental progression of general cognitive reasoning (see Chapter 3.6).

Health professionals need to be aware of the variety of ways to accomplish patient/family education. With clinic time often limited, it is important to realize that the doctor or nurse need not be the only disseminator of this knowledge. For example, at Children's Hospital San Diego, a parent of a child with JIA is included as part of the rheumatology team. The parent, with training in the diagnoses, medications, and psychological impacts of paediatric rheumatology, is available for all patients at every appointment. In addition to having first-hand knowledge of family needs, such a resource person can educate the medical team with many of the concerns parents have in raising a child with a JIA. Other sources of information may include specific lectures provided by the team for the family members about JIA, previously reviewed websites, books, brochures, educational camps for children with rheumatic diseases, parent support groups, national juvenile arthritis conferences, and local arthritis organizations (see Table 3.5.4).

Issues surrounding education of others involved with the family

Everyone who comes in contact with a child with JIA needs to be educated about the disease to some degree. Relatives and friends of the family can be a tremendous support, but without proper education they may jeopardize the child's treatment by giving fallacious and conflicting advice. Often, it is the responsibility of the parent to balance this education for the child. Parents need to be encouraged to discuss these issues with the rheumatology team so they may be provided additional factual information including written materials to distribute to interested family and friends. They may also need to be helped to develop techniques for diffusing well-intended but inappropriate advice. Immediate family should be encouraged to attend office visits with the patient. It is not uncommon for one of the parents (usually the father) to never attend an office visit. Having not

Table 3.5.3 Progression of educational needs

Early stages of disease	Basic information about disease and prognosis
	Identifying disease symptoms: adjusting activities accordingly
	When, why and how to take medications
	Potential side-effects of medications
	Comfort measures (warm baths, heat, rest versus activity)
	How to advocate for educational rights
	Managing time commitments: medications, physical therapy, frequent doctor's appointments, laboratory testing, and school advocacy
	Where to seek additional information (websites)
	Coping with chronic illness
	Resources available for support
Established disease	In-depth information about disease and treatment options
	Effectiveness of current treatment regimen
	Need for additional medications and their potential side-effects
	Psychosocial impact on child: peer/family relationships, school impact potential for rebellion
	How to educate others (classmates, extended family and friends) on disease and management
	Responding to others' "well intentioned" advice
	Coping with disease variability: good days/ bad days, flares, and remissions
	Child's changing needs as he/she progresses through the school system
	Transitioning from parent to patient responsibility and advocacy
	Transitioning to adulthood: college, career
Refractory disease	Deteriorating disease prognosis and possibility of significant impairment and handicap
	Explanation and rationale for more aggressive treatment: risks versus benefits
	Coping with decisions to start experimental medications with increased risks
	Coping with chronicity of disease: anger, depression, and rebellion
	Modifying life goals and plans: higher education, work, and sexual relationships, having children
	Supports available for family and child with significant impairment or handicap

been directly educated about the disease and rationale for treatment recommendations, the uninvolved spouse may be more likely to undermine the required treatment. The spouse may feel unsupported and isolated, and should be encouraged to participate in clinic visits, even if by telephone. Separated and/or divorced parents may have similar issues, and information must be disseminated to all appropriate family members to assure recommendations are followed. Even if parents cannot be physically present at an office visit, if they are educated and feel they are participating in decision making the likelihood of success and adherence is improved. Childcare providers or babysitters must similarly be informed, especially since they may be called upon to administer medication to the child.

Parents and children may be aware of discrimination and a lack of acceptance, because education about arthritis is lacking at a societal level. A major barrier that parents have identified is the teacher's lack of knowledge about the disease and particularly the fluctuating nature of the condition. Children spend a majority of their day at school, and it is imperative for teachers and other school personnel to understand the child's symptoms and limitations. It is difficult for adults and other children alike to understand why a child may have trouble moving in the morning, but is playing normally in the afternoon. Literature such as "When Your Student Has Arthritis" [10] can be a valuable resource for teachers and school staff. In addition, an Individualized Education Plan (see section on Advocacy), may provide an appropriate strategy for school personnel. The teacher, the parent, or the child himself can help educate classmates by preparing a report or lesson on JIA for incorporation into a science or health project.

Educational and support organizations

There are a number of organizations that provide education and information for families of children with JIA. Table 3.5.4 provides a list of organizations, printed materials, and websites for families. Most organizations provide a website containing a plethora of additional information including links to other organizations, bulletin boards, chat rooms, and materials for purchase. Internet searches yield many sites not included here. It is a rich source of information and more and more patients arrive at a doctor appointment armed with a wealth of information regarding symptoms, diagnoses, and potential treatments. It is important that families are cautious about accepting information from these sites without determining the expertise of the writer and credentials of the host. The family members researching information about JIA on the Internet must try to separate opinion from fact and information from misinformation—sometimes a nearly impossible task. The team members should all encourage patients and parents to bring any questions or questionable information to their attention.

Another area for caution is unmonitored bulletin boards and chat rooms; especially those designed by children themselves. Children (and their parents), can be sources of misinformation. A partially understood comment or hearsay from well-meaning friends and family may be confusing or even harmful. Parents should be encouraged to monitor their children's participation in an age-appropriate manner, and should seek chat rooms for themselves that are monitored by someone whom they feel is knowledgeable.

Advocacy

Parents advocate for their children on a daily basis and need to be provided with the tools necessary to advocate in the health care system, community, and especially, in the school system. After the child's needs in school are identified, parents need to gain a working knowledge of ways to help them meet those needs.

Parents need to become familiar with their child's legal rights in the school system by learning the laws protecting children with special needs (if they exist). In the United States, there are primarily two federal laws protecting children with arthritis. The "Individuals with Disabilities Education Act" (IDEA) provides children with special needs the right to a free, appropriate education in the least restrictive environment (children must be mainstreamed in a regular classroom) with an individualized education plan (IEP) based on the child's needs. For children to qualify under IDEA they must have been evaluated by a multidisciplinary team and designated as eligible for

special education. It is important to note that a child need not have a cognitive deficit to qualify for special education under IDEA, and it can be based solely on a physical disability. A child is eligible under this law only if the disability interferes with their ability to learn [11].

The other federal law protecting the majority of children with JIA in the United States is Section 504 of the Rehabilitation Act. This law establishes that students with disabilities have a right to a free appropriate education even if it *does not* interfere with his or her ability to learn. The disability must "substantially limit" one "major life activity" such as performing manual tasks or walking to qualify. The law requires schools to provide a 504 plan allowing for "reasonable accommodations" in the regular classroom. Parents have the right to be included in the process of developing a 504 plan or IEP and the right to due process if they disagree with the school's recommendations [12].

States also have their own laws addressing education in general and special education in particular. Parents can obtain a copy of their state's laws by contacting the state and/or school district's department of special education. Most states in the United States have parent advocacy networks to help families negotiate the school system. The local school district should provide this information, or the National Information Center for Children and Youth with Disabilities (www.nichy.org) can be contacted. The team social worker and other team members can often help the family negotiate this complex, confusing area.

In Canada, there are no federally mandated policies for the entire country. The provinces and territories each establish their own policies and the local school districts have the final decision-making power. In British Columbia, for example, the BC School Act of 1995 requires a school board to make an educational program available to everyone who lives and enrolls in a school in the district. An Individual Education Plan is also developed to accommodate the child's special needs. Most schools have a school-based team that plans and coordinates service in the school, and provides support for the teachers. In BC, the school principal is responsible for ensuring that the IEP is developed, implemented, and reviewed. An IEP may include services provided by physical and occupational therapists, school psychologists, and homebound education services among others.

The British counterpart to the IEP is a Statement of Special Educational Need, originally established under the Education Act of 1981. This Act was amended by the Education Act of 1993 and 1996, requiring local education authorities (LEA) to identify children with special needs, make an assessment of those needs, including educational, medical, and psychological needs, and make a formal statement of those needs. A parent, teacher, or health provider may alert the LEA of a child's needs, and a parent may request a formal evaluation. The earlier laws have been superceded by the Special Educational Needs and Disability Act (SENDA) 2001 which came into effect in January 2002. This new act strengthens the rights of children with special educational needs to be in mainstream schools, requires LEAs to provide parents of children with special needs with information on resolving disputes with schools and LEAs, and places a duty on LEAs to increase the accessibility of all schools' premises, the curriculum, and the way written information is provided to disabled students. In England, the Connexions Service (the guidance service for 13–19–year-olds) provides information on further education or employment when a young person leaves school.

In Italy, the 1992 frame law number 104 granted disabled children the right to an education at every level, including University, and

Table 3.5.4 Resource directory

Organization	Address	Description
American Juvenile Arthritis Organization (AJAO)	1330 West Peachtree Street Atlanta, GA 30309 800–282–7800 (toll free) 404–872–7100 x6271 404–872–0457 (fax) www.arthritis.org	The AJAO is a council of the Arthritis Foundation devoted to serving the needs of children, adolescents, young adults with rheumatic diseases and their families. The AJAO serves as a clearinghouse of information, sponsors a bi-annual national conference, promotes legislation that affects children with arthritis, sponsors research via the Arthritis Foundation, and offers training to parents and health professionals in skills such as promoting educational rights for children with arthritis
Arthritis Foundation	1330 West Peachtree St Atlanta, GA 30309 800–283–7800 www.arthritis.org	The Arthritis Foundation is a wealth of information regarding all forms of rheumatic illness for both children and adults.
National Institute of Arthritis and Musculoskeletal and Skin Diseases (NIAMS)	National Institutes of Health 1 AMS Circle Bethesda, MD 20892–3675 310–494–4484 (phone) www.nih.gov/niams	NIAMS provides free health information devoted to childhood rheumatic diseases. The organization has information about JIA, support groups, and paediatric rheumatology centres around the USA
Eurydice Organization	www.eurydice.org	The information network on education in Europe set up by the European Commision. Its database EURYBASE provides detailed information on the special education system in many European countries
British Society for Rheumatology	www.rheumatology.org.uk/	The UK organization for rheumatology professionals whose principal objective is to advance the science and practice of rheumatology
Arthritis Care	www.arthritiscare.org.uk	A voluntary organization in the United Kingdom that provides information, self-management and personal development courses, networking and advocacy for individuals with arthritis
The Arthritis Research Campaign (arc)	www.arc.org.uk/	A medical research charity in the United Kingdom that raises funds to promote research into the cause, treatment and cure of arthritis and related conditions, and to provide information about arthritis to the public and health professionals
The Children's Chronic Arthritis Association	www.ccaa.org.uk/	A charity in the United Kingdom run by parents and professionals that provides emotional and practical support for children with arthritis and their families through a support network, a newsletter, family weekends, and outings
National Dissemination Center for Children with Disabilities (NICHCY)	P.O. Box 1492 Washington, DC 20013–1492 www.nichcy.org.	Provides information to assist parents, educators, and others in helping children and adolescents with disabilities become participating members of the community
Multipurpose Arthritis and Musculoskeltal Disease Center (MAMDC)	David Glass, MD Children's Hospital Medical Center-PAV 2–129 University of Cincinnati, College of Medicine Cincinnati, OH 45229–2899 e-mail:glasdO@chmcc.org www.cinciMAMDC.org	MAMDC is a research centre funded by NIAMS that specializes in research on paediatric diseases including JIA
National Center For Youth with Disabilities	University of Minnesota Box 721–UMHC Minneapolis, MN 55455 Phone:800–333–6293 ncyd@gold.tc.wmn.edu	An information and resource centre focusing on adolescents with chronic illness and disabilities
Institute for Family-Centered Care	7900 Wisconsin Ave, Suite 405 Bethesda, MD 20814 www.familycenteredcare.org/	Provides leadership to advance the understanding and practice of family-centred care for all medical needs. Serves as a central resource for both family members and members of the healthcare field
Internet Resources for Special children Disability Links-Arthritis	www.irsc.org/arthritis.htm	Provides valuable information for parents, family members, caregivers, friends, educators, and medical professionals who interact with children who have disabilities

Additional printed resources are listed in References (Refs 14–21) determined regulations for the "diagnosis and certification of the handicap, and for a complete school integration." The act introduced the appointment of support teachers, accessible buildings, and "program agreements" with health, social, cultural, welfare services, local authorities, and specialized teaching consultants.

In France, the framework law number 75–534 of June 1975 of handicapped persons established the education of handicapped persons as a "national duty" preferably in mainstream classes. The latest inter-ministerial circular, number 98–004, from January 1998, viewed the school's objective as to provide adapted teaching methods to offer pupils the knowledge and aptitudes for attaining "level V qualifications in a school or via an apprenticeship contract." The ultimate purpose is to assist students in acquiring the skills to find a job.

Information on the special education laws and objective of several other European countries can be found on the EURYDICE database, EURYBASE (www.eurydice.org) [13]. EURYDICE is the information network on education in Europe, providing information on national education systems and policies. The Brussels-based European Unit set up by the European Commission is responsible for management of the network and coordination of activities.

The parent, the health professional, and school personnel, working together need to determine the complexity of the child's needs at school. If the child's needs are relatively simple, such as having one set of books for home and one set for school, use of an elevator, and/or participation in physical education as tolerated, it is not necessary to pursue the "formal approach" of a special education evaluation as the child can usually get his or her needs met through informal communications with the school via phone calls, school meetings, or letters from the medical team. If the child requires more extensive interventions at school including physical and occupational therapy and adaptive physical education, an IEP or 504 plan in the United States or equivalent if available in other countries may be indicated [11].

Various members of the rheumatology team may be required to provide information to school health personnel or representatives. In addition, health care professionals can promote and foster advocacy among families by having a basic working knowledge of educational laws and how to meet the child's needs in the school system. The family is often unaware that these services are available or that their child qualifies. It may also be necessary to assist the family with the stigma surrounding the association of a child requiring "special services" which could imply that the child has a cognitive disability. Parents must understand that availing themselves of such a program is not detrimental to the child's academic achievement record but rather a means to an end.

The importance of education for patients and families should continually be recognized as part of the treatment regimen for children diagnosed with JIA.

Conclusion

When their child is diagnosed with a chronic illness, parents often feel life will never again be the same. However, with education, support, and disease control, routines resume and life becomes quite manageable. In addition, as the family gains a better understanding of their situation, this information can be passed on to others who interact with the child, further easing the burden. Education, therefore, becomes a key ingredient allowing a child with JIA to progress physically, emotionally, and socially while enabling the family to live a positive and rewarding life.

References

1. Kroll, T., Barlow, J.H., and Shaw, K. Treatment adherence in juvenile rheumatoid arthritis—a review. *Scand J Rheumatol* 1999;28:10–8.

2. Thompson, S.M., Dahliquist, L.M., Koenning, G.M., and Bartholomew, L.K. Brief report: adherence-facilitating behaviors of a multidisciplinary pediatric rheumatology staff. *J Pediatr Psychol* 1995;20(3):291–7.

3. Kemper, K.J., Cassileth, B., and Ferris, T. Holistic pediatrics: a research agenda. *Pediatrics* 1999;103(4):902–9.

4. Astin, J.A. Why patients use alternative medicine. *JAMA* 1998;279(19):1548–53.

5. Szer, I.S. and Stebulis, J. Communication and health education for patients and families. In T.R. Southwood and P.N. Malleson (eds), *Bailliere's Clinical Paediatric International Practice and Research: Arthritis in Children and Adolescents.* London: Bailliere Tindall, 1993, pp. 745–67.

6. Tucker, L.B., De Nardo, B.A., Stebulis, M.A., and Schaller, J.G. *Your child with arthritis: a family guide for caregiving.* Baltimore, MD: The John Hopkins University Press, 1996, pp. 141–61.

7. Barlow, J.H., Shaw, K.L., and Harrison, K. Consulting the 'experts': children's and parent's perceptions of psycho-educational interventions in the context of juvenile chronic arthritis. *Health Educ Res* 1999;14(5):597–610.

8. Konkol,L., Lineberry, J., Gottlieb, J., Shelby, P.E., Miller, J.J., III and Lorig K. Impact of juvenile arthritis on families: an educational assessment. *Arthritis Care Res* 1989; 2(2): 40–8.

9. Hobbs, N.J., Perrin, J.M., and Ireys, H.T. *Chronically ill Children and their Families.* San Francisco,CA: Josey-Bass, 1985;62–101.

10. *When your Student has Arthritis: pp. Guide for Teachers.* Atlanta: Arthritis Foundation, 2002.

11. Wetherbee, L.L. and Neil, A.J. *Educational Rights for Children with Arthritis: Manual for Parents.* Atlanta: Arthritis Foundation, 1989.

12. deBettencourt, L.U. Understanding the differences between IDEA and Section 504. Council for Exceptional Children, 2002, 34,16–22.

13. EURYDICE: www.eurydice.org.

14. Arthritis Foundation (ed.) *Raising a Child with Arthritis: parent's guide.* Atlanta: Arthritis Foundation, 1998.

15. Brewer, E.J. and Cochran AK. Parenting a child with arthritis: a practical, empathetic guide to help you and your child live with arthritis. Michigan, MI: Lowell House, 1995.

16. Vadosy, P. and Meyer, D.J. *Living with a brother or sister with special needs: a book for sibs.* Seattle,WA: University of Washington Press, 1996.

17. Brewer, E.J. and Cochran, K.A. *The Arthritis Sourcebook.* New Jersey,NJ: McGraw Hill/Contemporary Books, 1994.

18. Furst, D.E., (ed.) *Arthritis and Rheumatology: An Internet Resource Guide.* New Jersey,NJ: Thomson Medical Economics, 2002.

19. Wallace, D.J. *The Lupus Book: A Guide for Patients and their Families.* Oxford: Oxford University Press, 2000.

20. Lahita, R.G. and Phillips, R.H. *Lupus: Everything you Need to Know.* New York: Avery Publishing Group, 1998.

21. Phillips, R.H., Carr, R.I., and Spiers, H. *Coping with Lupus: A Practical Guide to Alleviating the Challenge of Systemic Lupus Erythematosus.* New York: Avery Publishing Group, 2001.

3.6 Psychosocial aspects

Karen Shaw

Aims

Why some children and families with JIA cope well, and why others have social and emotional difficulties is discussed. How to recognize and address psychosocial problems so as to maximize the overall well-being, and minimize the disability of a child with JIA is explored.

Structure

- Introduction
- The challenges faced by families as a consequence of the disease course
- What impact do these challenges have on the psychosocial adjustment of families?
- What can be done to support the psychosocial needs of families?
- Summary

Introduction

Despite the difficulties associated with Juvenile Idiopathic Arthritis (JIA), psychosocial dysfunction is not inevitable. The majority of families manage with considerable skill. They develop new competencies and for some, the presence of arthritis can even result in strengthened family ties. This said, living with JIA is not easy. Families face a plethora of difficult challenges and, compared to 'healthy' families, are at an increased risk of developing serious social and emotional problems. As a result, most health professionals will find themselves caring for at least some families who are experiencing significant emotional crises. Unfortunately, failure to respond to these appropriately may not only jeopardize the child's immediate physical health, but also risk the family's quality of life and long-term development. Optimal treatment of adjustment to JIA, therefore, requires that health providers not only manage the medical aspects of disease, but also address the family's psychosocial needs.

To understand how and why families may be at risk of developing psychosocial problems, it is important to ask the following questions:

1. What social and emotional challenges do families face as a consequence of JIA?

2. What impact do these challenges have upon the psychosocial adjustment of families?

In answering these questions, it is useful to adopt a *developmental perspective*. Psychologists certainly agree that there are identifiable patterns of change and stability throughout the lifespan, and while there is some debate about the way in which these changes occur, development is largely assumed to occur in structured sequences that involve biological, cognitive, social, and psychological processes.

The intention of this section is to highlight the developmental processes that take place during childhood and adolescence. However, it is essential to remember that other family members are also undergoing change and face their own developmental tasks. So while JIA may compromise an adolescent's accomplishment of independence outside the family, their parents may find that the stability associated with middle adulthood (e.g. job-security) is equally threatened. Moreover, families do not experience arthritis in isolation, but in a social situation that includes the extended family, friends, and members of a wider community. As such, adjustment to JIA depends not only upon the individual characteristics of family members, but also upon the behaviour of other people, including those within the healthcare team.

In addition to child development, it is also important to understand the challenges associated with the different stages of disease. Indeed, the psychological responses displayed at diagnosis are likely to be much different to those exhibited after years of active disease.

The challenges faced by families as a function of the disease course

Pre-diagnosis

The early symptoms of JIA can be subtle and difficult to interpret [1]. It is not surprising therefore, that many families have felt the impact of arthritis long before they have been referred to a specialist. Indeed, the first outwardly signs of JIA are not always physical, especially in the very young who are less able to articulate their pain or stiffness. Instead, children may appear irritable, tearful, and withdrawn, display poor appetites, disturbed sleep or an avoidance of normal activities. Such behavioural changes can certainly increase the demands made upon families and in wondering why a previously happy child is now so discontent, many parents will doubt the adequacy of their parenting. Thus, even at this early stage, JIA can undermine the family environment and strain relationships between husbands and wives and between children and parents.

Even in the presence of physical symptoms, misinterpretation is common. Children and parents frequently attribute the causes of pain and stiffness to minor injury or accept the symptoms as 'growing pains'. This not only has implications for children's physical health, but may also threaten psychosocial development and quality of life.

Regrettably, even when it is apparent that something is physically amiss with the child, initial attempts to seek medical advice are not always successful [2]. The subtlety of symptoms and relative low incidence of JIA can make it difficult for family practitioners to provide an immediate diagnosis, especially when compounded by the developmental constraints of infancy and early childhood. Unfortunately, delays and diagnostic mistakes can have profound consequences for the family, leaving them feeling disbelieved, angry, and helpless. Professional insensitivity at this point can also thwart families' attempts to seek subsequent help and it is understandable that at least some parents may arrive at the consultant's doorstep feeling suspicious and hostile.

Diagnosis

The diagnosis of JIA brings about a new set of challenges for families and no matter how sensitively the news is broken, the experience is life-changing. JIA is a disease that has no understandable cause, no available cure, and no definite prognosis. Facing this can be deeply distressing and health professionals have to prepare themselves for a range of emotional reactions. Indeed, the response to such a diagnosis is frequently likened to the process of bereavement [3], in which children grieve for their loss of self, and families grieve for the loss of the 'normal child'. This process typically begins with feelings of (1) shock, followed by stages of; (2) disbelief, (3) depression, (4) anger, (5) guilt, and finally (6) resolution and adaptation.

Shock

For those families who have been without a diagnosis for a long time, being offered a firm disease label may come as a relief, validating their persistent beliefs that something is medically wrong and providing a direction for treatment. However, in the vast majority of cases, the first response to the diagnosis is one of shock. This is usually described as a feeling of 'numbness' and can last from a few seconds to several weeks. Shock typically impairs the family's ability to recognize the scale of the news, and can produce what appear to be inappropriate responses. Some individuals may exhibit feelings of great physical pain; others will appear very calm, even apathetic. At this point, families may struggle to digest new information, and it is crucial that important details of the consultation are given in written form and repeated on subsequent occasions.

Disbelief and denial

Shock is often followed by denial and manifests in a longer period of being unable to believe the news. In many instances, the denial is episodic and both children and their families may experience beliefs that they *are in a dream*, or that *the doctors are wrong*. However, while denial can impede the family's ability to manage the physical aspects of the condition, in these early stages of response it can represent a positive coping mechanism. Denial prevents the individual from experiencing more emotional distress than they can currently deal with and pressure to relinquish these feelings prematurely may result in loss of hope. Instead, health professionals should allow the family a little time to move through this stage, and offer alternative strategies with which to cope only if it appears persistent.

Anger

Anger is another defence mechanism that prevents people thinking excessively about themselves and guards against feelings of helplessness, guilt, and despair. In the absence of any legitimate causes for blame, families' anger can range from expressions of irritability directed towards family and friends, to outbursts of rage that are directed at health professionals, the health system, God, Fate, or Nature. Children may also blame their parents. However, whilst anger appears to be a negative emotion, if channelled positively it can provide the energy for effective action.

Depression and helplessness

As denial and anger break down, people can begin to feel great sadness. The family begins to experience an increasing realization that life may never be the same. Parents start to acknowledge that their once healthy child now has a disease for which there is no current cure and which may cause great pain and disability. In addition, children and families may have to let go of long held aspirations. Depression is an expression of these losses and results from feelings that they can do little to change the situation.

Guilt

Guilt is a common reaction to the diagnosis of JIA. Parents feel guilty that they somehow caused or contributed to the disease either through a lack of vigilance or by passing on a genetic weakness. They can also feel guilty that they did not recognize the symptoms earlier or act sooner in seeking medical assistance. Siblings can also feel culpable, wondering whether they did something to cause the arthritis and all members of the family may wonder whether they are being punished for past offences.

Resolution and adaptation

With time, these emotions begin to recede. Families begin to appreciate that a diagnosis of JIA does not discount the ordinary rewards of raising a child and that much of everyday life can be maintained. Families begin to re-appraise their priorities in life and realize that many of their aspirations remain intact. Resolution allows families to begin reorganizing their lives in which JIA has a place and, as each member becomes more skilled in the everyday tasks associated with managing JIA, the burden of care becomes less.

There are no time limits to any of these phases. Each one may last a matter of minutes, or years. Moreover, the persistent nature of chronic illness can make it exceedingly difficult for families to completely resolve their grief. Instead they are likely to suffer from 'chronic sorrow' in which periods of coping are interrupted by periods of distress [4]. It is important, therefore, that health professionals never assume that individuals are coping just because they have lived with JIA for a long time or adhere to treatment. New challenges, such as starting school, and additional life stresses can begin the grief cycle over again. Families' grief can also be triggered by interventions that are designed to be supportive. For instance, respites of care may allow families to remember how life used to be before the onset of arthritis.

Post diagnosis

Early arthritis

Following diagnosis, the responsibility for daily healthcare very quickly shifts from health-professional to the family. At this stage, the immediate focus for families, particularly parents, is to understand the disease and its treatment. While this thirst for knowledge is a positive step towards adjustment, families may still remain in a considerable state of emotional turmoil. Too much, too soon, can be overwhelming and leave families feeling inadequate and helpless. So although families should never be denied the information they seek, it is important that they are offered the support to deal with it.

The emotional consequences of JIA in this early stage can be extremely profound. All members of the family are forced to re-evaluate their lives in the context of JIA. It may be particularly difficult for them to accept that arthritis is a disease that has no cure and which may be felt over the long-term. This will be particularly true of individuals who have had little previous experience of chronic illness. Many of the grief experiences described previously will remain throughout the early stage of disease as children and other family members question why this awful thing has happened to them. The speeds at which individuals pass through these stages may vary and this lack of synchronicity may itself cause difficulties as each member finds it difficult to understand why others are acting in ways that they perceive as inappropriate or unhelpful. Conflicts are also likely to arise if family members have different priorities for the child's care.

At this stage in the course of disease, children are likely to be subject to many medical assessments and undergo a number of different treatments. These can be extremely stressful for both children and their families, particularly if they are ill-prepared about the procedures. Unfortunately, many of these interventions are unpleasant and painful and even with the best preparation, some children will experience considerable distress. For a few, this may develop into specific anxieties or phobias (e.g. 'needle-phobia') and make the long-term management of JIA significantly more difficult.

The medical management of JIA is equally challenging for parents, especial when they are forced to undertake procedures that go against their natural instincts [2]. It is not surprising, therefore, that many parents fear that their children will grow to hate them for the pain and discomfort that they may inflict. In this early stage it is common for parents to try and compensate the ill child for their condition, particularly in response to the pain and discomfort. All members of the family including grandparents, aunts, and uncles, will try hard to cheer up the child by buying gifts and allowing them to behave in ways that are normally deemed as unacceptable. While this is perfectly understandable in the short term, over the longer period this begins to create family difficulties and may impede the normal development of the sick child. Balancing the short-term needs of the child with their long-term development and the needs of other family members is likely to be extremely difficult in the early stages of disease and many parents will feel extremely guilty that they are not succeeding.

Siblings of chronically ill children are particularly vulnerable in the early stages of disease [5]. At a time of emotional upheaval, many can find themselves overlooked by families and medical staff alike. Understandably, many siblings will feel neglected and resentful about the special treatment that is afforded the sick child. The expression of these can manifest in a range of negative behaviours and they may become argumentative, feign illness, or become depressed [6]. Parental concern with the sick child and periods of hospitalization can also reduce the sibling's opportunities to discuss what is happening to their ill brother or sister. As a consequence, many will be extremely worried about their ill brother or sister, even believing that they may die. In the absence of information and comfort, siblings may also fear that they too will develop JIA or believe that they have somehow caused the JIA.

Established arthritis

With time, most families become proficient at managing the practical aspects of the child's healthcare and realize that not all the features of life are disrupted by arthritis and its treatment. As initial fears subside, the distress associated with diagnosis lessens. However, while these feelings are tempered with time, it is dangerously optimistic to assume that all families will cope consistently well. Instead, most families with established disease may experience 'chronic sorrow'.

One of the problems faced by families with established disease is the return to 'normal' life. Friendships outside the family are a common casualty of JIA, either because they have been neglected during the early stages of the disease or because friends no longer know how to respond to the ill child or their family. The presence of JIA also reduces their opportunities for new social contacts. Ill health, limited mobility, and the time-commitments of health regimens all conspire to make social activities difficult, particularly when compounded by financial hardship and a lack of personal transport.

Like all young people, children and adolescents with JIA face a number of developmental demands and challenges. Chronic illness, however, makes the attainment of these tasks much more difficult and there is a real possibility that they may lag behind their healthy peers. Children can certainly feel isolated from their friends and have a restricted access to many aspects of life that are considered important elements of their youth-culture. Difficulties in socializing can increase as children grow older, and friends begin to travel further afield. For many young people, accepting JIA as part of their identity can be a major challenge. Every aspect of JIA, including its treatment, can serve to make them look, feel, act, and be treated differently to their peers [7]. All this is at a time when peer conformity is at a premium. It is no wonder, therefore, that many children attempt to lessen their 'difference' by choosing to not adhere to their health-regimens [7]. Difficulties re-establishing their identity may also manifest in denial, loss of self-esteem, social withdrawal, and negative body image.

The demands on parents are equally difficult. In addition to the normal demands of parenting, parents are typically responsible for ensuring that the child adheres to treatment. They also have to respond to the child's new emotional needs. While JIA has the potential to strengthen family bonds [8], the additional stresses faced by families can also undermine relationships. Although there is little evidence to suggest that JIA leads to higher divorce rates among couples, the presence of arthritis can potentially affect the quality of relationships. It is common for couples to argue about disproportionate burdens of care, and conflicts can arise when parents differ in their attitudes towards healthcare, discipline, or the severity of the child's illness. Mothers appear to bear the major responsibility for the child's healthcare, and research does support that mothers tend to experience more anxiety, depression, and stress than fathers or than mothers of healthy children [9]. However, although fathers may not hold the main role in caring for their child, it is likely that they play a vital role in supporting their partners and positive spousal support does appear to be a major determinant of maternal adjustment. The extra demands of caring for a child with JIA also leave less time for parents to spend time with one another. Caring for a child with JIA may also restrict parents' opportunities to undertake full-time employment. This not only has implications for the family's financial welfare, but also reduces opportunities for social relationships.

The impact of established disease upon siblings is not well documented in the context of JIA. However, research in other chronic conditions suggests that siblings are likely to experience significant amounts of distress [6]. JIA certainly restricts the amount of time that siblings have available for leisure and peer activities [2]. Family activities can become limited by the ill child's functional limitations, and opportunities to spend time with peers may also be curtailed. For instance, parents can often ask siblings to take on a disproportionate number of tasks compared to the affected child or encourage them to join in home physical therapy to help motivate their brother or sister. Siblings can also feel embarrassed about the presence of JIA in the family, especially if the arthritis is visible and may even be teased because of it. As a consequence, they may hesitate to invite friends to their home, especially if the house is fitted with obvious aids and adaptations. Like their parents, siblings also feel helpless that they cannot relieve their brother or sister's pain, and can worry about the burden of care that is placed upon their parent's shoulders. However, while siblings are at risk of serious maladjustment, the experience of chronic illness within the family can also have a positive effect upon their attitudes and behaviours. Siblings can certainly provide the ill child with an invaluable source of emotional and practical support and living with a chronic condition may also promote the development of empathy, compassion, and helpfulness [10].

Refractory arthritis

The detrimental effect on the quality of life of refractory disease can be pronounced. Children may spend much of their waking time in pain or discomfort, and find themselves limited in many aspects of their everyday life. Opportunities for peer participation may be greatly reduced and prolonged school absenteeism may compromise academic achievement. Children may face periods of hospitalization and have to undergo treatments that are not only distressing and painful, but have potentially serious side-effects.

The impact on parents is no less significant. The demands on parents caring for children with refractory JIA rarely diminish and can be extremely arduous. The physical demands of care are particularly difficult for those parents whose children are older (and thus heavier) and may be compounded by their own increasing age. In meeting the demands of care, it is also probable that one, if not both parents, may have to give up work. As such, they may have fewer opportunities for social relationships outside of the immediate family circle and the impact upon financial stability can be considerable. The costs associated with frequent travelling to clinics and the purchase of necessary medications, aids, and adaptations may also undermine the families' financial stability.

Children and parents are likely to become inordinately despondent as little improvement is seen and in considering the future, many people have low expectations of what a child with refractory disease can achieve. This can be equally true of parents, schoolteachers, and health-professionals. Unfortunately, this lowering of expectations often occurs with little knowledge of what supports and possibilities actually exist for people with even the most limiting disease. Although it may be unrealistic to expect that children with uncontrolled disease have the same opportunities and choices as their healthy peers, appropriate support, and encouragement will allow them to participate meaningfully in most aspects of 'normal life'. Sadly, in the face of negativity and low expectation, it is likely that children themselves will believe that they have nothing valuable to offer or contribute.

The challenges faced by families as a function of the child's developmental status

In addition to the challenges faced as a consequence of disease stage, families also have to face challenges that are unique to the child's developmental level. The attainment of the skills and experiences necessary to achieve normal developmental tasks can be much more difficult for the child with arthritis. Support for children with JIA consequently requires an approach that is developmentally appropriate.

Children's understanding of JIA

Many attempts to understand children's adjustment to chronic illness have emphasized the role of cognitive development [11–13]. Proponents of this approach suggest that children's responses to disease will vary as a function of their cognitive status, and that children at different developmental levels will have substantially different conceptualizations of illness. From this viewpoint, awareness of children's cognitive development, allows us to predict and make sense of their responses to JIA and to offer more appropriate explanations of illness and treatment.

The works of Piaget [14,15] have been seminal in understanding children's development and propose that cognitive ability evolves systematically through four predictable stages.

The Sensorimotor stage (0–2 years): At the beginning of this stage, infants are unable to make distinctions between themselves and the rest of the world. However, between 18 and 24 months, infants are able to present objects as mental images, an ability that manifests in language, re-enacted actions from memory and simple problem solving behaviour.

The Pre-operational stage (2–7 years): Increases in toddlers' muscle control and fine motor skills lead to greater independence and wider opportunities for exploration. Their continued development of language, mental imagery, and memory also facilitate a growing sense of self-awareness. However, they continue to be influenced by how objects look and are egocentric (i.e. unable to see things from any perspective other than their own).

The Concrete-operational stage (7–11 years): Children begin to think logically and gain an understanding of concepts such as time, space, and quantity. They are now able to perform mental actions and understand the concepts of reversibility and 'conservation' (i.e. that things can stay the same despite changes in appearance). However, they are still unable to engage in hypothetical thought and remain egocentric.

The formal-operational stage (11–adult): The young person is now able to engage in abstract thought and hypothetical-deductive reasoning. This ability to deal with possibilities, rather than just actualities, enables the young person to consider alternatives to their existing circumstances and think about the future.

Although these stages are invariate, children's movement within and between them is thought to vary in relation to their genetic endowment and opportunities to interact with environmental stimuli.

It is within this framework that children's concepts of health and illness have been most commonly explored [12,13]. A summary of these findings is presented in Table 3.6.1.

While this classical staged approach remains influential and provides a useful framework to explore children's understanding of illness, there is increasing criticism that such structuralist theory fails to acknowledge the role of experience in children's conceptualizations [16].

Table 3.6.1 Children's conceptualizations of health and illness as a function of cognitive development

Pre-operational stage (2–7 years)

Illness described only in reference to external manifestations (e.g. having a cough)

Unable to understand that symptoms are caused by the body's response to foreign agents. Instead illness believed to be a consequence of some action that the child has (or has not) performed

Illness thought to be caused by something that happens near the body and which occurs directly before first visible signs of illness are observed

Causal link between the source of the illness and the child's body frequently described in terms of magic and punishment

Recovery from illness thought to occur by adhering to rules (e.g. taking medicine, keeping warm)

At end of stage, children begin to understand the concept of contagion, but often fail to appreciate that not all diseases are contagious

Concrete-operational stage (7–11 years)

Illness generally described in terms of physical symptoms

Demonstrate a basic understanding of contagion and appreciate that not all illnesses are contagious

Illness typically thought to be caused by 'germs' or 'dirt' transmitted to the body by physical contact or involvement in a particular activity

Recovery from illness typically conceptualized as involving topically applied medications, although children do perceive themselves to have some control over the cause and cure of illness by avoiding the sources of ill health

Recovery assumed to be based on adhering to doctor's or parental instructions

Formal–operational stage (11 years–adult)

Illness is associated with internal physiological processes that may involve an interaction of multiple causes and manifest in various ways

Recognize that physical disease can also result from psychological stress and dysfunction

Descriptions of illness no longer rely upon external symptoms. Instead, incorporate feelings of reduced well-being

Understand that medical intervention may be necessary to their recovery, but may not be sufficient

Indeed there is some evidence that children may have as much understanding as adults where their experience is similar [16]. This suggests that, where children's experience is high, explanations of JIA and treatments may not necessarily require an approach that is qualitatively different to that of adults. However, despite these divergences in theoretical positions, it is generally agreed that although individual adolescents of the same chronological age may vary in their level of understanding, older age is generally associated with more sophisticated thinking. This certainly appears true of children with JIA. For instance, Berry *et al.* [11] assessed the extent to which children with JIA, aged between 6 and 17 years, accurately understood their disease. Children's understanding did indeed follow a developmental progression, with older children offering more sophisticated and more accurate explanations of JIA than younger ones. However, although proportionately more of the older children were functioning at the formal operational level, compared to younger children, a substantial number of older children were actually still functioning at a concrete level. In addition, children displayed a number of misunderstandings about the causes of arthritis and this was despite the fact that many of the 6–17 year olds had lived with JIA for a considerable length of time and had received routine disease education during clinic visits.

Developmental challenges

Infancy and early (pre-school) childhood

Impact on the child During infancy, the main development tasks include (i) gaining a sense of control over the self and environment, and (ii) differentiating the self from others. These tasks are largely accomplished through the infants' exploration of their surroundings, manipulation of objects, and interaction with people. Much of this is achieved through 'play', which allows children to develop news competencies and consolidate previously acquired skills. However, for children with JIA, opportunities for play can be significantly reduced.

In part, this is attributable to the infant's reduced motor development, but is further constrained by the time-requirements of healthcare and parental fears of causing pain through physical contact.

Parent's reluctance to handle their children may also affect the formation of the 'primary social attachment'—the process by which infants develop selective relationships with their caregivers, and which enables them to feel secure in unfamiliar environments [17]. Attachment typically begins at 6 weeks of age and, by the age of 18 months, the securely attached child should be able to find comfort when needed and use the parent as a safe base from which to explore their environment. As such, attachment is pivotal for cognitive development.

Attachment may also be negatively affected by periods of hospitalization that result in prolonged separations between the infant and their parents. In addition to separation from parents, hospitalization is also likely to involve painful medical procedures and handling by numerous people, which may jeopardize the child's development of 'basic trust'. Reassuringly, however, the bulk of evidence suggests that although attachment can be temporarily affected, children appear to be extremely resilient, and in most cases, manage to develop normally over the longer-term. This said, it is important to understand the real impact that short-term separations (e.g. hospitalization) can have upon infants and younger children. Separations are likely to induce considerable distress and can manifest in three distinct phases [17]:

1. *Protest*: The immediate reaction to separation is evidenced by overt behaviours such as crying, screaming, and kicking. Children will often try to escape or cling vehemently to their parent to prevent the separation.

2. *Despair*: With time these protests give way to calmer behaviour and children may even appear apathetic. However, internally, children are likely to be very angry and fearful. At this point, children typically reject other people, including those trying to comfort them and do not appear to expect the return of their parents.

3. *Detachment*: With prolonged attachment, children may begin to
   interact with people, but tend to treat all people similarly, favouring
   no one. On the return of a parent, children often appear to reject
   them and in many cases, the relationship between them needs to
   be 're-learnt'.

Separations are thought to be most distressing between 6 and 36
months, peaking between 12 and 18 months. Infants do not have the
cognitive skills to hold mental images of their parents and children
may struggle to understand concepts such as 'tomorrow' or 'just a few
days'. Young children are likely to feel that they have been abandoned
altogether and may feel that they are some way responsible for their
situation (e.g. a punishment for misbehaviour). If parents are unable
to be with the child, it may be helpful, therefore, to provide the child
with some evidence of their parents' existence (e.g. photos, audio
recording of their voice or video). Distress may also be eased by the
presence of other people familiar to the child or by the provision of
familiar toys or objects.

A long-term consequence of hospitalization (or other separations
from the main attachment figure/s) is 'separation anxiety' [17]. At the
heart of this is a belief that the separation will happen again; it can
be evidenced in several ways. Children may display increased
aggressive behaviour and make excessive demands upon parents. They
may become clingy, refuse to stay alone at the homes of friends and
extended family or become detached. In severe cases, children may
also be unable to stay in a room alone or may develop school phobia.
In an attempt to remain at home, children will sometimes pretend to
be ill or feign an exacerbation of their JIA symptoms. They may even
develop psychophysiological disorders (i.e. where symptoms are real,
but are initiated by a psychological event). These can manifest in a
huge variety of conditions (e.g. headache, asthma) and range from the
innocuous to the serious.

Impact on the family Parenting during infancy and young childhood
is a demanding task, regardless of health status. However, when the
child has JIA, the daily requirements of caregiving can be dramatically
increased. Parents are likely to be faced with increased loss of sleep,
and the extra demands of health regimens can leave parents feeling
extremely fatigued. During infancy, parents may have to adapt
traditional methods of caregiving to suit their new circumstances and
can be forced to develop new priorities. They can easily find themselves feeling overwhelmed and many will undoubtedly question their
adequacy as parents. First-time parents may feel especially helpless; at
the same time as they are learning the usual parenting skills, they are
also having to develop other competencies to look after a child who
has special needs. Time given over to managing arthritis also leaves
less time for parents to engage in more pleasurable activities with their
children, such as playing together or day-time outings.

The limited linguistic abilities of infants and very young children
add extra complications for parents. They can find it difficult to gauge
children's pain and it is understandable that many parents may
become hyper-vigilant in monitoring their child's every moment. It is
also difficult for parents to prepare infants and toddlers for any
medical procedure, or to explain why temporary separations, such as
hospitalizations, are necessary.

Illness in a child's second year may be particularly stressful.
Whereas healthy children are undergoing rapid advancements in their
cognitive, social, and motor development, the development of
children with JIA may be much slower. The wider impact of JIA

becomes much more noticeable and parents may become acutely
aware of the differences between their child with JIA and other healthy
children. Such noticeable differences force parents to acknowledge the
significance of the disease and consider the implications it may have
for their child's future development. Two-year olds are also renowned
for their temper tantrums and as parents increasingly try to direct
their child's behaviour and impose healthcare activities upon them, it
is likely that conflicts will increase.

Middle (school-aged) childhood

Impact on the child During middle childhood, children's concerns
typically focus on their relationships with others, particularly their
peers. Children become increasingly aware of the differences between
themselves and others and realize the extent of their physical
limitations, especially as healthy friends become more independent
and engage in more demanding activities. Almost every aspect of JIA
and its treatment cause children to feel 'different' to their peers. It is
not surprising, therefore, that children can perceive their disease as a
massive threat to their quality of life and assign greater priority to
conforming to group identities than adhering to therapeutic regimens [7]. Children often go to extreme lengths to hide and deny their
disease, and despite apparently understanding the benefits of therapy
and the risks of certain behaviours, will commonly refuse to comply
with the requirements of their care. They will refuse to undertake their
programmes of exercise, resist wearing splints, spurn assistive aids, tell
friends that they are visiting the dentist rather than admit to a clinic
appointment and even deny a period of hospitalization by saying they
were on holiday!

Surprisingly the emotional impact on children towards the mild
end of the severity spectrum can be particularly pronounced. Unlike
those children whose disability is severe and therefore, have little
choice but to accept themselves as disabled, the invisibility of these
children's condition enables them to deny their disease (to themselves
and others). Unfortunately, children's attempts to keep up with their
healthy friends may not be successful and those with less visible
disease may find themselves on the margins of both the disabled and
the able-bodied, belonging fully to neither group. Inability to see the
visible signs of JIA can also reduce the empathy and support offered by
others, including health professionals and schoolteachers and can
contribute further to children's feelings of isolation [2].

School attendance is particularly important to child development.
In addition to the long-term socioeconomic benefits associated with
academic attainment, school also provides children with a sense of
social and cultural norms and offers opportunities to develop
relationships outside of the family [18]. In normal circumstances,
children spend most of their waking time at school, and it is within
this environment that they consolidate their social skills and develop
personal autonomy. In many respects, the need for young people to
gain a full education is of particular importance for children with JIA.
Current labour markets are highly competitive and despite recent
improvements in disability legislation, employers remain largely
prejudiced against those with disabilities. To compete in this environment, individuals with JIA may have an increased need to gain higher
qualifications [19].

Unfortunately, although school entry promotes social and intellectual
development, it can also heighten children's awareness of their
limitations and differences. Ill health and clinic appointments can
cause frequent non-attendance [20], and when at school, symptoms,

side-effects, and functional limitation can all compromise the child's classroom performance [21]. However, despite the increased absenteeism of children with JIA, poor school achievement is not inevitable. Although some authors suggest that children with JIA perform less well than their healthy peers [20,21] others report that they perform as well, if not better than their peers [22]. In the face of functional limitations, it may be that some children devote time to their studies that, in other circumstances, would be taken up with more physical activities.

The cumulative effects of poor attendance, and inability to participate in school activities such as physical education, may certainly disadvantage children's sense of belonging to their school, class, and peer group. Children with JIA may find themselves unable to participate in sporting activities and excluded from school trips and other extra-curricular activities such as fieldwork activities and school plays. As a consequence, children may have fewer opportunities to develop and consolidate friendships and may feel that they exist only on the periphery of class activity. Not being able to participate in school activities, such as sponsored walks to raise money for charities or take part in sports days also prevents children from contributing to collective goals and may reduce their opportunities to consolidate self-esteem. Children with JIA can become the targets of name-calling and physical bullying, especially when their arthritis is visible and reduced mobility and strength makes them particularly vulnerable. The effects of this can be devastating and may damage, perhaps irrevocably, children's confidence and feelings of self-worth.

School entry also forces the child to manage their condition outside of the home and without the support of parents. This necessitates that children assume more responsibility for their condition. The success of this will depend on many factors, not least the amount of preparation involved and the support of the school. Children certainly need to be taught the skills necessary to manage their symptoms independently within the classroom. They need to be able to manage their medication and adopt joint protection and energy-conservation techniques. In addition to taking responsibility for their symptom management, children also need to be given strategies to deal with the social situations that they may face including disclosure, seeking assistance, and bullying. One of the most difficult problems for children at school is explaining their condition to others and publicly asserting their needs; although most children with JIA agree that greater awareness about the disease in schools is warranted, they rarely want classmates to know that they, themselves, have arthritis. They worry that telling others will identify them as 'different' and fear that teachers will not believe them. Sadly the responses of other people frequently serve to confirm this fear. The common misconception that arthritis is a disease of old age means that people often find it difficult to believe that children can also have arthritis. Inappropriate responses may be compounded for children who have fluctuating symptoms [2]. Both parents and teachers may struggle to accurately judge the extent and genuineness of children's symptoms. Most teachers have a limited understanding of chronic illness and receive scant training in this field. Expectations of children at school can, therefore, be based on behaviour when they are relatively 'symptom free', rather than on behaviour and well-being during periods of pain, stiffness, or fatigue. As a consequence, the potential impact of JIA on a child's physical functioning, emotional well-being, and academic performance can be minimized and difficulties attributed to laziness or misbehaviour.

Impact on the family Managing treatment regimens may also become more complicated as children assume a greater role in their care and may impact on the family as a whole. Parents are typically responsible for explaining why a treatment is necessary and for encouraging their child's performance at home. Children may come to resent parental reminders and much of this frustration and anger may be directed at family members. Parents may find this resentment upsetting, and can feel guilty about the depriving children of their independence and personal freedom.

The family faces particularly difficult challenges as the child approaches school age. Often, with very little support, parents have to make educational choices for their children that balance their physical needs with those of their academic potential [2]. The child's entry into school also means that the parent can no longer be responsible for much of the child's immediate care. They have to teach the child to manage their arthritis outside the home and have to hand over responsibility to teachers. Letting go of these responsibilities can be a particularly stressful experience for parents, and trusting teachers to act appropriately can be difficult. School entry also requires that parents explain the condition to people other than their immediate family and friends. Parents do not always feel that they have sufficient knowledge and social confidence to do this and can fear the stigmatization that is so often associated with illness and disability.

Adolescence

Impact on the adolescent Traditional views of adolescence have characterized this period as a time of 'storm and stress' in which young people reject adult values and experience great emotional tensions. However, contemporary understanding of adolescence adopts a less problem-focused approach, acknowledging that most young people achieve their developmental goals with skill, and make valuable contributions to society [23]. Moreover, although adolescence is associated with increased intimacy with peers, parents generally retain a strong influence upon young people's behaviour. Nevertheless adolescence is a time of enormous physical, cognitive, and social change, during which young people attempt to meet externally defined expectations of adult behaviour, interpret the world, and evaluate their place within it.

The main goals of adolescence include the consolidation of identity, and acquisition of the skills necessary to undertake adult roles. Tasks include increased autonomy from parents, the development of adult relationships, and establishment of vocation; mastering these tasks can be particularly difficult for an adolescent with JIA.

Consolidation of identity may be particularly challenging. Subsumed within the notion of identity are *self-image* (the individual's description of the self) and *self-esteem* (the individual's evaluation of the self), both of which are likely to be affected by JIA. Arthritis and its treatment can have many adverse physical and body-altering effects; sexual maturation can be delayed and growth is frequently retarded. Smaller stature may not only cause adolescents to feel different from their peers, but, may also result in other people responding to them in a manner congruent with their younger looking appearance, rather than their chronological age. Adolescents may also experience local growth disturbances, such as limb-length inequalities, which may alter appearance and physical function. Gait and posture may be affected, joints may appear swollen, and the side-effects of medication (corticosteroids) may be very visible and disturbing. Much of a young person's identity (particularly their self-esteem) is influenced by reflected appraisals, social comparisons, and knowledge of member-ship to valued social groups. Adolescents with JIA now grow up in a world of stereotyping, where much premium is placed upon the 'body-beautiful' and disability is defined as 'different' [24]. In such circumstances, consolidation of identity can be extremely difficult.

Adolescence is perhaps the most emotionally difficult time to develop JIA. In evaluating their self-worth, not only do adolescents compare themselves with their peers, but also with their former healthy selves. In re-establishing their identity, adolescents have to reconsider their place in society and may have to give up long-held desires and aspirations. Many will also find that their existing friends fall away, often because they are unsure about how to respond to the adolescent's arthritis. Some adolescents will find their academic performance compromised at a particularly crucial stage in their education.

Cognitive advances in adolescence make it possible for adolescents to engage in hypothetical thought and so, concerns about the future become increasingly important. Issues of prognosis may be afforded considerable attention and adolescents can become particularly worried about the long-term implications of their current and previous treatments. Adolescents also begin to think about and act upon their sexuality. Concerns about sexual attractiveness, sexual performance, family planning, and parenthood are likely. Adolescents may also have anxieties about passing arthritis on to their children.

Having arthritis may also hamper independence from parents. Functional limitations may result in adolescents being dependent upon parents for self-care tasks and mobility. In some cases, parents may be reluctant to relinquish the long-held role of caregiver, with the result that parental overprotection can interfere with the transition to independence. For adolescents with JIA learning to take responsibility for their own healthcare is a major component of the move towards adulthood as well as being vital for optimal disease management both in adolescence and in later adult life.

Establishing adult relationships outside the family can also pose increased difficulties for adolescents with JIA. Functional limitations, especially restricted mobility, can render peer participation particu-larly difficult, also young people can be reluctant to accept those with disabilities into their peer group. This, in turn, may limit the adoles-cents' opportunities to develop or consolidate social skills and gain in social confidence. The importance of peer relationships, is not to be underestimated. Interactions with peers not only help the young person to develop an identity that is separate from their family role, but, may also offer important social, emotional, and practical support, and enable adolescents to learn about the development of relation-ships [25]. The effect of JIA upon children's social lives can often become more pronounced as they get older. With greater age, healthy peers go further afield and make spontaneous decisions about where they may go. For many adolescents with JIA, this may mean that they see friends less than they would like.

Having arthritis may also adversely affect the adolescent's ability to find a vocation. Arthritis can compromise some young people's educational attainment [20], and this has serious implications for their vocational aspirations. Lack of a definite prognosis, also makes it difficult for adolescents to plan for the future. In addition, the provisions for disabled school leavers are poor and the opportunities for employment are much reduced compared with healthy individuals. The vast majority of employers are unaware of the needs of disabled employees and are often unwilling to accommodate their special requirements.

Impact on the family As the cognitive development of a teenager with JIA increases they are increasingly able to contemplate their future. As a consequence, many parents will find themselves being asked questions that they are unable (or unwilling) to answer. As adolescents mature, parents are forced to consider new questions, including the adolescent's ability to move-away from home, enter employment, find a partner and start a family.

Adolescents' increasing needs for independence may be a major source of concern for parents, particularly when their young person has severe functional limitations. Parents may find themselves feeling deeply saddened that their children are often forced to sacrifice deep seated aspirations. Moreover, parents may also find themselves the targets of adolescents' frustrations as they face enforced dependency. For many parents, it can be exceptionally difficult to relinquish their role of care-giver, especially if this has been a long-held role. Not only will they worry about their child's abilities to manage alone, but they have to re-evaluate their own purpose in life. Many will have given up work to look after their children and their social networks may have been much reduced as a consequence. For these parents, the 'empty-nest' syndrome may be doubly felt (see also Part 3, Chapter 3.3).

What impact do these challenges have on the psychosocial adjustment of families?

Psychosocial adjustment is not a single parameter, but an umbrella term that subsumes dimensions that include *psychological adjustment* and *social adjustment*. In both cases, adjustment is usually defined as mental and behavioural functioning that is developmentally appro-priate and follows population norms. In contrast, maladjustment is evidenced in mental and behavioural functioning that is not age appropriate, does not conform to population norms and is particularly evidenced from pathological behaviour. In the context of childhood, adjustment is also considered to include *school performance* [26] and is defined as behaviour that progresses towards positive adult functioning [27].

As yet, attempts to understand the impact of JIA upon psychosocial adjustment are inconclusive. Some studies demonstrate an increased risk of social and emotional problems for families living with JIA [9], while others show their functioning to be comparable to levels found in the general population [28,29]. A minority even suggest that JIA can have a positive effect on families by strengthening aspects of the family environment [8].

Methodological issues

The disparate findings in families' psychosocial adjustment may, in part, be attributable to methodological issues, including the diverse ways in which the dimensions have been conceptualized and operationalized. For example, psychological adaptation to JIA has been studied in relation to self-esteem, specific mood (such as anxiety and depression), patterns of behavioural problems (internalizing or externalizing disorders) and psychiatric diagnosis. There are similar variations in respect to social adaptation and while school performance is considered an integral component of children's adjustment to chronic illness few studies have actually examined the school functioning of children with JIA. Those that have, have generally confined their assessments to academic attainment and absenteeism, with wider issues of school performance receiving scant attention.

Other methodological problems concern the choice of design and sample. Most studies have been cross-sectional which make it difficult to infer causality. The majority have also focused upon children attending tertiary centres and may consequently have included a disproportionate number of severe cases. Most have used small samples, limiting generalizability, and have provided insufficient details of participant characteristics to assess representativeness. In addition, many have failed to include control groups, although some have compared their findings with normative data. Unfortunately, those that have used control groups have often used siblings. As a control group, siblings are likely to match on important family and social–ecological characteristics. However, living with a chronically ill brother or sister may also place them at increased risk for psychosocial difficulties and as a result, differences in psychosocial functioning may be obscured.

Measures used to assess adjustment have also varied, ranging from the use of questionnaires to psychiatric diagnostic interviews. Studies have also used different informants, including children with JIA, their parents and professionals involved in their care. The use of such diverse methods makes it difficult to compare findings. Studies have generally demonstrated a relatively low concordance between children and other adult respondents and comparisons of alternative modes of assessment, such as checklists and clinical diagnoses, show less than optimal agreement. Potential bias can occur using measures not specifically designed for use with young people with chronic illness. For example the Child Behavior Checklist (CBCL) [30] developed to identify physically healthy children's behavioural problems and social competence has been very commonly used for studies of children with JIA. However, many of the CBCL items used to indicate maladjustment may actually reflect disease symptomatology and not psychopathology and therefore confound interpretation of the data [27].

Despite these many methodological limitations, a review of the literature suggests that JIA does place a considerable proportion of families at risk for psychosocial dysfunction, but the variability across findings indicates that psychosocial problems are not inevitable. In fact the majority of children with JIA and their families appear to manage their arthritis with aplomb. Unfortunately, for those who do experience difficulties, there is no evidence to suggest that these problems spontaneously resolve during adulthood, the limited data available indicating that adults who had JIA as children may be at increased risk for clinical depression, unemployment, relationship difficulties and functional problems compared to healthy peers [31–33].

Correlates of psychosocial adjustment

Attempts to delineate the variation in the functioning of children with JIA and their families have focused on examining correlates of psychological adjustment. For the most part, these studies have focused upon *disease/disability parameters*, *personal parameters*, and *social–ecological parameters*.

Disease/disability parameters

Examinations of disease and disability parameters in the context of psychosocial adjustment have included the *type of JIA onset, disease severity, disease duration, co-morbidity, intensity of pain*, and *functional status*. However, the number of studies is small and their findings are discordant. With respect to diagnostic group, the limited evidence suggests that psychosocial adjustment is unrelated to the type of JIA [34–36]. The relationship between disease severity and adaptation, however, is more difficult to interpret. Several authors have reported that children with severe JIA are at increased risk for experiencing psychological problems [35,36], poor social adaptation [37] and low school attendance [36] when compared to those with mild or inactive disease. Others, however, have found no significant differences between severity groups [34], and a small proportion of studies suggest that those with mild disease exhibit the poorest adjustment [38].

Co-morbidity remains a neglected variable in the context of children's adaptation to JIA. There is some limited evidence that the presence of a second condition may place them at increased risk for distressed mood and fewer good friends [37]. There is a similar paucity of studies examining disease duration. However, it does appear that newly diagnosed children may be at increased risk for poorer psychological and social adaptation [37,38].

The relationship between pain and adaptation is unclear. Several authors have found that increased pain places children at risk for anxiety, depression [39], and low social competence [40]. Others, however, have found no such relationships [41,34]. A study by Schanberg et al. [42] found that symptoms were predicted by daily mood and daily stressful events, but that children with JIA were not clinically depressed. The authors concluded that fluctuations in daily mood, rather than changes in clinical state, might exacerbate symptoms.

Few associations have been reported for functional status; there is modest evidence to suggest that greater disability in JIA may predict poorer social functioning, but may be unrelated to behavioural adaptation. In a 1-year longitudinal study of 165 children with juvenile arthritis, Timko et al. [43] found that patients' functional status provided little explanation regarding the variability in their psychosocial status. However, children with greater functional disability did have fewer good friends and poorer academic attainment 1 year later, even when significant baseline factors were controlled.

Personal parameters

Whether adaptation varies as a function of personal parameters is equally unclear. With respect to age, adolescents do appear to be particularly vulnerable for experiencing problems in psychosocial adaptation. Compared to younger children, they are more likely to exhibit emotional problems [44], high-risk behaviour [9], low social competence [38,44], increased school absence, and reduced participation in family and peer activities [36]. However, there is poor agreement about which particular groups of adolescents are at risk. For instance, Daltroy et al. [38] report that older age is associated with more behaviour problems only for males and that recently diagnosed adolescents, who have mild JIA, are most at risk for adaptation problems. In contrast, Billings et al. [36] suggest that adolescents with the most severe disease are most vulnerable.

There are similar disparities in relation to gender. A study by Ennett et al. [44] detected no significant differences in adaptation. In contrast, Timko et al. [9] found that girls engaged in less health risk behaviour than boys did and were more distressed.

The roles of intrapersonal variables in adjustment to JIA are largely unknown. However, Ennett et al. [44] have reported that perceived competence is significantly linked to how children experience their disease, independent of disease severity. Those with a more negatively perceived disease experience described themselves as less athletically competent, less popular among peers, less attractive, and exhibited lower self-worth when compared to participants with a more positive perceived experience. Ungerer *et al.* [35] have also demonstrated that adaptation may be significantly related to self-concept. Children with the lowest self-concept reported that they spent less time with peers than those with higher self-concept, had fewer close friends, dated less often, felt more lonely, were teased about their arthritis more frequently, had poorer health status and were more eager to leave school early.

Social–ecological parameters

With respect to social–ecological parameters, more adaptive functioning has been related to increased family cohesion and adaptability [45], fewer chronic life events and family stressors [45,46], better parental mood and emotional resources [9,26,38], and fewer parental health-risk behaviours [9].

A model of psychosocial adjustment

To understand why some individuals adjust better to JIA than others, it is useful to look at psychosocial adjustment within a 'risk and resistance' framework. Such approaches hypothesize that there are *risk factors* that place children at risk for developing adaptation problems but there are also *resistance factors* that have a protective effect.

One of the most comprehensive and sophisticated models of risk and resistance is proposed by Wallander *et al.* [47] and is presented in Figure 3.6.1. The authors adopt a 'non-categorical' approach. That is, they advocate that the psychosocial effects of chronic illness vary little as a function of the specific diagnostic condition, and believe, therefore, that attempts to understand psychosocial adjustment is more expediently achieved by considering different illnesses together. An underlying assumption of the model is that chronic illness does not necessarily represent an adverse event, but instead, presents the child and their family with potentially stressful situations that require successful management to avoid maladjustment. Sources of stress in

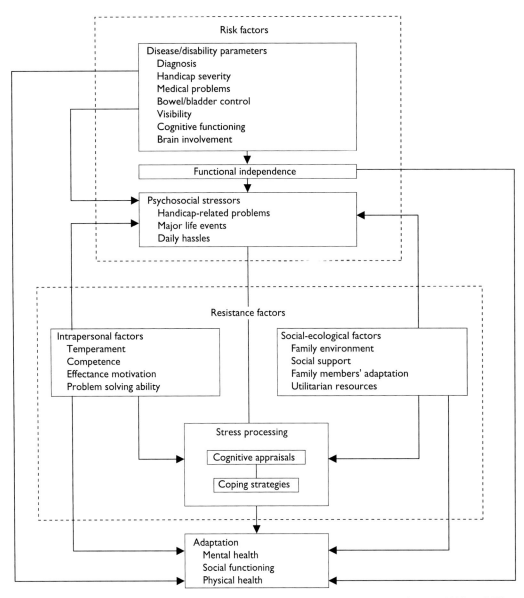

Figure 3.6.1 Disability-stress-coping model of adjustment to chronic illness. (From Wallander, Varni, Babani, Banis, and Wilcox [47])

JIA are varied. Some stressors emanate from the condition itself, such as disease parameters and functional limitations. Other stressors involve aspects of the individual's life, including daily hassles, major life events or transition points, such a going to school. These stressors may, or may not, be indirectly linked to their condition. For example, stresses normally associated with examinations may be exacerbated for adolescents with JIA, because other disease-related stressors already exist.

According to the model, an individual's adjustment to JIA is viewed as a function of the level of stress experienced (which is influenced by the nature of the stressors involved), and the effectiveness of their coping responses. Families not only have to cope with the practical demands of treatment, but must also cope with the social and emotional sequelae of the chronic arthritis.

The relationships between stressors, coping responses and adaptation are organized within a *risk* and *resistance* framework. The authors hypothesize that there are not only *risk factors* (i.e stressors) that place children at risk for developing adaptation problems, but that there are also *resistance factors* that have a protective effect. These include biological, psychosocial, and environmental variables, the interplay of which is thought to be continuous and occurs across the life span.

Resistance factors are hypothesized to influence adaptation in both direct and indirect ways. Resistance factors, thought to mediate the impact of stressors upon adaptation, include relatively stable intrapersonal factors (e.g. the child's temperament, competence, effective motivation, and problem solving ability), social–ecological factors (e.g. family environment and practical resources) and stress-processing (e.g. cognitive appraisal and coping strategies).

The individual's selection of relevant coping skills is influenced by the way in which they cognitively appraise the stressor, and involves judgements about the extent to which the stressor poses a threat to well-being and the individual's perceived ability to cope. The meaning attached to the stressor (i.e. the individual's appraisal) is mediated by intrapersonal characteristics, disease-related factors, and social–ecological factors. Once individuals have appraised the event and judged what resources are available, they endeavour to master the situation by selecting a coping strategy.

Support for the model

Psychosocial research, in the context of chronic illness, has been criticized as lacking a clear theoretical framework [48] and so, has provided an insufficient basis for theory-driven research. Theories of psychosocial adjustment, therefore, represent a welcome contribution to the field of JIA. However, the model proposed by Wallander *et al.* [47] is still in its infancy, and is descriptive rather than explanatory (i.e. it cannot explain the entire process of adjustment). Moreover, the model's complexity renders it difficult to validate as a whole, and preliminary support for the model is mixed and inconclusive. Nonetheless, the model remains one of the most sophisticated and comprehensive models of psychosocial adjustment that can be used to think about these issues in children and families with JIA, and despite these limitations, the model still possesses an important heuristic function. Not only does it integrate previously disparate and contradictory findings, but it also provides a framework in which to design studies and interpret data. The model has provided the conceptual framework for several studies in children's chronic illness [49,27,47], including JIA [9,37,43,46]. It provides a systematic framework in which to explore the relative risks for different groups of children with

JIA and family members and as such, may offer vital information about the appropriate targeting of interventions. Such theory-driven research will also help to test the model further, and where disparities occur, may provide important indications about how to revise the framework.

What can be done to support the psychosocial needs of families?

In addressing the psychosocial needs of families it is important to recognize that individuals' abilities to manage the challenges of JIA depend not only upon their own personal skills, but also upon services and social networks that support these behaviours. Central to this approach are the concepts of 'empowerment' and 'effective helping' [29], which advocate that (i) people have the capacity to become competent, and that, (ii) a person's level of competence is dependent upon the extent to which social systems provide opportunities for competencies to be displayed [50]. At the very minimum, health professionals need to provide families with a safe and friendly atmosphere in which concerns and emotional problems can be raised and recognized. While many of these can be addressed by members of the healthcare team, others will require support from other appropriately trained professionals (e.g. clinical psychologist, youth worker). Unfortunately, for those who do experience serious psychosocial difficulties, support of this kind is typically provided at a crisis point, if at all [51]. Elander and Midance [51] suggest this is often because suitable interventions have not been adequately developed, or because those responsible for referring families to other agencies are not fully aware of the availability of psychosocial services. As such, psychosocial interventions generally respond to maladjustment, rather than occur to help promote adjustment. It is more appropriate that approaches to healthcare focus upon prevention and anticipatory planning. Psychosocial adjustment to JIA is a dynamic process that unfolds over time in relation to changing disease status, individual variables and family and social environments, and therefore psychosocial interventions need to be routinely and recurrently offered to all families living with JIA, and to be delivered in response to their changing needs, life-events, and personal challenges. Appropriate targeting of intervention, therefore, necessitates an ongoing and highly individualized process of needs assessment that takes account of factors beyond the child's physical health.

In meeting families' needs, there are three approaches to psychosocial intervention that may be appropriate; the *problem-focused approach*; the *cognitive approach*, and the *social approach* [51].

The *problem-focused approach* targets behaviour relating to specific medical procedures (e.g. preparation for joint injections or surgery), specific behaviour problems (e.g. 'needle phobia') and symptoms (e.g. pain), using techniques such as relaxation, biofeedback and behavioural conditioning. Such interventions are particularly useful in helping children to manage their symptoms, treatments and functional limitations. Reductions in these potential risk factors may also serve to indirectly promote the child and families' psychosocial adjustment.

The *cognitive approach* aims to produce more general improvements in children's adaptation by modifying ineffective coping styles and maladaptive thoughts about the disease. This is often achieved through education and stress management.

The *social approach* intervenes at the socio-ecological level and aims to improve the child's adaptation by improving delivery of care, increasing children's social opportunities (e.g. through educational or vocational programmes), and supporting families. The social approach to psychosocial intervention might be directed at helping to develop a comprehensive system of care that recognizes the multifactorial nature of JIA and which promotes adjustment through anticipatory planning and the provision of inter-agency and multidisciplinary support. Central to this is a process of regular and individualized needs-assessments, which in addition to evaluating children's needs should also include the needs of the family. Maternal competence is posited as one of the most important influences upon children's psychosocial adjustment to JIA [52]. Work by Reisine [53] demonstrates that children in families characterized by greater cohesion and fewer stressful life events, display better adaptation. Parenting styles have also been associated with adherence with medication [45], with better adherence associated with mothers who had a greater variety of coping behaviours available to them, and fathers who reported higher satisfaction with life. A recent qualitative study of the experiences of parenting in JIA [2] also highlights a number of family-based interventions that may relieve some of the stresses encountered in caring for a child or adolescent with JIA. These included greater provision of information, increased support through self-help groups, more opportunities for discussion with health professionals, training in shared decision making for parents and the healthcare team, and assertiveness training for parents. The success of such an approach, however, is largely dependent on the extent to which the various medical, psychological, and community-based services can be integrated into a structured and coordinated system of care.

In reality, there is a great deal of overlap between these approaches. As Elander and Midance [51] note, theory in this field is extremely complex, interventions can have effects beyond their intended target and specific behavioural-changes may be elicited by more than one approach or depend upon a combination of strategies. For instance, social support can be an extremely useful coping mechanism in chronic illness. A study of 153 children and adolescents with various chronic diseases (including JIA) found that participants with high levels of social support from family and peers had significantly fewer behaviour problems than participants with high social support from just one of these sources [54]. Attempts to improve social support may include strategies that intervene at the level of the child, such as social skills training, which teaches children how to elicit and maintain social support using techniques such as modelling, coaching, behavioural rehearsal, and social–cognitive problem-solving strategies. Key objectives typically involve increased initiation of peer interactions, increased social participation, increased ability to express thoughts, wishes and concerns (assertiveness), increased ability to handle adverse encounters (such as name-calling) and greater problem-solving. However, social support may also be increased through social approaches, including interventions that support the family, particularly mothers [52,55], or raise awareness in schools by educating the child's teachers and classmates. Thus, while the divisions in psychosocial intervention may be somewhat heuristic in their function, they do emphasize the need for a system of care that targets different aspects of behaviour and intervenes at the level of the child, the family, and wider social-systems.

Despite the considerable potential to promote psychosocial adaptation in JIA, practical support for families remains under-developed [56]. As yet, the provision of rheumatology healthcare continues to mainly reflect the medical model of illness and accordingly, concentrates its efforts on managing the physical symptoms of arthritis through pharmaceutical, surgical, and rehabilitative interventions. The concept of health, however, incorporates much more than medical influences; a sentiment reflected by the World Health Organization [57], which defines health as, '*a state of complete physical, psychological and social well-being and not simply the absence of disease or infirmity*'. Strategies to truly meet health-needs in JIA therefore require a system of healthcare that recognizes the multi-factorial nature of arthritis and necessitate interventions that respond to the full spectrum of families' disease-experiences. From this stance, a comprehensive system of care requires an integrated and co-ordinated team-approach that, at the very least, includes health professional, psychologists, and social workers. In part, this requires sufficient allocation of fiscal resources, however, by far the greatest requirements are attitudinal, and begin with an appreciation of the demands made upon families, and a willingness to address them. Effective support requires that rheumatology professionals learn to recognize families at risk, and while specific psychological conditions, such as suicide risk, should always be dealt with by appropriately trained professionals, it is within the rheumatology clinic that psychosocial adaptation can be most usefully promoted. A rheumatology team has the most regular contact with children who have JIA and already performs ongoing assessments of their physical health; it is therefore probably in the best position to also monitor psychosocial health, and provide psychosocial support that not only responds to changes in the disease process, but also reflects the child's developmental status and the families' needs and dynamics.

In the absence of formal training, health professionals may benefit enormously by establishing close working relationships with local psychological services [48,51]. Not only may they able to provide direct therapeutic interventions, but early involvement of psychologists may also enable them to identify individuals at risk and minimize possible future crises. Psychologists (and other similarly qualified professionals) may also be able to offer the rheumatology team useful advice and training. Areas for potential input are given in Table 3.6.2.

However, even in the absence of psychological input, health professionals can still do much to address families' social and emotional needs. Support can be found at both local and national levels, with many organizations and mutual support groups offering professional advice about a range of psychosocial issues. So, while it may not be possible to directly provide psychosocial support to families, all health professionals should be able to signpost useful addresses, publications, helplines, and websites. This said, it is important to remember that some families will not have the sufficient skills and confidence to deal with other organizations; for these families health professionals may have to advocate for the family or actively connect them with the appropriate agency.

Summary

JIA is a chronic disease in which physical, psychosocial, and socio–ecological factors combine to influence the family's disease experience. It pervades every aspect of their lives. In addition to managing

Table 3.6.2 Suggested areas for psychological input

Child development

Understanding normative child development
Understanding the impact of illness on the attainment of developmental tasks
Understanding children's beliefs about the causes and treatment of illness

Needs-assessment

Creating supportive environments in which families can disclose fears and concerns
Developing effective child-centred and parent-centred communication/interviewing skills
Recognizing paediatric/adult symptoms of psychological maladjustment
Identifying risk and resilience factors
Using screening measures
Using appropriate multidisciplinary and inter-agency referral-routes

Interventions and health promotion

Promoting pain management
Preparing children and their families for medical procedures
Promoting adherence
Facilitating child and parent decision making
Providing developmentally appropriate disease education
Recognizing and promoting effective coping strategies
Providing social skills training (e.g. self-advocacy, dealing with bullying)
Developing basic counselling skills
Becoming an advocate for children and their parents

unpleasant symptoms and time-consuming treatments, families must also cope with the emotional impact of JIA, and a plethora of social barriers. It is not surprising therefore, that JIA places children and their families at risk of experiencing significant psychosocial problems. The reciprocal link between physical and psychosocial health means that failure to support the family's social and emotional needs may put the child's physical health at further risk. Optimal care in JIA therefore requires a family-centred approach that offers increased opportunities for psychological intervention and effective integration of health, psychological, and social services. Admittedly, there are no easy solutions to the issues raised and the feasibility and cost-effectiveness of many of the interventions are uncertain. Managing the psychosocial needs of families does involve utilizing resources that are often limited and difficult to access. However, while *resources* are important, being *resourceful* is equally valuable. Much can be achieved by understanding the psychosocial aspects of JIA, providing opportunities for families to discuss concerns, making links with local services and identifying existing resources. Rheumatology professionals are certainly in the best position to promote long-term healthy adaptation and by grasping this opportunity, families will have a much greater chance of meeting the challenges of JIA.

Useful reading

Bradford, R. *Children, Families and Chronic Disease*. London: Routledge, 1997.
Eiser, C. *Growing up With a Chronic Disease: the Impact on Children and Their Families*. London: Jessica Kingsley Publishers Ltd, 1993.
Thompson, R.J. and Gustafson, K.E. *Adaptation to Chronic Childhood Illness*. Washington DC: American Psychological Association, 1996.

References

1. Southwood, T.R. and Malleson, P.N. The epidemiology of arthritis: an overview. In T.R. Southwood and P.N., Malleson eds. *Arthritis in Children and Adolescents*. London: Bailliere's Clinical Paediatrics; *Int Pract Res* 1993;1:635–6.
2. Barlow, J.H., Harrison, K., and Shaw, K.L. The experience of parenting in the context of juvenile chronic arthritis. *Clin Child Psychol Psychiatry* 1998;3:445–63.
3. Taylor, D.C. Mechanisms of coping with handicap. In G.T. McCarthy, ed. *Physical Disability in Childhood. An Interdisciplinary Approach to Management*. London: Churchill Livingsone, 1992, pp. 53–64.
4. Worthington, R. The chronically ill child and recurring family grief. *J Fam Pract* 1989;29:397–400.
5. Eiser, C. *Growing up with a chronic disease: the impact on children and their families*. London: Jessica Kingsley Publishers Ltd, 1993, pp. 175–195.
6. Cadman, D., Goldsmith, C., and Bashim, P. The Ontario Child Health Study: Social adjustment and mental health of siblings of children with chronic health problems. *J Dev Bev Pediatri* 1988;9:117–21.
7. Kroll, T., Barlow, J.H., and Shaw, K. Treatment adherence in juvenile rheumatoid arthritis. A review. *Scand J Rheumatol* 1999;28:10–8.
8. Konkol, L., Lineberry, J., Gottlieb, J., Shelby, P.E., Miller III, J.J., and Lorig, K. Impact of juvenile arthritis on families: an educational assessment. *Arthritis Care Res* 1989;2:40–8.
9. Timko, C., Stovel, K.W., and Moos, R.H. Functioning among mothers and fathers of children with juvenile rheumatic disease. A longitudinal study. *J Pediatr Psychol* 1992;17:705–24.
10. Horwitz, W.A. and Kazak, A.E. Family adaptation to childhood cancer: sibling and family system variables. *J Clin Child Psychol* 1990;19:221–8.
11. Berry, S.L., Hayford, J.R., Ross, C.K., Pachman, L.M., and Lavigne, J.V. Conceptions of illness by children with juvenile rheumatoid arthritis: a cognitive developmental approach. *J Pediatr Psychol* 1993;18:83–97.
12. Bibace, R. and Walsh, M.E. Development of children's concepts of illness. *Pediatrics* 1980;66:912–7.
13. Burbach, D.J. and Peterson, L. Children's concepts of physical illness: a review and critique of the cognitive-developmental literature. *Health Psychol* 1986;5:307–25.
14. Piaget, J. Intellectual evolution from adolescence to adulthood. *Hum Dev* 1972;15:1–12.
15. Piaget, J. *The child's conception of the world*. London: Paladin, 1973.
16. Eiser, C. Children's concepts of illness: towards an alternative to the 'stage' approach. *Psyhol Health* 1989;3:93–101.
17. Bowlby, J. *Attachment and Loss*, Vol.1. New York: Basic Books, 1969.
18. Weitzman, M. School and peer relations. *Pediatr Clin North Am* 1984;31:59–69.
19. Kurtz, Z. and Hopkins, A. Services for young people with chronic disorders in their transition from childhood to adult life. London: Royal College of Physicians of London, 1996.
20. Lovell, D.J., Athreya, B., Emery, H.M. *et al.* (1990). School attendance and patterns, special services and special needs in pediatric patients with rheumatic diseases. *Arthritis Care Res* 1990;3:196–203.
21. Stoff, E., Bacon, M.C., and White, P. The effects of fatigue, distractibility and absenteeism on school achievement in children with rheumatic diseases. *Arthritis Care Res* 1989;2:49–53.
22. Hull, R.G. Outcome in juvenile arthritis. *Br J, Rheumatol* 1988;27:66–71.
23. Coleman, J. and Roker, D. Adolescence. *Psychologist* 1998;11:593–6.
24. Hurst, R. A disabled person's viewpoint. In Z. Kurtz, and A. Hopkins, eds. *Services for Young People with Chronic Disorders in their Transition from Childhood to Adult Life*. London: Royal College of Physicians of London, 1996, pp. 1–12.
25. Nutbeam, D. and Booth, M.I. Health behaviour in adolescence: risk and reasons. In G.H. Penny, P. Bennett, and M. Herbert, eds. *Health*

Psychology. A Lifespan Perspective. Reading, MA: Harwood Academic Publishers, 1994.

26. Thompson, R.J. and Gustafson, K.E. *Adaptation to Chronic Childhood Illness.* Washington DC: American Psychological Association, 1996.

27. Wallander, J.L. and Thompson, R.J. Psychosocial adjustment of children with chronic physical conditions. In M.C. Roberts, ed. *Handbook of Pediatric Psychology.* New York: Guidford Press, 1995, pp. 124–41.

28. Frank, R.G., Hagglund, K.J., Schopp, L.H *et al.* Disease and family contributors to adaptation in juvenile rheumatoid arthritis and juvenile diabetes. *Arthritis Care Res* 1998;11:166–76.

29. Huygen, A.C.J., Kuis, W., and Sinnema, G. Psychosocial, behavioral, and social adjustment in children and adolescents with juvenile chronic arthritis. *Ann Rheum Dis* 2000;59:276–82.

30. Achenbach, T. and Edlebrock, C. *Manual for the Child Behavior Checklist and Revised Behavior Profile.* Burlington, VT: University Associates in Psychiatry, 1983.

31. Martin, K. and Woo, P. Outcome in juvenile chronic arthritis. *Rev Rheumatol* 1997;10:S242.

32. Petersen, L.S., Mason, T., Nelson, A.M., O'Fallon, W.M., and Gabriel, S.E. Psychosocial outcomes and health status of adults who have had juvenile rheumatoid arthritis: a controlled population-based study. *Arthritis Rheum* 1997;40:2235–40.

33. David, J., Cooper, C., Hickey, L., *et al.* The functional and psychosocial outcomes of juvenile chronic arthritis. *Br J Rheumatol* 1994;33:876–81.

34. Vandvik, I.H. and Eckblad, G. Relationship between pain, disease severity and psychosocial function in patients with juvenile Chronic arthritis. *Scand J Rheumatol* 1990;19:295–302.

35. Ungerer, J.A., Horgan, B., Chaltow, J., and Hampion, G.D. Psychosocial functioning in children and young adults with juvenile arthritis. *Pediatrics* 1988;81:195–202.

36. Billings, A.G., Moos, R.H., Miller, J.J., and Gottlieb, J.E. Psychosocial adaptation in juvenile rheumatic disease: a controlled evaluation. *Health Psychol* 1987;6:343–59.

37. Timko, C., Stovel, K.W., Moos, R.H., and Miller, J.J. Adaptation to juvenile rheumatic disease: a controlled evaluation of functional disability with a one-year follow-up. *Health Psychol* 1992;11:67–76.

38. Daltroy, L.H., Larson, M.G., Eaton, H.M. *et al.* Psychosocial adjustment in juvenile arthritis. *J Pediatr Psychol* 1992;17:277–89.

39. Ross, C.K., Lavigne, J.V., Hayford, J.R., Berry, S.I., Sinacore, J.M., and Pachman, L.M. Psychological factors affecting reported pain in juvenile rheumatoid arthritis. *J Pediatr Psychol* 1993;18:561–73.

40. Thompson, K.L., Varni, J.W., and Hanson, V. Comprehensive assessment of pain in juvenile rheumatoid arthritis: an empirical model. *J Pediatr Psychol* 1987;1:24155.

41. Hagglund, K.J., Schopp, L.M., Alberts, R., Cassidy, J.T., and Frank, R.G. Predicting pain among children with juvenile rheumatoid arthritis. *Arthritis Care Res* 1995;8:36–42.

42. Schanberg, L.E., Sandstrom, M.J., Starr, K. *et al.* The relationship of daily mood and stressful events to symptoms in juvenile rheumatic disease. *Arthritis Care Res* 2000;13:33–41.

43. Timko, C., Stovel, K.W., Moos, R.H., and Miller III, J.J. A longitudinal study of risk and resistance among children with juvenile rheumatic disease. *J Clin Child Psychol* 1992;21:132–42.

44. Ennett, S.T., DeVellis, B.M., Earp, J.A., Kredich, D., Warren, R.W., and Wilhelm, C.L. Disease experience and psychosocial adjustment in children with juvenile rheumatoid arthritis: children's versus mother's reports. *J Pediatr Psychol* 1991;16:557–68.

45. Chaney, J.M., and Peterson, L. Family variables and disease management in juvenile rheumatoid arthritis. *J Pediatr Psychol* 1989;14:389–404.

46. Timko, C., Stovel, K.W., Baumgartner, M., and Moos, R.H. Acute and chronic stressors, social resources, and functioning among adolescents with juvenile rheumatic disease. *J Res Adolesc* 1995;5:361–85.

47. Wallender, J.L., Varni, J.W., Babani, L., Banis and H.T, Wilcox KT. Family resources as resistance factors for psychological maladjustment in chronically ill and handicapped children. *J Pediatr Psychol* 1989; 14:157–73.

48. Bradford, R. Children, Families and Chronic Disease. London: Routledge, 1997.

49. Brown, R.T., Doepke, K.L., and Kaslow, N.J. Risk-resistance-adaptation model for pediatric chronic illness: sickle cell syndrome as an example. *Clin Psychol Rev* 1993;13:119–32.

50. Dunst, C.J., Trivette, C.M., Davis, M., and Cornwell, J. Enabling and empowering families of children with health impairments. *Child Health Care* 1988;17:71–81.

51. Elander, J. and Midence, K. Children with chronic illness. *Psychologist* 1997;10:211–5.

52. Miller, J.J. Psychosocial factors related to rheumatic disease in childhood. *J Rheumatol* 1993;20:1–11.

53. Reisine, S.T. Arthritis and the family. *Arthritis Care Res* 1995;8:265–71.

54. Wallander, J.L. and Varni, J.W. Social support and adjustment in chronically ill and handicapped children. *Am J Community Psychol* 1989;17:185–201.

55. Lustig, J.L., Ireys, H.T., Sills, E.M, and Walsh, B.B. Mental health of children with juvenile rheumatoid arthritis: appraisal as a mediator. *J Pediatr Psychol* 1996;12:719–33.

56. Barlow, J.H., Shaw, K.L., and Southwood, T.R. Do psychosocial interventions have a role to play in paediatric rheumatology? *Br J Rheumatol* 1998;37:573–8.

57. World Health Organization. Final report, Regional Working Group on health needs of adolescents. Manilla, Philippines, 1980.

3.7 Pain assessment and management

David D. Sherry, James W. Varni, and Michael A. Rapoff

Aim

The aim of this chapter is to discuss the assessment of pain in children, pain coping, cognitive behavioral management, and medical management in the context of arthritis pain, and painful procedures.

Structure

- Introduction
- Pain assessment
- Comprehensive assessment of paediatric pain
- Health-related quality of life
- Pain coping
- Cognitive-behavioural treatment
- Cognitive-behavioural therapy in JIA
- Medical management
- Summary

Introduction

Arthritis, conjures up images of joint pain and, as expected, most children with arthritis have significant pain and stiffness associated with their disease. Children, on the whole, experience as much pain as do adults under similar circumstances although we recognize that some children report either no pain or less pain than do adults [1,2]. Pain is subjective and personal which makes the communication and treatment of this experience in children especially challenging. The issue is further clouded by the studies demonstrating that the degree of arthritis is not always correlated with the intensity of reported pain [1,3]. Part of the problem of adequately addressing the pain of childhood arthritis rests in the fact that pain has not been a focus of research of most rheumatologists or psychologists, and therefore is inadequately studied. Given the prevalence of childhood arthritis, this is an area sorely needing further research. In addition to the pain of arthritis, the pain of various procedures such as venepunctures and intra-articular corticosteroid injections, is a major issue for children.

Pain is an unpleasant sensory and emotional experience associated with actual or potential tissue damage or described in such terms [4]. In addition to the inflammatory damage, other factors that shape the pain experience include the child's developmental level, emotional and cognitive state, personality traits, cultural background, physical condition, and past pain experience [5]. Determining the meaning of the pain to the child and family and how it affects their daily lives will help the clinician understand the pain from the child's and family's perspective and is the first step in adequately addressing the pain. This chapter will deal with the assessment of pain in children, pain coping, cognitive-behavioural management, and medical management in the context of arthritis pain and painful procedures.

Pain assessment

The three types of paediatric pain assessment methods described in the literature are physiologic monitoring, behavioural observations, and self-report.

Physiological monitoring

Physiological monitoring captures indicators of sympathetic nervous system stimulation associated with pain and involves monitoring parameters such as heart rate, blood pressure, respiratory rate, and beta-endorphin levels. In clinical settings, pain is often associated with changes of 10–20% in noninvasively measured physiological parameters, such as heart rate [6]. This method of assessing pain is usually done for acute pain. For example, Leonard *et al.*, measured beta-endorphin levels in 10 adolescents receiving posterior spinal fusion surgery and found a significant but modest inverse correlation between beta-endorphin levels and pain ratings by patients ($r = -30$, $p = 0.014$) [7]. Physiological monitoring can be useful for patients who are unable to report their pain, and may elucidate mechanisms that underlie the experience of pain [8]. However, physiological responses tend to habituate over time with persistent pain and they may reflect general arousal associated with states other than pain, such as anxiety. Therefore, physiological monitoring would be more useful for acute pain and for experimental purposes.

Behavioural observation

Observing and coding pain behaviours is usually done for acute pain associated with invasive medical procedures [6]. However, Jaworski *et al.*, developed and validated an observation method for assessing pain behaviours in 30 children with JIA [9]. The children were videotaped over a 10-min session during which they performed a series of standard manoeuvres, including sitting, walking, standing, and reclining. The videotapes were then scored by trained observers to yield frequencies of individual pain behaviours (e.g. guarding, bracing, and rubbing) and total pain behaviours. The total pain behaviour scores were significantly and positively correlated with both child and parent ratings of pain, and with functional disability as rated by a trained observer. Behavioural observations may have a limited role in assessing pain in children with arthritis under standard conditions (such as performing physical manoeuvres or during physical examinations).

However, behavioural observations for chronic and recurrent pain are rarely utilized in the contemporary literature because of the lack of a significant relationship between pain behaviours and patient self-report of perceived pain intensity. A child can experience chronic and recurrent pain without necessarily exhibiting overt verbal and nonverbal pain behaviours. Consequently, behavioural observation techniques can result in considerable measurement error in assessing paediatric pain perception [10].

Self-report

Some investigators in the past questioned the validity of child pain self-report measures because adult observer estimates of child pain do not always correlate highly with child self-report. To doubt a child's pain self-report because of a lack of significant correlation with observer estimates of child pain is an erroneous concept. Pain is a subjective phenomenon; and other individuals cannot be expected to assess accurately another person's pain experience. Imperfect concordance, termed cross-informant variance [11] has been consistently documented among child/adolescent, parent, teacher, and healthcare professionals' reports in the assessment of children with chronic health conditions [12–14], as well as healthy children [15]. Agreement has been found to be lower for internalizing problems (e.g. depression) than for externalizing problems (e.g. hyperactivity). Given that pain derives from an individual's perceptions, the demonstration of cross-informant variance indicates an essential need in paediatric pain measurement for reliable and valid child self-report instruments for the broadest age range possible.

Assessment of self-reports of pain with children requires a full appreciation of the individual child's cognitive developmental stage in order to provide the appropriate measurement approach. Children's conceptualizations of pain mirrors Piaget's stages of cognitive development [16]. Support for the theory of developmental stages of pain perception has been found in a large-scale study of school-aged children's definitions of pain [17]. The pattern of responses given by the children followed a developmental sequence consonant with Piaget's theory of cognitive development. The children in the study showed a shift from concrete, perceptually dominated perspectives to more abstract, generalized, and psychologically oriented views with increasing age. In a second study, children's understanding of the causality of pain showed a developmental pattern similar to the pattern of development found in children's definitions of pain: Objective and abstract explanations of pain increased significantly with the children's age [17]. These findings emphasize the importance of children's conceptualizations of pain when conducting clinical assessments of pain perception in children across age groups.

The Paediatric Pain Questionnaire

In order to facilitate the incorporation of accurate pain measures in paediatric rheumatology, Varni and colleagues developed the Paediatric Pain Questionnaire (PPQ), designed to be sensitive to children's particular cognitive developmental stages and to include patient self-report as the major component. Although the PPQ is a comprehensive instrument, the three components that are most germane for assessment and intervention are the PPQ's age-appropriate visual analogue scale (VAS), body outline, and pain descriptor list.

Visual analogue scale

Present pain and worst pain intensity for the previous week are assessed in the PPQ by a VAS. Each VAS is a 10-cm horizontal line with no numbers, marks, or descriptive vocabulary words along the length of the line. The child VAS is "anchored" by developmentally appropriate pain descriptors (e.g. "not hurting," "hurting a whole lot") and by happy and sad faces at the beginning and end of the line, respectively. The adolescent and parent VAS are anchored by the phrases "no pain" and "severe pain," in addition to the pain descriptors "hurting" and "discomfort." The child, adolescent, or parent is asked to place a vertical line through the horizontal VAS line at the place that represents the intensity of pain along the continuum from no pain to severe pain.

The assessment of paediatric pain must fulfill the requirements for any measurement instrument, including reliability, validity, minimum inherent bias, and versatility [18]. The VAS, although deceptively simple, has demonstrated the reliability, validity, minimum inherent bias, and versatility necessary for an objective pain measure in a variety of experimental and clinical pain studies. Historically, the VAS has been used extensively with adult patients because of its sensitivity and reproducibility. As a continuous measurement scale, the VAS avoids the spurious clustering of pain reports that can occur with stepwise or categorical pain scaling methods. In both children and adults, the VAS has demonstrated excellent construct validity in postoperative medication studies, showing the expected reduction in pain subsequent to analgesia intake, and in studies of chronic musculoskeletal pain, demonstrating the expected increase in perceived pain intensity with greater rheumatic disease activity [19] and perceived stress and emotional distress [20,21]. The child VAS has been shown to be a reliable and valid measure of pain perception in children as young as 5 years of age [19,22].

Body outline

Body outline figures are very useful in helping children report the location of their pain. In the PPQ, age-appropriate body outlines are provided for children, adolescents, and parents. For children, a color-coded pain rating scale is used to measure both pain intensity and location. Four developmentally appropriate categories of pain descriptors are provided, along with eight standard crayons and the age-appropriate body outline. The child is instructed to color in the four boxes underneath each descriptive category representing pain intensity, and then to color in the body outline with the selected colour-intensity match. In this way, the child can communicate to the health professional not only the exact location of multiple painful joint sites, but four levels of pain intensity. Body outlines can be used effectively with children as young as 5 years of age [19].

Pain descriptors

The PPQ uses age-appropriate sensory, affective, and evaluative pain descriptors modified from the original McGill Pain Questionnaire [23]. The child is instructed to circle the words from the list that best describe his or her pain.

In the PPQ, children are given the opportunity to first write down words that describe their pain before being presented with the word list. However, for younger children, word recognition appears to be easier than generating their own words. Other investigators have shown that paediatric pain descriptors from a supplied word list correlated significantly with pain intensity scores and the number of pain sites (concurrent validity), and also demonstrated significant test–retest reliability [24].

Comprehensive assessment of paediatric pain

The degree of musculoskeletal pain experienced by a child with Juvenile Idiopathic Arthritis (JIA) is the result of the interaction between disease activity, tissue damage, and a number of factors specific to the individual child. Consequently, there is no "right" amount pain for any given amount of joint inflammation; the "right" amount is what the individual reports. The veracity of a child's pain report should not be questioned. Rather, a search for the factors that influence pain perception and report is a more meaningful clinical approach.

Pain assessment encompasses the measurement not only of pain intensity, location, and quality, but also of what exacerbates or ameliorates pain perception. Consequently, a comprehensive assessment of paediatric pain requires a multifactorial approach [25]. A multidimensional assessment battery provides a comprehensive basis for developing paediatric chronic and recurrent pain management interventions.

A conceptual biobehavioral model of the hypothesized predictors of paediatric pain has been proposed, in an attempt to account for the observed variability in paediatric pain perception and pain behavior (shown schematically in Figure 3.7.1) [26]. It has been developed in an effort to identify potentially modifiable constellations of factors to be targeted for intervention. In the model, the precipitants include disease (e.g. arthritis), physical injury, and psychological stress. Intervening factors are biological predispositions (e.g. behavioural genetics or temperament, age, gender, cognitive development), family environment (e.g. family functioning, family pain models, family reinforcement style), cognitive appraisal (e.g. meaning of pain), coping strategies (e.g. problem-focused or emotion-focused strategies), and perceived social support. Health-related quality of life (HRQOL) variables are hypothesized to be both affected by, and to affect pain perception and pain behaviour.

The theoretical framework can be further broken down into pain antecedents, factors having a casual role in pain onset or which exacerbate pain intensity; pain concomitants (e.g. depression, anxiety), which occur only during a painful episode and which may be reciprocal; and pain consequences, which persist beyond pain relief and include long-term psychological, social, and physical disability [20,21,26].

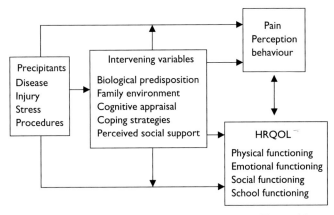

Figure 3.7.1 The biobehavioural model of paediatric pain. This model shows a variety of factors that may influence both the pain perception and pain behaviour.

For an individual child, the conceptual model can be used to help develop a tailored intervention. For example, if the child is experiencing a lack of family support or coping skills deficits, then interventions can be targeted for these problem areas. If the child is experiencing depressive symptoms associated with chronic pain, then an approach which combines both a direct intervention for pain, while also targeting the depressive symptoms, may most efficaciously ameliorate the child's distress. If a child is experiencing a great deal of stress, then interventions designed to problem-solve solutions for identified stressors are indicated (see also Part 3, Chapter 3.6). In the next sections, a fuller description of HRQOL and coping assessment will be presented since they are potentially modifiable components in the proposed model.

Health-related quality of life

Health-related quality of life measurement has increasingly been integrated into clinical trials, clinical practice improvement initiatives, and healthcare services research and evaluation as an essential health outcome [27–29]. While health status, functional status, and HRQOL are terms often used interchangeably, a recent meta-analysis suggests that a more parsimonious distinction between these terms is indicated [30]. Health status and functional status refer to physical functioning, whereas HRQOL additionally includes the psychosocial dimensions of emotional, social, and role functioning.

Measurement of HRQOL provides a more comprehensive assessment of the impact of paediatric chronic and recurrent pain than does traditional biomedical outcome tools. It is particularly useful in the comprehensive evaluation of chronic disease management, including pain management (see also Part 3, Chapter 3.4).

Paediatric quality of life and pain inventory

One option for HRQOL assessment is the PedsQL™4.0 (Paediatric Quality of Life Inventory™, Version 4.0) Generic Core Scales which have been tested in a range of chronic health conditions such as paediatric asthma, arthritis, diabetes, cystic fibrosis, cancer, as well as in physically healthy children. The PedsQL™Measurement Model is a modular approach to measuring HRQOL in children and adolescents, with both generic core scales and disease-specific modules [31]. The PedsQL™4.0 Generic Core Scales were designed as a generic HRQOL instrument to be utilized noncategorically (i.e. across multiple paediatric populations), and measure the core physical, mental, and social health dimensions as delineated by the World Health Organization (1948), and also include role (school) functioning [32]. Paediatric patient self-report (ages 5–18) and parent proxy-report (ages 2–18) forms are available for the 23-item PedsQL™4.0 Generic Core Scales that include the following domains: Physical Functioning (eight items), Emotional Functioning (five items), Social Functioning (five items), and School Functioning (five items). The PedsQL™4.0 distinguishes between healthy children and paediatric patients with arthritis and other rheumatological conditions, is responsive to clinical change over time in children with rheumatological conditions, and has demonstrated an impact on clinical decision making in paediatric rheumatology [33].

The 22-item PedsQL™ Arthritis Module includes scales measuring pain and hurt (four items), daily activities (five items), treatment problems (seven items), worry (three items), and communication (three items). The PedsQL™3.0 Arthritis Module scales have demonstrated acceptable internal consistency and reliability for group comparison construct validity, and responsiveness to individual patient change over time as a result of clinical intervention.

Pain coping

Interventions for children with chronic health conditions are often presented to children and their parents as opportunities to learn more effective coping strategies for handling the challenges of their condition. Standardized coping assessment provides a means for identifying coping strengths and deficits in a systematic manner.

The construct of "coping with pain" refers to the process whereby the child engages in cognitive and/or behavioural strategies to manage painful episodes. By definition, coping efforts may be either adaptive or maladaptive, depending on their outcomes in terms of pain relief, emotional adjustment, or functional status. Thus, coping is conceptualized as a process mechanism and not as an outcome measure. The assessment of both adaptive and maladaptive pain-coping strategies may help explain the variability in pain perception and pain behavior between children. Furthermore, the systematic study of paediatric pain-coping strategies may contribute substantially to the understanding of the individual differences observed in patients' responses to pharmacological and cognitive-behavioural treatment modalities.

Although coping has been studied to some extent in paediatric pain populations, research has focused mostly on the acute pain associated with painful procedures. In contrast, an extensive empirical literature in adult chronic pain patients has documented the effects of pain coping strategies on pain and adjustment [34].

Within the biobehavioural conceptual model of paediatric pain, coping strategies are hypothesized to be a vital intervening factor [26]. This theoretical framework served as the paradigm for the conceptual development of the Paediatric Pain Coping Inventory (PPCI). The PPCI was developed with the goal of facilitating research designed to further the understanding of the demonstrated individual differences in paediatric pain perception and pain behaviour, and potentially to give direction in the development and further refinement of cognitive-behavioural pain management treatment techniques for children.

Investigation of the psychometric properties of the PPCI in 187 children and adolescents with rheumatic disease revealed a five-factor multidimensional structure: Cognitive Self-Instruction (e.g. "Pretend I don't have any pain or hurt"), Seek Social Support (e.g. "Tell my mother or father"), Strive to Rest and Be Alone (e.g. "Go to bed"), Cognitive Refocusing (e.g. "Play a game"), and Problem-Solving Self-Efficacy (e.g. "Know that I can do something to make the pain or hurt feel better") [20]. Pain-coping strategies were significantly correlated with pain and adjustment outcome measures and depending on the direction of the correlation, they could be considered adaptive or maladaptive. For example, greater utilization of Cognitive Refocusing coping was associated with lower patient-reported worst pain and depressive symptoms, and lower parent-rated patient present pain, worst pain, and internalizing emotional problems. In contrast, greater utilization of Strive to Rest and Be Alone coping was associated with higher patient-reported and parent-rated patient present pain, worst pain, depressive symptoms, state and trait anxiety, internalizing emotional problems, and lower self-esteem.

Recently, a paediatric pain-coping measure, the Pain Coping Questionnaire (PCQ), has been developed and preliminary psychometric data from three samples has been reported in 258 healthy children, 28 children with arthritis, and 48 children with recurrent headaches [35]. Factor analysis supported eight hypothesized subscales: Information Seeking (e.g. "Ask a doctor or nurse questions"), Problem Solving (e.g. "Figure out what I can do about it"), Seeking Social Support (e.g. "Tell someone how I feel"), Positive Self-Statements (e.g. "Tell myself it's not so bad"), Behavioural Distraction (e.g. "Do something fun"), Cognitive Distraction (e.g. "Put it out of my mind"), Externalizing (e.g. "Say mean things to people"), and Internalizing/Catastrophizing (e.g. "Think that the pain will never stop"). Higher-order factor analysis yielded three overall factors: Approach coping (including Information Seeking, Problem Solving, and Seeking Social Support subscales), Problem-Focused coping (including Positive Self-Statements, Behavioural Distraction, and Cognitive Distraction subscales) and Emotion Focused coping (including Externalizing and Internalizing/Catastrophizing subscales). In children with arthritis, higher utilization of Emotion-Focused coping was associated with greater pain intensity, pain duration, and anxiety. Higher utilization of Approach coping was related to lower functional disability. Preliminary data on reliability and validity of a Danish translation of the PCQ has been reported on a sample of 352 healthy children and a sample of 40 children with arthritis for coping with experimentally-induced pain (cold pressor test) and clinical pain [36].

Cognitive-behavioural treatment

There is increasing evidence for the value of cognitive-behavioural therapy techniques in managing paediatric pain [37,38]. The primary cognitive-behavioural treatment techniques utilized in the management of paediatric pain and distress have been categorized as follows: *pain perception regulation* using such self-regulatory techniques as progressive muscle relaxation, meditation, and guided imagery; *pain behaviour modification* which identifies and modifies social and environmental factors that influence pain expression and rehabilitation [39].

Communicating the pain concept

In contrast to the rather extensive research literature on the assessment and management of pain in adult rheumatoid arthritis (RA), pain associated with JIA, and the other paediatric rheumatic diseases has not been as widely investigated. Given that there is not a one-to-one relationship between disease activity and pain intensity (psychological and social factors modifying the pain experience) focusing only on disease control may not provide adequate patient care. Measurement of pain should be considered as vital as measurement of disease activity parameters, and pain levels should be regularly assessed at all clinic visits as a routine part of patient care [10]. A comprehensive pain management approach in paediatric rheumatology should ideally combine appropriate pharmacological agents with cognitive-behavioural therapy and physical modalities to optimize patients' quality of life [10].

A comprehensive pain management approach requires that children and parents "buy in" to a biobehavioural or multidimensional model of pain. A careful and understandable presentation of the physiological and psychological components of pain needs to be made that avoids any suggestion that children's pain is psychogenic or "in their heads." A "puzzle" has been suggested as a descriptive visual metaphor for

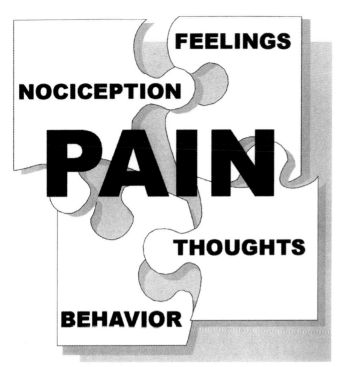

Fig. 3.7.2 The pain puzzle.

pain because pain is a "puzzling" phenomenon and the pain experience consists of various interlocking "pieces" that form a "whole." The pain puzzle (Figure 3.7.2) is a visual and conceptual metaphor that has been used clinically and in research studies with children having disease-related pain and their families [40].

Nociception

The "nociception piece" of the pain puzzle is the physiological, anatomical, and chemical properties of the nervous system that contribute to the perception of pain. Patients and their parents can be given a basic description of the nociceptive system with specific information about joint pain transmission and the role of chemical mediators of inflammation (e.g. prostaglandins) which sensitize joint afferent nerve fibres. Implications for pain treatment deduced from nociceptive factors include: early identification and aggressive pharmacological treatment of chronic arthritis (inverting the traditional therapeutic pyramid); the importance of strategies to maintain adherence to effective pharmacological therapies [41]; and the value of non-pharmacological therapies (e.g. cooling and resting an inflamed joint, relaxation exercises) in controlling nociceptive input and reducing peripheral and central sensitization mechanisms.

Feelings

The "feelings piece" of the pain puzzle captures the strong link between emotional distress (particularly anxiety and depression) and pain. Patients and parents can learn about the reciprocal link between distress and pain. For example, emotional distress can be a consequence of pain (e.g. increased pain results in reduction in social/recreational activities which contributes to depression) or distress can exacerbate pain (e.g. increased distress contributes to muscle tension and increased pain). Treatment based on affective factors include:

1. *Psychological interventions* (e.g. relaxation, problem-solving) which reduce general and disease-related stress and therefore can directly reduce pain intensity and pain interference.

2. *Emotional enhancement* (such as humour) which provide physiological and psychological benefits and may function as analgesics.

3. *Drug interventions* (e.g. antidepressants) which may help reduce depression and pain through common biological pathways (regulation of serotonin).

Thoughts

The "thoughts piece" of the pain puzzle is concerned with how people attend to and think about the experience of pain. The focus in the pain literature has been on nonadaptive thinking, rather than adaptive thinking. Cognitive processing of pain can be nonadaptive in at least two ways: children may fail to understand or pay attention to the information or may fail to generate self-talk that might be helpful in coping with pain, or they can actively engage in dysfunctional thinking that leads to maladaptive coping and greater pain. A particular "toxic" type of dysfunctional thinking consistently identified in the literature is "catastrophizing," which includes three components: rumination (preoccupation with pain-related thoughts); magnification (exaggeration of the threat value of pain); and helplessness (thinking that one cannot do anything about the pain).

Children who do not pay appropriate attention to their thoughts, can be helped to increase their awareness by the use of "thought diaries" as a first step in learning to cope with pain. Cognitive restructuring strategies can be taught to counter nonadaptive thinking (e.g. substitute "I can't do anything to make my pain better" with "I can do relaxation exercises to reduce my pain"). Distraction techniques (e.g. guided imagery, participate in engaging activities) can be learnt to help with the management of acute exacerbations of pain, and for painful procedures.

Behaviour

The "behaviour piece" of the pain puzzle refers to both verbal and nonverbal pain behaviours displayed by patients and the responses of significant others (e.g. parents, siblings, friends) to these behaviours. Pain behaviours, like any behaviours, are influenced by reinforcement and punishment (e.g. positively reinforced by attention from others or negatively reinforced by avoiding aversive events such as homework). Pain behaviours, such as guarding and malpositioning of affected joints, can be maladaptive for children with arthritis. Responses to a child's pain behaviours by other important individuals, may also be maladaptive, such as when parents allow children to avoid attending school, resulting in low academic performance and missed opportunities for social interaction. Observational learning or parental modelling is also an important determinant of how children learn to express their pain and about the consequences of pain expression. New observational measures need to be developed to capture pain behaviours and the responses of significant others' to these behaviours. Parents are important role models for their children and they need to be able to model appropriate coping strategies when they themselves experience pain. Parents and other important individuals (e.g. grandparents, teachers) need to be taught how to avoid being overly solicitous and attentive to pain behaviours, and how to reinforce the child's adaptive coping strategies.

Cognitive-behavioural therapy in JIA

One study applied cognitive-behavioural therapy techniques to 13 children aged 5–16 years with JIA [42]. The intervention was based on a previously developed self-regulation treatment package for chronic musculoskeletal pain in hemophilic arthropathy (43,44).

Instruction in the cognitive-behavioural self-regulation of joint pain perception consisted of three sequential phases:

1. Each child was first taught a 25-step progressive muscle relaxation sequence involving the alternative tensing and relaxing of major muscle groups.

2. The child was then taught meditative breathing exercises, consisting of medium–deep breaths inhaled through the nose and slowly exhaled through the mouth. While exhaling, the child was instructed to say the word "relax" silently to himself or herself, and to initially describe aloud and subsequently visualize the word "relax" in warm colors, as if written in coloured chalk on a blackboard.

3. Finally, the child was instructed in the use of guided imagery techniques consisting of pleasant, distracting scenes selected by the child. The child was instructed to imagine being in a scene previously experienced as pain-free. Initially, the child was instructed to imagine actually being in the scene, not simply to observe himself or herself there. The scene was evoked by a detailed multisensory description by the therapist and subsequently described out loud by the child. Such scenes depended on the child's preference, but could include detailed descriptions of the sound sights of ocean and beach. Once the scene was clearly visualized by the child, the child was instructed to experiment with other, different scenes to maintain interest and variety. Additional guided imagery techniques involved invoking images that represented a metaphor for the sensory pain experience, and then altering the metaphor and thus the perception of pain. Specific images were based on sensory descriptors endorsed on the PPQ, with elaboration through subsequent discussion in an attempt to generate a concrete metaphor. For example, if a child described the pain as "hot," a metaphoric image might be that "Someone is in my knee with a blowtorch." An image was then generated of a blowtorch in the knee that was subsequently extinguished. Another alternative involved the use of colours. Children generated images in which painful sites appeared in a particular colour that contrasted with pain-free tissue. They then imagined the coloured area shrinking and then disappearing. Finally, for some of the older children, sessions began with a simple review of the nervous system, and then images of "pain switches" were used to block the transmission of pain messages.

The children were instructed to practice these techniques on a regular basis at home, and were seen for a total of eight weekly individual sessions for maintenance problem solving. Parents were seen on two occasions. In the first session, a review of behavioural pain management techniques was provided. Specific suggestions for implementation with their children were made, including behaviour modification techniques to encourage adaptive activities and to discourage maladaptive pain behaviours [45]. The second session, held 4–6 weeks after the first,

served as a forum to discuss the implementation of behavioural pain management and to address questions that may have arisen.

To assess the immediate short-term effects on the intervention, the children were administered the PPQ's VAS for present pain just prior to engaging in the self-regulation techniques (taking about 20 min), and were immediately re-administered the VAS. Data collected in the clinic setting demonstrated excellent immediate short-term benefits of the self-regulation techniques. To assess more long-term effects, the children were reviewed at 6 and 12 months. At the 6-month assessment, the children's average home ratings of pain on the VAS were significantly lower. Although there was some increase of pain at the 12-month assessment relative to the 6-month assessment, the average pain intensity was still in the mild range. Parent VAS data essentially paralleled those of their children at the follow-up periods. Functional status, as measured by the Child Activities of Daily Living Index [46] also showed improvement at the 6- and 12-month evaluations relative to the pretreatment baseline [46].

The results of this study on the self-regulation of chronic musculoskeletal pain by children with JIA suggest the value of cognitive-behavioural techniques as components of the comprehensive management of children with chronic arthritis. The findings support the potential of combining these cognitive-behavioural techniques with disease-modifying pharmacological treatments in order to minimize the pain associated with JIA, and to maximize overall quality of life [10]. An identical cognitive-behavioural therapy treatment package has been successfully utilized for chronic musculoskeletal pain associated with hemophilic arthropathy [44]. Other studies have also successfully employed cognitive-behavioural therapy for pain management in adult RA [47,48] and in JIA [49]. The consistency of the findings across various paediatric and adult musculoskeletal pain populations supports the potential generalizability of these initial findings. These techniques provide children with skills in self-regulation as a means of reducing levels of pain intensity, which may hopefully lead to enhanced HRQOL.

Medical management

Pain is rarely used as an outcome for medical therapies although decreasing inflammation is one important factor in decreasing joint pain. However, even with optimal treatment of the arthritis and utilizing appropriate behavioural and cognitive techniques, pain can continue to cause distress and dysfunction particularly in those children with severely damaged joints. Such children should not be denied the benefit of other analgesic management including analgesic medications, physical and occupational therapy, and surgery.

Analgesic medication

One of the first treatments used is simple analgesia (Figure 3.7.3). Acetaminophen may be used alone or in addition to a nonsteroidal anti-inflammatory drug (NSAID). For more intense pain, if the child is not on a NSAID, ketorolac is a useful drug. Ketorolac is a potent analgesic but because it is an NSAID it is not advisable to add it to another NSAID. If this is inadequate then tramadol, hydrocodone (with acetaminophen), or oxycodone (with acetaminophen) may be added. Codeine is not advised as it has a high rate of side-effects and is relatively ineffective. For more intense chronic pain, long-acting opioids may be used. Pain is usually best controlled by using analgesics

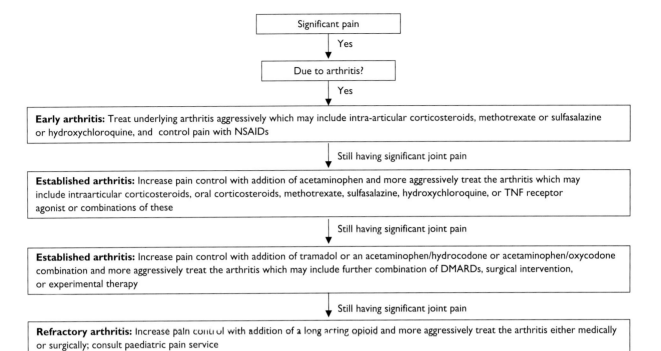

Fig. 3.7.3 An approach to the management of pain in children with JIA. In addition, physical and occupational therapy, and cognitive-behavioural treatments should be utilized Not every patient requires the same interventions, as mutiple factors influence the pain including the degree of the destruction, development age, coping strategies, and the preferences of parents, patient and the paediatric rheumatology team (Modified from American Pain Society.)

Table 3.7.1 Medications used for pain control

Generic	Proprietary[a]	Adult dose	Paediatric dose	Available forms[a]
Acetaminophen	Multiple	Up to 1 gm QID	10–15 mg/kg/dose q 4–6 h maximum 5 doses/24 hours	Drops, 100 mg/ml; Elixir 160 mg/5 ml Suspension 160 mg/5 ml Chewable 80 mg Tablet caplet 325 mg, 500 mg, 650 mg
Tramadol	Ultram	50–100 mg q 4–6 h 400 mg maximum	Not available	Tablet, 50 mg
Hydrocodone combinations				
Acetaminophen	Vicodin Lortab	5–10 mg[b] q 4 h 60 mg[b] maximum	0.2 mg/kg/dose[b] q 6–8 h (q 8 h if < 2 years old)	Tablets: acetaminophen/hydrocodone 500/5, 500/7.5, 500/10, 750/7.5, 660/10
ASA	Lortab ASA	1–2 tablets q 4 h		Tablet: 325 mg ASA, 5 mg hydrocodone
Ibuprofen	Vicoprofen	1 q 4–6 h		Tablet: 200 mg ibuprofen, 7.5 mg hydrocodone
Oxycodone				
Immediate release	OxyIR Roxicodone	1–2 tablets q 4–6 h	0.2 mg[b]/kg/dose q 3–4 h	Tablet 5 mg Liquid 1 mg/ml
Controlled release	OxyContin	10–40 mg q 12 h	Not available	Tablet, 10 mg, 20 mg
Combined with				
Acetaminophen	Percocet Tylox Roxicet	1–2 tablets q 4–6 h	0.2 mg[b]/kg/dose q 3–4 h Maximum 5 mg[b]/dose	Tablet: acetaminophen 325 mg, oxycodone 5 mg Liquid: 325/5 per 5 ml
Aspirin	Percodan	1–2 tablets q 4–6 h	0.2 mg[b]/kg/dose q 3–4 h maximum 5 mg[a]/dose	Tablet: ASA 325 mg, oxycodone 4.5 mg
Morphine SR	MS Contin Oramorph SR	15–30 mg q 8–12 h	0.5–0.75 mg/kg/dose q 8–12 h	Tablets 15 mg, 30 mg, 60 mg, 100 mg 200 mg

[a] Proprietary names and available forms may vary from country to country.

[b] Dose based on either the hydrocodone or oxycodone component.

on a regular, rather than "as needed basis," and this is certainly so once opioids are required. If available for children with chronic pain, the paediatric pain service, should be involved. When using an opioid one should anticipate side-effects especially constipation and initiate preventative treatment (Table 3.7.1).

Physical and occupational therapy

There are no studies that rigorously evaluate pain management using physical modalities in children. However, clinical experience suggests that an individual child reports less pain when treated with various physical and occupational interventions, including splinting, ice, heat, paraffin baths, massage, active exercise, and stretching. Joint protective techniques may help decrease the pain associated with daily living activities. Aerobic conditioning may also relieve pain, by improving the child's energy levels, and sense of wellbeing. This can be done safely; an 8-week program of structured physical conditioning improved the aerobic endurance of 25 children with Polyarthritis without exacerbating the arthritis or the pain [50].

Surgery

Surgery is sometimes an appropriate treatment for children with destroyed, painful joints or with refractory arthritis (see also Part 3, Chapter 3.12). Synovectomy of the elbow, knee, and proximal interphalangeal joints in children may result in a marked reduction of pain [51,52]. Soft-tissue release of the hips has decreased pain both in the short- and long-term [53,54]. As in adults, total joint replacement in children is usually very effective in relieving pain [55,56].

Complementary therapies

There are no studies of various complementary neutraceuticals and treatments that address the pain of arthritis in children. It seems probable that some of these therapies may provide pain relief, if only via a placebo effect.

Pain associated with procedures

Painful procedures including venepunctures and arthrocenteses need special attention in children since, for the most part, the child is not giving consent, and the procedures are often performed repeatedly. Therefore, they can be very distressing, especially for younger children who exhibit more distress during invasive procedures and rate procedure-related pain higher than older children [57,58]. Appropriate interventions to minimize pain and anxiety related to procedures should be an integral part of the management of children with arthritis. Interventions must be individually tailored to the child and the procedure.

Non-pharmacological interventions shown to be effective in helping children cope with painful procedures include: providing age-appropriate information about the procedure, distraction, relaxation exercises, guided imagery, and hypnosis [59]. The procedure should be explained in advance, and there should be discussion about what the child might experience. Allowing the child to role-play the procedure and practice effective coping strategies such as slow, deep breathing may help reduce anxiety and pain [60]. Anxiety can be diminished by allowing the parents to remain with the child to provide help with coping and distraction.

Topical anaesthetic agents, ice, and cognitive-behavioural techniques frequently help children who require repeated blood tests or subcutaneously administered medication. Lidocaine/prilocaine cream (EMLA®) has been shown to be safe and effective in decreasing the pain associated with venipuncture, vaccinations, lumbar puncture, subcutaneous drug reservoir injection, and neonatal circumcision [61]. Iontophoresis has also produced rapid, safe, and effective topical anaesthesia in children undergoing minor invasive procedures.

Intra-articular corticosteroid injections are the most frequent non-routine procedure performed on children with JIA. Repeated joint injections over the years may be required, so every effort should be made to reduce the pain and distress associated with the procedure. There are no studies of pain management of arthrocentesis in children, however, studies of other painful procedures in children indicate that cognitive-behavioural interventions and topical anaesthetics may be effective in minimizing arthrocentesis pain. In our experience, a calm environment, the presence of parents who have been educated how to help the child, the use of slow breathing, and other distraction techniques (such as bubble blowing), and the use of local anaesthesia with topical anaesthetic preparations (such as lidocaine/prilocaine cream or vapocoolant spray followed by buffered lidocaine), can help decrease the pain to the point that many children report only minimal discomfort. Lidocaine, is buffered by adding 2 ml of 1 mEq/ml sodium bicarbonate to 10 ml of 1% lidocaine.

For many children (and even adolescents) undergoing arthrocentesis, the use of "conscious sedation" with oral midazolam 0.2–0.3 mg/kg is often very helpful. This therapy is often associated with amnesia for the event, and therefore is extremely useful in minimizing anxiety if the child needs the arthrocentesis repeated in the future. If many joints need to be injected, or if the child is particularly upset at the idea of having an injection, general anaesthesia may be required. Post-injection pain is usually adequately managed with acetaminophen and ice but if many joints are injected ketorolac seems to be particularly helpful. When using conscious or deep sedation, the guidelines developed by the American Academy of Pediatrics for patient monitoring and resuscitative equipment should be followed [62].

Summary

Clearly, more research is needed on pain assessment and management strategies for children with arthritis. However, this should not hamper efforts to regularly assess and minimize acute and chronic pain in clinical rheumatology settings. We now know quite a lot about how to measure and manage pain in children. It is vital that physicians and other healthcare professionals looking after children with JIA use this knowledge effectively, so as to minimize pain, and thereby help the children to thrive even if the arthritis is difficult to control, and the joints are damaged.

References

1. Schanberg, L.E., Lefebvre, J.C., Keefe, F.J., Kredich, D.W., and Gil, and K.M. Pain coping and the pain experience in children with juvenile chronic arthritis. *Pain* 1997;73:181–9.
2. Hagglund, K.J., Schopp, L.M., Alberts, K.R., Cassidy, J.T, and Frank, R.G. Predicting pain among children with juvenile rheumatoid arthritis. *Arthritis Care Res* 1995;8:36–42.

3. Vandvik, I.H., and Eckblad, G. Relationship between pain, disease severity and psychosocial function in patients with juvenile chronic arthritis (JCA). *Scand J Rheumatol* 1990;19:295–302.

4. Merskey, D.M., and Bogduk N. (eds). *Classification of Chronic Pain. Descriptions of Chronic Pain Syndromes and Definitions of Pain Terms*, 2nd edn. Seattle, WA IASP Press, 1994.

5. Thastum, M., Zachariae, R., and Herlin, T. Pain experience and pain coping strategies in children with juvenile idiopathic arthritis. *J Rheumatol* 2001; 28:1091–98.

6. Franck, L.S., Greenberg, C.S., and Stevens, B. Pain assessment in infants and children. *Pediatr Clin N Am* 2000;47:487–512.

7. Leonard, T.M., Klem, S.A., Asher, M.A., Rapoff, M.A., and Leff, R.D. Relationship between pain severity and serum beta-endorphin levels in postoperative patients. *Pharmacotherapy* 1993;13:378–81.

8. Melzack, R., and Katz, J. Pain measurement in persons in pain. In: P.D., Wall, and R. Melzack (eds), *Textbook of Pain*, 3rd ed. New York: Churchill Livingstone, 1994:pp.37–51.

9. Jaworski, T.M., Bradley, L.A., Heck, L.W., Roca, A., and Alarcon, G.S. Development of an observation method for assessing pain behaviors in children with juvenile rheumatoid arthritis. *Arthritis Rheum* 1995;38: 1142–51.

10. Varni, J.W., and Bernstein, B.H. Evaluation and management of pain in children with rheumatic diseases. *Rheum Dis Clin N Am* 1991;17:985–1000.

11. Varni, J.W, Katz, E R , Colegrove, R., and Dolgin, M. Perceived physical appearance and adjustment of children with newly diagnosed cancer: a path analytic model. *J Behav Med* 1995;18:261–78.

12. Guyatt, G.H., Juniper, E.F., Griffith, L.E., Feeny, D.H., and Ferrie, P.J. Children and adult perceptions of childhood asthma. *Pediatrics* 1997;99:165–8.

13. Varni, J.W., Katz, E.R., Seid, M., Quiggins, D.J., Friedman-Bender, A., and Castro, C.M. The Pediatric Cancer Quality of Life Inventory (PCQL). I. Instrument development, descriptive statistics, and cross-informant variance. *J Behav Med* 1998;21:179–204.

14. Varni, J.W., and Setoguchi, Y. Screening for behavioral and emotional problems in children and adolescents with congenital or acquired limb deficiencies. *Am J Dis Child* 1992;146:103–7.

15. Achenbach, T.M., McConaughy, S.H., and Howell, C.T. Child/adolescent behavioral and emotional problems: implications of cross-informant correlations for situational specificity. *Psychol Bull* 1987;101:213–32.

16. Thompson, K.L., and Varni, J.W. A developmental cognitive-biobehavioral approach to pediatric pain assessment. *Pain* 1986;25:283–96.

17. Gaffney A, and Dunne, E.A. Developmental aspects of children's definitions of pain. *Pain* 1986;26:105–17.

18. McGrath, P.A. The measurement of human pain. *Endod Dent Traumatol* 1986;2:124–9.

19. Varni, J.W., Thompson, K.L., and Hanson, V. The Varni/Thompson Pediatric Pain Questionnaire. I. Chronic musculoskeletal pain in juvenile rheumatoid arthritis. *Pain* 1987;28:27–38.

20. Varni, J.W., Rapoff, M.A., Waldron, S.A., Gragg, R.A., Bernstein, B.H., and Lindsley, C.B. Effects of perceived stress on pediatric chronic pain. *J Behav Med* 1996;19:515–28.

21. Varni, J.W., Rapoff, M.A., Waldron, S.A., Gragg, R.A., Bernstein, B.H., and Lindsley, C.B. Chronic pain and emotional distress in children and adolescents. *J Dev Behav Pediatr* 1996;17:154–61.

22. McGrath, P.A., and de Veber, L.L. The management of acute pain evoked by medical procedures in children with cancer. *J Pain Sympt Manage* 1986;1:145–50.

23. Melzack, R. The McGill Pain Questionnaire: major properties and scoring methods. *Pain* 1975;1:277–99.

24. Wilkie, D.J., Holzemer, W.L., Tesler, M.D., Ward, J.A., Paul, S.M., and Savedra, M.C. Measuring pain quality: validity and reliability of children's and adolescents' pain language. *Pain* 1990;41:151–9.

25. Thompson, K.L., Varni, J.W., and Hanson, V. Comprehensive assessment of pain in juvenile rheumatoid arthritis: an empirical model. *J Pediatr Psychol* 1987;12:241–55.

26. Varni, J.W. *An Empirical Model for the Biobehavioral Investigation of Pediatric Pain*. Phoenix: American Pain Society, 1989.

27. Faryers, P.M., and Machin, D. *Quality of Life: Assessment, Analysis, and Interpretation*. New York: John Wiley & sons, 2000.

28. Spilker, B. *Quality of Life and Pharmacoeconomics in Clinical Trials*, 2nd edn. Philadelphia, PA: Lippincott-Raven, 1996.

29. Varni, J.W., Seid, M., and Kurtin, P.S. Pediatric health-related quality of life measurement technology: a guide for health care decision makers. *J Clin Outcomes Man* 999;6:33–40.

30. Smith, K.W., Avis, N.E., and Assmann, S.F. Distinguishing between quality of life and health status in quality of life research: a meta-analysis. *Qual Life Res* 1999;8:447–59.

31. Varni, J.W., Seid, M., and Rode, C.A. The PedsQL: measurement model for the pediatric quality of life inventory. *Med Care* 1999;37:126–39.

32. Varni, J.W., Seid, M., and Kurtin,. P.S. The PedsQL 4.0: reliability and validity of the Pediatric Quality of Live Inventory Version 4.0 generic core scales in healthy and patient populations. *Med Care* 2001;39: 800–12.

33. Varni, J.W., Seid, M., Smith, T.S., Burwinkle, T., Brown, J., and Szer, I.S. The PedsQL™ in pediatric rheumatology: reliability, validity and responsiveness of the Pediatric Quality of Life Inventory™ Generic Core Scales and Rheumatology Module. *Arthritis Rheum* 2002;46:714–25.

34. Jensen, M.P., Turner, J.A., Romano, J.M., and Karoly, P. Coping with chronic pain. a critical review of the literature. *Pain* 1991;47:249–83.

35. Reid, G.J., Gilbert, C.A., and McGrath, P.J. The Pain Coping Questionnaire: preliminary validation. *Pain* 1998;76:83–96.

36. Thastum, M., Zachariae, R., Scholer, M., and Herlin, T. A Danish adaptation of the Pain Coping Questionnaire for children: preliminary data concerning reliability and validity. *Acta Paediatr* 1999;88:132–8.

37. McGrath, P.A. *Pain in Children: Nature, Assessment, and Treatment*. New York: Guilford, 1990.

38. Holden, E.W., Deichmann, M.M., and Levy, J.D. Empirically supported treatments in pediatric psychology: recurrent pediatric headache. *J Pediatr Psychol* 1999;24:91–109.

39. Varni, J.W. *Clinical Behavioral Pediatrics: A Interdisciplinary Biobehavioral Approach*. New York: Pergamon Press, 1983.

40. Rapoff, M.A., and Lindsley, C.B. The pain puzzle: a visual and conceptual metaphor for understanding and treating pain in pediatric rheumatic disease. *J Rheumatol* 2000;27:29–33.

41. Rapoff, M.A. *Adherence to Pediatric Medical Regimens*. New York: Kluwer/Plenum, 1999.

42. Walco, G.A., Varni, J.W, and Ilowite, N.T. Cognitive-behavioral pain management in children with juvenile rheumatoid arthritis. *Pediatrics* 1992;89:1075–9.

43. Varni, J.W., Gilbert A, and Dietrich, S.L. Behavioral medicine in pain and analgesia management for the hemophilic child with factor VIII inhibitor. *Pain* 1981;11:121–6.

44. Varni, J.W. Behavioral medicine in hemophilia arthritic pain management: two case studies. *Arch Phys Med Rehabil* 1981;62:183–7.

45. Masek, B.J, Russo, D.C, and Varni, J.W. Behavioral approaches to the management of chronic pain in children. *Pediatr Clin N Am* 1984;31: 1113–31.

46. Varni, J.W, Wilcox, K.T, Hanson, V., and Brik R. Chronic musculoskeletal pain and functional status in juvenile rheumatoid arthritis: an empirical model. *Pain* 1988;32:1–7.

47. Bradley, L.A, Young, L.D., Anderson, K.O., *et al.* Effects of psychological therapy on pain behavior of rheumatoid arthritis patients. Treatment outcome and six-month followup. *Arthritis Rheum* 1987;30:1105–14.

48. Parker, J.C, Frank, R.G, Beck, N.C, *et al.* Pain management in rheumatoid arthritis patients. A cognitive-behavioral approach. *Arthritis Rheum* 1988;31:593–601.

49. Lavigne, J.V., Ross, C.K, Berry, S.L., Hayford, J.R., and Pachman, L.M. Evaluation of a psychological treatment package for treating pain in juvenile rheumatoid arthritis. *Arthritis Care Res* 1992;5:101–10.

50. Klepper, S.E. Effects of an eight-week physical conditioning program on disease signs and symptoms in children with chronic arthritis. *Arthritis Care Res* 1999;12:52–60.

51. Lonner, J.H., and Stuchin, S.A. Synovectomy, radial head excision, and anterior capsular release in stage III inflammatory arthritis of the elbow. *J Hand Surg [Am]* 1997;22:279–85.

52. Rydholm, U., Elborgh, R., Ranstam, J., Schroder, A., Svantesson, H., and Lidgren, L. Synovectomy of the knee in juvenile chronic arthritis. A retrospective, consecutive follow-up study. *J Bone Joint Surg Br* 1986;68:223–8.

53. Mogensen, B., Brattstrom, H., and Ekelund, L., Svantesson, H., Lidgren, L. Synovectomy of the hip in juvenile chronic arthritis. *J Bone Joint Surg Br* 1982;64:295–9.

54. Witt, J.D., and McCullough, C.J. Anterior soft-tissue release of the hip in juvenile chronic arthritis. *J Bone Joint Surg Br* 1994;76:267–70.

55. Witt, J.D., Swann, M., and Ansell, B.M. Total hip replacement for juvenile chronic arthritis. *J Bone Joint Surg Br* 1991;73:770–3.

56. Haber, D. and Goodman, S.B., Total hip arthroplasty in juvenile chronic arthritis: a consecutive series. *J Arthroplasty* 1998;13:259–65.

57. Kazak, A.E., Penati, B., Brophy, P., and Himelstein, B. Pharmacologic and psychologic interventions for procedural pain. *Pediatrics* 1998;102:59–66.

58. Wong, D.L. and Baker, C.M. Pain in children: comparison of assessment scales. *Okla Nurse* 1988;33:8.

59. Powers, S.W. Empirically supported treatments in pediatric psychology: procedure-related pain. *J Pediatr Psychol* 1999;24:131–45.

60. McCarthy, A.M., Cool, V.A., and Hanrahan, K. Cognitive behavioral interventions for children during painful procedures: research challenges and program development. *J Pediatr Nurs* 1998;13:55–63.

61. Miser, A.W., Goh, T.S., Dose, A.M., *et al*. Trial of a topically administered local anesthetic (EMLA cream) for pain relief during central venous port accesses in children with cancer. *J Pain Symptom Manage* 1994;9:259–64.

62. Anonymous. Guidelines for the elective use of conscious sedation, deep sedation, and general anesthesia in pediatric patients. Committee on Drugs. Section on anesthesiology. *Pediatrics* 1985;76:317–21.

Pharmacological treatment of early or established arthritis

Peter N. Malleson

Aim

The aim of this chapter is to discuss the usual pharmacological management of JIA in a manner that is practical, highlighting the benefits and disadvantages of the more commonly used drugs

Structure

- Introduction
- Management of early and established disease for each specific JIA subtypes with treatment algorithms.
- Management of refractory disease mentioned briefly
- Management of remission
- Discussion of specific anti-rheumatic drugs.
  NSAIDs
  DMARDs

Introduction

The treatment of Juvenile Idiopathic Arthritis (JIA) is challenging for both the physician and the patient. Although the goal of treatment is straightforward—to achieve remission of disease—without significant physical or emotional sequelae, there are no therapies that consistently and reliably achieve this result for all children. Some children with JIA have a mild disease course, and go into permanent remission, however, it is now recognized that JIA is not a benign disease for most children. Many will have disease well into adult life with significant morbidity (and occasionally mortality) [1,2]. There is also some evidence in adult rheumatoid arthritis that there is a "window of opportunity" early in the disease course during which time treatment may be significantly more effective than when used later in the disease [3]. The recognition of the non-benign nature of JIA, and the possibility that early disease may be more easy to treat than long-established disease, has led to increasingly early and more aggressive treatment strategies. The concept is to quickly and completely suppress the arthritis, so as to prevent, or minimize, any permanent structural damage to the joint, and to hopefully prevent the development of an irreversible self-perpetuating inflammatory process. Although as yet, there are no studies confirming the beneficial effects of this approach, there is general agreement among paediatric rheumatologists that they see less children with severely damaged joints and deformity than was the case even a decade ago. The decreasing need for surgery also supports this belief (see also Part 3, Chapter 3.12).

At present determining the optimal treatment for any individual patient is limited by uncertainty about whether that child will have a mild disease or a severe one. A child with apparently mild disease affecting only one joint at onset, may 10 years later have widespread erosive polyarthritis, whereas another child with Systemic Arthritis may be in complete remission with no evidence of joint damage several months later.

The lack of knowledge about the aetiopathophysiology of JIA, the variability of the disease, and uncertainty about the mechanism of action of the drugs used for its treatment (and in fact whether or not the drugs actually work) have also hindered the development of a consistent approach or approaches to the pharmacological management of JIA (see also Part 3, Chapter 3.13).

However, in recent years some factors predictive of poor outcome have been reported (4–6), and work is now underway to develop clinical treatment protocols of the kind used so successfully in childhood cancer. Furthermore the recognition of the central roles of certain cytokines (TNFα and IL-1), has led to the development of the "biologics," that are already being shown to have a dramatic effect in children with JIA resistant to the more conventional therapies (see also Part 3, Chapter 3.14).

This chapter initially discusses the present approach to drug treatment depending on the subtype of JIA, and whether or not it is early in the disease course, established disease, or disease refractory to usual therapy. The severity of the disease is also taken into account. Algorithms are presented to graphically demonstrate this approach, but it should be stressed that treatment needs to be tailored to the individual patient. Later in the chapter, individual drugs are discussed in more detail. Experimental approaches for children with refractory disease, failing conventional treatment are discussed in a later chapter (Part 3, Chapter 3.14). It should be emphasized that there is only fairly limited evidence that supports the approaches described here; they represent the authors' approach and are based largely on the cumulative experience of the paediatric rheumatology community. It is to be hoped, and expected, that these treatment approaches will be obsolete in a few years, due to improved drugs and well-designed clinical drug trials, and that some of the experimental approaches discussed later would have become standard therapies.

The importance of a thorough history, and careful examination at each visit cannot be overestimated if the child's treatment is to be optimal (see Part 1, Chapter 1.1). Children often do not complain of pain and dysfunction in the same way as adults do, and therefore clues such as mood and behavior changes, alteration in sleeping patterns, appetite and activity must be sought. A complete examination of all joints, as well as observation of function both in the examination room and also in the waiting room or play area can give important additional information on which to base treatment decisions. Routine repeat laboratory investigations may be needed to monitor for drug toxicity, but they are often not helpful in monitoring disease activity. Although persistently raised acute phase reactants (thrombocytosis, raised ESR, or CRP) are highly suggestive of ongoing active inflammation that may well be damaging joints, it is quite common for children to have active arthritis in the face of normal blood tests. The frequency of radiographic monitoring is also contentious. Radiographs are insensitive to change, and if the physician waits until radiographic changes such as joint space narrowing or erosions have occurred before making therapeutic changes, it is likely that the child will be treated too little too late. Although some authorities would recommend radiographs of the affected joint on a yearly basis; this may be excessive. It seems reasonable to recommend repeating radiographs at the time that a significantly new therapy is introduced, so as to act as a baseline for evaluation later in the disease course. Repeated radiographic imaging may become more important as drugs become available that are capable of causing radiographic "healing."

It should be remembered that it is of critical importance to involve the child as much as possible in the therapeutic decision making process, particularly as the child becomes an adolescent. There is a greater likelihood of adherence to therapy if the child has been routinely included in the discussions about the rationale for drug treatment and the various treatment options. Also issues such as illicit drug and alcohol use, and pregnancy risk, are more likely to be managed effectively if the adolescent is fully involved and informed (see also Part 3, Chapters 3.5 and 3.6).

It should also be stressed here that a critical component of the management of JIA is the screening for, and treatment of uveitis.

For the purposes of this discussion the term Disease Modifying Antirheumatic Drug (DMARD) will be used to describe drugs other than nonsteroidal anti-inflammatory drugs (NSAIDs) and corticosteroids, although for many of them there is really little evidence that they are either more or less disease modifying than NSAIDs or corticosteroids.

Oligoarthritis

Early disease (treatment Algorithm I)

In children who present with only a few involved joints, there is a choice of using either nonsteroidal anti-inflammatory agents (NSAIDs) [7–13] (Table 3.8.1), or intra-articular corticosteroid

ALGORITHM I Treatment of early Oligoarthritis

START TREATMENT AS SOON AS POSSIBLE.

If only one joint (or perhaps 2 joints) involved consider IACI alone.

If more than one joint involved or if unable to perform IACI in immediate future start NSAID.

If arthritis is either severe or has not improved significantly after 1–2 months, add IACI to treatment.

REMISSION

Continue NSAID for 6 months before discontinuation.

RELAPSE

If treated with IACI alone, and remission persisted for 4 or more months, repeat IACI.

If previously treated with NSAID reinstitute NSAID.

PERSISTENT ARTHRITIS

If arthritis persists or recurs within 4 months of IACI, or new joints become involved, the approach is that disease has become established (see Algorithm III).

Note: This approach is also appropriate for early Psoriatic Arthritis and early Enthesitis-Related Arthritis.

injections (IACI) [14–20] (see Appendix). If the patient has severe disease at the onset, serious consideration should be given to starting treatment with both an NSAID and IACI. If an NSAID alone is used, most patients should be subjectively improved by 1 month with decreased morning stiffness, increased activity, more normal movement and improved mood; almost all patients who are going to respond (about 60%) will have done so by 8–12 weeks [21]. If remission is achieved, the NSAID should be continued for another 3–6 months before considering its discontinuation. If IACI is used alone initially, the synovitis should resolve within a few days. If IACI results in complete resolution of the arthritis for 4–6 months, repeated injections would be an acceptable therapeutic option, as there is no evidence that repeated injections are associated with any deleterious effects [22]. However, if the disease extends to involve several joints, or if the recurrence rate is frequent then the management will need to be modified as for established disease.

The use of only NSAIDs and/or IACI is likely to be adequate for about 50–60% of patients with Oligoarthritis.

Established disease

Once the disease is established, a combination of NSAIDs with repeated IACI may still be appropriate, however, most patients with Persistent Oligoarthritis are candidates for all the treatments one would consider for patients with established Polyarthritis (see below). At this therapeutic decision point, consideration needs to be given to the specific joints involved and the functional disability (or potential disability) caused by persistent arthritis. One would be less inclined to aggressively treat a patient with multiple drugs who has synovitis in only one small toe joint, but would not hesitate to use this approach in a child developing multiple joint involvement, or in a child with persistent knee and ankle involvement.

Table 3.8.1 Nonsteroidal anti-inflammatory drugs (NSAIDs)

Drug	Dose (mg/kg/day)	Doses /day	Maximum daily adult dose (mg)	Toxicity ranking[a]	Comments
Naproxen	15–20	2	2400	2	Large experience of use in JIA. Highest risk of pseudoporphyria with this agent.
Ibuprofen	30–50	3–4	2400	1	Effective, well tolerated, but three/four times a day regimen may limit adherence and cannot continue indefinitely.
Tolmetin	30–40	3	1800	4	Frequently used for Enthesitis-Related Arthritis. Increasing difficulty obtaining 400 and 600 mg tablets in North America. Unavailable in UK.
Indomethacin	1–3	2 or 3	150	5	Effective for fever and serositis. Highest levels of toxicity, particularly headache. Long-acting drug available for twice daily administration.
Piroxicam	0.4	1–2	40	3	Second choice NSAID, studied but not labelled for use in JIA.
Diclofenac	2–3	2	225	3	Second choice NSAID, studied but not labelled for use in JIA.
Sulindac	3–4	2	400	3	Second choice NSAID, studied but not labelled for use in JIA.
Trisalicylate[b]	50–60	2	3000	2	A non-acetylating salicylate with less prolonged anti-platelet effect than ASA, and lower GI toxicity. Reye syndrome has been described, but actual risk unknown.
Rofexocib[c]	0.5[d]	1	25	ND	No evidence of improved toxicity compared with standard NSAIDs
Celecoxib[c]	8[d]	2	400	ND	As for Rofexcoxib. Pseudoporphyria in JIA has been described.
Nabumetone[c]	30	1–2	2000	ND	Some evidence for equal effectiveness as standard NSAIDs. Tablets can be suspended in warm water to create a slurry.

Drugs are listed in order of authors' estimate of relative frequency of use and importance in JIA. Frequency of use differs by country. Acetylsalicylic acid (ASA) is not included in this list as it is no longer recommended for use in JIA because of risk of Reye syndrome.

Some of these drugs are available in liquid, or chewable form in some countries. Drug availability varies between countries.

[a] Toxicity ranking is an estimate of toxicity based mainly on data from two publications (Fries et al. [45] in adults, and Flato et al. [48] in children), as well as a literature review, and clinical anecdote. Those drugs in which there is least experience of use in JIA are scored higher. The differences between lowest toxicity (1 and 2), and the highest toxicity (4 and 5) are clinically significant.

ND = No data on which to evaluate toxicity in children with JIA.

[b] Trisalicylate is choline magnesium trisalicylate.

[c] COX-2 selective NSAIDs.

[d] Drug dose extrapolated from adult dosage, as little if any published experience of the use of these drugs in children on which to base dosage. Calculation based on maximum daily adult dose divided by 50. Trials in children are ongoing.

Polyarthritis

Early disease (see treatment Algorithm II)

As with Oligoarthritis, the treatment of early Polyarthritis depends on its severity. Some patients may respond quickly to NSAIDs, but the great majority will need the early institution of methotrexate (MTX), or occasionally one of the other DMARDs, in combination with a NSAID. The addition of low dose prednisone (0.1–0.25 mg/kg/day) for the first 3 months, and then tapered over the next 3 months, can improve symptoms and speed resolution of synovitis. Intra-articular corticosteroid injections of target joints can also be very helpful.

ALGORITHM II Treatment of early Polyarthritis

START TREATMENT AS SOON AS POSSIBLE.

Start NSAID.

Start DMARD either immediately, or after 1–2 months if arthritis has not improved significantly. It is a mistake to delay institution of DMARD for more than a few weeks even if the arthritis seems mild, as remission is unlikely to occur.

Most effective DMARD is MTX. Use of hydroxychloroquine can be considered for very mild disease. Salazopyrine is not first choice DMARD.

Low dose corticosteroids may be very helpful to increase function and decrease pain. For very severe disease a larger dose followed by a rapid taper to a low dose may be beneficial. If corticosteroids are started this should always be in conjunction with a DMARD, with a plan to wean off corticosteroids over a few weeks.

REMISSION

A small percentage of patients will go into remission with NSAID only. Most require a DMARD.

If remission occurs continue NSAID for 6 months then discontinue. Continue DMARD for 1 year after induction of remission, then wean over a few months.

RELAPSE

If relapse occurs, reintroduce all drugs that patient was on when remission was induced.

PERSISTENT ARTHRITIS

Consider IACI for target joints.

If arthritis persists beyond 6 months the arthritis should be considered established (see Algorithm III)

Established disease (see treatment Algorithm III)

Once the disease is established, a combination of medications including an NSAID and one or more DMARDs, often with low dose prednisone (0.1–0.25 mg/kg/day) is required. From a starting dose of 0.3 mg/kg/week of MTX, monthly incremental increases in dose of 2.5 mg (equivalent to 1 tablet) should be considered for ongoing disease activity. Since a decreasing percentage of oral MTX is absorbed as the dose increases, it is usually appropriate to switch to subcutaneous administration if the arthritis is still active despite an oral dose of 0.5 mg/kg/week. It is reasonable to increase the subcutaneous MTX dose to 1 mg/kg/week (maximum dose about 40 mg) unless toxicity occurs before deciding that MTX is ineffective. MTX can also be combined with other DMARDs without a significant increase in toxicity and

ALGORITHM III Treatment of established Polyarthritis and established Oligoarthritis

Treatment of established disease requires a combination of drugs.
An NSAID.
One or more DMARDs.
Probably corticosteroids

The drug of choice is MTX, initially orally. The dose should be increased from a starting dose of about 0.3 mg/kg/week to about 0.5 mg/kg/week. Folic acid 1 mg daily helps minimize toxicity.

If the arthritis remains active after about 6 months then, unless it is very mild, switch to a subcutaneous route of administration, and increase in monthly stages to about 1 mg/kg/week.

If the patient does not want subcutaneous injections or if subcutaneous methotrexate is inefficacious or toxicity (usually nausea) is unacceptable, add a second DMARD. The dose of MTX may have to be lowered to allow toxicity to resolve, but ideally should be continued.

Second DMARD could be either hydroxychloroquine, or sulfasalazine. Use of MTX, hydroxychloroquine and sulfasalazine may be more effective than any combination of 2 of these drugs, without significantly increased toxicity.

The use of Etanercept instead of, or with MTX, rather than using 2 or 3 DMARDs in combination is increasingly common.

IACI and/or oral corticosteroids may be necessary to maintain function.

REMISSION

If remission occurs no change in therapy should be made for several months.

Corticosteroids should be weaned and discontinued first.

NSAIDs can be discontinued once corticosteroids have been stopped.

After at least 1 year of continuous remission the DMARDs can be weaned. It is probably reasonable to discontinue hydroxychloroquine first, followed by sulfasalazine, and lastly MTX.

RELAPSE

If relapse occurs, all the drugs being used at the time of established remission should be reinstituted.

PERSISTENT ARTHRITIS

If the arthritis persists despite the above approach, the disease should be considered refractory and the patient becomes a candidate for experimental therapies.

this approach may be more effective than using MTX as the sole DMARD, although good evidence to support this belief is lacking.

Systemic Arthritis

Early disease (see treatment Algorithm IV)

Systemic Arthritis is perhaps the most challenging form of JIA to treat. Patients with this disease may be only mildly symptomatic with nocturnal fever spikes, or may have life threatening disease with multiple organ involvement. Most patients have disease that falls somewhere between these two ends of the spectrum. The treatment algorithms provide a basic approach to the treatment of Systemic Arthritis. If the child is only mildly ill, treatment can start with an NSAID alone. Most children, however, are quite ill, requiring hospitalization and more intensive treatment. Indomethacin at a dose of 1–2 mg/kg/day may be particularly effective for the fever and serositis [23], but corticosteroids in high doses (prednisone 1–2 mg/kg/day) are usually required. Pulse

ALGORITHM IV Treatment of Systemic Arthritis

> MILD DISEASE (fevers, rash, arthritis only)
>
> Start treatment with a NSAID. Indomethacin may be more effective to treat fever than naproxen or tolmetin, but has higher toxicity (headache, liver enzyme abnormalities).
>
> Many children may require medium dose corticosteroids (prednisone 0.25–0.5 mg/kg/day in 2 or 3 divided doses).
>
> SEVERE DISEASE (systemic symptoms and serositis)
>
> Start treatment with indomethacin and high dose corticosteroids (prednisone 1–2 mg/kg/day in 2 or 3 divided doses).
>
> Intravenous pulses of methylprednisolone (30 mg/kg/day) for 3 consecutive days and then at weekly intervals may control disease, and allow more rapid weaning of oral corticosteroids.
>
> MACROPHAGE ACTIVATION SYNDROME (MAS)
>
> If features of MAS develop, intravenous methylprednisolone for several days, followed by high dose oral corticosteroids are required. Add cyclosporin if clinical and laboratory features do not improve within days.
>
> EARLY REMISSION
>
> A few children will remit with NSAIDs or/and corticosteroids alone after a few weeks, but most children will not.
>
> PERSISTENT DISEASE
>
> If the disease becomes established, a DMARD is required, although there is concern that MAS is more likely to occur with the addition of a DMARD if the systemic features are still present. The evidence for this is particularly strong for sulfasalazine, which is contraindicated during the systemic phase.
>
> MTX is probably the drug of choice, though cyclosporin or cyclophosphamide may also be used, alone or in combination. The role of anti-TNF agents is still unclear.
>
> In many children the systemic features remit, but the child continues to have active arthritis, and is treated in the same manner as a child with established Polyarthritis. If the systemic features persist for several months the child is considered refractory to treatment, and is a candidate for experimental therapies. Arthritis may be very persistent even after systemic features have resolved; again, in this situation the child is a candidate for experimental therapies.
>
> LATER REMISSION
>
> If remission occurs, the drugs are weaned as for Polyarthritis.

IV methylprednisolone (30 mg/kg/day) for at least 3 days is sometimes effective in quickly decreasing systemic features. Some clinicians will continue treatment with weekly IV pulse methylprednisolone in an attempt to avoid daily corticosteroid use, but others start daily prednisone at 2 mg/kg/day in three divided doses, and gradually taper the dose, as the systemic features come under control. Laboratory tests are helpful to monitor therapy, as increased WBC, platelets, ESR, CRP, and a decreased hemoglobin and albumin, are all associated with active disease. A very high ferritin level is also suggestive of active disease. The presence of low grade DIC (as evidenced by increased serum levels of D-dimers, and often abnormal PT and PTT), without overt hemorrhage or thrombosis is common [24]. Increasingly abnormal coagulation studies in association with a sudden drop in the ESR and platelet count, often with extraordinary high ferritin levels and raised triglycerides, are harbingers of the Macrophage Activation Syndrome [25]. This is a life-threatening event requiring high dose IV methylprednisolone pulses, and often cyclosporin (3.0–5.0 mg/kg BID IV) [26,27].

Established disease (see treatment Algorithm IV)

If Systemic Arthritis does not remit fairly quickly, and becomes established, it is often extremely hard to treat effectively. It is frequently difficult to wean corticosteroids to levels that do not cause cushingoid side effects but yet control the disease. How to treat persistently active systemic disease is controversial. There is some evidence suggesting that cyclophosphamide (2 mg/kg/day orally or weekly IV pulses of 10 mg/kg or monthly pulses of 500–1000 mg/m^2) is beneficial [28,29], but in view of its potential toxicity many paediatric rheumatologists would probably try anti-TNF therapy before using cyclophosphamide, even though evidence supporting anti-TNF use in this situation is limited to reports of a few cases only [30–32]. There is fairly good evidence that children with Systemic Arthritis are particularly prone to toxicity with sulfasalazine, therefore this drug should be avoided during the systemic phase of the disease [33]. Even when the systemic features resolve the arthritis may be very resistant to therapy. The use of thalidomide for recalcitrant Systemic Arthritis has been proposed [34]. It is this group of children with refractory disease who may be candidates for other experimental therapies such as stem cell transplant (see Part 3, Chapter 3.14).

Enthesitis-Related Arthritis

Early disease (see treatment Algorithm V)

Treatment of patients with this form of JIA is similar to that of patients with Oligoarthritis with the use of NSAIDs and IACI either alone or in combination. Occasionally enthesitis can be so incapacitating that oral

ALGORITHM V Treatment of Enthesitis-Related Arthritis

> START TREATMENT AS SOON AS POSSIBLE
>
> EARLY DISEASE
>
> Start NSAID. Some authorities use Tolmetin as the initial NSAID of choice for this form of JIA, but there is no evidence that it is more effective than other NSAIDs
>
> If disease is severe (enthesitis may be particularly incapacitating) high dose oral corticosteroid, rapidly tapering to low dose over 2–4 weeks, or intravenous methylprednisolone pulses can be very effective while waiting for the NSAID to take effect.
>
> ESTABLISHED DISEASE
>
> If the arthritis does not remit rapidly (over 2–4 months) with NSAIDs alone, add sulfasalazine, starting at about 25 mg/kg/day divided twice a day, and increase to 50 mg/kg/day if the drug is tolerated.
>
> If the disease persists, MTX may be added or substituted.
>
> There is early evidence that the anti-TNF agents may be very effective for established disease.
>
> REMISSION
>
> The arthritis sometimes comes under control quickly. If so the NSAID can be discontinued quite early, and the child continued on sulfasalazine alone for 6 months to 1 year of remission, before weaning it as well.
>
> RELAPSE
>
> Enthesitis-Related Arthritis seems to have a more episodic disease course than the other forms of JIA. Fairly short courses (4–6 months) of an NSAID and sulfasalazine may be adequate to obtain a prolonged remission, and these drugs can be re-introduced if, and when, the arthritis recurs.

prednisone at a dose of 1 mg/kg/day divided two or three times in a day, and tapered rapidly over 2–4 weeks is required.

Established disease (see treatment Algorithm V)

Many paediatric rheumatologists believe that sulfasalazine is the drug of choice for established disease, and there is some limited published evidence to support the proposition that it most effective for this subset of JIA [35–38]. Given the findings of asymptomatic gastrointestinal disease in children with this disease, and the fact that a proportion of patients will later develop overt inflammatory bowel disease (see also Part 1, Chapter 1.4), there seems to be a reasonable theoretical basis for this treatment.

The drug is usually given at a dose of about 50 mg/kg/day divided twice a day (to a maximum of 3 gm daily).

MTX alone, or in addition to sulfasalazine is probably helpful; whether MTX is more or less effective than sulfasalazine for Enthesitis-Related Arthritis is unknown.

Psoriatic Arthritis

Early disease

The treatment of early disease is similar to that of either Oligoarthritis or Polyarthritis depending on the extent of joint involvement. However, it is probable that children with oligoarticular onset Psoriatic Arthritis are more likely to have a severe disease course than children with Oligoarthritis, and therefore DMARDS usually need to be started soon after disease onset.

Established disease

The treatment of established Psoriatic Arthritis is the same as that for established Polyarthritis.

Refractory disease

A significant proportion of children with JIA continue to have active synovitis over many months and years despite early, aggressive, and consistent use of NSAIDs, DMARDs, and IACI. These children have refractory disease. The treatment of choice for refractory JIA is now anti-TNF therapy [39–40]. Although Etanercept and Infliximab are being used increasingly early in severe JIA, very little is known about long-term safety, so at the present time they should be reserved for children whose arthritis has failed to remit with methotrexate. The management of refractory disease is discussed in more detail in Part 3, Chapter 3.14.

Management of remission

Only some children with JIA go into a long-term full remission (as defined in the introduction to this section), and many of them relapse after obtaining remission [2]. The factors (other than JIA subtype) influencing whether or not a remission is obtained, and how long a remission is maintained, are largely unknown. There is little published evidence to guide the physician on how to discontinue medications once a drug-maintained remission has occurred. There is, however,

some quite convincing evidence that children on MTX are likely to relapse if MTX is discontinued soon after remission is obtained [41], and that they are more likely to remain in remission once MTX is discontinued if they are kept on the drug for at least one year after a drug-maintained remission has been achieved [42].

Most paediatric rheumatologists will wait until a patient has been in clinical remission with a normal ESR and platelet count for 4–6 months before discontinuing NSAIDs and for at least 1 year before weaning DMARDS (see Algorithm VI). Because of the risk of toxicity corticosteroids should be tapered to the lowest dose possible, as soon as possible. Given the evidence that MTX is the most efficacious drug, if a child is on MTX and a second DMARD, the latter drug is usually discontinued first, and another 4–6 months allowed to elapse before tapering the MTX. The best method for tapering MTX is not known—some physicians will gradually decrease the weekly dose, while others will steadily increase the dosage interval. In fact there is no good evidence that tapering the dose of MTX, or any DMARD, rather than simply discontinuing it in one step, is necessary.

ALGORITHM VI Remission management

DRUG-MAINTAINED REMISSION
Continue all medications for 4–6 months then discontinue NSAID

RELAPSE
Reinstitute NSAID

REMISSION MAINTAINED FOR FURTHER 6 MONTHS
If taking one DMARD, do not discontinue or begin taper until in drug-maintained remission for at least 1 year, then:

Hydroxychloroquine: Discontinue
Salazopyrine: taper over 3–6 months
Methotrexate: taper over 3–6 months

If taking 2 or more DMARDs, discontinue drugs in following order, waiting at least 3 months after discontinuation of one drug before tapering another:

Prednisone*
Hydroxychloquine
Sulfasalazine
Methotrexate

*It may be appropriate to continue low dose prednisone and discontinue one of the DMARDs first if it seems clinically likely that the DMARD had not contributed significantly to remission induction

RELAPSE
Immediately reinstitute last drug discontinued or increase most recently tapered drug back to full dose used to achieve drug-maintained remission.

REMISSION
Continue to observe for several years, as relapse rate is high, and may not be apparent, or may be ignored by the child and parents.

Specific anti-rheumatic drugs

Nonsteroidal anti-inflammatory drugs

Nonsteroidal anti-inflammatory drugs have been the mainstay of treatment for inflammatory arthritis for decades because of their analgesic as well as anti-inflammatory properties. One of the main actions of NSAIDs is the inhibition of cyclooxygenase (COX) with resultant decrease in the production of prostaglandins. Because these compounds are important for homeostasis as well as being involved in inflammation, inhibition of their function can result in side effects in addition to the desired effect of decreased inflammation. With the development of more powerful anti-rheumatic medications, the role of NSAIDs is not quite as central to the management of arthritis as it was a decade ago. Nevertheless, most children with arthritis are started on an NSAID. Although the efficacy of NSAIDs is similar between the different subtypes of JIA, individuals may vary in their responses to a specific NSAID [43]. Most NSAIDs inhibit both COX-1 (constitutive) as well as COX-2 (inducible). Newer NSAIDs (e.g. Celecoxib and rofecoxib), more selectively inhibit COX-2. Although these newer agents have been demonstrated in adults to cause less gastrointestinal toxicity than other NSAIDs, this has not yet been demonstrated in children. Furthermore they have other potential side-effects. In particular, because platelet function is not inhibited by selective COX-2 inhibition, there is concern that these drugs may be associated with an increased risk of thrombosis relative to nonselective COX inhibitors [44]. No study has been performed to demonstrate equivalent anti-inflammatory efficacy for the COX-2 selective NSAIDs compared with COX non-selective drugs in children with JIA, therefore at present there is no evidence to support their use in children. NSAIDs tend to share a similar toxicity profile, and there are some differences in toxicity between the drugs which may be important in clinical practice, with tolmetin and indomethacin having higher toxicity than Indomethacin and naproxen [45–48]. There are children who appear to have side effects with one NSAID, but not with another. It is therefore probably reasonable to substitute one NSAID for another if a child has a side effect with one agent, as this may well not recur with another NSAID. It is less clear, however, that if a child's arthritis fails to respond to one NSAID that it may respond to another NSAID; therefore failure of arthritis to respond adequately to an NSAID is usually indicates the need for IACI and/or a DMARD.

Acetyl salicylic acid (aspirin) is no longer used by the vast majority of paediatric rheumatologists because of strong evidence that it is a risk factor for the development of Reye syndrome [49].

Table 3.8.1 lists a number of the NSAIDs used in JIA with doses and relative toxicity. The COX-2 selective NSAIDs are also listed, but their role in JIA remains to be determined.

Specific toxicity

Bleeding

Inhibition of platelet function varies with each agent. Acetyl salicylate irreversibly inhibits platelet function for the life of the platelet. The selective Cox-2 inhibitors and choline-magnesium salicylate (Trilisate) have little or no effect on platelet adhesiveness. The other NSAIDs reversibly alter platelet adhesiveness and function to varying degrees. Although some increased bruising and epistaxis is common

with most NSAIDs, it is very rare that dangerous bleeding occurs in children.

Gastrointestinal side effects

Children are much less at risk from gastrointestinal (GI) toxicity than adults, and although abdominal pain does occur the frequency of severe side-effects such as gastrointestinal hemorrhage is low [50]. Abdominal pain is very common in children, and it is often difficult to determine if the pain is really due to NSAID therapy or not. If changing from one NSAID to another does not relieve the GI symptoms, the use of Misoprostol (a prostaglandin E_1 analogue) may be helpful [51]. The role and relative efficacy of other agents such as H_1 blockers and proton pump inhibitors in children with JIA is unknown.

Skin

Some children, particularly those with blue/grey eye color, blond hair or fair skin, treated with NSAIDs may develop multiple, shallow scars on their face and other sun exposed skin. This condition known as pseudoporphyria may be preceded by heavy sun exposure, or the lesions may appear insidiously as areas that fail to heal well following minor trauma such as scratches [52,53]. Naproxen is the most frequently implicated drug, with pseudoporphyria occurring in about 12% of children treated with this agent [53]. If these lesions occur the NSAID should be discontinued. Another NSAID can usually be substituted without further exacerbation of the lesions which usually heal over many months, but may be permanent [53].

A variety of other skin rashes have been described in children receiving NSAIDs [54].

Central nervous system

Reye syndrome has not been shown to be associated with any of the NSAIDs except acetyl salicylate. However, more subtle disturbances of Central Nervous System function, such as headache, mood change, and decreased school performance are sometimes attributed to the NSAIDs by the parent. It is difficult to know if this is complication of the drug, or a consequence of the chronic disease for which the child has been prescribed the NSAID, but it seems probable that this is a true, and under-recognized adverse event to NSAIDs [55].

Kidney disease

The NSAIDs can cause renal disease particularly in adults. In children the occurrence of clinically significant renal disease is rare [56]. Renal papillary necrosis and interstitial nephritis have been described, and may be more likely to occur if more than one NSAID is used concomitantly [57]. Subclinical evidence of renal disease in children with JIA has been demonstrated [58], but whether this is due to NSAID therapy, or the disease itself is unclear, and the clinical relevance of these findings is likely of limited importance.

Liver toxicity

Elevated liver enzymes may occur in a small percentage children with JIA [59]. It is probable that this is sometimes due to NSAID therapy, but may be found in untreated JIA, particularly of the systemic form. This enzymopathy is usually of questionable clinical significance, often resolving spontaneously. Severe liver disease is a feature of the Macrophage Activation Syndrome, and NSAIDs have been implicated as one of several factors causing this condition [24]. Although some authorities recommend routine monitoring for all children on

NSAIDs this is probably unnecessary, but is appropriate for children with Systemic Arthritis.

DMARDs

A number of second-line agents are considered to be disease modifying, as they appear, at least in some studies, to have a greater ability than NSAIDs to alter the disease course. The most commonly used DMARDs in the management of JIA are methotrexate, sulfasalazine, and hydroxychloroquine. Corticosteroids (both oral and intra-articular) are very effective agents and although not generally considered to be DMARDS, are discussed in this section.

Biologic agents are generally thought of separately from the classical DMARDs, even though they may well be disease modifying, and because of their relative newness, are presently mainly limited to children with refractory disease (see Part 3, Chapter 3.14). Although generally thought of as being more toxic than NSAIDs, this is probably not true [48,60], and delaying institution of DMARDs because of concerns about toxicity is often unwarranted.

Individual drugs are discussed below in an approximation of their importance in the management of JIA. The doses and toxicities of the DMARDs are listed in Table 3.8.2.

Corticosteroids

Systemic administration

Corticosteroids are commonly used in JIA. Their role when used systemically is controversial. There is no doubt that they can cause significant toxicity, but used judiciously they can be very helpful in children with severe arthritis who are unable to function adequately because of pain, morning stiffness, or systemic symptoms. In some situations such as the Macrophage Activation Syndrome they are life-saving. There is evidence in adult rheumatoid arthritis that corticosteroids are effective and decrease the rate of radiographic deterioration [61,62]. As a general rule, for the management of arthritis (as opposed to systemic features), they should be given orally in the lowest dose possible for the shortest length of time.

Intra-articular administration

Several studies have confirmed the efficacy, and relative safety, of intra-articular corticosteroids (particularly Triamcinolone hexacetonide) in the management of JIA [14,16,20,22,63–65,] . Their use is discussed in more detail in the Appendix.

Mechanism of action

Corticosteroids in physiologic or low-dose bind to cytosolic receptors and then translocate as a complex to the nucleus where the complex binds to DNA inducing mRNA transcription of some genes encoding for anti-inflammatory proteins, and decreasing the transcription of pro-inflammatory proteins. As the dose of corticosteroid increases it is likely that very rapid, non-receptor mediated events occur, causing other important effects including apoptosis (programmed cell death) of lymphocytes and other inflammatory cells [66].

Toxicity

The toxicity of corticosteroids is well known and includes obesity, short stature, hypertension, osteoporosis, and cataracts. Other side effects include mood changes, diabetes mellitus, avascular necrosis, and susceptibility to infection. Most of these effects are more prominent at high cumulative doses, but there is a great deal of variability in individual susceptibility to these problems.

Toxicity can be minimized by using the lowest possible dose, given either as a single daily dose in the morning, or even on alternate days. Although alternate dose corticosteroid therapy may be less toxic [67], it is also less effective at suppressing inflammation [68].

Role in JIA

Oral prednisone is often useful in the early stages of disease in a child who is quite functionally limited and/or in pain because of the severity of the arthritis. Low dose (0.05–0.2 mg/kg/day) given as a single morning dose is usually associated with significant improvement in symptoms while waiting for the other drugs (NSAIDs and DMARDs) to start working. If morning stiffness is marked, a small evening dose may also be helpful. For children who are severely limited by pain and stiffness, higher doses of prednisone (0.5–1.0 mg/kg/day) in two or three divided doses, tapering rapidly to a low-dose maintenance level over 1 or 2 weeks, is often very effective. Although the aim should be to discontinue the corticosteroid as soon as possible, it should be recognized that it is often difficult to discontinue corticosteroids once they are started, and it is not uncommon in practice for the child to remain on treatment for many months. A "burst" of oral prednisone as just described, or a bolus of very high dose intravenous methylprednisolone (30 mg/kg/dose) for 1–3 days, may be very beneficial for a child with moderate or severe established disease who has an upcoming important life event such as end of year examinations, or graduation.

Intravenous methylprednisolone given at intervals may be helpful to control the disease in children with severe Systemic Arthritis. The periodicity of the intervals may have to be established by trial and error, varying from weekly to every few weeks. The use of high dose alternate day oral prednisone (about 3 mg/kg/ alternate days) has been shown to be an effective and well-tolerated way of controlling the symptoms of Systemic Arthritis with minimal side effects [69].

The importance of preventing adrenal insufficiency in children on corticosteroids must be remembered. If a child has been on treatment for more than a few weeks, she is at risk of adrenal insufficiency if the prednisone is suddenly discontinued, either intentionally, or unintentionally due to vomiting and/or severe diarrhoea, or if corticosteroid requirements are increased because of stress from infection or surgery. Such a child requires corticosteroid administration intravenously. The child and family need to be made well aware of this risk, and if it seems probable that medium to long-term treatment with corticosteroids is going to be necessary, a card, bracelet, or necklace indicating that she is on such medication should be carried by the child at all time.

Methotrexate

Methotrexate is now the most important agent in the management of JIA. It is efficacious with low toxicity [70,71], and has the advantage of being administered only once a week.

Mechanism of action

Methotrexate is a folic acid analog that binds more tightly to dihydrofolate reductase (DHFR) than does folic acid. This results in marked reduction in the production of reduced folates, which are important cofactors for a variety of enzymatic pathways. When high doses of MTX (500–80,000 mg/m²/week) are used to treat malignancy,

Table 3.8.2 Disease modifying anti-rheumatic drugs

Drug	Dose (mg/kg/day)	Doses /day	Maximum daily adult dose (mg)	Toxicity ranking[a]	Comments
Prednisone	0.05–2	1–3	60	3	Low dose: 0.05–0.2 mg/kg for maintenance. Higher doses: 0.5–1 mg/kg for flares. Tablet has bitter aftertaste
IVMP[b]	30 mg/kg/dose	1	1000	2	Usually given for 1–3 days and repeated as necessary for severe flares, or poorly controlled Systemic Arthritis.
IACI[c]	1 mg/kg/large joint 0.5 mg/kg/small joint	NA	ND	2	Dose given is for triamcinolone hexacetonide. Large Joints: maximum dose ~40 mg, small joints ~20 mg. Mild systemic symptoms (mood change) may occur if several joints injected at once. Main toxicity is subcutaneous atrophy at injection site.
Methotrexate	0.3–1 mg/kg/week	NA	40 mg/week	2	Most commonly used and efficacious DMARD. Can be given orally or parenterally. Folic acid 1 mg daily minimizes toxicity.
Sulfasalazine	~50	2	3000	3	Allergy to sulfa drugs is contraindication. Desensitization can be performed.
Hydroxychloroquine	4–6	1	400	1	Low toxicity. Tablet has very bitter taste. For small children total weekly dose is calculated and 200 mg tablet given only on several days of the week.
Cyclophosphamide Oral IV	1–2 500–1000 mg/m²	1 1	100 1500	4	Give oral dose in morning and encourage fluids to prevent hemorrhagic cystitis. Use MESNA with IV treatment. IV dose is used 1–3 monthly.
Cyclosporin	3–5	2	200	4	Main use is for Macrophage Activation Syndrome May be used orally or intravenously.
Azathioprine	1–3	1	ND	3	
Etanercept[d]	0.4 mg/kg/twice a week	NA	25	3	Usually well tolerated with early onset of effect. Toxicity: Local reactions at injection site, headaches and upper respiratory symptoms. Long-term risks unknown. Screen for tuberculosis before starting treatment.
Infliximab[d]	3–10 mg/kg at 0,2,6 weeks, then 4–8 weekly	NA	ND	3	Usually well tolerated with early onset of effect. Use with MTX to prevent autoantibody formation. Must screen for tuberculosis.

Drugs are listed in order of author's estimate of relative frequency of use and importance in JIA, with the recognition that Etanercept and Infliximab are being used with increasing frequency, and often before the other DMARDS, but the evidence of long-term safety is still limited.

Maximum daily doses are conservative.

[a] Toxicity ranking is an estimate of toxicity based mainly on data from two publications (Fries et al. [60] in adults, and Flato et al. [48] in children), as well as a literature review, and clinical anecdote. Those drugs in which there is least experience of use in JIA are scored higher.

ND = no data.

[b] IVMP = intravenous methylprednisolone.

[c] IACI = intra-articular corticosteroid injection.

[d] Etanercept and Infliximab are discussed in Part 3, Chapter 3.14 on management of refractory JIA.

profound folate depletion halts the production of DNA and RNA, causing cell death, particularly in rapidly dividing cells. In the lower doses used in the treatment of rheumatic diseases (0.3–1.0 mg/kg/week or 10–30 mg/m^2/week), MTX has other important actions besides inhibiting DHFR. MTX administration results in increased adenosine release at sites of inflammation, due to an increase in the intracellular accumulation of 5-aminoimidazole-4-carboxamide ribonucleotide (AICAR) [72]. Adenosine is an intrinsic anti-inflammatory agent causing inhibition of neutrophil adherence to endothelial cells and fibroblasts. Other anti-inflammatory actions of low-dose MTX include: interference with the action of IL-1, inhibition of the production of IL-8 and leukotriene B$_4$, and decreased synovial collagenase gene expression (reviewed in Wallace)[73].

Pharmacology

After administration, methotrexate has a relatively short half-life in plasma; 80–90% of methotrexate is cleared by the kidneys in less than 24 h, the younger the child the more rapid the renal clearance. A decrease in glomerular filtration rate may increase the risk of toxicity. Methotrexate rapidly enters cells, where it is polyglutamated by hepatocytes, red cells, fibroblasts, bone marrow myeloid precursors, and possibly other cells. Polyglutamated methotrexate accumulates intracellularly and this may explain the emergence of nausea and vomiting in patients after months or even several years of treatment.

The route of administration is an important factor for children since the doses found to be effective in children (0.3–1 mg/kg/week) are in the range in which oral MTX becomes increasingly less well absorbed, although there is a wide individual variability [74]. Absorption has been demonstrated to be best when MTX is given without food [75]. For these reasons, subcutaneous (sc), or intramuscular administration may be more effective than oral MTX. Many clinicians change to sc MTX from oral administration at doses ≥ 0.5 mg/kg, and this often seems to be associated with improved efficacy and decreased gastrointestinal side-effects. Parents (or the older child) are usually easily taught to administer sc MTX.

The use of the parenteral solution of MTX (25 mg/ml) taken orally is a common practice, and is less expensive than tablets.

There is no role for measuring plasma MTX levels in the management of JIA.

Toxicity

MTX is well tolerated by children and is not more toxic than NSAIDs [48]. Relatively common side-effects include nausea and mouth sores. Headache, diarrhoea, hair loss, and mood changes are reported occasionally. On regular monthly screening transaminase abnormalities occur fairly commonly, but often resolve spontaneously without making an change to the methotrexate dose. Haematological abnormalities are uncommon. In adult RA some patients develop an increased number of subcutaneous nodules [76], which appear to resolve with discontinuation of MTX [77]. This condition of accelerated nodulosis appears to be very unusual in children but has been described [78,79]. There are many strategies for preventing or minimizing side-effects, in particular the addition of daily folic acid (1 mg) to the treatment regimen [80,81]. Increasing this dose to 2 mg or even 5 mg per day, is sometimes helpful in relieving side-effects without diminishing efficacy. Folinic acid, although not commonly used in JIA is also effective, though perhaps less so than folic acid [81,82]. It is also important to recognize the potential confounding or synergistic role of NSAIDs. Withholding a dose of NSAID before and/or after MTX administration, changing the NSAID, or discontinuing it may improve tolerance of MTX, and lead to resolution of transaminases elevation. When faced with nausea in an individual patient the following additional strategies might be helpful: taking MTX at bedtime, changing from oral to sc MTX, using an antiemetic before MTX administration, changing or discontinuing NSAIDs, or lowering the dose of MTX. A number of patients develop anticipatory nausea, and sometimes changing from the tablet to the parental liquid given orally can help minimize this.

Pneumonitis is rarely reported in children treated with MTX for rheumatic diseases. Its incidence may be similar to that of adults treated for RA—approximately 1%. The emergence of a new cough, or the development of dyspnea in a child recently started on MTX, should raise concerns of this serious side-effect. It usually responds to discontinuation of MTX and treatment with corticosteroids.

Hepatotoxicity is a potential concern with the use of long-term MTX. However, cirrhosis has not been reported in children using MTX for rheumatic diseases, and fortunately, several small studies have not revealed significant liver biopsy abnormalities in children with JIA after 2.3–6.0 years of treatment with MTX [83,84]. Adolescents taking MTX should be counselled against the use of alcohol, having said that, it is probable that many adolescent patients do in fact imbibe alcohol without any serious toxicity developing. Laboratory monitoring for possible toxicity should initially be monthly, but once the dosage is stable, it can be reduced to every 6–8 weeks. Evaluations should include a complete blood count, liver transaminases, and initially and then yearly plasma creatinine and urinalysis.

Prior to 1991, there were no published data to suggest oncogenicity of MTX in patients treated for rheumatic diseases. Since then, there have been multiple reports of the development of lymphoma in adult rheumatoid arthritis patients treated with MTX, and a few cases in children with JIA [85–87]. Some of these appear to be EBV-related, and may resolve after discontinuation of MTX. Any child with JIA on MTX (or any other immunosuppressive agent) who develops lymphadenopathy or splenomegaly should be investigated for the possibility of a lymphoma.

Gonadal function and reproduction are not altered by MTX. However, both males and females should wait for 3 months after discontinuing MTX before trying to conceive because MTX is a powerful teratogen. The use of effective birth control by young women receiving MTX needs to be repeatedly emphasized.

Role in JIA

At the present time MTX is the drug of choice in the management of any child with JIA who does not respond to NSAIDs alone, in fact a good argument could probably be made for its use as the initial drug instead of an NSAID, as it is more efficacious, and almost certainly no more toxic than an NSAID. Although the introduction of the biologics is an important advance, it is probably fair to say that no child should start such a drug until they have failed MTX given subcutaneously at a dose of between 0.5 mg and 1 mg/kg to a maximum of 50 mg/week, or unless intolerable side effects have occurred.

Sulfasalazine

Sulfasalazine (SASP) was developed in the late 1930s to treat inflammatory diseases, thought to be infectious in aetiology, by combining a sulfonomide antibiotic with a salicylate. Several studies have indicated that SASP is an effective treatment for JIA [35,37,38,88,89].

Mechanism of action

SASP has both antibacterial and anti-inflammatory effects. Less than 12% of the intact drug is absorbed from the stomach and small intestine. In the colon the drug is split into its two components by bacterial action. Absorption of 5-aminosalicylic acid is poor, however, sulfapyridine is well absorbed and is metabolized in the liver. One randomized controlled trial in adults with Ankylosing Spondylitis has indicated that it is probably the sulfapyridine component of the molecule that is the active ingredient [90]. SASP and its metabolites are weak inhibitors of cyclooxygenase (both COX-1 and COX-2). SASP (but not its metabolites) inhibits folate metabolizing enzymes (such as DHFR), and is a potent inhibitor of AICAR tranformylase. It is this effect on adenosine release that may largely explain its anti-inflammatory action [91].

Toxicity

As SASP is a sulfa-based molecule it should not usually be given to patients with a known allergy to sulfa; however, if the patient is desensitized (which usually takes a month), the drug may be tolerated. The most common side-effects occurring in 11–31% of children include: nausea, abdominal discomfort, diarrhoea, rash, elevated serum aminotransferase levels, fever, and cytopenias. These side-effects are generally mild and resolve when the medication is stopped. Orange coloured urine occurs in >50% of patients and does not require cessation of the drug. Stevens Johnson Syndrome is a rare but potentially very serious complication of this medication. Most physicians start the drug at a dose of about 10 mg/kg/day and increase to about 50 mg/kg/day divided twice a day. Laboratory monitoring (complete blood count, liver enzymes, and urinalysis), 1 month after starting SASP and every 3 months thereafter is necessary.

Role in JIA

There is fairly convincing evidence that SASP is efficacious in JIA, and perhaps particularly in Enthesitis-Related Arthritis. It might therefore be considered the first choice DMARD for use in Enthesitis-Related Arthritis, although there is no evidence to indicate whether it is actually better than MTX for this indication, and it is almost certainly more toxic than the latter agent. [46]. SASP is perhaps the drug of choice to add to MTX when JIA is not adequately controlled by MTX and an NSAID. SASP is contraindicated for use in Systemic Arthritis, at least during the acute phase of the disease, because of good evidence of increased toxicity in this situation [33].

Hydroxychloroquine

Hydroxychloroquine is an anti-malarial that has been used since 1951 to treat inflammatory arthritis. It has been used commonly in the management of JIA, and has generally been thought of as a mildly effective, but safe DMARD. However, the only placebo-controlled study of its use showed almost no benefit, with only pain on movement being statistically less in the hydroxychloroquine group than in the placebo group [92].

Mechanism of action

The exact mechanisms by which hydroxychloroquine works are not known, but it has been demonstrated to trap free radicals, impair cell movement, suppress prostaglandin production, and inhibit the release of IL-1 from monocytes [93,94].

Hydroxychloroquine is absorbed in the upper gastrointestinal tract and is excreted in both the urine and the faeces. It is completely absorbed when given by mouth and takes 3–4 months to reach steady-state levels. The anti-inflammatory effects usually take 2–4 months to occur [95].

Toxicity

Hydroxychloroquine can cause nausea, dyspepsia and abdominal discomfort in some patients, which seems to be helped by taking the medication at night, however, it is usually very well tolerated. Occasionally bleaching of the skin and hair can occur. The major concern about anti-malarial therapy is the risk of irreversible retinal damage. This occurs very rarely (if at all) with hydroxychloroquine if the dose is kept below 6.5 mg/kg/day. It is generally recommended that a patient on hydroxychloroquine have an ophthalmologic exam every 6 months, but this may be unnecessarily cautious, and some authorities think that yearly is sufficient.

Role in JIA

Hydroxychloroquine has a limited role in JIA. It is a drug that is perhaps worth considering in a child who has very mild synovitis, despite an adequate trial of an NSAID when the parent or child is anxious about the use of MTX. It is also a drug that is fairly safe to use in combination with MTX, or even with both MTX and Sulfasalazine [96]

Other DMARDs

The next few agents discussed here briefly are drugs that either have a very limited role in early or established disease (cyclophosphamide in Systemic Arthritis, cyclosporin in the macrophage activation syndrome), or have been used in the past prior to the recognition that MTX was such an effective drug, and are now occasionally still used in refractory disease (azathioprine), or are mainly of historical interest (gold salts and penicillamine). The biological agents are discussed in the chapter on the management of refractory JIA (Part 3, chapter 3.14).

Cyclophosphamide

Cyclophosphamide is a powerful alkylating agent, and is potentially a very toxic drug. There are significant risks of clinically important anorexia and nausea, alopecia, bone marrow suppression, immunosuppression, haemorrhagic cystitis, an increased malignancy rate, and most importantly for many families, sterility. Sterility increases in frequency with increasing age of the patient [97].

Clinical experience suggests daily oral therapy may be effective. The most convincing evidence of its efficacy is in severe Systemic Arthritis, given intravenously in combination with intravenous methylprednisolone and/or methotrexate [28,98].

Cyclosporin

Cyclosporin inhibits the early phase of T cell activation, and the production of several cytokines (IL-2, IL-3, IL-4, and IFNγ) important in modulating the immune response.

Cyclosporin has been shown to have some beneficial effects in JIA, but these are not dramatic [99–101]. When used to treat arthritis, it is most commonly combined with MTX. It had been hoped that cyclosporin might be particularly effective for refractory uveitis associated with JIA, but this has not turned out to be the case [99]. Cyclosporin's main role is probably in the treatment of the Macrophage Activation Syndrome [26,27]. Toxicity is significant and includes increased facial hair, gingivitis, hypertension, and nephrotoxicity.

Azathioprine

Azathioprine is an immunosuppressant, causing inhibition of T cell growth by interfering with DNA synthesis. It has been demonstrated to be an effective treatment for some patients with JIA [102]. Side-effects are fairly common and usually occur within the first 2 months of treatment. The most common adverse effects are abdominal pain, elevated transaminases, cytopenias, and rash. Adverse events are more common in patients with an inherited decreased activity of the enzyme that metabolizes azathioprine—thiopurine methyltransferase [103]. Data in RA patients suggesting a twofold increase in the risk of lymphoproliferative disease [104], but whether there is a significantly increased risk in children with JIA is unknown. There seems little doubt that it is much less effective than MTX, and its use is now restricted to children with methotrexate resistant arthritis.

Gold compounds

Prior to the recognition that MTX was such an effective drug, intramuscular gold injections were the main drug used for established JIA. Oral gold (auranofin) was never felt to be an effective agent in JIA [105]. Gold salts are hardly ever used now in JIA, and are not discussed further.

Penicillamine

Similar to gold, penicillamine's toxicity profile is high compared to its efficacy and now it is very rarely, if ever, used to treat JIA.

Chlorambucil

This drug is a potent alkylating agent. It is probably the drug of choice for the secondary amyloidoses that occasionally occurs in persistent JIA (see Part 2, Chapter 2.2).

Conclusion

Most children with JIA will have their disease adequately controlled by the use of the drugs mentioned in this chapter, using algorithms similar to the ones shown here. Failure of the above drugs to control inflammation indicates that the child has refractory disease and should be considered a potential candidate for more experimental approaches as is discussed in the chapter on the management of refractory JIA.

References

1. Levinson, J.E. and Wallace, C.A. Dismantling the pyramid [Review]. J Rheumatol Suppl 1992;33:6–10.
2. Oen, K., Malleson, P.N., Cabral, D.A., Rosenberg, A.M., Petty, R.E., and Cheang, M. Disease course and outcome of juvenile rheumatoid arthritis in a multicenter cohort. J Rheumatol 2002;29:1989–99.
3. Moreland, L.W. and Bridges, S.L.J. Early rheumatoid arthritis: a medical emergency? Am J Med 2001;111:498–500.
4. Oen, K., Malleson, P.N., Cabral, D.A., Rosenberg, A.M., Petty, R.E., Reed, M. et al. Early predictors of longterm outcome in patients with juvenile rheumatoid arthritis: subset-specific correlations. J Rheumatol 2003;30:585–93.
5. Oen, K., Reed, M., Malleson, P.N., Cabral, D.A., Petty, R.E., Rosenberg, A.M. et al. Radiologic outcome and its relationship to functional disability in juvenile rheumatoid arthritis. J Rheumatol 2003;30:832–40.
6. Wallace, C.A., Sherry, D.D., Mellins, E.D., and Aiken, R.P. Predicting remission in juvenile rheumatoid arthritis with methotrexate treatment. J Rheumatol 1993;20:118–22.
7. Makela, A.L. Naproxen in the treatment of juvenile rheumatoid arthritis. Metabolism, safety and efficacy. Scand J Rheumatol 1977;6:193–205.
8. Moran, H., Hanna, D.B., Ansell, B.M., Hall, M., and Engler, C. Naproxen in juvenile chronic polyarthritis. Ann Rheum Dis 1979;38:152–154.
9. Leak, A.M., Richter, M.R., Clemens, L.E., Hall, M.A., and Ansell, B.M., A crossover study of naproxen, diclofenac and tolmetin in seronegative juvenile chronic arthritis. Clin Exp Rheumatol 1988;6:157–60.
10. Giannini, E.H., Brewer, E.J., Miller, M.L., Gibbas, D., Passo, M.H., Hoyeraal, H.M. et al. Ibuprofen suspension in the treatment of juvenile rheumatoid arthritis. Pediatric Rheumatology Collaborative Study Group. J Pediatr 1990;117:645–52.
11. Levinson, J.E., Baum, J., Brewer, E., Jr, Fink, C., Hanson, V., and Schaller, J. Comparison of tolmetin sodium and aspirin in the treatment of juvenile rheumatoid arthritis. J Pediatr 1977;91:799–804.
12. Bhettay, E. Double-blind study of sulindac and aspirin in juvenile chronic arthritis. S Afr Med J 1986;70:724–726.
13. Williams, P.L., Ansell, B.M., Bell, A., Cain, A.R., Chamberlain, M.A., Clarke, A.K. et al. Multicentre study of piroxicam versus naproxen in juvenile chronic arthritis, with special reference to problem areas in clinical trials of nonsteroidal anti-inflammatory drugs in childhood. Br J Rheumatol 1986;25:67–71.
14. Allen, R.C., Gross, K.R., Laxer, R.M., Malleson, P.N., Beauchamp, R.D., and Petty, R.E. Intraarticular triamcinolone hexacetonide in the management of chronic arthritis in children. Arthritis Rheum 1986;29:997–1001.
15. Balogh, Z., Ruzsonyi, E. Triamcinolone hexacetonide versus betamethasone. A double-blind comparative study of the long-term effects of intra-articular steroids in patients with juvenile chronic arthritis. Scand J Rheumatol Suppl 1987;67:80–2.
16. Earley, A., Cuttica, R.J., McCullough, C., and Ansell, B.M. Triamcinolone into the knee joint in juvenile chronic arthritis. Clin Exp Rheumatol 1988;6:153–5.
17. Huppertz, H-I, Tschammler, A., Horwitz, A.E., and Schwab, K.O. Intraarticular corticosteroids for chronic arthritis in children: efficacy and effects on cartilage and growth. J Pediatr 1995;127:317–321.
18. Padeh, S., Passwell, J.H. Intraarticular corticosteroid injection in the management of children with chronic arthritis. Arthritis Rheum 1998; 41:1210–14.
19. Yang, M.H., Lee, W.I., Chen, L.C., Lin, S.J., and Huang, J.L. Intraarticular triamcinolone hexacetonide injection in children with chronic arthritis: a survey of clinical practice. Acta paediatr Taiwan 1999;40:182–5.
20. Ravelli, A., Manzoni, S.M., Viola, S., Pistorio, A., Ruperto, N., and Martini, A. Factors affecting the efficacy of intraarticular corticosteroid injection of knees in juvenile idiopathic arthritis. J Rheumatol 2001;28: 2100–02.
21. Lovell, D.J., Giannini, E.H., and Brewer, E.J., Jr. Time course of response to nonsteroidal antiinflammatory drugs in juvenile rheumatoid arthritis. Arthritis Rheum 1984;27:1433–7.
22. Sparling, M., Malleson, P., Wood, B., and Petty, R. Radiographic followup of joints injected with triamcinolone hexacetonide for the management of childhood arthritis. Arthritis Rheum 1990;33:821–6.
23. Sherry, D.D., Patterson, M.W., and Petty, R.E. The use of indomethacin in the treatment of pericarditis in childhood. J Pediatr 1982;100:995–8
24. Silverman, E.D., Miller, J.J., III, Bernstein, B., and Shafai, T. Consumption coagulopathy associated with systemic juvenile rheumatoid arthritis. J Pediatr 1983;103:872–6.

25. Hadchouel, M., Prieur, A-M., and Griscelli, C. Acute hemorrhagic, hepatic, and neurologic manifestations in juvenile rheumatoid arthritis: possible relationship to drugs or infection. *J Pediatr* 1985;106:561–6.

26. Mouy, R., Stephan, J.L., Pillet, P., Haddad, E., Hubert, P., and Prieur, A.M. Efficacy of cyclosporine A in the treatment of macrophage activation syndrome in juvenile arthritis: report of five cases. *J Pediatr* 1996; 129:750–4.

27. Ravelli, A., De Benedetti, F., Viola, S., and Martini, A. Macrophage activation syndrome in systemic juvenile rheumatoid arthritis successfully treated with cyclosporine. *J Pediatr* 1996;128:275–8.

28. Shaikov, A.V., Maximov, A.A., Speransky, A.I., Lovell, D.J., Giannini, E.H., and Solovyev, S.K. Repetitive use of pulse therapy with methylprednisolone and cyclophosphamide in addition to oral methotrexate in children with systemic juvenile rheumatoid arthritis-preliminary results of a longterm study. *J Rheumatol* 1992;19:612–16.

29. Wallace, C.A., and Sherry, D.D. Trial of intravenous pulse cyclophosphamide and methylprednisolone in the treatment of severe systemic-onset juvenile rheumatoid arthritis. *Arthritis Rheum* 1997;40:1852–55.

30. Elliott, M.J., Woo, P., Charles, P., Long-Fox, A., Woody, J.N., and Maini, R.N. Suppression of fever and the acute-phase response in a patient with juvenile chronic arthritis treated with monoclonal antibody to tumour necrosis factor-alpha (cA2). *Br J Rheumatol* 1997;36:589–93.

31. Prahalad, S., Bove, K.E., Dickens, D., Lovell, D.J., and Grom, A.A. Etanercept in the treatment of macrophage activation syndrome. *J Rheumatol* 2001; 28:2120–4.

32. Kimura, Y., Imundo, L.F., and Li, S.C. High dose infliximab in the treatment of resistant systemic juvenile rheumatoid arthritis. *Arthritis Rheum* 2001;44(9 Suppl):S272.

33. Cate, RH-T. and Cats, A. Toxicity of sulfasalazine in systemic juvenile chronic arthritis. *Clin Exp Rheumatol* 1991;9:85–8.

34. Lehman, T.J., Striegel, K.H., and Onel, K.B. Thalidomide therapy for recalcitrant systemic onset juvenile rheumatoid arthritis. *J Pediatr* 2002;140:125–7.

35. Ansell, B.M., Hall, M.A., Loftus, J.K., Woo, P., Neumann, V., Harvey, A. *et al.* A multicentre pilot study of sulphasalazine in juvenile chronic arthritis. *Clin Exp Rheumatol* 1991;9:201–3.

36. Huang, J.L. and Chen, L.C. Sulphasalazine in the treatment of children with chronic arthritis. *Clin Rheumatol* 1998;17:359–63.

37. Brooks, C.D. Sulfasalazine for the management of juvenile rheumatoid arthritis. *J Rheumatol* 2001;28:845–53.

38. Burgos-Vargas, R., Vazquez-Mellado, J., Pacheco-Tena, C., Hernandez-Garduno, A., and Goycochea-Robles, M.V. A 26 week randomised, double blind, placebo controlled exploratory study of sulfasalazine in juvenile onset spondyloarthropathies. *Ann Rheum Dis* 2002;61:941–2.

39. Lovell, D.J., Giannini, E.H., Reiff, A., Cawkwell, G.D., Silverman, E.D., Nocton, J.J. *et al.* Etanercept in children with polyarticular juvenile rheumatoid arthritis. *N Engl J Med* 2000;342:763–9.

40. Lovell, D.J., Giannini, E.H., Reiff, A., Jones, O.Y., Schneider, R., Olson, J.C. *et al.* Long-term efficacy and safety of etanercept in children with polyarticular-course juvenile rheumatoid arthritis: Interim results from an ongoing multicenter, open-label, extended-treatment trial. *Arthritis Rheum* 2003;48:218–26.

41. Ravelli, A., Viola, S., Ramenghi, B., Aramini, L., Ruperto, N., and Martini, A. Frequency of relapse after discontinuation of methotrexate therapy for clinical remission in juvenile rheumatoid arthritis. *J Rheumatol* 1995;22:1574–6.

42. Gottlieb, B.S., Keenan, G.F., Lu, T, and Ilowite, N.T. Discontinuation of methotrexate treatment in juvenile rheumatoid arthritis. *Pediatrics* 1997; 100:994–7.

43. Huskisson, E.C. Antiinflammatory drugs. *Semin Arthritis Rheum* 1977; 7:1–20.

44. Mukherjee, D., Nissen, S.E., and Topol, E.J. Risk of cardiovascular events associated with selective COX-2 inhibitors. *JAMA* 2001; 286:954–9.

45. Fries, J.F., williams, C.A., and Bloch, D.A. The relative toxicity of nonsteroidal antiinflammatory drugs. *Arthritis Rheum* 1991;34:1353–60.

46. Furst, D.E. Toxicity of antirheumatic medications in children with juvenile arthritis. *J Rheumatol* 1992;19 (Suppl 33):11–15.

47. Furst, D.E. Review: are there differences among nonsteroidal antiinflammatory drugs? Comparing acetylated salicylates, nonacetylated salicylates, and nonacetylated nonsteroidal antiinflammatory drugs. *Arthritis Rheum* 1994;38:1–9.

48. Flato, B., Vinje, O., and Forre, O. Toxicity of antirheumatic and anti-inflammatory drugs in children. *Clin Rheumatol* 1998;17:505–10.

49. Hurwitz, E.S., Barrett, M.J., Bregman, D., Gunn, W.J., Pinsky, P., Schonberger, L.B *et al.* Public Health Service study of Reye's syndrome and medications. Report of the main study. *JAMA* 1987;257:1905–11.

50. Dowd, J.E., Cimaz, R., and Fink, C.W. Nonsteroidal antiinflammatory drug-induced gastroduodenal injury in children. *Arthritis Rheum* 1995; 38:1225–31.

51. Gazarian, M., Berkovitch, M., Koren, G., Silverman, E.D., and Laxer, R.M. Experience with misoprostol therapy for NSAID gastropathy in children. *Ann Rheum Dis* 1995;54:277–80

52. Allen, R., Rogers, M., and Humphrey, I. Naproxen induced pseudoporphyria in juvenile chronic arthritis. *J Rheumatol* 1991;18:893–6.

53. Lang, B.A., and Finlayson, L.A. Naproxen-induced pseudoporphyria in patients with juvenile rheumatoid arthritis. *J Pediatr* 1994;124:639–42.

54. Lindsley, C.B. Uses of nonsteroidal anti-inflammatory drugs in pediatrics. *Am J Dis Child* 1993;147:229–36.

55. Duffy, C.M., Gibbon, W., Yang, J., *et al.* Non-steroidal anti-inflammatory drug-induced central nervous system toxicity in a practice-based cohort of children with juvenile arthritis. *J Rheumatol* 2000;27 (Suppl 58):73.

56. Szer, I.S., Goldenstein-Schainberg, C., and Kurtin, P.S. Paucity of renal complications associated with nonsteroidal antiinflammatory drugs in children with chronic arthritis. *J Pediatr* 1991;119:815–17.

57. Allen, R.C., Petty, R.E., Lirenman, D.S., Malleson, P.N., and Laxer, R.M. Renal papillary necrosis in children with chronic arthritis. *Am J Dis Child* 1986;140:20–22.

58. Malleson, P.N., Lockitch, G., Mackinnon, M., Mahy, M., and Petty, R.E. Renal disease in chronic arthritis of childhood. A study of urinary N-acetyl-beta-glucosaminidase and beta 2-microglobulin excretion. *Arthritis Rheum* 1990;33:1560–6.

59. Barron, K.S., Person, and D.A., and Brewer, E.J. The toxicity of nonsteroidal antiinflammatory drugs in juvenile rheumatoid arthritis. *J Rheumatol* 1982; 9:149–55.

60. Fries, J.F., Williams, C.A., Ramey, D., and Bloch, D.A. The relative toxicity of disease-modifying antirheumatic drugs. *Arthritis Rheum* 1993;36: 297–306.

61. Saag, K.G., Criswell L.A., Sems, K.M., Nettleman M.D., and Kolluri, S. Low-dose corticosteroids in rheumatoid arthritis. A meta-analysis of their moderate-term effectiveness. *Arthritis Rheum* 1996;39:1818–25.

62. Kirwan, J.R. and Arthritis and Rheumatism Council Low-Dose Glucocorticoid Study Group. The effect of glucocorticoids on joint destruction in rheumatoid arthritis. *N Engl J Med* 1995;333:142–6.

63. Honkanen, V.E., Rautonen, J.K., and Pelkonen, P.M. Intra-articular glucocorticoids in early juvenile chronic arthritis. *Acta Paediatr* 1993;82: 1072–4.

64. Padeh, S., and Passwell, J.H. Intraarticular corticosteroid injection in the management of children with chronic arthritis. *Arthritis Rheum* 1998; 41:1210–14.

65. Breit, W., Frosch, M., Meyer, U., Heinecke, A., and Ganser, G.A. subgroup-specific evaluation of the efficacy of intraarticular triamcinolone hexacetonide in juvenile chronic arthritis. *J Rheumatol* 2000;27:2696–702.

66. Buttgereit, F., Wehling, M., and Burmester, G.R. A new hypothesis of modular glucocorticoid actions: steroid treatment of rheumatic diseases revisited. *Arthritis Rheum* 1998;41:761–7.

67. Byron, M.A., Jackson, J., and Ansell, B.M. Effect of different corticosteroid regimens on hypothalamic-pituitary adrenal axis and growth in juvenile chronic arthritis. *J R Soc Med* 1983;76:452–7.

68. MacGregor, R.R., Sheagren, J.N., Lipsett, M.B., and Wolff, S.M. Alternate-day prednisone therapy. Evaluation of delayed hypersensitivity responses, control of disease and steroid side effects. *N Engl J Med* 1969;280:1427–31.

69. Kimura, Y., Fieldston, E., Devries-Vandervlugt, B., Li, S., and Imundo, L. High dose, alternate day corticosteroids for systemic onset juvenile rheumatoid arthritis. *J Rheumatol* 2000;27:2018–24.

70. Giannini, E.H., Brewer, E.J., Kuzmina, N., Shaikov, A., Maximov, A., Vorontsov, I. *et al.* Methotrexate in resistant juvenile rheumatoid arthritis. Results of the U.S.A.-U.S.S.R. double-blind, placebo-controlled trial. The Pediatric Rheumatology Collaborative Study Group and The Cooperative Children's Study Group. *N Engl J Med* 1992;326:1043–9.

71. Giannini, E.H., Cassidy, J.T., Brewer, E.J., Shaikov, A., Maximov, A., and Kuzmina, N. Comparative efficacy and safety of advanced drug therapy in children with juvenile rheumatoid arthritis. *Semin Arthritis Rheum* 1993;23:34–46.

72. Cronstein, B.N., Naime, D., and Ostad, E. The antiinflammatory mechanism of methotrexate. Increased adenosine release at inflamed sites diminishes leukocyte accumulation in an in vivo model of inflammation. *J Clin Invest* 1993;92:2675–82.

73. Wallace, C.A. The use of methotrexate in childhood rheumatic diseases. *Arthritis Rheum* 1998;41:381–91.

74. Ravelli, A., Di Fuccia, G., Molinaro, M., Ramenghi, B., Zonta, L., Regazzi, M.B. *et al.* Plasma levels after oral methotrexate in children with juvenile rheumatoid arthritis. *J Rheumatol* 1993;20:1573–7.

75. Dupuis, L.L., Koren, G., Silverman, E.D., and Laxer, R.M. Influence of food on the bioavailability of oral methotrexate in children. *J Rheumatol* 1995;22:1570–3.

76. Patatanian, E. and Thompson, D.F. A review of methotrexate-induced accelerated nodulosis. *Pharmacotherapy* 2002;22:1157–62.

77. Williams, F.M., Cohen, P.R., and Arnett, F.C. Accelerated cutaneous nodulosis during methotrexate therapy in a patient with rheumatoid arthritis. *J Am Acad Dermatol* 1998;39:359–62.

78. Muzaffer, M.A., Schneider, R., Cameron, B.J., Silverman, E.D., and Laxer, R.M. Accelerated nodulosis during methotrexate therapy for juvenile rheumatoid arthritis. *J Pediatr* 1996;128:698–700.

79. Falcini, F., Taccetti, G., Ermini, M., Trapani, S., Calzolari, A., and Franchi, A.C.M.M. Methotrexate-associated appearance and rapid progression of rheumatoid nodules in systemic-onset juvenile rheumatoid arthritis. *Arthritis Rheum* 1997;40:175–8.

80. Morgan, S.L., Alarcon, G.S., and Krumdieck, C.L. Folic acid supplementation during MTX therapy: It makes sense. *J Rheumatol* 1993;20:929–30.

81. Kotaniemi, K. Late onset uveitis in juvenile-type chronic polyarthritis controlled with prednisolone, cyclosporin A and methotrexate. *Clin Exp Rheumatol* 1998;16:469–71.

82. Ravelli, A., Migliavacca, D., Viola, S., Ruperto N., Pistorio A., and Martini, A. Efficacy of folinic acid in reducing methotrexate toxicity in juvenile idiopathic arthritis. *Clin Exp Rheumatol* 1999;17:625–27.

83. Kugathasan, S., Newman, A.J., Dahms, B.B., and Boyle, J.T. Liver biopsy findings in patients with juvenile rheumatoid arthritis receiving long-term, weekly methotrexate therapy. *J Pediatr* 1996;128:149–51.

84. Hashkes, P.J., Balistreri, W.F., Bove, K.E., Ballard, E.T., and Passo, M.H. The relationship of hepatotoxic risk factors and liver histology in methotrexate therapy for juvenile rheumatoid arthritis. *J Pediatr* 1999;134:47–52.

85. Cleary, A.G., McDowell, H., and Sills, J.A. Polyarticular juvenile idiopathic arthritis treated with methotrexate complicated by the development of non-Hodgkin's lymphoma. *Arch Dis Child* 2002;86:47–49.

86. Krugmann, J., Sailer-Hock, M., Muller, T., Gruber, J., Allerberger, F., and Offner, F.A. Epstein–Barr virus-associated Hodgkin's lymphoma and legionella pneumophila infection complicating treatment of juvenile rheumatoid arthritis with methotrexate and cyclosporine A. *Hum Pathol* 2000;31:253–5.

87. Londino, A.V., Jr., and Blatt, J., Knisely, A.S. Hodgkin's disease in a patient with juvenile rheumatoid arthritis taking weekly low dose methotrexate. *J Rheumatol* 1998;25:1245–6.

88. Van Rossum, M.A., Fiselier, T.J., Franssen, M.J., Zwinderman A.H., ten Cate, R., van Suijlekom-Smit, L.W. *et al.* Sulfasalazine in the treatment of juvenile chronic arthritis: a randomized, double-blind, placebo-controlled, multicenter study. Dutch Juvenile Chronic Arthritis Study Group. *Arthritis Rheum* 1998; 41:808–16.

89. Dougados, M., van der Linden, S., Leirisalo-Repo, M., Huitfeldt, B. *et al.* Sulfasalazine in the treatment of sponylarthropathy: a randomized, multicenter, double-blind, placebo-controlled study. *Arthritis Rheum* 1995; 38:618–27.

90. Taggart, A., Gardiner, P., McEvoy, F., Hopkins, R., and Bird, H. Which is the active moiety of sulfasalazine in ankylosing spondylitis? A randomized, controlled study. *Arthritis Rheum* 1996;39:1400–05.

91. Cronstein, B.N. The antirheumatic agents sulphasalazine and methotrexate share an anti- inflammatory mechanism. *Br J Rheumatol* 1995;34 (Supp2): 30–32.

92. Brewer, E.J., Giannini, E.H., Kuzmina, and N., Alekseev, L. Penicillamine and hydroxychloroquine in the treatment of severe juvenile rheumatoid arthritis. Results of the U.S.A.–U.S.S.R. double-blind placebo-controlled trial. *N Engl J Med* 1986;314:1269–76.

93. Miyachi, Y., Yoshioka A., Imamura S., and Niwa Y. Antioxidant action of antimalarials. *Ann Rheum Dis* 1986;45:244–8.

94. van den Borne, B.E., Dijkmans B.A., de Rooij, H.H., le Cessie, S., and Verweij, C.L. Chloroquine and hydroxychloroquine equally affect tumor necrosis factor-alpha, interleukin 6, and interferon-gamma production by peripheral blood mononuclear cells. *J Rheumatol* 1997;24:55–60.

95. van Kerckhove, C., Giannini, E.H., and Lovell, D.J. Temporal patterns of response to D-penicillamine, hydroxychloroquine, and placebo in juvenile rheumatoid arthritis patients. *Arthritis Rheum* 1988;31:1252–8.

96. O'Dell, J.R., Haire, C.E., Erikson, N., Drymalski, W., Palmer, W., and Eckhoff, P.J. *et al.* Treatment of rheumatoid arthritis with methotrexate alone, sulfasalazine and hydroxychloroquine, or a combination of all three medications. *N Engl J Med* 1996;334:1287–91.

97. Rivkees, S.A., and Crawford, J.D., The relationship of gonadal activity and chemotherapy-induced gonadal damage. *JAMA* 1988;259:2123–25.

98. Wallace, C.A., and Sherry, D.D., Trial of intravenous pulse cyclophosphamide and methylprednisolone in the treatment of severe systemic-onset juvenile rheumatoid arthritis. *Arthritis Rheum* 1997;40:1852–5.

99. Gerloni, V., Cimaz, R., Gattinara, M., Arnoldi, C., Pontikaki, I., and Fantini, F. Efficacy and safety profile of cyclosporin A in the treatment of juvenile chronic (idiopathic) arthritis. Results of a 10-year prospective study. *Rheumatology* 2001;40:907–13.

100. Pistoia, V., Buoncompagni, A., Scribanis R., Fasce, L., Alpigiani, G., Cordone, G., *et al.* Cyclosporin A in the treatment of juvenile chronic arthritis and childhood polymyositis-dermatomyositis. Results of a preliminary study [see comments]. *Clin Exp Rheumatol* 1993;11:203–8.

101. Reiff, A., Rawlings, D.J., Shaham, B., Franke, E., Richardson, L., Szer, I.S. *et al.* Preliminary evidence for cyclosporin A as an alternative in the treatment of recalcitrant juvenile rheumatoid arthritis and juvenile dermatomyositis. *J Rheumatol* 1997;24:2436–43.

102. Savolainen, H.A., Kautiainen, H., Isomaki, H., Aho, K., and Verronen, P. Azathioprine in patients with juvenile chronic arthritis: a longterm followup study. *J Rheumatol* 1997;24:2444–50.

103. Leipold, G., Schütz, E., Haas, J.P., and Oellerich, M. Azathioprine-induced severe pancytopenia due to a homozygous two-point mutation of the thiopurine methyltransferase gene in a patient with juvenile HLA-B27-associated spondylarthritis. *Arthritis Rheum* 1997;40:1896–8.

104. Silman, A.J., Petrie, J., Hazleman, B., and Evans, S.J. Lymphoproliferative cancer and other malignancy in patients with rheumatoid arthritis treated with azathioprine: a 20 year follow up study. *Ann Rheum Dis* 1988; 47:988–92.

105. Giannini, E.H., Barron, K.S., Spencer, C.H., Person, D.A., Baum, J., Bernstein, B.H., *et al.* Auranofin therapy for juvenile rheumatoid arthritis: results of the five-year open label extension trial. *J Rheumatol* 1991;18: 1240–2.

3.9 Physiotherapy and occupational therapy

Gay Kuchta and Iris Davidson

Aim

The aim of this chapter is to discuss the multiple roles of phyiotherapists and occupational therapists in the assessment and management of children with JIA as the disease evolves over time. The chapter emphasizes that the role of therapists is not only to address the physical functioning of the child, but working with other health care professionals to help optimize the child's overall wellbeing and psychosocial health.

Structure

- Introduction
- The management of early disease
  Pain and function
  Treatment goals
- The management of established disease
  Pain and function
  Identifying and managing impairments and functional limitations
  Teaching self-management and problem solving
  Advocating for the child
- The management of refractory disease
  Pain and function
  Treatment goals
- Summary

Introduction

Occupational therapists (OTs) and physiotherapists (PTs) complement the drug therapy of Juvenile Idiopathic Arthritis (JIA), by focusing on the symptoms of rheumatic diseases and attempting to prevent disability. It has been shown that patients with JIA despite good control of the inflammation often continue to have substantial problems with physical activity [1]. The exact role of these two disciplines varies greatly between countries and centres, however each discipline reinforces the other and engages the child and family in treatment decisions. In the early stages, pain is usually the underlying symptom leading the family to seek medical attention. Functional limitations both at home and at school, due to range of motion restrictions secondary to the pain and swelling, are also important early symptoms. Therapists identify, quantify, and address these issues with the family and child. The family must be engaged in managing the disease from the beginning. Engaging the child in self-management, and the family in supervising drug and exercise regimes is the most effective way to improve adherence [2].When the family and child are given support and education, their anxiety decreases and there is an improved

sense of hope leading to better adherence and improved outcomes. Psychological changes that take place in response to chronic disease lead to altered family relationships. Therapists (because of the extensive time spent with children and their families) are often in a unique position to identify and address these issues.

Given the chronic nature of arthritis, and the variety of responses to it, therapists are most effective when they are part of a multidisciplinary team of medical and allied health professionals including doctors, nurses, social workers, psychologists, nutritionists, and pharmacists. The literature supports this approach for many chronic diseases [3] (see Part 3, Chapter 3.2). Specifically for JIA, the multitude of affected domains that have been identified reinforces the need for this multidisciplinary approach [4,5].

Early assessments by OTs and PTs are very important; guides for why and when to refer children are shown in Tables 3.9.1 and 3.9.2. The more information provided by the physician to the therapist, the more timely and effective therapy will be (Table 3.9.3). The need for such information is particularly critical if the therapists do not meet regularly in team meetings to discuss patient management.

Table 3.9.1 Reasons for referral to physical and occupational therapy

Pain assessment and management
Assessment and management of impairments and functional restrictions
Reliable specific measurements for monitoring change and outcome
Reduction of disability using age-appropriate techniques to maintain optimal function
Evaluation and teaching of coping skills to improve self-efficacy
Education of disease process and management to improve compliance
Provision of ongoing support with referral to appropriate disciplines as needed

Table 3.9.2 Refer to physical and occupational therapy if:

Morning stiffness greater than half an hour
Avoidance of activity due to pain or fatigue
Asymmetry of movement in upper or lower limb
Decreased range of motion or muscle strength
Leg-length discrepancy
Regression of age-appropriate developmental behaviours
Marked mood or behavioural changes
Reduced productivity at school
Isolation from peers due to physical limitations
Poor sleep

Table 3.9.3 What the therapist needs to know from the physician

Clinic report containing

  Diagnosis: definite or possible, type of JIA
  Coexisting conditions
  Medication and date started
  X-ray, MRI, CT scan results
  Main problem areas from physician's perspective
  Time line for other therapeutic interventions planned, e.g. joint injection
    or DMARDS
  Restrictions to treatment, e.g. severe anaemia

The management of early arthritis

Pain and function (see Flow charts 3.9.1, 3.9.2(a) and (b))

In the early stage, before the diagnosis has been confirmed, the disease is not under control and pain is frequently the major symptom. It may be unremitting, and greatly interfere with function. The child may be fearful to move the involved joints and distrustful of anyone else attempting to move them. As a consequence, functional restrictions develop as the child assumes pain-relieving positions. Both the child and family are fearful of the cause of the pain and its implications for the future. Sleep is often disrupted and the child may exhibit pain behaviours such as moodiness and fatigue. Antalgic postures are common. For example, a varus hindfoot with a plantar flexed first ray and reduced weight-bearing on the first metatarsal head may develop due to foot involvement, but can also develop secondary to arthritis in the knee. Similarly, a child with arthritis of the wrist may hold the wrist in a neutral position with hyperextension of the proximal interphalangeal joints, rather than dorsiflexing at the wrist when weight-bearing getting up from a chair or the floor.

Once the pain is under control, a home programme can be initiated to address any joint restrictions or muscle weakness. Some patients whose daily function is more severely impaired will require more aggressive intervention with weekly, daily or twice daily therapy. Inpatient care is sometimes needed, but with earlier referral to paediatric rheumatology services, and earlier institution of appropriate treatement, this is now very uncommon. An overview of the therapist's role early in the disease is shown in Figure 3.9.1.

Treatment goals

Identification and control of pain

Physiotherapists and occupational therapists can help teach the child how to quantify pain. Methods such as the 'face' visual analogue scales [6] are used for the younger child and 10 cm visual analogue scales for the older children. Pain is quantified according to intensity, extent, duration, and character. The Varni/Thompson paediatric pain questionnaire is a useful outcome measure [7]. By using age-appropriate pain management techniques the therapists allow the child to lead them through the physical examination while maintaining a sense of control. This initiates the essential trust between the child and therapist that is so important for future treatment. Families are taught to identify pain behaviours which may be expressed as changes in mood, abnormal movement patterns, or withdrawal from customary activities. Once these behaviours are identified, the therapist is able to teach simple pain management techniques such as the use of ice, heat, contrast baths, and TENS. The positive role of exercise in pain reduction is explained and encouraged (see also Part 3, Chapter 3.7).

Cognitive strategies such as distraction, meditative breathing, visualization, and progressive relaxation have all been shown to reduce pain and muscle spasm in children with JIA. Adapting the environment at home and school can help reduce the mechanical stresses on the joints and with the other techniques, will reduce pain and improve function. For example, the use of a 'fat' pen or pencil reduces the pressure of

Flowchart 3.9.1 PT and OT interventions.

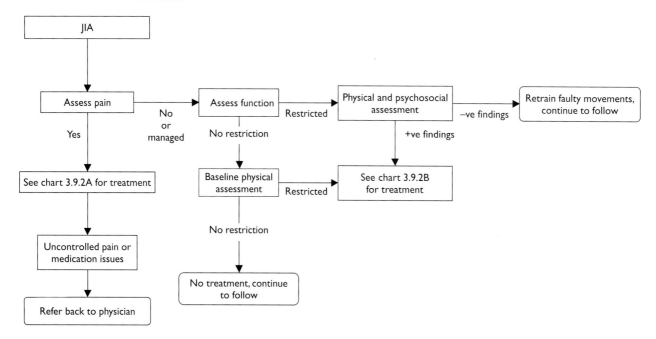

Flowchart 3.9.2 assessment, problem identification, and treatment related to pain (a) and functional limitations (b).

(a)

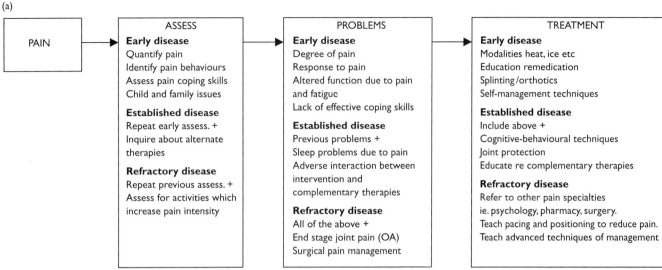

PAIN

ASSESS

Early disease
Quantify pain
Identify pain behaviours
Assess pain coping skills
Child and family issues

Established disease
Repeat early assess. +
Inquire about alternate
therapies

Refractory disease
Repeat previous assess. +
Assess for activities which
increase pain intensity

PROBLEMS

Early disease
Degree of pain
Response to pain
Altered function due to pain
and fatigue
Lack of effective coping skills

Established disease
Previous problems +
Sleep problems due to pain
Adverse interaction between
intervention and
complementary therapies

Refractory disease
All of the above +
End stage joint pain (OA)
Surgical pain management

TREATMENT

Early disease
Modalities heat, ice etc
Education remedication
Splinting /orthotics
Self-management techniques

Established disease
Include above +
Cognitive-behavioural techniques
Joint protection
Educate re complementary therapies

Refractory disease
Refer to other pain specialties
ie. psychology, pharmacy, surgery.
Teach pacing and positioning to reduce pain.
Teach advanced techniques of management

(b)

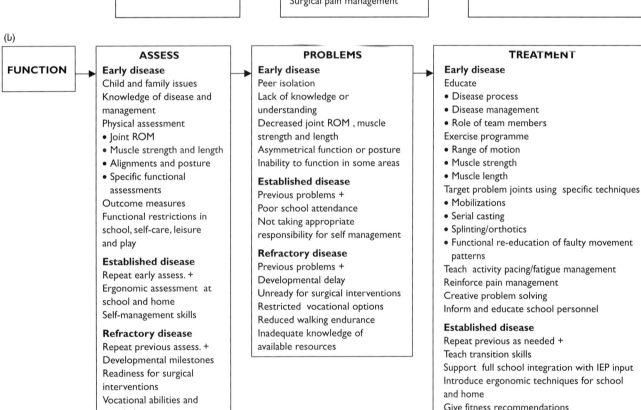

FUNCTION

ASSESS

Early disease
Child and family issues
Knowledge of disease and
management
Physical assessment
• Joint ROM
• Muscle strength and length
• Alignments and posture
• Specific functional
  assessments
Outcome measures
Functional restrictions in
school, self-care, leisure
and play

Established disease
Repeat early assess. +
Ergonomic assessment at
school and home
Self-management skills

Refractory disease
Repeat previous assess. +
Developmental milestones
Readiness for surgical
interventions
Vocational abilities and
restrictions
Need for mobility aids
Knowledge of funding
sources and vocational
planning support

PROBLEMS

Early disease
Peer isolation
Lack of knowledge or
understanding
Decreased joint ROM , muscle
strength and length
Asymmetrical function or posture
Inability to function in some areas

Established disease
Previous problems +
Poor school attendance
Not taking appropriate
responsibility for self management

Refractory disease
Previous problems +
Developmental delay
Unready for surgical interventions
Restricted vocational options
Reduced walking endurance
Inadequate knowledge of
available resources

TREATMENT

Early disease
Educate
• Disease process
• Disease management
• Role of team members
Exercise programme
• Range of motion
• Muscle strength
• Muscle length
Target problem joints using specific techniques
• Mobilizations
• Serial casting
• Splinting/orthotics
• Functional re-education of faulty movement
  patterns
Teach activity pacing/fatigue management
Reinforce pain management
Creative problem solving
Inform and educate school personnel

Established disease
Repeat previous as needed +
Teach transition skills
Support full school integration with IEP input
Introduce ergonomic techniques for school
and home
Give fitness recommendations
Provide adaptations to facilitate independence

Refractory disease
Repeat previous as needed +
Educate child, parents and school on age
appropriate milestones
Introduce preoperative treatment regimes
Educate for post-surgical care and expectations
Refer to appropriate resources for vocational
rehabilitation advice and funding sources
Prescribe mobility aides and teach use
Refer to driving schools for people with disabilities
for training and vehicle adaptation when needed
Prescribe structural adaptations to home, school,
work for independence
Consider assist dog for independent living

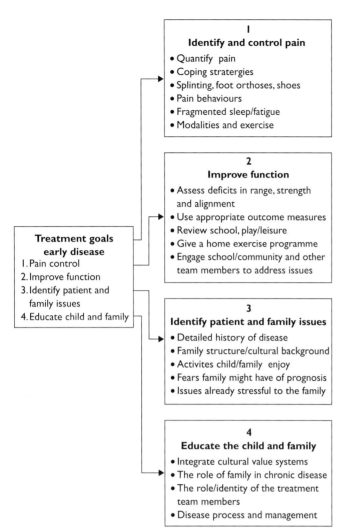

1
Identify and control pain
- Quantify pain
- Coping strartergies
- Splinting, foot orthoses, shoes
- Pain behaviours
- Fragmented sleep/fatigue
- Modalities and exercise

2
Improve function
- Assess deficits in range, strength and alignment
- Use appropriate outcome measures
- Review school, play/leisure
- Give a home exercise programme
- Engage school/community and other team members to address issues

Treatment goals early disease
1. Pain control
2. Improve function
3. Identify patient and family issues
4. Educate child and family

3
Identify patient and family issues
- Detailed history of disease
- Family structure/cultural background
- Activites child/family enjoy
- Fears family might have of prognosis
- Issues already stressful to the family

4
Educate the child and family
- Integrate cultural value systems
- The role of family in chronic disease
- The role/identity of the treatment team members
- Disease process and management

Fig. 3.9.1 An overview of the therapists' role in early arthritis

a tripod pinch on metacarpal joints, and decreases finger pain when writing. Using a wedged writing surface made out of a closed three-ring binder on the desk top often significantly decrease neck pain. These simple changes may improve school attendance and productivity without making the child conspicuous to their peers. Children are encouraged to use both shoulder straps and a waist strap on their back packs to give a more ergonomically balanced load and reduce stress on the shoulder girdle and back.

Splinting for pain management at night can improve the quality of sleep and such adherence is better than with daytime splinting particularly among adolescents in this early stage of the disease. Once the medications have started to work, the splinting should be re-evaluated. Well-made supportive, running shoes with a straight last and strong heel counter, and custom-made orthotics often lead to a significant improvement in function by decreasing pain in feet and knees. If appropriate techniques are used at the early stages of the disease it is believed that some of the adaptive abnormal movement patterns may be avoided, although there is little published evidence to support this belief.

Successful pain reduction is the first step in building a strong therapeutic relationship with the child and family. Pain and anxiety may cause poor-quality sleep; as a consequence the child may display poor concentration or behaviour problems at school, and be at risk for being labelled as learning disabled or disruptive [8]. Therapists may be very helpful in addressing this issue in the early stages of disease. By teaching sleep hygiene techniques together with pain management, therapists may greatly enhance the child's ability to cope with their arthritis and improve school performance. Teaching children how to pace their activities, so as to balance school work, sports, social activities, and the need for rest is extremely important. Fatigue management is also a priority at this stage of the disease, enabling children to continue functioning adequately and not becoming isolated from their healthy peers, as all too commonly occurs following the onset of arthritis.

Improving function and decrease impairment

Using validated assessment techniques the therapist measures range of joint motion, muscle strength and length, and functional alignments. Deficits are identified and recorded. Videotaping is a useful medium for recording gait assessments. Functional outcome measures such as CHAQ [9], JASI [10], JAQQ [11], JAFAR [12], CAHP [13] can be used when indicated (see Part 3, Chapter 3.4). Writing tests, pinch and grip strength measurements may demonstrate functional deficits of which the child or parent is not aware. Children learn to accommodate by using alternate patterns of motion which, if not identified can lead to deformity. Detailed information on these assessments can be found in recent therapy textbooks [14,15].

The OT focuses on school function, activities of daily living, as well as play and leisure to help the child maintain or regain independence. Reviewing the ergonomics of these activities often indicates the need for minor interventions, and occasionally more major changes. Encouraging normal activities that may often have been proscribed by well-meaning individuals with the mistaken belief that continuing such activities will in some way worsen the joint disease, is often necessary. It has been shown that short-term exercise does not exacerbate the disease [16]. In order to improve the child's level of social functioning at school, play, or leisure, the psychosocial aspects of chronic disease are addressed with the parents in this early stage. Parents who have this knowledge are more likely to report problems which can be dealt with before crises have developed. These interventions can help prevent isolation from peers and/or depression developing.

Physical therapy intervention is often quite limited until the anti-inflammatory medications have begun to diminish the extent of the synovitis. However, after an appropriate interval (usually not longer than 4–6 weeks) an extensive assessment of muscle strength, range of motion, pain, asymmetries, and gait, needs to be performed, and a home programme created. It is important to work with the child, the family, and team members to determine the functional priorities, as these determine the type of programme needed. Initially a daily programme restricted to a very few exercises, or a set amount of time (e.g. 10 min) is developed, which is modified over time. The relevance of the exercises to address each functional goal must be carefully explained to the child and family. However, not all families, particularly in the early stage of disease, can comfortably take on the responsibility of executing such a programme, and they may need the regular support of other healthcare providers.

Often families are faced with the decision of whether to attend therapy at the tertiary care centre where the paediatric rheumatology team works, or locally with therapists who will usually be less familiar with JIA. In some countries this decision may be made by their Health Insurance companies. The decision also has to take into account the effect of attending clinics and therapy appointments on the parent's ability to continue working, and on the child's school attendance. These factors determine where the child receives therapy. Occasionally, there are no local therapists who can become involved in the child's care and alternate arrangements must be considered; for example, a teacher's aide may be taught how to monitor the home programme. Close communication between therapists, both within the team, and between the team and the community, is needed to achieve realistic, attainable goals.

Parents are advised to encourage their children to participate in a wide variety of activities to the best of their abilities and to remain in physical education at school [17]. It is rare that any child even early in the disease course, needs to withdraw completely from physical education activities. However, school staff are usually worried about how to manage a child with chronic arthritis, and may either over-react and allow the child to stop all physical activities, or may ignore the problem and refuse to appropriately modify educational activities to accommodate the child's needs. The situation is further complicated by the fact that these needs will change as the disease fluctuates. The therapists can often play a vital role by educating the school staff about the child's disease status. Therapists may provide letters for school teachers which can be helpful in informing them about the disease, how it might impact on performance in school, and how this impact may change over time. Physical education teachers have to be encouraged to allow the child with JIA to participate to the extent that they are able to, and to grade the child appropriately on attitude and effort. Sometimes a new role can be found, such as coach or time-keeper, in order to keep the child involved with peers even at times of disease flare. It is very important that decreased performance in physical education is not allowed to inappropriately affect the school's assessment of the child's overall academic performance. This becomes particularly important when the older child is close to applying to institutions of higher education.

Recreational activities play an important role in establishing a child's positive self-esteem [14] and these activities constitute an important part of the work of childhood. The therapists encourage the child to respect her body and to become aware of the 'signals' it is sending. The child is taught to judge the level of activity which is appropriate for the disease state. The only activities which are relatively contraindicated are contact sports and gymnastic tumbling when there is C1–C2 joint laxity or severe osteoporosis. Almost all children with Polyarthritis and some with Oligoarthritis have cervical spine involvement, but only infrequently is it severe enough to warrant significant modification of activities [18].

Swimming is a good recreational activity that can be shared with family members and peers without causing increased pain to the child even during acute flares.

Not only is it important to engage the family in the child's treatment plan, but it is also essential that the school is actively involved. The OT and PT can sometimes help increase or improve this involvement by doing school visits. Establishing this community support as part of the treatment team is likely to lead to the quickest adaptation of the child and family to their new disease. Similarly, doing home visits may be useful in helping the family manage the disease.

Identifying child and family issues

Depending on the situation the therapists may take a detailed history from the child and family identifying attitudes, anxieties, family coping, communication skills, and value systems, particularly if the team lacks a social worker or psychologist. Understanding the family structure and cultural background will help the therapist to teach appropriate skills and to be realistic in expectations of care; ignoring these factors can be extremely detrimental [19]. Many families are immigrants, and may have a poor command of the primary language used by the clinicians, but are reluctant to admit they are having difficulty comprehending. The use of family members or friends as interpreters may be unhelpful, as the translation of what is being said may be modified by the untrained interpreter, leading to further miscommunication. It is preferable to arrange for professional interpreters to attend the initial clinic and therapy sessions to ensure that accurate information to the caregivers. One also needs to be aware that health care decisions may be made by a member of the extended family who is not attending the clinics or therapy sessions. A sensitivity to other concerns affecting the family and health issues in the extended family is important.

Educating the child and family

Although the primary role of OT and PT is to address the physical aspects of the management of JIA, many of the issues addressed by therapists are educational in nature, and therapy often has an important psychological component. A lot of therapy time is spent in reiterating and explaining what the physicians have told the family. This important role of emphasizing and clarifying the therapeutic 'message' can only occur effectively if the therapist and physicians are in close communication, and have regular team meetings. As the therapy progresses, the parents and other involved family members can share their concerns and misconceptions in an environment that may be more relaxed and less intimidating than the routine outpatient clinic. Using lay language to describe the mechanism of inflammation and the rationale for the medical regimen may help facilitate adherence to treatment. Explanation of the roles and expertise of the various team members during therapy sessions can often help implementation of the overall management plan. Educating the family about the importance of the family's role in developing and carrying through the treatment plan is integral to the success of the treatment. The therapist should explore with the family the impact of their cultural beliefs upon the medical management of the disease (and vice versa). The family needs to feel comfortable with any team member, trusting that their concerns will be passed on to the appropriate person. Identifying the key family member to facilitate care is critical given the wide variety of family structures in today's society. Therapists need to focus on building a solid, ongoing relationship with that pivotal person as well as the patient. Sometimes other family members will take on various aspects of care. Siblings are encouraged to understand the patient's care. They can be engaged in educational activities with the patient, especially if the activity is fun such as the use of educational computer games. Sibling involvement often helps address such concerns as 'Is this disease contagious? Is my sister going to die?', which are often otherwise left unanswered. Education is often directed by the questions from the parents or child rather than predetermined by the staff. Learning occurs best when the child or family member is at a stage when they are willing to learn.

The management of established arthritis

Pain and function (see Flow charts 3.9.1, 3.9.2(a) and (b))

In established disease, pain is usually under fairly good control but can be triggered by excessive physical activity or by a flare of synovitis. Ongoing assessment by therapists helps identify the reason for increased pain, and they may be able to alert the physician to the possible need for a change in medication in advance of the planned clinic visit. In established disease, joint restrictions may be present causing compensatory movement patterns. These patterns must be addressed before they become integrated into the child's neurophysiology and result in permanent misloading of the joint [20]. If joints are actively inflamed, it may be very difficult to regain and maintain normal joint function. The use of intra-articular corticosteroid injections is often a useful way of suppressing the inflammation in a particular joint allowing the therapist and child to effectively address tight joints and tendons and regain a normal joint range of movement and function. When multiple restrictions are present, a short period of inpatient rehabilitation may enable intensive therapy sessions to be undertaken within a short time frame.

An overview of the therapist's role in the established stage of the disease course is shown in Figure 3.9.2.

Identifying and managing impairments and functional limitations

Using the same assessment tools on a regular basis enables the therapist to identify changes in restrictions of range of motion, muscle strength and function, thereby facilitating early intervention and helping to prevent the development of fixed deformities. OTs and PTs working with the child plan a strategy for improvement of the deficits. They target those areas which are most significantly impacting daily function. It is probable that PTs and OTs working together rather than in parallel, leads to more effective interventions. For example, splinting by the OT is most effective immediately after pain stretching and pain-reduction techniques under the supervision of the PT. Teaching home exercise programmes necessary for maintaining range gained during splinting, is best done by both therapists together. Adherence to a home programme is particularly important when serial casting is being used to eliminate deformities [21]. Serial casting is an effective way to reduce contractures and is well tolerated if age-appropriate pain management is used [2,14]. The long-term outcome depends in part on the child and family's commitment to a home exercise programme. Without this commitment, it is sometimes not possible to regain the muscle strength and soft-tissue alignment in the new range.

Splinting and intensive therapy programmes will have only a limited effect, if the inflammation cannot be adequately suppressed by medications. Although therapists have a number of modalities that may help modify inflammation, such as splinting, icing, ultrasound, and exercise, there is no evidence that these techniques alone are adequate to control joint inflammation. Close collaboration between therapists and physicians is essential to achieve and maintain effective disease control. Children need regular re-assessments of their home physical therapy programme and splinting regime. Both have to be modified to reflect changes in the child's physical parameters and functional needs. Special attention should be paid to ensure that

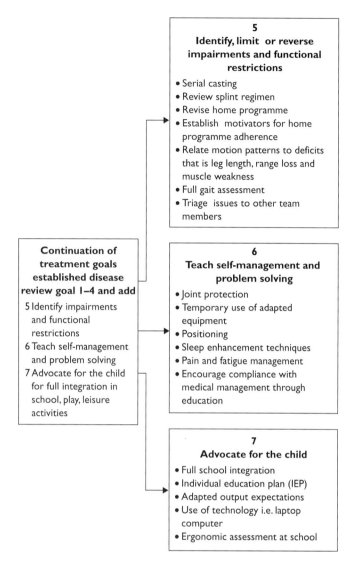

Fig. 3.9.2 An overview of the therapists' role in established arthritis

therapy programmes remain appropriate, respecting the time commitments needed for the social, physical, and academic functions that are part of the child's day-to-day life. Sensitivity to the individual child's need is critical for gaining compliance. For example, although night-time splinting is encouraged as it does not interfere with function or self-image, if its use causes sleep disturbance, almost as effective a response can be obtained by wearing a resting splint while reading or watching TV. School-aged children (particularly in the adolescent age group) may agree to wear working splints if their use is restricted to the home and not school; insisting on use at school may well lead to complete refusal to wear the splints, or removal as soon as the child is out of sight of the parents. Adherence with exercise and splinting regimes is often worse than for medication [21], therefore, it is important to build strategies for enhanced compliance. Engaging the child and family in setting realistic, achievable, short-term goals helps by giving them a sense of control, and has been shown to improve compliance [2]. Building on small successes is much easier than trying to regroup after the family and team have become frustrated by unrealistic and inappropriate expectations. Recognition of the effort required simply to maintain the status quo is also very important for both therapists and children to remember. Short-term, goal-specific contracts using stickers or rewards for success are often necessary when the child is unable to perceive the long-term goals of exercise or splinting regimes. Setting upper limits to the amount of time spent daily on therapy, and regularly re-evaluating progress helps to focus the family and child on the target goal. The therapeutic plan should be given to the child or family in writing, using language and diagrams that are both age and culturally appropriate. If available, videofilms of the therapists and child performing the home exercise programmes can be invaluable when language is an issue, or if the programme is to be supervised by an adult who is not present at the time the therapy programme is taught. There are many tips available in the literature to enhance adherence with therapy [14].

Hydrotherapy is often used in established disease to help improve cardiovascular functioning, muscle strength, joint range, and to re-educate functional movement patterns. At this stage the therapist must pay close attention to the alignment and quality of motion while in the pool working with the individual child. Unstructured playing in a group in the pool is useful as a social activity or to improve aerobic fitness, but it will not change faulty movement patterns or improve specific joint ranges or muscle strength.

Play is used in various ways by therapists, and can be divided into three categories: free or unstructured play, playfulness to enhance compliance with therapy, and play as therapy. Free or unstructured play is acknowledged as the work of childhood and allows the child to mature through the normal stages of development. However if a child is unable to complete a task in the 'normal' fashion, the child will adapt and use alternate movement patterns to achieve the desired outcome. Use of these alternate movement patterns because of pain, weakness, or loss of range of movement, leads to them becoming habitual. As a consequence weak muscles remain weak, and tight joints remain tight, despite the child participating in activities which would normally strengthen or stretch target areas in healthy children. Free play should be included in the therapeutic plan at all stages, but its role(s) as being either social, aerobic, or as a reward for doing specific exercises, needs to be clearly understood. Playfulness, however, is an extremely valuable tool for the paediatric therapist, allowing the execution of repetitive, and often boring exercises, especially with young children. For example, squeezing soap bubbles out of a sponge placed behind the knee achieves a specific exercise (using quadriceps contractions in end-range) in a playful manner. Imaginative play is possible with any specific exercise programme, and games can often be modified to achieve specific goals. If games and play are used as the focus of the therapeutic intervention, they are best utilized when the child has the required strength or range in the targeted areas. The child can then be taught how to use their newly regained range and strength effectively and efficiently in the activity.

If possible, both therapists should perform a gait assessment together at regular intervals to identify asymmetries caused by muscle imbalances, joint restrictions, leg-length discrepancies, or foot malalignments. This assessment includes walking, running, hopping, walking on tiptoes, walking on heels, and full flight stair climbing; the child needs to be in shorts and barefoot. In the young child, abnormal patterns develop quickly in response to inflammation and pain. Even when the inflammation is controlled, the pattern may continue and lead to further imbalances. Supportive shoes or orthotics are prescribed early to support the joints and prevent malalignments. It is important to educate the parents on selection of suitable shoes, and ways to promote normal gait at home. During these therapy sessions a close

therapeutic relationship often develops, and parents or children may mention other issues that are of concern to them. The therapist may be able to directly address these, or can refer to the appropriate team member.

Teaching self-management and problem solving

Joint protection is introduced at this stage of disease for the older interested child (Table 3.9.4). It has greatest impact if taught in a camp or retreat setting where the group dynamics help to reinforce the value of self care [5,14]. Children only use such strategies if they do not draw attention to themselves when with peers. The concept of using large joints and muscle groups to avoid stressing small joints is easily understood by the older child. Therapists ask the child to use a variety of small devices such as jar openers, pen grips, or reaching aides while explaining the principles of protection. If the family is engaged and supportive of this approach, the child will often be compliant. Not infrequently, adaptive devices are only required until a flare is controlled. It is useful for therapy departments to keep a selection of devices that can be loaned and returned as needed.

While the PT focuses mainly on motor function, the OT tends to focus on activities of daily living, such as time management, and how to balance activities to achieve maximum levels of function in leisure, self-care, play, and work. There is of course no strict demarcation of the role of the PT and OT in this area, and the roles may change depending on individual circumstances, both within the team structure, but also on the circumstances of the child and family.

The child who has been committed to activities whether in sport, the arts, or employment before developing arthritis needs to learn how to pay attention to her body, and respect pain and fatigue by pacing, and if necessary modifying the extent or frequency of the activity. Swimming or cycling are sports that can be substituted for contact sport—at least temporarily if need be—for example, during a flare of the arthritis. Because of restrictions in their physical abilities, students may choose to concentrate on academic pursuits. As the arthritis becomes better controlled the child is often able to resume most, if not all, aspects of his or her previous lifestyle. It has been recognized by paediatric rheumatologists that children who attend an educational retreat are often more adherent to treatment plans. They take responsibility for themselves and learn through interactions with other children with similar disease. Specifically, they learn to understand their symptoms, develop effective coping skills, and manage their disease better. They often appear to be more confident and hopeful about the future after attending such a retreat or camp.

An important role of the PT and OT is to work collaboratively with patients and their families so as to problem-solve around many of the issues that have been discussed above. The concept of patient-centred care addresses the fact that it is the patient's needs that are paramount, and empowers children with arthritis to increasingly identify their own needs, as they mature. Therapists play a critical role in helping the child develop the skills necessary for transitioning from a paediatric health care system to an adult-orientated system (see Part 3, Chapter 3.3).

Advocating for the child

Therapists continue to review, reassess, and modify the treatment programme established during early disease, adding or subtracting as appropriate. Schooling is always a priority, with daily attendance being

Table 3.9.4 Principles of joint protection and energy conservation for children with JIA

Symptom	Principle	Sample of management

Hand or wrist pain	Reduction of static work and mechanical forces on joints	At school
		   Use of a gel pen or mechanical pencil with a rubber grip on barrel to reduce tripod pinch forces
		   Use of a computer to relieve forces on finger joints
		   Mini-breaks during writing to rest joints
		
		At home
		   Use of tools such as jar openers
		   Use of a tray to carry objects, supported underneath by hands held in neutral position, slightly flexed at wrists
		   Asking for help

Knee and foot pain	Recognize pain, and reduce time spent in pain-inducing activity	At school
		   Permitting the child to move around the class (doing errands, etc.) to prevent gelling when sitting
		   Minimizing time sitting on floor
		   Minimizing distance between classrooms, allowing more time to get between classes. Self-pacing during PE classes. Grading PE on attitude, not performance
		Using supportive shoes and orthotics

Neck pain	Obtaining appropriate body postures	At school Revising height and angle of the desk to minimize persistent neck flexion. Lessening load in back pack, and wearing it across back rather than over a shoulder. Encouraging a short, non-obtrusive range of motion exercise of neck regularly throughout the day At home Setting up an ergonomic work space at home. Use of book rests. Reviewing use of soft collar. Avoiding reading on bed or floor with neck hyper-extended
Fatigue	Pacing activities improving sleep	Sleep hygiene education Reviewing patient's and family priorities, to maintain a balance between academic achievement and recreation

a primary goal of the whole team. In many countries full integration is a legal right for the child with a disability (see Part 3, Chapter 3.5). As parents may not know what help the child is entitled to, and what is available, the therapist is often the individual who can best coach them in advocating for their child. When necessary, the therapist can/will intervene with the school authorities on the child's behalf. An individual education plan developed by the school authorities in close collaboration with the family and the paediatric rheumatology team may be necessary for the child to access all the services they require. The fluctuating and commonly hidden nature of chronic arthritis is often a problem for educators who do not have a good grasp of the disease process, and the consequent disability. Productivity in writing, and performance in physical education may change from week to week, and the school staff will need to understand enough about the disease to be able to help the child cope with the educational requirements. Word processors or laptop computers, by substituting key boarding for writing, reduce the mechanical forces caused by a tripod pinch. Children prefer to use portable technologies such as a word processor or a laptop rather than a desktop PC which isolates them from their peers as the class moves between classrooms. Occasionally, ergonomic assessments are needed. This can be done as an outreach visit from the clinic, or by the school-based therapist. Children prefer not to draw attention to their disability and therefore often refuse aids and adaptations, choosing instead to make only minor adjustments to accommodate to pain or fatigue. Although such coping strategies are

not necessarily a bad thing, it is important that the therapists work closely with the child and teachers to ensure that this refusal to admit to problems, and accept help, does not become a hurdle to the long-term wellbeing of the child.

The management of refractory arthritis

Pain and function (see Flow charts 3.9.1, 3.9.2(a) and (b))

At this stage pain may be non-existent, well-controlled, or severe. Pain is commonly due to degenerative arthritis, but is often exacerbated by flares of continuing inflammation. Pain can also be due to tendon and muscle damage as a consequence of joint deformity or disease. Function is limited by pain, loss of range of motion, and/or muscle weakness. These functional restrictions may require intensive inpatient rehabilitation with or without surgical interventions. In this stage of the disease orthotics and splints may need to be accommodative rather than corrective, with the aim of reducing pain and providing stability to the joints, rather than regaining alignment or range of movement. Adaptive equipment may be necessary for activities of daily living. Unlike early and established disease in which the goal is often to correct compensatory movement patterns, in late refractory disease

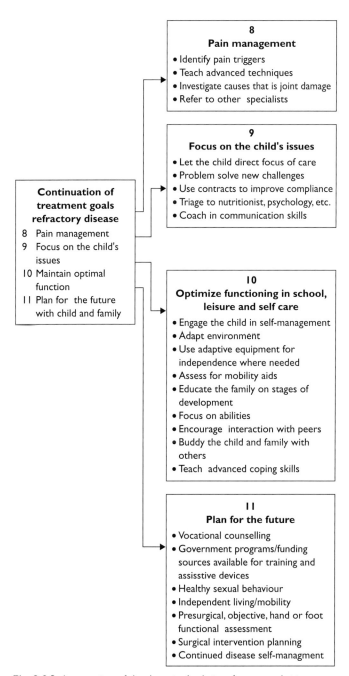

8
Pain management
- Identify pain triggers
- Teach advanced techniques
- Investigate causes that is joint damage
- Refer to other specialists

9
Focus on the child's issues
- Let the child direct focus of care
- Problem solve new challenges
- Use contracts to improve compliance
- Triage to nutritionist, psychology, etc.
- Coach in communication skills

Continuation of treatment goals refractory disease
8 Pain management
9 Focus on the child's issues
10 Maintain optimal function
11 Plan for the future with child and family

10
Optimize functioning in school, leisure and self care
- Engage the child in self-management
- Adapt environment
- Use adaptive equipment for independence where needed
- Assess for mobility aids
- Educate the family on stages of development
- Focus on abilities
- Encourage interaction with peers
- Buddy the child and family with others
- Teach advanced coping skills

11
Plan for the future
- Vocational counselling
- Government programs/funding sources available for training and assisstive devices
- Healthy sexual behaviour
- Independent living/mobility
- Presurgical, objective, hand or foot functional assessment
- Surgical intervention planning
- Continued disease self-managment

Fig. 3.9.3 An overview of the therapists' role in refractory arthritis

compensatory movement patterns may need to be taught so as to help overcome the disability of permanent deformities. An overview of the therapist's role in refractory disease is shown in Figure 3.9.3.

Treatment goals

Pain management

In this stage of the disease the child is often knowledgeable about their arthritis, what triggers pain, and what techniques to employ in order to best cope with the pain. However, children have different learning styles, and their readiness to learn and change varies as they mature. It is therefore important not to assume that previously taught information has been remembered or integrated into their daily life. Children who earlier were uninterested in knowing about their condition may a few years later become experts in understanding their disease. The ongoing, unremitting pain caused by joint damage is often under-reported to the physician. The child may be concerned that worsening symptoms will lead to painful treatments or investigations. Cognitive-behavioural techniques to help cope with the pain may be initiated by the therapist or psychologist in the team [22]. Pain due to end-stage joint disease may require surgical interventions including joint replacements surgery (see Part 3, Chapter 3.12). The therapist plays a critical role in helping plan for the surgery, ensuring that the child is as psychologically and physically prepared for the procedure as possible. The patient and family is encouraged to discuss the timing of the procedure, so that it causes as little interference with school or other major commitments as possible. Preoperatively, the therapist educates the child on the postoperative regime required to achieve maximum benefit from the intervention, with skills such as the use of walking aides, or one-handed self-care procedures, being taught when necessary. Occasionally, intensive therapy is required preoperatively in order to prepare the child for the rigours of the postoperative regimen. For example, upper body range and strength may need to be improved so that the child is capable of using crutches postoperatively. A coordinated plan between the surgical and rehabilitation treatment teams is necessary to ensure a smooth transition postoperatively. PT and OT involvement is often required intensely in the postoperative period to maximize the potential benefits of any surgical intervention.

Focusing on the child's issues

In the refractory stage, the child has lived with the disease long enough to know what are the major functional problems. Most children and adolescents strive to be independent. Older children usually have a good understanding of what each discipline offers and may attend follow-up clinics with a plan about what needs to be addressed. The younger child requires the therapist to uncover issues that have not been adequately addressed, perhaps because the child or the family think that the problem is insuperable. For example, sleepovers with friends may not have been possible in the early stages due to medication, splinting, or night pain, and the possibility that such an activity is now not only possible, but desirable, has been forgotten or rejected. The therapist is able to problem-solve with the child and parents to help make such an activity possible. Children may have issues with teasing at school, or may feel isolated from peers who spend hours walking in shopping malls. The therapist's role includes reviewing any adaptive equipment that may be necessary to enhance physical independence. The role also includes teaching communication skills, and coaching patients in advocating for themselves, so that they are as socially and psychologically capable of independent function as possible. The therapist may also intervene when necessary, with the child's permission, to arrange for appropriate ongoing support from adults.

Adherence to exercises and splinting may increasingly become an issue as the child and family gets tired of the daily routine. PT and OTs working in collaboration with the child decide the target areas to work on, arranging for 'therapy holidays' and other rewards, so as to make the therapy as sustainable and tolerable as possible. Contracts between the therapist or parents, and the patient have been found to be useful in enhancing adherence, especially in the 9–14-year-old age group. Older adolescents are often prepared to carry out an exercise programme in a community gym, or fitness centre that their friends may also attend.

Optimizing function in work, leisure, and self-care

As in the earlier disease stages, therapists continue to monitor range of motion, strength, and mobility, and prescribe appropriate exercises. Functional assessments are used to identify problem areas. The focus is always on the child's ability rather than disability. Adaptive equipment such as reaching aids, a bath bench or bidet toilet seat may be necessary to maintain independence in self-care.

In children with severe hand and wrist involvement the use of a validated hand assessment helps identify those children who require surgical intervention. The hand assessment will also provide information concerning the child's developmental readiness to comply with post-operative care. Based on this assessment, surgical intervention may be planned for the immediate future or may be postponed until the child is more mature.

Power mobility using scooters or chairs is generally avoided due to concerns that flexion contractures and osteoporosis will worsen with loss of ambulation. However, if the child is mature enough to understand these risks, having these may make it possible to join peers at the mall or to participate in other outdoor activities. Some patients use scooters or chairs for a year or two and then, often but not always after surgical interventions, become increasingly able to ambulate again. Other mobility aids such as canes, walkers, or crutches may be appropriate to enhance function, especially after surgery or during acute flares.

Therapists work with the families to help the child gain appropriate levels of independence as he or she matures, the amount of independence varying depending on the child's developmental level, the family values, and the child's perceived safety (see also Part 3, Chapters 3.3 and 3.6). Independence may be an issue for the children and adolescents with JIA, as they are frequently more physically dependant on their parents than their peers, but also because sometimes parents perceive children as being more dependent than they actually are. Therapists work with the family to enhance safe progression to independence, reinforcing input from the team psychologist or social worker in the process. Adaptations to the home or family care may be necessary for increasing independence. Adaptations at school may be more acceptable at this stage particularly in the adolescent years, as the child has had several years to come to terms with the condition, and peers are often able to accept the child for whom he or she is. The child may need to use the school elevator to reduce stair climbing, have notes photocopied, or use a laptop/word processor to reduce the mechanical stress on fingers and wrists. The therapist continues to work with the child and family to develop the communication skills necessary to educate peers and school staff in the disease and its management. When teasing or isolation from peers is an issue, the child can be taught how to be her own advocate, and therapists can also help by making the school staff aware of the problem. Learning how to cope with many of the normal adolescent issues, which are magnified by the presence of chronic arthritis can be enhanced by 'buddying' the child and family. Another child and family who has successfully negotiated similar issues can help the development of good coping skills.

If from the time of diagnosis, guidelines for attempting new activities have been taught, by the time the child is in the refractory stage of the disease she will have become increasingly confident in her ability to make wise choices. Each challenge successfully met increases the child's confidence and reinforces learning.

For a child with refractory arthritis effective, energy-efficient, compensatory movements patterns may need to be taught. For example, if the ankle joint is effectively fused and the patient descends stairs sideways, better alignment is achieved by placing the foot at the edge of the stair and rocking over to the next step, also a rocker bar can be added to the sole of both shoes to simulate a more normal gait pattern.

Planning for the future

Children with refractory disease as they approach adulthood may have many issues concerning their future careers. Therapists may need to refer the adolescent to the appropriate team member or agency for vocational counselling, and to provide information about physical abilities and limitations. Families applying for funding from government or private sources to cover the costs of assistive devices, mobility aides, splinting, or education often need a therapist to support the application with details of functional abilities and areas of restriction.

Chronic disease can affect both sensuality and sexuality in the adolescent. The therapist or social worker who is known to the child and adolescent can foster a non-threatening, non-judgemental atmosphere where they will feel comfortable discussing these issues confidentially. Creative problem solving around fatigue, positioning, pain, and range restrictions can be covered with the patient alone or with their partner. Risks of pregnancy both because of the disease, and because of the medications can be reviewed. The family perception of the adolescent's sexuality may need to be explored and communication facilitated by the therapist within the context of the family's religious and cultural value systems. Referral to a counsellor may be appropriate (see also Part 3, Chapter 3.6).

All the team members need to address transition issues regularly as the child matures. Self-management skills, such as knowing correct medication and dosage, preparing questions for the clinic visits or reporting symptoms are encouraged even with young children. Adolescents are encouraged to take responsibility from their parents when visiting the team. Both adolescents and their parents may need encouragement to enable the patient to be seen in the clinic without the parent being present. The adolescent will need to learn how to initiate visits and how to raise any issues they wish to discuss. Gradually, they become ready to enter the adult world, including the adult-orientated medical care system.

Independent living is a goal for all young adults. Occasionally, this requires careful planning and problem solving. The therapist is often able to organize home care or support independence with adaptive equipment, home-maker help, or by suggesting the removal of architectural barriers.

Adherence to treatment regimes may be more challenging to the newly independent young adult. Team members need to have a lot of patience as the young person learns to organize her own schedules. Close cooperation between team members, the adolescent, and the family helps to make the transition smooth.

The issues of transition are discussed in more detail in Part 3, Chapter 3.3.

Summary

Referral for physical and occupational therapy should occur soon after the diagnosis of JIA has been made, and pharmacological treatment has begun. Continued PT and OT reassessment and management is necessary for many children with JIA throughout their childhood, and into adult life. The type of help required differs widely between children, and an individual child may require different approaches at different times during the disease course. This chapter outlines many of the areas that need to be addressed as the disease evolves. The overall goals of PT and OT interventions are to promote age-appropriate independence, and as normal function as possible in all aspects of the child's life.

References

1. Miller, M.L., Kress, A.M., and Berry, C.A. Decreased physical function in juvenile rheumatoid arthritis. *Arthritis Care Res* 1999;12:309–13.

2. Rapoff, M.A. Evaluating and enhancing adherence to regimens for pediatric rheumatic diseases. In J.L. Melvin and F.V. Wright, (eds.), *Rheumatologic Rehabilitation*, Vol. 3. Bethesda, MD: AOTA Inc, 2000; pp. 127–40.

3. Petty, R.E. Juvenile rheumatoid arthritis. *Annals RCPSC* 1982;15:475–81.

4. Kuis, W., Heijnen, C.J., Hogeweg, J.A., Sinnema, G., and Helders, P.J.M. How painful is juvenile chronic arthritis? *Arch Dis Child* 1997; 77:451–3.

5. Emery, H.M. Rehabilitation of the child with juvenile chronic arthritis. In T.R. Southwood and P.N. Malleson, (eds.), *Bailliere's Clinical Paediatrics*, Vol. 1:3: London: Bailliere Tindall, 1993, pp. 803–23.

6. Unruh, A.M. and McGrath, P.J. Pain in children: psychosocial issues. In J.L. Melvin and F.V. Wright, (eds.), *Rheumatologic Rehabilitation*, Vol. 3. Bethesda, MD: AOTA Inc, 2000, pp. 141–68.

7. Varni, J.W., Thompson, K.L., and Hanson, V. The Varni/Thompson pediatric pain questionnaire. I. Chronic musculoskeletal pain in juvenile rheumatoid arthritis. *Pain* 1987;28:27–38.

8. Zamir, G., Press, J., Tal, A., and Tarashiuk, A. Sleep fragmentation in children with juvenile rheumatoid arthritis. *J Rheumatol* 1998;25:1191–7.

9. Singh, G., Athreya, B.A., Fries, J.F., and Goldsmith, D.P. Measurement of health status in children with juvenile rheumatoid arthritis. *Arthritis Rheum* 1994;37:1761–9.

10. Wright, F.V., Longo Kimber, J., Law, M., Goldsmith, C.H., Crombie, V., and Dent, P. The juvenile arthritis functional status index (JASI): a validation study. *J Rheumatol* 1996;23:1066–79.

11. Duffy, C.M., Arsenault, L., Duffy, K.N., Pacquin, J.D., and Strawcznski, H. The juvenile arthritis quality of life questionnaire: development of a new responsive index for juvenile rheumatoid arthritis and juvenile spondyloarthritides. *J Rheumatol* 1997;24:738–46.

12. Howe, S., Levinson, J., Shear, E., Hartner, S., McGirr, G., Schulte, M., and Lovell, D. Development of a disability measurement tool for juvenile rheumatoid arthritis; The Juvenile Arthritis Functional Assessment Report for children and their parents. *Arthritis Rheum* 1991;34:873–80.

13. Tucker, L.B., DeNardo, B.A., Abetz, L.N., Landgraf, J.M., and Schaller, J.G. The Childhood Arthritis Health Profile (CAHP): validity and reliability of the condition specific scales. *Arthritis Rheum* 1995; 38(Suppl. 9):S183.

14. Wright, F.V. and Smith, E. Physical therapy management of the child and adolescent with juvenile rheumatoid arthritis. In J. Walker and A. Helewa (eds.), *Physical Therapy in Arthritis*. Philadelphia, PA: W.B., Saunders, 1996, pp. 211–44.

15. Wright, F.V. Measurement outcome in juvenile rheumatoid arthritis. In J.L. Melvin and F.V. Wright, (eds.), *Rheumatologic Rehabilitation*, Vol. 3. Bethesda, MD: AOTA Inc, 2000, pp. 231–48.

16. Singsen, B.H. Physical fitness in children with juvenile rheumatoid arthritis and other chronic pediatric illnesses. *Pediatr Clin N Am* 1995; 42:1035–49.

17. Tucker, L.B., DeNardo, B.A., Stebulis, J., and Schaller, J.G. Creating a positive school environment. In *Your Child with Arthritis: A Family Guide for Care Giving*. Baltimore, MD: John Hopkins University Press, 1996, pp. 167–213.

18. Emery, H.M. and Bowyer, S.L. Physical modalities of therapy in pediatric rheumatic diseases. *Rheum Dis Clin N Am* 1991;17:1001–14.

19. Krefting, L.H., and Krefting, D.V. Cultural influences on performance. In C. Christiansen and C. Baumn (eds.), *Occupational Therapy: Overcoming Human Performance Deficits*. Thorofare: Slack Inc, 1991, pp. 101–24.

20. Hafner, R., Truckenbrodt, H., and Spamer, M. Rehabilitation in children with juvenile chronic arthritis. *Bailliere's Clini Rheumatol*. 1998;12:329–61.

21. Barden, W., Brooks, D., and Ayling-Campos, A. Physical therapy management of the subluxed wrist in children with arthritis. *Phys Ther* 1995;75:879–85.

22. McGrath, P.J. and Breau, L. Musculoskeletal pain. In P.J. McGrath and G.A. Finley, (eds.), *Chronic and Recurrent Pain in Children and Adolescents. Progress in Pain Research and Management*, Vol. 13. Seattle, WA: IASP Press, 1999, pp. 173–97.

3.10 Nutrition

Deborah Rothman

Aim

The aim of this chapter is to discuss the importance of nutrition and nutritional deficits in the morbidity of children with JIA.

Structure

- Introduction
- Growth failure

  Role of nutrition

  Role of corticosteroids.
- Osteoporosis
- Nutritional therapy for JIA
- Conclusion

Introduction

Protein–energy malnutrition as well as obesity, poor linear growth, anaemia, and osteoporosis are all common problems in children with Juvenile Idiopathic Arthritis (JIA). Dietary intake is only one of many contributing factors including the disease process itself, malabsorption, side-effects from drug therapy, and decreased physical activity.

Growth failure

Frederick Still was the first to describe the growth failure seen in untreated JIA:

'A remarkable feature in these cases is the general arrest of development that occurs when the disease begins before the second dentition. A child of 12 and one half years would easily have been mistaken for 6 or 7 years, while another of 4 years looked more like 2 and one half or 3 years' [1].

His original observations have been confirmed by studies that evaluated children at initial diagnosis, during treatment and into early adulthood. Greater than 30% had heights measuring less than either the 3rd or 5th percentiles at the time of diagnosis and during treatment[2–4]. Short stature continues into adulthood for many of these children, with one study finding that 50% of children with Systemic Arthritis and 16% with Polyarthritis had heights less than the 5th percentile [5].

The future may be different for children diagnosed with JIA since the advent of newer drug therapies such as methotrexate and etanercept. There is evidence that children show catch-up growth if disease control is achieved before skeletal maturation. This would suggest that the underlying inflammation is the main cause of poor growth.

Role of nutrition

The role that nutrition alone plays in the growth failure of Juvenile Idiopathic Arthritis (JIA) is controversial. Although children with active disease show decreased lean body mass, anaemia, and hypoalbuminaemia, all signs of malnutrition, they are also markers of a pro-inflammatory state and may not reflect dietary inadequacy.

Studies have shown conflicting results in terms of dietary adequacy in JIA, with reports of both suboptimal as well as adequate intakes. One study found that children with Systemic Arthritis, despite being overweight, consumed less than the recommended amount of calories for their age and weight [6]. Decreased physical activity, the use of corticosteroids, and inaccurate reporting of food intake may all be responsible for this.

Reports of adequate intake but poor growth could be explained by increased nutritional requirements in JIA. Studies reporting adequate intakes in children with poor growth have not taken this possibility into account. The hypothesis is that children with active disease are in a hypermetabolic state and therefore have increased energy and protein requirements. Earlier studies, which have shown adequate protein and caloric intakes, have based their findings on the needs of healthy children, but may have underestimated the needs of children with active disease. To study this, resting energy expenditure (REE) was measured in children with JIA as well as in healthy controls [7]. These children were not hypermetabolic, with no significant differences found in REE between children with active compared to non-active disease. The absolute fat-free mass (FFM) was decreased in children with Systemic Arthritis compared to the controls. However, when this was expressed as a percentage of bodyweight, these differences were no longer present. When REE was adjusted for both bodyweight and FFM, a significant increase in REE was seen in patients with Systemic Arthritis, but not in children with Oligoarthritis or Polyarthritis, compared to the controls. This may simply reflect less metabolically active tissue in patients with Systemic Arthritis, or may be the result of increased protein catabolism secondary to the disease process, or a result of corticosteroid therapy, which is known to cause catabolism of lean body mass and promote lipogenesis.

Although evidence suggests that caloric insufficiency is not the primary cause of poor growth in JIA, there are children with profound

Table 3.10.1 Nutritional screening

1. Plot weight for age, height for age, and weight for height on a growth chart at each clinic visit to identify children at risk. Standard growth curves are not appropriate for evaluating weight for height proportion in the pubescent child. For this group the Body Mass Index (BMI) should be used.

2. Assess current medications that could be causing anorexia, nausea, gastritis, diarrhoea, and mouth sores which could contribute to poor oral intake. Determine if there is TMJ involvement which may cause problems with chewing.

3. Any child with evidence of either obesity or malnutrition should be referred to a dietician. If there is no dietician available during clinic the parents are asked to keep a 72-h food diary and mail it back for review.

4. If the intake is either inadequate or excessive, the appropriate interventions are going to be dietary changes and/or increasing physical activity.

5. If the nutritional intake appears adequate and the child is not growing well then further evaluation is indicated. Poor growth is usually associated with active disease and may not improve until disease control is attained.

6. General laboratory testing may include CBC, ESR, serum iron, ferritin, TIBC, albumin, and pre-albumin levels.

anorexia, generally those with poorly controlled Systemic Arthritis, who appear to benefit from caloric supplementation with nocturnal nasogastric tube feedings. One study showed impressive gains in growth velocity and weight gain during a 6-month period in children who were unable to consume adequate protein and calories orally [5] Nutritional screening and monitoring is recommended for all children with JIA (Table 3.10.1)

Role of corticosteroids

Corticosteroids contribute to the linear growth failure of JIA. Intake of low dose corticosteroids is associated with suppression of linear growth [8]. The degree of suppression is variable, however, and also depends on other factors, such as disease activity and duration. Alternate day, compared to daily, corticosteroids, even at high doses, may cause less compromise in linear growth. A retrospective study of children with Systemic Arthritis who were treated in this fashion showed only slightly diminished linear growth in most children, and in two children who were initially at <5th percentile, an increase in growth velocity occurred over the course of a year [9].

However, even children who have not received corticosteroids may show significant growth failure. One investigation of short stature in patients with JIA who were followed into adulthood found that although prior corticosteroid use was greater in the group with growth failure, only 42% of those with growth failure had used corticosteroids, suggesting that the underlying disease process was primarily responsible (5).

Obesity

Although linear growth may often be compromised in children with JIA, obesity is also common, rarely at disease onset, but often after long-term daily corticosteroids. The prevalence of obesity in children with JIA is estimated to be 20% [10]. This can be chiefly attributed to

the ravenous appetite caused by corticosteroids although lack of exercise is also a contributing factor. Nutritional counselling is essential, beginning at the onset of corticosteroid therapy, and not after the child has become morbidly obese.

Changes may need to be made of both the type and quantity of food consumed.

General recommendations include increasing the intake of fresh fruits and vegetables, whole grains, and low fat dairy products. Consumption of highly processed foods should be discouraged as they are high in calories, fat, and sodium. Specific nutritional advice should include limiting saturated fat, increasing the amount of polyunsaturated and monounsaturated fat, limiting sodium intake to no more than 1.5 g/day, and ensuring that calcium and Vitamin D intakes are appropriate (Table 3.10.2) In addition, the child should be encouraged to get as much exercise as possible, working to a goal of one hour of physical activity every day. Given the amount of time children in the developed world now spend watching television and eating "junk food" these are daunting goals. However, without careful attention to these nutritional issues, an even more serious problem may arise, namely nonadherence to therapy. Although this has not been studied in a rigorous way, it is the experience of most paediatric rheumatologists that excessive weight gain is often the reason for failing to adhere to corticosteroid treatment. Adolescents may abruptly and covertly stop corticosteroids on their own, but parents of young children may also stop treatment without notifying their physician. Counselling about weight gain, and how to minimize it at the advent of corticosteroid therapy, may improve adherence. It is essential that a nutritionist well versed in paediatric rheumatic diseases be part of the multidisciplinary team (see Part 3, Chapter 3.2).

The role of anaemia

Children with JIA may have anaemia attributable to the chronic disease, to iron deficiency, or to a combination of both. Medications, including nonsteroidal anti-inflammatory drugs (NSAIDs) and corticosteroids, may further exacerbate the anaemia by causing an erosive gastritis with gastrointestinal blood loss.

The role of iron deficiency remains to be clarified. The serum transferrin receptor concentration, which is not influenced by inflammation, and is elevated in iron deficiency, may be a useful marker for this [11]. Haemoglobin levels were inversely related to circulating transferrin receptor levels in one study of anaemic children with JIA, suggesting that iron therapy would be effective [12]. Oral iron supplementation has resulted in improved haemoglobin levels according to some studies but not others [13]. A trial of oral iron supplementation is recommended as initial therapy. However, in cases where this is ineffective, one small study has shown that intravenous iron may be effective [14]. The use of erythropoietin in resistant anaemia is controversial (see Part 3, Chapter 3.11).

Osteoporosis

Osteopenia and osteoporosis are common in JIA [15]. Children with Systemic Arthritis and Polyarthritis are thought to have the most severe osteoporosis although one study found no difference in bone mineral densities between children with Systemic Arthritis and those with Oligoarthritis or Polyarthritis if they had not been treated with corticosteroids [16]. Aetiological factors include cytokine-mediated

Table 3.10.2 Parent handout on calcium, vitamin D, and prednisone

DRIs (Dietary Reference Intakes) for calcium

1–3 years: 500 mg/day
4–8 years: 800 mg/day
9–18 years: 1300 mg/day

Servings/day your child needs to get enough calcium

(300 mg = 1 serving)
1–3 year old: 2 servings (1⅔ cups milk)
4–8 year old: just under 3 servings (2⅔ cups milk)
9 and older: 4 servings/day (4⅓c milk)

One serving could be

8 oz calcium-fortified orange juice
8 oz milk or yogurt
1½ oz cheese
Most children love cheese, so any variation will do (macaroni and cheese, pizza, omelette, cheese on toast, or English muffin).

One-half serving

1 ounce calcium-fortified cereal
1 cup cooked spinach
1/2 cup pudding (not ready to eat)
1 string cheese stick

Foods that have some calcium but not a lot include ice cream, frozen yogurt, cottage cheese, and dry beans.
There are some fun products tailored to children such as squeezable and drinkable yogurt. These may vary in calcium content so read labels. Children usually like string cheese.
Many but not all cereals are enriched with calcium so take time to read labels. Cereal can be a good snack with a serving of milk. If your child does not tolerate cow's milk both soy milk and rice milk are fine as long as the label says they are enriched with calcium. There is a product called "Enriched Rice Dream" which comes in chocolate and has 300 mg of calcium per cup. If your child has a poor appetite she may do better with small, frequent meals throughout the day. Try to increase her calcium intake by hiding it in foods she likes, such as adding cheese to scrambled eggs and using milk instead of water to make oatmeal and hot chocolate.

Vitamin D

Everyone needs 200 IU of Vitamin D/day (5 ug/day). Only fluid milk is fortified with vitamin D so if your child is getting calcium from other dairy products she may need a daily multivitamin. Check with your paediatrician.

Foods that are a good source of calcium:

Food	Serving size	Calcium (in mg)
Milk, non-fat	1 cup	300 mg
Calcium-fortified orange juice	1 cup	300 mg
Yogurt, flavoured (low-fat)	1 cup	300 mg
Chocolate milk (1%)	1 cup	285 mg
Swiss cheese	1 ounce	270 mg
Tofu (processed w/calcium sulfate)	1/2 cup	260 mg
American cheese	1 ounce	170 mg
String cheese	1 ounce stick	150 mg
Frozen yogurt	1/2 cup	105 mg
Spinach	1/2 cup	120 mg
Dried figs	3	80 mg
Broccoli	1/2 cup	45 mg

bone loss (IL-1, IL-6, and TNF-α enhanced osteoclast activity), inadequate weight bearing activity, medications, chiefly corticosteroids and possibly methotrexate, and inadequate calcium and Vitamin D intake.

It is difficult to isolate the role of nutrition from the other causes of osteoporosis in JIA. There is a paucity of information on calcium and vitamin D requirements in healthy children and even less so for children with JIA. The RDAs (Recommended Daily Allowances), renamed the DRIs (Dietary Reference Intakes) in 1999, are based on the nutritional needs of healthy children and may not be applicable to children with JIA. The current DRIs are based on limited studies of calcium balance in healthy infants and children and several placebo-controlled trials of calcium supplementation. These recommendations do not take into account other dietary practices that may alter requirements for these nutrients, such as sodium and protein intake, nor do they consider racial differences in calcium metabolism. There are also few studies that include accurate dietary information. With these caveats in mind, several issues are discussed further.

Although most studies report normal serum calcium levels in children with JIA, this is not a good indicator of calcium status because serum calcium is tightly regulated. There is no biochemical assay that reflects calcium nutritional status. Dietary calcium intake is generally reported as either adequate or low but the DRIs were increased in 1999 for calcium, and earlier studies do not reflect this fact. Vitamin D levels have been normal in the few studies in which this was measured, with one exception [17]. In another study, supplementation with Vitamin D did not result in improvement in cortical bone density [18].

This raises the question of whether or not there is sufficient evidence to support calcium and Vitamin D supplementation in children with JIA to improve bone density. Several randomized controlled trials in healthy girls showed that increased calcium intake above 900 mg/day is associated with positive effects on bone mineral accretion [19]. Differences between prepubertal and pubertal girls were seen in one study [20]; prepubertal girls showed a greater response to calcium supplementation. In two other studies, no difference was found between these two age groups [19,21]. Increased bone densities were not maintained after the calcium supplementation was stopped.

There have been few studies of calcium and vitamin D supplementation in children with JIA. One crossover study in children with rheumatic diseases, six of whom had JIA, examined the effect of calcium and vitamin D supplementation on corticosteroid associated osteoporosis [22]. The study design included an initial 6-month period of supplementation of a minimum of 1 g/day of calcium and 400 IU of vitamin D followed by 6 months without supplementation. There was an increase in spine density in most children but inconsistent results were found in the radius after the first 6 months of supplementation. There was more complete dietary information in this study compared to most, and the authors reported a significant negative correlation of the spinal bone mineral density (BMD) with sodium and protein intakes. These data reflect the complexity of this issue, with many nutritional and non-nutritional variables influencing the BMD.

Given the paucity of data, only general recommendations can be made to optimize bone health in children with JIA. These include consuming at least the DRI's for calcium and vitamin D, minimizing

Table 3.10.3 General recommendations for children taking prednisone

Prednisone causes an increase in appetite. To prevent excessive weight gain please try to follow these guidelines:

1. Avoid salty, high fat foods.
2. Change all dairy products to skim or 1% fat
3. Make sure your child eats the recommended amounts of both calcium and Vitamin D. This is important to build strong bones.
4. Increase the amount of fresh fruits and vegetables that your child eats. Substitute these for cookies, chips, and candy.
5. REMOVE ALL JUNK FOOD FROM THE HOUSE.
6. Encourage your child to be active. One hour of exercise every day is ideal. This will help prevent excessive weight gain and increase the strength of your child's bones.

corticosteroid exposure, and encouraging weight-bearing physical activity (Table 3.10.3).

Nutritional therapy for JIA

One of the commonest questions asked by parents is whether there is a specific diet or food that would help their child with arthritis. One survey found that 70% of children with JIA have used unconventional remedies to treat their arthritis. Dietary manipulation was used by 43% of this group and included increased intake of fish and fish oil, megavitamins and herbal remedies [23]. Use of these alternative therapies probably reflects the frustration of living with poorly controlled chronic arthritis.

The idea of a more physiological or "natural" approach to treatment of arthritis is appealing. The adult literature is replete with studies of the effect of vegetarian diets, fasting, specific foods, minerals, and vitamins on arthritis. Results have been equivocal at best; studies are poorly controlled and many reports are anecdotal. Although fasting does appear to have modest effects on suppressing joint inflammation, it cannot be advocated for children who need calories to promote both brain and somatic growth. However, there is now evidence, supported by well-controlled clinical trials in adults, and one report in children, showing that certain dietary modifications may be helpful. Specifically, certain unsaturated fatty acids may be useful pharmacologic agents for the treatment of inflammatory arthritis. Unsaturated fatty acids serve as precursors for prostaglandins, thromboxanes, and leukotrienes—collectively termed eicosanoids—that participate in the initiation and modulation of immunological and inflammatory responses. By altering intake of particular fatty acids, it is possible to generate a unique eicosanoid profile with less inflammatory potential than ordinarily results from oxidation of arachidonic acid, the major eicosanoid precursor fatty acid in membranes of cells from people who eat a typical western diet [24]. For example, administration of fish oil, rich in eicosapentaenoic acid and docosahexaenoic acid suppresses formation of cyclooxygenase and lipoxygenase products derived from arachidonic acid and exerts a modest anti-inflammatory action in adult patients with rheumatoid arthritis (RA) [25].

A more recent development has been the use of certain botanical lipids to treat adults with RA. Administration of the fatty acid, gammalinolenic acid (GLA), found in the seeds of the borage (9%) and evening primrose (23%) plants, reduces joint pain and swelling in

RA patients with active synovitis [26]. One double-blind placebo controlled trial in which children with JIA were given 40 mg/kg/day of either borage or safflower oil for two 6-month periods in a crossover design found a small but significant improvement in both the number of joints with active arthritis and the physician's global assessment in the group treated with borage oil. No adverse effects were reported and the borage oil was well-tolerated. [27]. These promising results warrant further trials.

Conclusion

The main nutritional problems of children with JIA, particularly those with poorly controlled long-standing disease include malnutrition, poor linear growth, anaemia, obesity, and osteoporosis. It is hoped that with the advent of newer, more effective therapies, disease control may be achieved sooner, before these problems occur. However, with currently available therapies, and awareness of potential problems early in the disease course, it may be possible to at least minimize these nutritional complications if not eliminate them completely.

References

1. Still, G.F. On a form of chronic joint disease in children. *Trans Roy Med Chir Soc* 1897;80:47–50. Reprinted in *Arch Dis Childh* 1941;16:156–65.
2. Bernstein, B.H, Stobie, D., Singsen, B.H., Koster-King K., and Hanson V. Growth retardation in juvenile rheumatoid arthritis. *Arthritis Rheum* 1977;20 (Suppl.):212–16.
3. Henderson, C.J. and Lovell, D.J. Assessment of protein-energy malnutrition in children and adolescents with juvenile rheumatoid arthritis. *Arthritis Care Res* 1989;2:108–13.
4. Warady, B.D., McCammam, S.P., and Lindsley, C.B. Nutritional assessment of patients with juvenile rheumatoid arthritis. *Arthritis Rheum* 1988;31:S113.
5. Lovell, D.J., and White P.H. Growth and nutrition in juvenile rheumatoid arthritis. In P. Woo, White P. and Ansell B, ed. Pediatric rheumatology update. New York: Oxford University Press, 1990, pp.47–56.
6. Bacon, M.C., White, P.H., Raiten, D.J. *et al.* Nutritional status and growth in juvenile rheumatoid arthritis. Seminars *Arth Rheum.* 1990;20:97–106.
7. Knops, N., Wulffraat, N., Lodder, S., Houwen, R., and deMeer, K. Resting energy expenditure and nutritional status in children with juvenile rheumatoid arthritis. *J Rheumatol* 1999;26:2039–43.
8. Avioli, L.V. Glucocorticoid effects on statural growth. *Br J Rheumatol* 1993;32 (Suppl. 2): 27–30.
9. Kimura, Y., Fieldston, E., Devries-Vandervlugt, B., Li, S., and Imundo, L. High dose, alternate day corticosteroids for systemic onset juvenile rheumatoid arthritis. *J Rheumatol* 2000;27:2018–24.
10. Henderson, C.J. and Lovell, D.J. Nutritional aspects of juvenile rheumatoid arthritis. *Rheum Dis Clin N Am* 1991;17:403–13.
11. Kivivuori, S.M., Pelkonen, P., Verronen, P., and Siimes, M.A. Elevated serum transferrin receptor concentration in children with juvenile chronic arthritis as evidence of iron deficiency. *Rheumatology* (Oxford) 2000;39:193–7.
12. Cazzola, M., Ponchio, L., de Benedetti, F. *et al.* Defective iron supply for erythropoiesis and adequate endogenous erythropoietin production in the anemia associated with systemic-onset juvenile chronic arthritis. *Blood* 1996;87:4824–30.
13. Koerper, M.A., Stempel, D.A., and Dallman, P.R. Anemia in patients with juvenile rheumatoid arthritis. *J Pediatr* 1978;92:930–3.
14. Martini, A., Ravelli, A., Di Fuccia, G., Rosti, V., Cazzola, M., and Barosi, G. Intravenous iron therapy for severe anaemia in systemic-onset juvenile chronic arthritis. *Lancet* 1994;344:1052–4.

15. Rabinovich, C.E. Bone mineral status in juvenile rheumatoid arthritis. *J Rheum* 2000;(Suppl 58): 34–7.

16. Pereira, R.M.R., Corrente, J.E., Chahade, W.H., and Yoshinari, N.H. Evaluation by dual X-ray absorptiometry (DXA) of bone mineral density in children with juvenile chronic arthritis. *Clin Exp Rheum* 1998;16:495–501.

17. Bianchi, M.L., Bardare M., and Caraceni, M.P. *et al.* Bone metabolism in juvenile rheumatoid arthritis. *Bone Miner* 1990;9:153–62.

18. Reed, A., Haugen, M. Pachman, L.M., and Langman, C.B. 25-Hydroxyvitamin D therapy in children with active juvenile rheumatoid arthritis: short-term effects on serum osteocalcin levels and bone mineral density. *J Pediatr* 1991;119:657–60.

19. Lloyd, T., Andon, M.D., Rollings, N. *et al.* Calcium supplementation and bone mineral density in adolescent girls. *J Am Med Assoc* 1993; 270:841–44.

20. Johnston, C.C., Miller, J.Z., Slemenda, C.W. *et al.* Calcium supplementation and increases in bone mineral density in children. *N Engl J Med* 1992;327:82–7.

21. Chan, G.M. Dietary calcium and bone mineral status of children and adolescents. *Am J Dis Child* 1991;145:631–4.

22. Warady, B.D., Lindsley, C.B., and Robinson, R.G., and Lukert BP. Effects of nutritional supplementation on bone mineral status of children with rheumatic diseases receiving corticosteroid therapy. *J Rheum* 1994;21:530–5.

23. Southwood, T.R., Malleson, P.N., Roberts-Thomson P.J., and Mahy M. Unconventional remedies used for patients with juvenile arthritis. Pediatrics 1990;85:150–4.

24. Rothman, D., DeLuca, P., and Zurier, R.B. Botanical lipids: Effects on inflammation, immune responses, and rheumatoid arthritis. *Seminars Arth Rheum* 1995;25:87–96.

25. Kremer, J.M., Jubiz, W., Michalek, A. *et al.* Fish-oil fatty acid supplementation in rheumatoid arthritis. *Ann Intern Med* 1987;106:497–504.

26. Leventhal, L.J., Boyce, E.G., and Zurier, R.B. Treatment of rheumatoid arthritis with gammalinolenic acid. *Ann Intern Med* 1993;867–73.

27. Rothman, D., Nocton, J., Ostrov, B., *et al.* The treatment of juvenile rheumatoid arthritis with borage oil. *Arthritis Rheum* 1999;42:S229.

3.11 Adjunctive therapies

Marisa Klein-Gitelman

Aim

The aim of this chapter is to discuss therapies that are potentially important in managing the complications of JIA, including anaemia, growth failure, drug toxicity, and osteoporosis.

Stucture

- Introduction
- Erythropoietin
- Human growth hormone
- Folic acid
- Bisphosphonates
- Calcitonin

Children with Juvenile Idiopathic Arthritis (JIA) may develop secondary medical problems as a result of the initial disease process itself and/or the medical therapy used to control arthritis. Adjunctive therapies are interventions that treat symptoms associated with the underlying illness or its treatment but do not specifically alter the disease course. This chapter examines the use of several adjunctive therapies in the treatment of children with chronic arthritis.

Erythropoietin

The anaemia of chronic disease is a significant problem for the child with JIA. It is most profound in children with Systemic Arthritis. Anaemia in this setting is multifactorial. One important cause of the anaaemia is iron deficiency. Iron deficiency may be a result of decreased intake of iron, poor absorption of ingested iron, or increased iron losses due in part to medications. Most children respond to oral iron therapy while some may require parenteral infusions of iron. The anaemia of chronic disease which is not directly due to iron deficiency is less well-understood; however, it is a common finding in disorders associated with the increased production of cytokines such as tumor necrosis factor (TNF), interferon γ (INF-γ), and interleukin 1 (IL-1) which mediate the immune or inflammatory response [1]. Chronic inflammation may disturb the production, release, and life span of red blood cells (RBCs). For example, rats perfused with sub-lethal doses of TNF, IL-1α, or salmonella endotoxin for 7 days had a 25–31% decrease in total RBC mass and had a significant reduction in iron utilization demonstrated by low ^{59}Fe incorporation into newly synthesized RBCs [2]. Elevated IL-1 levels have also been correlated with shortened RBC survival in adults with rheumatoid arthritis [3].

Erythropoietin, a haematopoietic growth factor that has a mechanism of action similar to a hormone, regulates the production of RBCs. It is a 30–39 kD glycoprotein that binds to specific surface receptors on erythroid precursors. This binding stimulates differentiation and maturation of erythroid precursors into mature RBCs and promotes proliferation and maintenance of RBC viability. The production of erythropoietin and the response of erythroid progenitor cells may also be altered by chronic inflammatory states.

Data supporting abnormal erythropoietin production in chronic inflammation has been documented in adults with rheumatoid arthritis [4]. Although these patients had rising levels of erythropoietin associated with falling haemoglobin, the level of erythropoietin was higher in patients with iron deficiency anaemia than in patients with rheumatoid arthritis with the same degree of anaemia. This finding suggests that cytokines likely play a role in blunting the erythropoietin response to anemia in patients with persistent inflammation. This has also been seen in adults with other inflammatory conditions such as HIV [5] and cancer [6]. TNF, IL-1, and INFs reduce production of RBCs by erythroid colony forming units in a dose-dependent manner [7,8]. Exposure to IL-1, TNF α, or transforming growth factor beta (TGF β) decreases erythropoietin production both in cell lines and in isolated perfused rat kidney [9,10]. More recently, a study of patients undergoing renal dialysis who had a poor response to recombinant erythropoietin demonstrated higher levels of TNF and IL-1 production by the peripheral blood mononuclear cells of the poor responders when the cells were exposed *in vitro* to recombinant erythropoietin [11]. One possible mechanism for cytokine-mediated regulation of erythropoiesis is through CD45, a transmembrane protein tyrosine phosphatase highly expressed in all haematopoietic cell lines and a key regulator of antigen receptor signaling in lymphocytes. One function of CD45 is to suppress janus kinase (JAK), an intracellular signalling molecule, and negatively regulate cytokine receptor signaling. To better understand the role of CD45, a CD45-deficient mouse cell line was generated. In this model, interferon-receptor-mediated activation of JAK and STAT (signal transducer and activators of transcription) proteins was unchecked. One result was increased erythropoietin-dependent haematopoiesis. This model demonstrates the role of CD45 as a negative regulator of erythropoietin-dependent red cell production in mice [12].

Erythropoietin may also act as a growth factor or cytokine to protect cells beyond the haematopoietic lineage from apoptosis (programmed cell death), and may play an important role in muscle development and repair [13]. Blunted responses to erythropoietin in chronic inflammatory states may, therefore, not only alter erythropoiesis but also vascular endothelial and muscle repair mechanisms.

A recombinant form of human erythropoietin (rHuEPO) has been available since the mid-1980s. Its use in the treatment of profound anaemia associated with renal disease and a variety of illnesses including bone marrow transplantation has been highly successful. Although anaemia of chronic disease is a frequent problem in the patients with arthritis, and can be particularly severe in children with Systemic Arthritis, the use of erythropoietin in the management of anaemia of chronic disease in these populations is more limited. In 1989, Means et al. [14] reported that two patients with rheumatoid arthritis responded to rHuEPO. Pincus et al. [15] supported this finding in a randomized study followed by open label treatment of 17 adults with rheumatoid arthritis. The patients had a mean haematocrit of 31% with a mean erythropoietin level of 31 and range 10–69 mU/nl. (normal 5–25 mU/nl) prior to treatment. The increased level of erythropoietin in these anaemic patients supports the concept of a blunted response to erythropoietin. Treatment with rHuEPO improved the haematocrit by a mean of 4%. Patients, however, did not report symptomatic improvement. The use of rHuEPO has been helpful in the pre-surgical preparation of patients with rheumatoid arthritis undergoing hip replacement [16]. Patients had improved haematocrits allowing donation of autologous blood prior to surgery and the use of auto-transfusion in the operating room.

The use of rHuEPO in children has been reported by Fantini et al. in 1992 [17]. A group of 13 patients with active Systemic Arthritis and long-standing anaemia were treated with rHuEPO after a failed response to oral iron therapy. The patients received 2–5 weekly subcutaneous or intravenous injections of rHuEPO. This was supplemented with iron therapy. The mean haemoglobin prior to treatment was 7.0 gm/dl with a mean peak response of 12.3 gm/dl and a mean level of 11.4 gm/dl at last visit 4–13 months after rHuEPO was started. Serum iron levels rose concomitantly from 18.7 ug/dl to 46.5 ug/dl. The authors reported that the children also had an improvement in wellbeing, linear growth, muscle strength, and performance of daily activities as documented in a 10-item quality of life survey. Unfortunately, there have been no further studies specifically addressing the use of rHuEPO in children with chronic arthritis. In a child with early or mild disease, it is suggested that the physician observes the response of anaemia to the overall management of arthritis. Often, children who respond well to treatment of arthritis, will also have resolution of anaemia. In children with resistant arthritis despite intensive medical intervention and who are symptomatic secondary to anaemia despite a trial of iron therapy, the use of rHuEPO may be considered. The current suggested starting dose is 50–100 units/kg three times per week. The dose is increased after 8 weeks if the target haematocrit is not reached. The dose is reduced when the target haematocrit is reached or if the haematocrit rises greater than 4 points in a 2-week period. Maintenance dose is usually 25 units/kg, three times per week.

Human growth hormone

Poor linear growth in the child with JIA is usually a consequence of both persistent disease activity and chronic use of corticosteroid therapy. Chronic synovitis leads to widened epiphyses, early maturation, and early closure of growth plates. Recent studies have demonstrated that corticosteroids inhibit growth hormone receptor mRNA and may, therefore, affect the response to growth hormone at the cellular level [18]. Resolution of arthritis and discontinuation of corticosteroids before the adolescent growth spurt allows many patients the opportunity for significant catch-up growth. However, the child who requires corticosteroids during the pubertal growth spurt or who has chronic, persistent, active arthritis during adolescence is at significant risk of having permanent short stature. The pathophysiological causes of short stature in these children also interfere with the effectiveness of growth hormone therapy used to treat short stature making this intervention problematic.

Systemic inflammation interferes with the effectiveness of growth hormone signaling. In the normal host, growth hormone stimulates insulin-like growth factor I (IGF-1) production in the liver. IGF-1 mediates the anabolic actions of growth hormone, promotes growth of most cell types, and stimulates cellular differentiation and differentiated functions of specialized cells. It has insulin-like metabolic effects, decreasing blood glucose, and inhibiting lipolysis, as well as retarding protein breakdown. It provides negative feedback by inhibiting growth hormone release at the level of the pituitary gland. Chronic systemic inflammation leads to a catabolic state and the level of IGF-1 is decreased. The catabolic patient with low IGF-1 does not benefit from the growth effects listed above. Furthermore, the catabolic patient develops growth hormone resistance probably secondary to low IGF-1 levels. This may be one of the reasons why exogenous growth hormone is relatively ineffective in patients with inflammatory conditions [19].

There is a transgenic IL-6 mouse model; the animal has normal production of IGF-1 in the liver, decreased serum IGF-1, low insulin-like growth factor binding protein 3 (IGFBP-3) levels, increased serum IGFBP-3 proteolysis and growth retardation [20]. Non-transgenic littermates have normal levels of IGF-1 and IGFPB-3, but develop low levels when injected with IL-6. Growth hormone levels in children with Systemic Arthritis range from low to normal. While these patients typically have high levels of IL-6, the levels of IGF-1 and IGFBP-3 are low similar to growth hormone [20,21]. Decreased IGFBP-3 levels have been shown to correlate inversely with the number of active joints, the C-reactive protein level, and the erythrocyte sedimentation rate [22]. Reduction of IFGBP-3 plays a pivotal role in the regulation of IGF-1, and decreased levels probably play an important role in the IL-6-induced impairment of linear growth.

The growth hormone/ IGF-1 axis is also stimulated by exercise and may play a role in the body's adaptive changes to exercise and training. Growth hormone levels rise in response to both acute aerobic and anaerobic exercise. There is evidence that chronic resistive exercise or endurance training increases the circulating level of IGF-1. The effect of exercise on children is more pronounced during puberty than in prepubertal states. Patients with growth hormone deficiency have an associated impaired exercise capability [23]. Many children with JIA have decreased exercise tolerance and therefore lose the ability to stimulate growth hormone through exercise. However, children with arthritis who are able to participate in an exercise program may still not respond appropriately to exercise, due to the adverse effects of chronic inflammation on the growth hormone axis.

Growth hormones have been used to treat patients with growth hormone deficiency and related conditions for many years. Initially, growth hormone was isolated from cadaveric tissues. More recently, synthetic production of the hormone has decreased the risk of viral infections associated with the use of human products. Growth hormone therapy has been used in children with JIA. Simon et al. [24] published the results of growth hormone therapy in 14 children with chronic arthritis. Prior to treatment, the children studied had heights at least 2 standard deviations (SDs) below normal and growth velocity at least 1 SD below normal over the previous year while receiving a stable medical regimen over the previous 6 months. All patients had also received glucocorticoids for more than 2 years prior to treatment with growth hormone. During the study period, the patients received standard growth hormone therapy for 1 year and were monitored anthropomorphically (i.e. growth velocity, percentage of lean body mass, percentage of body fat) as well as with serologic tests. Growth velocity increased in nine patients and 3/9 had partial catch-up growth, however, growth velocity returned to base line when the therapy was discontinued. Of note, growth velocity was inversely correlated with the dose of glucocorticoids received by the patients. Lean body mass increased by 12% and fat mass fell by 20% during treatment, but fat mass increased dramatically again when growth hormone was discontinued. The children had no change in bone age to chronological age ratios, calorie intake did not change, and there was no significant hyperglycaemia although half of the patients had elevations in insulin levels and haemoglobin A_1C levels. There was no change in arthritis activity.

The effect of recombinant human growth hormone on bone metabolism in children with chronic arthritis and severe bone demineralization (a mean level of 3.7 SDs below normal for age) has also been studied [25,26]. After 1 year of growth hormone therapy, the patients had increased bone formation markers (serum levels of osteocalcin, C-terminal propeptide of type I collagen) and resorption markers (urinary hydroxyproline, pyridinoline, and deoxypyridinoline) but had no improvement in bone density as measured by bone density studies (DXA). The level of osteocalcin 1 month after the initiation of therapy was the best predictive marker of growth response to growth hormone treatment. The authors of this study suggested that a longer treatment period might be required to demonstrate an improvement in bone density.

Therefore, growth hormone therapy in chronic arthritis is feasible, but may be of limited benefit, and potential risks including the possibility of asymmetrical limb growth remain undefined. In order to confer the best risk to benefit ratio for the treatment candidate, the patient should have a complete growth hormone axis study before treatment to rule out other causes of growth failure. This usually includes IGF-1 and IGFBP-3 levels, stimulation of the growth hormone axis using clonidine, glucagon, or insulin and obtaining growth hormone, glucose, and cortisol levels at 20–30 min intervals over several hours, as well as anatomic imaging of the hypothalamus and pituitary gland. Baseline levels of IGF-1 and IGFBP-3 may be compared to levels after 4 days of a therapeutic trial of growth hormone and serve as an indicator of whether the growth hormone dose is likely to be of benefit. However, differences in levels are not predictive of total growth expected. It is important to note that children receiving chronic corticosteroids would not be expected to have a normal cortisol response. Although the literature suggests that many children with JIA have normal growth hormone secretion, some do have decreased growth hormone responses to stimulation, supporting the use of growth hormone therapy. The child who has well-controlled inflammation, and who can be maintained on alternate day or intermittent high-dose corticosteroids is likely to have the most optimal response to growth hormone therapy and is therefore a good candidate for treatment. It is particularly important to consider children for growth hormone therapy who have demonstrated growth retardation, have active disease, are entering the adolescent growth phase, and still have open epiphyses. Clearly, children with closing or closed epiphyses have missed the opportunity to have significant benefit from therapy. The recently diagnosed patient who has not had the benefit of an adequate trial of treatment to control arthritis should not be considered a candidate for treatment. The decision to give growth hormone should be made in concert with a paediatric endocrinologist who should be primarily be responsible for the treatment regimen.

IGF-1 has been used in the treatment of growth failure associated with primary IGF-1 deficiency and has been shown to be beneficial. Trials comparing recombinant growth hormone replacement in idiopathic growth hormone deficiency to recombinant IGF-1 replacement in growth hormone receptor-deficiency demonstrate benefit in both groups. It is hypothesized that 20% or more of the effect of growth hormone is secondary to a direct effect of growth hormone on bone bypassing IGF-1. This hypothesis has been supported by data from the comparative trials and supports the notion that the patient with growth failure who has IGF-1 responsiveness to rises in growth hormone may have greater benefit from the use of recombinant growth hormone than from the use of recombinant IGF-1 [27].

Folic acid

Since the introduction of methotrexate into the armementarium of the paediatric rheumatologist, there has been much discussion about the need for, and the role of folic acid as an appropriate adjunctive medication. It has been well established that methotrexate interferes with folic acid metabolism. Although it has not been demonstrated that patients who receive methotrexate have a folic acid deficiency that requires extra nutritional resources, it has been shown that patients have reduced side-effects from methotrexate when their diet is supplemented with folic acid [28], and more recently that paediatric patients benefit from the addition of leucovorin (folinic acid) to their methotrexate regimen [29]. Folinic acid is a tetrahydrofolic acid derivative of folic acid that bypasses the need for enzyme activation in order to participate in purine and pyrimidine synthesis.

Folic acid is converted to tetrahydrofolate (THF), a central component of folate-dependent pathways. Once formed, intracellular folate is polyglutamated to retain its presence within the cell. THF is an important cofactor for enzymes that are involved in the *de novo* synthesis of purines and pyrimidines, and is therefore important in the metabolism of proliferating cells such as bone marrow and liver [30]. The best measure of the availability of folate within the cell is the evaluation of the conversion between S-adenosyl-L-homocysteine and methionine, the latter being an important part of polyamine production. The ability of methotrexate to interfere with polyamine production results in decreased cellular activity and a loss of immunologic responsiveness. Structurally, methotrexate is very similar to dihydrofolate. It enters cells by active transport and is polyglutamated and retained within the cell. Once inside the cell, it interferes with dihydrofolate reductase resulting in high levels of dihydrofolate and decreased levels of THF. This leads to increased levels of homocysteine and elevated levels of adenosine. Inhibition of homocysteine remethylation, and adenosine release may be responsible for much of methotrexate's anti-inflammatory actions. The cytostatic effects of methotrexate leading to drug toxicity are seen most noticeably in organs with a high cell turnover, and a high requirement for purines and pyrimidines, including the bone marrow, the liver, and the gastrointestinal tract.

It is clear from the biochemistry of folic acid that blood levels of folic acid are not the best reflection of total THF since it is polyglutamated and remains within the intracellular environment. A surrogate measure to determine folic acid "deficiency" may be the serum level of homocysteine. It is important to note that interference with the homocysteine pathway leads to increased homocysteine levels or hyperhomocysteine-mia, a risk factor for vascular disease. It is also important to note that some patients with a methylene-tetrahydrofolate reductase gene mutation will have increased methotrexate toxicity with increased risk for thromboses both from methotrexate metabolism and the methylene-tetrahydrofolate reductase gene mutation [31].

Some studies of the benefit of folic acid and folinic acid supplementation in the adult treated with methotrexate have reported equivocal results. These studies are confounded by the baseline nutritional status of patients who are treated with methotrexate. For example, one study from New Zealand evaluated the dietary intake of folic acid, calcium, vitamin E, zinc, and selenium in adult patients with rheumatoid arthritis. Many individuals had poor folic acid intake at their initial evaluations; however, patients treated with methotrexate appeared to be more deficient in dietary intake of folic acid than those individuals who were not treated with methotrexate [32]. Ravelli *et al.* [29] studied the efficacy of folinic acid in reducing the side effects of methotrexate in children. The study population was a group of children who had known side-effects due to methotrexate treated with a dose no greater than 20 mg/m2/week of methotrexate. Children were given folinic acid (2.5–7.5 mg) as a single dose 24 h after methotrexate. Following the introduction of folinic acid, the frequency of elevated liver enzyme abnormalities fell from 2.3 to 0.32 episodes per patient-year ($p < 0.001$) and the number of episodes of gastrointestinal toxicity fell from 1.09 to 0.29 episodes per patient-year ($p = 0.002$). The concern that supplementation with folic acid would antagonize the benefit of methotrexate therapy while treating what is essentially an intracellular THF deficiency, has been addressed in this and other studies as there were no changes in the rate of remission and flare over the course of the study. It has also been suggested, but not proven, that administration of folic acid reduces the frequency of liver biochemical abnormalities and, perhaps, the risk of liver fibrosis due to long-term use of methotrexate [33]. An advantage of folinic acid over folic acid is the ease of use (weekly versus daily). However, the cost of folinic acid may exceed the cost of folic acid in some countries making folic acid supplementation more cost-effective. It is still controversial whether children should routinely receive folic acid or folinic acid with methotrexate or whether supplementation should be reserved for those children who display symptomatic or laboratory evidence of methotrexate toxicity. In practice, both methods are employed regularly. The usual dose of folic acid is 1 mg daily. The smallest recommended dose of folinic acid is 3 mg/m2, 24 h after methotrexate is given. The smallest oral tablet is 5 mg and 2.5 mg is the smallest recommended dose.

Bisphosphonates

Osteoporosis is a high-profile condition. Information about what it is, how to diagnose it, and how to treat it has become readily available to the public. This information, however, appears to have had little effect on the adolescent diet. Most adolescents do not have an adequate dietary intake of calcium. This is of great concern in the child with arthritis who already has increased risks for osteoporosis due to both arthritis disease activity itself, and corticosteroid therapy. The additive risks of poor intake of calcium, arthritis and corticosteroid therapy occur at the time of greatest bone growth. The use of calcium and vitamin D to combat osteoporosis is discussed in Part 3, Chapter 3.10. These nutritional interventions are critical and the reader should be

familiar with the nutritional requirements for children and adolescents. However, nutritional interventions alone may not be enough for many children with JIA; DXA studies have demonstrated significant bone loss in children with JIA despite nutritional education and intervention. For a subset of these patients, adjunctive therapy with bisphosphonates may be appropriate. There is a large body of literature describing the benefits of bisphosphonates in the adult population. Drug development is evolving and new bisphosphonates have been created with improved safety profiles, as well as improved treatment regimens to decrease side-effects.

Osteoclasts arise from the monocyte/macrophage cell lineage. In the individual with JIA, there is an increase in the number and activity of osteoclasts at the trabecular surface of cancellous bone. The ruffled border of the osteoclast cell membrane leaches mineral from bone and removes collagen matrix by acidification of the bone edge and secretion of lysosomal enzymes. The leftover matrix proteins are endocytosed and moved to the opposing surface of the bone resulting in osteoporosis and increased risk of fracture. Therapy that blocks osteoclastic bone resorption has utility in the management of osteoporosis from arthritis. Bisphosphonates are a class of medication that were originally designed to treat the hypercalcaemia of cancer, pathologic heterotopic ossification, and Paget disease. Bisphosphonates consist of two phosphonate groups attached to a single carbon. Bisphsophonate adsorbs to bone mineral and inhibits bone resorption due to its physicochemical effects on hydroxyapatite crystals. Bisphosphonates appear to preferentially bind to the bone at the site of osteoclastic activity. They do not alter the presence or attachment of osteoclasts; however, in the presence of bisphosphonate, the ruffled border of the osteoclast disappears. One possible mechanism for the inhibition of the ruffled border is the effect of bisphosphonates internalized by the osteoclast. For example, the nitrogen-containing bisphosphonates may inhibit the biosynthesis of compounds that are essential for post-translational modification of small GTPases needed for ruffling the osteoclast membrane [34]. Normal bone forms over the area where bisphosphonate binds and it appears to become pharmacologically inactive. Therefore, continuous administration of bisphosphonate is required for the benefit of osteoclast inhibition allowing for increased bone mass over time. In animal models of inflammatory arthritis, bisphosphonates maintain bone volume, tensile strength, or fracture toughness, and the articular cartilage appears to be protected by decreased loss of subchondral bone [35].

There is little accumulated experience of treating children with bisphosphonates for corticosteroid-induced osteopenia or osteopenia associated with JIA. Wolfhagen *et al.* [36] found that seven children with severe corticosteroid-induced osteopenia responded well to bisphosphonate therapy; however none of the patients had chronic arthritis as a primary disease. Bianchi *et al.* [37] demonstrated improved bone mass in children with a variety of connective tissue diseases treated with the bisphosphonate alendronate. In this group of 38 patients, 18% had Polyarthritis, 24% had Systemic Arthritis, 29% had lupus, and 16% had juvenile dermatomyositis. Most of the children did not achieve the recommended daily allowance for calcium in their diets. Physical activity was low in 42%, moderate in 47%, and high in 11%. Baseline bone mineral density (BMD) Z scores ranged from −1.6 to −5.3. Bone mineral metabolism studies revealed high levels of type 1 collagen telopeptides, mild elevation of alkaline phosphatase, and normal levels of calcium, phosphorus, and vitamin D. The children under 20 kg were treated with 5 mg of alendronate daily while children over 20 kg received 10 mg of alendronate daily. Families were educated and encouraged to increase dietary calcium to the RDA but no supplements were prescribed. After 1 year, BMD had improved by 14.9 ± 9.8%; 13 patients (34%) achieved BMD in the normal range. Patients achieving puberty during the study had the greatest improvements in BMD. There were improvements in type 1 collagen telopeptide and alkaline phosphatase levels. In a related study, 45 patients treated with alendronate for 12 months for corticosteroid-induced osteoporosis were evaluated for biochemical parameters of bone turnover [38]. Patients with high baseline levels of bone-specific alkaline phosphatase and matrix metalloproteinase 3 had the greatest benefit from therapy. The benefit of therapy did not persist after the medication was withdrawn.

Therefore, limited evidence suggests that bisphosphonates may be beneficial in children with osteopenia. It is important to note that bisphosphonates are rated category C for pregnancy risk. Category C defines drugs in which an unknown risk to pregnancy cannot be ruled out. There have been no studies of bisphosphonates in pregnant women and the risk to the fetus in women previously treated with bisphosphonates is unknown. There is a chance of fetal harm if the drug is administered during pregnancy but the potential benefit may outweigh the potential harm. The evidence that bisphosphonates become pharmacologically inactive after binding to bone suggests that there would not be significant amounts of pharmacologically active bisphosphonate available in a previously treated woman to be dangerous, but this is not known. This uncertainty is a concern when considering the use of bisphosphonates in young females, who will grow up and may have children of their own. It is also unknown if the drug has adverse effects on bone growth and remodelling after many years, nor whether there could be future unknown side-effects from taking this medication in childhood. For children with high fracture risk, the potential future side effects of this drug are probably outweighed by the proven benefit of the drug in the treatment of osteoporosis.

Alendronate has been the bisphosphonate used in the paediatric studies described above. Based on this experience, the following treatment guidelines are suggested when considering treatment of chronic arthritis associated osteopenia with bisphosphonates. The patient should have a baseline BMD study ideally using DXA, which has become the standard measurement of bone mass. Criteria for treatment would include a BMD Z score of at least −1.5 or −2.0 at the lumbar spine plus either a history of fracture or the requirement of extended glucocorticoid therapy for at least 6 months. Five milligrams of alendronate is recommended for the patient under 20 kg while 10 mg daily is recommended for the patient over 20 kg. A more recent and popular alternate regimen of 35 mg or 70 mg weekly can be considered. Patients should have baseline bone metabolic profiles prior to treatment including, ideally, measurements of ionized calcium, phosphorus, magnesium, uric acid, vitamin D levels, PTH, osteocalcin, bone-specific alkaline phosphatase, collagen propeptide, collagen telopeptide, urine collagen X-links, and a 24-h urine for calcium, creatinine, citrate, and oxalate. This evaluation should be repeated a few weeks after the therapeutic intervention has begun to assess potential toxicity and to evaluate the biochemical response to the medication. Since there are alternative bisphosphonates including intermittent intravenous therapy with pamidronate, it is useful to determine the biochemical effects of alendronate in an individual in case there is a poor or limited response to the intervention. The family and patient require counselling regarding how to take alendronate. It must be given after an overnight fast, an hour before eating, and the patient must sit or stand for at least 30 min after swallowing the medication. This maximizes absorption and reduces the risk of gastroesophageal irritation that may frequently occur. The patient and family must also be counselled regarding the recommended daily allowance of calcium and vitamin D in the child's diet (see Part 3, Chapter 3.10). The recommended laboratory investigations and BMD measurements should be obtained at 6-month intervals to observe any toxicity or benefit of therapy. Other side-effects, most notably gastrointestinal intolerance should be monitored.

Calcitonin

Calcitonin is a polypeptide hormone that inhibits bone resorption by blocking osteoclast activity. The physiologic role of calcitonin is to fine-tune extracellular calcium and may be confined to times of stress such as growth, pregnancy, lactation, and high calcium intake. Calcitonin therapy can induce loss of calcitonin receptors resulting in hormone-induced resistance. This feature of the hormone is difficult to overcome when planning a therapeutic intervention for osteoporosis [39] Calcitonin has been used in the treatment of osteoporosis in adults. It has been particularly useful in post-menopausal osteoporosis. The experience in children has been more limited. Calcitonin has been used with some success in the treatment of juvenile idiopathic osteoporosis, thalassaemia, osteogenesis imperfecta as well as acute hypercalcaemia, and osteoporosis associated with malignancy. Intranasal calcitonin and vitamin D therapy were also used with benefit to treat five children with corticosteroid-induced osteoporosis associated with treatment of nephrotic syndrome [40]. There is one report of a child with systemic lupus erythematosus (SLE) and severe osteoporosis who responded to combination therapy of calcitonin and vitamin D [41]. Calcitonin has potential therapeutic benefit for children with JIA; however, there are no data at present to demonstrate this.

Summary

The pharmacological management of JIA is primarily aimed at suppressing joint inflammation. If such suppression is effective, the majority of children need no other therapeutic interventions. However, a significant number of children have refractory disease and persistent, inadequately controlled inflammation despite aggressive management. For these children a number of adjunctive therapies as discussed above may have a role in minimizing the morbidity associated with JIA.

References

1. Means, R.T. Jr. Pathogenesis of the anemia of chronic disease: a cytokine-mediated anemia. *Stem Cells* 1995;13:32–7.
2. Moldawer, L.L., Marano, M.A., Wei, H., *et al.* Cachectin/tumor necrosis factor-alpha alters red blood cell kinetics and induces anemia in vivo. *FASEB* 1989;3:1637–43.
3. Salvarani, C. Casali, B. Salvo, D., *et al.* The role of interleukin 1, erythropoietin and red cell bound immunoglobulins in the anaemia of rheumatoid arthritis. *Clin Experim Rheumatol* 1991;9:241–6.

4. Baer, A.N., Dessypris, E.N., and Krantz, S.B. The pathogenesis of anemia in rheumatoid arthritis: a clinical and laboratory analysis. *Sem Arthritis Rheum.* 1990;19:209–23.

5. Spivak, J.L., Barnes, D.C., Fuchs, E., and Quinn, T.C. Serum immunoreactive erythropoietin in HIV-infected patients. *JAMA* 1989;261:3104–7.

6. Miller, C.B., Jones, R.J., Piantadosi, S., Abeloff, M.D., and Spivak, J.L. Decreased erythropoietin response in patients with the anemia of cancer. *N Engl J Med* 1990;322:1689–92.

7. Means, R.T. Jr. and Krantz, S.B. Inhibition of human erythroid colony forming units by tumor necrosis factor requires beta interferon. *J Clin Invest* 1993;91:416–9.

8. Means, R.T. Jr. and Krantz, S.B. Inhibition of human erythroid colony forming units by interferons alpha and beta: differing mechanisms despite a shared receptor. *Exp Hematol* 1996;24:204–8.

9. Faquin, W.C., Schneider, T.J., and Goldberg, M.A. Effect of inflammatory cytokines on hypoxia-induced erythropoietin production. *Blood* 1992;79:1987–94.

10. Jelkmann, W., Pagel, H., Wolff, M., and Fandrey, J. Monokines inhibiting erythropoietin production in human hepatoma cultures and in isolated perfused rat kidneys. *Life Sci* 1992;50:301–8.

11. Takemasa, A., Yorioka, N., Ueda, C., Amimoto, D., Taniguchi, Y., and Yamakido, M. Stimulation of tumour necrosis factor-alpha production by recombinant human erythropoietin may contribute to failure of therapy. *Scand J Urol Nephrol* 2000;34:131–5.

12. Irie-Sasaki, J., Sasaki, T., Matsumoto, W., *et al.* CD45 is a JAK phosphatase and negatively regulates cytokine receptor signalling. *Nature* 2001; 409:349–54.

13. Ogilvie, M., Yu, X., Nicolas-Metral, V., Pulido, S.M., *et al.* Erythropoietin stimulates proliferation and interferes with differentiation of myoblasts. *J Biol Chem* 2000;275:39754–61.

14. Means, R.T. Jr., Olsen, N.J., Krantz, S.B., *et al.* Treatment of the anemia of rheumatoid arthritis with recombinant human erythropoietin: clinical and in vitro studies. *Arthritis Rheum* 1989;32:638–42.

15. Pincus, T., Olsen, N.J., Russell, I.J., *et al.* Multicenter study of recombinant human erythropoietin in correction of anemia in rheumatoid arthritis. *Am J Med* 1990;89:161–8.

16. Mercuriali, F., Gualtieri, G., Sinigaglia, L., *et al.* Use of recombinant human erythropoietin to assist autologous blood donation by anemic rheumatoid arthritis patients undergoing major orthopedic surgery. *Transfusion* 1994;34:501–6.

17. Fantini, F., Gattinara, M., Gerloni, V., Bergomi, P., and Cirla, E. Severe anemia associated with active systemic-onset juvenile rheumatoid arthritis successfully treated with recombinant human erythropoietin: a pilot study. *Arthritis Rheum* 1992;35:724–6.

18. Beauloye, V., Ketelslegers, J.M., Moreau, B., and Thissen, J.B. Dexamethasone inhibits both growth hormone (GH) induction of insulin-like growth factor –1 (IGF-1) mRNA and GH receptor (GHR) mRNA levels in rat primary cultured hepatocytes. *Growth Hormone Igf Res.* 1999;9:205–11.

19. Thissen, J.P., Underwood, L.E., and Ketelslegers, J.M. Regulation of insulin-like growth factor-I in starvation and injury. *Nutrition Rev* 1999;57:167–76.

20. De Benedetti, F., Meazza, C., Oliveri, M. *et al.* Effect of IL-6 on IGF binding protein-3: a study in IL-6 transgenic mice and in patients with systemic juvenile idiopathic arthritis. *Endocrinology* 2001;142:4818–26.

21. Davies, U.M., Jones, J., Reeve, J., *et al.* Juvenile rheumatoid arthritis. Effects of disease activity and recombinant human growth hormone on insulin-like growth factor 1, insulin-like growth factor binding proteins 1 and 3, and osteocalcin. *Arthritis Rheum* 1997;40:332–40.

22. Pignatti, P., Vivarelli, M., Meazza, C., Rizzolo, M.G., Martini, A., and De Bnedetti, F. Abnormal regulation of interleukin 6 in systemic juvenile idiopathic arthritis. *J Rheumatol* 2000;28:1670–6.

23. Jenkins, P.J. Growth hormone and exercise. *Clinical Endocrinol* 1999;50:683–9.

24. Simon, D., Touati, G., Prieur, A.M., Ruiz, J.C., and Czernichow, P. Growth hormone treatment of short stature and metabolic dysfunction in juvenile chronic arthritis. *Acta Paediat* 1999;88(Suppl.):100–5.

25. Touati, G., Ruiz, J.C., Porquet, D., Kindermans, C., Prieur, A.M., and Czernichow, P. Effects on bone metabolism of one year recombinant human growth hormone administration to children with juvenile chronic arthritis undergoing chronic steroid therapy. *J Rheumatol* 2000;27:1287–93.

26. Rooney, M., Davies, U.M., Reeve, J., Preece, M., Ansell, B.M., and Woo, P.M. Bone mineral content and bone mineral metabolism: changes after growth hormone treatment in juvenile chronic arthritis. *J Rheumatol* 2000;27:1073–81.

27. Guevara-Aguirre, J., Rosenbloom, Al., Vasconez, O., *et al.* Two-year treatment of growth hormone (GH) receptor deficiency with reconminant insulin-like growth factor I in 22 children: comparison of two dosage levels and to GH-treated Gh deficiency. *J Clin Endocrinol Metabol* 1997;82:629–33.

28. van Ede, A.E., Laan, R.F.J.M., Rood, M.J., *et al.* Effect of folic or folinic acid supplementation on the toxicity and efficacy of methotrexate in rheumatoid arthritis: a forty-eight week, multicenter, randomized, double-blind, placebo-controlled study. *Arthritis Rheum* 2001;44:1515–24.

29. Ravelli, A., Migliavacca, D., Viola, S., Ruperto, N., Pistorio, A., and Martini, A. Efficacy of folinic acid in reducing methotrexate toxicity in juvenile idiopathic arthritis. *Clin Exp Rheumatol* 1999;17:625–7.

30. van Ede, A.E., Laan, R.F., Blom, H.J., De Abreu, R.A., and van de Putte, L.B. Methotrexate in rheumatoid arthritis: an update with focus on mechanisms involved in toxicity. *Sem Arthritis Rheum* 1998;27:277–92.

31. van Ede, A.E., Laan, R.J.M., Blom, H.J., *et al.* The C677T mutation in the methylenetetrahydrofolate reductase gene: a genetic risk factor for methotrexate-related elevation of liver enzymes in rheumatoid arthritis patients. *Arthritis Rheum* 2001;44:2525–30.

32. Stone, J., Doube, A., Dudson, D., and Wallace, J., Inadequate calcium, folic acid, vitamin E, zinc, and selenium intake in rheumatoid arthritis patients: results of a dietary survey. *Sem Arthritis Rheum* 1997;27:180–5.

33. Hashkes, P.J., Balistreri, W.F., Bove, K.E., Ballard, E.T., and Passo, M.H. The relationship of hepatotoxic risk factors and liver histology in methotrexate therapy for juvenile rheumatoid arthritis. *J Ped* 1999; 134:47–52.

34. Russell, R.G., and Rogers, M.J. Bisphosphonates: from the laboratory to the clinic and back again. *Bone* 1999;25:97–106.

35. Bogoch, E.R. and Moran, E. Abnormal bone remodelling in inflammatory arthritis. *Canadian J Surg* 1998;41:264–71.

36. Wolfhagen, F.H., Van Buuren, Hr., den Ouden, J.W., Hop, *et al.* Cyclical etidronate in the prevention of bone loss in corticosteroid-treated primary biliary cirrhosis. A prospective, controlled pilot study. *J Hepatol* 1997;26:325–30.

37. Bianchi, M.L., Cimaz, R., Bardare, M., *et al.* Efficacy and safety of alendronate for the treatment of osteoporosis in diffuse connective tissue diseases in children: a prospective multicenter study. *Arthritis Rheum* 2000;43:1960–6.

38. Cimaz, R., Gattorno, M., Pia Sormani, M.P., *et al.* Alendronate treatment in pediatric patients. How does it work? Who will respond? How long should we treat? *Arthritis Rheum* 2000;43:S381.

39. Rodan, G.A. and Martin, T.J. Therapeutic approaches to bone diseases. *Science* 2000;289:1508–14.

40. Nishioka, T., Kurayama, H., Yasuda, T., Udagawa, J., Matsumura, C., and Niimi, H. Nasal administration of salmon calcitonin for prevention of glucocorticoid-induced osteoporosis in children with nephrosis. *J Ped* 1991;118:703–7.

41. Ozaki, D., Shirai, Y., Nakayama, Y., Yoshihara, K., and Huzita, T. Multiple fish vertebra deformity in child with systemic lupus erythematosus: a case report. *J Nippon Med School* (Nihon Ika Daigahu Zasshi) 2000;67:271–4.

3.12 Surgical interventions

Ann Hall

Aim

The aim of this chapter is to discuss the role of surgical procedures in the management of JIA.

Structure

- Introduction
- Preparation for surgery
- Surgery of the axial skeleton and jaw
- Surgery of the upper limb
- Surgery of the lower limb
- Summary

Introduction

Surgery has an established place in the management of juvenile idiopathic arthritis (JIA) although this role is diminishing because of improved medical management. However, a proportion of children will require surgery during the course of their illness. In one centre [1] 10% of all patients with JIA had at least one surgical procedure; 50% of these patients had Rheumatoid Factor positive Polyarthritis. First reports of surgery for JIA began to appear in the literature in the 1960s. Griffen *et al.* reported their results of prophylactic synovectomy of the knees [2] and this report was followed by other reports of upper limb synovectomies and multiple osteotomies [3]. In the 1970s, capsulotomy and tenotomy of the knee were performed. Wiles in 1957 [4] was probably the first person to perform a total hip replacement in a patient with 'Still disease', using a prosthesis of his own design. Later, surgery on temporomandibular joints [5], osteotomy to correct mandibular deformity, and atlantoaxial fusion to stabilise the upper cervical spine were reported. In the 1960s at the Canadian Red Cross Hospital, Taplow, UK, pioneering work by Ansell, Arden, and colleagues established the value of total hip replacement in JIA [6]. In addition, they performed realignment osteotomies at the hip and knee and Girdlestone pseudarthroses. Later they began to replace knees and upper limb joints.

Preparation for surgery

There can be no doubt that the management of JIA is best conducted in a specialist centre as Swann *et al.* have described [7]. The team approach to management is nowhere more important than when surgery is being considered and it is advisable that the surgical programme is planned well ahead by the paediatric rheumatologist and orthopaedic surgeon, ideally in combined clinics at quaternary centres, with support from the full paediatric rheumatology team. (See Part 3, Chapter 3.2) Surgical procedures should always complement medical management and should be supported by appropriate physiotherapy and splinting. The timing of surgery should be arranged so that there is as little disruption to the life of the child and family as possible, taking into account schooling, and important family events.

When surgery is being planned and it is obvious that more than one reconstructive procedure will be necessary, it is important to ensure the operations are performed in the most appropriate order, for example, hip replacement should precede knee surgery, otherwise the surgery becomes more difficult and the postoperative rehabilitation is compromised. Similarly, a knee replacement should be performed before ankle or foot stabilization, as the realignment of the knee which takes place at arthroplasty can alter the stance of a stiff foot. Lower limb surgery should take precedence over upper limb surgery because the use of crutches postoperatively may cause damage to an upper limb joint on which surgery has been previously performed.

Adolescents particularly may have unrealistic expectations of surgery and it is essential that they are accurately aware of the expected outcome of the procedure. This is critically important when the young person is about to undergo prosthetic joint replacement; the causes of prosthetic joint failure and its functional limitations must be made clear.

The anaesthetist should be involved in surgical planning too and must be aware of problems with the cervical spine and of temporomandibular joint involvement. A rigid neck, a small airway, micrognathia, and limited mouth opening may make conventional intubation impossible, although the use of the fibreoptic laryngoscope and the laryngeal mask have reduced the risks [8]. When patients have upper limb surgery, a brachial plexus block may be used to avoid a general anaesthetic, while for lower limb procedures, it is appropriate to consider a spinal anaesthetic.

Indications for surgery

Surgery should be considered when medication and appropriate physiotherapy and splints have failed to control pain and deformity, when severe joint instability has developed or when function is significantly impaired.

It is important at all times to avoid damage to the epiphysis, so surgical intervention is best limited to prophylactic soft-tissue procedures in the growing child. Such prophylactic procedures include intra-articular corticosteroid injections (Part 3, Appendix) tenosynovectomy, joint synovectomy, epiphyseal stapling, and soft-tissue release operations. Reconstructive procedures, such as osteotomies, arthrodeses, and arthroplasties are not usually required until late adolescence when skeletal growth has ceased. Nevertheless, the general aim of surgery is to restore function and to relieve pain, so if function is poor and pain is severe it may be appropriate to consider reconstructive surgery even in a younger child.

The preoperative work-up

The initial consultation and planning by the paediatric rheumatologist and orthopaedic surgeon in the clinic, should always be combined with advice from the therapists regarding the pre-, peri-, and post-operative physiotherapy programme. A visit to the occupational therapist to optimise splints may be required and it is essential for the paediatric rheumatologist, often with back-up from other members of the team, to fully explain the operative procedure and postoperative plans to the patient and the parents.

For younger children, the play therapists or the paediatric rheumatology nurses can help allay fears using play therapy and explanatory drawings.

A visit to the hospital to see, and have explained, any apparatus to be used postoperatively, such as traction equipment or a walking frame, is also important. Support from the psychologist or psychiatrist may be necessary for particularly anxious children and parents. The preoperative evaluation includes a full, general examination of the child and any imaging procedures relevant to the planned surgery. In all patients, an X-ray of the cervical spine in flexion and extension should be performed, to assess the extent of neck involvement likely to cause problems for the anaesthetist. A full blood count, and erythrocyte sedimentation rate (ESR) or

C-reactive protein (CRP), are important to aid assessment of disease activity and, blood cross-matching may be necessary. Occasionally, as part of the pre-operative evaluation, examination under anaesthetic may be helpful to assess the full extent of the available passive joint movement when pain-induced muscle spasm is abolished by the anaesthetic.

While overall growth failure, growth anomalies, and deformities are evident to the surgeon, osteoporosis may not be, and a bone mineral density measurement may provide helpful information.

Surgery of the axial skeleton and jaw

The cervical spine

Cervical spine involvement in JIA is common, occurring in up to 66% of patients [9]; it is frequently painful. Neck movement becomes limited and a torticollis is not uncommon. The apophyseal joints bear the brunt of the disease in the neck in JIA and facet joint fusion occurs, classically at the C2/3/4 level. Sometimes, fusion may involve the whole of the cervical spine producing the characteristic 'rat tail' neck on X-ray [10]. In addition, due to reduced growth, the cervical vertebrae may be shorter and narrower than in the physically healthy child.

Atlantoaxial and subaxial subluxation (Figure 3.12.1(a) and (b)) are more likely to develop in Rheumatoid Factor Positive Polyarthritis and Enthesitis Related Arthritis, but significant subluxation is rare before late adolescence as this complication is invariably associated with long-standing severe disease. In one review of adult patients with JIA, 35% had radiological evidence of atlantoaxial subluxation in varying degrees [11].

This subluxation may be completely asymptomatic. Symptoms, when they occur, vary from mild neck pain and limitation of

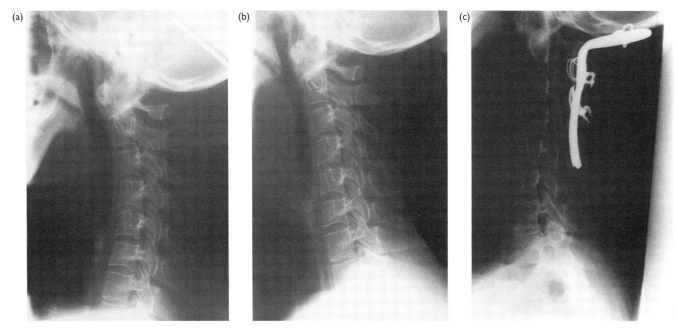

Figure 3.12.1 A young woman with a 10-year history of Rheumatoid Factor Positive Polyarthritis complained of severe neck pain and parasthesiae in both arms and hands. Examination revealed hyper-reflexia, sustained ankle clonus, and an equivocal plantar response. The preoperative radiographs (a) flexion and (b) extension show destructive changes in the atlantoaxial region and significant atlantoaxial shift. After occipitocervical fusion (c) the symptoms remitted.

movement to intractable pain with neurological deficit. Physical signs may be absent or there may be sensory dysfunction, motor weakness, hyper-reflexia, clonus, extensor plantar responses, and bladder and bowel dysfunction. However, the plantar response may be difficult to interpret in a patient with forefoot damage and it is not advisable to rely on an extensor plantar response before considering the diagnosis.

Although a firm cervical collar may stabilize the neck and prevent further subluxation, if the subluxation is associated with neurological deficit or intractable pain, surgical fusion is indicated.

Posterior fusion using metal plates, wires, and bone grafts with or without laminectomy is the usual procedure (Figure 3.12.1(c)). However, if the dens is impacted and requires removal, an anterior approach may be necessary as well and, depending on the degree of subluxation, atlantooccipital fusion may also be required.

The lumbar and thoracic spine

A structural scoliosis occurs more commonly in JIA than in the normal population [12] and arises from a postural curve. It is usually associated with pelvic tilting due to asymmetrical lower limb overgrowth, unilateral hip involvement, or both. Very rarely the scoliosis is severe enough to require surgical correction by conventional methods of stabilization.

The temporomandibular joint

Though temporomandibular joint disease is common, pain is rare and involvement is often missed until obvious overbite, micrognathia, and reduced mouth opening occur. In addition, facial asymmetry due to unilateral disease can be seen in children with Oligoarthritis [13].

The typical 'bird' facies of JIA is due mainly to undergrowth and a backward rotational growth pattern of the mandible. This results in an anterior open bite, decreased mandibular ramus height and length, and a steep mandibular plane with crowding of the lower incisors [14]. Condylar changes range from minor erosion to flattening of the articular surface with severe destruction of the condylar head.

Conservative treatment includes daily exercises aimed at promoting jaw development, orthoses worn at night to improve occlusion, and intra-articular steroid injection into the temporomandibular joint (TMJ) [15]. When growth has ceased, mandibular surgery for severe micrognathia will significantly enhance facial appearance. Synovectomy and discectomy has been performed in patients with JIA with benefit. In one study, 73% of patients experienced pain relief, and significant improvement in mouth opening and lateral mandibular movement was achieved [16]. Costochondral implants have been used to replace mandibular condyles and anecdotal reports are encouraging showing improved function and pain relief. There is a risk of asymmetrical mandibular overgrowth if surgery is performed before skeletal maturity has been obtained [17].

Surgery of the upper limb

The shoulder joint

The shoulder joint is rarely affected in Oligoarthritis but may be involved in as many as half the patients with Polyarthritis [18]. Not uncommonly the involvement only comes to light when the child starts to use crutches for lower limb problems. The earliest sign of involvement is usually some loss of internal rotation followed by reduced abduction with pain. Swelling is rarely obvious clinically. As the disease progresses, radiographs show a decreased glenohumeral joint space with some erosive damage and deformity. The humeral head becomes square-shaped and in addition subluxes superiorly due to stretching, though rarely, rupture of the rotator cuff (Figure 3.12.2(a)). When medical treatment, including exercises and corticosteroid injection fail, particularly if florid synovitis can be demonstrated by ultrasound or magnetic resonance imaging (MRI) and if there is only little radiological damage, it is worth considering debulking synovectomy. It would seem appropriate to perform this procedure through the arthroscope but to date there are no reports in the literature of its use in the shoulder affected by JIA. The procedure is helpful for pain relief [19] but does not influence the long-term outcome for the joint in adults with rheumatoid arthritis.

When severe pain and gross destructive changes are present, reconstructive surgery should be considered. An osteotomy of the humeral neck combined with an osteotomy of the glenoid neck, provides good relief of pain though only rarely improvement in range of movement [20]. This procedure has become less popular since the advent of shoulder arthroplasty.

Arthroplasty may be considered for relief of intractable pain in patients with a destroyed glenohumeral joint. Almost invariably patients have reached adulthood by this stage, and skeletal growth has ceased; however because of the small size and deformity of the humeral head and glenoid, a custom made prosthesis may be required. There are no published series of results in patients with JIA, but in patients with adult rheumatoid arthritis the results of arthroplasty are good, with excellent pain relief, improvement in range, and over 90% 10-year survival of the prosthesis [21]. In one study, 11 hemi arthroplasties (Figure 3.12.2(b)) have been performed in 9 young adults, all of whom have improved range of movement and adequate pain relief, but the follow-up time is short, with a mean of 32 months [22]. Arthrodesis, as a salvage procedure after failed arthroplasty, will relieve pain but at the expense of glenohumeral movement, though scapular movement will remain [23].

The elbow joint

Just under half of all children with JIA develop elbow involvement. Early signs include some reduction of extension followed by soft-tissue swelling and reduction of pronation and supination. The involvement of the joint is characterized by overgrowth of the radial head and not uncommonly this is the only radiological change for many years. When conservative measures, including intra-articular corticosteroids and aggressive medical management of the underlying disease, fail to suppress persistent inflammation, a limited synovectomy with radial head excision and anterior capsular release may be quite effective in improving range of movement (particularly pronation/supination), and relieving pain. This intervention is of benefit if there is no, or only minimal, radiological damage, apart from an overgrown radial head [24]. Instability of the joint has been reported after this procedure [25]. In addition, if the patient later requires an elbow arthroplasty, the prior removal of the radial head may adversely affect this procedure. For the destroyed elbow with intractable pain nothing short of a prosthetic joint replacement is suitable, but surgery is difficult because of soft-tissue contractures, and small bones with

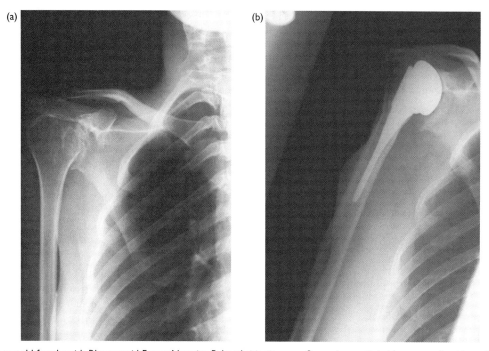

Figure 3.12.2 A 19-year-old female with Rheumatoid Factor Negative Polyarthritis since age 8, was incapacitated by severe shoulder pain. (a) Note the osteoporosis and gross erosive changes in the glenohumeral joint. The humeral head has risen upwards because of an incompetent rotator cuff mechanism. (b) Hemiarthroplasty relieved her pain completely and this was associated with a marked improvement in function. There has been no deterioration at 3-year follow-up.

narrow intramedullary cavities. There is little information regarding elbow arthroplasty in children in the literature. In the only published series to date, 19 children with JIA (24 elbows) who had undergone total elbow replacement were reviewed [26]. At a mean follow-up of 7.4 years the majority of patients (96% of the elbows) had little or no pain but the improvement in range of movement was less encouraging. A complication rate of 50% was reported including fracture of the olecranon, problems with wound healing, prosthetic loosening, and joint instability. Eight young adults, in one study, have had 11 elbows replaced with both reduction in pain and improved function (personal observation) (Figure 3.12.3(a) and (b)). Early complications have included: short-lived parasthesia in the ulnar nerve distribution, a triceps rupture in one patient, and surgical correction for malalignment of the prosthesis in another.

The wrist

Wrist involvement is common in JIA, and in the majority of cases is detectable within 1 year of onset [27].

Deformity and loss of movement occur frequently in the hand and relate to the age of onset and specific diagnosis. Children with early onset disease show most growth anomalies and bony fusion while those with Rheumatoid Factor Positive Polyarthritis have more destructive erosive changes (Figure 3.12.4(a)).

Early signs of activity in the wrist include reduced extension followed by soft-tissue swelling, and the wrist is often held in a few degrees of flexion. Later, more marked flexion deformity develops with ulnar deviation. Rarely, the deformity progresses to complete subluxation of the carpus, giving rise to the so-called, 'bayonet deformity'. Growth failure at the wrist is common and may give rise to a shortened hand and forearm [28].

Soft-tissue swelling and narrowing of the inter-carpal joint spaces are early radiological changes. Later, the carpal epiphyses change shape becoming angular, and early maturation and fusion of the ulnar epiphysis occurs. The carpus may show signs of ulnar translocation, the lunate shifting ulnar-wards in relation to the radius. Also the carpal bones may fuse together.

Wrist deformity may be an important factor in the development of more distal deformities in the hand, with hyperextension at the metacarpophalangeal (MCP) joints and flexion at the proximal interphalangeal joints being a fairly common occurrence when there is marked flexion deformity of the wrist.

The role of synovectomy in a child with severe wrist involvement is not clearly established. There are no published results of series large enough to accurately assess its value, but when synovitis is marked and persistent despite appropriate medical management it is reasonable to consider synovectomy to relieve pain and improve movement. This procedure will not, however, influence the long-term outcome for the joint and may result in some loss of range of movement [29].

A soft-tissue release procedure should be considered to correct a flexion deformity of the wrist resistant to splinting and repeated intra-articular corticosteroid therapy, provided the radiocarpal joints are well preserved on X-ray. The volar wrist joint capsule is divided and the wrist flexors lengthened.

When an ulnar growth defect is pronounced it may lead to ulnar deviation and translocation of the carpus ulnar-wards. Occasionally, even complete dislocation of the carpus off the radius and ulna is seen despite regular splinting. As the ulna shortens, attempts at splintage may be fruitless and indeed may increase pressure across the wrist increasing the likelihood of fracture of the radial epiphysis. This length discrepancy between radius and ulna can be corrected by surgical

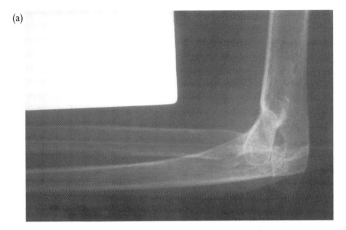

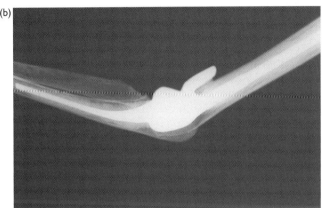

Figure 3.12.3 (a) Radiograph showing a destroyed left elbow in a 40-year-old female with a 30-year history of Systemic Arthritis. (b) After replacement surgery, her pain was relieved and she was able to move the elbow through a 90° arc.

ulnar distraction lengthening leading to improvement in the alignment of the radiocarpal joint (Figure 3.12.4(b)) [30].

More invasive reconstructive procedures for the wrist may inhibit local bone growth and are therefore delayed until growth has ceased, bearing in mind that early epiphyseal fusion due to disease, may bring that date forward in the patient with JIA. These procedures include arthroplasty and arthrodesis. Arthroplasty should be considered in wrists with severe symptomatic destruction without ankylosis (Figure 3.12.5(a) and (b)). In general, arthroplasty should be reserved for wrists with destruction of the joint surface but maintained joint stability; these requirements generally preclude its use in JIA. In one study the indications were extended to include patients with a subluxing wrist joint. Many of their patients had very poor hand function and the maintenance of some stable wrist mobility enhanced function significantly. The altered wrist posture after surgery improved the effectiveness of the long finger flexors and extensors [31]. At follow-up evaluation of eight wrist arthroplasties in seven patients, six arthroplasties were considered to be successful by the surgeon and patients reported significantly enhanced mobility and function. Two prostheses had been removed, one because of infection, the other due to carpal collapse around the prosthesis. Arthrodesis will rarely be necessary but is indicated for uncorrectable ulnar translocation, radiocarpal dislocation, or for salvage of a failed arthroplasty.

The fingers

The most common deformity seen in the fingers is a mild fixed flexion deformity involving the proximal interphalangeal (PIP) joints and distal interphalangeal (DIP) joints. Flexion at MCP joint level can also occur but if there is significant fixed flexion of the wrist, some degree of MCP hyperextension is likely. Radial deviation of the fingers is common and may be secondary to ulnar deviation at the wrist.

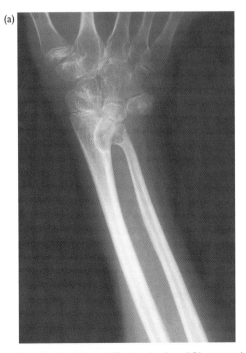

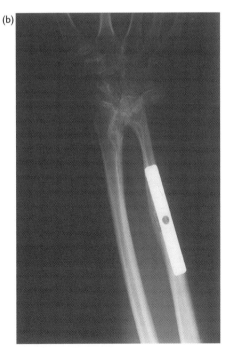

Figure 3.12.4 (a) Hand radiograph of a girl aged 13 who developed Rheumatoid Factor Positive Polyarthritis at age 8. The gross ulnar growth defect and erosive damage at the radioulnar joint had resulted in ulnar deviation and instability in the wrist. (b) An ulnar distraction lengthening procedure improved the stability and alignment.

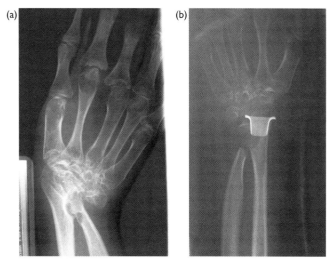

Figure 3.12.5 (a) After 15 years of active disease, a girl with Rheumatoid Factor Positive Polyarthritis had a painful, unstable wrist due to gross destruction of the carpus and radioulnar joint. (b) Wrist arthroplasty relieved her pain and improved the wrist posture and grip strength and at follow-up 5 years later there was no deterioration.

Bony enlargement of both PIP and DIP may occur and periostitis of the proximal phalanges may be obvious on X-ray. Boutonnière deformities (the result of extensor tendon dislocation producing fixed flexion of the PIP joint and hyperextension at the DIP joint) are not as common as in adult rheumatoid arthritis, reported in 26% of patients in one paediatric series [29]. Swan neck deformities (the result of flexor tendon dislocation producing hyperextension at the PIP joint and flexion at the DIP joint) are quite rare in children, seen in 3.3% in the same series. Similarly, 'main-en-lorgnette' or opera glass deformity, with telescoping of the fingers due to marked bone resorption is very uncommon in JIA. Growth of all fingers and the metacarpals may be uniformly reduced resulting in a small hand, or more commonly, one digit may be shorter than the rest due to premature fusion of a single metacarpal epiphysis. Synovectomy of the small joints of the hand has no long-term benefit and in the short term, particularly in young children, may produce further loss of range of movement and is therefore not recommended [29].

The MCP joints

Surgery of the MCP joints is rarely undertaken as there is generally less severe involvement of these joints in JIA. In Rheumatoid Factor Positive Polyarthritis such involvement may lead to volar subluxation and ulnar drift similar to that seen in adult rheumatoid arthritis. MCP joint arthroplasty is rarely necessary before adulthood and should always be delayed until skeletal maturity has been reached.

The PIP joints

For early Boutonnière deformities a combination of static rest splints and dynamic splintage for exercise may be attempted to correct the deformity. Synovectomy is inappropriate because when synovial proliferation is profuse it is invariably accompanied by severe damage to the articular surfaces, and any surgical intervention usually results in further significant loss of movement. For a fixed flexion deformity of the PIP joint which is hampering hand function, the choice lies

between arthrodesis and arthroplasty; always after growth has ceased. Arthrodesis is an unattractive option for the young person, and although the range of movement achieved after Swanson arthroplasty in these patients is not great, it is the more appropriate choice. Mild swan neck deformity may be controlled by small restraining ring splints for each affected finger. If deformity is disabling and becoming fixed, surgical treatment is directed at limiting extension with a tenodesis of the extensor mechanism.

Flexor tendons

Limitation of flexion or extension may be due to flexor tenosynovitis, and be responsive to corticosteroid injections. However, if triggering or entrapment due to nodules has not responded to corticosteroid injection localized tenosynovectomy and removal of the nodule is indicated [32,33].

Extensor tendons

Isolated extensor tendon synovitis leading to rupture is rare in childhood but prophylactic synovectomy to prevent rupture at the wrist should be considered when very florid synovitis persists despite repeated intra-articular steroid injection, particularly in children with Rheumatoid Factor positive disease.

Surgery of the lower limb

The hip

Hip involvement is common in JIA [34] and is the single most frequent cause of reduced mobility. Usually, the inflamed hip is held in flexion, adduction, and external rotation, often associated with the development of an excessive lumbar lordosis (Figure 3.12.6(a) and (b)). Overgrowth of the femoral capital epiphysis associated with an under-developed acetabulum not uncommonly causes lateral subluxation of the femoral head, and in addition, premature fusion and overgrowth of the capital epiphysis produces a short, broad neck which is valgus and anteverted. The trochanters are enlarged, the enlargement of the lesser trochanter being specifically related to traction from the psoas muscle. The femoral shaft is often bowed. If femoral anteversion is pronounced, the femoral head tends to sublux anteriorly leading to further hip flexion and because of this, abnormal development of the abductor lever occurs, manifesting as a waddling gait [35,36]. An uninflamed hip may develop deformities secondary to a flexed knee or scoliosis of the spine.

The exact pattern of deformities relates to the age of onset and duration of the disease [37], but in general the earlier the onset the more overgrowth of the femoral head and the shorter and broader the femoral neck with more pronounced anteversion and bowing of the femoral shaft. In the child who has disease onset after 10 or 11 years, the hip architecture remains normal but a protrusio acetabuli pattern of deformity may develop later.

As the disease progresses, cartilage destruction, bony erosion and not uncommonly, avascular necrosis of the femoral head occurs, the latter complication is probably due to tamponade of the joint resulting from synovitis, effusion, and associated muscle spasm.

When there is no or only minimal radiographic change and when deformities and loss of range are due to muscle spasm, demonstrated by the presence of a full range of movement under anaesthetic,

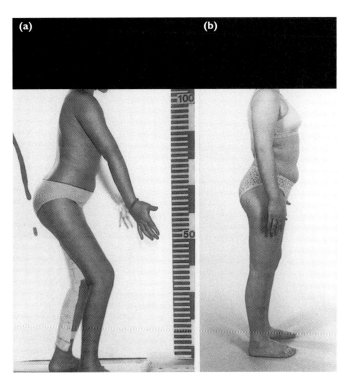

Figure 3.12.6 (a) A girl with Extended Oligoarthritis onset immediately prior to soft-tissue release operation of the right hip at age 11. The knee contractures were treated with intra-articular corticosteroid and splinting. (b) Two years post-hip surgery the improved posture is maintained.

long-acting intra-articular corticosteroid, combined with hydrotherapy, prone lying, and night traction in extension and abduction, are usually sufficient to control pain, prevent significant deformity, and maintain function. Intra-articular pressure in the hip is at its highest with the leg in extension, amd the benefit of night traction has been questioned [38]. Therefore, if the flexion deformity is largely due to muscle spasm, a soft-tissue release procedure may be considered before extensive traction and prone lying is used. Similarly, in more advanced disease when there is an established flexion contracture which persists under anaesthetic provided the joint space on X-ray is not grossly narrowed, a soft-tissue release procedure may be appropriate. The adductor and psoas tendons are divided through a small incision in the groin and postoperatively rehabilitation includes traction in abduction and extension [39]. Until the wounds are healed and stitches are removed, traction is maintained around the clock with breaks for twice daily exercise focusing particularly on the hip and knee flexors and the hip abductors. Hydrotherapy commences when the stitches are removed and the wounds are dry and clean and the patient is mobilized using either a pulpit frame or crutches. Cycling may be encouraged at this stage as well. It is best to use bilateral traction even if a unilateral release has been performed, to maintain symmetry of the pelvis and prevent adaptive shortening on the newly lengthened side. After discharge from the hospital, the exercise programme continues at home, and night traction is maintained for 12 months to prevent recurrence of the contractures.

This procedure not only improves the range of movement in the joint and reduces the degree of contractures, but in addition there is almost universally a dramatic relief of pain, probably due to reduction in the intra-articular pressure. Radiographic improvement with widening of the joint space, reduced osteoporosis, and a clearer definition of the joint line, has also been demonstrated, suggesting that repair is taking place. The long-term results at 3 or more years of follow-up tend to reflect the activity of the disease and the benefit of surgery is partially lost in those patients with continuing active synovitis [40].

For children with the most severe fixed flexion deformities and little passive movement in the joint, a more extensive release procedure has been described with the muscles being stripped from their attachments to the ilium [41].

Even in patients with severe destructive change soft-tissue release may be beneficial, as pain relief is almost invariable. Also, the improved hip posture will help the surgeon if an arthroplasty is required at a later date. Soft-tissue release procedures may be effective in delaying a seemingly imminent arthroplasty for several years. The role of synovectomy for hip disease is unclear. The procedure may reduce pain but at the expense of movement; this procedure is no longer often performed.

For the child with a marked valgus femoral neck and associated lateral subluxation of the hip, a varus osteotomy to reposition the femoral head is indicated. However, because of osteoporosis in these severely affected youngsters, internal fixation is often not possible, and external immobilization in a plaster cast usually leads to further loss of movement in the hip. Fortunately, over the last decade, with improved medical management of JIA, this procedure has become virtually obsolete.

Total hip replacement is indicated for the patient with severe pain who is wheelchair dependent with a destroyed hip joint (Figure 3.12.7(a) and (b)) [42–44]. Most of these patients are adults or in their late teens, but a wheelchair bound child should not be refused hip arthroplasty simply on grounds of age. Growth retardation at the hip as a consequence of surgery is always a concern, but in reality there will be little growth at the hip if the capital epiphysis is destroyed or has fused prematurely; fortunately most growth in the leg occurs at the knee. Although most patients are adults at the time of arthroplasty, a custom-made prosthesis may be necessary because of the abnormal growth of the femur and acetabulum. The operation is often technically difficult for the same reason. It should be made clear to the patient that the procedure is performed primarily for pain, and particularly in a hip where fibrous ankylosis has occurred, there may be little gain in movement, but there will be a major improvement in function due to pain relief. Follow-up studies have shown that a high proportion of these hips fail either due to loosening or rarely following late infection [45–47]. In one series a quarter of hips had been revised at 10 years or less due to complications; however despite this disappointing result all but one patient in this series considered that the operation had been worthwhile [48]. Revision arthroplasty is usually possible though difficult, particularly because of the poor bone stock and the abnormal architecture; for an occasional patient a Girdlestone pseudarthrosis, as a salvage procedure, enables mobilisation, albeit usually on crutches.

The knee

The knee is the most commonly affected joint in JIA; invariably if inflammation is untreated a flexion deformity develops. Initially, the

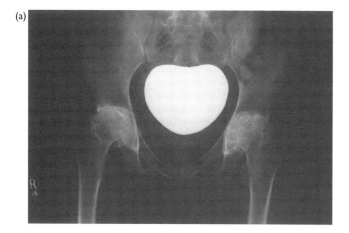

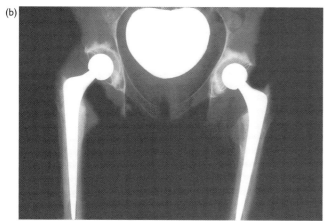

Figure 3.12.7 (a) Pre- and (b) Postoperative radiographs of a 20-year-old woman with Psoriatic Arthritis since age 9 years. Small size standard cemented prostheses were implanted with subsequent relief of pain, enabling her to return to her job to which she cycled.

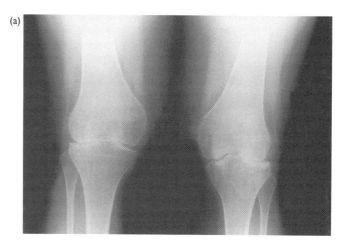

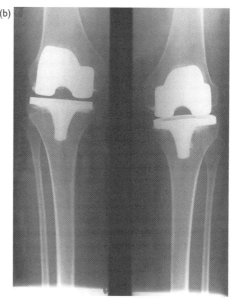

Figure 3.12.8 (a) Pre knee surgery radiographs of a 21-year-old wheelchair bound woman who was diagnosed with Systemic Arthritis at age 4. The typical overgrown medial femoral condyles with depression of the medial tibial plateau and osteoporosis are seen. (b) Bilateral replacements with press fit condylar prostheses relieved her pain and enabled her to walk comfortably.

joint is held in a flexed position for comfort, and subsequently, hamstring shortening prevents straightening of the knee. In time, resistant flexion contractures develop as periarticular structures fibrose and intra-articular adhesions develop. The knee commonly also develops a valgus deformity; in addition significant fixed flexion of the knee will produce flexion in an ipsilateral uninvolved hip. Occasionally, posterior subluxation of the tibia develops and tibial torsion may be a feature. When the knee involvement is unilateral, leg length discrepancy, due to overgrowth of the affected side, is common [49].

The medial side of the growth plate usually grows to a greater extent than the lateral and on X-ray a large bulbous medial femoral epiphysis is characteristic and this overgrowth may contribute to the valgus deformity. As the disease progresses there is increasing loss of joint space (Figure 3.12.8(a)).

The patella enlarges and may become square and deep. In early disease, a programme of exercise and night rest splints prevent deformity and maintain movement. Intra-articular corticosteroid is particularly valuable in the knee to reduce the degree of inflammation and to help correct fixed flexion and to limit overgrowth [50]. There is good evidence that intra-articular corticosteroid is more effective in early disease [51]. Because of the effectiveness of intra-articular corticosteroid therapy, synovectomy (ideally arthroscopic) of the knee is rarely necessary, but may be considered for the child in whom repeated

intra-articular corticosteroid injections have failed to reduce synovitis. In the past, the results of open synovectomy, particularly in young children, were frequently poor as the child was unable to cooperate in the physiotherapy programme in large part because of postoperative pain. Arthroscopic synovectomy is now recommended (even though it is not possible to completely remove synovium from the back of the knee through the arthroscope), because there is minimal morbidity and the child can easily exercise postoperatively [52].

A soft-tissue release of the hamstring tendons and posterior capsule of the knee joint is rarely necessary but may straighten a knee previously unresponsive to conservative therapy [53,54]. The hamstring tendons are lengthened and the posterior capsule incised. Plaster of Paris is applied to the knee which is bivalved after 2–3 days and exercise and hydrotherapy may begin. The bivalved cast is usually worn for 4–5 weeks and exercises and hydrotherapy continue until the deformity is corrected.

The patella in children with JIA is often misshapen and overgrown and is mechanically unsound. A fibrous ankylosis of the patellofemoral joint may cause fixed deformity of the knee, requiring a soft-tissue release. When a fixed flexion and valgus deformity is associated with more advanced disease and radiological damage, a supracondylar femoral osteotomy to correct gross valgus deformity has been used with success [55]. Supracondylar osteotomy will make any future knee replacement technically more difficult, therefore if knee arthroplasty is considered inevitable, this procedure is best avoided. Stapling of the knee epiphysis can be used to arrest growth, thereby reducing a leg length discrepancy [56]. Stapling may also correct a valgus deformity, but again, since better medical management this is rarely needed. For the patient with severe knee pain, limited function and a destroyed knee joint, total knee replacement is the treatment of choice (Figure 3.12.8(b)). It is rarely necessary in childhood and if at all possible should not be undertaken before skeletal maturity, so as to allow maximal growth in the limb. A custom-made prosthesis may be necessary.

Results of total knee arthroplasty in JIA are encouraging. Although loosening and late infection may occur, published studies have suggested that less loosening and infection is seen than occurs after hip replacement. One study [57] reported that only 1 of 29 knees became infected and none were revised because of loosening of the prosthesis; others have reported similarly positive results [58–61].

The foot and ankle

The majority of children have some foot or ankle involvement within 1 year from onset of the disease. The ankle is most commonly affected and this is almost invariably associated with subtalar and midtarsal inflammation. Growth anomalies and deformities are common and may assume many forms, either due to foot joint involvement per se, or secondary to knee involvement. A pronation deformity of the foot with a valgus heel is the most frequent finding and clawing of the toes is common. A varus hind foot with hallux valgus and hammer toes is also seen. Radiological change tends to occur late in the foot, with narrowing of the tibiotalar joint space, flattening and sometimes avascular necrosis of the talus, overgrowth of the navicular bone, and premature fusion of one or more metatarsal epiphyses resulting in shortened toes [62].

Careful attention to footwear and provision of appropriate orthoses is essential to the maintenance of good function and the relief of discomfort. Because ankle involvement is almost invariably associated with the involvement of the subtalar and midtarsal joints, better results using intra-articular corticosteroids are obtained if injections of these joints are performed at the same time, ideally using imaging techniques [63].

When injection of corticosteroid alone fails to improve foot posture, it is worth repeating the procedure combined with resting the hind foot in a neutral position in plaster for 4–5 weeks. It may be necessary to maintain the improved position once the plaster is removed by the use of a brace. Splints should be worn to support the hind foot in neutral at night. Corticosteroid injections into tendon sheaths reduce tenosynovitis and relieve pain. In particular, the peroneal tendons are involved in early disease and an early corticosteroid injection may dramatically reduce the flat foot which occurs secondary to peroneal muscle spasm.

When conservative measures fail to prevent deformity, a soft-tissue release may be considered. A fixed equinus deformity of the ankle may be corrected by lengthening the Achilles tendon accompanied by a capsulotomy of the ankle and sub-talar joints. Varus deformities of the hind foot may be corrected by a posteriomedial release, similar to the procedures used for the treatment of congenital club foot.

If soft-tissue releases fail to correct severe valgus or varus deformity of the hind foot, a calcaneal or midtarsal osteotomy may be performed to realign the foot. A wedge of bone is removed from the medial side of the calcaneum to correct a varus deformity and from the lateral side to correct valgus. A midtarsal osteotomy may be preferred if there is significant midtarsal damage. The metatarsal bases are removed, the opposing surfaces debrided, and a wedge of bone is taken from the cuboid to correct a valgus deformity and from the first cuneiform to correct varus. A cast is applied for 5–6 weeks while bony union develops. When severe destructive change produces intractable pain, arthrodesis of the ankle, subtalar, or talonavicular joints may be necessary. Fusion of all three joints causes unacceptable limitation of movement and it is therefore expedient to fuse only the most affected joint. If there is uncertainty as to which joint is the most painful, an injection of local anaesthetic into the suspected joint may be diagnostically helpful. The long-term results of arthroplasty of the ankle in adult patients are uncertain, and this procedure is not recommended for the paediatric patient at the present time. It is rarely necessary to operate on the forefoot in the child with JIA. Most forefoot problems can be managed with suitable footwear and/or orthoses. Once growth has ceased a hallux valgus deformity, if severe and symptomatic, may be corrected by a realignment osteotomy of the first metatarsal although if the other toes are severely deformed an arthrodesis of this joint is a better alternative. An excision forefoot arthroplasty should be considered when metatarsophalangeal joints are subluxed and painful although the deformity may recur [64].

Summary

Long-term outcome studies in JIA highlight the destructive nature of the disease. Between 17% and 55% of patients have limited physical function and independence after 10–15 years [65–70]. Even in more recent reports arthritis is present 10 years or more after onset in up to 55%, particularly in children with a polyarticular course [71,72]. In one centre, 50% of adult patients with JIA had had at least one prosthetic joint replaced [73].

The need for reconstructive surgery should be regarded as a negative outcome measure in JIA and the eventual goal must be to make surgery for JIA obsolete. Improved medical treatment programmes over the last decade have meant that the number of referrals to the surgeon are falling but for the foreseeable future there will still be a need for carefully planned surgical intervention in the well-evaluated patient.

References

1. Swann, M. The surgery of juvenile chronic arthritis, an overview. *Clin Orthop* 1990;219:38–49.

2. Griffen, P.P., Tachdjian, M.O., and Green, N.T. Pauciarticular arthritis in children. *J Am Med Assoc* 1963;182:23–8.

3. Garrett, A.L. and Campbell, C.A. Synovectomy in children. In R.L. Cruess and N. Mitchell (eds), Chapter 16 III. Philadelphia, PA: JP Lippincott & Co, 1971.

4. Wiles, P. The surgery of the osteoarthritic hip. *Br J Surg* 1957;45:488–97.

5. Martis, C.S. and Karakasis, D.T. Ankyloses of the temperomandibular joint caused by Still's disease. *Oral Surg* 1973;35:462–6.

6. Arden, G.P., Ansell, B.M., and Hunter, M.J. Total hip replacement in juvenile chronic arthritis. *Clin Orthop* 1972;84:130–6.

7. Swann, M. Modern trends in the surgical management of juvenile chronic arthritis. In *Paediatric Rheumatology Update*. P. Woo, P.H. White, and B.M. Ansell (eds), Oxford University Press, 1990, pp. 107–16.

8. Smith, B.M. Anaesthesia for juvenile chronic arthritis. P. Woo, P.H. White, and B.M. Ansell (eds), In *Paediatric Rheumatology Update*. Oxford University Press, 1990, pp. 124–30.

9. Ansell, B.M. and Bywaters, E.G.L. The cervical spine in juvcnile rheumatoid arthritis (Still's Disease). *Paed Clin N Am* 1963;10:921–39.

10. Fried, J.A., Athreya, B., Gregg, J.R., Das, M., and Doughty, R. The cervical spine in juvenile rheumatoid arthritis. *Clin Orthop* 1983;179:102–6.

11. Laiho, K., Hannula, S., Savolainen, A., Kantiainen, H., and Kauppi, M. The cervical spine in patients with juvenile chronic arthritis and amyloidosis. *Clin Exper Rheum* 2001;19:345–8.

12. Ross, A.C., Edgar, M.A., Swann, M., and Ansell, B.M. Scoliosis in juvenile chronic arthritis. *J Bone Joint Surg* 1987;69B:175–82.

13. Walton, A.G., Welbury, R.R., Foster, H.E., and Thomason, J.M. Juvenile chronic arthritis; a dental review. *Oral Dis* 1999;5:68–75.

14. Pedersen, T.K., Gronhoj, T., and Melsen, B. Condylar condition and mandibular growth during functional treatment of children with juvenile chronic arthritis. *Eur J Orthodon* 1995;17:385–94.

15. Larheim, T.A., Haanes, H.R., and Ruud, A.F. Mandibular growth tempero-mandibular joint changes and dental occlusion in juvenile rheumatoid arthritis. *Scand J Rheumatol* 1981;10:225–33.

16. Bjornland, T. and Larheim, T.A. Synovectomy and diskectomy of the temperomandibular joint in patients with chronic arthritic disease compared with diskectomies in patients with internal derangement. *Eur J Oral Sci* 1995;103(I):2–7.

17. Svensson, B. and Adell, R. Costochondral grafts to replace mandibular condyles in juvenile chronic arthritis patients; long-term effects on facial growth. *J Craniomaxillofac Surg* 1998;26(5):275–85.

18. Libby, A.K., Sherry, D.D., and Dudgeon, B.J. Shoulder limitation in juvenile rheumatoid arthritis. *Arch Phys Med Rehabil* 1991;72:382–4.

19. Ovregard, T., Hoyeraal, H.M., Pahle, J.A., and Larsen, S. A three year retrospective study of synovectomies in children. *Clin Orthop* 1990; 259:76–82.

20. Benjamin, A. Double osteotomy of the shoulder. *Scand J Rheumatol* 1987;3:65–70.

21. Stewart, M.P.M. and Kelly, I.G. Total shoulder replacement in rheumatoid disease. *J Bone Joint Surg (Br)* 1997;79:68–76.

22. Thomas, M., Price, A.J., Wexler, D.M., and Hall, M.A. Shoulder arthroplasty in juvenile chronic arthritis. *J Shoulder Elbow Surg* 1999;8:529 (Abs 103).

23. Mah, J.Y. and Hall, J.E. Arthrodesis of the shoulder in children. *J Bone Joint Surg Am* 1990;72(4):582–6.

24. Lonner, J.H. and Stuchin, S.A. Synovectomy, radial head excision and anterior capsular release in Stage III inflammatory arthritis of the elbow. *J Hand Surg Am* 1997;22(2):279–85.

25. Gendi, N.S.T., Axon, J.M.C., Carr, A.J., Pile, K.D., Burge, P.D., and Mowat, A.G. Synovectomy of the elbow and radial head excision in rheumatoid arthritis. *J Bone Joint Surg (Br)* 1997;79:918–23.

26. Connor, P.M. and Morrey, B.F. Total elbow arthroplasty in patients who have juvenile rheumatoid arthritis *J Bone Joint Surg (Am)* 1998;80(5):678–88.

27. Weinberger, A., Ansell, B.M., and Evans, D. Wrist involvement in juvenile chronic arthritis five years after the onset of the disease. *Israel J Med Sci* 1982;18:653–4.

28. Chaplin, D., Pulkki, T., Saarimaa, A., and Vainio, K. Wrist and finger deformities in juvenile rheumatoid arthritis. *Acta Rheumatol Scand* 1969;15:206–23.

29. Granberry, W.M. and Mangum, G.L. The hand in the child with juvenile rheumatoid arthritis. *J Hand Surg* 1980;5:(2): 105–13.

30. Mink van der Molen, A.B., Hall, M.A., and Evans, D.M. Ulnar lengthening in juvenile chronic arthritis. *J Hand Surg (Br)* 23 (4):438–41.

31. Evans, D.M., Ansell, B.M., and Hall, M.A. The wrist in juvenile arthritis. *J Hand Surg (Br)* 1991;16B:293–304.

32. Harrison, S.H., Ansell, B.M., and Hall, M.A. Value of flexor tendon synovectomy in juvenile chronic polyarthritis. *The Hand* 1976;8:1:13–16.

33. Laxer, R.M. and Clarke, H.M. Rheumatic disorders of the hand and wrist in childhood and adolescence. *Hand Clinics N Ame* 2000;16:4:659–71.

34. Isdale, J.C. Hip disease in juvenile rheumatoid arthritis. *Ann Rheum Dis* 1970;29:603–8.

35. Jacqueline, F., Boujot, A., and Canet, L. Involvement of the hips in juvenile rheumatoid arthritis. *Arthritis Rheum* 1961;4:500–13.

36. Rombouts, J.J. and Rombouts-Lindemans, C. Involvement of the hips in juvenile rheumatoid arthritis. *Acta Othop Scand* 1971;17:248–67.

37. Ansell, B.M. and Kent, P.A. Radiological changes in juvenile chronic arthritis. *Skeletal Radiol* 1977;1:129–44.

38. Rydholm, U., WingstrandH, Egund, N., Elborgh, R., Forsberg, L., and Lidgren, L. Sonography, arthroscopy and intracapsular pressure in juvenile chronic arthritis of the hip. *Acta Othop Scand* 1986;57:295–8.

39. Swann, M. and Ansell, B.M. Soft-tissue release of the hips in children with juvenile rheumatoid arthritis. *J Bone Joint Surg (Br)* 1986;68:404–8.

40. McCullough, C.J. Surgical management of the hip in juvenile chronic arthritis. *Br J Rheumatol* 1994;33:178–83.

41. Witt, J.D. and McCullough, C.J. Anterior soft tissue release of the hip in juvenile chronic arthritis. *J Bone Joint Surg (Br)* 1994;76:267–70.

42. Scott, R.D. Total hip and knee arthroplasty in juvenile rheumatoid arthritis. *Clin Orthop Rel Res* 1990;259:83–91.

43. Chmell, M.J., Scott, R.D., Thomas, W.H., and Sledge, C.B. Total hip arthroplasty with cement for juvenile rheumatoid arthritis. Results at a minimum of ten years in patients less than thirty years old. *J Bone Joint Surg (Am)* 1997;79(1):44–52.

44. Rahimtoola, Z.O., Finger, S., Imrie, S., and Goodman, S.B. Outcome of total hip arthroplasty in small-proportioned patients. *J Arthroplasty* 2000;15(1):27–34.

45. Haber, D. and Goodman, S.B. Total hip arthroplasty in juvenile chronic arthritis; a consecutive series. *J Arthroplasty* 1998;13(3):259–65.

46. Lehtimaki, M.Y., Lehto, M.U., Kautiainen, H., Savolainen, H.A., and Hamalainen, M.M. Survivorship of the charnley total hip arthroplasty in juvenile chronic arthritis. A follow-up of 186 cases for 22 years. *J Bone Joint Surg (Br)* 1997;79(5):792–5.

47. Kumar, M.N. and Swann, M. Uncemented total hip arthroplasty in young patients with juvenile chronic arthritis. *Ann R Coll Surg Engl* 1998;80(3):203–9.

48. Witt, J.D., Swann, M., and Ansell, B.M. Total hip replacement for juvenile rheumatoid arthritis. *J Bone Joint Surg (Br)* 1991;73:770–3.

49. Simon, S., Whiffen, J., and Shapiro, F. Leg-length discrepancies in monar-ticuar and pauciarticular juvenile rheumatoid arthritis. *J Bone Joint Surg (Am)* 1981;63(2):209–15.

50. Sherry, D.D., Stein, L.D., Reed, A.M., Schanberg, L.E., and Kredich, D.W. Prevention of leg length discrepancy in young children with pauciarticular juvenile rheumatoid arthritis by treatment with intra articular steroids. *Arthritis Rheum* 1999;42 11:2330–4.

51. Allen, R., Gross, K., Laxer, R., Malleson, P., Beauchamp, R., and Petty, R. Intra articular triamcinolone hexacetanonide in the management of chronic arthritis in children. *Arthritis Rheum* 1986;29:997–1001.

52. Vilkki, P., Virtanen, R., and Makela, A-L. Arthroscoopic synovectomy in the treatment of patients with juvenile rheumatoid arthritis. *Acta Universitatis Carolinae Medica* 1991;37:84–6.

53. Moreno Alvarez, M.J., Espada, G., Maldonado-Cocco, J.A., and Gagliardi, S.A. Longterm follow up of hip and knee soft tissue release in juvenile chronic arthritis. *J Rheumatol* 1992;19:1608–10.

54. Rydholm, U., Brattstrom, H., and Lidgren, L. Soft tissue release for knee flexion contracture in juvenile chronic arthritis. *J Pediatr Orthop* 1986;6:448–51.

55. Swann, M. Juvenile chronic arthritis. *Clin Orthop* 1987;219:38–49.

56. Rydholm, U., Brattstrom, H., Bylander, B., and Lidgren, L. Stapling of the knee in juvenile chronic arthritis. *J Pediatr Orthop* 1987;7:63–8.

57. Sarokhan, A.J., Scott, R.D., Thomas, W.H., Sledge, C.B., Ewald, F.C., and Cloos, D.W. Total knee arthroplasty in juvenile rheumatoid arthritis. *J Bone Joint Surg (Am)* 1983;65:1071–80.

58. Carmichael, E. and Chalin, D.M. Total knee arthroplasty in juvenile rheumatoid arthritis. A seven year follow up study. *Clin Orthop* 1986;210:192–200.

59. Stuart, M.K., and Rand, J.A. Total knee arthroplasty in young adults who have rheumatoid arthritis. *J Bone Joint Surg (Am)* 1988;70(1):84–7.

60. Boublik, M., Tsahakis, P.J., and Scott, R.D. Cementless total knee arthroplasty in juvenile onset rheumatoid arthritis. *Clin Orthop* 1993;286:88–93.

61. Lyback, C.O., Belt, E.A., Hamalainen, M.M., Kauppi, M.J., Savolainen, H.A., and Lehto, M.U. Survivorship of AGC knee replacement in juvenile chronic arthritis. 13 year follow up of 77 knees. *J Arthroplasty* 2000;15(2):166–70.

62. Truckenbrodt, H., Hafner, R., and Von Altenbockum, C. Functional joint analysis of the foot in juvenile chronic arthritis. *Clinical Exper Rheum* 1994;12(Suppl. 10):591–6.

63. Remedios, D., Martin, K., Kaplan, G., Mitchell, R., Woo, P., and Rooney, M. Juvenile chronic arthritis, diagnosis and management of tibio-talar and sub-talar disease. *Br J Rheumatol* 1997;36(11):1214–17.

64. Tillman, K. Surgery of the rheumatoid forefoot with special reference to the plantar approach. *Clin Ortho* 1997;340:39–47.

65. Svantesson, H., Akesson, A., Eberhardt, K., and Elborgh, R. Prognosis in juvenile rheumatoid arthritis with systemic onset. A follow up study. *Scand J Rheumatol* 1983;12:139–44.

66. Laaksonen A. A prognostic study of juvenile rheumatoid arthritis: analysis of 544 cases. *Acta Paediatr Scand* 1966;166 (Suppl. 1):23–30.

67. Stoeber, E. Prognosis in juvenile chronic arthritis: follow up of 433 chronic rheumatic children. *Eur J Pediatr* 1981;135:225–8.

68. Calabro, J.J., Marchesano, J.M., and Parrino, G.R. Juvenile rheumatoid arthritis: longterm management and prognosis. *J Musculoskeletal Med* 1989;6:17–32.

69. Ansell, B.M. and Wood, P.H.N. Prognosis in juvenile chronic polyarthritis. *Clin Rheum Dis* 1976;2:397–412.

70. Wallace, C.A. and Levinson, J.E. Juvenile rheumatoid arthritis; outcome and treatment for the 1990s. *Rheum Dis Clin N Am* 1991:17:891–905.

71. De Inocencio, J. and Lovell, D.J. Clinical and functional monitoring, outcome measures and prognosis of juvenile chronic arthritis. *Bailliere's Clin Paediatr* 1993;1:769–801.

72. Flato, B., Aasland, A., Vinje, O., and Forre, O. Outcome and predictive factors juvenile rheumatoid arthritis and juvenile spondyloarthropathy. *J Rheumatol* 1998;25:366–75.

73. Packham, J. and Hall, M.A. Longterm follow up of 246 adults with juvenile idiopathic arthritis (JIA). Functional outcome. *Rheumatology* 2002;41:1428–35.

Further reading

Swann, M. Surgery for juvenile idiopathic arthritis. In P.J. Maddison, D.A. Isenberg, P. Woo, and D. Glass (eds) *Oxford Textbook of Rheumatology*, 2nd edn. Oxford Medical Publications, Oxford, 1998, pp. 1713–22.

Drew, J., Cohen, B., and Witt, J.D. Surgical management of adolescents with rheumatic disease. In D.A. Isenberg and J.J. Miller *Adolescent Medicine*. Martin Dunitz. 1999, pp. 243–72.

Swann, M. Juvenile idiopathic arthritis. In M.K.D. Benson, J.A. Fixsen, M.F. Macnicol, and K. Parsch, *Clinical orthopaedics and fractures*, 2nd edn. Churchill Livingstone, London 2002, pp. 177–89.

3.13 Clinical trials

Brian Feldman

Aim

The aim of this chapter is to explain the rationale for the use of clinical trials in Juvenile Idiopathic Arthritis (JIA). Some important clinical issues that dictate the need for clinical trials are discussed. The clinical trials that have been performed in JIA are detailed, with their strengths and weaknesses. The overriding concept presented in this chapter is that in order for the most rapid, and effective advance in the treatment of JIA to occur the great majority of all children with JIA should be routinely enrolled in clinical trial protocols.

Structure

- Introduction
- Clinical trials primer
- A short history of clinical trials in medicine and in JIA
- Clinical trials in JIA

Introduction

Clinical trials have not yet been well developed for the treatment of Juvenile Idiopathic Arthritis (JIA). Many of our mainstay treatments are supported by only a single randomized controlled trial (RCT). This is quite a different state of affairs when compared to other clinical specialties. For example, there are over 10,000 randomized studies examining the usefulness of interventions in adult cardiology.

The purpose of this chapter is to introduce the reader to the necessity of proper therapeutic research for JIA, to discuss what has already been done in establishing the efficacy of our current treatments, and to suggest some future areas for research. Accordingly the chapter is split into three sections—a clinical trial primer, the history of drug trials for JIA, and a short section discussing future directions.

Clinical trials primer

In this section several issues concerning the development of clinical trials for children with JIA are discussed. The need for clinical trials, the basic elements of a good clinical trial (and why these elements are necessary) and the history of how clinical trials came about are reviewed. Particular difficulties that arise in using clinical trials to study therapy in children, are discussed, as are some possible solutions that have been, or should be used.

Why are clinical trials needed?

The emperor's new clothes

There are some situations in which it is difficult to maintain equanimity and objectivity. A clinical interaction with a patient (and perhaps even more so when the patient is a child) is one such situation. Health care professionals all want their therapies to work, and for their patients to get better. In a normal clinical practice (in which one gets to observe hundreds or thousands of patients and their response to treatment) a practitioner should certainly get the opportunity to evaluate what works and what doesn't. The problem is that medical professionals have a vested interest in their therapies, and maintaining objectivity is very difficult. It has been convincingly argued that health care professionals get entrapped into seeing what they want to see when it comes to their patients. The clinical trial formalizes the kinds of observations that one might make in practice in a way that allows for more objectivity.

Regression to the mean

There has been much discussion in clinical trials about the so-called 'placebo response'. In drug trials for adult arthritis, between 20% and 40% of subjects assigned to a placebo treatment show an objective response. In arthritis (and this applies to many other chronic processes) regression to the mean accounts for a large portion of this placebo response.

Regression to the mean is a formal statistical term. However, it is easy to conceptualize regression to the mean as it applies to JIA. JIA is characterized by an up and down course—periods of worsening alternating with periods of improvement. Most new therapies began at a time when a patient's condition is poor. In a disease like JIA, it can be expected that many patients who are doing poorly will improve over time, whether they receive treatment or not. Unless one formally incorporates methods to objectify observations, any new treatment that is introduced for JIA will seem effective, simply because of regression to the mean. This is why there are so many positive case reports and case series for treatments that do not hold up to further study.

Elements of a clinical trial

There are certain elements of the clinical trial that have been developed to obtain objectivity. Some of these elements are discussed below: prospective data collection, representative sampling, random allocation to experimental or control treatments, blinding and statistical analysis.

Prospective data collection

A prospective study is one which is designed and begun *before* the outcomes have occurred.

There are several advantages of prospective, as opposed to retrospective, designs. First, investigators can ensure that patients who are being studied have important data (for instance, how well they are doing on the study treatment) rigorously and accurately recorded. Retrospective studies—for example chart reviews—suffer from the poor quality of the recorded data. Second, in a prospective study, investigators can make sure that all the outcomes of importance are measured. Data that are available for retrospective studies may not include all the relevant outcomes. Finally, investigators can plan a prospective study so that objectivity is maintained (see below) and there is no systematic bias favouring one treatment over another.

When analysing retrospective data, consider that there often was a *reason* why some patients were given the treatment of interest as opposed to any other treatment; this preceding reason may have more to do with the eventual outcome than the actual treatment under study.

Representative sampling

Readers want to know to whom they can apply the results of a clinical trial. Investigators can use a *representative sampling scheme* to make sure that the results of their trial are generalizable. For example, using a random number list, investigators can select a truly random sample of subjects from the target population. Using this example, randomly selected subjects from a national JIA registry would well represent the overall registry.

When carrying out a drug study there are a number of issues that work against generalizability. Samples of patients for a study are often selected because of convenience (they all attend the large tertiary care clinic at which the investigators work) and because of certain features that make them desirable patients (they are compliant volunteers that are likely to see the study through). While this type of sampling helps to get a study done, it may not be clear at all that the effect of a drug in local volunteers is the same as the effect in other types of patients.

Random allocation to experimental and control groups

The major threat to understanding the truth about treatments comes when one unwittingly compares 'apples to oranges'. These comparisons can be explicit or implicit. The regression to the mean concept given above can be considered an example of an invalid implicit comparison. Take the case of children with JIA treated with a new anti-inflammatory drug. Should investigators be impressed if 40% show an improvement in pain and morning stiffness? One should always ask 'compared to what?'. The investigators would be impressed if they expected none of these children to respond without treatment (an implicit comparison). Sophisticated readers know that all or part of that 40% may be due to regression to the mean or a placebo response. In this case, the implicit comparison probably should be to how a similar group of children would be expected to respond if they were not treated with the new anti-inflammatory drug. The trouble of course is that one does not really know how a similar group of children would have responded if not treated. That is why investigators planning clinical trials must include explicit comparison (control) groups.

Including control groups does not, by itself, eliminate the apples versus oranges problem. Ideally, the treatment group (sometimes called the experimental group) and the control group should be identical in all aspects with the exception of the treatment under study. If not, it may be characteristics of the groups other than the experimental treatment that determine which has a better outcome.

The best way to make sure that the control and experimental groups are similar is to randomly allocate patients (using a table of random numbers) to the two groups. Very honest and objective researchers might try to match up the groups without using randomization; they might try to form two similarly composed groups. In that case, however, children can only be matched for prognostic factors that the researchers *already know about*. Random allocation (on average) makes sure that *all* prognostic factors (known and unknown) are evenly distributed between the two study groups. An even bigger problem in some studies is that the researchers have difficulty maintaining objectivity. For example, a compassionate researcher may unconsciously assign patients who are sicker to the experimental group, and those who are less sick to the placebo group. Any process that allows the investigator control over which study group a patient ends up in, is open to 'allocation bias'. Allocation bias (comparing apples and oranges) is probably the biggest threat to validity in studying treatments.

Blinding and the nature of outcome measurement

In a clinical trial, the results of treatment are called outcomes. Outcomes can be good (e.g. decreased disease activity) or bad (e.g. side effects). Statisticians call these outcomes the 'dependent variables' in the sense that they are dependent on the effect of the treatments that the researcher introduces. (The 'independent variable' in a clinical trial is whether a subject is in the experimental or control group.) Clinical trials are designed (or should be) in a way that makes measurement of the outcomes objective and similar between the experimental and control groups.

'Measurement bias' is the term used when outcomes are measured in a systematically different way for the experimental and control groups.

Measurement bias can occur because of design faults in the trial. For example, a researcher may design a study in which subjects in the experimental group get weekly blood tests looking for side effects, while the control group patients only get blood tests at the beginning and end of the trial (since they are on placebo). In this situation, by chance alone, it is much more likely that an experimental group subject will have an abnormal blood test result—the experimental group is being checked so much more often!

Measurement bias can also occur because of subconscious human error. Certain types of outcomes are especially susceptible to human error. Subjective evaluations (e.g. disease severity, extent of skin rash) and physical examination findings (e.g. joint count, muscle strength) can be strongly influenced by the manner in which they are done, and by interpretation on the part of the examiner. In some situations, interpretation can depend on what the examiner knows about the patient. For example, if the examiner knows that a study patient is taking placebo, the examiner may be more prone to call a questionable joint as being inflamed.

The best defense against measurement bias is to ensure that outcomes are measured according to a protocol in which all subjects are evaluated similarly. In addition, when subjective outcomes are being measured, they should be measured blindly. In this case blinding means that the evaluator (and often the patient also) must not be allowed to know whether a given study patient belongs to the experimental or control group.

An important issue that an investigator must decide about is which outcomes are the important ones. Sometimes the most important outcomes are difficult to measure (e.g. quality of life) or occur too late to be measured in a reasonable time (e.g. long-term disability). In cases like these, investigators might be forced to settle for *surrogate measures* (e.g. joint count, ESR). All things being equal, it is better to measure outcomes that are important to (i) patients, (ii) treaters and (iii) society.

Improvement criteria for clinical trial outcomes

In an effort to standardize clinical trial outcomes for adult rheumatoid arthritis, the American College of Rheumatology (ACR), Outcome Measures in Rheumatoid Arthritis Clinical Trials committee (OMERACT) developed the ACR outcome criteria [1]. The OMERACT committee reasoned that clinical trials in rheumatoid arthritis suffered from too many different outcomes; the committee felt that using a core set of outcomes in all subsequent trials would facilitate comparison across studies. In addition, the committee defined a way to combine the measures into a single index of improvement. Using this improvement index offered two advantages. Clinicians may now use study data to determine the likelihood that a given individual would respond to a new treatment. Also, combining a number of measures into an overall index improves the ability to differentiate those study subjects who respond from those who do not; this in turn allows fewer subjects to be studied saving on the monetary and time costs of treatment studies. More recently this same approach has been applied to Juvenile Idiopathic Arthritis [2]. Using a complex, multi-stage consensus process, an international group of investigators developed the "JRA core set "outcome criteria and determined an index of improvement. The core set is: (i) patient global assessment of overall well being, (ii) MD global assessment of overall disease activity, (iii) functional ability, (iv) number of joints with active arthritis, (v) number of joints with limited range of motion, (vi) erythrocyte sedimentation rate.

An 'improver' is a patient who has "at least a 30 % improvement in at least 3 of the 6 core set variables (listed above) with no more than 1 remaining variable worsening by >30%" [2]. This is now recognized as the official measure of improvement by the American College of Rheumatology and is known as the ACR paediatric 30 (see www.rheumatology.org/publications/classification/ped30.asp).

Analysis of results and sample size calculation

A clinical trial is a true experiment—the investigator controls the design of the study in order to answer a hypothesis. Like all branches of science, in clinical science it is philosophically difficult to *prove* an assertion. The trialist, like all scientists tries to *disprove* the null hypothesis. For example, it would be very difficult for a scientist to prove that all clover has three leaves. Even after collecting thousands of samples of three-leafed clover, the assertion is still not proved. However, finding only 1 four leafed clover disproves the hypothesis.

For most clinical trials the null hypothesis is considered disproved if the results suggest that it is extremely unlikely that the two study groups show the same clinical response. How does one tell whether it is extremely unlikely? Formal statistical analysis should be part of all clinical trials.

There are a few statistical concepts that are necessary in order to understand the design of clinical trials and these are discussed below. They are (i) variability, (ii) type I error, (iii) type II error, and (iv) sample size calculation.

Variability

All clinical phenomena are variable. People with the same disease have widely different prognoses; patients given the same treatments have widely different responses, and so on. How then can a study demonstrate that one treatment is better than another? Some patients fail despite even the best treatments. Others show a good response to placebo. In general, to solve these problems researchers try to characterize the average patient's response on an experimental treatment and compare this response to the average response on a control treatment.

The average response to treatment has to be considered along with the variability in that response. For example, an investigator might design a treatment trial with a new anti-arthritis drug. It is possible that on one of the experimental treatments, treatment A, the average improvement might be 2 fewer joints with active arthritis, and almost everyone getting treatment A has 2 fewer active joints. It is also possible, though, that another experimental treatment, treatment B, results in a similar average response—also of 2 fewer active joints— but with treatment B some patients end up with 15 fewer active joints and others end up with 13 more active joints.

If, in this study, no subjects have a change in joint count when taking placebo, then when one compares treatment A to placebo one gets excited! Almost everyone improves with treatment A and no one improves with placebo.

If the study were of treatment B, though, one would be far from excited. There is so much variability in the response to treatment B that it is very difficult to know whether the average improvement in the joint count of two is just a fluke.

Understandably, an investigator is much more confident that a clinical phenomenon is true if it is consistently repeated many times. For example, when considering the case of loaded dice—a die that rolled a six, 600 times out of 700 would give one much more cause to worry than a die that rolled six, 3 times out of 3. Even with the imaginary treatment B, if it were studied in a very large number of patients, one would be much more comfortable that the average improvement in joint count of two is in fact true.

In general, in a clinical trial, statistical tests compare the average response between treatments and compare that response to the precision of the responses. The precision is based on the variability in the response and the number of people who have been treated. The more variable the response, the less precise—the more people who have been treated, the more precise.

Type I error (False positive error)

As mentioned above, investigators who plan a clinical trial are interested in showing how unlikely it is that their study groups are responding in a similar fashion. How unlikely is unlikely? The choice of how unlikely is arbitrary. For many decades, it has been considered 'statistically significant' if there is less than a 5% chance that the study groups are similar. This is what is meant by '$p < 0.05$' in a paper. The formal meaning of '$p < 0.05$' is roughly:

> If the study were repeated a countless number of times, and the treatment and placebo responses, in fact, were not different, one would get the results *seen in this study*, or results more extreme, less than 5% of the time.

This level of 5%, then, can be considered the false positive error rate. That is, the community of scientists has accepted that a difference between study groups that would occur as a fluke less than 5% of the time is an unlikely enough difference to be considered true. However, it also means that 5% of positive clinical trials are falsely positive. This false positive rate is also called the 'type I error' rate.

Type II (False negative error)

The false negative rate works the other way around. It is the likelihood that a true difference between treatments is missed and falsely called statistically insignificant. This false negative rate is also called the type II error rate.

As noted above, one considers treatments in a clinical trial to be different if it is highly unlikely, based on statistical tests, that the two treatments *are not different*. The statistical tests are based on the average difference in response, and on the precision of the response. (In turn, the precision is based on variability and importantly on the number of study subjects.) If a new treatment is truly better than placebo, but the response to the new treatment is somewhat variable, and too few subjects are studied, the clinical trial will be falsely negative.

The acceptable level of type II error is also arbitrary. In clinical medicine it is usually assumed that it is *more dangerous* to falsely conclude that a useless treatment is beneficial (false positive), than to conclude that a helpful treatment does not work (false negative). For this reason, the false negative rate is usually a bit more relaxed than the false positive rate—acceptable levels being in the range of 0.10–0.20.

Sample size calculation

Investigators consider the need to reduce false positive and false negative results when planning a clinical trial. They take into account what is known about the precision of the treatment response when calculating the size of the sample that is needed. However, the most important consideration when deciding on a sample size is the 'minimal clinically important difference' between the experimental and control groups.

For example, a study is designed to test whether a new biologic agent is superior—in terms of the response criteria listed above—to placebo. One must consider how many more responses would be needed in the experimental group before the experimental treatment would be considered useful. This is not at all straightforward. The efficacy of the new biologic—that is, how many more responses the new agent will produce than placebo—has to be balanced against its potential toxicity and cost when considering its usefulness. The minimal clinically important difference is a judgement call; different clinicians, and different patients may disagree about what the minimal clinically important difference should be.

Armed with a reasonable idea of the minimal clinically important difference and the precision of the treatment response, the trialist can easily calculate how many subjects must be studied—so that there is an acceptable false negative and false positive rate.

There is some tension that the researcher must resolve when determining the size of the study. A small study is easier, but may lead to greater error (false positive or false negative). A large study is likely to reduce error but is more costly and more difficult.

Problems with clinical trials in children

Rarity of diseases

It should now be obvious that to avoid false positive and false negative results in clinical studies, researchers must be able to enroll adequate numbers of subjects. The problem with the various forms of childhood rheumatic diseases is that they are all rare. Only about 1 per thousand children come to medical attention because of JIA. Dermatomyositis in children is even more rare—affecting only about 2 or 3 per million children each year. Similarly, most hospitals see only a few children with SLE, scleroderma, Kawasaki disease, and so on—too few to perform clinical trials that have adequate power.

Lack of acceptability

Doctors and patients alike are often not receptive to controlled studies, especially those with placebo controls. The physician's primary role is as an advocate for the individual patient—and not as an advocate for the health of society at large. As such, it can be very difficult to accept the basic clinical trial requirement, which is that an individual's therapy is chosen by a play of chance.

This ethical dilemma is thought to be defensible if the medical community is in a state of 'equipoise'. That is, there is *no good reason* to choose one treatment arm of a clinical trial over another. Some have argued that true equipoise rarely or never exists. The argument is as follows—the only reason to study a new therapy is that investigators expect it to be better, safer, or cheaper than the existing therapies; therefore investigators are not in a true state of equipoise. More recently, the principle of uncertainty (a less stringent requirement) has been used as a defense of clinical trials.

In any case, it is clear from studies of individuals with cancer, that most clinical trial participants do so to please their physicians; they are older, less well educated, and have not understood the consent forms as well as patients who refuse participation [3]. Moreover, it also seems clear that most physicians recommend studies with the hope that their patients will get the best new therapy, rather than to further scientific enquiry. These issues are probably compounded when the study subjects are children who are unable to even provide proper informed consent. Certainly, there is evidence from parents, that when they do enter their children into studies, it is often for a variety of reasons that suggest little understanding of the scientific process [4].

However, a reluctance to perform clinical trials in children has meant that many children must use medications that are unlicensed and unstudied. For example, about two-thirds of children who are hospitalized and 90% of sick neonates receive off-label drugs [5].

There is therefore a state of ambivalence. We all want to treat children only with known, safe, and effective treatments—which goes against entering children into trials—yet if clinical trials are not done we will end up treating children with drugs of unknown efficacy and toxicity.

Developmental differences in response

Pharmacokinetics

Children are not just small adults. The clinical specialty of paediatrics has developed, based on this theme. What is true clinically is also true in the field of research.

Children metabolize medications differently at different stages of development, and often quite differently than adults. The potential differences in physiology are at all levels, including absorption, distribution, metabolism, excretion, and pharmacodynamics [6]. For example NSAIDs, which seem mostly harmless in children, are a significant cause of morbidity in the elderly. Studying new treatments in children can be difficult since the dose and timing might be different than the adult dosing, and indeed may differ between different childhood age groups.

Compliance

Compliance with medical therapies is poor in most chronic diseases—even in adult patients. Poor compliance in a clinical trial leads to imprecise outcomes, and sometimes to an inability to detect a true treatment effect. Children may not understand the importance of the research that they volunteer for, and may therefore have very poor compliance.

Ethical difficulties with consent

One of the axioms of clinical trial research involving volunteers is that the participants have to understand what they are volunteering for. Young children may not be capable to fully consent to take part in a clinical trial. Even those children who are capable may not legally be able to consent. Issues of consent for children (and the related issue of parental proxy consent) have plagued researchers and ethics review boards—the international community has yet to develop suitable regulations [7].

Innovative solutions and future directions

The biggest of the problems facing investigators who wish to study new treatments for JIA, is the problem of lack of acceptability. Poor acceptability means that children and their families are often reluctant to enter into studies, and often physicians are reluctant to take part. This, in turn, leads to poor accrual, poor study power, and an inability to detect if a treatment is truly effective or not (for an example see Silverman *et al.* [8]).

A potential solution is to use clinical trial designs that differ from the standard randomized, controlled, parallel groups trial. Some of these designs are more acceptable and can potentially increase accrual; some are more powerful and need fewer subjects to be studied.

More acceptable trial designs

In general, studies in which fewer patients are enrolled in a placebo arm, or in which placebo is given for as short a time as possible, are more acceptable to physicians and patients. A number of different trial designs might be suitable for the study of JIA.

One such design involves 'adaptive randomization'. With adaptive randomization, the ratio of subjects allocated to experimental or control arms of a trial changes to favour the study arm that (to that point in the study) is most successful. This approach is rarely used however. It is quite complex and may be difficult for subjects to understand. Also, bizarre things can happen—in one study of extracorporeal membrane oxygenation (ECMO) in preterm neonates, all the subjects but one ended up in the ECMO arm.

A second option is to allow all subjects to be treated with the experimental therapy after a standard randomized controlled trial is finished. This approach has been used in many adult studies of new arthritis therapies. The disadvantage of this approach is that children assigned to a placebo treatment must still take placebo for the whole length of the clinical trial before being eligible for the experimental therapy.

Recently, the 'randomized withdrawal' approach has been used in studying JIA [9]. In this design all subjects begin the study on the experimental treatment. Only those that show a defined response go on to the randomized portion of the study. The responders are then randomly assigned to continue taking the experimental treatment or to switch to a placebo. The subjects are then followed to compare the rate of relapse in the two arms.

One final option to consider is the newly developed 'randomized placebo phase design' (RPPD) [10]. In the RPPD, all subjects start the trial on a short course of placebo. The length of time on placebo is randomly varied—at a randomly determined time each individual subject is blindly switched to the experimental treatment. The research question answered by the RPPD is 'do those subjects who are treated with experimental therapy sooner respond sooner (on average) than those who are treated later'?

More powerful trial designs

In order to improve the power of clinical studies one can either study more subjects, or get more information from each subject studied.

Multi-centre clinical trial networks

Because juvenile rheumatic diseases are relatively uncommon, the best way to study more subjects is to involve more centres. Clinical trial networks (e.g. the Paediatric Collaborative Study Group (PRCSG), the Paediatric Rheumatology International Trials Organization (PRINTO), and the Childhood Arthritis and Rheumatology Research Alliance (CARRA)) provide an administrative framework to allow multi-centre studies to come to fruition. Multi-centre studies are difficult to implement—quality control becomes more difficult as the number of centres increases. However, collaborative networks have been strikingly successful in the field of childhood cancer. There are currently strong efforts to get funding agencies to provide more support for North American and European collaborative clinical trials.

Crossover studies

One way to get more information from each studied subject, is to study each subject under both the experimental and control situation. Each subject can be randomly exposed to both experimental and control treatments once (a single crossover) or many times (multiple crossovers). This design can be so powerful that a clinical trial may be successfully performed using only one subject ('n-of-1 design'). There is a trade-off, though. When fewer subjects are studied, one is less certain that the results can be generalized widely. A single successful n-of-1 study is unlikely to convince anyone, besides the subject of the study, that the treatment works.

Crossover designs all require that the treatment be reversible. A permanent experimental treatment, if given first to a patient in a crossover study, would carry over into the control period.

For very rare chronic diseases, in which there is a reversible treatment, a multi-centre registry of n-of-1 trials is a very appealing way to study therapy.

A short history of clinical trials in medicine [11] and in JIA

Pierre Louis (1787–1872) and the end of leeches

Until the time of Pierre Louis (the French clinician who practised in the late eighteenth and early nineteenth centuries) the one absolute certainty in clinical medicine was that the best treatment for uncomplicated lobar pneumonia was the application of medical leeches. Louis turned the medical world upside-down with his application of his so-called 'numerical method'. The numerical method—hailed in Louis' time as either revolutionary or heretical—meant simply counting up the number of patients who lived or died treated by different methods. Louis was able to show that leeches, in fact, led to an increased mortality rate—and it was not until the late twentieth century that medical leeches again found uses in therapy.

Many physicians in his time censured Louis. They felt that the subtleties of clinical medicine made each case entirely unique, and that any comparison between patients was invalid. Similar arguments have resurfaced in the late twentieth and early twentyfirst centuries in response to the concept of 'evidence based medicine'. However, Louis' arguments proved persuasive and adaptation of the numerical method blossomed into the rich field of clinical science that we now know.

Ronald Fisher (1890–1962) and plant genetics

Sir Ronald A. Fisher was an extremely influential statistician whose work was directed towards plant genetics experiments at the University of Cambridge. Fisher's experiments led to theories of genetic inheritance, and as a statistician he developed some of the most important techniques—for example, analysis of variance. However, perhaps the most influential of his ideas (at least in clinical medicine) came from his understanding of the potential biases that came about when planting different batches of seeds into different plots of land. Fisher needed to overcome the problem that soil quality might influence growth potential as much as the genetics of the seed. To get around this problem he introduced the concept of randomization.

Following Fisher's lead, the principle of random allocation has been widely adopted in medical research. He was knighted in 1952 in recognition of his contributions to the scientific method.

Austin Bradford Hill (1897–1991) and the randomized trial

Sir Austin Bradford Hill is probably best known for his collaboration with William Richard Doll, in which they were the first to link cigarette smoking with lung cancer. However, Hill has a special place in the history of clinical trials, as he was the first to apply and promote Fisher's principle of randomization to the study of therapeutics in humans. His early study of the use of Streptomycin in tuberculosis was one of the first randomized controlled trials. Since then, over 150,000 randomized trials have been reported in the medical literature.

Archie Cochrane (1909–88) and science in medicine

Professor Cochrane was a physician, trained in London, who spent much of his career practicing epidemiology in Cardiff. His early experiences tending wounded soldiers in a German Second World War prisoner of war camp convinced him that there was very little evidence from which to choose therapies. He was a great promoter of guiding health care with knowledge and saw the randomized trial as the best method for doing so.

His influence led to the science of combining the knowledge accumulated through clinical trials, first with the Oxford Database of Perinatal Trials in the 1980s, and more recently with the Cochrane Collaboration, formed in 1993. The Cochrane Collaboration is a multinational collaborative effort. Researchers around the world use formal techniques (such as meta-analysis) to combine the knowledge gained from all clinical trials in order to best guide therapy.

David Sackett (1934–) and evidence based medicine

Dave Sackett, along with Archie Cochrane (and Alvan Feinstein at Yale) is considered one of the founding fathers of modern clinical epidemiology. He founded the Department of Clinical Epidemiology and Biostatistics at McMaster University (in Hamilton, Canada) in 1969. As a researcher he has been tremendously productive and has done some of the landmark clinical trials in stroke care and prevention, treatment of hypertension, and many other fields. He has also done very important work in the development of the methods used by clinical trialists.

Perhaps Sackett's most influential work, though, has been in the education of others in applying the methods of critical appraisal and evidence-based medicine. He authored a series of articles, first in the Canadian Medical Association Journal, and later (with his students and colleagues) in the Journal of the American Medical Association, which described the principles of critical appraisal. These articles, and his introductory textbook, have formed the curriculum for evidence-based medicine courses at medical schools throughout the world.

Pediatric Rheumatology Collaborative Study Group

The Pediatric Rheumatology Collaborative Study Group (PRCSG) was formed in 1973. The group was formed to begin to study therapies for children with rheumatic diseases. The specific objectives were (i) to develop a methodology for collaborative drug trials in JIA and (ii) to investigate the efficacy and safety of anti-inflammatory drugs used in the treatment of children with JIA [12]. It was recognized that studying relatively uncommon diseases, like JIA, needed more subjects than could be gathered at any one hospital.

The group's first study was the study comparing Tolmetin Sodium with ASA in childhood arthritis [12]. In 1982 the PRCSG published standards for running clinical trials for juvenile arthritis [13]. Since then, many clinical trials have been published, which have provided evidence for many of the treatments used in JIA today. By 2002, the PRCSG had 94 members in North America and was still growing.

Paediatric Rheumatology International Trials Organization

PRINTO (Paediatric Rheumatology International Trials Organization) was formed in 1996, initially as a European clinical trials group. The group originally represented 14 countries—that number has now grown to over 30. The PRINTO group now includes centres in South and Central America, as well as North Africa and Asia. The group has done important work in standardizing outcome measures for clinical trials, and has started studies looking at the effectiveness of different doses of methotrexate and the usefulness of cyclosporine.

Childhood Arthritis and Rheumatology Research Alliance (CARRA)

In North America the PRCSG has been very successful at studying new agents with the support of the pharmaceutical industry. However, many new ways of giving old medications have not been studied. Recently a new network—CARRA (Childhood Arthritis and Rheumatology Research Alliance)—has been formed specifically to carry out 'investigator initiated' clinical trials. CARRA has been modelled on other successful clinical trial networks like the Children's Oncology Group and the Cystic Fibrosis Network. CARRA will hopefully enable the development of treatment registries, and the use of innovative study designs (such as the ones discussed above). The eventual hope is to change the North American therapeutic climate so that all patients with arthritis (and indeed other rheumatic illnesses) are treated with a clinical trial protocol; this would be similar to the current climate for the treatment of childhood cancer.

Clinical trials in JIA

In this section some of the research studies that have had a major impact on treatments used for childhood arthritis will be described.

NSAID

Some of the earliest studies were done to confirm the usefulness, and safety of nonsteroidal anti-inflammatory medications (NSAIDs).

Tolmetin sodium [12]

This was the first study performed by the PRCSG (see above). At the time of the tolmetin study, acetylsalicylic acid (ASA) was the first line treatment of choice for JIA. However, it was widely recognized that ASA had a narrow therapeutic index (i.e. medication levels just slightly above the therapeutic range caused salicylate toxicity), was inconvenient to dose (it was given 3 or 4 times daily) and frequently had to be discontinued because of adverse events including gastrointestinal discomfort and elevation of liver transaminases. The PRCSG group, in an effort to find an alternative to ASA, initially studied 30 patients in an open-label trial of tolmetin sodium. Following their perception that the drug was safe, the investigators initiated this double blind study.

Trial design

One hundred and nine patients were enrolled in this study, but two were dropped from the analysis due to protocol violations. The study was blinded (by using identical medication capsules) so that the investigators, patients, and parents did not know to which group the subjects were assigned. The assignment to the alternate treatments was made randomly, but the exact method is not detailed in the paper, and it is unclear whether the allocation was hidden. The experimental treatment was tolmetin sodium. The initial dose was 15 mg/kg/day. The dose was then escalated by 5 mg/kg/day at weekly intervals until efficacy was seen or toxicity developed. The maximum dose was 30 mg/kg/day (up to 1800 mg). The control treatment for this study was ASA. The dose of ASA was escalated in a similar manner. The baseline ASA dose was 50 mg/kg/day and it was increased weekly, in the same manner, by 16.7 mg/kg/day. The maximum ASA dose allowed was 100 mg/kg/day (up to 5900 mg).

Populations studied

The specific inclusion and exclusion criteria for this study were not as well documented as would be expected today. However, all subjects were required to have juvenile rheumatoid arthritis (JRA) (any onset subtype). The enrolled subjects were all between the ages of 2 and 16 and had an average illness length of about 3.5 years.

Outcomes measured

Subjects were examined at baseline, and at 2, 4, 8, and 12 weeks. The reported outcomes mostly were related to adverse events and to articular findings. Basic laboratory screening was done at each study visit.

Results

Both drugs seemed to perform as well, and there were no adverse event differences between the drugs that were statistically significant. However, six of the ASA treated subjects were withdrawn due to side effects of the treatment. One tolmetin sodium treated subject had transient proteinuria (thought at the time to be unrelated to therapy, although it is now known that proteinuria may be a false positive result).

Comments

This first study came at a time when no drug was approved in North America for the treatment of childhood arthritis; the results led to approval of tolmetin sodium for use in JRA. The authors suggested that due to the tolerability of tolmetin sodium, and its similar efficacy to ASA, tolmetin sodium might be used for those who were intolerant of ASA, and they suggested that it might be tried for those children who did not have an adequate response to ASA. They did not suggest that tolmetin sodium could replace ASA.

Diclofenac sodium [14]

By the early 1980s, ASA was still a mainstay therapy for JIA. Other NSAIDs, including diclofenac, were being more widely used in adults with other types of arthritis. Early uncontrolled promising studies of diclofenac in JIA prompted Finnish investigators to study the medication against ASA and placebo.

Trial design

Following a pharmacokinetic study in seven subjects, a three group, 2-week controlled study was done. The method of allocation was described as being randomized, however, the group sizes ended up being exactly even—a highly unlikely event if simple randomization was used. The three groups were (i) diclofenac 2–3 mg/kg/day, (ii) ASA 50–100 mg/kg/day, and (iii) placebo diclofenac. Although it is described as a double-blind study, the trial was really single blind; the medications were all packed into identical bottles so that investigators did not know which medication was being taken, but patients did.

Populations studied

Forty-five subjects were enrolled—15 into each group. The subjects all had JRA (including all three onset subtypes). They were eligible if they were between 3 and 15 years. All subjects were hospitalized for arthritis care at the time of study. Equal numbers of subjects were being given concomitant gold, chloroquine, and corticosteroid therapy in the three groups.

Outcomes measured

Subjects were examined at baseline and again at day 7 and 14. A number of articular, laboratory, and global assessments were carried out.

The investigators did not indicate which outcome was to be considered the primary study outcome.

Results

There were more dropouts due to side-effects in the ASA group (4 of 15 compared to 0 in the diclofenac and placebo groups). Morning stiffness improved in all three groups, but joint tenderness was only improved in the diclofenac and ASA groups—it worsened in the placebo group. More subjects in the diclofenac group were rated as improved or in remission (73%) than in the ASA group (50%) or the placebo group (27%).

Comments

Typical of earlier clinical trials, this study lacks some of the refinements that are currently expected. There was a potential for unblinding, it is unclear if allocation was done blindly and using a true random process, and patients who dropped out were not included in the efficacy analysis. Nonetheless, taken with other NSAID studies, diclofenac is now seen as a safe and effective anti-inflammatory treatment for JIA.

Naproxen [15]

Naproxen is now one of the most widely prescribed NSAIDs for the treatment of JIA. In the late 1970s, though, it had only been studied in short-term crossover studies, and in uncontrolled case-series investigating safety. Kvien and colleagues in Oslo used the PRCSG trial format to study the efficacy of naproxen when compared to the then-standard first line therapy, ASA.

Trial design

This study was a randomized, double blind study. The randomization was done in blocks, with the groups balanced for disease course (pauciarticular or polyarticular) and for disease duration. The subjects were assigned either to naproxen, 10 mg/kg/day divided into two doses (with a placebo tablet given at mid-day) or to microencapsulated ASA at a dose of 75 mg/kg/day divided into three doses. The study was kept double blind by the use of specially prepared medications that were identical between the groups. A third party monitored the ASA levels to preserve the blind.

Populations studied

The inclusion criteria for this study specifically excluded those children with the systemic form of arthritis. All subjects were between the ages of 3 and 16 years and had at least one active joint. Eligible children were not allowed to use concomitant second line agents, so children with mild disease were preferentially enrolled. Of 80 subjects initially accrued, 2 dropped out at the beginning due to protocol violations. Twelve of the 80 subjects were HLA-B27 positive, and 1 of 80 was rheumatoid factor positive.

Outcomes measured

The study was for 24 weeks. Subjects were examined and had basic laboratory screening done monthly by their local physicians, and were seen for study visits at baseline, 12 and 24 weeks by the study team. Subjective assessments of symptoms and adverse events, physician, and physical therapy assessments and laboratory assessments were done at these study visits.

Results

As would be expected, both patient groups improved, and efficacy seemed similar with both treatments. The most interesting result from this study was that ASA was considerably more toxic than naproxen. The average platelet count rose in the ASA group, and the liver transaminases increased in the ASA group but not the naproxen group. Moreover, 20 of 38 ASA group subjects were withdrawn for adverse effects compared to only 5 of 40 in the naproxen group. The withdrawals were mostly for gastrointestinal complaints and for central nervous system effects compatible with salicylate toxicity.

Comments

The doses used in this study, both for naproxen and ASA, were likely lower than the doses that would be used in many centres today. However, this study clearly demonstrated the advantages of naproxen over ASA; naproxen has a higher therapeutic index and is easier for patients to take (as it is prescribed only twice daily).

Ibuprofen [16]

In the early 1980s, most NSAIDs were formulated as tablets or capsules. Ibuprofen was available as a suspension and therefore offered an appealing alternative for children. The PRCSG published a report in which they describe two studies—a controlled 12-week comparison of ibuprofen suspension with acetylsalicyclic acid (ASA), and a 24-week 'open-label' case series of children treated with ibuprofen.

Trial design

The first study was a multi-centre, randomized double blind study in which subjects were allocated to either ibuprofen (30 mg/kg/day divided into three doses) and placebo ASA, or ASA (60 mg/kg/day divided into three doses) and placebo ibuprofen. The randomization scheme was given as a list of consecutive numbers; it is difficult to know if the allocation was hidden from the investigators. For the open-label study, children were given ibuprofen between 30 and 50 mg/kg/day.

Populations studied

The eligible children were between the ages of 2 and 15 years (minimum age of 1 year for the open-label study). They all had JRA based on ACR criteria and could have any of the three onset types. Ninety-two subjects were enrolled in the double-blind study and 84 in the open-label study.

Outcomes measured

A number of clinical indices of joint activity were measured every 2 weeks or so for the controlled study and at weeks 16 and 24 for the open-label study. The primary analysis was based on the physician global categorical score (i.e. proportion of children who were rated as better or much better). For the sample size calculation, it was determined that about 60% of the ASA treated group would be rated as better or much better, and that an additional 30% of the ibuprofen group would have to improve for the study to be positive. This means that, given the sample size, a difference between the group of less than 30% might have been missed.

Results

Both groups showed an improvement in the controlled study. About 80% of the subjects in both groups were listed as globally improved by the physicians at 12 weeks. There were more dropouts in the ASA group due to side effects (6 of 47 compared to none in the ibuprofen group).

Comments

Although the study was not large enough to rule out a modest difference in efficacy between the groups, there does not appear to be a striking difference in efficacy between ibuprofen and ASA. The higher number of adverse events in the ASA group, and the availability of ibuprofen as a suspension might suggest that it is a superior treatment. At some centres higher doses of both ASA and ibuprofen are routinely prescribed. Nonetheless, studies like this one have certainly led to a reduced usage of ASA in JIA.

Piroxicam [17]

Piroxicam has a long half-life and only needs to be given once daily. Once daily dosing is one of several factors that is associated with improved medication adherence. For this reason, in the mid-1980s two groups studied the efficacy of piroxicam compared to the then standard, naproxen. The first study was done in Argentina and presented in 1985. It was published after a similar British study that showed equal efficacy between the two treatments [18]. The Argentinian study, while small, actually showed a benefit to piroxicam when compared to naproxen.

Trial design

The Argentinian study was a single centre, randomized study in which the treatments were compared in a double blind fashion. The study lasted 3 months. The experimental treatment, piroxicam, was given in a dose depending on weight as follows: children weighing 15–30 kg were given 5 mg once daily, those weighing 31–45 kg were given 10 mg, and those weighing 46–55 kg were given 15 mg. After 1 week, there was a dosage increase (by 5 mg/day) if the therapy was thought to be inefficacious and no side effects had occurred. The control therapy (naproxen) was given in a dose of 12.5 mg/kg/day divided into 2 doses. To ensure blinding, those in the piroxicam group also received naproxen placebo, while those in the naproxen group received piroxicam placebo.

Populations studied

Twenty-six children were studied. The children were between 3 and 16 years of age and all had JRA with polyarticular course and active joint disease of at least 3 months duration.

Outcomes measured

Subjects were studied at baseline, and then again at 2, 4, 8, and 12 weeks. The main outcome measures included a physician global assessment of improvement as well as articular examination indices. In addition basic laboratory screening was done.

Results

In this study both groups improved, but there was a statistically significant greater improvement in both painful joint count and swollen joint count in the piroxicam group. In addition more patients were considered improvers in the piroxicam group (67% versus 38%). Side-effects were not different between the groups.

Comments

This is a small study; moderate differences in side effects between piroxicam and naproxen might have been missed. The randomization scheme was not detailed and it is possible that the allocation was not hidden. Nonetheless, taken together with the British study it is likely that piroxicam is a useful NSAID for the treatment of JIA.

Corticosteroids

Corticosteroid therapy has been studied in a variety of forms for the treatment of JIA. In general, although the studies have been small, the well-known efficacy of steroids has been confirmed [19–22] (Table 3.13.1)

Disease modifying anti-rheumatic drug

Traditional (DMARDs) that have been used in adult rheumatoid arthritis have been studied in controlled trials in children. These studies have mainly shown little effect. [23–34] (Tables 3.13.2–3.13.4)

Azathioprine [31]

Azathioprine had been widely used (with reported success) in some European centres by the mid-1970s. Controlled studies in adult rheumatoid arthritis had demonstrated efficacy; this led to a randomized study of azathioprine in children with arthritis.

Trial design

This study was a randomized, single centre study. The duration of the study was 16 weeks. Using a double-blind design, the investigators allocated subjects to either azathioprine (2.5 mg/kg/day) or to matching placebo tablets. All subjects were concomitantly taking prednisolone; the dose was to be tapered during the study in 5–8 steps if possible.

Populations studied

The subjects in this study all had active and progressive JRA. They were consecutively enrolled if they required immunomodulatory therapy for severe systemic features or for severe progressive joint disease (that was thought to be leading to irreversible deformities). Thirty-two subjects were enrolled over a 4-year period (17 azathioprine, 15 placebo).

Outcomes measured

Patients were seen weekly for examinations and blood tests to evaluate safety. Study outcomes were measured at 8 and 16 weeks. A variety of subjective, articular, laboratory, and functional measurements were taken.

Results

At 16 weeks, the azathioprine group seemed to be doing somewhat better, but most of the comparisons were not statistically significant. For example, the number of affected joints decreased from 17 to 11 in the azathioprine group compared to no change in the placebo group, but this was not statistically significant.

Comments

Three of the azathioprine patients were withdrawn due to side-effects (compare to 0 in the placebo group); the side effects were mostly haematologic. Considering the available options, azathioprine should likely not be considered a useful treatment for JIA until it has been proven in a larger study with adequate power.

Methotrexate [32]

Methotrexate is now the most widely used 'second-line' agent in the treatment of JIA. Its popularity mirrors its widespread use in adult rheumatoid arthritis, and is largely due to the international, PRCSG run study that was published in 1992.

Table 3.13.1 Corticosteroid therapy

	Prednisolone [19]	Methylprednisolone mini-pulses (IVMP) [20]	Deflazacort [21,22]
Trial design	Placebo-controlled trial 7-day duration Unclear allocation scheme Double-blind Prednisolone (0.4 mg/kg/d) versus placebo (P)	RCT 6-and 12-month endpoints Blinded observer IVMP 5mg/kg × 3 d, then 2.5 mg/kg × 3 d, then prednisone 1 mg/kg po od versus prednisone 1 mg/kg po od	RCT 12 months duration (with later follow-up at 2 yrs.) Unblind Deflazacort versus prednisolone (dose as needed)
Populations studied	N = 20 JRA (9 pauci, 11 poly) Hospitalized for this study Functional class I and II	N = 22 (20 were analysed) 'Severe' systemic onset JCA (unresponsive to 3–6 months of NSAIDs)	N = 34 (31 analyses) JCA with active poly course All had beem on prednisolone at least 5 mg/day × 1 year
Outcomes measured	Patient subjective (e. g. pain, fatigue) Articular indices Laboratory Observed function (Lee index)	Clinical outcomes Steroid dose Steroid side-effects as measured by BMI	New vertebral fractures (radiograph) Bone mineral content by dual photon absorptiometry (DPA) Growth parameters Clinical outcomes
Result	Prednisolone group improved subjectively but not for pain 'Weighted' (for severity and size of joint) active joint count improved the most No improvement in labs or function	IVMP group had quicker control of symptoms/signs and lower cumulative steroid dose No difference in steroid dose at 12 mos. Subjectively less Cushing syndrome in IVMP group, but no difference in BMI	Two new spinal fractures in Deflazacort group vs. 1 in prednisolone group Better preservation of bone by DPA in deflazacort group (when) adjusted for somatic growth Height gain similar but decreased weight gain in deflazacort group
Comments	This study was designed to test which measures were most useful for clinical trials in JRA, rather than to test the efficacy of prednisolone		2 year follow-up confirmed safety of deflazacort, with good somatic growth

Trial design

This placebo-controlled, randomized, double blind study was carried out at 18 American, and 5 USSR centres. The study was 6 months in duration. Participants were randomly allocated to 1 of 3 groups: placebo, methotrexate 5 mg/m^2/week, or methotrexate 10 mg/m^2/week (maximum 15 mg/week).

Populations studied

All of the 127 enrolled children met criteria for JRA and had at least three active joints despite therapy with NSAIDs. Thirty-two of the subjects had had a systemic course.

Outcomes measured

Subjects who met criteria similar to the ACR response criteria were considered to be improved. They must have had a decrease of 25% or more in the articular-severity score and must have been improved according to the MD and parent global assessment.

Results

More patients in the 10 mg/m^2 group were improved (63%) than in the 5 mg/m^2 group (32%) or the placebo group (36%). Systemic features of the illness, in those affected, improved to the same degree

for all three treatment groups. Side-effects were few and comparable between the treatment and placebo groups.

Comments

In this study those who were poorly compliant or who dropped out early were specifically excluded from the analysis (i.e. not intention-to-treat) so in actual practice results from methotrexate are likely to be poorer than those presented.

A second, more recent, comparative trial of methotrexate and placebo was done to specifically study the effect in the JIA subgroups of Systemic Arthritis and Extended Oligoarthritis [33].

Trial design

This second study was a randomized crossover study in which the participants were assigned to either methotrexate (15 mg/m^2/week with an option to increase to 20) or placebo for 4 months and then switched to the opposite treatment for another 4 months. There was a 2-month period between the two treatments for washout purposes.

Populations studied

In this study two groups of subjects participated—children with Extended Oligoarthritis (N = 43) and children with Systemic

Table 3.13.2 Studies of gold compounds

	Auranofin [23]	**Gold sodium thiomalate [24,25]**	**Gold sodium thiomalate [26]**
Trial design	RCT 6 months duration 24 centres Double-blind Auranofin (A) 0.15–0.2 mg/kg/d versus placebo (P)	RCT 50 weeks duration unblinded Gold(G) 0.7 mg/kg weekly × 20 then monthly versus hydroxychloroquine (HCQ) 5 mg/kg/d versus D-Penicillamine (Pen) 10 mg/kg/d No placebo	RCT 50 weeks. Duration unblinded Gold vs. D-Penicillamine Extension of previous study
Populations studied	N = 231 JRA At least 3 active joints	N = 72 JRA (-1/3 with pauci course)	N = 77 47 from previous study and 30 new subjects
Outcomes measured	MD global Active joint count Joint severity scores	Number with 50% improvement in subjective global, number of active joints, joint index, MD global, or ESR TMJ radiographs	Same as previous study
Results	Over 60% improved in both groups No difference between A and P	1/3 to 1/2 in each group improved by over 50% in important outcomes No difference between the groups	More patients improved in G Number needed to treat = 8 for 50% improvement in active joint count at 50 weeks Overall the groups were similar
Comments	Auranofin was relatively safe although there was an increase in diarrhoea and skin rash	3 G subjects withdrew, compared to 6 Pen and 0 HCQ No real difference between groups for TMJ progression	

Table 3.13.3 Studies of D-Penicillamine

	D-Penicillamine [27]	**Penicillamine and hydroxychloroquine [28]**
Trial design	RCT 6 months. duration Double blind D-Penicillamine (Pen) 5 mg/kg/d × 2 months then 10 mg/kg/d versus placebo (P)	RCT 18 centres Double blind 12 months duration D-Penicillamine (Pen) 5 mg/kg/d × 2 mos. then 10 mg/kg/d versus hydroxychlorroquine (HCQ) 3 mg/kg/d × 2mos. Then 6 mg/kg/d versus placebo
Populations studied	N = 74 JCA with active arthritis and inflammatory labs	N = 162 JRA 'severe, active' 142 poly, 11 pauci, 9 systemic
Outcomes measured	Global subjective Articular Laboratory	25% improvement in global subjective and articular indices Safety measures including ocular exams
Results	Pen was better with larger decrease in painful joints (3 versus 2) but not inflamed joints More Pen subjects had improved global scores (MD 21 versus 10, patient 22 versus 12)	No difference between the groups Marked, but similar, improvement in all the groups
Comments	Two Pen subjects withdrawn for side-effects Overall eight subjects dropped out	This study highlights the importance of regression to the mean

Table 3.13.4 Controlled trials of sulfasalazine

	Sulfasalazine and chloroquine [29]	Sulfasalazine [30]
Trial design	RCT 6 months duration Sulfasalazine (SSZ) 20–30 mg/kg/d versus chloro- quine (c) 3–4 mg/kg/d Unclear if blinded	RCT 6 months duration Double blind Sulfasalazine (SSZ) 50 mg/kg/d in two doses versus placebo
Populations studied	N = 39 Juvenile arthritis (local criteria) Mostly poly	N = 69 JCA (poly and pauci with fairly mild disease)
Outcomes measured	Improvement in 5 of 6; number of clinical criteria present, number of affected joints, duration of AM stiffness, pain, ESR, functional capacity	Improvement by two grades in the severity of joint swelling score JRA core set improvement criteria
Results	No difference in number of improvers C group improved in AM stiffness duration compared to SSZ group	SSZ group improved more often (~50%) compared to P (~25%)
Comments		Almost 1/3 of the SSZ group dropped out due to side-effects

Arthritis (N = 45). During the course of the study two children with Extended Oligoarthritis and seven children with Systemic Arthritis withdrew.

Outcomes measured

The 'core' clinical outcomes measured, and used to decide response, were physician and parent/child global assessments of disease activity, active joint count, and number of joints with limited range of move- ment—these were based on the JRA core set. Laboratory measures were also obtained.

Results

In the extended oligoarticular group more children responded when taking methotrexate (48%) than when taking placebo (18%). They improved mostly in the subjective scores and labs, rather than in joint counts. The systemic onset group, though, did not have more improvers when taking methotrexate than placebo (25% versus 16%).

Comments

When analysed together, the overall study results show a benefit for methotrexate. The effect was certainly much more limited in those patients with Systemic Arthritis who really only improved in the global subjective measures.

An additional issue to consider when prescribing methotrexate is whether or not to concomitantly prescribe folic acid. Folic acid in adult patients has been shown to reduce side effects of methotrexate, especially oral ulcers and gastrointestinal distress. One small paediatric study—a randomized crossover study—suggested that folic acid, 1 mg/d, is safe and does not interfere with the action of methotrexate [34].

Intra-articular corticosteroids

Although widely used, intra-articular steroids have not been well studied in children with arthritis. There have been a few studies that

do support the efficacy of joint injections [35–38]. Although the stud- ies are limited in the rigour of their design, it is likely that injections are beneficial, that injections may limit leg length discrepancy, and that long acting corticosteroids (like triamcinolone hexacetonide) are more beneficial than short acting ones (Table 3.13.5).

Intravenous immunogloblin

Intravenous immunoglobulin (IVIG) is an indicated therapy for autoimmune thrombocytopenia and Kawasaki disease. A controlled trial has suggested that IVIG is useful in adult dermatomyositis, and several case-series were reported in the 1980s and 1990s to suggest a potential usefulness in other rheumatic disorders. Two randomized trials have been done by the PRCSG to examine the efficacy in JIA.

In the first study children with Systemic Arthritis were targeted [8].

Trial design

Nine centres participated in this study. The investigators randomly allocated children separately based on whether or not they were taking corticosteroids at the outset. The IVIG group were given 1.5 gm/kg every 2 weeks for 2 months and then monthly for an additional 4 months. The other group was given a blinded placebo.

Populations studied

To be eligible for this study, children had to have active articular and systemic features of their disease. Thirty-one children were studied, although the investigators note that 60 were required for adequate power. Two children could not be assessed because of protocol violations, and a further seven dropped out of each group.

Outcomes measured

The primary outcome was the physician global score. To be improved, subjects had to have responded by greater than 30% for the number of active joints, physician global score, or by greater than 25% for laboratory outcomes.

Table 3.13.5 Studies investigating intra-articular corticosteroids

	Triamcinolone hexacetonide (IATH) versus betamethasone (B) [35]	Triamcinolone acetonide (IATA) [36]	Triamcinolone hexacetonide [37]	Triamcinolone hexacetonide [38]
Trial design	RCT Double blind Knee injections with IATH (dose not reported) versus B (dose not reported) Follow up to 42 days	Retrospecti case-series (no control group) Unblinded IATA 20 mg for knee injections	Retrospective case-series (no controls) Unblinded IATH 10–40 mg.	Retrospective cohort Compared children followed at Seattle (16 of 16 got IATH) to those followed at Duke/UNC (3 of 14 got IATH)
Populations studied	N = 23 JCA (pauci)	N = 21 of 56 eligible JCA (pauci)	N = 71 JRA (61), reactive arthritis [6], other arthritis [4]	N = 30 JRA (pauci) with onset <7 years
Outcomes measured	Subjective global Knee flexion Joint size	Duration of remission	Duration of remission Resolution of Baker cysts	Leg length discrepancy Thigh circumference discrepancy
Results	Global measures better even at 7 days for IATH IATH was longer lasting (at least 42 days versus about 7 days for B)	70% had >6 months Remission Mean remission length was 15 months	82% had >6 months Remission 11 of 11 Baker cysts resolved 61% able to stop oral meds	Seattle group had no leg length discrepancy versus 7 to 14 at UNC/Duke No difference in thigh circumference discrepancy
Comments	Only side effects were 1 case of skin atrophy in IATH group	Skin atrophy in two subject, no other side-effects	Skin atrophy in three subjects, no other side-effects	

Results

The groups did not differ statistically. One-half of the IVIG group showed a greater than 30% response by physician global score compared to 27% in the placebo group, but this was not statistically significant.

Comments

The authors of the study acknowledge the high likelihood of a type II (false negative) error due to the inadequate sample size.

The second study applied a slightly different design and studied children with polyarticular JRA. This study was labelled as a pilot study rather than a definitive clinical trial [39].

Trial design

This study, classed a 'blinded withdrawal' design, was a randomized trial with an open (everyone was given IVIG) run in phase. Seven centres participated. Those children who responded to IVIG in the open phase were than randomly assigned to a group that continued to receive IVIG, and a group that switched to placebo.

Populations studied

Three groups of children (total N = 25) with polyarticular JRA were included and randomized separately. The first group was made up of children of older onset who were rheumatoid factor positive and relatively newly diagnosed. The second group was also made up of children who were relatively newly diagnosed, but who were of younger onset. The third group was made up of children who had had a longer duration of disease.

Outcomes measured

Response and worsening were defined by a 25% change in 2 of (i) active joint count, (ii) joint index, and (iii) physician global assessment.

Results

Nineteen of the 25 children responded in the open phase. In the randomized phase 8 of 10 assigned to IVIG and 4 of 9 assigned to placebo maintained their response. This was not statistically significant, however, the effect for most of the outcomes was large.

Comments

While not definitive, this study does suggest some efficacy. A larger study is warranted based on the apparently large effect sizes seen.

Other agents

Etanercept [9]

Etanercept (recombinant tumour necrosis factor (TNF) receptor fusion protein) was the first of the so-called biological agents studied for JIA in clinical trial. The investigators had high hopes for this new agent, given its success in adult rheumatoid arthritis. For this reason, a new study design was used—similar to the open-label run in design used in the IVIG study (above). The reason for using this design was to limit the amount of time that children were exposed to placebo.

Trial design

All children were initially started on etanercept at a dose of 0.4 mg/kg (maximum 25 mg) subcutaneously twice weekly. This therapy was carried on for 3 months. Those children that met predefined responder criteria were then randomly assigned to either continuing with etanercept, or switching to placebo in a double blind fashion. The subjects were followed for an additional 4 months. They were followed until they flared (using predefined criteria) at which point they were dropped from the study and given the option of continuing with open-label (unblinded) etanercept.

Populations studied

Children in this study all had polyarticular course arthritis and had either failed methotrexate, or were intolerant of it. Sixty-nine subjects entered the study, and 51 were included in the randomized part of the study.

Outcomes measured

Response and flare criteria were based on the JRA core set.

Results

The response rate in the open phase was quite high (74%). Responders then took part in the double blind phase. In the placebo group 81% of the subjects flared, while only 28% flared in the etanercept group. The average (median) time it took to flare in the placebo group was 28 days.

Comments

From this study, it became apparent that etanercept is a potent and safe treatment for JIA. Following the publication of the results, etanercept has become widely used despite its extremely high cost.

Cyclosporin

Although cyclosporin A (CyA) has been used in many centres for the treatment of resistant JIA (especially for Systemic Arthritis form) it has never been studied in a clinical trial. Several retrospective case series have suggested that CyA may have some effect with significant, but acceptable, toxicity [40–42] (Table 3.13.6).

Cyclophosphamide in Systemic Arthritis

Despite advances in the therapy of other forms of JIA, Systemic Arthritis continues to be difficult to control. In the late 1980s, cyclophosphamide was studied in the USSR in children with systemic JRA. Patients in the USSR with this condition had a high degree of amyloidosis that justified an aggressive treatment approach [43].

Trial design

This study was an open study with no control group. The outcomes were assessed without blinding. Subjects were given treatments every 3 months for 1 year along with weekly methotrexate (10 mg/m^2 by mouth). The 3 monthly treatments consisted of intravenous methylprednisolone (30 mg/kg/d × 3 days) and intravenous cyclophosphamide (0.4 gm/m^2). The cyclophosphamide was only continued while systemic features of the disease were still present.

Populations studied

Eighteen children with systemic JRA were studied; all had active systemic disease an average of 2 years following diagnosis. None had used methotrexate in the past.

Outcomes measured

A variety of end points were examined in this study including frequency of remission (by ACR criteria), systemic signs and symptoms, functional ability, and laboratory measures.

Results

The treatment seemed quite successful in this group. Two-thirds of the subjects met remission criteria. The number of subjects with severe disability (ACR functional class III or IV) decreased from two-thirds to one quarter. Rash and fever disappeared in all the subjects, and 17 of 18 subjects were able to decrease their daily dose of corticosteroid.

Comments

Given that there were no concomitant control subjects, regression to the mean may explain a significant amount of the response seen in this study.

Subsequently a series of American patients treated with a similar regimen was published [44].

Trial design

The children in this study continued to receive their usual doses of daily NSAID, and prednisone. They were given weekly methotrexate (1 mg/kg subcutaneously). Intravenous methylprednisolone was given at a dose of 30 mg/m^2 × 1 each month, and cyclophosphamide was given, also monthly, at a dose of 500 to 1000 mg/m^2. The cyclophosphamide was continued monthly for 6–10 months and then spread out to every 2–3 months for a few more treatments.

Populations studied

All four children in this study had severe destructive systemic onset JRA and were corticosteroid dependent with growth failure. Unlike the study from the USSR, these children had been on methotrexate and did not have active systemic features at the time of study.

Outcomes measured

Like the USSR study, remission using the ACR criteria was measured. In addition growth and corticosteroid dose reduction were examined.

Results

Three of the four subjects met criteria for remission, and all four showed subjective improvement. There was a considerable reduction in corticosteroid dose, and eventually all subjects were able to completely discontinue prednisone. Growth parameters showed improvement as demonstrated by growth charts.

Comments

This study suffers from the same concerns as the USSR study.

Oral type II collagen [45]

Oral tolerance was seen as an attractive mechanism for treating arthritis in the early 1990s following its successful use in preventing arthritis in animal models, and following suggestive evidence of efficacy in a randomized trial in adult rheumatoid arthritis.

Table 3.13.6 Case series of response to CyA

	CyA [40]	CyA [41]	CyA [42]
Trial design	Case series CyA 4–15 mg/d At least 6 months duration	Case series CyA 3.5–10 mg/kg/d 9–48 months duration	Case series CyA 2 to 7 mg/kg/d 6 to 32 month duration
Populations studied	$N = 14$ JRA, with active arthritis and refractory to other treatments 10 of 14 were systemic onset	$N = 9$ (also 3 patients with JDM) JCA, active with failure of previous treatment 7 of 9 were systemic onset	$N = 17$ (also five patients with JDM) JRA, refractory to other treatments with active synovitis or uncontrolled systemic features 14 of 17 were systemic onset
Outcomes measured	Remission	Fever Joint inflammation score Corticosteroid reduction	Fever Active joint count Corticosteroid reduction
Results	1 of 14 went into remission after 17 months No real effect on the others	Fever gone (in 6 of 6 who were febrile) within 1 month Improvement in joint score 4 of 9 reduced prednisone by> 50%	Fever gone in 10 of 11 Swollen joint count Improved in 12 of 17 11 of 14 had significant reduction in prednisone (discontinued in 5)
Comments	Side-effects included increased creatinine and anaemia	No anaemia, nor change in creatinine seen in this series	Creatinine increased in 11 of 17 No hypertension, hirsutism or gum hypertrophy

Trial design

This was an open (uncontrolled) pilot study. Subjects were given type II oral collagen in a dose of 100 mcg/day for one month and then 500 mcg/day. The study was 3 months in duration.

Populations studied

Children in this study had active JRA with three or more swollen joints. They were not allowed to continue with DMARD therapy, but were allowed stable doses of NSAID and low dose prednisone.

Outcomes measured

Laboratory data, joint counts, and subjective global scores were collected monthly.

Results

The type II collagen was well tolerated. Most measures improved in most patients over the course of the study. One patient with systemic onset JRA went into remission.

Comments

Similar to other uncontrolled studies, this one must be interpreted with caution. Regression to the mean (spontaneous improvement) may account for all of the effects seen. The authors rightly suggested that proper controlled studies were warranted.

Synovectomy

All of the clinical trials that have been discussed thus far have been of pharmacological therapies. There have been very few clinical trials of physical or occupational therapy, and only one trial of surgery for childhood arthritis. Surgical trials have inherent difficulties (e.g. it is difficult to provide a placebo operation). Synovectomy, though, has been studied in JRA [46].

Trial design

Investigators enrolled children and randomly assigned them to open synovectomy or to no therapy. Subjects were followed to 24 months following the procedure.

Populations studied

All eligible children had arthritis that was considered to be at high risk to lead to deformities. They were consecutively sampled from a tertiary care centre. The joints operated on were 18 wrists, 8 ankles, and 4 knees. By chance, the non-operated group had more children with polyarticular course, an older age, and a longer duration of arthritis.

Outcomes measured

A variety of measures, including joint swelling, joint activity, pain, range of motion, and function were measured at 3, 6, 12, 18, and 24 months following the procedure.

Results

There were more subjects with a reduction in swelling (87% versus 7%) and a reduction in joint activity (53% versus 0) in the synovectomy group at 24 months. However, function was not different between the groups and range of motion was decreased in the operated joints (especially early in the follow-up).

Comments

With the current widespread use of corticosteroid injections the indications for synovectomy have become quite limited, and it is rarely practised at most centres.

The future of clinical trials in JIA

With the impressive advances that have already been made in the study of therapies for JIA, one can be confident that further progress will occur rapidly in the immediate futre. New ways of collaboration (e.g. the PRCSG, PRINTO, and CARRA) will allow a new culture to develop in paediatric rheumatology in which every patient can provide an objective lesson—improving our understanding and our treatments of JIA. New powerful agents (like the anti-cytokine biologics) will provide the opportunity—the substrate—for researchers to advance the therapeutic field. Finally, new more powerful, and more acceptable, clinical trial designs will provide the methods needed to support a clinical trials/evidence-based culture in paediatric rheumatology.

References

1. Felson, D.T., Anderson, J.J., Boers, M. *et al.* American College of Rheumatology preliminary definition of improvement in rheumatoid arthritis. *Arthritis Rheum* 1995;38(6):727–35.
2. Giannini, E.H., Ruperto, N., Ravelli, A., *et al.* Preliminary definition of improvement in juvenile arthritis. *Arthritis Rheum* 1997;40(7):1202–9.
3. Gotay, C.C. Accrual to cancer clinical trials: Directions from the research literature. *Soc Sci Med* 1991;33(5):569–77.
4. Glogowska, M., Roulstone, S., Enderby, P., Peters, T., and Campbell, R. Who's afraid of the randomised controlled trial? Parents' views of an SLT research study. *Int J Lang Comm Disorders* 2001;365:499–504.
5. Choonara, I. Clinical trials of medicines in children. *BMJ* 2000; 321:1093–4.
6. Berlin, C.M.J. Challenges in conducting pediatric drug trials. *J Allerg Clin Immunol* 2000;106:S127–7.
7. Rosato, J. The ethics of clinical trials: A child's view. *J Law Med Ethics* 2000;28:362–78.
8. Silverman, E.D., Cawkwell, G.D., Lovell, D.J. *et al.* Intravenous immunoglobulin in the treatment of systemic juvenile rheumatoid arthritis: A randomized placebo controlled trial. Pediatric Rheumatology Collaborative Study Group. *J Rheumatol* 1994;21(12):2353–8.
9. Lovell, D.J. Giannini, E.H., Reiff, A., *et al.* Etanercept in children with polyarticular juvenile rheumatoid arthritis. Pediatric Rheumatology Collaborative Study Group [see comments]. *N Eng J Med* 2000; 342(11):763–9.
10. Feldman, B.M., Wang, E., Willan, A., and Szalai, J.P. The Randomized Placebo-Phase Design for Clinical Trials. *J Clin Epi* 2001;54(6):550–7.
11. White, K.L. Health care research: Old wine in new bottles. Pharos Alpha Omega Alpha Honor Med Soc. 1993;56:12–6.
12. Levinson, J.E., Baum, J., Brewer, E., Jr. *et al.* Comparison of tolmetin sodium and aspirin in the treatment of juvenile rheumatoid arthritis. *J Pediatr* 1977;91(5):799–804.
13. Giannini, E.H., and Brewer, E.J., Jr. Standard methodology for Segment I, II, and III Pediatric Rheumatology Collaborative Study Group studies. II. Analysis and presentation of data. *J Rheumatol* 1982;9(1):114–22.
14. Haapasaari, J., Wuolijoki, E., and Ylijoki, H. Treatment of juvenile rheumatoid arthritis with diclofenac sodium. *Scand J Rheumatol* 1983;12(4):325–30.
15. Kvien, T.K., Hoyeraal, H.M., and Sandstad, B. Naproxen and acetylsalicylic acid in the treatment of pauciarticular and polyarticular juvenile rheumatoid arthritis. Assessment of tolerance and efficacy in a single-centre 24-week double-blind parallel study. Scandinavian *J Rheumatol* 1984;13(4):342–50.
16. Giannini, E.H., Brewer, E.J., Miller, M.L., *et al.* Ibuprofen suspension in the treatment of juvenile rheumatoid arthritis. Pediatric Rheumatology Collaborative Study Group. *J Pediatr* 1990;117(4):645–52.
17. Garcia-Morteo, O., Maldonado-Cocco, J.A., Cuttica, R., and Garay, S.M. Piroxicam in juvenile rheumatoid arthritis. *Eur J Rheumatol Inflam* 1987;8(1):49–53.
18. Williams, P.L., Ansell, B.M., Bell, A., *et al.* Multicentre study of piroxicam versus naproxen in juvenile chronic arthritis, with special reference to problem areas in clinical trials of nonsteroidal anti-inflammatory drugs in childhood. *Br J Rheumatology* 1986;25(1):67–71.
19. Kvien, T.K., Hoyeraal, H.M., and Sandstad, B. Assessment methods of disease activity in juvenile rheumatoid arthritis—evaluated in a prednisolone/placebo double-blind study. *J Rheumatol* 1982;9(5):696–702.
20. Picco, P., Gattorno, M., Buoncompagni, A., Pistoia, V., and Borrone, C. 6-methylprednisolone 'mini-pulses': A new modality of glucocorticoid treatment in systemic onset juvenile chronic arthritis. *Scand J Rheumatol* 1996;25(1):24–7.
21. Loftus, J., Allen, R., Hesp, R., *et al.* Randomized, double-blind trial of deflazacort versus prednisone in juvenile chronic (or rheumatoid) arthritis: A relatively bone-sparing effect of deflazacort. *Pediatrics* 1991,88(3):428–36.
22. Loftus, J.K., Reeve, J., Hesp, R., *et al.* Deflazacort in juvenile chronic arthritis. *J Rheumatol*—Supplement 1993;37:40–2.
23. Giannini, E.H., Brewer, E.J., Jr., Kuzmina, N., Shaikov, A., and Wallin, B. Auranofin in the treatment of juvenile rheumatoid arthritis. Results of the USA–USSR double-blind, placebo-controlled trial. The USA Pediatric Rheumatology Collaborative Study Group. The USSR Cooperative Children's Study Group [see comments]. *Arthritis Rheum* 1990; 33(4):466–76.
24. Kvien, T.K., Larheim, T.A., Hoyeraal, H.M., Sandstad, B. Radiographic temporomandibular joint abnormalities in patients with juvenile chronic arthritis during a controlled study of sodium aurothiomalate and D-penicillamine. *Br J Rheumatol* 1986;25(1):59–66.
25. Kvien, T.K., Hoyeraal, H.M., and Sandstad, B. Slow acting antirheumatic drugs in patients with juvenile rheumatoid arthritis—evaluated in a randomized, parallel 50-week clinical trial. *J Rheumatol* 1985;12(3):533–9.
26. Kvien, T.K., Hoyeraal, H.M., and Sandstad, B. Gold sodium thiomalate and D-penicillamine. A controlled, comparative study in patients with pauciarticular and polyarticular juvenile rheumatoid arthritis. *Scand J Rheumatol* 1985;14(4):346–54.
27. Prieur, A.M., Piussan, C., Manigne, P., Bordigoni, P., and Griscelli, C. Evaluation of D-penicillamine in juvenile chronic arthritis. A double-blind, multicenter study. *Arthritis Rheumat* 1985;28(4):376–82.
28. Brewer, E.J., Giannini, E.H., Kuzmina, N., and Alekseev, L. Penicillamine and hydroxychloroquine in the treatment of severe juvenile rheumatoid arthritis. Results of the U.S.A.–U.S.S.R. double-blind placebo-controlled trial. *N Eng J Med* 1986;314(20):1269–76.
29. Hoza, J., Kadlecova, T., Nemcova, D., and Havelka, S. Sulphasalazine and Delagil—a comparative study in patients with juvenile chronic arthritis. *Acta Universitatis Carolinae—Medica* 1991;37(1–2):80–3.
30. van Rossum, M.A., Fiselier, T.J., Franssen, M.J., *et al.* Sulfasalazine in the treatment of juvenile chronic arthritis: a randomized, double-blind, placebo-controlled, multicenter study. Dutch Juvenile Chronic Arthritis Study Group. *Arthritis Rheumat* 1998;41(5):808–16.
31. Kvien, T.K., Hoyeraal, H.M., and Sandstad, B. Azathioprine versus placebo in patients with juvenile rheumatoid arthritis: A single center double blind comparative study. *J Rheumatol* 1986;13(1):118–23.
32. Giannini, E.H., Brewer, E.J., Kuzmina, N., *et al.* Methotrexate in resistant juvenile rheumatoid arthritis. Results of the U.S.A.–U.S.S.R. double-blind, placebo-controlled trial. The Pediatric Rheumatology Collaborative Study Group and The Cooperative Children's Study Group [see comments]. *N Eng J Med* 1992;326(16):1043–9.

33. Woo, P., Southwood, T.R., Prieur, A.M., et al. Randomized, placebo-controlled, crossover trial of low-dose oral methotrexate in children with extended oligoarticular or systemic arthritis. *Arthritis Rheumat* 2000; 43(8):1849–57.

34. Hunt, P.G., Rose, C.D., McIlvain-Simpson, G., and Tejani, S. The effects of daily intake of folic acid on the efficacy of methotrexate therapy in children with juvenile rheumatoid arthritis. A controlled study. *J Rheumatol* 1997;24(11):2230–2.

35. Balogh, Z., and Ruzsonyi, E. Triamcinolone hexacetonide versus betamethasone. A double-blind comparative study of the long-term effects of intra-articular steroids in patients with juvenile chronic arthritis. *Scand J Rheumatol-Supplement* 1987;67:80–2.

36. Hertzberger-ten Cate, R., de Vries-van der Vlugt, B.C., van Suijlekom-Smit, L.W., and Cats, A. Intra-articular steroids in pauciarticular juvenile chronic arthritis, type 1. *Eur J Pediatr* 1991;150(3):170–2.

37. Padeh, S. and Passwell, J.H. Intraarticular corticosteroid injection in the management of children with chronic arthritis. *Arthritis Rheum* 1998; 41(7):1210–4.

38. Sherry, D.D., Stein, L.D., Reed, A.M., Schanberg, L.E., and Kredich, D.W. Prevention of leg length discrepancy in young children with pauciarticular juvenile rheumatoid arthritis by treatment with intraarticular steroids. *Arthritis and Rheum* 1999;42(11):2330–4.

39. Giannini, E.H., Lovell D.J., Silverman, E.D., et al. Intravenous immunoglobulin in the treatment of polyarticular juvenile rheumatoid arthritis: A phase I/II study. Pediatric Rheumatology Collaborative Study Group [see comments]. *J Rheumatol* 1996;23(5):919–24.

40. Ostensen, M., Hoyeraal, H.M., and Kass, E. Tolerance of cyclosporine A in children with refractory juvenile rheumatoid arthritis. *J Rheumatol* 1988;15(10):1536–8.

41. Pistoia, V., Buoncompagni, A., Scribanis, R. et al. Cyclosporin A in the treatment of juvenile chronic arthritis and childhood polymyositis-dermatomyositis. Results of a preliminary study [see comments]. *Clini Experi Rheumatol* 1993;11(2):203–8.

42. Reiff, A., Rawlings, D.J., Shaham, B., et al. Prliminary evidence for cyclosporin A as an alternative in the treatment of recalcitrant juvenile rheumatoid arthritis and juvenile dermatomyositis. *J Rheumatol* 1997;24(12):2436–43.

43. Shaikov, A.V., Maximov, A.A., Speransky, A.I., et al. Repetitive use of pulse therapy with methlprednisolone and cyclophosphamide in additioin to oral methotrexate in children with systemic juvenile rheumatoid arthritis—preliminary results of a longterm study. *J Rheumatol* 1992; 19(4):612–6.

44. Wallace, C.A. and Sherry, D.D. Trial of intravenous pulse cyclophosphamide and methylprednisolone in the treatment of severe systemic-onset juvenile rheumatoid arthritis. *Arthritis Rheum* 1997;40(10):1852–5.

45. Barnett, M.L., Combitchi, D., and Trentham, D.E. A pilot trial of oral type II collagen in the treatment of juvenile rheumatoid arthritis. *Arthritis Rheum* 1996;39(4):623–8.

46. Kvien, T.K., Pahle, J.A., Hoyeraal, H.M., and Sandstad, B. Comparison of synovectomy and no synovectomy in patients with juvenile rheumatoid arthritis. A 24-month controlled study. *Scandinavian J Rheumatol* 1987;16(2):81–91.

3.14 Pharmacological treatment: Approach to the management of refractory arthritis

Nico M. Wulffraat and Berent J. Prakken

Aim

The aim of this chapter is to provide a thorough discussion of the role of aggressive, and largely experimental treatment options for children with severe and refractory Juvenile Idiopathic Arthritis (JIA) who have failed conventional therapies.

Structure

- Introduction
- High dose methotrexate
- Biologicals
- Leflunomide
- Autologous hemopoietic stem cell transplantation
- Novel therapeutic horizons for JIA
- The hierarchy of experimental treatment options
- Summary

Introduction

In recent years, because of the recognition of the relatively poor outcomes of Juvenile idiopathic arthritis (JIA), treatment of these conditions has been intensified considerably. Potent immunosuppressive drugs have been introduced early in attempts to suppress joint inflammation in those children who do not respond rapidly to nonsteroidal anti-inflammatory drugs (NSAIDs) [1,2]. However, despite the use of a variety of pharmacological agents including high-dose intravenous methylprednisolone, methotrexate (MTX) given parenterally in increasingly higher doses, and cyclophosphamide both orally and intravenously, most paediatric rheumatologists have looked after children with JIA, particularly with Systemic Arthritis, who have not responded adequately to such treatments [1]. Early experience with the anti-TNF drugs also suggests that a significant proportion of children with Systemic Arthritis is likely to remain resistant to these therapies. Children with this refractory disease not only develop severe morbidity and significantly impaired quality of life, both from the disease and from drug toxicities, but they also have a significantly increased mortality rate [3,4].

If a child with JIA continues to have poorly controlled joint inflammation, despite consistent pharmacological interventions provided by physicians with experience in determining when a child has failed an adequate trial of standard therapies, and assuming that the child has been compliant with the prescribed drug regimen, then the child is a candidate for experimental therapies. However, the outcome of such therapies is very difficult to assess unless the child's treatment is undertaken in a centre that can provide the multidisciplinary approach necessary to adequately and carefully monitor response (or lack of response) to treatment. Given the relatively small number of children with refractory disease that any one centre will be caring for at any one time, such experimental therapies need to be undertaken using standardized clinical protocols, as part of international trials or consensus workshops. The Paediatric Rheumatology International Trials Organization (PRINTO), the Paediatric Rheumatology Collaborative Study Group (PRCSG), and the Childhood Arthritis and Rheumatology Research Alliance (CARRA) are three such international organizations working together to enable treatment protocols to be designed so as to most efficiently determine which are the most effective therapies under different circumstances, particularly when children with JIA are refractory to standard first and second line therapies [5,6]. Many of the therapeutic advances documented in the last few decades in childhood cancers have come about by the use of such well-organized international multicentre clinical research protocols. Although the clinical endpoints are somewhat more difficult to assess for children with arthritis than for those with cancer, the measurement tools, the number of trained paediatric rheumatologists worldwide, and the increasing variety and number of new drugs make a similar approach not only feasible, but essential [5,6].

High-dose methotrexate

Long-term observational studies have documented that active disease persists in a significant percentage of patients with Systemic and Poly arthritis, and that functional status frequently deteriorates as the disease persists. Most of the mortality associated with JIA also occurs in these children [3]. A number of studies have looked specifically at the role of MTX in Systemic Arthritis; however, although it has had a major impact on control of disease activity, many treatment failures with oral, low-dose regimens have been reported [2,7–10]. Anecdotal experiences have suggested continuing treatment failures in Systemic Arthritis when using higher-dose regimens, even if combined with cyclophosphamide and corticosteroids [1,10,11]. Recently, the PRINTO has conducted a multicentre randomized open label trial to assess the safety and efficacy of parenteral MTX in medium (15 mg/m^2/week to a maximum of 20 mg/week) or higher doses (30 mg/m^2/week to a maximum of 40 mg/week) in children who had failed standard low-dose oral MTX (8–12.5 mg/m^2/week) [12].

Thirty percent (161 of 534) of the children in this study did not improve after 4–6 months treatment with standard dose oral MTX and were randomized to higher doses of MTX. These data suggest that parenteral MTX is more efficacious than oral MTX, that there is no statistically significant difference in clinical outcome between the medium dose (15 mg/m^2/week) and the higher dosage (30 mg/m^2/week), and that a proportion of children are probably resistant to even high-dose MTX [12]. Those children who have failed high-dose MTX will be invited to enroll in further studies using newer biologicals and immunomodulatory drugs such as etanercept, infliximab, anti-Interleukin-1 Receptor antagonist (IL1-Ra), and leflunomide [13].

Biologicals

Etanercept

Etanercept is a fusion protein consisting of the extracellular ligand-binding portion of the human tumour necrosis factor receptor (TNFR-p75) linked to the Fc portion of human IgG1. It binds to tumor necrosis factor (both alpha and beta) and blocks its interaction with cell surface TNF receptors (Table 3.14.1). Recently, it has been demonstrated that treatment with etanercept has a major beneficial effect on children with refractory JIA [14,15]. In this study of children with Polyarthritis and Systemic Arthritis who had failed standard dose MTX, 74%, 64%, and 36% demonstrated improvements of 30%, 50%, and 70% improvement, respectively, using core set outcome measures [14].

Etanercept is administered subcutaneously twice weekly as its median half-life is 115 h. After 3 months of treatment with 0.4 mg/kg subcutaneously twice weekly, most children respond if they are going to do so. Continued improvement with longer treatment is reported in both children and adults; unfortunately relapse rates are high when the drug is discontinued early. To date, there are no studies of discontinuation of the drug after one or more years of remission of disease.

The most common side-effects seen in children are mild and include headache, nausea and vomiting, abdominal pain, injection site reactions, and upper respiratory tract infections (Table 3.14.1). Infections seen in children are generally mild and consistent with those commonly seen in paediatric clinic populations. Reported adverse reactions have included varicella, diarrhoea, depression, skin ulcers, Type I diabetes, Group A streptococcal sepsis, and esophagitis with gastritis. Serious infections and death from sepsis have been reported in adult patients with rheumatoid arthritis (RA) and there have been rare reports of cytopenias. There are no long-term studies available using etanercept in adults with RA to assess carcinogenesis, mutagenesis, or possible impairment of fertility. It is recommended that children receiving etanercept be tested for varicella immune status and previous exposure to tuberculosis and if not immune, etanercept should be temporarily discontinued when there is significant exposure to varicella or tuberculosis. Reports of adverse effects of etanercept have not as yet shown an increased incidence of TB, in contrast to infliximab [16]. Responses to immunizations have not been studied in children receiving etanercept. The use of live vaccines is contraindicated. Adult patients enrolled in clinical trials of etanercept who received influenza vaccines did not have any unexpected problems.

The use of anti-TNF treatment in children with Systemic Arthritis has been discussed extensively at several paediatric rheumatology meetings and the general impression (reflecting experience in some 40 patients with Systemic Arthritis, treated for more than 4 months) is that in active systemic disease this treatment is less effective than in the other forms of JIA, with a clear response occurring in only a minority of patients [17–22].

Infliximab

Infliximab (Remicade) is a chimeric human/mouse anti-TNF monoclonal antibody, which binds to TNF alpha and blocks its binding to cell surface receptors (Table 3.14.1). It is given intravenously and has a half-life of about 10 days. In combination with MTX, infliximab has been shown to be effective in adult RA with halting of radiographic progression of disease. MTX (oral dose up to 15 mg/week) must be given with infliximab to decrease the possibility of antibodies developing to infliximab, or the risk of autoantibody formation. Some small case series report favourable effects in JIA [23,24]. At present a

Table 3.14.1 Biologicals and immunomodulating drugs

Drug name	Mechanism of action	Indication	Side-effects
Soluble TNF-receptor (etanercept)	Binds to TNFα	MTX resistant JIA with polyarticular course	Headache, nausea, abdominal pains, injection site reactions; mild infections
Chimeric anti-TNF antibody (infliximab)	Binds to TNFα and prevents binding to TNFr	MTX resistant JIA with polyarticular course (under evaluation)	Increased incidence of infections (TB); human anti-chimeric antibodies; autoantibodies (anti ds-DNA); possibly congestive heart failure
Humanized anti-TNF antibody (adalimumab)	Binds to TNFα and prevents binding to TNFr	MTX resistant JIA with polyarticular course or MTX toxicity (under evaluation)	Possibly less antibody formation (under study)
IL-1 receptor antagonist (anakinra)	Blockade of the pro-inflammatory effects of cytokine IL1 on endothelial cells, lymphocytes, chondrocytes and macrophages	MTX resistant JIA with polyarticular course (under evaluation)	Injection site reactions
Leflunomide	Inhibits pyrimidine synthesis and T cell proliferation	MTX resistant JIA with polyarticular course or MTX toxicity (under evaluation)	Possibly liver toxicity, diarrhoea, abdominal pain, gastritis, rash, headache, alopecia

3.14 PHARMACOLOGICAL TREATMENT: REFRACTORY ARTHRITIS

randomized, placebo controlled multicenter trial is being conducted to establish its effectiveness in children with MTX resistant polyarticular course JIA. Infliximab is usually infused over several hours at a dose of 3–10 mg/kg at 0, 2, and 6 weeks, followed by every 4–8 weeks thereafter, as indicated by the patient's disease and response to treatment. Many investigators report patients with RA feeling improved after the first dose, and anecdotal reports have indicated similar very rapid symptomatic improvement in some children with JIA. If there has been no response by the 4th dose it is reasonable to discontinue further infusions.

Adverse events include infections, nausea, diarrhoea, and rash. Hypersensitivity reactions including fever, chills, urticaria, dyspnoea, congestive heart failure, and hypertension have been reported. Some patients have developed human anti-chimeric antibodies as well as autoantibodies, especially anti-ds-DNA antibodies. Severe infections have been reported. Particularly concerning have been reports of tuberculosis and it is unclear if these are reactivations or new cases [35,98]. All children starting anti-TNF drugs should be carefully screened for tuberculosis. There are no data regarding immunizations of patients on this drug; nor are long-term toxicities or the possibility of oncogenicity, or effects on fertility known.

Infliximab and etanercept have also been studied for other conditions characterized by chronic inflammation, including resistant uveitis, Crohn disease, and Behçet disease [26–29]. However, it remains unclear if anti-TNF therapies are efficacious in uveitis [30,31].

There are two important unresolved questions with the use of anti-TNF therapies in JIA. First, as both etanercept and infliximab have been well documented to halt progression of joint damage in early adult RA, should such apparently effective agents be given at the onset of treatment for JIA, rather than being saved for use in refractory disease, as is current practice? If indeed there is a window of opportunity when treatments are maximally efficacious, should these agents be part of an early aggressive treatment plan? Second, how and when should these treatments be discontinued? Early studies demonstrated flare of disease in most patients (treated less than 1 year) within 1 month of discontinuing etanercept (longer for infliximab). There are a few reports of patients with JIA successfully stopping etanercept without a flare of disease, but the optimal length of treatment after attaining remission and how best to discontinue anti-TNF therapy are unknown.

IL-1r antagonist

Another approach involving the blockade of inflammatory cytokines involves the use of Interleukin-1 Receptor antagonist (IL-1RA) (anakinra). An animal model employing mice that were genetically manipulated to prevent the production of IL-1RA, showed a chronic arthritis resembling RA [32]. IL-1RA prevents IL-1 binding to its target cells (Table 3.14.1). The actions of IL-1 include stimulation of the release of platelet-activating factor (endothelial cells), lymphocyte growth factors (lymphocytes), collagenases (chondrocytes), and activation of osteoclast precursor cells (macrophages) [33]. Therefore IL-1 is a potential target for therapeutic intervention in diseases with chronic joint inflammation [34]. Several placebo-controlled double blind studies have proven the clinical efficacy and safety of IL1-RA in adults with RA [35,36]. IL-1RA was studied in combination with MTX

for 6 consecutive months as daily single subcutaneous injections in a dose range of 0.04–2.0 mg/kg [36]. Responses to the IL-1RA/MTX combination therapy were significantly greater than to MTX alone [36]. In addition, IL-1RA reduced the rate of radiological progression when compared with placebo [35]. This biological agent was registered at the end of 2001 for use in RA. A multicentre study is presently being performed in the United States to assess efficacy and safety in JIA. There is anecdotal evidence to suggest that Systemic Arthritis patients respond more readily to anti-IL1 treatment than to anti-TN treatments.

Leflunomide

Leflunomide (Arava) is a novel isoxazol drug. *In vitro* studies have shown it is a pro-drug and is quickly metabolized to an active metabolite. This metabolite reversibly inhibits the enzyme dihydroorotate dehydrogenase, which is required for pyrimidine nucleotide synthesis (Table 3.14.1). This drug has an anti-proliferative effect on T cells *in vitro*, but little is known about its mechanism of action in patients. After absorption, leflunomide is metabolized to its active metabolite which reaches peak levels between 6 and 12 h. The site of metabolism is unknown, although studies suggest a role for both the gastrointestinal wall and the liver. Due to the very long half-life of the metabolite (about 2 weeks) a loading dose of 100 mg per day for 3 days is used to facilitate rapid attainment of steady-state levels.

The active metabolite is eliminated by further metabolism and excretion by both the kidneys and the biliary system. It is important to note that neither the pro-drug nor the active metabolite are dialyzable. Elimination can be hastened by the use of activated charcoal (reported in one patient) or cholestyramine (three patients). The active metabolite is extensively bound to albumin and can cause a 13–50% increase in free serum NSAID levels. It has been used with methotrexate and is thought not to have significant pharmacokinetic interactions. However, recent data from post-marketing reports from the European Agency for the Evaluation of Medicinal Products reveals reports of serious liver toxicity including 2 patients with cirrhosis, and 15 with liver failure. Most of these events occurred in the first 6 months of treatment; contributing factors included: NSAIDs and MTX use, alcohol ingestion, and hepatitis and renal disease.

The onset of leflunomide's effects have been evident as early as 4 weeks and improvement continues until about 5 months. Thereafter, the benefit appears to plateau but can be maintained. Adults with RA treated with leflunomide for 12 months have been shown to have retardation in progression of X-ray damage [37].

The most common adverse reactions have been gastrointestinal symptoms: diarrhoea, anorexia, abdominal pain, dyspepsia, gastritis, and elevation of transaminases. Other problems occurring in approximately 5–10% of patients include rash/allergic reactions, headache and reversible alopecia. Less common are weight loss and hypophosphatemia. Leflunomide is teratogenic; there are no long-term studies to assess its carcinogenicity or effect on fertility.

Studies of leflunomide use in children show a similar activity to MTX [99]. The lack of experience of its use in other diseases, its long half-life and non-dialyzable formulation are reasons for the clinician to be cautious at present about its use in children with JIA.

Autologous haemopoietic stem cell transplantation

Introduction

Since the 1970s, several case reports of patients with malignancy and coincidental autoimmune disease reported prolonged remission of the autoimmune disease after stem cell transplantation (SCT) performed as a treatment for the malignancy; however, continuing autoimmune disease has also been reported [38,39]. This observation of remission of the autoimmune disease was further supported by experimental evidence demonstrating that Lewis rats with adjuvant arthritis could be cured by autologous SCT (Auto-SCT) using Total Body Irradiation (TBI) as a conditioning regimen [41]. It is hypothesized that the immunosuppressive conditioning of Auto-SCT erases putative autoreactive T cells. After reinfusion of stem cells, the T cell repertoire is regenerated "de novo". In addition, the reconstituted T cells may be tolerized by presented antigens derived from the damaged synovial and cartilage tissues. It is at present not clear if this reinfusion of autologous stem cells is necessary for healthy immune reconstitution, or simply allows for more rapid recovery from immunosuppression and aplasia.

Clinical experience

Autologous haemopoietic stem cell transplantation (Auto-SCT) has been performed in adults with multiple sclerosis, systemic sclerosis, rheumatoid arthritis, and systemic lupus erythematosus, and in children with JIA [39,42–45]. The first reported use of Auto-SCT in JIA included children with the most severe and long-standing systemic disease, with much erosive and irreversible joint destruction already present [44,46]. Since this report, more than 45 cases have been reported by 9 paediatric bone marrow transplant units registered in the database of the Working Party for Autoimmune diseases of the European Blood and Marrow Transplantation group (EBMT). Thirty-two of these have been analysed in detail (Figures 3.14.1–3.14.3, and Table 3.14.2) [47–49]. All children were corticosteroid dependant, resistant to high-dose parenteral MTX and failed etanercept (when available). The results of Auto-SCT were striking with a prolonged drug free follow-up of 6–60 months. Fifty percent are still in drug free remission [49,50]. One quarter of the patients showed a transient or mild relapse of active arthritis, and 13% developed a persistent relapse of arthritis. No new cases of macrophage activation syndrome (MAS) have occurred. Seventeen of 32 children (53%) showed a drug free improvement of more than 50% after a follow up of 4–60 months, with a marked decrease in the scores of the Childhood Health Assessment Questionnaire, the physicians global assessment and in swollen joint count (Figures 3.14.1 and 3.14.2) [47,48]. The measurement of limitation of movement which largely reflects permanent joint destruction did not, as expected, change (Figure 3.14.3). The ESR, CRP, and haemoglobin levels returned to near normal values within 6 weeks.

A relapse was noted in seven children 18 months after ASCT. Some of these relapses have been mild with oligoarthritis and sporadic fever, which could be controlled easily with a 3-month course of low dose prednisone and NSAIDs. Even these seven patients showed a 30% improvement in their disease. Four children were refractory to ASCT and showed a persistent recurrence of disease that was as severe as before the ASCT.

Prior to the onset of their arthritis the Dutch children in this study had heights between −0.2 and +2 SD of the mean length for their age. During the course of their disease they lost 3–5 SDS. After ASCT some (mostly the younger children) showed a catch up growth of 1–2 SDS.

Four patients died. Causes of death were mostly due to infection associated with bone marrow suppression. In three of these children MAS, a well-known complication of Systemic Arthritis [60,61], reflecting

Table 3.14.2 General outcome of 31 children after ASCT for JIA

Complete remission	17 (7 no TBI)
Partial response	7 (3 no TBI)
No response	2
Transplant related mortality (MAS)	3
Nontransplant related mortality	1
Other	1

Data obtained from: Utrecht and Leiden, The Netherlands; Brussels, Belgium; Jena and Halle, Germany: Paris, France; Newcastle and London, England.

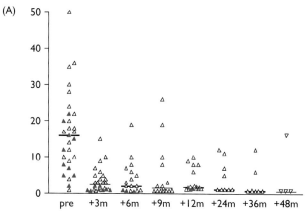

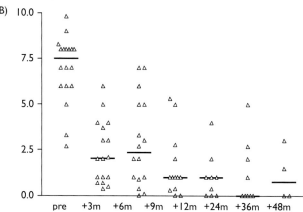

Fig. 3.14.1 Swollen joint counts (A) and Global Physician's assessment (B) (given as a Visual Analogue Scale (VAS)) ranging from 0 (healthy) to 10 (most severely affected) of disease severity in 32 patients before and after Auto-SCT. Patient data were obtained from 8 European paediatric transplant centres. Solid triangles represent children transplanted without use of TBI as part of the conditioning regimen.

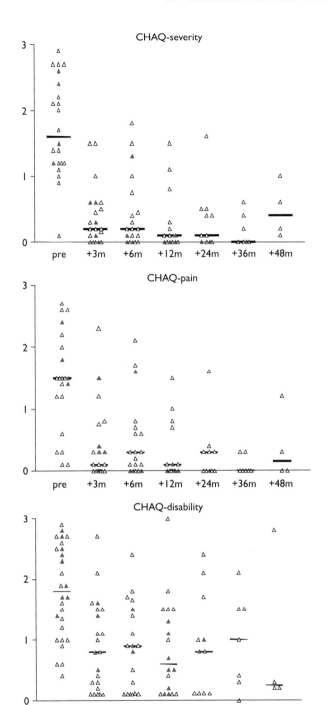

Fig. 3.14.2 Child Health Assessment Questionnaire (CHAQ) in 32 children after Auto-SCT. Solid triangles represent children transplanted without use of TBI as part of the conditioning regimen.

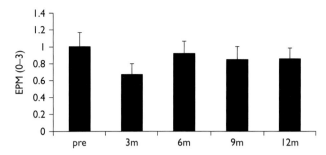

Fig. 3.14.3 Limitation of movement (EPM-ROM) in 32 children after Auto-SCT.

Immunological reconstitution

Post-ASCT the neutrophils recovered ($> 0.5 \times 10^9$/l) between day 12–30, and the platelet count reached 20×10^9/l between days 16–35. Five to nine months after ASCT the numbers of circulating T cells were normal, with normal *in vitro* mitogenic responses at 6–18 months after ASCT. Patients with JIA who were transplanted after conditioning with high dose cyclophosphamide, ATG and low dose TBI, showed a prolonged lymphopenia, especially of CD4 + lymphocytes, persisting for 6–12 months after ASCT [46]. The hypothesis for the efficacy of ASCT in the treatment of an autoimmune disease is that it induces immunological tolerance. In the absence of putative autoreactive T cells, the T cell repertoire is regenerated "*de novo*". The use of such a conditioning regimen inducing a profound lymphopenia of at least 6 months may increase the likelihood of permanently ablating autoreactive T cells, but also puts the patient at increased risk of opportunistic infections and immunological imbalance, which may precipitate MAS.

The role of auto-SCT in understanding the pathogenesis of MAS in JIA

The unexpected occurrence of MAS after auto-SCT remains unexplained. This complication resembles the active phases of familial haemophagocytic lymphohistiocytosis (FHL), in which an immunological imbalance between regulatory T cells and macrophages has been postulated [54]. This similarity has directed research for evidence of macrophage activation during active disease and after ASCT.

Decreased expression of perforin on the cell surface of cytotoxic T cells and NK cells

Familial haemophagocytic lymphohistiocytosis is an autosomal recessive disorder characterized by uncontrolled activation of T cells and macrophages and excessive production of inflammatory cytokines. The clinical features include fever, hepatosplenomegaly, pancytopenia, disseminated intravascular coagulation, and haemophagocytosis. Recently a defect in the perforin gene was described as an underlying cause of this disease [55]. The perforin protein is involved in the immunoregulatory process of target cell killing.

marked macrophage activation due to loss of T cell control, and perhaps an underlying abnormality of macrophage function, was also present [51–53]. This complication was preceded by infections including Epstein–Barr Virus reactivation and disseminated toxoplasmosis. The presently available follow-up data are still limited, and as yet only permit a global analysis of the changes of the core set criteria [47].

The Macrophage Activation Syndrome that occurs in patients with Systemic Arthritis is clinically very similar to FHL. Therefore the perforin expression levels on cytotoxic T cells and NK cells were determined in patients with Systemic Arthritis before and after auto-SCT. Both cell types from patients with Systemic Arthritis expressed significantly lower levels of perforin than cells from healthy controls or from children with other forms of JIA [50]. In four patients with Systemic Arthritis who were treated with auto-SCT, perforin expression was analysed both before and 12 months after Auto-SCT (Figure 3.14.4). In all four patients a clear increase in perforin expression was found both in NK cells as well as in cytotoxic effector cells [50]. In another patient, treated with auto-SCT, a similar response of perforin expression was also seen after SCT; this patient developed a full and persistent relapse of disease activity 7 months after SCT, and the relapse was associated with a recurrence of the decreased perforin expression in both NK and cytotoxic T cells.

Therefore perforin expression appears to often be severely reduced in Systemic Arthritis, and this finding may explain why Systemic Arthritis is sometimes complicated by MAS and haemophagocytosis. Auto-SCT leads to a reconstitution of the (T cell) immune system with a normal expression of perforin. This fact rules out the possibility that there is a mutation of the perforin gene in JIA; however, other factors controlling gene transcription could account for this phenomenon [56].

Myeloid-related protein secretion parallels disease activity before and after ASCT

We have recently found a correlation between serum concentrations of myeloid-related proteins 8 and 14 (MRP8 and MRP14) and disease activity in 12 patients with refractory JIA who underwent ASCT [57]. ASCT induced a remission of disease in 10 of these 12 patients, as measured by a decrease in at least 3 out of 6 of the core set criteria, and there was a concomitant decrease in MRP8 and MRP14 serum concentration. MRP8 and MRP14 are released at sites of local inflammation and are reliable markers for monitoring local activity of the phagocyte system during inflammatory processes [58,62]. Conventional markers such as the ESR and CRP lack the required sensitivity and specificity due to the fact that these parameters reflect systemic rather than local inflammatory activity. Transient relapses in three patients after ASCT was accompanied by an increase in MRP8/MRP14 serum concentrations [57,59]. One child with a persistent relapse post-ASCT showed an increase in MRP8/MP14 serum concentrations exceeding pre-transplant levels. The significant increase in MRP8/MRP14 concentration during active disease, and the correlation with disease activity, supports the hypothesis that phagocytes excreting MRP8 and MRP14 play an important role in the pathogenesis of JIA. As MRP8/MRP14 is a macrophage activation marker we expected its serum concentration to rise during or before

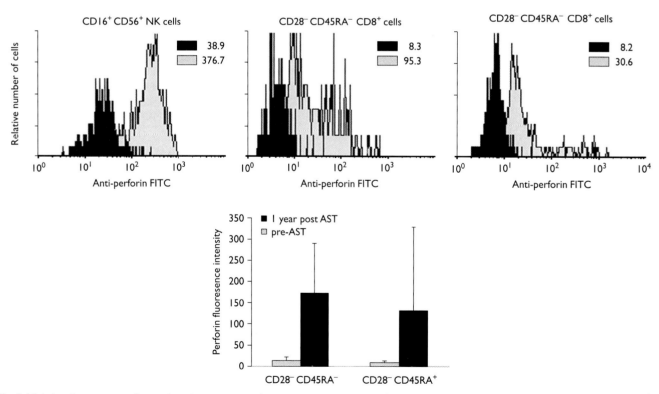

Fig. 3.14.4 Autologous stem cell transplantation restores perforin expression in systemic JIA. Upper panel: FACS analysis on NK cells (left), CD28−CD8+ (middle) and CD28−RA+CD8+ (right) shows reduced expression before auto-SCT (black histogram) that normalizes 1 years after SCT (grey histogram). Lower panel: Mean fluorescence Intensity of CD28−CD8+ and CD28−RA+CD8+ lymphocytes (vertical bars represent SEM of four patients).

MAS. However, in one patient who developed MAS 5 months post-ASCT there were persistently low MRP8/MRP14 serum concentrations prior to and during the episode of MAS. The fact that this patient did not show an increase in MRP8/MRP14 concentration suggests that MRP8/MRP14 is not a reliable marker for the detection of early MAS. Another JIA patient who developed MAS shortly after auto-SCT had persistently high MRP8/MRP14 serum concentrations that did not differ from pre-transplant levels found in other patients. Since MRP8 and MRP14 expression is restricted to neutrophils and the early differentiation stages of monocytes, the lack of an increase in serum MRP8/MP14 seems to point to an involvement of mature or resident tissue macrophages in the pathogenesis of MAS [63,64]. These resident nondividing tissue macrophages are relatively resistant to low dose TBI, and this may perhaps explain the occurrence of MAS shortly after auto-SCT when the normal feedback control of T cells is lacking.

Two of the patients with MAS shortly after ASCT had high systemic activity, with spiking fever, lymphadenopathy, thrombocytosis, anaemia, and high serum ferritin levels, just prior to and during conditioning. Removing the control of T cells by the conditioning regimen may have contributed to the occurrence of MAS. We therefore plan not to transplant future patients during phases of high systemic activity, but to try and induce a temporary remission with high dose intravenous corticosteroids before performing the auto-SCT. We also would propose performing auto-SCT at a younger age in children who are becoming refractory to treatment; however, unfortunately, there are at present no very specific predictors available that reliably indicate a poor outcome [4]. Infection may also be the trigger for MAS in some patients [65,66].

Allogeneic versus autogeneic transplantation

Allogeneic stem cell transplantation has been proposed as an alternative to Auto-SCT because healthy, HLA identical donors will probably not carry putative disease susceptibility genes or autoreactive T lymphocytes. The limited available data, however, do not yet favor allogeneic over autologous transplantation [67]. Although remission of autoimmune disorders in patients receiving allogeneic transplantation for malignancies has been noted, relapses of the autoimmune disease have also been observed, even in patients with 100% donor lymphocytes [38]. In general, allogeneic transplantation is associated with a higher treatment related mortality, especially for patients in a poor general condition.

Novel therapeutic horizons in juvenile idiopathic arthritis

Although treatment options for JIA have improved significantly with the introduction of novel immune response modifiers, it still remains questionable whether these treatment regimens are safe for the long-term treatment of JIA. The short-term side-effects of TNF-α blockade are limited, but significantly more side-effects might be expected when children are treated for significantly longer periods of time; it is also clear that these drugs are not effective in all patients. Therefore, there is a need for the development of more specific immune-based interventions in JIA. Over the last decade rapid progress has been made in our understanding of the molecular mechanisms underlying immunological processes leading to self-recognition and autoimmunity [68,69]. Based on this growing knowledge, novel avenues for the

therapy of autoimmune diseases have been explored in animal models of autoimmunity [70,71]. As a consequence, in the next decade new possibilities for immune intervention in JIA will probably arise, including gene therapy and antigen-specific tolerance induction.

Traditionally gene therapy is directed at replacing a missing gene or gene product. This type of gene therapy may be of value for the treatment of conditions like type 1 diabetes, but will probably not be applicable for autoimmune diseases with a heterogeneous genetic background such as JIA. Gene therapy may, however, be used for local delivery of immune-modulatory molecules such as suppressive cytokines, or for targeting signaling pathways involved in ongoing arthritis [72–74]. Interference with the NF-kB pathway may be an especially powerful option leading to down regulation of the production of pro-inflammatory cytokines such as IL-1 and TNF-α.

In addition to gene therapy, various options are being developed for antigen-specific tolerance induction in arthritis. These options all have in common the fact that they are based on attempts to induce antigen-specific changes in the immune system instead of generalized immune suppression [75–77]. For that reason they are expected to more specifically target the "deranged" immune cells, and leave the general immune system intact and capable of mounting an adequate defense against microbial pathogens and tumors.

Different methods and routes for antigen-specific immune therapy have been explored for the treatment of autoimmune diseases, such as intravenous administration of a soluble antigen (both in its innate form and as altered peptide ligands), or antigen administration in combination with a second tolerogenic signal.

At present, by far the most promising avenue for antigen-specific immune therapy is the mucosal route of immune tolerance induction [76]. In animal models of autoimmunity, oral or nasal administration of the disease inducing auto-antigens is an extremely effective way to prevent and even treat ongoing autoimmune disease [78–80]. The striking efficacy of mucosal tolerance induction in animal models has already led to clinical trials in adult RA and multiple sclerosis using, respectively, type II collagen and myelin basic protein [81–83].

One of the main issues remaining to be solved if such an approach is to be effective in JIA is the choice of antigen used for tolerance induction in JIA. Although in many human autoimmune diseases, including JIA, disease-triggering auto-antigens are not known, this does not necessarily preclude the possibility for antigen-specific immune therapy.

Due to bystander activation during ongoing inflammation, many epitopes become recognized by the activated immune system through a process called epitope spreading [84]. One or more of these epitopes could be used for antigen-specific immune therapy. An antigen that is to be used for antigen-specific immune therapy should fulfill at least the following prerequisites: (1) Be present and up-regulated at the site of inflammation. (2) Be immunologically recognized in the majority of patients. Both type II collagen and Heat Shock proteins (HSPs) fulfill these prerequisites, and are considered strong potential candidates for antigen-specific immune therapy in JIA.

In patients with JIA, autoantibodies against type II collagen can be detected. In animal models of arthritis, type II collagen is an important disease-triggering auto-antigen, and it has been used effectively for immune therapy in such experimental models [85,86]. Oral administration of type II collagen has been used with some success in adults with RA [83,87]. More recently, oral treatment with type II collagen has been attempted in patients with JIA with encouraging preliminary results; a majority of patients showing significant improvement without any side-effects [88,89].

Heat shock proteins are also prime candidates for antigen-specific immune therapy in JIA. HSPs are highly conserved cellular proteins that are produced in increased amounts when cells are exposed to any kind of environmental form of stress [90]. Interestingly, HSPs from microbial origin are immunodominant and serve as key targets for immune responses towards invading microorganisms. HSPs could therefore be involved in so-called antigen mimicry in arthritis; an immune response first directed against a microbial HSP being redirected towards a self-HSP expressed on inflamed synovial tissue [91]. An increased expression of human (self) HSP 60 has been demonstrated in lining cells of inflamed synovial tissue from patients with JIA (Figure 3.14.5) [92].

Several groups have reported a specific T cell response directed against both human and microbial HSPs in JIA [93–95]. The role of this natural immune response towards HSPs in JIA is still debated, but it is clear that HSPs may form an excellent target for immune therapy in this condition [96]. In animal models, immunization or mucosal administration of HSPs or HSP-derived peptides induces protection in virtually all forms of experimental arthritis [96,97]. To date, a few clinical trials are being performed with HSP-peptides in adults with RA. Depending on the results of these studies, new trials in patients with JIA will be considered.

The hierarchy of experimental treatment options

The difficulty with any experimental therapy is deciding when to introduce such a therapy, and which treatment to use. Clearly, one should avoid experimental therapies until conventional, proven therapies have been shown to have failed in an individual. However, it is also obvious that there is no point in waiting to try such therapies (particularly if there is a theoretical rationale, and some clinical evidence of efficacy), until the child has such damaged joints that no useful recovery can be expected.

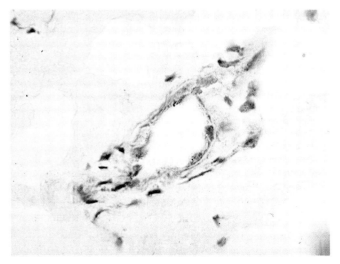

Fig. 3.14.5 Synovial lining cells of a patient with JIA stained with monoclonal; antibody LK1, specific for human hsp60 from Graeff–Meeder et al. [82].

Given our present state of knowledge, the biologics directed against TNF and IL-Ra are drugs that should be used quite early in refractory disease. It seems probable that other biologic agents (such as IL-6 related agents in Systemic Arthritis) will also supplement these therapies. Leflunomide and other newer immunomodulatory agents are likely to be less toxic that auto-SCT, and might reasonably be expected to be tried prior to proceeding to transplantation. Immunization approaches are also probably going to be less toxic than transplantation, and if available are probably warranted. At present, although auto-SCT is clearly very efficacious, its toxicity is such that it should only be recommended as a therapy when other less toxic (albeit less efficacious therapies) have failed. The caveat to this statement being the necessity of performing auto-SCT in children whose joints have recoverable function and whose general health is not so debilitated by long-term persistent disease that the risks of the procedure are unduly increased. If there were measures that accurately predicted a very poor outcome, it would perhaps be justified to undertake auto-SCT earlier than is presently the case. Unfortunately such measures are not available concurrently.

Recent developments

Due to the rapid progress that has been made in the management of JIA a number of drugs are being used with increasing frequency for refractory Systemic Arthritis. These include IL-1r antagonist, thalidomide, and anti IL-6 receptor which have been proposed in small series as effective therapies for this indication.

IL-1r antagonist

This agent (discussed in greater detail earlier in this chapter on p433) has been reported as effective for Systemic Arthritis [100–104]. In these studies approximately 24 to 27 (89%) patients (the exact number is not clear as some subjects may be reported more than once) with refractory Systemic Arthritis had a significant beneficial response with about one third going into complete remission. These exciting results though uncontrolled and open to a number of biases, strongly suggest that IL-1 is an important cytokine in the pathogenesis of Systemic Arthritis, and that therapies directed against IL-1 are effective for this form of JIA.

Humanized anti IL-6 receptor antibody (MRA)

IL-6 probably plays a primary role in the cytokine cascade responsible for the inflammatory features of Systemic Arthritis [105,106]. Studies in both adult onset Still's disease and Systemic Arthritis (which are probably the same conditions) suggest that antibodies to the IL-6 receptor are very effective in suppressing both the systemic features and the arthritis [107–109]. Of 29 children with severe refractory Systemic Arthritis studied in open label phase II trials [108,109] over 70% achieved at least 30% improvement in their arthritis and 62% achieved 50% improvement. As these trials are more formally designed than those described for IL-1r antagonist it is probable that these very impressive results are more likely to accurately represent "reality" than are the results reported for the IL-1r antagonist studies.

Thalidomide

Thalidomide has anti-TNF activity [110]. There is increasing interest in its use as an immunosuppressive therapy in a number of conditions, and some limited data suggest, it may be a useful drug in refractory Systemic Arthritis [111,112]. Of the 21 children reported in these two studies. 18 (86%) had significant improvement. These data are intriguing, but somewhat surprising given the relative inefficacy of anti-TNF therapy in Systemic Arthritis, and suggest either that the data are biased due to the open nature of the studies, or that thalidomide exerts an effect through other mechanisms than TNF modulation alone.

Summary

A number of novel avenues for immune therapy in JIA such as gene therapy and antigen-specific immune therapy hold great promises for the future. The translation from basic animal models towards real life human autoimmunity may still prove to be a difficult undertaking. However given the rate of advance in this area it seems probable that several new approaches and new agents will become available in the next few years and that they will be used earlier in the disease course, as their relative effectiveness in the various types of JIA becomes clear.

References

1. Wallace, C.A. and Sherry, D.D. Trial of intravenous pulse cyclophosphamide and methylprednisolone in the treatment of severe systemic-onset juvenile rheumatoid arthritis. *Arthritis Rheum* 1997;40:1852–55.

2. Cassidy, J.T. Medical management of children with juvenile rheumatoid arthritis. *Drugs* 1999;58:831–50.

3. Petty, R.E. Prognosis in children with rheumatic diseases: justification for consideration of new therapies. *Rheumatology* 1999;38:739–42.

4. Spiegel, L.R., Schneider, R., Lang, B.A., Birdi N., Silverman E.D., Laxer R.M., *et al.* Early predictors of poor functional outcome in systemic-onset juvenile rheumatoid arthritis: a multicenter cohort study. *Arthritis Rheum* 2000;43:2402–09.

5. Ruperto, N., Ravelli, A., Falcini, F., Lepore, L., De Sanctis, R., Zulian, F., *et al.* Performance of the preliminary definition of improvement in juvenile chronic arthritis patients treated with methotrexate. Italian Pediatric Rheumatology Study Group. *Ann Rheum Dis* 1998;57:38–41.

6. Giannini, E.H., Ruperto, N., Ravelli, A., Lovell, D.J., Felson, D.T., and Martini, A. Preliminary definition of improvement in juvenile arthritis. *Arthritis Rheum* 1997;40:1202–09.

7. Speckmaier, M., Findeisen, J., Woo, P., Hall, A., Sills, J.A., Price, T. and *et al.* Low-dose methotrexate in systemic onset juvenile chronic arthritis. Clin *Exp Rheumatol* 1989;7:647–50.

8. Ravelli, A., Migliavacca, D., Viola, S., Ruperto, N., Pistorio, A., and Martini, A. Efficacy of folinic acid inreducing methotrexate toxicity in juvenile idiopathic arthritis. *Clin Exp Rheumatol* 1999;17:625–27.

9. Reiff, A., Rawlings, D.J., Shaham, B., Franke, E., Richardson, L., Szer, I.S. *et al.* Preliminary evidence for cyclosporin A as an alternative in the treatment of recalcitrant juvenile rheumatoid arthritis and juvenile dermatomyositis. *J Rheumatol* 1997;24:2436–43.

10. Wallace, C.A. On beyond methotrexate treatment of severe juvenile rheumatoid arthritis. *Clin Exp Rheumatol* 1999;17:499–504.

11. Gottlieb, B.S., Keenan, G.F., Lu, T., and Ilowite, N.T. Discontinuation of methotrexate treatment in juvenile rheumatoid arthritis. *Pediatrics* 1997;100:994–7.

12. Ruperto, N., Murray, K., Gerloni, V., Wulffraat, N.M., Oliveira, S., Falcini, F., *et al.* A Randomized Trial of Methotrexate (MTX) in Medium Versus Higher Doses in Children with Juvenile Idiopathic Arthritis (JIA) Who Failed on Standard Dose. *Arthritis Rheum* 2002;46(suppl. 9)S195.

13. Fleischmann, R., Iqbal, I., Nandeshwar, P., and Quiceno, A. Safety and efficacy of disease-modifying anti-rheumatic agents: focus on the benefits and risks of etanercept. *Drug Saf* 2002;25:173–97.

14. Lovell, D.J., Giannini E.H., Reiff, A., Cawkwell, G.D., Silverman, E.D., Nocton, J.J., *et al.* Etanercept in children with polyarticular juvenile rheumatoid arthritis. Pediatric Rheumatology Collaborative Study Group. *N Engl J Med* 2000;342:763–69.

15. Kietz, D.A., Pepmueller, P.H., and Moore, T.L. Therapeutic use of etanercept in polyarticular course juvenile idiopathic arthritis over a two year period. *Ann Rheum* Dis 2002;61:171–3.

16. Keane, J., Gershon, S., Wise, R.P., Mirabile-Levens, E., Kasznica, J., and Schwieterman, W.D. Tuberculosis associated with infliximab, a tumor necrosis factor alpha-neutralizing agent. *N Engl J Med* 2002;345:1098–04.

17. Takei, S., Groh, D., Bernstein, B., Shaham, B., Gallagher, K., and Reiff, A. Safety and efficacy of high dose etanercept in treatment of juvenile rheumatoid arthritis. *J Rheumatol* 2001;28:1677–80.

18. Ten Cate, R., Suijlekom-Smit, L.W., Brinkman, D.M., Bekkering, W.P., Jansen-van Wijngaarden, C.J., and Vossen and J.M. Etanercept in four children with therapy-resistant systemic juvenile idiopathic arthritis. *Rheumatology* (Oxford) 2002;41:228–9.

19. Schmeling, H., Mathony, K., John, V., Keysser, G., Burdach, S., and Horneff, G. A combination of etanercept and methotrexate for the treatment of refractory juvenile idiopathic arthritis: a pilot study. *Ann Rheum Dis* 2001;60:410–12.

20. Prahalad, S., Bove, K.E., Dickens, D., Lovell, D.J., and Grom, A.A. Etanercept in the treatment of macrophage activation syndrome. *J Rheumatol* 2001;28:2120–4.

21. Arkachaisri, T. and Lehman, T.J. Use of biologics in the treatment of childhood rheumatic diseases. *Curr Rheumatol Rep* 2000;2:330–6.

22. Kimura, Y., Imundo, L., and Li, S.C. High dose infliximab in the treatment of resistant Systemic Juvenile Rheumatoid *Arthritis*. *Arthritis Rheum* 2001;44 (Suppl 9) S272.

23. Billiau, A.D., Cornillie, F., and Wouters, C. Infliximab for systemic onset juvenile idiopathic arthritis: experience in 3 children. *J Rheumatol* 2002;29:1111–14.

24. Lahdenne, P., Vahasalo, P., and Honkanen, V. Infliximab or etanercept in the treatment of children with refractory juvenile idiopathic arthritis: an open label study. *Ann Rheum Dis* 2003;62:245–7.

25. Lim, W.S., PRJI. Tuberculosis and treatment with infliximab. *N Engl, J Med* 2002;346:623–6.

26. Fries, W., Giofre, M.R., and Catanoso, M., Lo, G.R. Treatment of acute uveitis associated with Crohn's disease and sacroileitis with infliximab. *Am J Gastroenterol* 2002;97:499–500.

27. Reiff, A., Takei, S., Sadeghi, S., Stout, A., Shaham, B., Bernstein, B., *et al.* Etanercept therapy in children with treatment-resistant uveitis. *Arthritis Rheum* 2001;44:1411–15.

28. Smith, J.R., Levinson, R.D., Holland, G.N., Jabs, D.A., Robinson, M.R., Whitcup, S.M., *et al.* Differential efficacy of tumor necrosis factor inhibition in the management of inflammatory eye disease and associated rheumatic disease. *Arthritis Rheum* 2001;45:252–7.

29. Munoz-Fernandez, S., Hidalgo, V., Fernandez-Melon, J., Schlincker, A., and Martin-Mola E. Effect of infliximab on threatening panuveitis in Behcet's disease. *Lancet* 2001;358:1644.

30. Schwartzman, S., Flynn, T., Barinstein, L., Gartner, S., and Onel, K. Infliximab Therapy for Resistant Uveitis. *Arthritis Rheum* 2002;46(Suppl 9)S326.

31. Smith, J.A., Smith, S., Whitcup, S.M., Suhler, E., Clarke, G., Thompson, D *et al.* The Treatment of JRA-associated Uveitis with Etanercept. *Arthritis Rheum* 2002;46(suppl 9):S482.

32. Horai, R., Saijo, S., Tanioka, H., Nakae, S., Sudo, K., Okahara A *et al.* Development of chronic inflammatory arthropathy resembling rheumatoid arthritis in interleukin 1 receptor antagonist-deficient mice. *J Exp Med* 2000;191:313–20.

33. Dinarello C.A. The role of the interleukin-1-receptor antagonist in blocking inflammation mediated by interleukin-1. *N Engl J Med* 2000;343:732–4.

34. Dayer, J.M., Feige, U., Edwards, C.K., III, and Burger, D. Anti-interleukin-1 therapy in rheumatic diseases. *Curr Opin Rheumatol* 2001;13:170–6.

35. Jiang, Y., Genant H.K, Watt, I., Cobby, M., Bresnihan B., Aitchison, R, *et al.*, A multicenter, double-blind, dose-ranging, randomized, placebo-controlled study of recombinant human interleukin-1 receptor antagonist in patients with rheumatoid arthritis: radiologic progression and correlation of Genant and Larsen scores. *Arthritis Rheum* 2000;43:1001–9.

36. Cohen, S., Hurd E., Cush, J., Schiff, M., Weinblatt, M.E., Moreland, L.W. *et al.* Treatment of rheumatoid arthritis with anakinra, a recombinant human interleukin-1 receptor antagonist, in combination with methotrexate: results of a twenty-four-week, multicenter, randomized, double-blind, placebo-controlled trial. *Arthritis Rheum* 2002;46:614–24.

37. Prakash, A. and Jarvis B. Leflunomide: a review of its use in active rheumatoid arthritis. *Drugs* 1999;58:1137–64.

38. Snowden, J.A., Kearney, P., Kearney, A., Cooley, H.M., Grigg, A., Jacobs P *et al.* Long-term outcome of autoimmune disease following allogeneic bone marrow transplantation. *Arthritis Rheum* 1998;41:453–59.

39. Tyndall, A. and Gratwohl, A. Bone marrow transplantation in the treatment of autoimmune diseases. *Br J Rheumatol* 1997;36:1–3.

40. Burt, R.K., Fassas, A., Snowden, J., van Laar, J.M., Kozak, T., Wulffraat, N.M., *et al.* Collection of hematopoietic stem cells from patients with autoimmune diseases. *Bone Marrow Transplant* 2001;28:1–12.

41. van Bekkum, D.W. Effectiveness and risks of total body irradiation for conditioning in the treatment of autoimmune disease with autologous bone marrow transplantation. *Rheumatology* (Oxford) 1999;38:757–61.

42. Joske, D.J., M.a. D.T., Langlands, D.R., and Owen, E.T. Autologous bone-marrow transplantation for rheumatoid arthritis. *Lancet* 1997;350:337–8.

43. Jantunen, E. and Myllykangas-Luosujarvi and R. Stem cell transplantation for treatment of severe autoimmune diseases: current status and future perspectives. *Bone Marrow Transplant* 2000;25:351–6.

44. Wulffraat, N.M., van Royen, A., Bierings, M., Vossen, J., and Kuis, W. Autologous haemopoietic stem-cell transplantation in four patients with refractory juvenile chronic arthritis. *Lancet* 1999;353:550–3.

45. Tyndall, A., Black, C., Finke, J., Winkler, J., Mertlesmann, R., Peter, H.H. *et al.* Treatment of systemic sclerosis with autologous haemopoietic stem cell transplantation. *Lancet* 1997;349:254.

46. Wulffraat, N.M., Sanders, L.A., and Kuis, W. Autologous hemopoietic stem-cell transplantation for children with refractory autoimmune disease. *Curr Rheumatol Rep* 2000;2:316–23.

47. de Kleer, I., Brinkman, D., Rijkers, G.T., Prakken, B.J., ten Cate, R., Kuis, W., *et al.* 18 Children after autologous stem cell transplantation for refractory juvenile idiopathic arthritis: 1 to 51 months of follow up. *Ann Rheum Dis* 2001;60(suppl II):11.

48. Wulffraat, N.M., Brinkman, D., Ferster, A., Opperman, ten Cate, R., Wedderburn, L.R., *et al.* Long term follow up of autologous Stem Cell Transplantation for refractory Juvenile Idiopathic Arthritis (JIA). *Bone Marrow Transplant* 2003;32 suppl 1:s61–4.

49. Wulffraat, N.M., de Kleer, I., Brinkman, D., ten Cate, R., vanderNet, J.J., Rijkers, G.T., *et al.* Autologous stem cell transplantation for refractory juvenile idiopathic arthritis: current results and perspectives. *Transplantation Proc* 2002;34:2925–26.

50. Wulffraat, N.M., Rijkers, G.T., Elst, E.F., Brooimans, R.A., and Kuis, W. Reduced perforin expression in systemic juvenile idiopathic arthritis is restored by autologous stem cell transplantation. *Rheumatology* (Oxford) 2003;42:375–9.

51. Wulffraat, N.M., Kamphuis, S.S., van der Net, J., Brinkman, D., ten Cate, R., and Kuis W. Autologous stem-cell transplantation in 12 cases with refractory juvenile arthritis. *Osteological Bull* 2000;5:62–5.

52. Quartier, P., Prieur, A.M., and Fischer, A. Haemopoietic stem-cell transplantation for juvenile chronic arthritis. *Lancet* 1999;353:1885–6.

53. Mouy, R., Stephan, J.L., Pillet, P., Haddad, E., Hubert, P., and Prieur, A.M. Efficacy of cyclosporine A in the treatment of macrophage activation syndrome in juvenile arthritis: report of five cases. *J Pediatr* 1996;129:750–4.

54. Stepp, S.E., Mathew, P.A., Bennett, M., de Saint, B.G., and Kumar, V. Perforin: more than just an effector molecule. *Immunol Today* 2000;21:254–5.

55. Stepp, S.E., Dufourcq-Lagelouse, R., Le Deist, F., Bhawan, S., Certain, S., Mathew, P.A., *et al.* Perforin gene defects in familial hemophagocytic lymphohistiocytosis. *Science* 1999;286:1957–9.

56. Yu, C.R., Ortaldo, J.R., Curiel, R.E., Young, H.A., Anderson, S.K., and Gosselin, P. Role of a STAT binding site in the regulation of the human perforin promoter. *J Immunol* 1999;162:2785–90.

57. Wulffraat, N.M., Haas, P.J., Frosch, M., De Kleer, I.M., Vogl, T., Brinkman, D.M., *et al.* Myeloid related protein 8 and 14 secretion reflects phagocyte activation and correlates with disease activity in juvenile idiopathic arthritis treated with autologous stem cell transplantation. *Ann Rheum Dis* 2003;62:236–41.

58. Frosch, M., Strey, A., Vogl, T., Wulffraat, N.M., Kuis, W., Sunderkotter, C., *et al.* Myeloid-related proteins 8 and 14 are specifically secreted during interaction of phagocytes and activated endothelium and are useful markers for monitoring disease activity in pauciarticular-onset juvenile rheumatoid arthritis. *Arthritis Rheum* 2000;43:628–37.

59. Haas, P.J.M., Frosch, M., de Kleer, I., Vogl, T., Brinkman, D., Quartier, P. *et al.* Increased myeloid related protein 8 and 14 secretion reflects phagocyte activation and correlates with disease activity in juvenile idiopathic arthritis treated with autologous stem-cell transplantation. *Ann Rheum Dis* 2001;60(Suppl II):29.

60. Stephan, J.L., Zeller, J., Hubert, P., Herbelin, C., Dayer, J.M., and Prieur, A.M. Macrophage activation syndrome and rheumatic disease in childhood: a report of four new cases. *Clin Exp Rheumatol* 1993;11:451–6.

61. Ravelli, A., De Benedetti, F., Viola, S., and Martini, A. Macrophage activation syndrome in systemic juvenile rheumatoid arthritis successfully treated with cyclosporine. *J Pediatr* 1996;128:275–8.

62. Odink, K., Cerletti, N., Bruggen, J., Clerc, R.G., Tarcsay, L., Zwadlo, G., *et al.* Two calcium-binding proteins in infiltrate macrophages of rheumatoid arthritis. *Nature* 1987; 330:80–2.

63. Roth, J., Goebeler, M., van den, B.C., and Sorg, C. Expression of calcium-binding proteins MRP8 and MRP14 is associated with distinct monocytic differentiation pathways in HL-60 cells. *Biochem Biophys Res Commun* 1993;191:565–70.

64. Roth, J., Goebeler, M., Wrocklage, V., van den, B.C., and Sorg, C. Expression of the calcium-binding proteins MRP8 and MRP14 in monocytes is regulated by a calcium-induced suppressor mechanism. *Biochem J* 1994;301:655–60.

65. Vlieger, A.M., Brinkman, D.M., Quartier, P., Prieur, A.M., ten Cate, R., Bierings, M., *et al.* Infection associated macrophage activation syndrome in 3 patients receiving autologous stem cell transplantation (ASCT) for refractory JCA. *Bone Marrow Transplant* 2000;25(Suppl 1):81.

66. Wulffraat, N.M. and Kuis, W. Treatment of refractory juvenile idiopathic arthritis. *J Rheumatol* 2001;28:929–31.

67. Barron, K.S., Wallace, C., Woolfrey, C.E.A., Laxer, R.M., Hirsch, R., Horwitz, M., *et al.* Autologous stem cell transplantation for pediatric rheumatic diseases. *J Rheumatol* 2001;28:2337–58.

68. Shevach, E.M. Certified professionals: CD4(+)CD25(+) suppressor T cells. *J Exp Med* 2001;193:F41–6.

69. Kreuwel, H.T. and Sherman, L.A. The T-cell repertoire available for recognition of self-antigens. *Curr Opin Immunol* 2001;13:639–43.

70. Taneja, V. and David, C.S. Lessons from animal models for human autoimmune diseases. *Nat Immunol* 2001;2:781–84.

71. Martin, R., Sturzebecher, C.S. and McFarland, H.F. Immunotherapy of multiple sclerosis: where are we? Where should we go? *Nat Immunol* 2001; 2:785–88.

72. Tarner, I.H. and Fathman, C.G. Gene therapy in autoimmune disease. *Curr Opin Immunol* 2001;13:676–82.

73. Nakajima, A., Seroogy, C.M., Sandora, M.R., Tarner, I.H., Costa, G.L., Taylor-Edwards, C., *et al.* Antigen-specific T cell-mediated gene therapy in collagen-induced arthritis. *J Clin Invest* 2001;107:1293–301.

74. Morita, Y., Yang, J., Gupta, R., Shimizu, K., Shelden, E.A., Endres, J., *et al.* Dendritic cells genetically engineered to express IL-4 inhibit murine collagen-induced arthritis. *J Clin Invest* 2001;107:1275–84.

75. Harrison, L.C. and Hafler, D.A. Antigen-specific therapy for autoimmune disease. *Curr Opin Immunol* 2000; 12:704–11.

76. Weiner, H.L., Friedman, A., Miller, A., Khoury, S.J., al Sabbagh, A., Santos, L., *et al.* Oral tolerance: immunologic mechanisms and treatment of animal and human organ-specific autoimmune diseases by oral administration of autoantigens. *Annu Rev Immunol* 1994;12:809–7.

77. Wraith, D.C. Antigen-specific immunotherapy of autoimmune disease: a commentary. *Clin Exp Immunol* 1996;103:349–52.

78. Metzler, B. and Wraith, D.C. Inhibition of experimental autoimmune encephalomyelitis by inhalation but not oral administration of the encephalitogenic peptide: influence of MHC binding affinity. *Int Immunol* 1993;5:1159–65.

79. Zhang, Z.Y., Lee, C.S., Lider, O., and Weiner, H.L. Suppression of adjuvant arthritis in Lewis rats by oral administration of type II collagen. *J Immunol* 1990;145:2489–93.

80. Prakken, B.J., van der, Z.R., Anderton, S.M., van Kooten, P.J., Kuis, W., and van Eden, W. Peptide-induced nasal tolerance for a mycobacterial heat shock protein 60 T cell epitope in rats suppresses both adjuvant arthritis and nonmicrobially induced experimental arthritis. *Proc Natl Acad Sci U S A* 1997;94:3284–89.

81. Trentham, D.E., Dynesius-Trentham, R.A., Orav, E.J., Combitchi, D., Lorenzo, C., Sewell, K.L., *et al.* Effects of oral administration of type II collagen on rheumatoid arthritis. *Science* 1993;261:1727–30.

82. Weiner, H.L., Mackin, G.A., Matsui, M., Orav, E.J., Khoury, S.J., Dawson, D.M., *et al.* Double-blind pilot trial of oral tolerization with myelin antigens in multiple sclerosis. *Science* 1993;259:1321–4.

83. Choy, E.H., Scott, D.L., Kingsley, G.H., Thomas, S., Murphy, A.G., Staines, N., *et al.* Control of rheumatoid arthritis by oral tolerance. *Arthritis Rheum* 2001;44:1993–7.

84. Vanderlugt, C.L. and Miller, S.D. Epitope spreading in immune-mediated diseases: implications for immunotherapy. *Nat Rev Immunol* 2002;2:85–95.

85. Trentham, D.E., Townes, A.S., and Kang, A.H. Autoimmunity to type II collagen an experimental model of arthritis. *J Exp Med* 1977;146:857–68.

86. Thompson, H.S. and Staines, N.A. Gastric administration of type II collagen delays the onset and severity of collagen-induced arthritis in rats. *Clin Exp Immunol* 1986;64:581–6.

87. Sieper, J., Kary, S., Sorensen, H., Alten, R., Eggens, U., Huge, W., *et al.* Oral type II collagen treatment in early rheumatoid arthritis. A double-blind, placebo-controlled, randomized trial. *Arthritis Rheum* 1996;39:41–51.

88. Barnett, M.L., Combitchi, D., and Trentham, D.E. A pilot trial of oral type II collagen in the treatment of juvenile rheumatoid arthritis. *Arthritis Rheum* 1996;39:623–8.

89. Myers, L.K., Higgins, G.C., Finkel, T.H., Reed, A.M., Thompson, J.W., Walton, R.C., *et al.* Juvenile arthritis and autoimmunity to type II collagen. *Arthritis Rheum* 2001;44:1775–81.

90. Welch, W.J. How cells respond to stress. *Sci Am* 1993;268:56–64.

91. Cohen, I.R. Autoimmunity to chaperonins in the pathogenesis of arthritis and diabetes. *Annu Rev Immunol* 1991;9:567–89.

92. Graeff-Meeder, E.R., Voorhorst, M., van Eden, W., Schuurman, H.J., Huber, J., Barkley, D., *et al.* Antibodies to the mycobacterial 65-kd heat-shock protein are reactive with synovial tissue of adjuvant arthritic rats and patients with rheumatoid arthritis and osteoarthritis. *Am J Pathol* 1990;137:1013–17.

93. Prakken, A.B., van Eden, W., Rijkers, G.T., Kuis, W., Toebes, E.A., Graeff-Meeder, E.R., *et al.* Autoreactivity to human heat-shock protein 60 predicts disease remission in oligoarticular juvenile rheumatoid arthritis. *Arthritis Rheum* 1996;39:1826–32.

94. Graeff-Meeder, E.R., van Eden, W., Rijkers, G.T., Prakken, B.J., Kuis, W., Voorhorst-Ogink, M.M., *et al.* Juvenile chronic arthritis: T cell reactivity to human HSP60 in patients with a favorable course of arthritis. *J Clin Invest* 1995;95:934–40.

95. Life, P., Hassell, A., Williams, K., Young, S., Bacon, P., Southwood, T., *et al.* Responses to gram negative enteric bacterial antigens by synovial, T. cells from patients with juvenile chronic arthritis: recognition of heat shock protein HSP60. *J Rheumatol* 1993;20:1388–96.

96. van Eden, W., van der, Z.R., Paul, A.G., Prakken, B.J., Wendling, U., Anderton, S.M., *et al.* Do heat shock proteins control the balance of T-cell regulation in inflammatory diseases? *Immunol Today* 1998;19:303–7.

97. Anderton, S.M., van der, Z.R., Prakken, B., Noordzij, A., and van Eden, W. Activation of T cells recognizing self 60-kD heat shock protein can protect against experimental arthritis. *J Exp Med* 1995;181:943–52.

98. Armbrust, W., Kamphuis, S.S., Wolfs, T.W., *et al.* Tuberculosis in a nine-year-old girl treated with infliximab for systemic juvenile idiopathic arthritis. *Rheumatology* (Oxford) 2004;43:527–9.

99. Silverman, E., Mouy, R., Spiegel, L., *et al.* Leflunomide or methotrexate for juvenile rheumatoid arthritis. *N Engl JMed* 2005;352:1655–66.

100. Irigoyen, P.I., Olson, J., Hom, C., Ilowite, N.T. Treatment of systemic onset juvenile rheumatoid arthritis with anakinra. *Arthritis Rheum* 2004; 50(9 suppl): S437.

101. Henrickson, M. Efficacy of anakinra in refractory systemic arthritis. *Arthritis Rheum* 2004;50(9 suppl):S438.

102. Verbsky, J.W., White, A.J. Effective use of the recombinant interleukin-1 receptor antagonist anakinra in therapy resistant systemic onset juvenile rheumatoid arthritis. *J Rheumatol* 2004; 31:2071–5.

103. Pascual, V., Allantaz, F., Arce, E., Punaro, M., Banchereau, J. Role of Interleukin-1 (IL-1) in the pathogenesis of systemic onset juvenile idiopathic arthritis and clinical response to IL-1 blockade. *J Exp Med* 2005;201:1479–86.

104. Weiss, J., Henrickson, M., Walco, G., Feinstein, A., Kimura, Y. Combination therapy with anakinra and anti-TNF agents in refractory Systemic JIA (SJIA). *Arthritis Rheum* 2005:52(9 suppl):S84.

105. De Benedetti, F. and Martini, A. Is systemic juvenile rheumatoid arthritis an interleukin 6 mediated disease? *J Rheumatol* 1998:25:203–7.

106. Fishman, D., Faulds, G., Jeffery, R., Mohamed-Ali, V., Yudkin, J.S., Woo, P. The effect of novel polymorphisms in the interleukin-6 (IL-6) gene on IL-6 transcription and plasma IL-6 levels, and an association with systemic-onset juvenile chronic arthritis. *J Clin invest* 1998;102:1369–76.

107. Iwamoto, M., Nara, H., Hirata, D., Minota, S., Nishimoto, N., Yoshizaki, K. Humanized monoclonal anti-interleukin-6 receptor antibody for treatment of intractable adult-onset Still's disease. *Arthritis Rheum* 2002;46:3388–9.

108. Yokota, S., Miyamae, T., Imagawa, T., Iwata, N., Katakura, S., Mori, M. *et al.* Therapeutic efficacy of humanized recombinant anti-interleukin-6 receptor antibody in children with systemic-onset juvenile idiopathic arthritis. *Arthritis Rheum* 2005;52:818–25.

109. Woo, P., Wilkinson, N., Prieur, A.M., Southwood, T., Leone, V., Livermore, P. *et al.* Open label phase II trial of single, ascending doses of MRA in Caucasian children with severe systemic juvenile idiopathic arthritis: proof of prinicple of the efficacy of IL-6 receptor blockade in this type of arthritis and demonstration of prolonged clinical improvement. *Arthritis Res Ther* 2005;7:R1281–8.

110. Calabrese, L. and Resztak, K. Thalidomide revisited: pharmacology and clinical applications. *Expert opin Investig Drugs* 1998;7:2043–60.

111. Lehman, T.J., Striegal, K.H., Onel, K.B. Thalidomide therapy for recalcitrant systemic onset juvenile rheumatoid arthritis. *J Pediatr* 2002: 140:125–7.

112. Badot, V., Debandt, M., Job Deslandre, C., Lê, Q.P., Wouters, C., Hatron, P.-Y. Efficacy and tolerance of thalidomide in refractory systemic onset juvenile idiopathic arthritis (So-JRA): A retrospective study in 19 patients. *Arthritis Rheum* 2005;52(9 suppl):S85.

Appendix

Clive A.J. Ryder, Taunton R. Southwood, and Peter N. Malleson

Intra-articular corticosteroid injections

Introduction

Intra-articular corticosteroids are being used increasingly as first and second line treatment for chronically inflamed joints. In early disease they produce rapid symptom control, reducing pain, stiffness and swelling, facilitating early physiotherapy and potentially preventing growth disturbance. In addition they help avoid the need for oral or intravenous corticosteroids and "buy time" for second line therapies such as methotrexate to have their beneficial effects. Many patients who respond well to joint injection may not even need to use non-steroidal anti-inflammatory drugs. Although often not "curative", there can be long periods (months or even years) of remission of arthritis, particularly with triamcinolone hexacetonide (TH) [1,2]. Corticosteroid joint injection is also useful in established disease where it may allow clinicians to better gain control of the disease if it has not responded fully to second line agents. Some centres now use multiple joint injections as a routine part of the management of children with polyarthritis.

Children with Rheumatoid Factor Positive Polyarthritis and Systemic Arthritis perhaps respond less well to intra-articular corticosteroids than do children with Oligoarthritis, but even in these children remission of inflammation in the injected joint can be long lasting [3]. In a recent study a high ESR was the only variable associated with a sustained clinical response [4]

Anesthesia and analgesia

Joint injections are most easily performed under general anaesthesia. This can be done as a day case and provides a relaxed, immobile patient; there is very little psychological trauma and there is no limit to the number of joints that can be done at any one time. The use of a general anaesthetic also allows careful examination of joints to assess involvement, particularly range of movement when muscle spasm is abolished. It also allows splinting, with or without prior stretching to be performed painlessly.

For even young children having only one or two joints injected, benzodiazapine sedation can be very effective. Midazolam is probably the most useful as it has the shortest half life and therefore the quickest recovery time. Despite this, the recovery process will often take longer than following a general anaesthetic. Realistically a maximum of 2 or 3 joints can be done under sedation before the patient wakes or starts to complain about the procedure.

Some centres are now using self-administered nitrous oxide either as an adjunct to sedation or on its own, and initial reports are

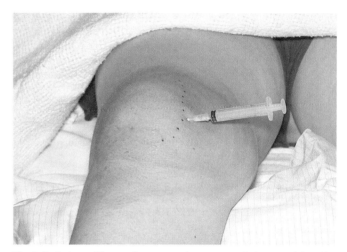

Fig. 1 Right knee: The needle is inserted approximately 1 cm medial to the patella, at about the junction of the upper and lower halves. The needle is directed slightly caudally.

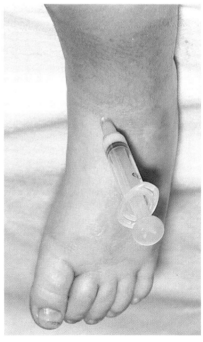

Fig. 2 Left ankle: The needle is inserted anteriorly just lateral to the hallucis extensor longus tendon.

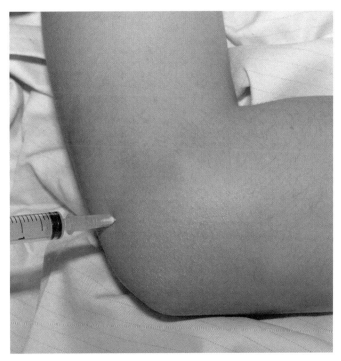

Fig. 3 Right elbow: With the elbow flexed at about 90° the needle is inserted from the posterior aspect lateral to the olecranon.

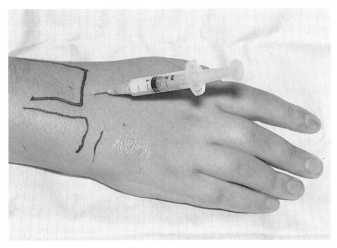

Fig. 4 Right wrist: The needle is inserted just distal to the end of the radius angled proximally at about 60° to the dorsal aspect of the forearm, with the wrist slightly palmar flexed.

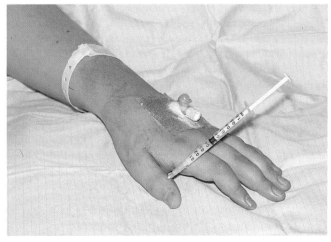

Fig. 5 Left thumb, Inter-phalangeal joint: The joint is entered from the ulnar aspect. Palpating the joint while passively flexing and extending the joint will help localize the joint space.

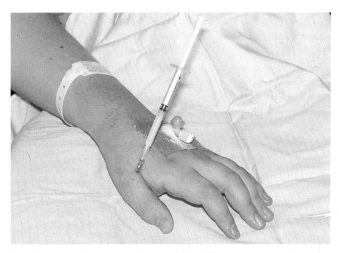

Fig. 6 Left thumb, metacarpophalangeal joint: The joint is entered from the ulnar aspect near the webspace.

encouraging, but again this approach is really only suitable for older children or adolescents who are having a maximum of 2 or 3 joints injected.

Older children and adolescents will tolerate having some joints injected with only local analgesia. Knees and shoulders are particularly easy to do with local anaesthetic only, but wrists, ankles and fingers may be more difficult and quite uncomfortable. A recent potential advance is the use of dermal anaesthesia using lidocaine iontophoresis. Early anecdotal evidence (communication from Dr Kimura) using a commercially available product (see www.iomed.com/prod-numby.html) suggests efficacy even in very young children, negating the need for sedation in some.

It is important to stress that when sedation is used, trained nursing staff, all appropriate monitoring procedures (including ideally pulse oximetry), and resuscitation equipment must be in place. If undue sedation or paradoxical hyperactivity occurs with midazolam it can be reversed with flumazenil. It should not be used routinely to reverse sedation.

Dosage of midazolam

• 0.5mg/kg orally 30 minutes to one hour prior to joint injection.

Dosage of flumazenil

• 0.01mg/kg intravenously. Can be repeated twice if needed.

Which corticosteroid preparations?

TH is the best corticosteroid to use for intra-articular injection, but at the present time availability of this preparation is very limited. Triamcinolone acetonide (TA) is a reasonable alternative but is not nearly as effective even in larger doses [2]. Its lesser efficacy is due to the fact that it is a much more soluble drug, and diffuses out of the joint more rapidly, than the poorly soluble TH. There is also anecdotal evidence that corticosteroid toxicity, such as mood change, is more common with the acetonide salt. It is generally agreed among paediatric rheumatologists that more soluble short acting agents such as methylprednisolone acetate and hydrocortisone do not have a role in joint injections in children.

Dosage of triamcinolone hexacetonide

There is no convincing evidence about the optimal dose of TH, but the following doses have become generally accepted:

- Large joints (knees, shoulders, hips): 1 mg/kg/joint.
- Medium joints (ankles, wrists, subtalars): 0.5 mg/kg/joint.
- Temporomandibular joint: 0.25mg/kg/joint.
- Small joints (PIPs, MCPs): 0.2–0.4 mg *total dose* per joint .

These dosages can safely be rounded up or down and should be doubled when using TA. Although some paediatric rheumatologists restrict the total dose injected into any given joint, there is some limited evidence that smaller doses are less effective than larger doses [1]. No absolute limit to the total dose that should be used is therefore recommended at present, but it should be appreciated that the more corticosteroid that is injected the more will be absorbed, and therefore potentially cause systemic side-effects [5]. This problem however is always likely to be less with intra-articular injection than with oral or intravenous administration. Also larger volumes may possibly contribute to leak into the subcutaneous tissues and the development of subcutaneous atrophy.

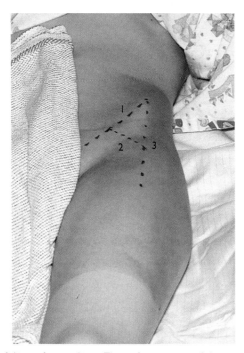

Fig. 7 Left hip surface markings: The surface anatomy of the joint is marked as follows: (1) Line 1 is drawn between the pubic tubercle and anterior superior iliac spine. (2) At the midpoint of line, 1 line 2 is dropped perpendicularly. (3) Line 3 is drawn from the anterior superior iliac spine along the axis of the femur to join line 2.

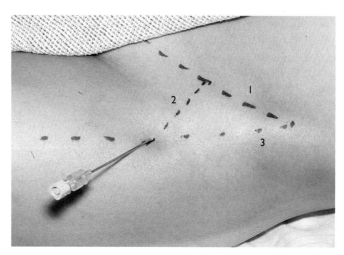

Fig. 8 Left hip needle insertion: (1) The junction of line 2 and 3 is where the needle is inserted angled at about 60° to the skin and directed towards the midpoint of line 1. (2) The needle is pushed until it just touches the bone, and is then withdrawn about a millimetre. (3) The needle position should be checked with fluoroscopy or plain X-ray.

Side-effects

Systemic corticosteroid side-effects.

Facial flushing, increased appetite, and mild dysphorias, are seen occasionally. Less commonly weight gain and striae formation can occur. These side-effects are seen more commonly when a large number of joints are injected. Long-term side-effects such as interference with growth and osteoporosis are extremely unusual.

Subcutaneous atrophy

This will occasionally occur even in the hands of the most skilled operator (studies quote rates between 2.3% and 8.3%) [1,2,6]. Ensuring correct needle placement and limiting the volume of drug given into an individual joint will reduce the occurrence of this side-effect. The atrophic areas will remain abnormal for several years but 4–5 years after injection areas of atrophy have usually resolved, though there may be a persistent depigmentation.

Sepsis

There is a potential risk of introducing sepsis into the joint but as long as sterile precautions are taken this is an extremely rare occurrence. Two large centres have not seen this occur in over 8 years of regular joint injection programmes.

Chemical synovitis

The crystalline structure of the injected corticosteroids uncommonly triggers a chemical synovitis. This may result in pain and swelling of the affected joint for 12–24 hours after the injection. The differential diagnosis includes joint sepsis, but symptoms usually occur earlier with chemical synovitis and fever is not present.

Calcification

Intra or periarticular calcification occurs as a late complication of intra-articular corticosteroid injection in about 5% of injected joints [6,7]. It only very rarely causes any symptoms.

Cartilage growth disturbance

If the needle is incorrectly placed, an injection of corticosteroid directly into cartilage can cause significant interference with cartilage growth and its development. This is an extremely rare occurrence.

Avascular necrosis

There are reports that avascular necrosis may result from intra-articular injections into hip joints. Our own experience of over 400 injected hips and other recently published data has failed to demonstrate that this is a significant risk [8]. In the original reports patients were put into traction following joint injection and this may, perhaps, have been a contributing factor for the avascular necrosis.

Frequency of re-injections

There is some controversy about how often joints may be injected. The adult literature suggests that there should be a 3–6 month gap between injections and that any single joint should only be done 4–5 times. We have not followed this practice and we have injected joints whenever they have been swollen. If the response is of little clinical benefit then we have not repeated the procedure but for some patients even 2–3 months short term relief is worthwhile. We have injected some joints over 15 times without any obvious side-effects, and others have published similar results [7].

Procedure

- Patients and their parents/guardian should always have the procedure explained to them in detail so they are enabled to give properly informed consent.

- All children receiving sedation should be fasting for at least 5 hours prior to sedation. Clear fluids may be given up to 2 hours prior to sedation.

- 1 hour prior to joint injection Eutetic Mixture of Local Anaesthetics (EMLA) or similar should be applied to the injection site.

- 30 minutes to 1 hour prior to the injection midazolam should be given orally.

- If sedation or local anesthesia alone is being used, the environment should be "child friendly" and conducive to minimizing the child's distress. The presence of a child life worker (play therapist) is very helpful. The presence of parents is usually valuable, but they should be coached in how to be supportive to the child and not increase the child's anxiety.

- The skin should be adequately sterilized usually with chlorhexadine or poviodine containing preparation. Operators should have properly clean hands and be wearing sterile gloves. Gowns and masks are not necessary.

- Local anaesthesia with 1% lidocaine is helpful for children not having a general anesthetic. It is not necessary to add local anaesthetic to the corticosteroid preparation, and in fact the increased injection volume may increase the risk of subcutaneous atrophy.

- The smallest sized needle should be used whilst still able to obtain appropriate access to the joint, for example this means:
  1. 21 gauge needles for knees, ankles and subtalar joints
  2. 23 gauge needles for wrists, temporomandibular joints
  3. 25 gauge or smaller for PIPs and MCPs

- It is preferable to aspirate the joint prior to injection of the corticosteroid but it is not essential. Obtaining synovial fluid does confirm that the needle is appropriately situated in the joint. It is probably preferable not to have the joint completely dry as a small amount of residual fluid helps to distribute the steroid preparation around the joint.

- As the corticosteroid is being injected into the joint we would recommend giving about 10% of the total volume, waiting for a few seconds and then giving a further 10%, waiting a few seconds again, etc., until the full dose has been given. An injection should never be forced, because if force is necessary it is likely that the needle placement is incorrect. Once the injection has been completed the needle

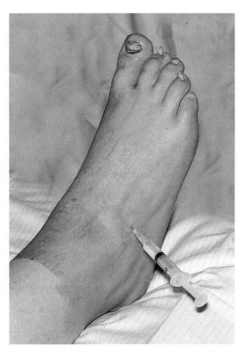

Fig. 9 Right subtalar joint: The needle is inserted just distal to the lateral malleolus and angled towards the base of the first toe. There is often a distinct feeling of decreased resistance as the joint is entered.

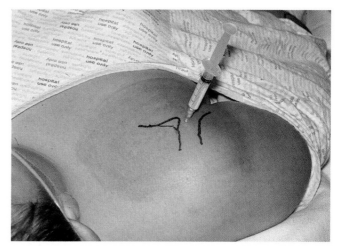

Fig. 10 Right shoulder: The humeral head and coracoid process are marked. The needle is inserted from the anterior position just lateral to the coracoid process.

should be left *in situ* for 30 seconds to allow some of the drug to be absorbed thus reducing the risk of leakage. Once the needle has been removed it may be helpful to gently rub the tissues around where the needle was placed to try and obliterate the track.

· Image intensifiers or ultrasonography can be used to ensure correct needle placement. This is particularly useful in deep joints such as hip or sub-talar and small joints such as PIPs and MCPs. With experience this is not always necessary.

· If several joints are being injected mild opiates can be added to the anaesthetic so the patient does not wake with any pain. Some centres routinely give acetaminophen both pre-injection and for one or two doses post-injection to help minimise any pain as a consequence of the procedure.

Post-injection management

Our current practice is to suggest that the patient rest the injected joints for 12–24 hours post injection. In the past we have splinted joints for 48 hours but no longer do so, unless we have applied a splint to help correct a flexion contracture. With our change of practice we have not noticed any diminution of the efficacy of the joint injection or an increase in side effects. In adult practice, patients often have their joints injected in outpatient clinic and then return to normal activity immediately afterwards; this may in fact be appropriate for children as well, thus minimizing disruption to their schooling and/or social life. Families should have clear instructions on who to contact if they have any concerns post injection.

References

1. Allen, R.C., Gross, K.R., Laxer, R.M., Malleson, P.N., Beauchamp, R.D., Petty, R.E. Intraarticular triamcinolone hexacetonide in the management of chronic arthritis in children. *Arthritis Rheum* 1986;29:997–1001.

2. Zulian, F., Martini, G., Gobber, D., Plebani, M., Zacchello, F., Manners, P. Triamcinolone acetonide and hexacetonide intra-articular treatment of symmetrical joints in juvenile idiopathic arthritis: a double-blind trial. *Rheumatology* (Oxford) 2004;43:1288–1291.

3. Breit, W., Frosch, M., Meyer, U., Heinecke, A., Ganser, G. A subgroup-specific evaluation of the efficacy of intraarticular triamcinolone hexacetonide in juvenile chronic arthritis. *J Rheumatol* 2000;27:2696–2702.

4. Ravelli, A., Manzoni, S.M., Viola, S., Pistorio, A., Ruperto, N., Martini, A. Factors affecting the efficacy of intraarticular corticosteroid injection of knees in juvenile idiopathic arthritis. *J Rheumatol* 2001;28:2100–2102.

5. Huppertz, H.I., Pfüller, H. Transient suppression of endogenous cortisol production after intraarticular steroid therapy for chronic arthritis in children. *J Rheumatol* 1997;24:1833–1837.

6. Job-Deslandre, C., Menkes, C.J. Complications of intra-articular injections of triamcinolone hexacetonide in chronic arthritis in children. *Clin Exp Rheumatol* 1990;8:413–416.

7. Sparling, M., Malleson, P., Wood, B., Petty, R. Radiographic followup of joints injected with triamcinolone hexacetonide for the management of childhood arthritis. *Arthritis Rheum* 1990;33:821–826.

8. Neidel, J., Boehnke, M., Kuster, R.M. The efficacy and safety of intraarticular corticosteroid therapy for coxitis in juvenile rheumatoid arthritis. *Arthritis Rheum* 2002;46:1620–1628.

Index

Note: Page numbers in *italics* refer to figures and tables

acetaminophen 362, *363*
acetylsalicylic acid 50, 373, 420, 421, 422
Achilles tendon 14, *15*, 140
   see also Enthesitis-Related Arthritis
achondroplasia 191, *192*
acne 61, 71, 123
ACR Pediatric Outcome Variables 332–3
   see also core outcome variables
acro/acromesomelic dysplasia *193*, 197–8
Activities of Daily Living (ADL) 362, 384, 387–8
active arthritis, defined 301
active joint count 330
acute haemorrhagic oedema of infancy (AHE) 54, *55*
acute inflammatory rheumatic syndromes 49–62, *50*
acute lymphoblastic leukaemia (ALL) 155–6, *156*
acute phase reactants 20
acute rheumatic fever (ARF) *32*, *33*, 49–51, *50*, *51*
Addison disease 162
adenosine deaminase deficiency 196–7
adherence 313, 319–20, *320*, 337, *338*, 418
adhesion molecules 274
adjunctive therapies 397–402
adjuvant arthritis (AA) 292, 294
adolescent rheumatology services 315–29
   adherence 319–20, *320*
   administrative support 325
   advocacy issues for parents 322
   collaboration of adult and paediatric services 325
   confidentiality issues 319
   consultation dynamics 322
   cost implications of transitionalm care 326
   essentials of transitional care service 323–6, *323*
   exercise 318
   health education/promotion 317–18, *318*
   involvement of young people 325
   need for 316–17, *317*
   nutrition 318–19
   primary care involvement 325
   school issues 320
   self-determination and self-advocacy 321–2
   sexuality issues 319
   substance use 319
   transition and disease characteristics 325–6
   transition clinic models 322–3
   transition concept 315–16, *316*
   work issues 320–1
advocacy 321–2, 340–2, 387–8
affected sibling pairs studies 280–1
agammaglobulinemia 74, 168
AIDS *82*
   see also HIV
air-borne pollution 290
alcaptonuria 166
alendronate 400–1
algorithms 24–8, *25–31*
   child with back pain 28, *29–30*
   child with fever and musculoskeletal pain/dysfunction
      24, *25–6*
   child with musculoskeletal pain/dysfunction following
      trauma 28, *31*

child with musculoskeletal pain/dysfunction without
   fever 24–8, *27–8*
   pharmacological treatment of *368*, *370*, *371*, *372*
allergic diseases, hygiene hypothesis293–4
allodynia 150
allogeneic stem cell transplantation 437
alopecia 91, *92*
ALPS 168, 170
amoxicillin 77
amyloidosis 118, 119, 122, 171, 217, 241,286
amyopathic dermatomyositis (JDM sinemyositis) 104–5
anakinra *432*, 433
analgesics 362–4, *363*
ancillary health care professionals 306,*306*
anaemia 92–3, 393, 397–8
aneurysms 58, *59*, 108
angiitis *see* vasculitis
angioneurotic oedema 55–6
ankle
   examination 14–16, *14*, *15*
   imaging *67*, *71*
   injection 442
   subtalar joint 15,140, 411, 445
   surgery 411
   see also foot
ankylosing spondylitis (AS) 53, 206–8, 214
   see also Enthesitis-Related Arthritis
antalgic postures 382
anterior knee pain syndrome (patello-femoral syndrome)
   13, *14*, 138
anticardiolipin antibodies 88, 100
antigen-specific immune therapy 437–8
anti-DEK antibody 227, 248
anti-IL1 agent 119, 122, 123
anti-malarial *see* hydroxychloroquine
antineutrophilic cytoplasmic antibodies (ANCA) 109
antinuclear antibodies (ANA) 21, 95–6, 100, 226,
   246–7, 248
antiphospholipid antibody syndrome 100, *100*
antistreptococcal antibodies *see* streptococcus
anti-TNF therapy 302, 371, 372, 432–3
anxiety 315–28, 343–56, 357–66
apophyseal ring fracture 142
apophysitis
   of foot 140
   of hip 134
apoptosis 170, 275
arachnodactyly 181, 186
arteritis *see* vasculitis
arthrocentesis 19, 364
arthrodesis 405, 407, 411
arthrogryposis multiplex congenita *182*, 186
arthroplasty 405–6, 407, 408, 409, 411
arthroscopy 405, 410
   articular disease activity, measurement 330
ASOT *see* streptococcus
aspirin *36*, 49, 100, 373
atlanto-axial subluxation 404–5, *404*
attachment (psychosocial) 347
avascular necrosis *35*, 132—4

and Cushing syndrome 162
and Gaucher 166
and haemoglobinopathies *159*
   see also osteonecrosis
auranofin 378, *424*
autoimmune lymphoproliferative syndrome(ALPS) 168,
   170, *170*
autoimmunity, mechanisms of 291–3, *291*
autoinflammatory diseases 116–29
   defined 116
autologous haematopoietic stem cell transplantation
   (auto-SCT) 434–7,438
   clinical experience 434–5, *434*, *435*
   immunological reconstitution 435
   and pathogenesis of MAS 435–7, *436*
autosomal dominant periodic fever with amyloidosis 122
axial skeleton, surgery 404–5, *404*
azathioprine 375, 378, 422

B cells 276–7, *276*
back
   examination of cervical spine 7, *8*
   examination of lumbar spine 16, 17
   musculoskeletal syndromes localized to 140–2
   pain, child with 28, *29–30*, 140–2
bacterial DNA 292
Baker cyst 12, 139, *139*, 175, 218
band keratopathy 122, 124, 164
   see also uveitis
Bartonella Henselae see cat-scratch disease
bayonet deformity 406
Beau lines 56, *58*
Beal Syndrome 182
Behçet syndrome *34*, 110–11, *215*
Beighton Score 131, *132*
benign limb pains 131–2, *131*, *132*
benign viral myositis *33*, 80
beta-2-microglobulin amyloidosis 171
biceps tenosynovitis *219*
biological agents 374, *375*, 426–7, 432–3, *432*, 438
bipartite patella 136–7
birth control 240, 376
bisphosphonates 400–1
Blau syndrome (familial granulomatous arthritis) 125,
   125, *215*
blindness *120*, 123, 195, 257
   see also uveitis
Bloomstrand dysplasia 197
blood disorders 159–61, *159*
bone age 191
bone cyst 172, *173*
bone density
   decreased *179*, 198–9
   increased 180, *193*, 199
   measurement of 214, 237, 394, 399
bone disease
   congenital and inherited 179–201
   metabolic 162–4, *163*
bone dysplasia *29*, *36*, 133
   see also osteochondrodysplasias

bone formation *180*, 181
bone infections
    acute and chronic 63–85
    less common 80–4, *82*
bone marrow biopsy 155
bone marrow transplant *see* allogenic and autologous
    stem cell transplant
bone mass 318, 399, 400–1
bone scan 66, *66*, *73*, 150
bone tumours, primary 171–5
    benign 171–4, *171*, *172*, *173*, *174*
    malignant *171*, 174–5, *175*
Borage seeds 395
Borrelia burgdorferi 75, 151, 292
boutonniere deformity 88, *89*, 408
brittle bone disease *see* Ostogenesis Imperfecta (OI)
Brighton criteria 132, *132*
Brodie abscess 70, *70*, *71*
brucellosis 80
Bruton agammaglobulinemia 168
bunion bursitis *see* Hallux Valgus
bystander activation 291, *291*, 292
bystander suppression 291, *291*

C-reactive protein (CRP) 20, 50, 64, 212
    see also erythrocyte sedimentation rate
CACP 186–7, *187*, *188*
Caffey disease *see* infantile cortical hyperostosis
Caffey-Silverman syndrome 125–7, *126*
calcaneus 14, 65, 140, 411
    see also enthesis; enthesitis related arthritis
café-au-lait spots 172, 175
CAHP *see* Childhood Arthritis Health Profile
calcific periarthritis 171
calcinosis 103, *104*
calcitonin 401
calcium intake 393–4, *394*, 400
camptodactyly 186
camptodactyly-arthropathy-coxa vara-
    pericarditis syndrome (CACP, arthropathy-
    campodactyly syndrome) 186–7, *187*, *188*
Campylobacter 32, 260
Camurati–Engelman syndrome 199
cancer *see* malignancies
carpal-tarsal osteolysis 199–200
carpal tunnel syndrome 171, 187, 240
CARRA *see* Childhood Arthritis and Rheumatology
    Research Alliance
cartilage *180*, 181
    disorganized development *194*
cartilage-hair hypoplasia 197
cartilage tumours 171–5
cataracts
    and CINCA 122
    and Conradi–Hunermann syndrome 198
    and corticosteroids *96*, 374
    and Fabry disease 167
    and idiopathic osteolysis 194
    and Lowe oculocerebrorenal syndrome 166
    and MPS 182
    and multicentric reticulohistiocytosis 167
    and oligoarthritis 124, *230*,
    and pseudoHurler 190
    and rhizomelic chondrodysplasia 198
    and Stickler dysplasia 195
    and stippled epiphyses *193*
    and Winchester syndrome 200
    and uveitis 230, 257
'catcher's crouch' 79
cat-scratch disease 69, 81, *82*
ceftriaxone 77
cerebrovascular accident (CVA)
cervical spine
    examination 6, *7*
    surgery 404–5, *404*
Charcot disease *see* congenital indifference to pain
CHAQ *see* Childhood Health Assessment Questionnaire
chemokines 274, 284

child abuse 145, *145*, 152
Childhood Arthritis and Rheumatology
    Research Alliance (CARRA) 420
Childhood Arthritis Health Profile (CAHP) 331,
    334–5, *334*
Childhood Health Assessment
    Questionnaire (CHAQ) 331
chlorambucil 217, 378
chondrodysplasia punctata 198
chondrolysis of hip 134, *135*
chondroma 172–3
chondromalacia patellae *see* anterior knee painsyndrome;
    patellofemoral syndrome
chorea 49–51, 95, 100
chronic cutaneous lupus erythematosus
    (CCLE) 98–9, *98*
chronic fatigue syndrome (CFS) 151, *151*
chronic infantile neurological cutaneous
    and articular syndrome (CINCA)
    (neonatal onset multisystem inflammatory disease
    (NOMID)) 120, 122–3, *123*, *124*, 215
chronic non-bacterial osteomyelitis (CNO) *see*
chronic recurrent multifocal osteomyelitis
chronic recurrent multifocal osteomyelitis (CRMO) 33,
    71, *71*, *72*
Churg–Strauss syndrome 35, 111
CIAS1 mutations 119–123, *120*
CINCA *see* chronic infantile neurological cutaneous and
    articular syndrome
classification of childhood arthritis 205–9
clavicle
    in CRMO *33*, 71–2, *126*
    osteomyelitis 65
clear-cell sarcoma 176
clinical remission, defined 301–2
clinical trials 313, 414–30
    adaptive randomization 418
    allocation bias 415
    analysis of results 416–17
    blinding 415–16
    and compliance 418
    cross-over studies 418
    developmental differences in response 417
    disease evaluation 332–3
    elements 414–17
    ethical difficulties with consent 418
    and experimental therapies 431
    future 429
    history of in medicine 418–19
    improvement criteria for outcomes 332–3, 416
    in JIA 420–9, 431
    lack of acceptability 417, 418
    measurement bias 415
    more acceptable designs 418
    more powerful designs 418
    multi-center networks 418, 419–20, 431
    need for 414
    objectivity 414
    outcome measurement 415–16
    and pharmacokinetics 417
    problems with 417–18
    prospective data collection 415
    random allocation to experimental/controlgroups 415
    randomized placebo phase design 418
    and rarity of diseases 417
    and regression to mean 414
    representative sampling 415
    sample size calculation 417
    type I error (false positive error) 416–17
    type II error (false negative error) 417
    variability in response 416
clinodactyly 186
Clutton joints *32*, *82*, 83
clotting factors 160, 216
coagulation 160, 161, 180
    see also macrophage activation syndrome
CNO *see* chronic recurrent multifocal osteomyelitis
coccidiomycosis 60, 83

Cochrane, Archie 419
Cochrane collaboration 419
codeine 363
coeliac disease *36*, 157–9
Cogan syndrome 111
cognitive-behavioural treatment 360–2
cognitive development 317, 346–7, *347*, 358
colchicine 118
colitis 3, 4
    see also ulcerative colitis
collagen, type II 195–6, 427–8, 437–8
common variable immunodeficiency (CVID) 167–9
complement
    and acute phase reactants 20
    drug reactions, serum sickness 55–6
    and hepatitis viruses 79
    in HSP 53
    in SLE 20, 34, 87, 90, 92–6,
    in Systemic Arthritis 212
    in Oligoarthritis 227, 229
complement deficiencies 168, *168–9*
complementary/alternative medicine 337, 364, 395
compliance *see* adherence
concrete operational stage 317, 346, *347*
confidentiality issues 319
congenital contractural arachnodactyly (Beal syndrome)
    182, 186
congenital indifference to pain (Charcot disease)
    36, 143, *143*, *144*
conjunctival hyperemia 56, *56*, *57*
conjunctivitis 3
    and adenovirus *78*
    and ADPF 122
    and Behçet syndrome 110
    and ERA 261, 263
    and Kawasaki disease *33*, *59*
    and reactive arthritis *41*, 52
    and relapsing polychondritis 112
    and SLE 95
    and TRAPS 119, *120*, 121, *121*
    and Wegener granulomatosis *101*
connective tissue disorders, congenital
    and inherited 179–201
    see also major rheumatic diseases
Conradi–Hunermann syndrome 198, *198*
contractures 4, *4*, 6, 186–201
    in Blau syndrome 124
    in CINCA 123
    in diabetic cheiroarthropathy 161–2, *161*
    of elbows 9
    in eosinophilic fasciitis 108
    in Farber disease 167
    of hips *11*, 17
    in juvenile dermatomyositis 104
    in Kashin–Beck and Mselini joint disease 161–2
    in localized scleroderma 107
    in metabolic storage disease 166
conversion disorder 152
core set outcome variables 332––3, *332*, 416
corticosteroids 372, 374
    in acute inflammatory rheumatic syndromes 54, 61
    clinical trials 422, *423*, 425, *426*
    and growth failure 219–20, *220*, 393, 398, 399
    intra-articular injections,
    in major rheumatic diseases 91–2, 96–7, *96*, *97*
    mechanism of action 374
    and osteonecrosis 89, 133–4, *133*
    in periodic fever syndromes 117
    role in JIA 374
    systemic administration 374
    toxicity 374
    see also specific drugs
contraception 240, 318, 376
contraceptives *see* oral contraceptives
corneal opacities *see* cataracts
costochondritis 93
coup de sabre 107–8, *107*
COX inhibitors 373, 377

coxa vara
  and CACP 186–7
  and Schmid type metaphyseal dysplasia 197
  and Schwachman–Diamond syndrome *192*, 197
  and slipped capital femoral epiphysis 134
CpG motifs 292
cracking joints 145
C-reactive protein (CRP) 20, 64, 212
CREST syndrome 35, 108
cryoglobulins *21, 106*
cryoglobulinemia *32*, 79, *106*
CRMO *see* chronic recurrent multifocal
  osteomyelitis
Crohn disease 53, 111, 125, 263
  see also inflammatory bowel disease
cryopyrin *120*, 127
CT scan *20*, 21–2
  in child with fever and musculoskeletal pain *26*
  in child with musculoskeletal pain and trauma *31*
  in ERA *261, 262*
  in Ewing sarcoma *175*
  in osteoid osteoma *36*, 174, *174*
  in psoas abscess 80
  in rhabdomyosarcoma 176, *177*
  in systemic sclerosis *35*
  in tarsal coalition 140, *140*
Cushing syndrome 162
cutaneous lupus
  chronic cutaneous lupus 98–9
  subacute cutaneous lupus *37, 42*, 99
cutis laxa 185, *185*
CVID *see* common variable immunodeficiency
cyclic neutropenia 117, *120*
cyclooxygenase (COX) 373, 377
cyclophosphamide 371, *375*, 377, 427
cyclosporin 371, *375*, 377–8, 427, *428*
cystic fibrosis (CF) 157, *159*
cysts
  Baker 12, *22*, 23, 139, 175, 218, *219, 247*
  biceps *219*
cytokines
  balance within network in inflammation 284, *284*
  and erythropoietin 397
  genes 283–5
  imbalance and T cells 275
  see also IL-1, IL-2 etc.

dactylitis 160, 252, *253*
deafness
  and Cogan syndrome 86, 111
  and CINCA *120*, 122
  and immune mediated hearing loss *111*
  and Muckle Wells syndrome *37*, 119, *120*, 122
  and mucopolysaccharidoses *182, 183*
  and osteochondrodysplasias 191, *192*, 195
  and osteogenesis imperfecta *199*
DEK 227, 248
dendritic cells 276, *276*
depression 147, 148, 344
dermatographism *see* Koebner phenomenon
dermatomyositis *34*, 100–4, *101*
  amyopathic 104–5
  clinical manifestations *45*, 89–91, 102–3, *102*
  course, treatment, and prognosis 103–4
  diagnosis 100, *102*
  laboratory findings 103
  late complications 103, *104*
  sine myositis (amyopathic dermatomyositis) 104–5
desquamation 56, *58*
dermatosis, inflammatory 61, *61*
diabetes mellitus 161–2, *161*
diabetic cheiroarthropathy 161–2, *161*
diagnostic tests 19–21, *20–1*
  positive and negative predictive value 19–20
  sensitivity 19
  specificity 19
dialysis-related arthritis 171
diclofenac sodium 420–1

diet *see* nutrition
dieticians 306
differential diagnosis, arthritis 24–48
diffuse idiopathic pain *36*, 147, 148–50, *148, 149*
DiGeorge syndrome 169–70
discitis *33*, 69–70, *69, 70*
discoid lupus erythematosus (DLE) 98–9, *98*
discoid meniscus 138, *138*
disease activity
  defined 302
  measurements 330–2
disease damage
  defined 302
  measurements 332, *332*
disease evaluation 330–6
disease improvement/worsening,
  quantification 332–3, *332*
disease modifying anti-rheumatic drugs (DMARDs)
  368, 372, 374–8, *375*, 422–5, *424–5*
disease-specific clinics 311, *311*
disk herniation 142
distal arthrogryposis 186
distal inter-phalangeal joints,
  examination 7, *8*
DMARDs 239, 240, *363*, 367–380
doxycycline 77, 169
drug-induced lupus (DIL) 99–100, *99*
drug reactions 55–6
dry synovitis 247–8, *248*
dual-energy X-ray absorptiometry 214, 237, 394, 399
dwarfism 191, 192
Duchenne muscular dystrophy
dysostosis multiplex 189
dysplasias See bone dysplasias
DXA scan 214, 237, 394, 399

ear
  in polychondritis *35, 86*, 111–2
  see also deafness
early disease, defined 302
educational issues 337–42
  and advocacy 340–2
  educational and support organizations 340, *341*
  education of others involved with family 339–40
  health education/promotion 317–18, *318*
  importance of education for patient and family
    337–42, *338*
  and physiotherapy and occupational therapy 385
  progression of educational needs 339, *339*
  special needs 340–2
Ehlers–Danlos syndrome (EDS) *34*, 161, 181–5, *182, 184, 185*
elbow
  corticosteroid injection *443*
  examination 8–9, *9, 10*
  little leaguer's elbow 142–3
  musculoskeletal syndromes localized to 142–3
  overuse injuries 142–3
  surgery 405–6, *407*
electromyography (EMG) 20, 21, 98, 102–3
emboli
  pulmonary 93–4
  septic 64
  thromboembolism 92, 167, 189
  see also antiphospholipid syndrome
embryopathy 198
EMG *see* electromyography
Emery–Dreifus muscular dystrophy *182*, 187–8
enchondroma 172–3, *173*
endochondral bone formation 181
endocrine disorders 161–2
Enthesitis Related Arthritis (ERA) *35*, *148*, 259–64
  acute anterior uveitis 263
  aortic valve insufficiency 263
  arthritis 260–1, *261*
  classification 208, 259, *259*, *260*, 268
  clinical features 260–1, *260*
  complications 262–3, *262*

enthesitis 260
  epidemiology 259–60, *260*
  etiology and pathogenesis 260
  examination of foot and ankle 14
  investigations 261–2, *261, 262*
  monitoring 262
  pharmacological treatment 371–2, *371*, 377
  prognosis 263
  spinal fusion 262, *263*
  systemic manifestations 261
environmental factors in pathogenesis 290–8
  climate 290
  evidence from animal models 294
  gut microbial environment 294, 295
  heat shock proteins as regulators 294–5
  hygiene hypothesis 293–4
  immunizations 292–3
  interactions between microbial environment and
    immune system 291–3, *291*
  nutrition 290
  socioeconomic factors 290
eosinophilic fasciitis 108
eosinophilic granuloma 173, *173*
eosinophilic synovitis 139
epiphyseal dysplasia *192*, 196, *196*
epithelioid sarcoma 176
epitope spreading 437
Epstein–Barr virus (EBV) 20, 77, *78*, 435
  and lymphoma 376
  and molecular mimicry 273, 291–2
episcleritis 95, 121, 240
ERA *see* Enthesitis Related Arthritis
erythema
  marginatum *33, 37, 38*, 49–51, 224
  migrans 76–7, *76*
  multiforme *42*, 55–6
  nodosum (EN) *43*, 60, *60*
erythrocyte sedimentation rate (ESR) 20, 58, 212
erythropoietin 397–8
ESR *see* erythrocyte sedimentation rate
established disease, defined 302
etanercept *375*, 426–7, 432, *432*, 433
evaluation
  clinical skills 3–18
  disease evaluation 330–6
  investigations and imaging 19–23
EULAR (European League against Rheumatism)
  classification *206*, 282
  and Oligoarthritis 223
  and Polyarthritis 234, *234*
  and Systemic Arthritis 213
  and Undifferentiated Arthritis 265–6
Evans syndrome 93
evening primrose 395
Ewing sarcoma 174–5, *175, 176*
eye
  in Behçet disease *34*
  in enthesitis related arthritis 263
  and hypermobility *132*
  in juvenile dermatomyositis 100
  in Kawasaki disease *57*
  and periodic fever syndromes *120*, 122, 124–5
  ophthalmologist 307, 312
  and polyarthritis 240, 248
  see also uveitis
exercise 318, 398
exostosis 174, *193, 194*, 198
experimental therapies 431–41

Fabry disease 167, *167*
familial cold autoinflammatory syndrome (FCAS) 119, *120*
familial expansile osteolysis 200
familial haemophagocytic
  lymphohistiocytosis (FHL) 435–6
familial joint laxity *182*, 185
familial Mediterranean fever (FMF) *34*, 117–18, *117, 118, 120*, 215

family
    challenges faced by 343–50
    education for 337–42, *338*, 385
    'enmeshment' 150
    history 4
    impact of challenges on 350–3
    psychosocial adjustment 343–56
    support for psychosocial needs 353–4
Farber disease 167, *167*
FAS *see* fetal alcohol syndrome
fascia
    plantar 14, 260, *261*, 262, *262*
fasciitis
    eosinophilic 108
fatigue
    adolescent 317–8
    in chronic fatigue syndrome 147, 151, *151*
    in fibromyalgia *28*, 148–50
    in HIDS 119
    in idiopathic pain syndromes *28, 36*, 148–50
    in juvenile dermatomyositis *101*
    in JIA *79, 87*, 261
    in Lyme disease *76, 77*, 151
    and psychological aspects 348–9
    in rheumatic disease evaluation 3, *30*
    in SLE 86, *87*, 92
    in vasculitis *101*, 108, 110
    see also physiotherapy and occupational therapy
fatty acids, unsaturated 395
Felty syndrome 93, 240
ferritin *20, 36, 59*, 92
    and MAS 212, 216, *217*, 331
fetal alcohol syndrome (FAS) *182*, 186
fever
    acute fever and rash *51*
    febrile syndromes 116–23, *120*
    and musculoskeletal pain/dysfunction, child with 24,
        25–6
fibrillin gene *see* Marfan syndrome
fibroblast growth factor 23,164
fibroblast growth factor receptor genes 191
fibroblasts *276, 277*
fibrocortical defects 172
fibrodysplasia ossificans progressiva *182*, 188–9, *188, 189*
fibromyalgia (FMS, diffuse idiopathic pain) 147, 148–50,
    148, 149
fibromatosis, juvenile *see* juvenile hyaline
fibrous dysplasia 171–2
fifth disease *see* parvovirus arthritis
fingers
    acroosteolysis 199, *200*
    arachnodactyly
        and Beal syndrome *182*, 186
        and Marfan syndrome 181, *182*
        definition *183*
    Boutonnière deformity 88, 125, *236*, 408
    camptodactyly
        see also CACP; fetal alcohol syndrome
    clubbing
        and cystic fibrosis 157
        definition *183*
        and hypertrophic osteoarthropathy *36, 107*, 157
        and hyperthyroidism 162
    flexion contractures
        and Beal syndrome 186
        and carpal-tarsal osteolysis 199
        and diabetes mellitus 161–162, *161*
        and JIA 6, 77, *248*
        and mucopolysaccharidoses 190
        and SLE 88
        and Williams syndrome 187
    frost bite *106, 107*, 143–4, *144*
    joints *see specific joints*
    nail fold capillaroscopy *20*, 103
    Raynaud phenomenon *3, 4, 106*
    and CREST *35*, 108
    and frostbite arthropathy 144, *144*
    and MCTD *34*, 97–8

and SLE *87*, 89, 91
and systemic sclerosis *35, 39, 40, 46*, 105–6, *105*
sausage *107 see* dactylitis
surgery 407–8
Swan neck deformity 88, *236*, 408
tenosynovitis *132*, 235, 245, 252, 408
trigger finger 408
fish oil *see* nutrition
Fisher, Ronald 419
flare, defined 302
flat feet
    and accessory bones 140
    and hypermobility 132
    in JIA 411
    in Marfan syndrome 181
    and tarsal coalition 140
flexibacteria infections 83–4
flexion contractures *see* contractures
flumazenil 443
fluoresence 164–5
FMF *see* Familial mediterranean fever
folic acid 376, 399–400, 425
folinic acid 399, 400
foot
    accessory bones 140
    examination 14–16, *15*
    flat foot *see* flat feet
    musculoskeletal syndromes localized to 139–40
    pain 139–40, *140*, 388
    pes cavus *182*
    pes planus *see* flat feet
    tarsal coalition 140
    surgery 411
foreign-body synovitis 81–3, *81, 83*
formal operational stage 317, 346, *347*
fractures *see* stress fractures, trauma, back pain
Freiberg disease 139
frostbite arthropathy 144, *144*
functional state
    assessment measures 331–2, *332*
    evaluation 17–18, *18*
    and physiotherapy and occupational therapy 382,
        382, 383, 386, 388–9, 390
    and psychosocial adjustment 351
fungal arthritis 83

gait
    antalgic 9
    assessment 9, 387
Gallium scan *26*, 69, 159, 213
gammalinoleic acid (GLA) 395
ganglion 175
gangrene 100, *106*
Gaucher disease *36*, 166, *166*
genes *see* genetic factors
gene therapy 437
genetic factors 280–9
    affected sibling pairs studies 280–1
    association studies 281
    candidate genes 282–6
    cytokine genes 283–5
    evidence for 280–1
    HLA class I associations 282–3
    HLA class II associations 283
    HLA linkage 283
    importance of clinical and biological homogeneity
        281–2
    investigatory methods 281–2
    linkage studies 281
    non-MHC genes 286
    and oligoarthritis 226, 229, 282–3, 285
    positive associations with non-HLA MHC genes
        285–6
    and statistical power 282
    transmission disequilibrium test 281
    twin studies 280
    whole genome scans 286
glaucoma 167, 189, 230, 257

glenohumeral joint *see* shoulder
glomerulonephritis
    and acute rheumatic fever 50
    and Henoch–Schönlein purpura (HSP) 54
    and microscopic polyarteritis 109
    and Wegener's granulomatosis *34*, 109
glucocorticoid *see* corticosteroids
glycogen storage disease 165
gold compounds 378, *424*
Goldbloom syndrome 125–6, *126*, 157
gonococcal arthritis–dermatitis–
    tenosynovitis syndrome *32*, 74–5
Gottron papules *102*, 103
gout 165–6, *165*
Gower sign 4, *5*, 103
granulocytopenia 93
granulomatous diseases 123–5
groin pain *see* hips
growing pains 131, *131, 148*
growth hormone 398–9
growth retardation 219–20, *220*, 318,
    392–3, 398–9
gut microbial environment 294, 295

haematuria 54, *55, 101*, 238
haemarthrosis 160–1, *160*
haemochromatosis 161
haemoglobin 21
haemoglobinopathy *see* sickle cell disease and
    thalassemia
haemophagocytosis *see* MAS; familial haemophagocytic
    lymphohistiocytosis)
haemophilia *34*, 160–1, *160*
Haemophilus influenzae 74
haemosiderin 160, 176, *34*
haemoptysis 109
hair loss *see* alopecia
hallux valgus 411
hamstring tightness 16, *17*
hand
    assessment 390
    examination 6–8, *8*
    musculoskeletal syndromes localized to 143–5
    surgery 407–8
    swelling 106, *107*
    see also finger
HAQ 213, *220*, 221, 240
    See also CHAQ
health assessment tools *see* CHAQ
health-related quality of life (HRQOL)
    measurement 333–5, *333, 334*, 359–60
hearing loss, autoimmune 111, *111*
    see also deafness; Cogan syndrome
heat shock proteins (HSP) 294–5, 437, 438, *438*
heel pain *3, 4, 41*, 140
heliotrope rash *38, 101, 102*
Henoch–Schönlein purpura (HSP) *33, 44*, 53–4, *53, 54,*
    55
hepatitis
    autoimmune *32*, 92
    A, virus 293
    prodrome *32*, 79
    and viral arthritis 79
hereditary febrile syndromes 116–23, *120*
HIDS *see* hyperimmunoglobulinemia D
Hill, Austin Bradford 419
hip
    apophysitis 134
    chondrolysis 134, *135*
    coxa vara 134, 186, 197
    examination 9–10, *11, 12*
    femoral epiphysis 132, 134, 410
    injection *144*
    Legg–Calve–Perthes *35*, 132, 133, *133*
    musculoskeletal syndromes localized
        to 132–5
    osteoarthritis 135, *135*
    osteonecrosis 132–4, *132, 133*

pain, child with 31, *40–1*, 132–5
  septic arthritis 72, 73, *73*
  snapping 135
  stress fractures 134–5
  surgery 403, 408–9, *409*
  transient demineralization 134
  transient synovitis (irritable hip, toxic synovitis of hip) 53
histocompatibility antigens (HLA)
  and enthesitis related arthritis 259, 260, 261
  HLA genes 282–3
  and Oligoarthritis 226, 229, 282–3
  and Psoriatic Arthritis 254
  and Rheumatoid Factor Negative Polyarthritis 245, 283
  and Rheumatoid Factor Positive Polyarthritis 239, 283
history-taking interview 3–4, *3, 4*
'hit and run' hypothesis 294
HIV 74, 80, *82, 169*
  see also AIDS
HLA-B27 259–260, *260*, 261, *261*, 266, 267, 269, 282, 283, 286
homocystinuria 181, *182*, 189
hospitalization 347–8
human growth hormone 398–9
Hunter syndrome *182*
Hurler syndrome *182*, 190, *190*
hydrocodone 362, *363*
hydrotherapy 307
hydroxychloroquine *375*, 377
hygiene hypothesis 293–4
hypercalcemia 162, *162*
hyperimmunoglobulinemia D syndrome (HIDS) 118–19, *118, 120*, 215
hyperlipoproteinemia, type II (familial hypercholesterolemia) 166
hypermobility syndromes, benign 35, 131–2, *131, 132, 148*
  see also joint laxity
hyperostosis syndromes 125–7, *126*
hyperparathyroidism 162
hypersensitivity vasculitis (HV) 55, *55*
hypertension 35, 94–5, 108, 374, 378
  pulmonary 93, 98, 100, 106
hyperthyroidism 162
hypertrophic osteoarthropathy 36, 157, *159*
  hereditary 157
  secondary 157
hyperuricemia 165–6, *165*
hypochondroplasia 191
hypogammaglobulinemia *see* immunodeficiency disorders
hypothyroidism 36, 162

ibuprofen *369*, 421–2
idiopathic multicentric osteolysis 200
idiopathic osteolysis *194*, 199–200, *199, 200*
idiopathic pain syndromes 147–54, *148*
idiopathic periosteal hyperostosis with dysproteinemia (Goldbloom syndrome) 125, *126*, 157
IL-1 284
IL-1 receptor antagonist (anakinra) *432*, 433
IL-6 285
IL-10 284–5
ILAR (International League of Associations for Rheumatism)
  classification 205–9, 233, *233*, 244, 252–3, *253*, 265, 268–70, *269*
iliac lymphadenitis, suppurative 80
iliopsoas abscess *see* retroperitoneal abscess
iliotibial band 139
imaging techniques 21–3, *22*
immune-stimulatory DNA sequences (ISS) 292
immune system, interactions with environment 291–5, *291*
immunizations 292–3
immunodeficiency disorders 36, 74, 167–70, *168, 169*, 196–7
immunopathology of joint 272–9
immunosuppressive agents 217, 376, 431

inactive disease, defined 301
indomethacin *369, 370*
infantile cortical hyperostosis (Caffey disease, Caffey–Silverman syndrome) 125–7, *126*
infantile systemic hyalinosis *182*, 188
infections
  arthritis syndromes associated with 28, *32*
  of bones and joints, acute and chronic 63–85
  and pathogenesis 291–4
  reactive arthritis
infertility 218
inflammatory bowel disease (IBD) 35, 52–3, 60, 89, *216*
inflammatory dermatoses associated with arthritis *61*
inflammatory rheumatic syndromes, acute 49–62, *50*
infliximab *375*, 432–3, *432*
inpatient service 308
  consultations 308
  facilities 308
  rheumatology inpatients 308
insulin-like growth factor I (IGF-1) 398, 399
insulin-like growth factor binding protein 3 (IGFBP-3) 398, 399
integrins 274
interferon 275, 283, 285, 292, 397
interleukin 260, 282, 284
intervertebral disc 22, 69, *70*
intra-articular corticosteroid
  injections *375*, 442–6
  anaesthesia and analgesia 442–3
  choice of preparation 443–4,
  clinical trials 425, *426*
  dosage 444
  frequency of re-injections 445
    in specific joints 410
  in oligoarthritis 368
  outpatient service 311–12
  pain management 364
  post injection management 446
  procedure 445–6
  side effects 444–5
intravenous immunoglobulin (IVIG) 169, 425–6
intravenous infusions 311–12
investigations 19–21, *20–1*
iridocyclitis *see* uveitis
iritis *see* uveitis
iron supplementation 393

Jaccoud arthropathy 88
Jansen dysplasia 197
jaw 227–228, *278*, 307, 403–405
  see also TMJ or temporomandibular joint
joint
  adaptive immune system and persistence of inflammation 274–5
  B cells 276–7
  cytokine imbalance and T cells 275
  dendritic cells 276
  fibroblasts 277
  histopathology 272–4, *273*
  immunopathology 272–9
  injection *see* intraarticular corticosteroid injection
  innate immunity and initiation of inflammation 274
joint aspiration 64, 73, 445
joint chart/mannequin 6, *6*
joint effusions, in osteomyelitis 64
joint infections
  acute and chronic 63–85
  less common 80–4, *82*
  macroscopic pathology 272, *272*
  mediators of damage 274–5
  monocytes and neutrophils 276
  role of immunoregulation 275–6
  T cell abnormalities 274–5
joint laxity
  benign hypermobility syndromes 35, 131–2, *131, 132, 148*

congenital and family syndromes 181–6, *182*, 191–200
joint pain and symptom patterns 31, *33–6*
joint protection 387, *388*
joints, physical examination 5–16, *5*
  inspection 5
  palpation 5
  range of motion 6, *6*
  strength 4, *5*
joint stiffness/contractures, congenital and familial syndromes *182*, 186–200
joint tumors, primary 171, 175–7
juvenile ankylosing spondylitis (JAS) 259–60, 263
Juvenile Arthritis Functional Assessment Scale and Report (JAFAS) 331–2
Juvenile Arthritis Quality of Life Questionnaire (JAQQ) 331, 334, *334*
Juvenile Arthritis Self-Report Index (JASI) 331
juvenile chronic arthritis (JCA) 206, *206*, 234, *234*
juvenile dermatomyositis (JDM) 100–4, *101*
juvenile hyaline fibromatosis 188
Juvenile Idiopathic Arthritis (JIA) 203–446
  classification 205–9, *206*
  defined 207
  and environmental factors 290–8
  genetic and cytokine associations 280–9
  immunopathology of joint 272–9
  novel therapeutic horizons 437–8
  treatment approach 299–446
juvenile rheumatoid arthritis (JRA) 206, *206*, 233–4, *234*
juvenile systemic hyalinosis 188

Kashin–Beck disease 161
Kawasaki disease *33*, 51, 56–60, *56, 57, 58, 59*, 215
keratic precipitates 135, *229*
keratoconjunctivitis sicca 240
keratitis 95, 111, 112, 233
keratoderma blenorrhagicum 224, 261
ketorolac 362, 364
knee
  examination 11–14, *12, 13, 14*
  injection *442*
  Baker cyst 12, 139, 175, 218, *247*
  cruciate ligament 138
  genu valgum *see* knock knee
  osteomyelitis 64
  ligament injury 138–9
  meniscal problems 138, *138*
  musculoskeletal syndromes localized to 135–9
  pain secondary to bone problems 136–7
  pain secondary to patella tracking/alignment problems 138
  pain secondary to soft tissue injuries 138–9
  stress fractures 137
  surgery 409–11, *410*
Kniest dysplasia *193*, 195–6
knock knee *183*
Koebner phenomenon 211, *36, 45, 59*
Kohler disease 139
kyphosis 141, *142*

laboratory evaluation 19–21, *20–1*, 331
Langer–Gideon syndrome 198
Langerhans cell histiocytosis 173
Langer mesomelic dwarfism 197
Larsen syndrome *182*, 185–6
leflunomide *432*, 433, 438
Legg–Calvé–Perthes 35, 132, 133, *133*
leg length discrepancy 11–12, *13*
leg length measurement 11–12, *13*
Leri pleonosteosis *182*, 187
Leri–Weill syndrome 197
Lesch–Nyhan disease 165
leukaemia 155–6, *156*
leukocytoclastic vasculitis *33, 60*, 54, 55
leukopenia 93
lidocaine 364, 445
linear scleroderma *47*, 107–8, *107*

lipodystrophy 103, *104*
lipopolysaccharide (LPS) 285
Little Leaguer's elbow 142–3
Little Leaguer's shoulder 142
livedo reticularis 4, *4, 44,* 38, 99, 100
LMP2 gene 285–6
LMX1B transcription factor 186
localized idiopathic pain *35,* 147, *148,* 150–1, *150, 151*
Louis, Pierre 418–19
Lowe oculocerebrorenal syndrome 166
lubricin *see* CACP
lumbar lordosis 9–10, *11*
lumbar spine
    examination 16, *16, 17*
    surgery 405
lupus
    chronic cutaneous 98–9, *98*
    discoid 98–99, *98*
    drug induced 99–100, *99*
    neonatal 97, *97*
    subacute cutaneous 99, *99*
    systemic, erythematosus *39,* 86–97
Lyme disease *32, 33,* 75–7, *76*
    chronic 151–2
    and molecular mimicry 292
    post-Lyme syndrome 151–2
lymphadenopathy *50,* 56, 58, *59,* 78, 92, 119–122, 155, 170, *170,* 211, *215, 220*
lymphocytes *see* T cell; B cell
lymphopenia 93
lymphoedema 217, *219,* 229, 240
lymphoma 156–7, 376

McCune–Albright syndrome 171–2, *172*
macrophage activation syndrome (MAS) 216, *217,* 275, 331, 371, 373–4, 434–7
macrophage inhibitory factor (MIF) 285
Madelung deformity 197
Maffucci syndrome 172–3
MAGIC syndrome 112
magnetic resonance imaging (MRI) 21–23, *22,* 66, 67, 103, *103, 111*
malar rash 89, *90*
malignancies *33,* 155–7, 171, 174–5, 176–7, *215*
Marfan syndrome 181, *182, 183, 184*
MAS *see* macrophage activation syndrome
mevalonic acid 119, 127, *215*
medial tibial stress syndrome (shin splints) 137
MEFV gene 118
melorheostosis 199
meningococcus *132,* 75, 93
mesomelic dysplasia *193,* 197
metabolic bone disease 162–4, *163*
metabolic storage disorders 166–7
metacarpo-phalangeal joints
    examination 7, *8*
    surgery 408
metaphyseal dysplasia *192*–3, 196–7, *197*
metatarsalgia 16
metatarsophalangeal joints *234*
methotrexate (MTX) 374–6, *375,* 432
    clinical trials 422–5
    folic acid supplementation 376, 399–400, 425
    high-dose 431–2
    mechanism of action 374–6
    pharmacology 376
    in polyarthritis 370
    and remission 372
    role in JIA 376
    toxicity 376
methylprednisolone 370–1, 374, *375*
Meyer dysplasia 133, *133*
MHC *see* HLA genes
microbial environment 291–5
    animal models 294
    bystander activation 291, *291,* 292
    bystander suppression 291, *291*
    in gut 294, 295

interactions with immune system 291–3
    molecular mimicry 291, *291,* 292–3, 294, 438
    persisting microbial antigens 291–2
    persisting microbial DNA 292
micrognathia *193,* 307, 403, 405
microscopic polyangiitis (MPA) 109
midazolam 364, 443, 445
mixed connective tissue disease (MCTD) *34,* 97–8, *98*
mobility aids 390
molecular mimicry 291, *291,* 292–3, 294, 438
monocytes 276, *276*
mononeuritis multiplex 109, 111
mononucleosis *see* EBV
morphea *46,* 107
Morquio syndrome 189, 190
mouth ulcers *101,* 110
    see also oral ulcers
MRI 22–3, *22,* 66, *67*
Mselini joint disease 161
Mucha–Habermann disease (acute parapsoriasis, PLEVA) 60–1, *60, 61*
Muckle–Wells syndrome (MWS) 119–22, *120, 122, 215*
mucocutaneous lesions *90,* 91
mucolipidoses *183,* 189–90
mucopolysaccharidoses *182*–3, 189–90
multicentric reticulohistiocytosis 167
multiple epiphyseal dysplasia 196, *196*
multiple exostoses 198
Munchausen syndrome 152
Munchausen syndrome by proxy 152
muscle strength testing 4, *5*
muscular dystrophy *179,* 187
MVK gene mutation *see* HIDS
myalgia 16–17, 76, 80, 89, 147–50, 212
mycobacteria 25, 70, 283, 292–7
    see also tuberculosis
Mycoplasma pneumoniae infections 291–3
myeloid-related protein secretion 436–7
myositis
    dermatomyositis 100–4
    in MCTD 89
    polymyositis 104
    viral, benign 80
myxedema 162

nails
    nailfold capillaroscopy 91, *101,* 103, 106
    nail patella syndrome *182,* 186
    nail pitting *253, 255, 256*
    onycholysis *208,* 252, *253, 256*
    clubbing *4,* 157
naproxen *369,* 373, 421
natural killer cells (NK) 435–6
neck flexor strength 4
neonatal lupus erythematosus (NLE) 97, *97*
neonatal onset multisystem inflammatory disease (NOMID) *120,* 122–3, *123*
neoplasia *see* malignancy; cancer; tumour
nephritis *108,* 373
    see also glomerulonephritis
neuroblastoma 156, 157, *158*
neurofibroma 175
neurofibromatosis 175
neurogenic arthropathy 143
neutrophils 276, *276*
neutropenia
    due to DMARD or drug 432
    in Felty syndrome 240
    see also granulocytopenia
night pain 131, 171
NK cells 435–6
nocturnal pain 131, 171
NOMID *see* neonatal onset multi-inflammatory disorder
non-accidental injury *see* child abuse
non-inflammatory musculoskeletal disorders 130–46
non-ossifying fibroma 172, *172*

non-rheumatic disorders, musculoskeletal and autoimmune manifestations 155–78
nonsteroidal anti-inflammatory drugs (NSAIDs) *369,* 373–4
    clinical trials 420–2
    and remission 372
    toxicity 373–4 *see also* naproxen, ibuprofen, tolmetin, indomethacin
numerical method 418–19
nutrition 392–6
    and adolescents 318–19
    and growth failure 392–3
    nutritional therapy 395
    and osteoporosis 393–4, *394, 395*
    and pathogenesis 290
    Rheumatoid Factor Positive Polyarthritis 239–40
    screening *393*

obesity 393
occupational therapy 381–91
ocular disease *see* eye
oedema 4, 53–56, 100, 108, 119, *121,* 122, 150 *see also* lymphoedema
Oligoarthritis 223–32, *224,* 266–7
    clinical features 224–5, *225,* 229
    complications 228, 229–30
    defined 207
    and early-onset, ANA positive polyarthritis 247
    epidemiology 223–4, 228
    extended 228–9, 244
    genetics 226, 229, 282–3, 285
    and histocompatibility antigens 226, 229, 282–3
    immunopathology 226–7
    investigations 225–6, *226,* 229
    jaw involvement 227–8, *228*
    and molecular mimicry 292
    monitoring 227–8, *227, 228*
    persistent 223–8, 275–6
    pharmacological treatment 368, *368, 370*
    prognosis 228, 229
    and T cells 227, 275–6
    and uveitis 229–30, *229, 230*
Ollier disease 172
oncogene 286
ophthalmologists 307
opioids 362–4
oral ulcers *34*–35, 52, 87, 99, 110, *425*
oral contraceptives 20, 60
orthodontists/oral surgeons/oral hygienists 307
orthopaedic surgeons 307
Osgood-Schlatter disease 136, *136*
ossifying fibroma 172
osteoarthritis
    hip 135, *135*
    knee 137
osteoblast 180, 181
osteoclast 180, 191, 276, 394, 400–1, 433
osteoblastoma 174
osteochondritis dissecans (OD)
    elbow 143
    foot 140
    knee 137, *137*
osteochondrodysplasias 157, 189, 191–200, *192–4*
    with decreased bone density 198–9
    with increased bone density *193,* 199
osteochondroma 174, *175*
osteochondroses, of foot 139
osteogenesis imperfecta (OI) 198–9, *199*
osteoid osteoma *36,* 173–4, *174*
osteolysis, idiopathic *194,* 199–200, *199, 200*
    carpal-tarsal *194,* 199–200, *200*
    familial expansile 200, *200*
    Winchester syndrome 200, *200*
osteomalacia 163
osteomyelitis 63–71
    acute haematogenous 63–8, *63, 66*
    after puncture wound of foot 70
    bone examination 63–4, *65*

chronic 70
chronic recurrent multifocal (CRMO) *33*, 71, *71*, *72*
discitis *33*, 69–70, *69*, *70*
infections mimicking 79–80
laboratory studies 64
of patella, subacute 68, *68*
presentation 63, *64*
radiographic studies 66, *66*, *67*
in sacroiliac area 68
significance of adjacent joint effusions 64, *64*, *65*
subacute 70, *70*, *71*
systemic manifestations 64
treatment 68, *68*
vertebral 68–9, *69*
osteonecrosis
and corticosteroids 133–4, *133*
of hip 132–4, *132*, *133*
and systemic lupus erythematosus 89
osteopenia 142, 163, *163*, 400–1
osteopetrosis 199
osteoporosis 163, 400–1
and back pain 142
nutrition 318, 393–4, *394*
and Rheumatoid Factor Positive Polyarthritis 240
and Systemic Arthritis 219
osteosarcoma 174, *175*
outpatient service 308–12
clinic coordination and personnel 308–9, *308*
clinic facilities 309, *309*
integration of extended team into clinic 311
new consultations 309–10, *310*
outpatients with established rheumatic diseases 311, *311*
outpatients without established rheumatic diseases 310–11, *311*
technical procedures 311–12
outreach clinics 313
overuse injuries 131, 142–3
oxycodone 362, *363*

pachydermoperiostosis 157
Paediatric Pain Coping Inventory (PPCI) 360
Paediatric Pain Questionnaire (PPQ) 358
paediatric radiologists 307
paediatric rheumatologists 304, *305*, 313
Paediatric Rheumatology Collaborative Study Group (PRCSG) 419
Paediatric Rheumatology International Trials Organization (PRINTO) 419
paediatric rheumatology nurses 305–6, *305*
paediatric rheumatology team 304–7, *305*
consultants to 307, *307*
dynamics 307–8
paediatric rheumatology trainees 306–7
pain assessment 330–1, 357–60
behavioural observation 357–8
and biobehavioural model of paediatric pain 359
body outline figures 358
health-related quality of life 359–60
pain descriptors 358
physiologic monitoring 357
and physiotherapy and occupational therapy 382, *382*, *383*, 386
self-report 358
visual analogue scales 358
pain coping 360
Pain Coping Questionnaire (PCQ) 360
pain management 360–4
cognitive-behavioural treatment 360–2
communication of pain concept 360–1
complementary therapies 364
emotional distress 361
medical 362–4, *363*
nociception 361
nonadaptive thinking 361
pain associated with procedures 364
pain behaviour modification 360
pain behaviours 361–2

pain perception regulation 360
and physiotherapy and occupational and pain puzzle 360–1, *361*
surgery 364
pamidronate *see* bisphosphonates
pancreatitis *61*, 93–94, *97*
panniculitis *see* Weber–Christian syndrome; erythema nodosum
Panner disease 142–3
pannus *246*, 273
PAPA (pyogenic sterile arthritis, pyodermagangrenosum and acne) 123, *124*, 127
see also streaking leukocyte factor
paracetamol *see* acetaminophen
parasitic arthritis 83
parents
advocacy issues for 322, 340–2
importance of education for 337–42
psychosocial adjustment 343–56
parotid swelling 124–125
Parry Romberg syndrome *107*, 108
pars planitis *see* uveitis
parvovirus associated arthritis *32*, 78–9, *79*, 291
patella
bipartite 136–7
'patella apprehension' sign 13
recurrent dislocation and subluxation 138
subacute osteomyelitis 68, *68*
tracking/alignment problems 138–9
patellofemoral pain syndrome 13, *14*, 138
pathergy 111
pathological fractures 172, 173, *238*
patient-centred care, and team approach 303–14
pattern recognition 4
PedsQL *334*, 335, 359–60
penicillamine 378, *424*
penicillin 47, 50, 52, 77, 83
peptic ulcer *see* ulcer, peptic
perforin 216, 275, 435–6
pericarditis 50, *87*, 88, 91, 98, 99, 106, *108*, 118, 124–5, 186, 211, 214
peripheral neuropathy *76*, 88
periodic fever, aphthous stomatitis, pharyngitis, adenitis (PFAPA) *34*, 116–17, *117*, *120*, 215
periodic fever syndromes (PFS) 116–19,*120*
periostitis 157
Perthes *see* Legg–Calve–Perthes
pes cavus *182*
pes planus (flat feet) 132
petechiae *38*, 91, 93
see also purpura
PFAPA *see* periodic fever
phagocytes 436–7
phalangeal microgeodic syndrome 144–5, *145*
pharmacological treatment
adjunctive therapies 397–402
clinical trials 414–28, 431
of early or established arthritis 367–80
of refractory arthritis 372, 431–41
pharyngitis 49, *78*, 116, 117, *117*, *20*
phospholipid antibodies 88, 89, 93, 94, 96, 98, 100, *100*, *132*
see also anti-phospholipid
photosensitive rash 89–91, *90*
physical education at school 385
physical examination 4–17
of joints 5–16, *5*
lower extremity 9–16
lumbar spine 16
tender points 16–17
upper extremity 6–9
physiotherapy and occupational therapy 381–91
advocating for child 387–8
child and family issues 385, 389
education of child and family 385
management of early arthritis 382–5, *382*, *383*, *384*
management of established arthritis 386–8, *386*, *388*
management of functional limitations

and impairments 384–5, 386–7
management of refractory arthritis 388–90, *389*
optimization of function in work, leisure and self-care 390
pain management 364, 382–4, *383*, 389
planning for future 390
referrals 381–2, *381*, *382*
teaching self-management and problem-solving 387
and team approach 306, *306*
treatment goals 382–5, 389–90
pigmented villonodular synovitis (PVS) *34*, 176
piroxicam 422
placebo response 414
plant-thorn synovitis 81–3, *81*, *83*
platelets *see* thrombocytopenia; thrombocytosis; thrombosis
play 387
plica syndrome 139
pleural effusion *88*, 211, 240
pleuritis 55, *88*, *98*,*101*
pneumonitis 93, *94*, *97*, 376
polyarteritis nodosa (PAN) *34*, *101*, 108–9, *109*
polyarthritis *148*
classification *234*
pharmacological treatment 370, *370*
see also Rheumatoid Factor Negative Polyarthritis; Rheumatoid Factor Positive Polyarthritis
polychondritis *35*, 111, *112*
polymyositis 104
popliteal cyst 139, *139*, 175, 218
post-Lyme syndrome 151–2
post-streptococcal reactive arthritis (PSRA) *32*, 51
posture evaluation 17
PRDG ix, xi
prednisolone 422, *423*
prednisone 370, 371–2, 374, *375*, *395*
pre-operational stage 346, *347*
prepatellar bursitis, suppurative 79–80, *79*
presenting problems 24–48
primary hypertrophic osteoarthropathy without pachyderma 157
prognosis *see individual sections in disease chapters*
propylthiouracil 162
proximal inter-phalangeal joints
examination 7–8, *8*
surgery 408
proteinuria *34*, 54, 55, *88*, 94, *101*, 109, 217, *238*, 420
proteoglycans *180*, 187, 294
protrusio acetabulae *236*, *184*, 486
pseudoachondroplasia 196
pseudo-Hurler polydystrophy 190
Pseudomonas 70
pseudoporphyria 373
pseudo tumour *76*, 95, *97*, *107*, 164
Psoriatic Arthritis 252–8
arthritis 254–5
clinical features 254–5, *255*, *256*
complications 257
criteria and classification 207–8, 252–3, *253*, 268
dactylitis *253*, 254–5
enthesitis 255
epidemiology 253–4
historical considerations 252–3, *252*, *253*
investigations and monitoring 256
nail lesions 255, *256*
pathogenesis 254
pharmacological treatment 372
prognosis 257
psoriasis 255, *255*, *256*
uveitis 257
Vancouver Criteria 252–3, *253*
psychogenic rheumatism *36*
psychologists 306, 354, *355*
psychosocial adjustment 343–56
adolescents 349–50, 351
anger 344
children's understanding of JIA 346–7, *347*
correlates of 351–2

psychosocial adjustment (*cont.*)
  depression and helplessness 344
  developmental perspective 343
  and diagnosis 344
  disbelief and denial 344
  and disease/disability parameters 351
  and early arthritis 344–5
  and established arthritis 345–6
  family challenges and child's developmental status
    346–50
  guilt 344
  impact of challenges on families 350–3
  and infancy/early childhood 347–8
  methodological issues 350–1
  and middle childhood 348–9
  model of 352–3, *352*
  and pain 351
  and personal parameters 351–2
  post-diagnosis challenges 344–6
  pre-diagnosis challenges 343–4
  and refractory arthritis 346
  resolution and adaptation 344
  risk and resistance factors 352–3
  shock 344
  and social–ecological parameters 352
  support for families 353–4
PTPN22 gene 286
pulmonary hypertension 93, 98, 100, 106
purpura 50, 53, *53, 54*, 55, *55*, 93, 100, *101*, 118, 162
pyoderma gangrenosum 123, *124*, 170–1
pyogenic sterile arthritis, pyoderma gangrenosum, and
  acne syndrome *see* PAPA; streaking leukocyte factor)
  123, *124*
pyomyositis 80, *80, 81*
pyrin 127

quality assurance 313
quality of life, health-related 333–5, *333*,
  334, 359–60

radiographic studies *20–1*, 21–3
    see also imaging
range of motion 5, *5, 6, 6*, 7, 10, *10*, 13, 14
rash and acute fever *51*
Raynaud phenomenon *48*, 91, *92*, 105–6, *106*
reactive arthritis *32, 33*, 51–2, *52*
  BCG-induced 293
  and enthesitis related arthritis 263
  post-streptococcal (PSRA) 51
  viral associated 51–2
recombinant human erythropoietin 398
reconstructive surgery 404
recreational activities 385
reflex sympathetic dystrophy (RSD, localized idiopathic
  pain) 147, *148*, 150–1, *150, 151*
refractory disease
  defined 302
  pharmacological treatment 372, 431–41
Reiter syndrome *see* reactive arthritis
rehabilitation 306, 308, 386, 387, 403, 409
relapsing polychondritis (RP) *35*, 111–12, *112*
remission
  defined 301–2
  management 372, *372*
renal biopsy 54, 94, 109
renal disease 54–5, *88*, 88, 94, 109, 373, 398
retroperitoneal (psoas) abscess 80
Reye syndrome *369*, 373
rhabdomyosarcoma 176–7, *177*
rheumatic diseases, major 86–115
rheumatic fever *33*, 49–51, *50, 51*
rheumatoid arthritis (RA) 233, 234, *234*,
  235, 247, 290
rheumatoid factor (RF) 21, 239, *239*, 331
Rheumatoid Factor Negative Polyarthritis 244–51
  age and sex distribution 245
  classification 207, 244, *244*, 267–8
  clinical features 245–8, *246, 247*

clinical subgroups 246–8, *246*
  complications 248
  dry synovitis 247–8, *248*
  early-onset, ANA positive 246–7
  epidemiology 244–5
  ethnic differences 245
  genetics 283
  HLA associations 245, 283
  investigations 248
  monitoring 248
  prognosis 248, *249*
  prolific symmetric synovitis 247
Rheumatoid Factor Positive Polyarthritis *101*, 233–43
  classification 207, 233–4, *233, 234*, 268
  clinical features 234–5, *235, 236*
  complications 240
  epidemiology 234, *235*
  extra-articular features 235
  eye involvement 240
  functional outcome 240
  genetics 283
  growth, development and nutritional status 239–40
  HLA DR4 239, 283
  investigations 238–9, *238*
  monitoring 239–40
  mortality 241
  osteoporosis 240
  pattern of joint involvement 235, *235, 236*
  prognosis 240–1
  psychosocial development 240
  puberty and fertility 240
  reticuloendothelial system involvement 240
  rheumatoid factor 239, *239*
  rheumatoid nodules 235, *236, 237*
  surgical interventions 403, 404, 406, 408
  vasculitis 240
rheumatoid nodules 233, 234, *234, 236, 237*, 290
rheumatologic disease checklist *3, 4*
rhizomelic chondrodysplasia punctata 198
rickets 163–4, *163*
  hypocalcemic 163–4, *163*
  hypophosphatemic *163*, 164
rubella arthropathy *32*, 79
rubella vaccination 293

Sackett, David 419
sacroiliac joint, examination 16
sacroiliitis
  in ERA 259
  in FMF 118
  and HLA B27 282
  in JIA *208, 214*
  in Psoriatic Arthritis 252, *253*, 254–5
  and Undifferentiated Arthritis *265*
sacrum 16, 135, 141
saddle nose deformity 109, *110*
salicylates *see* acetylsalicylic acid
salivary glands 3
    see also parotid swelling
Salmonella 74, *74*, 81
salmonellosis 81
SAPHO syndrome *38*, 71, *72*
sarcoidosis *35*, 60, 123–5, *124*
  early onset *35*, 123–4
  late onset 125
sarcoma 131–2, *159*, 171–6, *175–7*
Scheie syndrome 190
Scheuermann disease (juvenile kyphosis) 141, *142*
Schimke immuno-osseous dysplasia 195
Schmid dysplasia 197
Schober's test 16, *17*, 261
Schwachmann—Diamond syndrome 197
scleroderma 105–8
  morphea 39, *46*, 77, 106–8
  linear *47*, 107–8, *107*
  localized 106–8, *107*
  systemic sclerosis 97, 105–6, *105, 106, 107*

scoliosis
  congenital *185*
  painful *29*
  in disc herniation 142
  in joint laxity syndromes 181, *182*
  in JIA 405
  in Marfan syndrome 183, *182, 184*
  in neurofibromatosis 175
  in osteoid osteoma 173
  in pseudo-Hurler polydystrophy 190
  in osteochondrodysplasias *192*, 196, 198
  in Scheuermann disease 141
screening clinics 309–10
scurvy 161
selective IgA deficiency 167, 169
selenium 161, 400
self-determination and self-advocacy 321–2
self-esteem 349–50
sensorimotor stage 346
separation anxiety 348
separations, effects of 347–8
septic arthritis *33*, 71–9
  acute 66, 71–4, *72, 73, 74*
  CpG motifs 292
  immunodeficiencies 74, 168
  infections mimicking 79–80
  tuberculous 75, *75*
serial casting 386
seronegative enthesitis arthritis (SEA)
  syndrome 206, 259–60, *259*, 263
serositis
  disease activity 208, 213, 266
  FMF *34*, 118
  JIA classification 207, 208, 405
  pharmacological treatment *369*, 370, *371*
  SLE *88*, 93, 96
  Systemic Arthritis 211, 213, *214,*
serum sickness *33*, 55–6
Sever disease 140
sexuality issues 319, 390
shigella *32*, 360
short stature 191–200
shoulder
  examination 9, *10*
  images of *156, 177, 406*
  injection *445*
  musculoskeletal syndromes localized to 142–3
  surgery 405, *406*
siblings 345, 346
Sicca syndrome 95, 240
sickle cell disease *34*, 74, *74*, 81, 159, *160*
Sinding-Larsen-Johansson 136
single-handed physician practices 313
sitosterolemia 167
Sjogren syndrome 21, *32, 82*, 95, 97, 100
skin manifestations associated with rheumatic diseases
  31, *37–40, 42–8, 61*
SLE *see* systemic lupus erythematosus
slipped capital femoral epiphysis 132, 134, *134*
slow acting anti-rheumatic drugs *see* disease modifying
  anti-rheumatic drugs
small-centre practices 313
smoking 290
social workers 306
socioeconomic factors 290
soft-tissue release procedures 403–4, 409, 410, 411
special educational needs 340–2
splenomegaly 3
  and ALPS 170
  and CINCA 122, *123*
  and Cogan syndrome 111
  and common variable immunodeficiency 168
  and EBV 78
  and FMF 118
  and Felty syndrome 240
  and Gaucher disease
  and HIDS 118–9
  and malaria *82*

and MAS *217*
and methotrexate 376
and mucopolysaccharidoses *182–3*
and sarcoidosis 125
and Systemic Arthritis *36, 207,* 211, 213, *214*
and SLE *34,* 92
spine *see* back; cervical spine; lumbar spine
splinting 384, 386, 406
spondyloarthropathies *see* ERA
spondyloepiphyseal dysplasia (SED) 191, *192,* 195–6
spondyloepiphyseal dysplasias congenital (SEDC) 191
spondyloepiphyseal dysplasias tarda 191–5
spondyloepiphyseal dysplasias tarda with progressive
    arthropathy (pseudorheumatoid arthritis of
    childhood) 195
spondylolisthesis 141, *141*
spondylitis *see* ankylosing spondylitis
spondylolysis 141
sports injuries *see* overuse injuries
Staphylococcus aureus 68, 69, 70, 74, 80
Steinbrocker classification system 332, *332*
stem cell transplant *see* allogenic and antologous stem
    cell transplant
sternum 65
Stevens—Johnson syndrome *51,* 56, 377
Stickler dysplasia *193,* 195–6, *195*
Still disease 206, 210, *214*
stippled epiphyses *193,* 198
streaking leukocyte factor 170–1, *171*
    see also PAPA
streptococcus
    and acute rheumatic fever *32,50*
    and antiphospholipid syndrome 100
    and antistreptococcal antibodies *20, 50*
    and erythema nodosum 60, *237*
    and post-streptococcal reactive arthritis *32, 50,* 51
    and psoriasis 254
    and streptococcal cell wall model of arthritis 294
stress fractures
    of elbow 143
    of foot 140
    of hip 134–5
    of knee 137
subacute cutaneous lupus erythematosus (SCLE) 99, *99*
substance use 319
subtalar joint 15, *15,*
    injections *445*
    surgery *411*
    and tarsal coalition 140
sulfasalazine (SSA) 372, *375,* 376–7, *425*
supra-patellar bursa 12, *13*
surgical interventions 403–13
    axial skeleton and jaw 404–5, *404*
    clinical trials 428–9
    indications 403–4
    lower limb 408–11, *409, 410*
    for pain management 364
    preoperative work-up 404
    preparation 403
    upper limb 405–8, *406, 407, 408*
swan neck deformity 408
Sweet syndrome 61, *61, 215*
symptom patterns 4, 31, *33–6*
synovectomy 406, 408, 410, 428–9
synovial chondromatosis 176
synovial fluid analysis 19
synovial haemangioma *34, 36,* 176
synovial plica syndrome 139
synovial sarcoma 176
synovium
    inflamed 272–4, *273*
    normal 272
syphilis *32,* 83
synovitis *see* arthritis
Systemic Arthritis *36, 51,* 210–22
    classification 207, 266
    clinical features 211–13
    diagnosis 213, *214, 215–16*

epidemiology 210–11, 291–2
extra-articular manifestations 211
ferritin levels 212
fever 211, *211*
genetics 283, 285
growth retardation 219–20, *220,* 392–3
imaging 213–14, *216*
investigations at initial evaluation 212–13
joint destruction 217, *217, 218*
laboratory testing 212, 331
leukocytosis with neutrophilia 212
lymphadenopathy 211
lymphedema 217, *219*
macrophage activation syndrome (MAS) 216, *217,*
    275, 331, 371, 373–4, 434–7
monitoring 213–14
monocyclic course 213
musculoskeletal complications 217, *217, 218*
musculoskeletal manifestations 212, *212*
organomegaly 211
osteoporosis 219
pathogenesis 291–2
pharmacological treatment 370–1, *371,* 427, 431, 432
polycyclic course 213
prognosis 220–1, *220*
rash 211, *211*
secondary amyloidosis 217
serositis and other visceral manifestations 211, *212*
synovial cysts 218, *219*
systemic complications 216–17, *217*
thrombocytosis 212
unremitting course 213
vs. autoinflammatory diseases 116–29
vs. dermatomyositis *101*
vs. idiopathic pain syndromes *148*
systemic lupus erythematosus (SLE) *34,* 86–97
    cardiac manifestations 91–2
    constitutional manifestations 89
    diagnosis 86–8, *87, 88*
    endocrine manifestations 95
    gastrointestinal manifestations 93–4
    haematological manifestations 92–3
    hepatic manifestations 92
    investigations *20, 21,* 95–6
    musculoskeletal manifestations 88–9, *89*
    neuropsychiatric manifestations 95, *95*
    pulmonary manifestations 93, *94*
    renal manifestations 94
    reticuloendothelial manifestations 92
    skin manifestations 89–91, *90, 91, 92*
    treatment and prognosis 96–7, *96, 97*
systemic sclerosis (SSc) 97, 105–6, *105, 106, 107*
systemic vasculitis 108–12, *108*

T cells 273, 274–5, *276*
    and adjuvant arthritis 294
    and auto-SCT 434, 435–6
    and cytokine imbalance 275
    death 275
    division 274
    polarization and cytokines 283–4
    recruitment 274
    regulatory 275–6, 293, 295
    responses to heat shock proteins 294–5
    retention 274–5
Takayasu arteritis *35,* 110
tarsal coalition 140, *140*
tarsitis *see* ERA
teachers 340
team approach 301, 303–14
    and communication 304
    consultants to paediatric rheumatologyteam 307, *307*
    delivery of comprehensive clinical service 308–12
    in early disease 312
    in established disease 312
    and family support 354
    importance 304
    incorporation of academic

responsibilities 312–13
    inpatient service 308
    objectives of delivery of care 304, *304*
    outpatient service 308–12
    paediatric rheumatology team 304–7, *305*
    and patient-centred care 303–14
    in refractory disease 312
    and research 312–13
    school issues 308
    team dynamics 307–8
    and trainee education 312
temporomandibular joint (TMJ)
    examination 6, *7*
    surgery 405
tenascin X 185
tender points
    examination 16–17
    in fibromyalgia 149, *149*
tendonitis *see* tenosynovitis
tenosynovitis
    ankle 14, *14,* 246
    in congenital indifference to pain 143
    in disseminated gonococcal disease 74, 75
    in Marfan disease 181
    in Polyarthritis 445, *246*
    in Psoriatic Arthritis 252
    in syphilis 83
    in Systemic Arthritis *219*
    treatment 408, 411
    wrist 9
    see also Charcot disease
TGF-Beta 276, 294
thalassaemia 160
thalidomide 371
Thiemann disease 143
thoracic spine, surgery 405
thrombasthenia 161
thrombocytosis *38, 88,* 91, 93, *96,* 96–100, 110,
    156, 170, *170*
thrombocytopenia 93 *see also* SLE
thrombosis 94, 100, 108, 111, *102, 182,* 189, 212, 371
thumb examination 7, *9*
thyroid acropachy 162
thyroid disease 162
Tim1 gene 293
TMJ 6, *6, 228, 246,* 393, 405
TNF-receptor-associated periodic syndrome (TRAPS)
    119, *120, 121*
TNF-alpha
    mechanism of action 216, 275–6, 283–5
    therapy 292, 302, 367–8, 426, 431–3, 437–8
    TRAPS 119
tolerance 293, 295, 427, 435
toll-like receptors 274
total body irradiation 434
tolmetin sodium 420
toxic shock syndrome (TSS) *51, 59*
trainee education 312
tramadol *149,* 362, *363*
transient synovitis of hip (irritable hip, toxic synovitis
    of hip) 53
transition 315–16, *316*
    clinics 313, 322–3
    components 315
    cost implications of transitional care 326
    defined 315
    disease-based model 323
    and disease characteristics 325–6
    essentials of transitional care service 323, *323*
    evidence of need for transitional care services 316–17
    medical transition 316, 317, *317*
    and physiotherapy and occupational therapy 390
    plan 315, 323–5, *324–5*
    primary care based model 323
    vs. transfer 316
transplantation 398, 434, 437–8
transporters associated with antigen processing (TAP)
    genes 286

TRAPS *34*, 118, 119, *120, 121*
trauma 28, *31*
treatment approach 299–446
Trendelenberg sign 9
triamcinolone acetonide *426*, 443–4
triamcinolone hexacetonide *426*, 444
trichorhinophalangeal dysplasia I 197–8
trigger finger 187, *187*
Tropheryma whippelii 83–4
tuberculosis *32*, 75, *75*, 226, 432, 433
tuberculous vertebral osteomyelitis (Pott disease)
      69, *69*, 75
tuberosity
      calcaneal 140
      ischial 10, *14*, 260,
      tibial 10, *14*, 136, *136*,
tumour *see* malignancy, cancer
tumour necrosis factor 284
      see also TNF α
twin studies 280

ulcerative colitis *3*, 53, 94, 263
ulcers
      aphthous *see* oral
      cutaneous
            in HIDS *118*
            in PAPA 171, *171*
      genital
            in MAGIC syndrome 112
            in Behcet 110
      oral 111
            in Behcet 110
            in HIDS *118*
            in IBD 35, *35*
            in methotrexate toxicity 425
            in SLE 86–7, *90*, 98–9,
            in vasculitis syndromes 101
      oesophageal
            in Behcet 111
ulnar distraction lengthening 406–7, *407*
ultrasound 21–2, *22*
Undifferentiated Arthritis 265–71

classification 208, 254, *267*, 268–70, *269*
      clinical patterns 266–8
      defined 265, *265*
      epidemiology 265–6, *266*
unemployment 316
upper-to-lower body segment ratio 181, *184*, 191
urethritis 4, *33*, *41*, 52
      in ERA 261, 263
urinalysis 20, 25, 27, 29, 94, 149, 151, 238, 376–7
urticaria *42*, 56, 119, *122*
uveitis
      and enthesitis related arthritis 263
      and Kawasaki disease 59
      and oligoarthritis 229–30, *229, 230*
      and Psoriatic Arthritis 257
      and Rheumatoid Factor Negative Polyarthritis 246–7,
            248

vaccinations *see* immunizations
varicella reactive arthritis *32*
vasculitis 108–12, *108*, 240
velocardiofacial syndrome 169–70
vertebrae
      in discitis 16, *25*, 69, *69*, 70, 140
      in hypochondroplasia 191–2
      in JIA 404
      in osteomyelitis 69, *70*, 82
      in osteoid osteoma 173
      in osteoporosis *219*
      in Scheuermann disease 141
viral arthritis 77–9, *78*
viral myositis, benign *33*, 80
vitamin A poisoning 164, *164*
vitamin D
      deficiency 163–4
      intake 393–4, *394*
      poisoning 164

weakness *3, 4, 5, 34*, 80
      in Camurati-Endelman syndrome 199
      in dysplasia 193, 195
      in dermatomyositis 100–3

in hyperparathyroid disease 162
      in hyperthyroid disease 162
      in JIA 382, 386–8
      in mixed connective tissue disease 97–8
      in muscular dystrophy 187
      in SLE 89
Weber–Christian *37, 39*
      see also panniculitis
Wegener granulomatosis (WG) *34*, *101*,
      109–10, *110*
      diagnosis 109
      laboratory findings 109
      limited 110
weight gain 392–5,
weight loss *34*, 74
      in Cogan syndrome 111
      in IBD 50, 52
      in malignancy 156, 175
      in nutrition 392–395
      in SLE 86, 89, 90, *101*
      in sarcoid 125
      in vasculitis syndromes 108–10, 216
      in Whipple disease 84
Weill–Marchesani syndrome *182*, 189
Whipple disease *32*, 83–4
white blood cell (WBC) count 19, 20–1
Williams syndrome *182*, 187
Winchester syndrome 200
Wiskott–Aldrich syndrome 170, *170*
work issues 320–1
wrist
      examination 6–8, *7, 8*
      musculoskeletal syndromes localized to 143–5
      physeal injuries 143
      surgery 406–7, *407, 408*
      synovial swelling 6, *7*

Yersinia sp. *32*, 60
      in ERA 260

X-ray *see* imaging

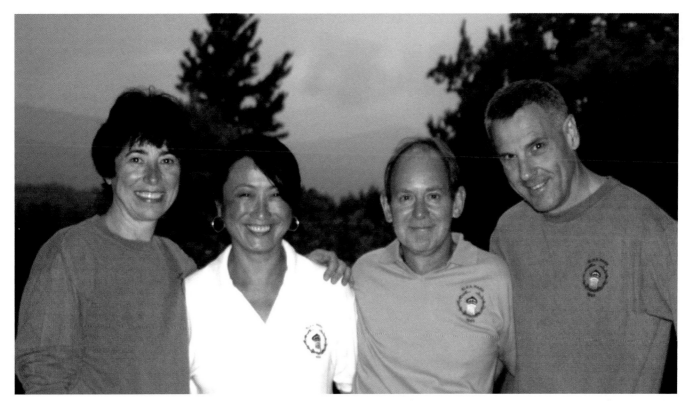

Elka Park, New York, August 14, 2005 (photo by Annie Kurtin).